W9-BRX-905

CECIL
ESSENTIALS
OF
MEDICINE

Editors

THOMAS E. ANDREOLI, M.D.

Edward Randall III Professor and Chairman,
Department of Internal Medicine,
University of Texas Medical School at Houston;
Chief of Medicine, Hermann Hospital, Houston, Texas

CHARLES C.J. CARPENTER, M.D.

Professor of Medicine, Brown University; Physician-in-Chief,
The Miriam Hospital, Providence, Rhode Island

FRED PLUM, M.D.

Anne Parrish Titzell Professor and Chairman, Department of Neurology,
Cornell University Medical College; Neurologist-in-Chief,
The New York Hospital, New York, New York

LLOYD H. SMITH, Jr., M.D.

Professor of Medicine and Associate Dean, University of California,
San Francisco, School of Medicine, San Francisco, California

W. B. SAUNDERS COMPANY

Philadelphia, London, Toronto, Mexico City, Rio de Janeiro, Sydney, Tokyo, Hong Kong

W. B. Saunders Company: West Washington Square
Philadelphia, PA 19105

Listed here is the latest translated edition of this book together
with the language of the translation and the publisher:

Portuguese—DISCOS CBS Industria e Comercio Ltda., Rio de Janeiro, Brazil

Library of Congress Cataloging in Publication Data
Main entry under title:

Cecil essentials of medicine.

   1 Internal medicine.   I. Cecil, Russell L.
(Russell La Fayette), 1881–1965.   II. Andreoli,
Thomas E., 1935–   .   III. Title: Essentials of
medicine.   [DNLM: 1. Medicine.   WB 100 C3882]
RC46.C42   1986   616   85-11959
ISBN 0-7216-1433-7

Editor: John Dyson

Designer: Lorraine B. Kilmer

Production Manager: Frank Polizzano

Manuscript Editor: Donna Walker

Cecil Essentials of Medicine   ISBN   0-7216-1433-7

Last digit is the print number: 9   8   7   6   5   4

CONTRIBUTORS

CARDIOVASCULAR DISEASES

WILLIAM M. MILES, M.D.

Assistant Professor of Medicine, Indiana University School of Medicine; Krannert Institute of Cardiology, Indianapolis. Attending Physician, Indiana University Hospital and Richard L. Roudebush Veterans Administration Hospital, Indianapolis, Indiana.

DOUGLAS P. ZIPES, M.D.

Professor of Medicine, Indiana University School of Medicine; Senior Research Associate, Krannert Institute of Cardiology, Indianapolis. Attending Physician, Indiana University Hospital, Richard L. Roudebush Veterans Administration Hospital, and Wishard Memorial Hospital, Indianapolis, Indiana.

RESPIRATORY DISEASES

DAVID R. DANTZKER, M.D.

Professor of Internal Medicine and Director , Division of Pulmonary Medicine, University of Texas Medical School at Houston. Attending Physician, Hermann Hospital, Houston, Texas.

MARTIN J. TOBIN, M.D.

Assistant Professor of Internal Medicine, University of Texas Medical School at Houston. Attending Physician, Hermann Hospital, Houston, Texas.

RALPH E. WHATLEY, M.D.

Clinical Instructor of Internal Medicine, University of Texas Medical School at Houston, Texas. Fellow, Department of Pulmonary, Occupational and Critical Care Medicine, University of Utah School of Medicine, Salt Lake City, Utah.

RENAL DISEASE

THOMAS E. ANDREOLI, M.D.

Edward Randall, III Professor and Chairman, Department of Internal Medicine, University of Texas Medical School at Houston. Chief of Medicine, Hermann Hospital, Houston, Texas.

R. MICHAEL CULPEPPER, M.D.

Assistant Professor of Internal Medicine, University of Texas Medical School at Houston. Attending Physician, Hermann Hospital, Houston, Texas.

CATHERINE S. THOMPSON, M.D.

Assistant Professor of Internal Medicine, University of Texas Medical School at Houston. Attending Physician, Hermann Hospital, Houston, Texas.

EDWARD J. WEINMAN, M.D.

Professor of Internal Medicine and Director, Division of Nephrology, University of Texas Medical School at Houston. Attending Physician, Hermann Hospital, Houston, Texas.

GASTROINTESTINAL DISEASE

NATHAN M. BASS, M.D., Ph.D.

Assistant Professor of Medicine, University of California, San Francisco, School of Medicine. Attending Physician, University of California, San Francisco Hospitals and Clinics, San Francisco, California.

LLOYD H. SMITH, JR., M.D.

Professor of Medicine and Associate Dean, University of California, San Francisco, School of Medicine, San Francisco, California.

REBECCA W. VAN DYKE, M.D.

Assistant Professor of Medicine, University of California, San Francisco, School of Medicine. Attending Physician, University of California, San Francisco Hospitals and Clinics, San Francisco, California.

HEMATOLOGY

MARGARET LEWIN, M.D.

Assistant Adjunct Physician, Lenox Hill Hospital, and Courtesy Staff Physician, Doctors Hospital, New York, New York.

ANNE MOORE, M.D.

Associate Professor of Clinical Medicine, Cornell University Medical College, New York. Associate Attending Physician, The New York Hospital–Cornell Medical Center, New York, New York.

BABETTE B. WEKSLER, M.D.

Professor of Medicine, Cornell University Medical College, New York. Attending Physician, The New York Hospital–Cornell Medical Center, New York, New York.

ONCOLOGY

MARGARET LEWIN, M.D.

Assistant Adjunct Physician, Lenox Hill Hospital, and Courtesy Staff Physician, Doctors Hospital, New York, New York.

ANNE MOORE, M.D.

Associate Professor of Clinical Medicine, Cornell University Medical College, New York. Associate Attending Physician, The New York Hospital–Cornell Medical Center, New York, New York.

BABETTE B. WEKSLER, M.D.

Professor of Medicine, Cornell University Medical College, New York. Attending Physician, The New York Hospital–Cornell Medical Center, New York, New York.

METABOLIC DISEASES

DONALD HRICIK, M.D.

Assistant Professor of Medicine, Case Western Reserve University School of Medicine, Cleveland. Attending Physician, University Hospitals of Cleveland, Ohio.

JAY WISH, M.D.

Assistant Professor of Medicine, Case Western Reserve University School of Medicine, Cleveland. Attending Physician, University Hospitals of Cleveland, Ohio.

ENDOCRINE DISEASES

KENNETH R. FEINGOLD, M.D.

Assistant Professor of Medicine, University of California, San Francisco, School of Medicine. Attending Physician, Veterans Administration Medical Center, San Francisco, California.

LAURENCE A. GAVIN, M.D.

Associate Professor of Medicine, University of California, San Francisco, School of Medicine. Attending Physician, Veterans Administration Medical Center, San Francisco, California.

MORRIS SCHAMBELAN, M.D.

Professor of Medicine, University of California, San Francisco, School of Medicine. Associate Director, General Clinical Research Center, San Francisco General Hospital, San Francisco, California.

ANTHONY SEBASTIAN, M.D.

Professor of Medicine, University of California, San Francisco, School of Medicine. Co-Director, General Clinical Research Center, Moffitt Hospital, San Francisco, California.

DISEASES OF BONE AND BONE MINERAL METABOLISM

LLOYD H. SMITH, Jr., M.D.

Professor of Medicine and Associate Dean, University of California, San Francisco, School of Medicine, San Francisco, California.

INFECTIOUS DISEASES

CHARLES C. J. CARPENTER, M.D.

Professor of Medicine, Brown University; Physician-in-Chief, The Miriam Hospital, Providence Rhode Island

JERROLD J. ELLNER, M.D.

Professor of Medicine, Case Western Reserve University School of Medicine, Cleveland. Attending Physician, University Hospitals of Cleveland, Ohio.

MICHAEL LEDERMAN, M.D.

Assistant Professor of Medicine, Case Western Reserve University School of Medicine, Cleveland. Attending Physician, University Hospitals of Cleveland, Ohio.

MUSCULOSKELETAL AND CONNECTIVE TISSUE DISEASES

GARY M. KAMMER, M.D.

Associate Professor of Medicine, Case Western Reserve University School of Medicine, Cleveland. Attending Physician, University Hospitals of Cleveland, Ohio.

NEUROLOGIC DISEASE

FRED PLUM, M.D.

Anne Parrish Titzell Professor and Chairman, Department of Neurology, Cornell University Medical College, New York. Neurologist-in-Chief, The New York Hospital, New York, New York.

JEROME F. POSNER, M.D.

Professor of Neurology, Cornell University Medical College, New York. Attending Neurologist, Memorial Sloan-Kettering Cancer Center and The New York Hospital, New York, New York.

PUBLISHER'S FOREWORD

The first edition of Russell L. Cecil's **Textbook of Medicine** was published by the W. B. Saunders Company in 1927. For many editions, first alone and later with the skilled and sensitive collaboration of Robert F. Loeb, Dr. Cecil guided the famous **Textbook** through a distinguished career of unquestioned authority and unique service to the ever more complex specialty of internal medicine and to those who would practice its art and master its science. This tradition has been carried forward by subsequent editors and authors, and the seventeenth edition of the classic **Cecil Textbook** was published by Saunders in 1985, a monumental lexicon of over two thousand pages representing the dedicated efforts of eleven internationally recognized editors and scores of superbly qualified contributing authors.

As work on this most recent edition of the **Cecil Textbook** progressed, it became ever more apparent to editors and publisher alike that in achieving its goal of completeness and authority another important goal had been to a degree eclipsed. The **Textbook** could no longer offer a fluid account of modern medicine to those members of its audience whose need was for either a teaching instrument in key general subjects or a reintroduction to the practice of general medicine. From this recognition, our new book, **Cecil Essentials of Medicine**, was developed.

It is important to understand that **Cecil Essentials** is a wholly new work—not an abridgement of the ancestor volume. **Cecil Essentials** quite properly shares editorship with the **Textbook**, but the editors now have set themselves different tasks. In **Cecil Essentials** their aim has been to provide a "reader-friendly" yet comprehensive review that describes all important medical disorders in a way that both the student and the nonspecialist will find readily understandable. Many sections can, in fact, be read at one sitting. The striking new two-color diagrams enhance the text without descending into mere decoration.

Its long history of success has demonstrated beyond argument that the **Cecil Textbook of Medicine** serves its specialty well. As we present our new **Cecil Essentials** to its ultimate judge—you, the reader—we hope you will find that it, too, fulfills successfully its own special role.

W. B. SAUNDERS COMPANY

PREFACE

We take pleasure in introducing a new idea in the teaching of general internal medicine—a short introductory textbook, **Cecil Essentials of Medicine**, to serve as a companion to the encyclopedic **Cecil Textbook of Medicine**.

The scope of medicine has enlarged greatly during recent years. As a consequence, the **Cecil Textbook of Medicine** has necessarily grown considerably, continuing to provide comprehensive accounts of both "traditional" medical disease states and the many "new" disorders appearing on the medical scene. These pressures have made the **Cecil** editors increasingly aware of the need for a smaller **Essentials** that would serve two principal purposes. One is to present the fundamental principles and practice of medicine that all medical graduates must know—at a length that can be digested within the framework of the standard undergraduate medical clerkship. The second, through regular revision of the **Essentials**, will be to offer a readable and succinct reintroduction for general physicians and other nonmedical specialists who wish to renew their knowledge of the constant advances that mark the progress of general medicine.

The twelve sections in **Cecil Essentials** focus on different organ systems. Each section begins with pertinent anatomic and physiologic considerations and a description of the cardinal clinical and laboratory manifestations of disease. The sections then provide a series of chapters describing major clinical disorders. The content of **Cecil Essentials** thus represents an appropriate "core" of internal medicine that a student of medicine can reasonably be expected to grasp during the traditional undergraduate medical clerkship.

This book relates closely to the **Cecil Textbook** in its editors, who have designed it so that the larger text, now in its seventeenth edition, can be employed easily for reference. The text and illustrations of **Cecil Essentials**, however, are original contributions by the small number of authors who assisted in preparing the twelve individual sections. We thank these contributors for their participation in this new venture. We also thank the residents, fellows, and faculty members at our institutions for their help in determining the content of the **Essentials** and for criticizing our early drafts.

At the W. B. Saunders Company, Mr. J. Dereck Jeffers and Mr. John Dyson provided valuable editorial assistance, and Mrs. Lorraine B. Kilmer gave inspirational help in the design and format of this book, assisting us at every stage of its preparation. We also thank those at our institutions who provided invaluable assistance in the preparation of **Essentials**: Ms. Clementine M. Whitman (Houston); Ms. Carol Bennett (Cleveland); Ms. Nancy Marmor (New York); and Ms. Judith A. Serrell (San Francisco).

THOMAS E. ANDREOLI

CHARLES C. J. CARPENTER

FRED PLUM

LLOYD H. SMITH, JR.

TABLE OF CONTENTS

VI ONCOLOGY

VII METABOLIC DISEASES

VIII ENDOCRINE DISEASES

IX DISEASES OF BONE AND BONE MINERAL METABOLISM

X INFECTIOUS DISEASES

XI MUSCULOSKELETAL AND CONNECTIVE TISSUE DISEASES

XII NEUROLOGIC DISEASE

SECTION

I

CARDIOVASCULAR DISEASES

1

STRUCTURE AND FUNCTION OF THE NORMAL HEART AND BLOOD VESSELS

GROSS ANATOMY

The human heart is located in the middle mediastinum just above the diaphragm between the left and right lungs. About two thirds of the heart is left of the midline, resulting in an apical impulse normally palpated in the fourth to fifth left intercostal space at the midclavicular line. Two relatively thin-walled upper chambers termed the right and left atria and two thicker-walled lower chambers, the right and left ventricles, compose the heart (Fig. 1–1). The interatrial septum, the thinnest portion of which is the foramen ovale, separates the left and right atria. The ventricles are muscular structures that pump blood through the pulmonary arteries to the lungs (right ventricle) and through the aorta and the entire systemic circulation to the body (left ventricle). The left ventricle has walls significantly thicker than those of the right ventricle because of the considerably higher systemic arterial pressure into which it pumps blood. The interventricular septum separates the two ventricles. The lower and much larger part of the interventricular system is

termed the muscular interventricular septum and is composed of muscle the same thickness as that of the left ventricular free wall. The uppermost portion of the septum, termed the membranous interventricular septum, also forms a portion of the right atrial wall. The thin inner layer of the heart wall that is in contact with the blood is the endocardium. Between the endocardium and the epicardium, or outer layer, is the heart muscle, or myocardium.

The tricuspid valve separates the right atrium and right ventricle. It is a three-leaflet structure that allows blood to flow from the right atrium to the right ventricle when right atrial pressure exceeds right ventricular pressure (diastole). When the right ventricle contracts (systole), the valve closes, preventing retrograde flow of blood into the right atrium. The mitral valve separates the left atrium from the left ventricle and has only two leaflets, a large anteromedial and a small posterolateral leaflet. A fibrous ring called the annulus supports each valve and forms a portion of the fibrous structural skeleton of the heart. Chords of fibrous tissue, the chordae tendineae, extend from the ventricular surfaces of both atrioventricular (AV) valves and attach to the papillary muscles. Papillary muscles are bundles of cardiac muscle (myocardium) arising from the interior of the ventricular walls. As the ventricles contract, the papillary muscles also contract, pulling taut the chordae tendineae and preventing the AV valves from prolapsing back into the atria and leaking. There are two papillary muscles in the left ventricle (anteromedial and posterolateral) and three in the right ventricle, connected via the chordae tendineae to each valve leaflet.

A somewhat different type of valve, the semilunar valve (meaning half moon, an indication of its shape), separates the ventricles from their respective outflow tracts. The pulmonic valve is the arterial valve of the right ventricle and is composed of three fibrous leaflets or cusps that are forced open against the walls of the pulmonary artery during ventricular ejection of blood but fall back into the pulmonary outflow tract during diastole, their free edges coapting to prevent blood from returning into the right ventricle. The aortic valve is a thicker but similar three-valved structure and lies between the left ventricle and the aorta. The aortic wall behind each aortic valve cusp bulges outward, forming three structures known as sinuses of Valsalva. The left and right coronary arteries emerge from the aortic wall of two of these sinuses of Valsalva. The two most anterior aortic cusps are known as the left and right coronary cusps because of the respective origins of the left and right coronary arteries,

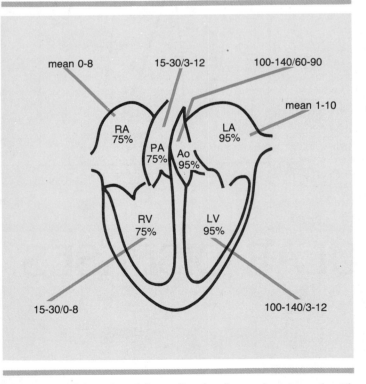

FIGURE 1–1. Orientation of the cardiac chambers and great vessels with normal intracardiac pressures (mm Hg) and oxygen saturations (%).

while the remaining posterior cusp is known as the noncoronary cusp.

The pericardium, a double-layered fibrous structure, encloses the heart. The visceral layer is immediately adjacent to the heart and forms part of the epicardium (outer layer) of the heart. The parietal layer is exterior to the heart and is separated from the visceral layer by a thin film of lubricating fluid (10 to 20 ml total) that allows the heart to move freely within the pericardial sac.

Venous blood returning from the body enters the right atrium through the inferior vena cava from below and the superior vena cava from above (Fig. 1–2). Most venous blood returning from the coronary circulation enters the right atrium via the coronary sinus. Blood from these three sources mixes and enters the right ventricle during diastole, when the triscupid valve is open. The right ventricle subsequently contracts (systole), closing the tricuspid valve to prevent retrograde blood flow, and ejects blood through the pulmonic valve into the pulmonary artery. The right ventricle is anterior to the left ventricle, and the pulmonary artery is anterior to the aorta. The pulmonary artery bifurcates into left and right branches that travel to the left and right lungs. The pulmonary artery has thinner walls than the aorta, and pulmonary arterial pressure is normally much less than aortic pressure. The pulmonary artery progressively divides into smaller and smaller arteries, arterioles, and eventually capillaries, where carbon dioxide is exchanged for oxygen via the pulmonary alveoli. The capillaries lead to pulmonary veins that coalesce to form the four larger pulmonary veins entering the left atrium posteriorly. Oxygenated blood from the pulmonary veins passes from the left atrium through the mitral valve to the left ventricle, which ejects blood during systole across the aortic valve into the aorta. The aorta divides into branches that deliver blood to the entire body (Fig. 1–3). The division continues to form smaller arteries, arterioles, and eventually capillaries that deliver oxygen and metabolic substrates to the tissues in exchange for CO_2 and other waste products. Blood collected from the peripheral capillaries is returned to the right atrium via the venous system.

The right and left coronary arteries course over the epicardial surface of the heart to distribute blood to the myocardium (Fig. 1–4). The left main coronary artery bifurcates within a few centimeters of its origin into two major vessels. The left anterior descending coronary artery proceeds anteriorly in the anterior interventricular groove (between both ventricles) toward the apex of the heart, supplying the anterior free wall of the left ventricle and the anterior two thirds of the septum. The circumflex coronary artery travels posteriorly in the atrioventricular groove (between left atrium and ventricle) and usually supplies a portion of the posterolateral surface of the heart. The right coronary artery courses in the right atrioventricular groove (between right atrium and ventricle) and distributes several branches to the right ventricle before reaching the left ventricle, where the atrioventricular grooves meet the pos-

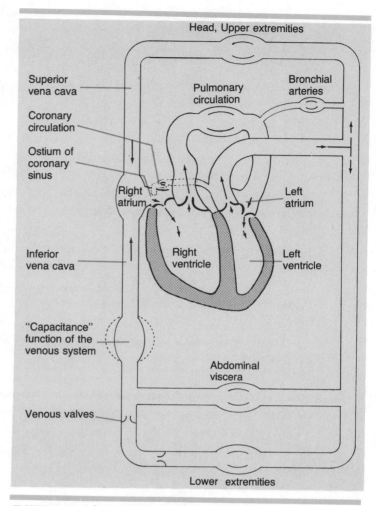

FIGURE 1–2. Schematic representation of the systemic and pulmonary circulatory systems. The venous system contains the greatest amount of blood at any one time and is highly distensible, accommodating a wide range of blood volumes (high capacitance).

terior interventricular groove (the "crux" of the heart). In 90 per cent of patients the right coronary artery reaches the crux of the heart and supplies the branches to the AV node and the inferobasal third of the septum (posterior descending artery). This pattern is termed "right dominant distribution" (even though the left coronary artery supplies the majority of the coronary circulation). In approximately 10 per cent of patients, a relatively large circumflex coronary artery reaches the crux of the heart and gives rise to the posterior descending coronary artery and the branch to the AV node. This situation is termed "left dominant," and the diminutive right coronary artery supplies only the right ventricle. Blood is supplied to the sinus node via a branch of the right coronary artery (55 per cent of cases) or the circumflex coronary artery (45 per cent). Most of the venous network of the heart coalesces to form the coronary sinus. Some of the right ventricular and atrial venous drainage occurs via much smaller anterior car-

	Vessel Diameter	Cross-sectional Area of Entire System (sq cm)	Per Cent of Total Blood Volume in System at Any Time	Mean Pressure (mm Hg)	Resistance
Aorta	25 mm	2.5		100	low
Artery	4 mm	20	15%	96	low
Arteriole	30 μ	40		85→30	high and variable
Capillary	8 μ	2500	5%	30→10	medium
Venule	20 μ	250		10	low
Vein	5 mm	80	59%	5	low
Vena cava	30 mm	8		0	low

FIGURE 1–3. Major components of the systemic vascular tree. Although the capillaries are smallest in diameter, their total cross-sectional area is largest because of their tremendous numbers. The velocity of flow through any portion of the system is inversely proportional to the total cross-sectional area; therefore the flow of blood is slowest in the capillaries, allowing for exchange of fluid and nutrients. The greatest pressure decrease occurs across the arterioles because of their high resistance to flow; this resistance is variable and regulates blood flow to each vascular bed.

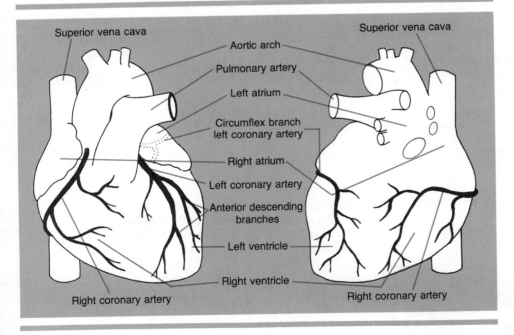

FIGURE 1–4. Major coronary arteries and their branches.

diac veins and tiny thebesian veins, most of which drain directly into the right atrium.

ELECTRICAL CONDUCTION SYSTEM (Fig. 1–5)

Cardiac electrical impulses originate in the sinus node, a spindle-shaped structure 10 to 20 mm long located near the junction of the superior vena cava and the right atrium. Even though various specialized tissues have been postulated to conduct the electrical impulse from the sinus node to the AV node, electrical transmission is probably cell-to-cell via working atrial muscle. The AV node provides the only normal conduction pathway between the atria and the ventricles. It is situated just beneath the right atrial endocardium above the insertion of the septal leaflet of the tricuspid valve and anterior to the ostium of the coronary sinus. After conduction delay in the AV node, the electrical impulse travels to the His bundle, which descends posteriorly along the membranous interventricular septum to the top of the muscular septum. The His bundle gives rise to the right and left bundle branches. The right bundle branch is a single group of fibers that travels down the right ventricular side of the muscular interventricular septum. The left bundle branch is a larger, less discrete array of conducting fibers located on the left side of the interventricular septum. The left bundle branch may divide into two somewhat distinct pathways that travel toward the anterolateral (left anterior fascicle) and posteromedial (left posterior fascicle) papillary muscles. The left posterior fascicle is larger and more diffuse than the anterior fascicle and usually has a more reliable vascular supply than either the left anterior fascicle or the right bundle branch. The left and right bundle branches progressively divide into tiny Purkinje fibers that arborize and finally make intimate contact with ventricular muscle tissue.

MICROSCOPIC ANATOMY

In general, two functional cell types are present in cardiac tissue: those responsible for electrical impulse generation and transmission and those responsible for mechanical contraction. Nodal cells are thought to be the source of normal impulse formation in the sinus node and are richly innervated with adrenergic and cholinergic nerve fibers. Like the sinus node, the AV node and His bundle regions are innervated with a rich supply of cholinergic and adrenergic fibers. Purkinje cells are large clear cells found in the His bundle, bundle branches, and their arborizations. They have particularly well-developed end-to-end connections that may facilitate rapid longitudinal conduction.

Atrial and ventricular myocardial cells, the contractile cells of the heart, contain numerous cross-banded bundles termed myofibrils that traverse the length of the fiber. Myofibrils are composed of longitudinally repeating sarcomeres (Fig. 1–6). Thick filaments composed of myosin comprise the A band, while thin filaments composed primarily of actin extend from the Z line through the I band into the A band, ending at the edges of the central H zone, which is the central area of the A band where thin filaments are absent. Thick and thin filaments overlap in the A band, and interaction between the thick and thin filaments provides the force for contraction of the heart.

The surface membrane of the cell is termed the sarcolemma, and adjacent myocardial cells are connected end to end by a thickened portion of the sarcolemma termed the intercalated disc. Near the Z lines of the sarcolemma are wide invaginations called the T system that traverse the cell. Not continuous with the T system is the sarcoplasmic reticulum that surrounds each myofibril and participates in the excitation of the muscle. When the sarcolemma is depolarized electrically,

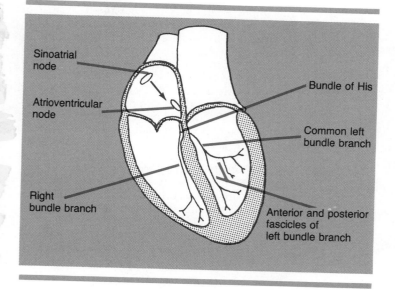

FIGURE 1–5. Schematic representation of the cardiac conduction system.

FIGURE 1–6. *A,* A sarcomere as it appears under the electron microscope. *B,* Schematic of the location and interaction of actin and myosin (see text).

the impulse conducts through the T system to cause calcium release from the sarcoplasmic reticulum and therefore activates the myofibrils to contract. The thick fibers in the myofibrils are composed of myosin molecules that have the ability to split ATP and interact with the thin actin filaments when activated by calcium. Regulatory proteins, troponin and tropomyosin, inhibit the interaction of actin and myosin unless a calcium-troponin complex is present that then allows the actin-myosin interaction to proceed. The sarcolemma possesses the ability to control the flux of various ions (especially sodium, potassium, and calcium) into and out of the cell via specific ionic channels located within the membrane. The selective permeability of the membrane establishes ionic gradients and the electrical forces that create and maintain the resting transmembrane potential and generate the action potential (see below).

CARDIAC DEVELOPMENT

Congenital heart disease results from altered embryonic development or failure of the rudimentary portion of a structure ever to be formed. Abnormal development of one structure in turn may hinder the development of another portion of the circulatory system (for example, abnormal development of the mitral valve may lead to abnormal formation of the left ventricle).

The fetus' circulation essentially places the pulmonary and systemic systems in parallel rather than in series as in the adult. Oxygenated blood from the umbilical vein passes into the portal venous system and subsequently into the inferior vena cava and is shunted preferentially across the patent foramen ovale to the left heart to perfuse the coronary arteries, head, and upper trunk. Blood returning from the upper portions of the body arrives at the right atrium via the superior vena cava, and most proceeds through the tricuspid valve to the right ventricle and pulmonary artery. However, only a small proportion of this blood goes into the pulmonary arterial tree; most is shunted via the patent ductus arteriosus to the

descending aorta. Note that many congenital lesions that cause intracardiac shunts (for example, tetralogy of Fallot) or markedly abnormal cardiac outflow (for example, transposition of the great arteries) would not cause any difficulty during fetal development.

At birth the pulmonary vascular resistance decreases markedly owing to the inflation of the lungs and the increase in oxygen tension to which the pulmonary vessels are exposed. Systemic vascular resistance rises when the umbilical cord is clamped, removing the low-resistance placental circulation. Left atrial pressure rises, which in turn closes the foramen ovale. The increase in arterial Po_2 along with alterations in prostaglandins causes the ductus arteriosus to close functionally within 10 to 15 hours. Many congenital heart lesions may not become apparent until cyanosis develops after closure of the foramen ovale or ductus arteriosus.

MYOCARDIAL METABOLISM

The heart uses ATP, created by metabolism of carbohydrates or fatty acids, to derive energy for contraction and electrical activity. Energy for electrical activity is minimal compared to that required for contraction. Stored energy reserves are scarce, and the heart must continually have a source of energy in order to function. The principal oxidative substrate for ATP production is fatty acid, but if it is not available, a variety of carbohydrates can be used. Myocardial metabolism is aerobic, and a constant supply of oxygen must be available. The heart, unlike skeletal muscle, is unable to acquire an "oxygen debt" because of its inability to utilize anaerobic metabolism.

CIRCULATORY PHYSIOLOGY

The interaction between myosin and actin, coupled with ATP produced by oxidative phosphorylation, is thought to be the basis for the contraction of each myofibril and therefore the contraction of the whole muscle. Each myofibril exhibits a property called contractility (or inotropic state) that represents the ability of the fiber to develop contractile force. The force exhibited by the fiber is influenced not only by its contractile state but also by its initial length, or preload, according to the Starling curve (Fig. 1–7). This concept can be expanded from the single fiber to describe the function of the entire ventricle. Thus, the abscissa, formerly preload or fiber length, becomes left ventricular filling pressure or volume (i.e., the amount of stretch on the myocardial fibers in diastole); and the ordinate, formerly tension, becomes stroke volume or stroke work (i.e., the ability of the heart to generate tension). Note that as diastolic pressure increases, the normal heart is able to increase its stroke volume, up to a point. This relationship is referred to as a ventricular function curve and, given identical states of contractility and afterload (see below), defines the amount of work that a heart is able to perform. Several factors determine left ventricular filling pressure (Table 1–1).

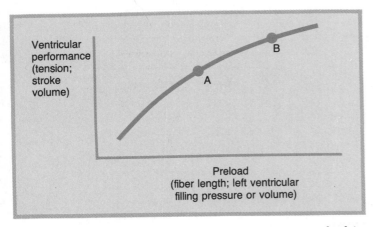

FIGURE 1–7. The normal ventricular function curve. As preload increases from A to B, the curve defines the resultant increase in developed tension or overall cardiac performance.

The term afterload describes the "impedance" or resistance against which the heart must contract. Like preload, afterload also can refer either to a single myofibril or to the heart as a whole. The afterload is approximated by the arterial pressure, the major determinant of the impedance to left ventricular contraction. In the intact heart, the afterload determines the amount of blood the heart can pump given a fixed preload and fixed state of contractility; that is, the higher the workload against which the heart must function, the less blood it can eject, and vice versa. Therefore, the ventricular function curve will be shifted up and to the left with decreasing afterload and shifted down and to the right with increasing afterload. Shifts in ventricular function with changes in afterload are minimal in normal ventricles but prominent in failing ventricles.

Heart rate is another determinant of cardiac performance. Even though an increased demand for cardiac output increases contractility and stroke volume via sympathetic nervous system activation, the most important response to sympathetic stimulation serving to increase cardiac output is the rise in heart rate (cardiac output = stroke volume × heart rate). A decrease in the cardiac output or blood pressure increases sympathetic and decreases parasympathetic discharge via baroreceptor mechanisms to increase heart rate. Likewise, an elevated blood pressure will activate the carotid baroreceptors, augment vagal activity, and slow the heart rate.

Four phases of the cardiac cycle can be identified upon initiation of ventricular myocardial contraction (Fig. 1–8). (1) During "isovolumic contraction," the intramyocardial pressure rises with no ejection of blood or change in ventricular volume. (2) When left ventricular pressure reaches that of the aorta, the aortic valve opens and blood is ejected from the contracting ventricle. (3) As the ventricle relaxes and left ventricular pressure decreases, the aortic valve closes, and "isovolumic relaxation" occurs. (4) Upon sufficient decrease in left ventricular pressure, the mitral valve opens and ventricular filling from the atrium occurs. The ventricle fills most rapidly in early diastole and again in late diastole when the atrium contracts. Loss of atrial contraction (e.g., atrial fibrillation or AV dissociation) can impair ventricular filling, especially into a noncompliant ("stiff") vehicle.

Normal intracardiac pressures are shown in Figure 1–1. Atrial pressure curves are composed of the a wave, which is generated by atrial contraction, and the v wave, which is an early diastolic peak caused by filling of the atrium from the peripheral veins. The x descent follows the a wave and the y descent follows the v wave. A small deflection, the c wave, occurs after the a wave in early systole and probably represents bulging of the tricuspid valve apparatus into the left atrium during early systole. Ventricular pressures are described by a peak systolic pressure and an end-diastolic pressure, which is the ventricular pressure immediately before the onset of systole. Note that the minimum left ventricular pressure occurs

TABLE 1–1. FACTORS AFFECTING CARDIAC PERFORMANCE

Preload (left ventricular diastolic volume)	Total blood volume Venous tone (sympathetic tone) Body position Intrathoracic and intrapericardial pressure Atrial contraction Pumping action of skeletal muscle
Afterload (impedance against which the left ventricle must eject blood)	Peripheral vascular resistance Left ventricular volume (preload, wall tension) Physical characteristics of the arterial tree (for example, elasticity of vessels or presence of outflow obstruction)
Contractility (cardiac performance independent of preload or afterload)	Sympathetic nerve impulses Circulating catecholamines Digitalis, calcium, other inotropic agents } increased contractility Increased heart rate or post-extrasystolic augmentation
	Anoxia, acidosis Pharmacological depression } decreased contractility Loss of myocardium Intrinsic depression
Heart Rate	Autonomic nervous system Temperature, metabolic rate

in early diastole. Aortic and pulmonary artery pressures are represented by a peak systolic and a minimum diastolic value.

Cardiac output is a measure of the amount of blood flow in liters/minute. The cardiac index is the cardiac output divided by the body surface area and is normally 2.8 to 4.2 L/min/sq m. Cardiac output can be measured by either indicator dilution or the Fick technique (see Chapter 2). The pulmonary and systemic vascular resistances are also important parameters of circulatory function. Resistance is defined as the difference in pressure across a capillary bed divided by the flow across that capillary bed, usually the cardiac output: $R = (P_1 - P_2)/flow$ (Fig. 1–3). For example, the pulmonary vascular resistance is the difference between the mean pulmonary arterial pressure and mean pulmonary venous pressure, divided by the pulmonary blood flow. Similarly, systemic vascular resistance is the difference between mean arterial pressure and mean right atrial pressure, divided by the systemic cardiac output. Note that an increase in arterial pressure may occur without necessarily causing an increase in vascular resistance. For example, if both pulmonary arterial and venous pressures are elevated to the same degree, pulmonary vascular resistance will be unchanged; if pulmonary blood flow and pulmonary arterial pressure increase while pulmonary venous pressure remains the same, resistance will be unchanged.

The most widely used parameter for quantitating overall ventricular function is the ejection fraction, defined as the diastolic volume minus the systolic volume (stroke volume), divided by

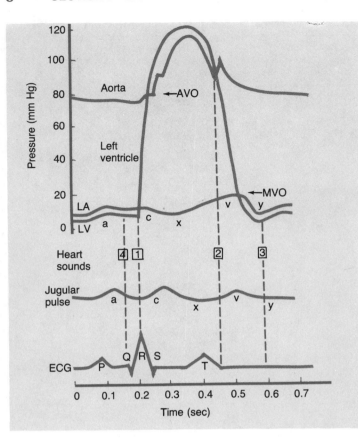

FIGURE 1–8. Simultaneous ECG, pressures obtained from the left atrium, left ventricle, and aorta, and the jugular pulse during one cardiac cycle. For simplification, right-sided heart pressures have been omitted. Normal right atrial pressure closely parallels that of the left atrium, and right ventricular and pulmonary artery pressures time closely with their corresponding left-sided heart counterparts, only being reduced in magnitude. The normal mitral and aortic valve closure precedes tricuspid and pulmonic closure, respectively, whereas valve opening reverses this order. The jugular venous pulse lags behind the right atrial pressure.

During the course of one cardiac cycle, note that the electrical events (ECG) initiate and therefore precede the mechanical (pressure) events and that the latter precede the auscultatory events (heart sounds) they themselves produce. Shortly after the P wave, the atria contract to produce the a wave; a fourth heart sound may succeed the latter. The QRS complex initiates ventricular systole, followed shortly by left ventricular contraction and the rapid build-up of left ventricular (LV) pressure. Almost immediately LV pressure exceeds left atrial (LA) pressure to close the mitral valve and produce the first heart sounds. When LV pressure exceeds aortic pressure, the aortic valve opens (AVO), and when aortic pressure is once again greater than LV pressure, the aortic valve closes to produce the second heart sound and terminate ventricular ejection. The decreasing LV pressure drops below LA pressure to open the mitral valve (MVO), and a period of rapid ventricular filling commences. During this time a third heart sound may be heard. The jugular pulse is explained under the discussion of the venous pulse.

the diastolic volume: (DV–SV)/DV. These volumes may be estimated from either invasive (e.g., left ventriculography) or noninvasive (e.g., echocardiography or radionuclide ventriculography) tests. The ejection fraction may be a useful gross evaluation of ventricular function, but there are situations (for example, when a large left ventricular aneurysm is present) in which the ejection fraction can give a misleading impression of overall ventricular function.

PHYSIOLOGY OF THE CORONARY CIRCULATION

Three major determinants of myocardial oxygen consumption are contractility, heart rate, and wall tension. Myocardial wall tension is directly proportional to the pressure within the ventricular chamber and the radius of the ventricular chamber (Laplace relationship). The myocardial mass is a determinant of wall tension and therefore myocardial oxygen consumption; the larger the muscle mass, the more oxygen needed.

The coronary vascular bed is able to autoregulate, enabling myocardial oxygen and substrate delivery to equal the demand. Coronary vascular resistance is normally determined by the arterioles and is influenced by neural and metabolic factors. Both the sympathetic and parasympathetic nervous systems innervate the coronary arteries. Alpha receptor stimulation causes vasoconstriction while stimulation of the beta-2 receptor as well as the vagus causes vasodilation. Metabolic factors regulate regional perfusion. Several mediators including oxygen, carbon dioxide, and metabolites such as adenosine are probably important. However, when coronary perfusion pressure falls to below 60 to 70 mm Hg, the vessels become maximally dilated and flow depends on perfusion pressure alone, since capability for further autoregulation is lost. The normal coronary vascular bed has a capacity to increase its blood flow four- to five-fold during maximal exercise. Hemodynamic factors that affect coronary perfusion include arterial pressure (especially diastolic pressure, since coronary flow occurs primarily in diastole), the time spent in diastole, and the intraventricular pressure (which exerts tension on the myocardial walls and diminishes coronary flow).

PHYSIOLOGY OF THE SYSTEMIC CIRCULATION

The aortic wall contains elastic fibers that allow it to expand with the expulsion of blood from the left ventricle, somewhat damping the pulse pressure generated and aiding diastolic flow to the coronary arteries with its recoil. The aorta successively branches into smaller and smaller vessels until arterioles, the major determinants of resistance in the systemic circulation, are reached (see Fig. 1–3). The arterioles contain a vascular sphincter that modulates blood flow dependent on regional metabolic needs; for example, acidosis and decreased oxygen tension increase regional perfusion, and vice versa. The capillaries consist of a single endothelial cell layer and allow diffusion of oxygen, nutrients, CO_2, and waste products. The capillaries lead into the venous system, where blood is eventually delivered back to the right atrium. The flow of blood returning to the heart is aided by the valves in the venous system, which prevent reverse flow, particularly in the larger veins of the legs. The "milking" action of the muscles of the arms and legs and the pressure changes in the thoracic cavity also help to return blood to the heart. The veins have considerably thinner walls than the arteries and can accommodate a larger blood volume under low pressures (capacitance vessels). Vasoconstriction or vasodilation of the venous system can control the amount of blood returning to the heart. More of the total blood volume is located in the venous than in the arterial portion of the circulation. The lymphatic vessels also contribute to the return of fluid from the periphery. The major terminal vessel of the lymphatic system is the thoracic duct, which usually empties into the left brachiocephalic vein.

PHYSIOLOGY OF THE PULMONARY CIRCULATION

The pulmonary circulation has a rich capillary network similar to that of the systemic circulation. The pulmonary alveoli are adjacent to the capillaries, permitting oxygen to diffuse into and carbon dioxide out of the capillary blood. Oxygen is the major mediator of pulmonary autoregulation. In regions where the partial pressure of oxygen is high, pulmonary vasodilation occurs and blood flow is directed preferentially toward well-oxygenated areas of the lung. When the partial pressure of oxygen is low, pulmonary vasoconstriction occurs, preventing the perfusion of areas of the lung that have relatively poor oxygen availability. These vasodilatory effects of oxygen are opposite to those in the systemic circulation. Acidemia potentiates the pulmonary vasoconstrictive effect of hypoxemia, also opposite to its effect on systemic arterioles.

The lungs receive blood through the bronchial arteries as well as the pulmonary arteries (dual blood supply). The bronchial arteries supply arterial blood to the pulmonary tissue and drain into the bronchial veins, some of which drain into the systemic venous bed. Some bronchial veins drain into the pulmonary veins, creating a small physiological right-to-left shunt.

Pulmonary vascular resistance is normally one tenth that of systemic vascular resistance and accounts for the small pressure gradient required to propel blood across the pulmonary vascular bed. Because the pulmonary vasculature is very distensible (compliant), a relatively large left-to-right intracardiac shunt may exist with only a minimal rise in pulmonary arterial pressure.

CARDIOVASCULAR RESPONSE TO EXERCISE

The heart responds to exercise principally by adrenergic stimulation and vagal withdrawal, which increase heart rate and contractility, and by peripheral circulatory alterations (Table 1–2). The increase in heart rate usually accounts for the majority of the increase in cardiac output. Increased contractility contributes to the increase in cardiac output by increasing the stroke volume.

TABLE 1–2. PHYSIOLOGIC RESPONSES TO EXERCISE

RESPONSE	MECHANISM
↑ Heart rate	↑ Sympathetic stimulation ↓ Parasympathetic stimulation

↑ Stroke volume
  ↑ Contractility
  ↑ Venous return
	↑ Sympathetic stimulation
	Sympathetic-mediated venoconstriction
	Pumping action of skeletal muscles
	↓ Intrathoracic pressure with deep inspirations
	Arteriolar vasodilation in exercising muscle

↓ Afterload	Arteriolar vasodilation in exercising muscle (mediated chiefly by local metabolites)
↑ Blood pressure	↑ Cardiac output Vasoconstriction (sympathetic stimulation) of nonexercising vascular beds
↑ O_2 extraction	Shift in oxyhemoglobin dissociation curve due to local acidosis

Vessels supplying exercising muscles dilate, whereas the remaining vascular beds vasoconstrict. Isometric and isotonic exercises affect the cardiovascular system somewhat differently. The predominant response to isometric exercise (e.g., weight lifting) is an increase in peripheral vasoconstriction with a subsequent increase in arterial pressure. In contrast, isotonic exercise (e.g., jogging) reduces systemic vascular resistance primarily in exercising muscles, which improves cardiac output. Those who exercise regularly obtain a cardiac training effect, with a lower resting heart rate and a greater capacity to increase cardiac output during exercise.

CARDIOVASCULAR PHYSIOLOGY DURING PREGNANCY

See Chapter 16.

ELECTROPHYSIOLOGY

If a microelectrode is introduced into a single myocardial cell, an action potential (Fig. 1–9) can be recorded by measuring the potential difference between the inside and the outside of the cell (inside negative). The resting membrane potential of a normal Purkinje cell is approximately −90 millivolts (mv) with respect to the outside of the cell. When the membrane potential is depolarized to a certain threshold level, an action potential occurs with a rapid upstroke (phase 0); a return toward zero from the initial overshoot or early rapid repolarization (phase 1); a plateau (phase 2); final rapid repolarization (phase 3); and resting membrane potential and diastolic depolarization (phase 4). The normal resting potential is maintained by the active (i.e., energy-requiring) exclusion of sodium and the accumulation of potassium inside the cell. Phase 0 or rapid depolarization is due chiefly to the opening of the sarcolemmal channels to sodium entrance in atrial and ventricular muscle and cells in the His-Purkinje system. Calcium is important in the maintenance of the action potential plateau of fast

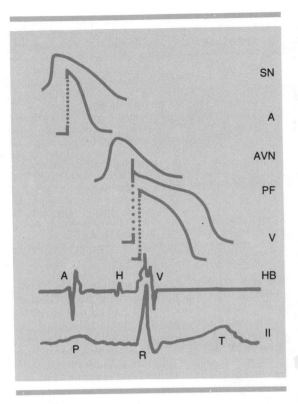

FIGURE 1–9. Action potentials recorded from different tissues in the heart remounted with a His bundle recording and scalar ECG from a patient to illustrate the timing during a single cardiac cycle. SN = Sinus nodal potential; A = atrial muscle potential; AVN = atrioventricular nodal potential; PF = Purkinje fiber potential; V = ventricular muscle potential; HB = His bundle recording; II = lead II. The A-H interval measured in the His bundle recording approximates AV nodal conduction time, and the H-V interval approximates His-Purkinje system conduction time.

sodium channel–dependent cells and in the generation of the action potential upstroke in slow calcium channel–dependent cells such as the sinus and AV nodes. Phase 3 is mediated chiefly by an outward potassium current, and the membrane returns to its negative resting potential during electrical diastole.

Automaticity is a property of some cardiac tissues to undergo gradual phase 4 depolarization spontaneously until threshold potential is reached and the cell initiates an action potential that is propagated from one cell to another. Normal automaticity is present in sinus nodal tissue, some atrial and junctional tissues, the bundle branches, and Purkinje fibers. The sinus node discharges more rapidly than the other cells and is the normal pacemaker of the heart. *Conduction* is the propagation of a cardiac impulse and is most closely influenced by the amplitude and upstroke velocity of phase 0 of the action potential. *Refractoriness* is a property of cardiac tissue during which a stimulus occurring soon after a previous action potential fails to elicit another normal action potential; it is most closely related to the duration of phase 3 of the cardiac action potential in most tissues.

The genesis of the normal electrocardiogram is from electrical activity recorded by skin electrodes that is the sum of all the cardiac action potentials of its component cells. The P wave represents atrial depolarization. The PR interval is a measure of the time necessary to travel from the sinus node through the atrium, AV node, and His-Purkinje system to activate ventricular myocardial cells. The QRS complex represents the sum of all ventricular muscle cell depolarizations (phase 0), the ST segment represents the plateau phase, and the T wave represents the rapid repolarization (phase 3) of the heart as a whole.

Although the autonomic nervous system may affect atrial and ventricular tissue to a small extent, the most prominent autonomic effects are observed on the sinus and the AV nodes. Sympathetic stimulation increases the rate of automaticity and increases conduction velocity, whereas parasympathetic (vagal) activation does the opposite. Baroreceptors in the carotid sinus, located at the bifurcation of the internal and external carotid arteries, activate the vagus nerve when blood pressure increases and reflexively decrease heart rate and AV nodal conduction velocity.

REFERENCE

Berne RM, and Levy MN: Cardiovascular Physiology. 4th ed. St. Louis, The CV Mosby Co, 1981.

2 EVALUATION OF THE PATIENT WITH CARDIOVASCULAR DISEASE

HISTORY

The history is the most important tool in the evaluation of a patient (Table 2–1). *Chest pain* is the most common presenting symptom of cardiovascular disease and must be characterized carefully. Chest pain may be cardiac (myocardial or pericardial) or noncardiac in etiology (Tables 2–2 and 2–3).

Ischemic myocardial pain is a visceral discom-

TABLE 2–1. CARDINAL SYMPTOMS OF CARDIAC DISEASE

Chest pain or discomfort
Symptoms of heart failure
Palpitation
Syncope, presyncope

fort caused by insufficient oxygen delivery to an area of the heart. A transient oxygen supply/demand mismatch causes angina pectoris, whereas ischemia followed by myocardial necrosis is termed myocardial infarction. Angina pectoris is typically evoked by emotion, exertion, or a heavy meal, but more severe episodes can occur at rest or awaken the patient from sleep. It generally lasts only a few minutes and diminishes after exertion is stopped. When it is due to fixed coronary obstruction, the same degree of activity tends to reliably reproduce the pain. When due to coronary arterial spasm, with or without fixed obstruction, the level of activity that causes pain may vary. Nitroglycerin typically relieves the pain in about 5 minutes. Pain of a prolonged duration (>30 minutes) suggests either myocardial infarction or noncardiac pain. Respiration does not influence ischemic chest pain. The pain of both angina pectoris and myocardial infarction can be atypical in some patients and difficult to diagnose. Many patients describe a chest discomfort or fullness that they do not consider pain. Any patient who

TABLE 2–2. CARDIOVASCULAR CAUSES OF CHEST PAIN

CONDITION	LOCATION	QUALITY	DURATION	AGGRAVATING OR RELIEVING FACTORS	ASSOCIATED SYMPTOMS OR SIGNS
Angina	Retrosternal region; radiates to or occasionally isolated to neck, jaw, epigastrium, shoulder or arms—left common	Pressure, burning, squeezing, heaviness, indigestion	<10 minutes	Aggravated by exercise, cold weather, or emotional stress, or occurs after meals; relieved by rest or nitroglycerin; atypical (Prinzmetal's) angina may be unrelated to activity and caused by coronary artery spasm	S_4, paradoxical split S_2, or murmur of papillary muscle dysfunction during pain
Rest or crescendo angina	Same as angina	Same as angina	>10 minutes	Same as angina, with gradually decreasing tolerance for exertion	Same as angina
Myocardial infarction	Substernal, and may radiate like angina	Heaviness, pressure, burning, constriction	Sudden onset, 30 minutes or longer but variable; usually goes away in hours	Unrelieved	Shortness of breath, sweating, weakness, nausea, vomiting, severe anxiety
Pericarditis	Usually begins over sternum or toward cardiac apex and may radiate to neck and down left upper extremity; often more localized than the pain of myocardial ischemia	Sharp, stabbing, knifelike	Lasts many hours to days	Aggravated by deep breathing, rotating chest, or supine position; relieved by sitting up and leaning forward	Pericardial friction rub, cardiac tamponade, pulsus paradoxus
Dissecting aortic aneurysm	Anterior chest; radiates to thoracic area of back; may be abdominal; pain may move as dissection progresses	Excruciating, tearing, knifelike	Sudden onset, lasts for hours	Unrelated to anything	Lower blood pressure in one arm, absent pulses, paralysis, murmur of aortic insufficiency, pulsus paradoxus, myocardial infarction

TABLE 2–3. NONCARDIAC CAUSES OF CHEST PAIN

CONDITION	LOCATION	QUALITY	DURATION	AGGRAVATING OR RELIEVING FACTORS	ASSOCIATED SYMPTOMS OR SIGNS
Pulmonary embolism (chest pain often not present)	Substernal or over region of pulmonary infarction	Pleuritic (with pulmonary infarction) or angina-like	Sudden onset; minutes to < hour	May be aggravated by breathing	Dyspnea, tachypnea, tachycardia, hypotension; signs of acute right heart failure and pulmonary hypertension with large emboli; rales, pleural rub, hemoptysis with pulmonary infarction; clinically present in minority of cases
Pulmonary hypertension	Substernal	Pressure; oppressive		Aggravated by effort	Pain usually associated with dyspnea; signs of pulmonary hypertension (Table 4–3)
Pneumonia with pleurisy	Localized over area of consolidation	Pleuritic, well-localized		Painful breathing	Dyspnea, cough, fever, dull to percussion, bronchial breath sounds, rales, occasional pleural rub
Spontaneous pneumothorax	Unilateral	Sharp, well-localized	Sudden onset, lasts many hours	Painful breathing	Dyspnea; hyper-resonance and decreased breath and voice sounds over involved lung
Musculoskeletal disorders	Variable	Aching	Short or long duration	Aggravated by movement; history of muscle exertion	Tender to pressure or movement
Herpes zoster	Dermatomal in distribution		Prolonged	None	Rash appears in area of discomfort
Gastrointestinal disorders (e.g., esophageal reflux, peptic ulcer, cholecystitis)	Lower substernal area, epigastric, right or left upper quadrant	Burning, colic-like, aching		Precipitated by recumbency or meals	Nausea, regurgitation, food intolerance, melena, hematemesis, jaundice
Anxiety states	Often localized to a point	Sharp burning, commonly location of pain moves from place to place	Varies; usually very brief	Situational anger—very brief	Sighing respirations, often chest wall tenderness

has chest discomfort provoked by exertion and relieved by rest and any patient who has chest discomfort similar to the pain of a previous myocardial infarction should be suspected of ischemic myocardial chest pain.

The pain of pericardial inflammation (Table 2–3) may be difficult to differentiate from ischemic pain in a patient with pericarditis following myocardial infarction.

Patients with mitral valve prolapse sometimes present with a chest pain syndrome that may or may not resemble ischemic myocardial pain. The etiology of this chest pain is unclear.

Dyspnea is a subjective sensation of shortness of breath and often is a symptom of cardiac disease, especially in patients with congestive heart failure (Table 2–4). When left ventricular failure occurs, left atrial and subsequently pulmonary venous pressures rise. Pulmonary compliance decreases (stiff lungs) and causes a subjective sensation of air hunger before hypoxia, hypercapnia, or low cardiac output occur. As congestive heart failure worsens, transudative fluid accumulates in the alveoli and hypoxemia results. Because the supine position compared with the upright position augments venous return, patients with congestive heart failure demonstrate orthopnea, i.e., shortness of breath in the supine position relieved by sitting up. They also may demonstrate paroxysmal nocturnal dyspnea, i.e., awakening with shortness of breath two to three hours after falling asleep. It usually occurs only once nightly, is relieved by sitting or standing, and is probably related to central redistribution of fluid upon assuming the reclining position.

Occasionally, dyspnea can represent the anginal equivalent, a symptom of acute myocardial ischemia. Dyspnea is also a prominent feature of pulmonary disease, and at times the differentiation between pulmonary and cardiac causes of dyspnea are difficult (see Table 3–2). For example, patients with pulmonary dyspnea can exhibit orthopnea, whereas wheezes may be heard in patients with cardiac dyspnea (e.g., congestive heart failure). Sudden dyspnea is a common presentation of a pulmonary embolus.

Cyanosis is a bluish discoloration of the skin caused by an increased amount of nonoxygenated hemoglobin in the blood. Central cyanosis, often best seen on the oral mucous membranes, is due to right-to-left shunting of blood or impaired pulmonary function. Peripheral cyanosis, best seen in the extremities, may be due to shunting or to local discoloration due to vasoconstriction (e.g., low cardiac output, peripheral vascular disease, or exposure to cold). Cyanosis is more difficult to see in dark-skinned than in light-skinned individuals. Since cyanosis becomes apparent when ≥4 grams/100 ml of reduced hemoglobin is present, polycythemia tends to accentuate cyanosis and anemia tends to minimize it.

Syncope has multiple origins, including circulatory (e.g., volume depletion from a variety of causes) and neurological (e.g., seizures) as well as cardiac (see Chapter 8).

Palpitation refers to an awareness of heart beat, usually either irregular or rapid (see Chapter 8).

Fatigue is a common cardiac symptom but is extremely nonspecific. Patients who have a reduced cardiac output often complain of fatigue that may be exacerbated by drugs (for example, beta-adrenergic blocking drugs).

Edema is common in patients with congestive heart failure. Edema of the lower extremities (or the sacral area in bedridden patients) often is a symptom of right ventricular failure. Other causes of peripheral edema include the nephrotic syndrome, cirrhosis, and venous insufficiency. Peripheral edema may increase at the end of the day and decrease overnight as the dependent part is elevated and the fluid resorbed. Fluid within the peritoneal cavity is referred to as *ascites* and within the chest cavity as *pleural effusion*. Patients who have severe edema secondary to congestive heart failure may develop ascites, and ascites is especially frequent in patients who have constrictive pericarditis. Noncardiac causes of ascites such as cirrhosis, nephrosis, and peritoneal tumor must be excluded.

Cough and *hemoptysis* may be associated with cardiac disease, but it may be difficult to differentiate cardiac from pulmonary disease on the basis of these two symptoms alone. A cough, often orthostatic in nature, may be the primary complaint in some patients with pulmonary congestion. They tend not to bring up thick purulent sputum as do patients with chronic bronchitis. Hemoptysis occurs in congestive heart failure and

TABLE 2–4. SYMPTOMS AND SIGNS OF CARDIAC FAILURE

	SYMPTOMS	SIGNS
Left heart failure	Dyspnea Orthopnea Paroxysmal nocturnal dyspnea	Tachypnea Left ventricular S_3 gallop Left ventricular S_4 gallop (nonspecific) Rales Wheezes (cardiac asthma) Functional mitral regurgitation Pulsus alternans
Right heart failure	Peripheral edema Nocturia Abdominal fullness	Jugular venous distention Peripheral edema Ascites Anasarca Hepatomegaly Splenomegaly Hepatojugular reflux Right ventricular S_3, S_4 gallops Tricuspid regurgitation (holosystolic murmur, pulsatile liver, large jugular V wave) Signs of pulmonary hypertension if present (Table 4–3)
Either left or right heart failure	Fatigue Weakness Anorexia	Tachycardia Blood pressure often elevated Narrow pulse pressure Sweaty, cool extremities Pleural effusion (usually bilateral or isolated right) Cardiomegaly Cheyne-Stokes (periodic or cyclic) respiration Mental confusion

is especially common in patients with mitral stenosis. Massive hemoptysis is generally not a cardiac symptom.

Nocturia, secondary to resorption of edema at night, is common in patients with congestive heart failure. Anorexia, abdominal fullness, right upper quadrant tenderness (secondary to hepatomegaly), and weight loss are also symptoms of advanced heart failure. Hoarseness may occasionally result from recurrent laryngeal nerve compression by an aortic aneurysm, dilated pulmonary artery, or large left atrium.

A history of rheumatic fever, prolonged febrile illnesses, sore throats, or any rheumatic complaints as a child should be sought. The patient should be asked about any past history of a heart murmur or other cardiac abnormalities noted in a previous examination. Childhood activity levels may be important in evaluating patients suspected of having congenital or rheumatic heart

TABLE 2–5. NEW YORK HEART ASSOCIATION FUNCTIONAL CLASSIFICATION

Class I	No limitation	Ordinary physical activity does not cause symptoms
Class II	Slight limitation	Comfortable at rest. Ordinary physical activity causes symptoms
Class III	Marked limitation	Comfortable at rest. Less than ordinary activity causes symptoms
Class IV	Inability to carry on any physical activity	Symptoms present at rest

disease. Females should be asked about problems during pregnancy, a state that stresses the cardiovascular system. The presence of risk factors for coronary artery disease (see Chapter 7) should be determined. The New York Heart Association's functional classification of patients with cardiac disease is useful (Table 2–5).

GENERAL PHYSICAL EXAMINATION

The patient's general appearance and vital signs are important in the overall evaluation of suspected cardiac disease (see Table 2–4). In mild to moderately severe heart failure, the blood pressure is usually elevated; hypotension is a sign of advanced myocardial failure. Cheyne-Stokes respirations, thought to be related to a delay in baroreceptor sensing of oxygenation due to poor perfusion of the baroreceptors, may be noted in patients with either advanced heart failure or primary central nervous system disease. Certain distinct syndromes may suggest a congenital anomaly; for example, Down's syndrome is associated with several congenital cardiac malformations (most commonly ventricular septal defect and endocardial cushion defect), and Marfan's syndrome is associated with disease of the aorta and aortic valve.

Examination of the lungs is generally normal in patients with heart disease unless left heart failure with pulmonary congestion is present (see Table 2–4). Pulmonary rales are fine, discrete sounds produced by fluid within alveoli. They occur first at the bases and may be heard toward the pulmonary apices as congestive heart failure worsens; they are not specific for heart failure. Hepatic systolic pulsations along with large jugular venous v waves may occur with tricuspid regurgitation. Hepatojugular reflux, an increase in cervical venous distention when pressure is applied over the liver during normal respiration, is a sign of right heart failure. Ascites and splenomegaly may occur in patients with tricuspid valve disease (especially tricuspid stenosis) or chronic constrictive pericarditis. Splenomegaly may also occur in patients with endocarditis. Cutaneous manifestations of endocarditis are discussed in Chapter 10.

EXAMINATION OF THE NECK VEINS

The purpose of neck vein examination is to estimate the right atrial pressure (central venous pressure) and to evaluate abnormalities in the venous pulse waveform. To estimate central venous pressure, the patient's torso should be at an angle so that the top of the internal jugular pulsation can be visualized. The vertical height of this column from the angle of Louis plus 5 cm (the distance from the angle of Louis to the right atrium at most angles is about 5 cm) approximates the actual venous pressure. Normal venous pressure is between 5 and 9 cm H_2O. Therefore, the normal vertical height of the jugular venous column is less than 3 to 5 cm above the sternal angle. Elevated jugular venous pressure occurs in patients who have right ventricular failure or an abnormality of right ventricular filling (e.g., tricuspid valve abnormality, constrictive pericarditis, or tamponade). The normal jugular venous pressure falls with inspiration and increases with expiration. If the opposite occurs (Kussmaul's sign), constrictive pericarditis or restrictive cardiomyopathy should be suspected.

The jugular venous pulse is composed of two large deflections (the a and v waves) and two negative deflections (the x and y descents) (Fig. 2–1). Even though not usually appreciated on physical examination, a second positive deflection after the a wave, the c wave, is recordable. The a wave results from atrial contraction and is accentuated in patients with right ventricular hypertrophy, tricuspid or pulmonic stenosis, or contraction of the atrium against a closed tricuspid valve as occurs in heart block (cannon a wave). Irregular cannon a waves occur with AV dissociation. Regular cannon a waves may occur in a junctional or ventricular rhythm that conducts retrogradely to the atrium or during some supraventricular tachycardias (see Chapter 8). The a wave is absent if atrial fibrillation is present. The c wave is due to transmitted pressure from the closed tricuspid valve thrust upward during right ventricular systole. The v wave is normally smaller than the a wave and is due to blood returning from the periphery to the right atrium during ventricular systole when the tricuspid valve is closed. The v wave may be the only visible positive deflection in patients with atrial fibrillation. Tricuspid regurgitation results in a large v wave with attenuation of the x descent. The y descent, representing atrial emptying, is decreased in the presence of tricuspid stenosis. Restricted filling of the right heart (e.g., constrictive pericarditis or restrictive cardiomyopathy) produces a venous pulse with distinctive steep x and y descents.

ARTERIAL PRESSURE AND PULSES

Arterial pressure is measured with a sphygmomanometer. Deflation of the arm cuff previously inflated above the systolic arterial pressure tole and diastole. Spurious blood pressure measurements can be obtained if a cuff of incorrect diameter is used; a narrow blood pressure cuff used on an obese arm gives falsely elevated blood pressure readings, and vice versa. In such a patient, blood pressure can be obtained in the forearm with a regular sized cuff, listening over the radial artery. Blood pressure must be measured in the lower extremities when excluding coarctation of the aorta as a cause for upper extremity hypertension. The normal blood pressure in the leg is approximately 10 mm higher than that in the arm.

Arterial pulses can be palpated over the carotid, axillary, brachial, radial, femoral, popliteal, dorsalis pedis, and the posterior tibial arteries. The carotid pulses are most closely related to the aortic pressure in both timing and contour and provide the most information concerning cardiac function. Representative carotid pulse contours are shown in Figure 2–2. Note that the normal upstroke is brisk and that the end of ejection is signified by the dicrotic notch, usually not palpable.

Arterial pulses are symmetrical bilaterally. Inequalities may be explained by chronic atherosclerosis or more acute processes involving regional circulation, for example, dissection of the aorta, peripheral emboli, or vasculitis (e.g., Takayasu's disease). In supravalvular aortic stenosis, there is streaming of the jet toward the right innominate artery, and the carotid and brachial arterial pulses may be stronger on the right than the left. Strongly palpable pulses in the upper extremities with weakly palpable pulses in the lower extremities may suggest coarctation of the aorta. The amplitude of the carotid pulse increases with anemia, thyrotoxicosis, and aortic insufficiency because of the increased stroke volume and rate of left ventricular ejection. The carotid pulse amplitude is attenuated (pulsus parvus) in conditions associated with decreased left ventricular stroke volume, for example, myocardial failure, tachycardia, hypovolemia, severe mitral stenosis, and constrictive pericarditis. Severe myocardial failure may result in pulsus alternans, an alternating intensity of the arterial pulse. Pulsus tardus et parvus is a slowly rising, low-amplitude, late-peaking arterial pulse due to severe aortic outflow tract obstruction (Fig. 2–2). In addition, severe aortic stenosis may be associated with a carotid shudder, coarse palpable carotid arterial vibrations associated with ejection. Pulsus tardus et parvus may not be present in older patients with aortic stenosis and a stiff, noncompliant arterial system or in patients with concomitant aortic insufficiency. Aortic insufficiency is associated with a high-amplitude pulse with a very rapid upstroke, referred to as a Corrigan or water-hammer pulse. Severe aortic insufficiency with or without aortic stenosis may be associated with a bisferiens pulse, a carotid arterial pressure contour with two palpable systolic peaks. A bisferiens pulse is also associated with hypertrophic obstructive cardiomyopathy (Fig. 2–2). In this condition, a rapid initial upstroke of the carotid

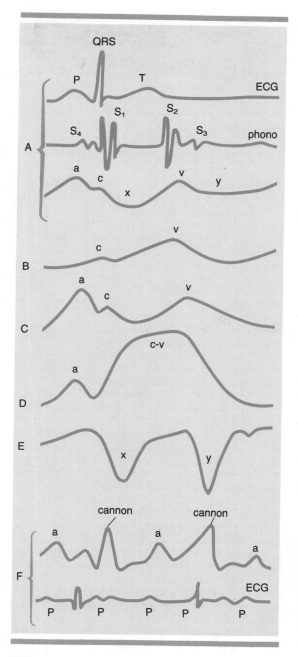

FIGURE 2–1. Normal and abnormal jugular venous pulse tracings. *A,* Normal jugular pulse tracing with simultaneous electrocardiogram and phonocardiogram. *B,* Loss of a waves in atrial fibrillation. *C,* Large a waves in tricuspid stenosis. *D,* Large c-v waves in tricuspid regurgitation. *E,* Steep x and y descents in constrictive pericarditis. *F,* Jugular venous pulse tracing and simultaneous electrocardiogram during complete heart block demonstrating cannon a waves occurring when the atrium contracts against a closed tricuspid valve during ventricular systole.

results in the sound of blood intermittently entering the artery (Korotkoff sounds) when cuff pressure falls to less than systolic pressure. As the cuff is progressively deflated to the diastolic pressure, the Korotkoff sounds disappear, signifying that blood is flowing within the artery in both sys-

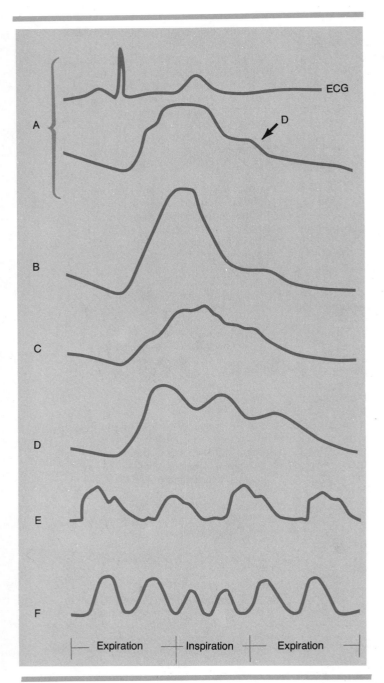

FIGURE 2–2. Normal and abnormal carotid arterial pulse contours. *A*, Normal arterial pulse with simultaneous electrocardiogram. The dicrotic wave (D) occurs just after aortic valve closure. *B*, Wide pulse pressure in aortic insufficiency. *C*, Pulsus parvus et tardus (small amplitude with a slow upstroke) associated with aortic stenosis. *D*, Bisferiens pulse with two systolic peaks, typical of hypertrophic obstructive cardiomyopathy or aortic insufficiency, especially if concomitant aortic stenosis is present. *E*, Pulsus alternans characteristic of severe left ventricular failure. *F*, Paradoxical pulse (systolic pressure decrease of greater than 10 mm Hg with inspiration), most characteristic of cardiac tamponade.

pressure with inspiration, characteristically occurs in pericardial tamponade but may also be present in other conditions such as airway obstruction (acute exacerbation of chronic obstruction pulmonary disease or asthma). The mechanism of pulsus paradoxus is complex and multifactorial. A pulse of irregular intensity may occur in atrial fibrillation or other irregular arrhythmia.

PRECORDIAL EXAMINATION

Before auscultation, the precordium should be inspected and palpated. With good lighting, the point of maximal cardiac impulse may be visible. Cardiac impulses are not normally observed in any other area. The normal apical impulse occurs in early systole and is located within an area of approximately one square centimeter in the fourth to fifth left intercostal space near the midclavicular line. Inspection of the precordium should reveal any abnormalities of the bony structures (for example, pectus excavatum) that may displace the heart to produce unusual findings on physical examination. Precordial palpation should begin with the point of maximal impulse and progress across the precordium, searching for abnormal impulses, palpable sounds, and thrills.

An abnormally prolonged and diffuse left ventricular impulse with increased amplitude is termed a left ventricular heave and is associated with left ventricular hypertrophy. Displacement of the left ventricular impulse downward and to the left indicates left ventricular dilation, common in left ventricular failure or valvular lesions associated with volume overload, such as aortic or mitral regurgitation. A palpable S_4 gallop is associated with pressure overload states, for example, aortic stenosis or long-standing hypertension. A double systolic apical impulse is characteristic of obstructive hypertrophic cardiomyopathy. A systolic bulge medial to the point of maximal impulse is sometimes felt after a recent myocardial infarction and probably represents an area of left ventricular asynergy. A left parasternal lift generally indicates right ventricular dilation and/or hypertrophy and is observed in patients with mitral stenosis or other causes of right ventricular stress. Occasionally, late systolic expansion of the left atrium in patients with severe mitral regurgitation can be palpated in the left parasternal area. Vibrations (thrills) associated with the murmurs of valvular or congenital lesions may be palpable, for example, in aortic stenosis or ventricular septal defect. Occasionally, pulmonic closure (P_2) is markedly accentuated and palpable in patients with severe pulmonary hypertension. Systolic retraction of the apical impulse is a characteristic finding in constrictive pericarditis.

CARDIAC AUSCULTATION

Both patient and examiner should be physically comfortable to ensure adequate cardiac auscul-

artery is attenuated in midsystole and followed by a second late systolic peak, indicative of a late systolic attempt by the ventricle to completely expel its blood. Pulsus paradoxus, a greater than normal decrease (>10 mm Hg) in systolic arterial tation. A good stethoscope has a diaphragm for auscultating relatively high-frequency sounds and a bell for low-frequency sounds. The diaphragm is applied with moderate pressure to the chest, whereas the bell should be applied very lightly, just enough to create a seal. The patient should be auscultated while supine and sitting. Certain sounds (for example, the murmur of aortic insufficiency and the rub of pericarditis) are best heard with the patient sitting upright and leaning forward in end-expiration to bring the heart as close to the chest wall as possible. Gallop rhythms are best heard at the apex with the patient supine or in the left lateral decubitus position. The murmur and opening snap of mitral stenosis are best heard with the patient in the left lateral decubitus position, and sometimes leg or arm exercises are needed to make the murmur audible. The click and late systolic murmur of mitral valve prolapse may be accentuated by standing.

There are four major auscultatory zones. The aortic listening area is the second intercostal space just to the right of the sternum, while the pulmonic area is opposite, at the second intercostal space just to the left of the sternum. The tricuspid area is the fourth intercostal space just to the left of the sternum and the mitral area is at the point of maximum impulse. These areas provide general guidelines to auscultate pathology for each valve, but exceptions exist.

The normal heart sounds consist of a first heart sound (S_1) and a second heart sound (S_2) (see Fig. 1–8). S_1 occurs at the onset of systole and is generated by mitral and tricuspid valve closure. The closure of the aortic (A_2) and pulmonic (P_2) valves at end-systole generates S_2. A_2 and P_2 occur almost simultaneously at end-expiration. Upon inspiration, venous return increases to the right heart because of decreased intrathoracic pressure and decreases to the left heart because of increased pulmonary vascular capacitance. These changes delay P_2 and slightly advance A_2 so that A_2 and P_2 separate temporally during inspiration, becoming superimposed during expiration. P_2 is normally less intense than A_2 and is best heard at the second intercostal space to the left of the sternum.

An early diastolic gallop rhythm (S_3) is a low-pitched sound heard best with the bell of the stethoscope placed lightly over the point of maximal impulse, especially with the patient in the left lateral decubitus position. It is generated by rapid filling of the left ventricle in early diastole and is a physiologically normal sound in young people into the early twenties. Heard in older age groups, an S_3 signifies left or right ventricular failure. An S_3 must be differentiated from other early diastolic sounds, for example, a widely split S_2, the opening snap of mitral stenosis, a tumor plop from a left atrial myxoma, or the pericardial knock of constrictive pericarditis.

A soft, early-peaking systolic ejection murmur at the second left intercostal space can be a normal finding in some people, especially younger people and patients with high circulatory flow states, for example, anemia, thyrotoxicosis, exercise, and

pregnancy. It is probably generated by flow across the pulmonic outflow tract. Diastolic murmurs are never physiological. Systolic and diastolic sounds can sometimes be heard over the cervical venous system (venous hums). These venous hums disappear with a change in position or light pressure over the vein. They are not pathological but must be differentiated from cardiac murmurs or bruits.

ABNORMAL HEART SOUNDS
(Fig. 2–3)

Variation in the intensity of S_1 may have diagnostic importance (Table 2–6). After a short PR interval, the mitral and tricuspid valves are wide open at the onset of systole (louder S_1), whereas after a long PR interval they are already almost closed at the onset of systole (softer S_1). S_1 may vary in intensity in patients with atrial fibrillation or some types of heart block, when the mitral and tricuspid valves are in various stages of closure at the onset of ventricular systole. S_1 is loud in patients who have mitral stenosis and a relatively pliable valve (the mitral valve is wide open at the onset of left ventricular ejection). Splitting of S_1 is rarely of any diagnostic significance.

Abnormalities in S_2 may be related to abnormal intensity or abnormal timing (Tables 2–6 and 2–7). A single S_2 is present in any condition in which the intensity of A_2 or P_2 is markedly attenuated. Persistent splitting of S_2 retaining normal respiratory variation occurs when P_2 is delayed, or occasionally when A_2 is early, as in patients with mitral regurgitation or ventricular septal defect. Fixed splitting of S_2 is characteristic of atrial septal defect or lesions in which the right ventricle is unable to augment its stroke volume, for example, severe pulmonic stenosis. Paradoxical splitting of S_2 (P_2 preceding A_2 during expiration and coincident with A_2 on inspiration) is usually caused by conditions that delay A_2.

TABLE 2–6. ABNORMAL INTENSITY OF HEART SOUNDS

	S_1	A_2	P_2
Loud	Short PR interval	Systemic hypertension	Pulmonary hypertension
	Mitral stenosis with pliable valve	Aortic dilation Coarctation of aorta	Thin chest wall
Soft	Long PR interval	Calcific aortic stenosis	Valvular or subvalvular pulmonic stenosis
	Mitral regurgitation	Aortic regurgitation	
	Poor LV function		
	Mitral stenosis with rigid valve		
	Thick chest wall		
Varying	Atrial fibrillation		
	Heart block		

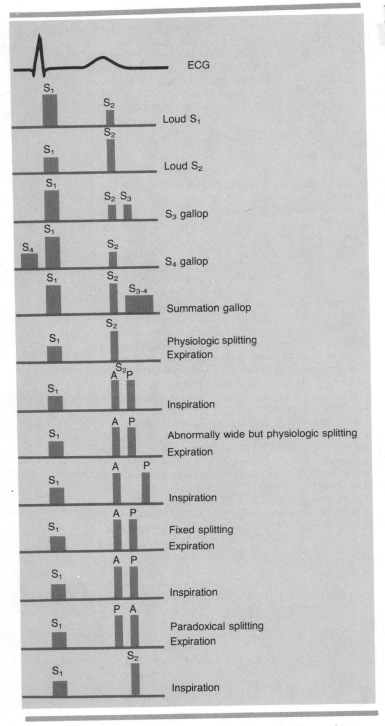

FIGURE 2–3. Abnormal heart sounds can be related to abnormal intensity, abnormal presence of a gallop rhythm, or abnormal splitting of S_2 with respiration.

The fourth heart sound (S_4 gallop) occurs during late diastolic ventricular filling due to atrial contraction. An S_4 is usually abnormal, but occasionally it may be heard in a healthy adult. Inspiration enhances an S_4 originating from the right ventricle but has little effect on a left ventricular S_4. An S_4 gallop is associated with an elevated left ventricular end-diastolic pressure due to decreased left ventricular compliance, secondary to either left ventricular hypertrophy or ischemia. It is characteristically found in patients with aortic stenosis, hypertrophic cardiomyopathy, acute mitral regurgitation, and myocardial infarction. A right ventricular S_4 is heard in pulmonary hypertension and pulmonic stenosis. An S_4 is not present in atrial fibrillation. A transient S_4 gallop coincident with chest pain may be suggestive of ischemia. The auscultatory rhythm of an S_4 is likened to pronouncing "Tenn´ (S_4) - e (S_1) - see (S_2)."

An early diastolic filling sound (S_3 gallop) may be physiological in older children and young adults (see above) but in adults occurs with impaired ventricular function of any cause and is the most sensitive and specific physical sign of ventricular dysfunction. It may be heard in chronic aortic or mitral insufficiency, where it probably also represents some degree of left ventricular dysfunction. Left ventricular gallop sounds are not heard in the presence of significant mitral stenosis. A right ventricular S_3 may be heard at the left lower sternal border or sometimes the epigastrium and is accentuated with inspiration. The auscultatory cadence of an S_3 is likened to pronouncing "Ken (S_1) - tuck´ (S_2) - y (S_3)."

When tachycardia is present and a diastolic gallop cannot be separated into a distinct S_3 and S_4, it often represents the summation of both and is termed a summation gallop. It has a distinct cadence likened to that of a galloping horse.

Normal valves make no sound as they open. However, an abnormal but pliable aortic or pulmonic valve may generate an opening sound called an ejection sound or click (Fig. 2–4, Table 2–8). Ejection sounds are high-pitched and occur early in systole, immediately upon completion of isovolumic contraction. More severe stenosis causes the ejection sound to occur earlier in systole, i.e., closer to S_1. The cause of ejection sounds in pulmonary or systemic hypertension is unclear but probably relates to the dilation of the aortic or pulmonary arterial root.

Mid to late systolic clicks, often followed by a late systolic murmur, occur in patients with mitral valve prolapse. The clicks are thought to result from sudden tensing of the mitral valve apparatus as the valve prolapses. The clicks may be single or multiple and may occur at any time during systole, although they are generally later than ejection sounds. The behavior of these clicks and associated murmurs during physiological maneuvers is summarized in Table 2–11.

The mitral and tricuspid valves also do not normally make an opening sound. However, with mitral or tricuspid stenosis, an early diastolic opening sound is heard if the valve is still pliable (Fig. 2–4). The opening "snap" (OS) of mitral stenosis is earlier in diastole, is of higher pitch than an S_3 gallop, and is located somewhat medial to the point of maximum impulse. More severe stenosis causes the opening snap to occur earlier, i.e., closer to S_2; the higher the left atrial pressure, the earlier the valve opens after the onset of isovol-

TABLE 2–7. ABNORMAL SPLITTING OF S_2

SINGLE S_2	WIDELY SPLIT S_2 WITH NORMAL RESPIRATORY VARIATION	FIXED SPLIT S_2	PARADOXICAL SPLITTING OF S_2
Aortic stenosis Pulmonic stenosis	Right bundle branch block Left ventricular pacing	Atrial septal defect Severe RV dysfunction	Left bundle branch block Right ventricular pacemaker
Systemic hypertension Coronary artery disease Any condition that can lead to paradoxical splitting of S_2	Pulmonic stenosis Pulmonary embolus Idiopathic dilation of the pulmonary artery Mitral regurgitation Ventricular septal defect		Angina, myocardial infarction Aortic stenosis Hypertrophic obstructive cardiomyopathy Aortic regurgitation

umic relaxation. Opening snaps disappear as the stenotic AV valve calcifies and becomes immobile.

A pericardial knock is an early diastolic sound, sometimes difficult to distinguish from an S_3 gallop, heard in patients with constrictive pericarditis. Another abnormal early diastolic heart sound is the tumor "plop" of an atrial myxoma.

ABNORMAL MURMURS

Heart murmurs are vibrations of longer duration than the heart sounds and represent turbulent flow across abnormal valves caused by congenital or acquired cardiac defects (Fig. 2–4). Murmurs are termed diastolic or systolic, and their intensity is graded (Table 2–9). The length of the murmur and its radiation (e.g., to the back, neck, axilla, or listening areas other than that of the valve primarily involved) should be described along with the quality of the murmur (e.g., blowing, harsh, rumbling, musical, or high- or low-pitched).

TABLE 2–8. EJECTION CLICKS

AORTIC	PULMONIC
Noncalcific congenital aortic stenosis Systemic hypertension Dilation of the aorta	Valvular pulmonic stenosis Pulmonary arterial hypertension Idiopathic dilation of the pulmonary artery
No change with respiration Loudest second right intercostal space and apex	Increased intensity with *expiration* (opposite to other right-sided events) Loudest left upper sternal border

Systolic murmurs are usually divided into ejection and holosystolic types (Table 2–10). Systolic ejection murmurs are generated either by abnormalities within or increased flow across the aortic or pulmonary outflow tracts. The systolic ejection

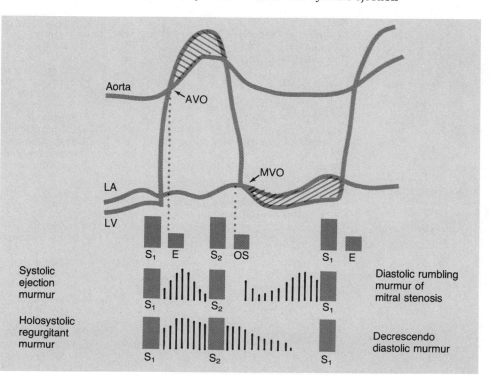

FIGURE 2–4. Abnormal sounds and murmurs associated with valvular dysfunction displayed simultaneously with left atrial (LA), left ventricular (LV), and aortic pressure tracings. AVO = Aortic valve opening; MVO = mitral valve opening; E = ejection click of the aortic valve; OS = opening snap of the mitral valve. The shaded areas represent pressure gradients across the aortic valve during systole or mitral valve during diastole, characteristic of aortic stenosis and mitral stenosis, respectively.

TABLE 2–9. GRADING SYSTEM FOR INTENSITY OF MURMURS

Grade 1	Barely audible murmur
Grade 2	Murmur of medium intensity
Grade 3	Loud murmur, no thrill
Grade 4	Loud murmur with thrill
Grade 5	Very loud murmur, stethoscope must be on the chest to hear
Grade 6	Murmur audible with stethoscope off the chest

murmur of coarctation of the aorta is late in systole compared to valvular ejection murmurs.

Mitral regurgitation due to the syndrome of mitral valve prolapse may be associated with a late systolic murmur that is often preceded by a systolic click. It may be somewhat atypical for mitral regurgitation in quality as well as timing and is often best heard more toward the left sternal border than at the traditional mitral listening area.

Early diastolic decrescendo murmurs are heard with aortic and pulmonic regurgitation. Aortic regurgitation can be due to valvular leaks or secondary to dilation of the valve ring (for example, after aortic dissection). Pulmonic regurgitation also can be valvular or secondary to dilation of the valve ring associated with pulmonary hypertension (Graham Steell murmur).

In addition to mitral and tricuspid stenosis, rumbles across AV valves can be heard in conditions in which there is increased diastolic flow across a nonstenotic valve (for example, tricuspid regurgitation or atrial septal defect) or nonvalvular obstruction to flow (for example, atrial

myxoma). A diastolic rumbling murmur may be heard in patients with severe chronic aortic insufficiency (Austin-Flint murmur, see Chapter 5).

Continuous murmurs or "machinery murmurs" are caused by lesions that generate turbulent flow in both systole and diastole due to a pressure gradient present throughout the cardiac cycle.

A pericardial friction rub is created when two inflamed layers of pericardium slide over one another. It is a scratchy sound having from one to three components. If all three components are present, one occurs during atrial systole, one during ventricular contraction, and one during rapid early diastolic ventricular filling. Pericardial friction rubs are usually best heard along the left sternal border while the patient is leaning forward in held expiration. Frequently only a single systolic component is audible and may be confused with a systolic mumur. A pleuropericardial friction rub involves not only the pericardial but also the pleural surfaces and varies with respiration.

PROSTHETIC VALVE SOUNDS

Metal valves of the ball and cage variety (e.g., Starr-Edwards valves) demonstrate loud, metallic opening and closing sounds that may be audible without a stethoscope. Tilting disk valves (e.g., the Bjork-Shiley valve) demonstrate a closing metallic sound but only a very soft opening sound. Porcine valves may generate no abnormal sounds; however, a porcine valve in the mitral position sometimes has an opening snap as well as a soft diastolic rumble. Since there is a persistent gra-

TABLE 2–10. CLASSIFICATION OF HEART MURMURS

CLASS	DESCRIPTION	CHARACTERISTIC LESIONS
Ejection	Systolic Crescendo-decrescendo Often harsh in quality Begin after S_1 end before S_2	Valvular, supravalvular, and subvalvular aortic stenosis Hypertrophic obstructive cardiomyopathy Pulmonic stenosis Aortic or pulmonary artery dilation Malformed but nonobstructive aortic valve ↑ transvalvular flow (e.g., aortic regurgitation, hyperkinetic states, atrial septal defect, physiological flow murmur)
Holosystolic	Extends throughout systole, up to and sometimes past S_2; relatively uniform intensity	Mitral regurgitation Tricuspid regurgitation Ventricular septal defect
Late systolic	Variable onset and duration, often preceded by a nonejection click	Mitral valve prolapse
Diastolic decrescendo	Begins with A_2 or P_2 Decrescendo with varying duration Often high-pitched, "blowing"	Aortic regurgitation Pulmonic regurgitation

Mid-diastolic	Begins after S_2, often after an opening snap
	Low-pitched "rumble" heard best with bell of stethoscope
	With exercise or left lateral decubitus position
	Loudest in early diastole and upon atrial contraction (presystolic accentuation)
		Mitral stenosis
		Tricuspid stenosis
		↑ flow across AV valves:
		  tricuspid regurgitation
		  mitral regurgitation
		  atrial-septal defect
		Atrial myxoma
		Austin Flint murmur

Continuous	Systolic and diastolic components "Machinery murmurs"	Patent ductus arteriosus Coronary AV fistula Ruptured sinus of Valsalva aneurysm into right atrium or ventricle

dient across any prosthetic valve, there is a systolic murmur across a prosthetic aortic valve and a soft diastolic rumble over a prosthetic mitral or tricuspid valve.

PHYSIOLOGICAL AND PHARMACOLOGICAL MANEUVERS

Various physiological and pharmacological maneuvers are sometimes useful in augmenting the intensity or delineating the etiology of heart sounds and murmurs (Table 2–11). Noting the effects of respiration on murmurs is the simplest test. With inspiration right heart filling is increased, and therefore the intensity of most sounds and murmurs generated from the right heart tends to increase. An exception to this rule is when right ventricular failure is present and the right ventricle is unable to increase its output during inspiration.

SPECIAL TESTS AND PROCEDURES

CARDIAC RADIOGRAPHY

From the routine PA and lateral chest x-ray, the size of the heart can be estimated. Cardiomegaly

is said to be present radiographically if the diameter of the heart exceeds more than half of the thoracic diameter (cardiothoracic ratio). Enlarged hearts not meeting this criterion are not uncommon, however. The structures comprising the cardiac borders can be seen in Figure 2–5. Dilation of the right atrium causes bulging of the right heart border, while dilation of the left atrial appendage straightens or bulges the left heart border between the left ventricle and pulmonary artery. In addition, an enlarged left atrium may cause a double density shadow on the right heart border and may elevate the left main stem bronchus. Dilation of the posteriorly situated left atrium may be highlighted by barium in the esophagus, used to delineate the posterior cardiac border. Dilation of the right ventricle is seen best on the lateral chest x-ray as an encroachment of the anterior clear space between the heart and the sternum. Left ventricular dilation causes prominence of the lower portion of the left heart border. Enlargement of the central pulmonary arteries can be detected by a bulging of the pulmonary artery segment of the left heart border; enlargement of the aorta can be detected by aortic dilation. On many occasions, the particular chambers responsible for cardiomegaly may not be identifiable on routine PA and lateral chest x-rays.

Fluoroscopy or plain films of the chest may be used to detect calcification in valves, pericardium, or aorta. The chest x-ray can be used to identify prosthetic valves. Cardiac fluoroscopy

TABLE 2–11. EFFECTS OF PHYSIOLOGICAL AND PHARMACOLOGICAL MANEUVERS ON AUSCULTATORY EVENTS

MANEUVER	MAJOR PHYSIOLOGICAL EFFECTS	USEFUL AUSCULATORY CHANGES*
Respiration	↑ venous return with inspiration	↑ right heart murmurs and gallops with inspiration splitting of S_2 (Table 2–7)
Valsalva (initial ↑ BP, phase I; followed by ↓ BP, phase II)	↓ BP, ↓ venous return, ↓ LV size (phase II)	↑ HOCM ↓ AS, MR MVP click earlier in systole, murmur prolongs
Standing	↓ venous return ↓ LV size	↑ HOCM ↓ AS, MR MVP click earlier in systole, murmur prolongs
Squatting	↑ venous return ↑ systemic vascular resistance ↑ LV size	↑ AS, MR, AI ↓ HOCM MVP click delayed, murmur shortens
Isometric exercise (e.g., hand grip)	↑ arterial pressure ↑ cardiac output	↑ gallops ↑ MR, AI, MS ↓ AS, HOCM
Post PVC or prolonged RR interval	↑ ventricular filling ↑ contractility	↑ AS little change in MR
Amyl nitrate	↓ arterial pressure ↑ cardiac output ↓ LV size	MVP click earlier in systole, murmur prolongs ↑ HOCM, AS, MS ↓ AI, MR, Austin Flint murmur
Phenylephrine	↑ arterial pressure ↓ cardiac output ↑ LV size	↑ MR, AI ↓ AS, HOCM MVP click delayed, murmur shortens

HOCM = hypertrophic obstructive cardiomyopathy
AS = aortic stenosis
MR = mitral regurgitation
MVP = mitral valve prolapse

AI = aortic insufficiency
MS = mitral stenosis
* ↑ = increased intensity; ↓ = decreased intensity

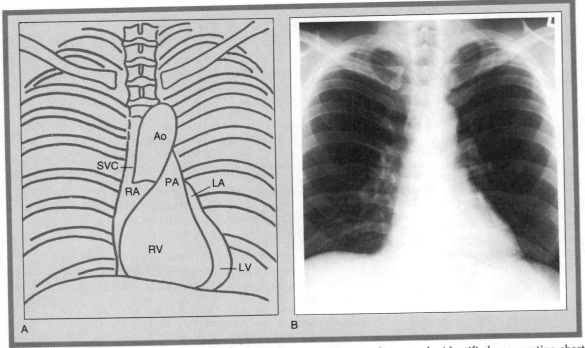

FIGURE 2–5. *A*, Schematic illustration of the parts of the heart whose outlines can be identified on a routine chest x-ray (*B*). AO = Aorta; SVC = superior vena cava; RA = right atrium; PA = pulmonary artery; LA = left atrium; RV = right ventricle; LV = left ventricle. *B*, Routine posteroanterior x-ray of the normal cardiac silhouette.

can determine if a ball valve or tilting disk valve opens and closes properly.

Specific radiographic signs of congenital and valvular lesions will be discussed in their respective sections.

The pulmonary vasculature is evaluated from the PA chest x-ray. *Decreased pulmonary blood flow* can be identified by a paucity of vascular shadows throughout the lung and may occur in patients with significant right-to-left shunts such as tetralogy of Fallot. *Increased pulmonary blood flow* can be detected by a generalized increase in pulmonary vascular markings throughout the lung fields and is typical of left-to-right shunts such as atrial septal defect. An *increase in pulmonary vascular resistance* causing pulmonary hypertension may be suspected if the central large pulmonary vessels are dilated but the peripheral pulmonary markings are attenuated. *Pulmonary venous hypertension* can be diagnosed by the radiographic signs of pulmonary edema; interstitial edema causes the small pulmonary vessels to become indistinct; engorged lymphatics cast discrete horizontal shadows in the outer portions of the lung bases called Kerley B lines; redistribution of pulmonary flow from the bases to the apices occurs; as pulmonary congestion worsens, alveolar edema causes confluent bilateral hilar infiltrates with a "butterfly" distribution, usually bilaterally symmetrical but occasionally somewhat atypical in appearance, especially in patients with pre-existing lung disease.

ELECTROCARDIOGRAPHY

It is beyond the scope of this text to provide a comprehensive discussion of electrocardiography; however, some basic principles will be reviewed (see Chapter 1). Impulses are initiated by the sinus node, travel through the atria initiating atrial contraction, and experience conduction delay through the AV node. The impulse travels from the AV node through the common bundle of His, down the right and left bundle branches, and through the Purkinje fibers to ventricular myocardium (see Fig. 1–5). No ventricular activation (QRS complex) is inscribed until ventricular muscle tissue is activated. The ventricular septum is activated from left to right before any other part of the ventricle. Subsequently, the bulk of the ventricular muscle is activated simultaneously, followed lastly by activation of the base of the heart superiorly. Myocardial electrical activity can be represented with a vector, a value with both magnitude and direction, at any time during the cardiac cycle. The mean QRS vector during depolarization is termed the electrical axis and can be identified using the surface electrocardiogram.

A diagrammatic representation of an electrocardiographic complex is seen in Figure 2–6. The vertical axis represents amplitude in millivolts (10 mm = 1 millivolt). The horizontal scale represents time (5 mm = 0.20 second, 1 mm = 0.04 second). Routine ECG paper speed is 25 mm/sec, and thus one can determine the heart rate by measuring the RR interval in millimeters and dividing that number into 1,500, or the RR interval in milliseconds divided into 60,000.

The first relatively low-amplitude and low-frequency deflection of the electrocardiogram, the P wave, represents atrial depolarization. The isoelectric portion of the electrocardiogram between the P wave and the next rapid deflection (QRS complex) is termed the PR segment. The PR interval is measured between the onset of the P wave and the onset of the QRS complex and is normally between 0.12 and 0.20 second in duration. A PR interval greater than 0.20 second is termed first-degree AV block. The rapid, high-amplitude deflections following the PR segment are termed the QRS complex and represent ventricular depolarization. Atrial repolarization usually is not visible on the electrocardiogram, since it is a low-amplitude, low-frequency event and occurs simultaneously with ventricular depolarization. An initial negative deflection of the QRS is termed the Q wave; the initial positive deflection is termed the R wave; and if a subsequent negative deflection is present, it is called the S wave. A positive deflection subsequent to the S wave is termed an R' wave. The duration between the onset and the termination of the QRS complex is called the QRS interval and is normally less than 0.10 second. Upper and lower case letters are used to indicate the relative size of QRS deflections; for example, qRs refers to a small Q wave, large R wave, and small S wave. The isoelectric portion of the electrocardiogram following the QRS complex is the ST segment, followed by a low-frequency deflection, the T wave, which represents ventricular repolarization. The QT interval is measured from the beginning of the QRS complex to the end of the T wave and represents the time required for ventricular electrical systole. The QT interval is a measure of ventricular muscle refractoriness and varies with heart rate, decreasing as the heart rate increases. The QT interval is usually 0.35 to 0.44 second for heart rates between 60 and 100 beats per minute, and one can estimate a corrected QT interval (normally less than 0.42 second in men and 0.43 second in women) by the Bazett formula, $QT_c = QT / \sqrt{RR}$ interval. In some patients, a broad, low-amplitude deflection follows the T wave and is called a U wave. The genesis of the U wave is not clear. The junction between the QRS and the ST segment is the J point.

Figure 2–7 illustrates the Einthoven triangle and the polarity of each of the six limb leads. Electrodes are connected to the left arm, right arm, and left leg (the right leg lead is a ground). Lead I displays the potential difference between the left and right arms (left arm positive); Lead II, the potential difference between the right arm and left leg (left leg positive); and lead III, the potential difference between the left arm and left leg (left leg positive). Likewise, the augmented limb leads aV$_L$, aV$_R$, and aV$_F$ are positive toward the left arm, right arm, and left leg, respectively. They are unipolar leads; that is, they measure the potential difference between the limb lead and a central point. When these six leads are taken together, they describe a full circle in the frontal plane at 30-degree intervals. Using this "hexaxial" frontal plane lead reference system, the frontal axis of any cardiac vector can be estimated. The most important axis is that of the mean QRS vector, normally between −30 degrees and +90 degrees. Mean QRS axes more superior than −30 degrees are termed left-axis deviation, and more rightward than +90 de-

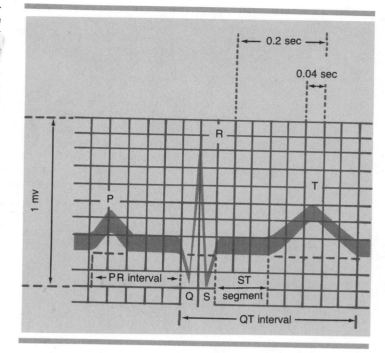

FIGURE 2–6. Normal electrocardiographic complex with labeling of waves and intervals.

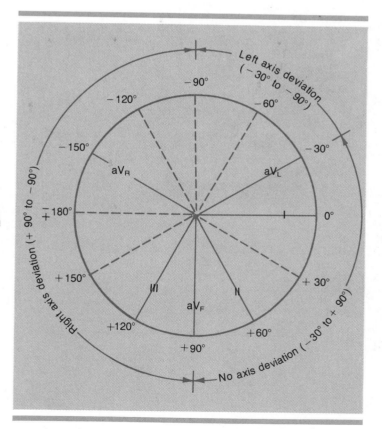

FIGURE 2–7. Hexaxial reference figure for frontal plane axis determination, indicating values for abnormal left and right QRS axis deviation.

grees, right-axis deviation. The T-wave axis is normally within 30 to 45 degrees of the QRS axis. Leads displaying large positive or negative QRS deflections are generally parallel to the mean QRS axis; leads that are isoelectric, or have equal negative and positive deflections, are perpendicular to the QRS axis.

In addition to the six frontal plane leads, there are six standard precordial leads, V_1 through V_6, that are unipolar leads placed across the anterior chest. The precordial leads are considered positive, and a central reference point serves as the negative pole (unipolar lead). Leads V_1 and to

some extent V_2 are close to the right ventricle and interventricular septum of the heart; leads V_4, V_5, and V_6 are close to the lateral wall of the left ventricle. Lead V_1 normally has a small R wave and large S wave, the midprecordial leads have equal R and S waves, and leads V_5 and V_6 have a large R wave and small S wave (often preceded by a small Q wave), reflecting the normal left ventricular predominance in the adult. If the right precordial leads (V_1, V_2) have relatively equal R and S waves with no other abnormality, counterclockwise rotation is said to be present; if V_5 and V_6 have relatively equal R and S waves, clockwise rotation is present. These can be normal variants.

A vectorcardiogram is a two-dimensional recording of the vector loop generated by atrial and ventricular depolarization. Vectorcardiograms are infrequently used today.

TABLE 2–12. ECG MANIFESTATIONS OF CHAMBER ENLARGEMENT

Left atrial enlargement
P wave duration ≥ 0.12 sec
Notched, slurred P wave in leads I and II (P mitrale)
Biphasic P waves in V_1 with a wide, deep, negative terminal component
Mean P wave axis shifted to the left (between +45 and −30 degrees)
Right atrial enlargement
P wave duration ≤ 0.11 sec
Tall, peaked P waves of ≥2.5 mm in amplitude in leads II, III, or aV_F (P pulmonale)
Mean P wave axis shifted to the right (≥ +70 degrees)
Left ventricular enlargement
Voltage criteria:
    R or S wave in limb lead ≥ 20 mm
    S wave in V_1, V_2, or V_3 ≥ 30 mm
    R wave in V_4, V_5, or V_6 ≥ 30 mm
Depressed ST segments with inverted T waves in lateral leads ("strain" pattern); more reliable in the absence of digitalis therapy
Left axis of −30 degrees or more
QRS duration ≥ 0.09 sec
Left atrial enlargement
Time of onset of the intrinsicoid deflection (time from beginning of QRS to peak of R wave) ≥ 0.05 sec in lead V_5 or V_6
Right ventricular enlargement
Tall R waves over right precordium and deep S waves over left precordium (R:S ratio in lead V_1 > 1.0)
Normal QRS duration (if no right bundle branch block)
Right axis deviation
ST-T "strain" pattern over right precordium
Late intrinsicoid deflection in lead V_1 or V_2

TABLE 2–13. ECG MANIFESTATIONS OF BUNDLE BRANCH BLOCK

Left Bundle Branch Block
QRS duration ≥ 0.12 sec
Broad, slurred, or notched R waves in lateral leads (I, aV_L, V_5-V_6)
QS or rS pattern in anterior precordium
Secondary ST-T wave changes (ST and T wave vectors opposite to terminal QRS vectors)
Late intrinsicoid deflection in leads V_5 and V_6
Right Bundle Branch Block
QRS duration ≥ 0.12 sec
Large R' wave in lead V_1 (rsR')
Deep terminal S wave in V_6
Normal septal Q waves
Inverted T waves in lead V_1 (secondary T wave change)
Late intrinsicoid deflection in leads V_1 and V_2

ABNORMAL ELECTROCARDIOGRAPHIC PATTERNS

The normal P wave vector is positive in leads I, II, and aV_F and negative in aV_R. Criteria for left and right atrial enlargement are described in Table 2–12.

The electrocardiogram can be used to diagnose left ventricular hypertrophy but is relatively insensitive. The hypertrophied ventricle generates increased electrocardiographic voltage that may meet any of several voltage criteria to qualify for left ventricular hypertrophy. However, normal young people may have high ECG voltage, and these criteria are not useful for patients under 35 years of age. At least one additional criterion must be present to diagnose left ventricular hypertrophy (Table 2–12).

The ECG findings in right ventricular hypertrophy are summarized in Table 2–12. The degree of right axis deviation correlates somewhat with the degree of right ventricular hypertrophy, as do certain QRS configurations (e.g., a qR complex in V_1 is associated with right ventricular pressure exceeding left ventricular pressure).

Acute pulmonary embolus may be associated with transient and nonspecific ECG changes. These include right atrial abnormality, right axis deviation with clockwise rotation, incomplete or complete right bundle branch block, S waves in leads I, II, and III ($S_1 S_2 S_3$ pattern), and T-wave inversion in the right precordial leads. Atrial arrhythmias are not uncommon.

Electrocardiographic manifestations of chronic obstructive pulmonary disease are due to both changes in lung volumes and right ventricular hypertrophy. Right atrial abnormality, right axis deviation, and clockwise rotation are often present. An $S_1 S_2 S_3$ pattern may be seen, and QRS voltage may be low. Right ventricular hypertrophy is sometimes present.

The common bundle of His divides into left and right bundle branches. Conduction delay or block in either of these bundle branches results in characteristic electrocardiographic patterns (Fig. 2–8, Table 2–13). In each of these, the QRS duration is 0.12 second or more. Left bundle branch block usually is an indicator of organic heart disease. During left bundle branch block, initial septal activation is abnormal; therefore, the diagnosis of myocardial infarction, dependent upon Q waves in the first 0.04 second of the QRS, usually cannot be determined. Left ventricular hypertrophy cannot be diagnosed in the presence of left bundle branch block.

Right bundle branch block can be associated with organic heart disease but is sometimes seen in apparently normal hearts. The right ventricle is activated late, and therefore there is a terminal unopposed QRS vector directed rightward and anteriorly. Initial ventricular activation is normal (septal activation occurs normally from the left bundle branch), and thus myocardial infarction can be diagnosed in the presence of right bundle branch block.

The left bundle branch in many hearts appears to divide into two major divisions (fascicles), the left anterior (superior) fascicle and the left posterior (inferior) fascicle. A delay in conduction in either fascicle is termed a hemiblock or fascicular block and changes the sequence of left ventricular depolarization, reflected in a frontal axis shift. Since the left anterior fascicle is smaller and more

TABLE 2–14. ECG MANIFESTATIONS OF FASCICULAR BLOCKS

Left Anterior Fascicular Block
 QRS duration ≤ 0.10 sec
 Left axis deviation (− 45 degrees or greater)
 rS pattern in leads II, III, and aV_F
 qR pattern in leads I and aV_L

Left Posterior Fascicular Block
 QRS duration ≤ 0.10 sec
 Right axis deviation (+ 90 degrees or greater)
 qR pattern in leads II, III, and aV_F
 rS pattern in leads I and aV_L
 Exclusion of other causes of right axis deviation (e.g., COPD, RVH, lateral MI)

discrete than the left posterior fascicle, left anterior hemiblock is much more common than left posterior hemiblock; in fact, the presence of left posterior hemiblock is unusual without concomitant right bundle branch block. The ECG criteria for left fascicular blocks are listed in Table 2–14. The term bifascicular block refers to a right bundle branch block associated with a left anterior or left posterior fascicular block. If evidence of conduction delay or block exists in all three fascicles, trifascicular block is said to be present (e.g., al-

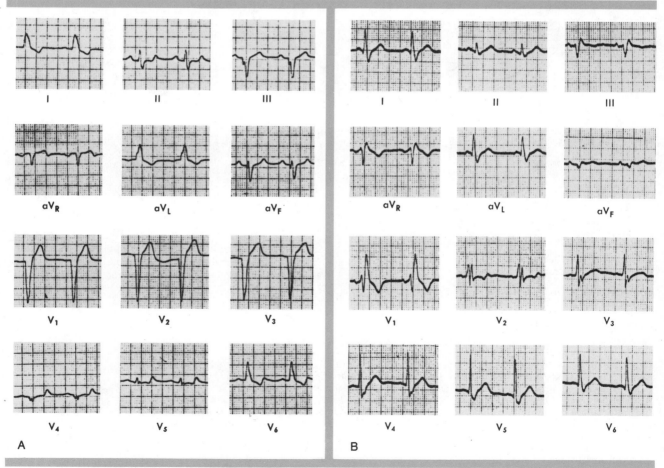

FIGURE 2–8. *A*, Left bundle branch block. *B*, Right bundle branch block. Criteria for bundle branch block are summarized in Table 2–13.

ternating bundle branch block, LBBB with infra-His first-degree AV block or complete infra-His heart block).

Preexcitation syndromes are discussed in Chapter 8.

The ECG is very useful in evaluating patients with ischemic heart disease. Nontransmural ischemia is manifested by downsloping or horizontally depressed (at least 1 mm) ST segments, which is the classic ischemic ST segment response seen with exercise testing. Symmetrical T wave inversion with or without ST depression may also indicate ischemia. ST depression and T wave changes, however, are nonspecific and must be correlated with the clinical setting. On the other hand, ST segment elevation is more specific and evokes a fairly narrow differential diagnosis. ST elevation may occur with acute transmural myocardial infarction, ventricular aneurysm after myocardial infarction, pericarditis, variant angina (Prinzmetal's angina, secondary to coronary artery spasm), and as a normal variant (early repolarization). ST elevation caused by acute ischemia is referred to as a "current of injury" (Fig. 2–9).

Infarctions are localized electrocardiographically to different areas of the heart (Table 2–15). Transmural myocardial infarction is usually characterized by the development of Q waves of at least 0.04 sec in duration, and by a typical electrocardiographic evolution (Table 2–16), the time course of which is extremely variable. Leads reflecting areas of the heart opposite the infarction will demonstrate ST depression (reciprocal changes). Persistence of ST elevation past the first few weeks implies the development of a ventric-

FIGURE 2–9. Evolutionary changes in a posteroinferior myocardial infarction. Control tracing is normal. The tracing recorded 2 hours after onset of chest pain demonstrated development of early Q waves, marked ST segment elevation, and hyperacute T waves in leads II, III, and aV$_F$. In addition, a larger R wave, ST segment depression, and negative T waves have developed in leads V$_1$ and V$_2$. These are early changes indicating acute posteroinferior myocardial infarction. The 24-hour tracing demonstrates evolutionary changes. In leads II, III, and aV$_F$ the Q wave is larger, the ST segments have almost returned to base line, and the T wave has begun to invert. In leads V$_1$ to V$_2$ the duration of the R wave now exceeds 0.04 second, the ST segment is depressed, and the T wave is upright. (In this example, ECG changes of true posterior involvement extend past V$_2$; ordinarily only V$_1$ and V$_2$ may be involved.) Only minor further changes occur through the 8-day tracing. Finally, 6 months later the ECG illustrates large Q waves, isoelectric ST segments, and inverted T waves in leads II, III, and aV$_F$ and large R waves, isoelectric ST segment, and upright T waves in V$_1$ and V$_2$, indicative of an "old" posteroinferior myocardial infarction.

ular aneurysm. The presence of Q waves and T wave inversion consistent with a myocardial infarction on a single electrocardiogram permits the diagnosis of a myocardial infarction, but of indeterminant age. Electrocardiographic patterns of subendocardial (also called nontransmural, or non-Q wave) myocardial infarctions include ST depression and T wave inversion that are often nonspecific in themselves. Clinical correlation with cardiac isoenzyme determinations is necessary to verify the infarction.

Abnormal Q waves may be present in the absence of myocardial infarction. These situations include myocarditis, cardiac amyloidosis, neuromuscular disorders such as muscular dystrophy, myocardial replacement by tumor, sarcoidosis, chronic obstructive lung disease, hypertrophic cardiomyopathy, and certain varieties of Wolff-Parkinson-White syndrome.

Many patients have electrocardiograms with nonspecific abnormal ST and T wave changes that preclude a definitive diagnosis. These are interpreted as "nonspecific ST and T wave changes" and must be correlated with the clinical status.

Primary T wave changes are those that occur in the absence of depolarization (QRS) abnormalities, whereas secondary T wave changes are those that result from abnormal QRS depolarization. Thus, secondary T wave changes may be due to bundle branch block or ventricular pre-excitation. Various drugs, electrolyte abnormalities, and ischemia may produce primary T wave changes.

Abnormalities of U waves include either increased amplitude of positive U waves or inverted U waves. Prominent positive U waves may be present normally in patients with bradycardia. They may also occur in hypokalemia and with some drugs, particularly digitalis and antiarrhythmic agents such as amiodarone. Negative U waves occur in left ventricular hypertrophy and ischemia. A large U wave may sometimes be a manifestation of the delayed repolarization (prolonged QT) syndrome (see Chapter 8).

Electrical alternans refers to alternation of QRS voltage and sometimes even P wave and T wave voltage. The most common cause of electrical alternans is a large pericardial effusion.

Metabolic and drug influences on the electrocardiogram are enumerated in Table 2–17. Electrocardiographic manifestations of pericarditis are discussed in Chapter 9.

LONG-TERM AMBULATORY ECG RECORDING

Long-term ambulatory ECG recording (Holter monitor) is used to detect rhythm disturbances in patients with symptoms suggestive of arrhythmia or to document the efficacy of therapy for arrhythmias. Arrhythmia frequency and complexity can be quantitated and correlated with patient symptoms. This test allows documentation of arrhythmias that occur infrequently or occur during a patient's normal daily activities. In addition, long-term ECG recording can document alterations in QRS morphology, ST segment, and T waves, and

TABLE 2–15. LOCALIZATION OF MYOCARDIAL INFARCTION

AREA OF INFARCTION	ECG CHANGES
Inferior	II, III, aV_F
Anteroseptal	V_1-V_3
Anterior	V_3-V_4 — Q waves, ST elevation, T wave inversions
Anterolateral	V_4-V_6
Extensive anterior	V_1-V_6, I, aV_L
Posterior	V_1-V_2: tall broad initial R wave, ST depression, tall upright T wave; usually occurs in association with inferior or lateral MI
Right ventricular	V_1 and V_{4r}: ST elevation; usually occurs in association with inferior MI

TABLE 2–16. TYPICAL ELECTROCARDIOGRAPHIC EVOLUTION OF A TRANSMURAL MYOCARDIAL INFARCTION

ECG ABNORMALITY	ONSET	DISAPPEARANCE
Hyperacute T waves (tall, peaked T waves in leads facing infarction)	immediately	6–24 hours
ST segment elevation	immediately	1–6 weeks
Q waves > 0.04 sec	immediately or in several days	years to never
T wave inversion	6–24 hours	months to years

TABLE 2–17. METABOLIC AND DRUG INFLUENCES ON THE ECG

Hyperkalemia	mild to moderate (K = 5–7 mEq/L): Tall, symmetrically peaked T waves with a narrow base more severe (K = 8–11 mEq/L): QRS widens, PR segment prolongs, P wave disappears; ECG resembles a sine wave in severe cases
Hypokalemia	ST depression T wave flattening large positive U wave
Hypercalcemia	shortened QT interval due to a shortened ST segment
Hypocalcemia	prolonged QT interval due to a prolonged ST segment; T wave duration normal
Hypothermia	Osborne or J waves: J point elevation with a characteristic elevation of the early ST segment. Slow rhythm, baseline artifact due to shivering often present.
Digitalis	ST depression T wave flattening or inversion shortened QT interval, increased U wave amplitude
Quinidine procainamide disopyramide phenothiazines tricyclic antidepressants	prolonged QT interval, mainly due to prolonged T wave duration with flattening or inversion QRS prolongation increased U wave amplitude
CNS insult (e.g., intracerebral hemorrhage)	diffuse, wide, deeply inverted T waves with prolonged QT

thus may be useful for evaluation of ischemia that produces ECG changes; however, the efficacy of ambulatory ECG recordings for this purpose is controversial.

Two electrocardiographic leads are usually recorded simultaneously via electrodes attached to the patient's skin. A small box containing the tape recorder is carried for the period of recording, usually 24 hours, and the patient is encouraged to maintain his normal activities and to perform any activity that he feels may precipitate the arrhythmia. In patients whose arrhythmia is infrequent and difficult to document on tape, recording for several days using a patient-activated recorder at the time of symptoms or transtelephonic transmission of the ECG may be useful. The tapes are scanned with a high-speed system with which a technician interacts, and examples are printed on electrocardiographic paper for physician interpretation.

STRESS TESTING

Since symptoms of cardiovascular disease may not be evident in the resting state, exercise stress testing is sometimes necessary to demonstrate an abnormality and assess its severity. The most common type of exercise testing consists of walking on a treadmill at increasing speeds and degree of incline. The test is continued until the patient has reached 90 per cent of his predicted maximal heart rate, has anginal chest pain that is progressive during exercise, has an excessive degree of ischemic ST segment depression or elevation during exercise, or has various arrhythmias (especially ventricular tachycardia or heart block) precipitated by exercise. The test is stopped if there are any signs of circulatory failure (for example, exhaustion, staggering gait, diminished pulse, or a decrease in systolic blood pressure). In addition to treadmill testing, patients can be stressed with bicycle or arm exercise. Exercise testing may be combined with the nuclear medicine techniques of thallium scanning or radionuclide ventriculography (see below).

Exercise testing can aid in the differential diagnosis of chest pain. In addition, it can be used to evaluate prognosis and/or functional capacity in patients with known coronary heart disease or following myocardial infarction. In patients with coronary artery disease, an exercise test that is positive (see below) in the first two stages (six minutes) carries a relatively poor prognosis, and further evaluation to include cardiac catheterization may be considered.

The normal response to exercise is an increase in heart rate and both systolic and diastolic blood pressure. The heart rate times maximum blood pressure may be calculated to estimate the work load obtained (double product).

The normal ECG response to exercise is a normal T wave polarity with either no change in the ST segment or mild depression of the J point with a rapidly upsloping ST segment. Abnormal electrocardiographic responses include at least 1 mm depression of the J point and downsloping or horizontal depression of the ST segment similar to the ECG findings of ischemia. ST elevation is a markedly abnormal response to exercise unless it occurs in an area of old transmural infarction, in which case it may be related to regional wall dysfunction rather than ischemia. It may also occur in patients with significant, usually three-vessel, coronary artery disease or with variant angina. The precipitation of negative U waves with exercise is a positive ischemic response and usually indicates disease of the left anterior descending coronary artery. Arrhythmias occurring with exercise may be due to ischemia. In addition to the reproduction of chest pain and ischemic electrocardiographic changes, nonelectrocardiographic signs may be important; for example, the patient may develop an S_4 or S_3 gallop, a systolic murmur of papillary muscle dysfunction, or pulmonary congestion with exercise. A sustained decrease in blood pressure with exercise is a particularly grave finding indicative of extensive coronary artery disease.

The ECG cannot be considered diagnostically reliable in patients with pre-existing nonspecific ST-T wave abnormalities, left ventricular hypertrophy, left bundle branch block, digoxin administration within the past 10 days, electrolyte abnormalities (e.g., hypokalemia), and labile ST-T changes (abnormal ST-T changes occurring with hyperventilation or position changes).

Many physicians perform a limited treadmill test in patients one to two weeks following myocardial infarction. In this situation, the end point is a heart rate of 70 per cent rather than 90 per cent of predicted maximum, or the production of symptoms. The prognosis of patients after infarction who have early exercise symptoms or ECG changes is poorer than it is in those with good exercise capacity. Patients with the following conditions should not be exercised: unstable angina or acute myocardial infarction; severe aortic stenosis; severe hypertension; congestive heart failure; uncontrolled cardiac arrhythmias; acute myocarditis or pericarditis; any acute, noncardiac systemic illness; and known severe coronary artery disease such as left main coronary stenosis.

PHONOCARDIOGRAPHY AND EXTERNAL PULSE RECORDING

Phonocardiography and external pulse recording are techniques for graphically recording heart sounds, murmurs, arterial and venous pulses, and the cardiac apical impulse for careful analysis of timing and quality. Clinical uses include the measurement of systolic time intervals, which can be used as gross indices of left ventricular function; assessment of jugular venous pulse tracings, which can be helpful in the evaluation of right ventricular function or pericardial constriction; quantitation of the interval between the closure of the aortic valve and the opening snap of mitral stenosis to estimate the severity of mitral stenosis; and noninvasive quantitation of aortic stenosis. Except for low-frequency sounds such as gallops, the phonocardiogram does not record cardiac

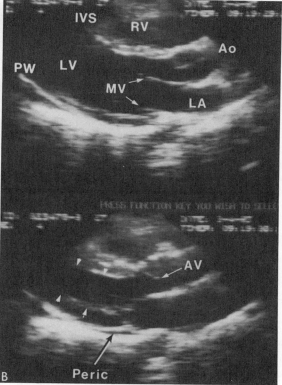

FIGURE 2–10. Portions of normal M-mode (A) and two-dimensional (B) echocardiograms. RV = Right ventricle; LV = left ventricle; MV = mitral valve; IVS = interventricular septum; AV = aortic valve; Ao = aorta; PW = posterior LV wall; Peric = pericardium; LA = left atrium. (Courtesy of William F. Armstrong, M.D.)

sounds not heard with the stethoscope. The function of prosthetic valves can be examined serially with phonocardiography to assure that opening and closing sounds do not change with time. Simultaneous M-mode echocardiography and phonocardiography can be performed to correlate valve motion with the etiology of specific sounds.

ECHOCARDIOGRAPHY

It is beyond the scope of this text to describe echocardiography in detail. Abnormal echocardiographic findings in specific disease states will be discussed with each disease.

Ultrasound consists of sound frequencies greater than those audible by the human ear that are directed toward the desired structures by a transducer placed on the chest wall. The sound waves are reflected at the interface of structures with differing acoustic densities and return to the transducer where they are recorded. Changes in tissue planes are generally strong reflectors of ultrasound, whereas body fluids such as blood reflect very little ultrasound. The depth of the structure reflecting the ultrasonic signal back to the transducer can be displayed as a one-dimensional "ice-pick" view against time on a strip chart recorder (M-mode) or can be displayed on an oscilloscope in real time as a two-dimensional cross-sectional "slice" of the heart (two-dimensional echocardiography) (Fig. 2–10).

Echocardiography can be used to diagnose mitral stenosis with high reliability, and two-dimensional echocardiography can quantitate mitral orifice area in most patients. In addition, concomitant lesions (for example, aortic insuffi-

ciency or tricuspid stenosis) and hemodynamic aberrations (for example, pulmonary hypertension or right ventricular failure) can be identified in patients with mitral stenosis. Patients with left ventricular outflow obstruction can be evaluated for either aortic valvular, supravalvular, or subvalvular stenosis. Even though quantitation of aortic stenosis is difficult, echocardiography may be useful to exclude significant aortic stenosis in many patients. Echocardiography is the technique of choice to diagnose mitral valve prolapse, hypertrophic cardiomyopathy, and atrial myxoma. Echocardiography is the most sensitive test for the detection of pericardial effusion, and certain echocardiographic signs are useful clues of hemodynamic compromise (tamponade). Echocardiography may be useful to visualize the vegetations of bacterial endocarditis, but smaller vegetations (<2 mm in diameter) are not usually identified. Even when the vegetations themselves are not seen, echocardiography may detect the structural complications of endocarditis (for example, flail mitral leaflet), the hemodynamic alterations due to valvular dysfunction (for example, the elevated left ventricular end-diastolic pressure in patients with acute aortic regurgitation), or the pre-existing valvular abnormality that predisposed the patient to endocarditis. Echocardiography may help detect pulmonic valve stenosis or pulmonary hypertension via abnormal motion of the pulmonic valve. The internal dimensions of the left atrium and left ventricle can be accurately measured, and an estimate of right ventricular and atrial size can be ascertained. The thickness of the septum and the posterior left ventricular wall can be measured accurately. Certain hemodynamic information can be ascertained, for example, pulmonary hypertension, decreased flow across the mitral valve, and elevated left ventricular end-diastolic pressure. Conduction abnormalities in left bundle branch block and some cases of the Wolff-Parkinson-White syndrome can be detected. Segmental wall motion abnormalities characteristic of coronary artery disease are detectable. Dilation of the aorta and occasionally an aortic dissection can be noted. The function of prosthetic valves can be evaluated grossly; however, detailed examination of prosthetic valves is often difficult because of their high echogenicity. In patients with congenital heart disease, echocardiography can often establish the diagnosis or complement cardiac catheterization in unraveling complex malformations. Thrombi in the left ventricle and atrium can be detected, but the sensitivity of echocardiography for this purpose is not clear. Mitral and aortic regurgitation are often not detectable directly and are inferred indirectly from their effects on wall motion, chamber size, and motion of other valves.

Two-dimensional echocardiography is superior to M-mode for most indications. M-mode echocardiography is preferred in certain situations in which higher resolution and careful timing of motion of certain structures is desired, for example, the identification of systolic anterior motion of the mitral valve in hypertrophic cardiomyopathy; detection of notching of the aortic valve in subaortic stenosis or of the pulmonic valve in pulmonary hypertension or pulmonic stenosis; detection of fluttering of the anterior mitral valve leaflet caused by the regurgitant jet in aortic insufficiency; and detailed evaluation of wall motion in patients with conduction abnormalities.

Contrast echocardiography can be useful in detecting atrial or ventricular intracardiac shunts or tricuspid regurgitation. Contrast agents include agitated saline, indocyanine green dye, and Renografin. Tiny bubbles in agitated solutions are echocardiographically opaque and produce bright echoes. After injection via an antecubital vein, the contrast can be traced through the right atrium and ventricle. The bubbles are absorbed by the pulmonary capillaries and normally do not opac-

ify the left side of the heart. A right-to-left shunt is detected by the appearance of contrast in the left atrium or ventricle. A left-to-right shunt is detected by a negative contrast effect in a right-sided chamber. Tricuspid regurgitation is detected by regurgitation of contrast into the inferior vena cava.

Echocardiography during or immediately following exercise may detect regional wall motion abnormalities not present in the resting state.

Doppler ultrasound is a newer technique currently being evaluated for the noninvasive detection and quantification of valvular lesions and blood flow.

NUCLEAR CARDIOLOGY

Three techniques using radioactive tracers are useful in clinical cardiology: radionuclide angiography, perfusion scintigraphy, and infarct-avid scintigraphy (Fig. 2–11, Table 2–18).

The first-pass study and the equilibrium study are two basic techniques employed in radionuclide angiography. In the first-pass study, a high-speed scintillation camera follows the transit of isotope injected into a peripheral vein through the right heart, pulmonary vasculature, and left heart, much as a radiopaque dye injection is recorded during a cardiac catheterization. The equilibrium method involves labeling the "blood pool" by introducing human serum albumin or red cells labeled with technetium-99. Images are acquired with a camera that times or "gates" acquisition according to the electrocardiogram; that is, the cardiac cycle is divided into multiple segments, each of which is counted repeatedly and individually, and the final average is displayed as one cardiac cycle that can be visualized over and over in an endless loop format.

Perfusion scintigraphy, "cold spot scanning," employs a radioactive potassium analog, thallium-201. Cells must be both perfused and metabolically intact in order to accumulate thallium-201. Therefore, nonperfused or dead myocardium appears as a "cold spot" on the scan. When exercise thallium imaging is performed, the patient

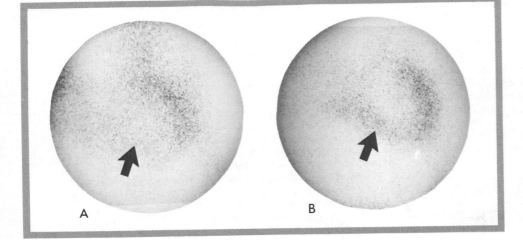

FIGURE 2–11. Thallium perfusion scans obtained immediately (A) and four hours (B) after exercise, showing a reversible perfusion defect. (Courtesy of J. Vannoy Faris, M.D.)

A   B

TABLE 2–18. SELECTED NONINVASIVE CARDIAC LABORATORY TESTS

TEST	REASON FOR TEST	ABNORMAL RESULT	MEANING
Long-term ECG	Palpitations Syncope	Brady- or tachyarrhythmias	Needs correlation with symptoms
Stress testing	Chest pain	ST depression with pain	Ischemia (false-positive and false-negative tests occur)
	Evaluate functional capacity and prognosis in patients with known heart disease	Positive for ischemia within first two stages	High-risk patient, should possibly undergo further evaluation
Radionuclide angiography	LV function	↓ ejection fraction; regional wall motion abnormalities	Abnormal resting ventricular function
	Exercise evaluation of chest pain or ventricular reserve (e.g., aortic regurgitation)	Exercise-induced regional or global wall motion abnormality; inability to ↑ EF with exercise	Ischemia or decreased cardiac reserve
	Intracardiac shunts	Abnormal lung time/activity curve	Left-to-right or right-to-left shunt
Perfusion scintigraphy (exercise)	Chest pain (especially in patients with abnormal baseline ECG); or to evaluate the functional significance of a known coronary lesion	Defect on exercise and reperfusion scans	Myocardial scar
		Defect on exercise scan that reverses on reperfusion scan	Myocardial ischemia
Infarct-avid scintigraphy	Document acute MI, especially if ECG and enzyme evidence are inconclusive	Myocardial uptake of isotope; focal area of uptake is most specific	Acute MI (false-positive scans sometimes occur with older MI's, myocarditis, pericarditis, LV aneurysm, breast lesion, rib fractures, calcified cartilages or valve structures; smaller infarctions can be missed)

is exercised to the usual stress testing end points and a scan is performed immediately after exercise and again four hours later, allowing thallium to redistribute into areas of myocardium that are reperfused after recovery from exercise. An area without thallium uptake (cold) on both exercise and reperfusion scans is considered infarcted, scarred, or irreversibly damaged. An area that is cold on the exercise scan but reperfused four hours later is considered "ischemic," with a reversible lesion.

In infarct-avid scintigraphy or "hot spot scanning," an isotope (usually technetium-99 stannous pyrophosphate) that accumulates in irreversibly damaged myocardial cells is administered intravenously to detect acute myocardial infarction. Technetium pyrophosphate scans are negative during the first few hours after infarction and usually become positive after about 12 hours. The probability of a positive scan decreases the first week after infarction and is low after two weeks. It is most sensitive in patients with transmural myocardial infarctions; however, these are the infarctions that are usually diagnosed with clinical electrocardiographic and enzyme determinations, so the usefulness of infarct-avid scintigraphy for questionable small infarcts is unclear.

NEWER TECHNIQUES

Computerized axial tomography (CAT scanning) is useful to detect dissecting aortic aneurysms and is probably the most sensitive method for detecting the pericardial thickening associated with constrictive pericarditis. CAT scanning may be useful for assessing the patency of saphenous vein grafts used in coronary artery bypass surgery.

Nuclear magnetic resonance can produce high-resolution tomographic images of the heart without employing ionizing radiation. It also has the potential for generating metabolic information about the heart. Future applications may be noninvasive angiocardiography and possibly characterization of diseased tissue.

Digital subtraction angiography is a technique whereby small concentrations of iodinated contrast material introduced in a vascular bed can be detected, analyzed by computer, and displayed as a high-quality angiogram, thus eliminating the need for direct injection of contrast into an artery or cardiac chamber. Venous contrast injections may provide left ventriculograms of good quality. The carotid circulation and coronary bypass grafts may be well visualized by this technique. Venous contrast injection does not usually provide adequate visualization of coronary arteries, but digital subtraction techniques can improve the quality of coronary angiograms obtained by selective coronary catheterization.

CARDIAC CATHETERIZATION

Cardiac catheterization involves introduction of hollow, fluid-filled catheters via the arterial and/or venous system into the heart to measure intracardiac pressures, blood flow, and oxygen saturation, and to inject dye to perform cardiac angiograms. The complexity of the procedure depends on the particular patient and lesion being investigated and ranges from extensive studies in patients with complex congenital and valvular heart disease to straightforward measurement of left heart pressures, ventriculography, and coronary arteriography in patients with coronary artery disease.

Fluid-filled catheters transmit pressure waves obtained in each chamber entered back to a transducer, and pressure waveforms are displayed on an oscilloscope and recorded. Intracavitary pressures are used to judge the performance of the right and left ventricles, and pressure differences across valves (gradient) are used to evaluate valvular stenosis. The pulmonary capillary wedge pressure is measured by wedging the pulmonary arterial catheter as far into the pulmonary arterial tree as possible or inflating a balloon in a distal pulmonary artery, thus blocking out pulmonary arterial pressure and allowing the catheter to record pulmonary capillary or venous pressure. This pressure, given a patent pulmonary venous system, reflects left atrial pressure, which in turn, given a normal mitral valve, reflects the left ventricular diastolic pressure. This measurement is useful not only in the catheterization laboratory but also during bedside right-heart (Swan-Ganz) catheterization to estimate the left-sided filling pressures.

The cardiac output may be measured during catheterization by one of two basic techniques. Using the *Fick method*, the oxygen consumption of the patient is measured by collecting the expired air over a known period of time and simultaneously measuring arterial and mixed venous (pulmonary artery) oxygen content. The Fick equation states:

$$\text{Cardiac output} = \frac{\text{oxygen consumption (ml/min)}}{\substack{\text{arterial } O_2 \\ \text{content}} - \substack{\text{mixed venous} \\ O_2 \text{ content (ml/L)}}}$$

Cardiac output is expressed in liters/minute and cardiac index in liters/min/sq m of body surface. In addition, cardiac output may be measured by an *indicator dilution technique*, using either a dye that is detected by colorimetric methods or temperature (thermodilution) as the indicator. When an indicator is injected into the circulatory system and detected downstream, a curve can be generated. The area under the curve is proportional to the cardiac output.

Intracardiac shunts can be detected by measuring oxygen saturations in various cardiac chambers. For example, an increase in oxygen saturation between the right atrium and right ventricle would occur in a ventricular septal defect in which oxygenated blood is shunted from the left to the right ventricle (oxygen "step-up"). If the cardiac output is known, the shunt can be quantitated. Secondly, indicator dilution methods similar to that used for cardiac output determination may be used to detect shunts. For example, if an indicator is introduced into the right atrium and detected sooner than expected in a systemic artery, a right-to-left shunt is present. In addition, indicator dilution methods can detect valvular regurgitation.

Cardiac catheterization can be used to detect and quantitate the severity of a stenotic valvular lesion. Valves that are regurgitant can be established (but are difficult to quantitate) by cardiac angiography, which involves injecting radiopaque contrast into various chambers of the heart. Upon coronary injection of contrast, atherosclerotic lesions appear as narrowings of the internal caliber of the vessels and are expressed in terms of per cent diameter narrowing, for example, a 70 per cent diminution in the luminal diameter. Lesions producing narrowings of 70 per cent or greater are definitely hemodynamically significant, and lesions of 50 to 70 per cent diameter narrowing are probably hemodynamically significant.

Cardiac catheterization is usually indicated in patients with congenital heart disease or acquired valvular heart disease in whom surgery is contemplated (Table 2–19). A few instances exist in which the value of routine preoperative cardiac catheterization has been questioned; for example, echocardiography is very reliable for diagnosing and quantifying mitral stenosis, and the likelihood of concomitant coronary artery disease in a young patient is small. Therefore, if there is no clinical evidence of significant aortic or tricuspid disease, some physicians would operate on such a patient without catheterization.

The indications for performing cardiac catheterization specifically for the purposes of coronary angiography are summarized in Table 2–19. Emergency coronary arteriography may be necessary in patients with unstable angina or myocardial infarction in whom maximal medical therapy fails to alleviate pain. Cardiac catheterization may be indicated to provoke coronary spasm with ergonovine in a patient suspected of having Prinzmetal's angina. Left heart catheterization with coronary arteriography is a relatively safe procedure, with a mortality of between 0.1 and 0.2 per cent. The risk is higher for patients with significant stenosis of the left main coronary artery.

TABLE 2–19. GENERAL INDICATIONS FOR CARDIAC CATHETERIZATION

1. Congenital or acquired defects for which surgical correction is contemplated:
   a. Establish the diagnosis
   b. Assess the hemodynamic severity of the lesion
   c. Exclude unsuspected additional lesions (for example, concomitant coronary artery disease)
2. Coronary artery disease:
   a. Patients with chest pain in whom the etiology remains unclear after noninvasive evaluation
   b. Patients with coronary artery disease and angina refractory to medical management
   c. Patients at high risk for having left main or severe three-vessel stenosis who may have improved survival with surgical therapy (see Chapter 7)
   d. Patients in whom an acute intervention (i.e., angioplasty or intracoronary thrombolysis) is contemplated in the first four to six hours after infarction

SPECIAL TECHNIQUES

Biopsies of the left or right ventricular endomyocardium can be obtained at the time of catheterization and are useful to diagnose myocardial rejection in patients with cardiac transplants and sometimes useful in the diagnosis of hypertrophic and congestive cardiomyopathies, especially if amyloid or other infiltrative processes are present.

Percutaneous transluminal coronary angioplasty involves passing balloon catheters into the coronary arteries and across stenotic lesions, where the balloon is inflated. This technique is effective in relieving obstruction in patients who have single vessel disease and in some situations multivessel disease. Left main coronary stenosis is generally not safe to dilate with angioplasty. Long-term results of this technique are still being evaluated.

The infusion of thrombolytic agents (e.g., streptokinase or urokinase), either intravenously or directly into the coronary system, can reopen an acutely occluded coronary artery in 60 to 80 per cent of patients suffering an acute transmural myocardial infarction. Complications appear to be low from either intravenous or intracoronary administration, although the risk of serious bleeding from any recent arterial punctures or surgical procedures is high. Long-term results are under investigation.

Bedside right heart catheterization with a balloon flow-directed catheter (Swan-Ganz catheter) can be accomplished in an intensive care unit, and the catheter can remain in place from several hours to several days to guide drug therapy or fluid administration. Serial measurements of pulmonary arterial pressure, pulmonary capillary wedge pressure, right atrial pressure, and cardiac output using the thermodilution technique can be obtained (Table 2–20).

REFERENCES

Berger HJ, and Zaret BL: Nuclear cardiology. N Engl J Med 305:799, 855, 1981.

Davis K, Kennedy JW, Kemp HG, Judkins MP, Gosselin AJ, and Killip T: Complications of coronary arteriography from the collaborative study of coronary artery surgery (CASS). Circulation 59:1105, 1979.

TABLE 2–20. INDICATIONS FOR BEDSIDE CATHETERIZATION WITH A BALLOON FLOW-DIRECTED CATHETER (SWAN-GANZ)

Management

Cardiogenic, septic, and other forms of shock

Intraoperative and postoperative management of patients with significant cardiac disease

Patients with multiorgan failure in whom the fluid and hemodynamic management is complex

Serial evaluation of pharmacological or other interventions in patients with various cardiopulmonary abnormalities

Diagnosis

Differential diagnosis of cardiac vs. noncardiac pulmonary edema

Differential diagnosis of ventricular septal vs. papillary muscle rupture in acute MI

Evaluation of hypotension unresponsive to fluid administration

Diagnosis of right heart abnormalities; for example, pericardial tamponade or constriction, right ventricular infarction

Ellestad MH, Cooke BM, and Greenberg PS: Stress testing: Clinical application and predictive capacity. Prog Cardiovasc Dis 21:431, 1979.

Feigenbaum H: Echocardiography. 3rd ed. Philadelphia, Lea & Febiger, 1981.

Goldschalager N: Use of the treadmill test in the diagnosis of coronary artery disease in patients with chest pain. Ann Intern Med 97:38, 1982.

Grossman W: Cardiac Catheterization and Angiography. 2nd ed. Philadelphia, Lea & Febiger, 1980.

Gruntzig AR, Senning A, and Seigenthaler W: Non-operative dilation of coronary artery stenosis. N Engl J Med 301:61, 1979.

Health and Public Policy Committee, American College of Physicians: Percutaneous transluminal angioplasty. Ann Intern Med 99:864, 1983.

Lipman BS, Dunn M, and Massie E: Clinical Electrocardiography. 7th ed. Chicago, Year Book Medical Publishers, 1984.

Marriott HJL: Practical Electrocardiography. 7th ed. Baltimore, Williams and Wilkins, 1983.

Perloff JK: Physical Examination of the Heart and Circulation. Philadelphia, WB Saunders Co, 1982.

Perloff JK: The physiologic mechanisms of cardiac and vascular physical signs. J Am Coll Cardiol 1:184, 1983.

Popp RL, Rubenson DS, Tucker CR, and French JW: Echocardiography: M-mode and two-dimensional. Ann Intern Med 93:844, 1980.

Strauss HW, and Pitt B (eds): Cardiovascular Nuclear Medicine. St. Louis, The CV Mosby Co, 1979.

Tavel ME: Clinical Phonocardiography and External Pulse Recording. 3rd ed. Chicago, Year Book Medical Publishers, 1978.

CIRCULATORY FAILURE 3

Heart failure refers to a state in which the heart cannot provide sufficient cardiac output to satisfy the metabolic needs of the body. It is commonly termed "congestive" heart failure, since symptoms of increased venous pressure (pulmonary congestion with left heart failure and peripheral edema with right heart failure) are often prominent.

Heart failure can result from several underlying diseases, most commonly in industrialized nations from atherosclerotic coronary artery disease with myocardial infarction. Myocarditis, various cardiomyopathies, and valvular and congenital defects may result in heart failure. Mitral and aortic regurgitation, ventricular and atrial septal defects, and patent ductus arteriosus cause volume overload states; aortic and pulmonic stenosis and systemic hypertension cause pressure overload states. Conditions that restrict ventricular filling, e.g., mitral stenosis, constrictive pericarditis, or restrictive cardiomyopathies, cause heart failure.

Patients with previously compensated heart failure may decompensate as a result of dietary indiscretion (increased sodium intake) or failure to take prescribed medications. Exposure to excess heat or humidity, excess exertion, anemia, pregnancy, hyperthyroidism, or infection may exacerbate heart failure by increasing the metabolic needs of the body. Systemic hypertension, acute myocardial infarction, pulmonary embolus, and endocarditis should be excluded. Recurrence of the primary etiology, e.g., acute rheumatic fever, must be considered. The sudden onset of an arrhythmia, e.g., atrial fibrillation, may cause decompensation in a previously well-compensated patient.

By adjusting stroke volume and heart rate, the normal heart can increase cardiac output from approximately 5 L/min at rest to as much as 20 L/min during strenuous activity. The stroke volume is dependent upon the inotropic state of the ventricle, the preload (the ventricular filling or end-diastolic pressure), and afterload (the resistance into which the ventricle empties) (see Chapter 1). The inotropic state or contractility does not limit cardiac output in the normal heart but is the limiting parameter in patients with cardiac muscle dysfunction. In heart failure, the resting cardiac output may be normal, but the ability to increase cardiac output with exercise is abnormal. The autonomic nervous system is important in regulating cardiac function in normal hearts. As heart failure ensues, sympathetic nervous system output increases to help maintain cardiac output via positive chronotropic and inotropic effects (Table 3–1), accounting for some of the clinical features of heart failure (tachycardia, diaphoresis, cool or cyanotic extremities due to peripheral vasoconstriction). However, excessive sympathetic nervous system activity also may be detrimental to cardiac function, most specifically by increasing myocardial oxygen requirements and increasing peripheral vascular resistance (afterload) against which the heart must pump. A downward spiral may occur: increased systemic vascular resistance causes diminished cardiac output which, in turn, leads to increasing sympathetic tone and even higher peripheral vascular resistance. Therefore, the autonomic nervous system plays an important role in both compensatory and decompensatory responses in congestive heart failure.

In addition to sympathetic augmentation of heart rate and stroke volume, the failing heart may attempt to compensate by either dilating to increase cardiac output via the Starling mechanism or hypertrophying in patients with pressure overload states. Normal and abnormal ventricular function curves are illustrated in Figure 3–1. The curve is shifted downward to the right and has a flattened contour in the patient with decreased cardiac contractility. In both the normal or decreased inotropic states, an increase in the left ventricular end-diastolic volume or pressure (LVEDP) increases cardiac output. The amount of increase in cardiac output for any given increase in LVEDP is greater in the normal than in the failing heart. In addition, elevation of LVEDP increases pulmonary venous pressures; once the pulmonary capillary wedge pressure exceeds approximately 20 mm Hg, pulmonary edema results. Therefore, augmentation of cardiac output by increasing LVEDP is limited by the relatively flat Starling curve in the failing heart and occurs at the expense of possibly precipitating pulmonary edema. Cardiac dilation increases myocardial oxygen consumption via the increased wall tension.

The mechanism of fluid retention and elevation of LVEDP in patients with heart failure is multifactorial. Two important mechanisms involve (1) sympathetic venoconstriction to decrease the capacitance of the venous system and increase venous return to the heart, and (2) chronic renal salt

TABLE 3–1. COMPENSATORY MECHANISMS IN HEART FAILURE

MECHANISM	FAVORABLE EFFECTS	UNFAVORABLE EFFECTS

↑ Sympathetic activity	↑ heart rate
	↑ contractility
	↑ venoconstriction→
	  ↑ venous return (preload)
		↑ arteriolar constriction →
		  ↑ afterload
		↑ O_2 requirements

Cardiac hypertrophy	↑ working muscle mass	↑ wall tension ↓ coronary flow ↑ O_2 requirements abnormal systolic and diastolic properties of hypertrophic muscle
Frank-Starling mechanism	↑ stroke volume for any given amount of venous return	Pulmonary and systemic congestion ↑ LV size → ↑ wall tension and O_2 requirements
Renal salt and water retention	↑ venous return	Pulmonary and systemic congestion ↑ renin-angiotension → ↑ vasoconstriction (afterload)
Increased peripheral O_2 extraction	↑ O_2 delivery per unit cardiac output	

↑ = increase
↓ = decrease

and water retention because of decreased perfusion.

Cardiac hypertrophy, which is an increase in the number and size of cardiac cells as a compensatory mechanism, also involves trade-offs: the increased muscle mass increases oxygen consumption. The hypertrophic ventricular muscle is not normal and its contractility is decreased. The hypertrophied ventricle maintains adequate cardiac output for some time via the increase in muscle mass, the Starling relation, and augmented sympathetic stimulation.

Abnormal systolic and diastolic (compliance) function are both features of heart failure due to ischemic heart disease and hypertrophic states. Compliance refers to the pressure required to fill a ventricle to a certain volume. Hypertrophied or ischemic ventricles become "stiff" or relatively noncompliant, requiring a higher LVEDP to achieve diastolic filling adequate to maintain cardiac output. Generally, in a patient with congestive heart failure and a relatively noncompliant ventricle, a pulmonary capillary wedge pressure of 15 to 18 mm Hg is usually optimal to maintain adequate left ventricular filling and output but to avoid pulmonary edema.

It is critical to distinguish valvular and congenital etiologies of congestive heart failure from those due to myocardial damage. In the former, corrective or palliative surgery is often possible. In the latter, however, therapy is imperfect and compensates only partly for the decrease in myocardial function. Patients with myocardial dysfunction unrelated to a correctable lesion have a relatively poor long-term prognosis, with a 50 per cent five-year mortality in some studies.

Left heart failure refers to decreased function of the left ventricle with resultant low systemic cardiac output and pulmonary vascular congestion. Right heart failure is characterized by the manifestations of elevated right ventricular end-diastolic pressure, jugular venous distention, hepatomegaly, and peripheral edema. Right heart failure may occur in severe lung disease and congenital or acquired defects involving the right-sided chambers or valves. The most common cause of right ventricular failure is chronic left ventricular failure; this probably occurs both because there is a chronic increase in pulmonary pressures in patients with left ventricular failure and because the failing septum is a structure common to both the left and right ventricle.

Low-output heart failure occurs when myocardial dysfunction prevents normal metabolic requirements from being met. High-output failure refers to inability of the heart to meet elevated circulatory demands in conditions such as arteriovenous fistula, Paget's disease, anemia, hyperthyroidism, and beriberi.

Backward versus forward heart failure are old terms that refer to the more prominent symptoms in any particular patient. The patient who presents with fatigue and weakness due to decreased cardiac output and azotemia due to decreased renal perfusion would be considered to have predominantly forward failure. On the other hand,

FIGURE 3–1. Normal and abnormal ventricular function curves. When the left ventricular end-diastolic pressure is greater than 20 mm Hg (A), pulmonary edema often occurs. The effect of diuresis or venodilation is to move leftward along the curve from A to B, with a resultant improvement in pulmonary congestion with minimal decrease in cardiac output. The stroke volume is poor at any point along this depressed contractility curve, and thus therapeutic maneuvers that would raise it more toward the normal curve would be necessary to significantly improve cardiac output (for example, inotropic agents or arterial vasodilators—see Figure 3–3).

the patient who presents with pulmonary or systemic congestive symptoms would be considered to have backward failure.

Acute and chronic heart failure are different clinical entities. A patient has acute heart failure when sudden circulatory decompensation occurs, for example, secondary to an acute myocardial infarction or ruptured chordae tendineae. Chronic compensatory mechanisms do not have time to occur, and the patient may experience acute pulmonary edema. A patient with chronic myocardial dysfunction of the same degree may have adequate compensatory mechanisms to make him less symptomatic. Patients with chronic congestive heart failure may develop superimposed acute congestive heart failure if one of the precipitating factors listed above occurs.

The patient's history is important to help establish the diagnosis of congestive heart failure and sometimes to identify its etiology (see Table 2–4). The most common symptoms of left heart failure are respiratory. If heart failure is chronic, dyspnea on exertion occurs before dyspnea at rest, and as the disease progresses, less and less exertion is necessary to provoke dyspnea. Some patients may not complain of shortness of breath but have restricted their activities significantly to avoid it. The patient should be questioned carefully about previous cardiac disease, cardiac medications, and the existence of precipitating factors for congestive heart failure. The physical examination should confirm the physician's suspicion of heart failure (see Table 2–4).

Arterial P_{O_2}, relatively normal in mild heart failure even though pulmonary stiffness due to interstitial edema may cause a sensation of dyspnea,

FIGURE 3–2. Posteroanterior (A) and lateral (B) chest x-ray showing cardiomegaly and pulmonary vascular congestion typical of pulmonary edema.

falls as alveolar edema occurs. In early heart failure, the patient hyperventilates and the P_{CO_2} decreases; when pulmonary edema becomes severe, carbon dioxide retention occurs. Hepatic congestion may elevate liver enzymes. Increased sympathetic stimulation may increase slightly the white blood cell count. The blood urea nitrogen and to some extent the creatinine may be elevated owing to low cardiac output (prerenal azotemia) without necessarily indicating intrinsic renal disease. No electrocardiographic changes are specific for heart failure but may reflect underlying cardiac disease (for example, myocardial infarction, left or right ventricular hypertrophy, or rhythm disturbances).

Radiographic signs of left heart failure depend on its severity and chronicity (Fig. 3–2). Manifestations of pulmonary venous hypertension are discussed in Chapter 2. Cardiomegaly is common in patients with chronic heart failure but is often absent in acute forms (for example, acute severe aortic regurgitation). The radiographic manifestations of pulmonary edema resolve 12 to 24 hours after hemodynamic improvement.

Noninvasive tests may be used to estimate ventricular function. Echocardiography demonstrates segmental or global wall motion abnormalities and provides chamber dimensions. Echocardiography may also suggest the etiology of the congestive heart failure. Radionuclide ventriculography reveals chamber size, regional wall motion abnormalities, and ejection fraction. The left ventricular filling pressure and the cardiac output form the two limbs of the ventricular function curve and may be obtained in unstable patients via Swan-Ganz catheterization.

Since many of the clinical manifestations of cardiac failure involve the lungs, the differentiation between heart failure and pulmonary disease is sometimes difficult (Table 3–2). Noncardiac pulmonary edema (adult respiratory distress syndrome, ARDS) must be distinguished from cardiogenic pulmonary edema. A variety of processes can cause ARDS (for example, infection, shock, neurological injury, and drug toxicity). ARDS results from leakage of plasma into the aveoli because of leaky capillaries; pulmonary venous (capillary wedge) pressures are normal (see Chapter 22).

Chronic congestive heart failure with peripheral edema must be differentiated from other edematous states, for example, the nephrotic syndrome, cirrhosis, and severe peripheral venous disease.

MANAGEMENT OF HEART FAILURE

The ideal treatment of congestive heart failure is to remove or correct the underlying cause, for example, replacing a stenotic aortic valve. Next, removing or correcting any factors exacerbating chronic compensated heart failure should be achieved, for example, correcting anemia. Finally, medical therapy should be aimed at treating the congestive heart failure itself in order to improve the pumping function of the heart, reduce its work load, and reduce excessive salt and water retention (Table 3–3).

ACTIVITY AND DIET

An acute exacerbation of congestive heart failure should be treated with bed rest and adequate oxygenation. Control of excessive salt and water retention can be obtained by salt restriction. The normal American diet contains 10 grams of salt

TABLE 3–2. DIFFERENTIAL DIAGNOSIS OF LEFT HEART FAILURE AND PULMONARY DISEASE

	LEFT HEART FAILURE	PULMONARY DISEASE
Dyspnea	+ + +	+ + +
Orthopnea	+ + +	+
Paroxysmal nocturnal dyspnea	+ + +	+
Chest pain	+ +	+
Sputum production	+	+
Hemoptysis	+	+ + +
Cyanosis	+ +	+ + +
Concomitant right heart failure	+ +	+ +
Use of accessory muscles	+	+ +
Barrel chest	0	+ + +
Clubbing	+	+ +
Rales	+ + +	+ +
Wheezes	+ +	+ + +
S₃ gallop	+ + +	0 unless right heart failure occurs
Hypoxemia	+ + +	+ + +
Chest x-ray	cardiomegaly, pulmonary congestion	normal heart; hyperexpansion; chronic interstitial changes
Abnormal pulmonary function tests	+ + (acutely)	+ + +
Echocardiogram	abnormal LV	often technically difficult; LV normal if visualized adequately
Radionuclide angiogram	abnormal LV	normal LV
LVEDP (pulmonary wedge pressure)	increased	normal

0 = absent
+ = occurs infrequently
+ + = occurs occasionally
+ + + = occurs frequently

daily. While the usual patient with heart failure does not require rigid salt restriction, a 4-gram salt diet can be obtained by avoiding salty foods and not adding salt at the table. For patients with more severe heart failure, a 2-gram salt diet can be prescribed which requires food to be cooked and prepared without salt. In particularly refractory cases, diets of 0.5 to 1 gram can be prescribed, but only the most compliant patients adhere to these diets, and diuretic therapy may be used instead of restricting salt intake so stringently. Salt substitutes are available that contain potassium chloride instead of sodium chloride. It is unusual to have to restrict water intake except when severe congestive heart failure with dilutional hyponatremia occurs. One of the most common causes for exacerbation of congestive heart failure is failure to adhere to a low-salt diet after hospital discharge.

DIGITALIS

Digitalis augments cardiac output in patients with myocardial failure by increasing the inotropic state of the heart, possibly by inhibiting the activity of sodium-potassium ATPase. It may act by altering the membranes of the sarcoplasmic reticulum and the mitochondria so that they release calcium ions more readily. In addition to its inotropic effects, digitalis has significant electrophysiological effects, the most prominent of which at therapeutic doses is an increase in AV nodal conduction time and refractoriness. Sinus rate may slow owing to sympathetic withdrawal as heart failure improves.

Digitalis is available in several different preparations, the most common of which are digitoxin and digoxin (Table 3–4). Digitoxin is less frequently used than is digoxin but is useful in patients with renal insufficiency and appears to control the ventricular response in some patients with atrial fibrillation better than digoxin, possibly because of less fluctuation in plasma drug levels due to the long half-life. The bioavailability of several digoxin preparations appears to differ markedly. Patients with malabsorption syndromes may absorb digoxin poorly, and nonabsorbed substances such as cholestyramine, kaopectate, nonabsorbable antacids, and neomycin may interfere with digoxin absorption. Excretion of digoxin is propor-

TABLE 3–3. MANAGEMENT OF CONGESTIVE HEART FAILURE

OBJECTIVE	THERAPY
Reduce cardiac work load	Physical and psychological rest
	Remove exacerbating factors (e.g., infection, anemia, heat, humidity, obesity)
	Vasodilators
	Intra-aortic balloon pump
Improve cardiac performance	Digitalis
	Other positive inotropic agents
	Correct any rhythm abnormality
	Correct underlying defect if possible (e.g., valve malfunction)
Control excess salt and water	Dietary sodium restriction
	Diuretics
	Mechanical fluid removal (e.g., phlebotomy, dialysis)

TABLE 3-4. THE USE OF DIGOXIN

Intravenous Administration

INITIAL DOSE	SUBSEQUENT DOSAGE	ONSET OF ACTION	PEAK EFFECT	ELIMINATION HALF-LIFE ($T_{1/2}$)
0.5-1.0 mg	0.25 mg every 2-4 hr for total dose ≤ 1.5 mg/24 hr	10-15 min	30 min-4 hr	36 hr

Oral Administration

LOADING DOSE (IN 24 HR)	MAINTENANCE DOSE (IN 24 HR)	GASTROINTESTINAL ABSORPTION	ELIMINATION HALF-LIFE ($T_{1/2}$)	PRINCIPAL ROUTE OF ELIMINATION	THERAPEUTIC SERUM LEVELS
1.0-1.5 mg	0.125-0.5 mg	60-85%	36 hr	Renal	0.7-2.0 ng/ml

tional to the creatinine clearance, and maintenance doses must be reduced in patients with renal failure. Digoxin has a high degree of protein binding and is not removed from the body by dialysis. Digoxin serum concentrations increase when conventional doses of quinidine or an experimental antiarrhythmic agent, amiodarone, are added; therefore, the dose of digoxin should be lowered by approximately half when these drugs are added. Digitalis serum concentrations are only guidelines of either adverse or favorable digitalis effects and should be interpreted in the context of the clinical setting. Digoxin serum concentrations should be drawn at least 6 hours after a dose to avoid the peak levels.

Ouabain is a rapidly acting digitalis glycoside with unreliable gastrointestinal absorption that is rarely used today.

The end point of digitalis administration in patients with heart failure is not always clear. Digitalis or any other positive inotropic agent shifts the ventricular function curve (Fig. 3-3) up and to the left; that is, for any given left ventricular end-diastolic pressure, ventricular function is increased. The improvement in ventricular function increases ventricular emptying, promotes a diuresis and, in turn, reduces the filling pressures in the failing ventricle. This shifts the ventricular function along the new curve to the left and reduces pulmonary venous congestion. Even though increased contractility increases oxygen consumption, this may be offset by reducing diastolic pressure and volume, leading to decreased wall tension and decreased net oxygen consumption. Digitalis is useful in myocardial failure due to ischemic, hypertensive, valvular, congenital, or pulmonary heart disease and idiopathic dilated cardiomyopathy. It is not useful in isolated mitral stenosis if normal sinus rhythm and normal right ventricular function are present and is not useful in restrictive states such as pericardial tamponade or constriction. In patients who have dynamic outflow obstruction (obstructive hypertrophic cardiomyopathy), digitalis is contraindicated because the increase in contractility may increase the outflow gradient. A hypertrophied but vigorously functioning ventricle probably does not need digitalis. The need for prophylactic use of digitalis in patients with decreased cardiac reserve about to undergo major surgery is controversial. Use of digitalis in arrhythmias often has a more distinct end point, especially in patients with atrial fibrillation, because the rate of ventricular response reflects the adequacy of digitalization. Digitalis is also useful in many patients with paroxysmal supraventricular tachycardias and atrial flutter.

Digitalis toxicity is one of the most common adverse drug reactions, encountered in 5 to 15 per cent of hospitalized patients receiving digitalis. Elderly individuals are more prone to digitalis toxicity than younger patients. Manifestations include cardiac arrhythmias of almost any type, commonly ventricular premature complexes and ventricular tachycardia, junctional escape rhythms, nonparoxysmal junctional tachycardia, paroxysmal atrial tachycardia with AV block, and type I (Wenckebach) second-degree atrioventricular block. Digitalis toxic rhythms have in common the combination of increased automaticity of ectopic pacemakers and impaired conduction. Noncardiac manifestations include anorexia, nausea, vomiting, disorientation, confusion, and seizures. Visual symptoms are not uncommon and include scotomas, halos, and changes in color perception (yellow-green halo commonly occurs). Massive overdoses of digitalis can cause a refractory hyperkalemia. Despite digitalis plasma levels, the diagnosis of digitalis toxicity requires clinical and electrocardiographic correlation. Hypokalemia exacerbates digitalis intoxication.

The treatment of digitalis intoxication depends on the degree of intoxication and specific manifestation. Mild rhythm abnormalities (occasional ectopic beats, first- and second-degree AV block, slow ventricular response to atrial fibrillation) require withdrawal of the drug and electrocardiographic monitoring. Ventricular tachycardia and marked bradyarrhythmias must be treated aggressively. Bradyarrhythmias may respond to atropine or if more severe may require temporary pacing. Phenytoin and lidocaine are effective drugs to

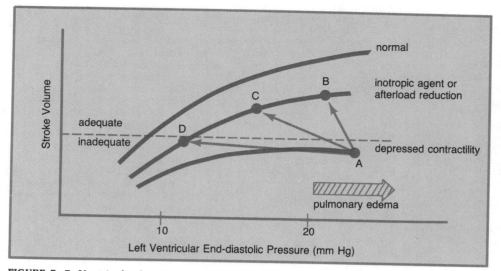

FIGURE 3–3. Ventricular function curve illustrating the effect of inotropic agents or arterial vasodilators. Unlike diuretics, the effect of digitalis or arterial vasodilator therapy in a patient with heart failure is to move onto another ventricular function curve intermediate between the normal and depressed curves. When the patient's ventricular function moves from A to B by the administration of one of these agents, his left ventricular end-diastolic pressure may also decrease because of improved cardiac function; further administration of diuretics or venodilators may shift him further to the left along the same curve from B to C and eliminate the risk of pulmonary edema. A vasodilating agent that has both arteriolar and venous dilating properties (for example, nitroprusside) would shift this patient directly from A to C. If this agent shifts the patient from A to D because of excessive venodilation or administration of diuretics, the cardiac output may fall too low even though the left ventricular end-diastolic pressure would be normal (10 mm Hg) for a normal heart. Thus, left ventricular end-diastolic pressures between 15 and 18 mm are usually optimal in the failing heart to maximize cardiac output but avoid pulmonary edema.

treat ventricular tachyarrhythmias and have little effect on conduction. Correction of a low serum potassium may suppress ectopic rhythms but must be done cautiously in patients with conduction disturbances, since potassium administration can exacerbate AV block. DC cardioversion is avoided if possible in digitalis intoxication because it may precipitate refractory ventricular fibrillation or cardiac standstill. If a life-threatening ventricular arrhythmia with hemodynamic collapse occurs, it must be employed with as low an energy level as possible. Since quinidine increases digoxin levels, it probably should be avoided in digitalis intoxication. The use of antibodies specific for digoxin has been reported to be effective for the treatment of severe digitalis intoxication.

DIURETICS

Diuretics are drugs that promote the excretion of sodium and water from the kidney and thus affect predominantly preload. They play a very important role in the treatment of heart failure.

VASODILATORS

Vasodilator therapy was introduced initially to treat refractory, severe heart failure, but it is now often used earlier in the treatment of congestive heart failure. Vasodilating agents can be divided into two broad categories: venodilators decrease preload by increasing venous capacitance, and the

arterial dilators reduce systemic arteriolar resistance and decrease afterload. Many vasodilators dilate both venous and arterial beds (Table 3–5).

The effect of arteriolar vasodilators on the ventricular function curve is demonstrated in Figure 3–3. Changes in afterload have little effect on normally functioning myocardium, since reflexes adapt the heart rate and stroke volume accordingly. However, elevated afterload can detrimentally affect the failing myocardium, markedly decreasing the ability of the heart to eject blood. The lower the resistance to the outflow of blood, the more blood is ejected with each beat. Since the heart is able to pump more blood with each stroke when afterload is decreased, the ventricular function curve is shifted upward and to the left, just as it is with an increase in contractility. The shift in the curve due to decrease in afterload is not associated with the increased demand for oxygen that an increase in contractility requires. As ventricular function moves from the failing curve to the afterload-reduced curve, the improvement in ventricular emptying subsequently also decreases preload and left ventricular dimensions, shifting down on the new curve to the left. This decrease in left ventricular dimension decreases left ventricular wall tension and myocardial oxygen consumption. Since failing myocardium is more sensitive to changes in afterload than normal myocardium, afterload reduction is particularly effective in patients with poorer myocardial function, whereas therapy to increase contractility de-

TABLE 3-5. COMMONLY USED VASODILATING AGENTS

AGENT	PREDOMINANT SITE OF ACTION	ROUTE OF ADMINISTRATION	USUAL DOSE	DURATION OF EFFECT	SIDE EFFECTS
Nitroprusside	A,V	IV	Initially 10 µg/min; titrate upward at 5-min intervals to desired hemodynamic effect	minutes	hypotension thiocyanate toxicity (fatigue, nausea, muscle spasm, psychosis, hypothyroidism)
Nitroglycerin	V	IV	Initially 10 µg/min; titrate upward at 5-min intervals to desired hemodynamic effect	minutes	postural hypotension, dizziness, syncope, headaches, nausea, ischemia upon abrupt withdrawal
		SL	0.3-0.6 mg	minutes	
		topical	1-2 inches of 2% ointment q4-6h; or controlled release topical patch q24h	hours	
Isosorbide dinitrate	V	SL	2.5-10 mg q2-3h	hours	same as nitroglycerin
		oral	10-40 mg q3-6h	hours	
Hydralazine	A	oral	40-400 mg/day in 2-4 divided doses	hours	reflex tachycardia, fluid retention, headache, nausea, lupus erythematosus—like syndrome (usually with doses ≥ 200 mg/day)
Prazosin	A,V	oral	1 mg initially; up to 21 mg/day in 2-3 divided doses; small initial test dose	hours	hypotension, especially after first dose; fluid retention, headache, nausea, rash; first dose: impairment of renal function, proteinuria, rash, neutropenia
Captopril	A,V	oral	6.25-25 mg t.i.d. initially; titrate upwards	hours	hypotension, especially after first dose; agranulocytosis; proteinuria; hyperkalemia

A = arterial dilator   V = venous dilator   IV = intravenous   SL = sublingual

---

pends on the availability of some residual functioning myocardium and is less effective as myocardial function declines.

Pure venodilators, preload-reducing agents, shift ventricular function along the same curve to the left as does diuretic therapy. Thus, preload reduction lowers left ventricular filling pressures; even though it does not directly affect forward cardiac output, the diminished left ventricular size decreases wall tension (one of the determinants of afterload) and oxygen consumption, possibly improving forward cardiac performance somewhat. Since the ventricular function curve for the failing myocardium is relatively flat, decreasing the left ventricular end-diastolic pressure to 15 to 20 mm Hg from higher values does not usually decrease cardiac output significantly.

Note that there are end points beyond which one cannot expect vasodilators to be effective. When agents are administered to reduce preload, the filling pressures must be kept high enough so that cardiac output can be maintained. It is especially important in states associated with decreased ventricular compliance (for example, acute ischemic heart disease and hypertrophic cardiomyopathy) that ventricular filling pressures be maintained higher than normal (15 to 20 mm Hg, normal being approximately 10 mm Hg). When arterial vasodilators are used to attempt to

increase forward output, arterial blood pressure may be a limiting factor. In patients whose blood pressure is high, lowering blood pressure by arterial vasodilators may have a beneficial effect. Patients who have relatively low arterial pressure may still benefit from afterload reduction because blood pressure depends not only upon arteriolar resistance, but also upon cardiac output (blood pressure = cardiac output × resistance). Patients may have low normal arterial pressure but still have elevated systemic vascular resistance; therefore, if cardiac output is low; therefore, if cardiac output improves as peripheral vascular resistance is decreased by arterial vasodilators, blood pressure may not fall. Once blood pressure falls below acceptable limits (approximately 90 mm systolic) during arteriolar vasodilator therapy, one has reached the limits of such therapy unless the decrease in blood pressure is due to an excessive fall in preload induced either by the afterload decrease or by venodilation from the drug itself. In that case, the hypotension can be corrected by fluid administration or decreasing preload-reducing agents. At times afterload reduction therapy may be tolerated only after the addition of an inotropic agent such as dopamine or dobutamine. Because of these limitations, it is often advisable to employ invasive hemodynamic monitoring in patients who are acutely ill and require intravenous vasodilator therapy. Indications for vasodilator therapy in congestive heart failure are listed in Table 3–6. Chronic administration of vasodilators has not been shown to increase longevity in patients with chronic heart failure. Afterload reduction must be used with caution in patients with aortic or mitral stenosis.

Sodium nitroprusside is a commonly used parenteral, short-acting vasodilator that has a direct smooth muscle relaxant effect on both arteriolar and venous systems. Hypotension, the most common adverse effect, is reversed within 10 minutes after discontinuation of the infusion. A metabolite of nitroprusside, thiocyanate, may accumulate after several days of administration, especially in patients with renal insufficiency. Serum levels of thiocyanate should be measured if the infusion is prolonged and should be kept below 6 mg/dl.

Nitroglycerin preparations are primarily venous dilators with lesser effects on the arterioles. Thus, they relieve pulmonary venous congestion with only a modest increase in cardiac output. An arteriolar dilator such as hydralazine may be combined with nitroglycerin to provide a balanced arteriolar and venous dilation.

Tolerance to the favorable hemodynamic effects of oral vasodilators appears to develop in some patients. Captopril has been reported to be the oral vasodilator to which tolerance is least likely to develop. Increased fluid retention during chronic vasodilator therapy may respond to an increase in diuretic.

SYMPATHOMIMETIC AMINES

Potent, parenteral inotropic agents other than digitalis are sometimes required in severe heart failure, the two most common being dopamine and dobutamine. These are sympathomimetic agents producing less tachycardia and fewer peripheral vascular effects than the older drugs norepinephrine, epinephrine, and isoproterenol. Dopamine stimulates the myocardium by activating $beta_1$-adrenergic receptors directly and indirectly by releasing norepinephrine from sympathetic nerve terminals. Dopamine at low doses (2 μg/kg/min) activates dopaminergic receptors in the renal, mesenteric, coronary, and cerebral vascular beds and causes vasodilation. This is partially responsible for dopamine-induced diuresis in patients with severe congestive heart failure (renal vasodilator plus inotropic effects). With larger doses of dopamine (5 to 10 μg/kg/min), alpha-adrenergic agonism similar to that of norepinephrine causes peripheral vasoconstriction. Thus, with infusion of 2 to 5 μg/kg/min, renal blood flow, cardiac contractility, and cardiac output all increase with little change in the heart rate and possibly a small decrease in peripheral vascular resistance. Higher doses (5 to 10 μg/kg/min) begin to increase arterial pressure, peripheral vascular resistance, and heart rate. In patients with hypotension, the vasoconstrictor effects of doses up to 20 μg/kg/min may be desired. The elevation of heart rate, contractility, and blood pressure associated with dopamine may increase oxygen de-

TABLE 3–6. INDICATIONS FOR VASODILATOR THERAPY OF HEART FAILURE

Heart failure refractory to conventional therapy with inotropic agents and diuretics

Treatment of earlier stages of heart failure in:
1. Patients intolerant to digitalis
2. Patients with other indications for vasodilators (e.g., nitrates or nifedipine for angina, hydralazine for hypertension)

Acute severe heart failure after myocardial infarction or transient myocardial contractile depression after cardiac surgery

Aortic or mitral regurgitation (acute or chronic) or ventricular septal defect (afterload reduction decreases regurgitant volume)

PREDOMINANT HEART FAILURE SYMPTOM	CAUSE	VASODILATOR OF CHOICE
Dyspnea	LV filling pressure	preload reduction (e.g., nitrates)
Fatigue	cardiac output	afterload reduction (e.g., hydralazine)
Dyspnea and fatigue	LV filling pressure and cardiac output	balanced vasodilation (e.g., hydralazine plus nitrates; prazosin)

mand, but if cardiac performance is improved and cardiac size decreases, the net oxygen consumption may not be adversely affected.

Dobutamine increases cardiac contractility but has less effect on the peripheral vasculature than dopamine. It is useful when the vasoconstrictive effects of higher dopamine doses are to be avoided. Dobutamine does not have the renal vasodilatory effects of dopamine. It is administered intravenously in a dose of 5 to 10 μg/kg/min.

Amrinone is a noncatecholamine, nondigitalis positive inotropic agent with vasodilator activity. It is available for short-term intravenous use in patients with severe congestive heart failure. Milrinone is an orally active inotropic agent under investigational use in the United States.

NONPHARMACOLOGICAL MANAGEMENT OF HEART FAILURE

Mechanical support of the failing heart by intra-aortic balloon counterpulsation is sometimes useful. The balloon is inserted either surgically or percutaneously into a femoral artery and advanced to the descending aorta. Timed from the electrocardiogram, the balloon is deflated immediately before ventricular ejection to decrease aortic pressure (afterload) during ventricular systole and inflated in early diastole to increase aortic pressure and to maintain coronary perfusion. Thus, the hemodynamic benefits of balloon counterpulsation are greater than those of vasodilatory drugs alone. Balloon counterpulsation is useful to stabilize patients before an intervention designed to provide long-term benefit (PTCA or surgical revascularization; surgical correction of acute mitral regurgitation or ventricular septal defect). It may be used prophylactically during cardiac catheterization in severely ill patients, as an aid during or after open heart surgery, during treatment of some life-threatening ventricular arrhythmias, and for relieving angina pectoris in patients in whom medical therapy has been unsuccessful.

The role of surgery in patients with congestive heart failure depends on the etiology; surgically correctable lesions should be identified and corrected if possible. In patients with end-stage myocardial dysfunction, the results with cardiac transplantation have recently improved with the introduction of cyclosporine and other improved immunological support. In addition, development of mechanical cardiopulmonary apparatus is promising.

MANAGEMENT OF ACUTE PULMONARY EDEMA

The general management of acute cardiogenic pulmonary edema is summarized in Table 3–7. Furosemide and morphine comprise standard first-line drug therapy. Digitalis is not necessary acutely unless atrial fibrillation or other supraventricular tachyarrhythmia is contributing to the pulmonary edema. Reversible causes or exacerbating factors of pulmonary edema should be sought (e.g., anemia, arrhythmia, etc.).

If initial measures fail to correct pulmonary edema, or if drug administration is limited by the development of hypotension, more aggressive management to include invasive hemodynamic monitoring is usually indicated. Parenteral inotropic and vasodilating agents may be administered. If adequate ventilation cannot be maintained, intubation with mechanical ventilation may be required to maintain oxygenation and decrease the work of breathing. In cases refractory to the above measures in whom a reversible pro-

cess is present, intra-aortic balloon counterpulsation may be employed.

SHOCK

Shock is acute severe circulatory failure. Regardless of etiology, shock is associated with marked reduction of blood flow to vital organs, and therefore profound arterial hypotension, impaired mentation, and diminished urinary output usually occur. The common denominator of all four broad categories of shock (Table 3–8) is eventual cellular damage and death. Shock may be divided into three stages. The first is a stage of "compensated hypotension"; that is, the fall in cardiac output or in delivery of cardiac output to the tissues stimulates a variety of compensatory mechanisms that alter myocardial function and peripheral resistance to maintain circulation to vital organs such as the brain and the heart. The clinical symptoms during this stage are minimal. In stage 2, the compensatory mechanisms for dealing with the low delivery of nutrients to the body are overwhelmed and tissue perfusion is decreased. Early signs of cerebral, renal, and myocardial insufficiency and of excessive sympathetic discharge are present. In stage 3, severe ischemia occurs along with damage to tissues by toxins, antigen-antibody reactions, or complement activation. Especially prone to damage are the capillary endothelia in the kidneys, the liver, and the lungs. Ischemic damage to the gastrointestinal tract allows invasion by bacteria. Renal ischemia may lead to acute renal insufficiency. Damage to capillary endothelia throughout the body allows transudation of fluid and protein into the extracellular space, exacerbating hypotension. The se-

TABLE 3–7. MANAGEMENT OF ACUTE PULMONARY EDEMA

INTERVENTION	PURPOSE	COMMENT
Sitting position	Decreases venous return and work of breathing; increases lung volumes	
Oxygen	Increases arterial P_{O_2}; pulmonary vasodilation	Humidify oxygen to prevent drying of secretions; mask may make patient feel like he is suffocating
Furosemide 10-20 mg IV; if no response within 30 minutes, administer progressively larger doses; usual max dose 200 mg, but occasional patient requires more	Decreases pulmonary congestion	Rapid pulmonary vasodilatory effect; diuretic effect onset in 5-10 min, peaks in 30 min
Morphine sulfate 1-4 mg IV q5-10 min as needed	Decreases venous return (venodilator); decreases anxiety	Respiratory depression can be reversed with naloxone
Vasodilators e.g., sublingual or IV nitroglycerin	Decreases venous return; relieves ischemia	
Aminophylline IV	Dilates bronchioles	Relieves "cardiac asthma"; can exacerbate arrhythmias
Phlebotomy	Decreases intravascular volume	Used only if the above fail
Rotating Tourniquets applied to three of the four extremities at a time and inflated above venous but below arterial pressure	Reduces venous return from the extremities	Used only if the above fail
Dialysis	Decreases intravascular volume	Useful in renal patients in whom diuretics have been ineffective

vere acidosis and toxins released into the blood contribute to further myocardial depression.

The etiology of hypoperfusion is evident in cardiogenic and hypovolemic shock. Septic shock is most commonly caused by gram-negative bacterial infections but can occur with infections by other agents. The mechanism of shock appears to be related to the release of an endotoxin (part of the bacterial cell wall) that interacts with substances from the blood and causes increased vascular permeability, intravascular coagulation, depression of myocardial contractility, and other adverse reactions. It is manifest by an abnormality in the distribution of blood flow to the tissues; that is, arteriovenous shunting of blood occurs and causes decreased delivery of nutrients to tissues despite an increase in cardiac output early in the course of the disease. Increased capillary permeability from the toxic products of infection allows fluid to leak into the interstitium, leaving the intravascular space relatively hypovolemic. Therefore, septic shock often involves the therapeutic paradox of needing to administer large quantities of fluid to a patient who is massively edematous in order to maintain adequate filling pressures. The only definitive therapy for this syndrome is control of the infection, but temporizing therapy includes maintaining intravascular volume via fluid administration, often directed by hemodynamic monitoring. One must remember that myocardial dysfunction may be prominent in stage 3 of septic shock. "Leaky" pulmonary capillaries can cause pulmonary edema without myocardial dysfunction (noncardiogenic pulmonary edema or adult respiratory distress syndrome) in which left ventricular filling pressures are normal or low (see Chapter 22).

Signs and symptoms of shock are summarized in Table 3–9 and its management in Table 3–10. Invasive hemodynamic monitoring is often required. Measurement of central venous pressure is sufficient in patients with known hypovolemic shock and good myocardial function; however, in patients with cardiac and lung disease, the central venous pressure may reflect poorly left ventricular filling pressures, and Swan-Ganz catheterization to measure pulmonary arterial and pulmonary capillary wedge pressures should be used in the more critically ill patients.

HIGH-OUTPUT STATES

If the circulatory system cannot meet a heightened demand for oxygen, high-output cardiac failure is said to occur. In high-output states, the heart must pump abnormally large volumes of blood, and the myocardial failure that ensues is similar to that caused by regurgitant valvular lesions. Disease entities associated with high-output heart failure include severe anemia, hyperthyroidism, systemic arteriovenous fistulae and other left-to-right shunts, e.g., patent ductus arteriosus, beriberi heart disease (vitamin B_1 deficiency), and Paget's disease. Increased workloads on the normal heart usually do not result in cardiac failure (e.g.,

TABLE 3–8. ETIOLOGIES OF SHOCK

CATEGORY OF SHOCK	CAUSES
Cardiogenic or vascular obstructive	Arrhythmias Obstructive outflow (valvular and peri-valvular) lesions Atrial myxoma Acute myocardial infarction Severe congestive heart failure Cardiac tamponade Massive pulmonary embolism
Hypovolemic	Hemorrhage Vomiting Diarrhea Dehydration Diabetes (mellitus or insipidus) Addison's disease Burns Peritonitis, pancreatitis
Septic	Gram-negative or other overwhelming infections
Miscellaneous	Anaphylactic Neurogenic Drug overdose Hepatic or renal failure Myxedema

TABLE 3–9. CLINICAL MANIFESTATIONS OF SHOCK

FINDING	SIGNIFICANCE
Hypotension	BP is normal in early shock (stage I) because of effective compensatory mechanisms
Tachycardia	Early manifestation
Increased respiratory rate	May represent compensation for metabolic acidosis or pulmonary congestion; may be an early sign
Fever	Septic shock
Cool, pale, moist skin	Sympathetic-mediated vasoconstriction
Warm skin	Septic shock or late shock of any cause when compensatory mechanisms fail
Elevated neck veins	Cardiogenic shock, cardiac tamponade
Collapsed neck veins	Hypovolemic or septic shock
Rales	Pulmonary edema; adult respiratory distress syndrome
Arrhythmias, murmurs, gallops	Suggest cardiac etiology
Abnormal abdominal exam	Source of sepsis, hemorrhage
Blood on rectal exam	Source of hemorrhage
Abnormal neurological status	Neurogenic shock or manifestation of cerebral hypoperfusion
Oliguria	Sign of renal hypoperfusion
Metabolic acidosis (anion gap)	Early sign of hypoperfusion

TABLE 3–10. MANAGEMENT OF SHOCK

General Measures
Assure adequate oxygenation
Bladder catheter to monitor urine output
Hemodynamic monitoring to optimize fluid management and cardiac output: indwelling arterial catheter, central venous pressure catheter, and/or Swan-Ganz catheter
Vasopressors as temporizing measures if necessary (e.g., dopamine, norepinephrine)

Specific Types

Cardiogenic	Diuretics
	Inotropic agents
	Vasodilators (if possible)
	Intra-aortic balloon pump
	Correction of underlying lesion (if possible)
Hypovo-lemic	Fluids/blood products
	Correction of underlying etiology
Septic	Identify source of infection
	Antibiotics
	? Steroids
	Support with fluids (massive edema may develop from leaky capillaries)
Neurogenic	Correct neurological abnormality (if possible)
Anaphy-lactic	Epinephrine
	Antihistamines
Addisonian	Fluids
	Mineralocorticoids
	Glucocorticoids
	Correct hypoglycemia

pregnancy, hepatic and renal disease, pulmonary disease, and obesity); however, if superimposed on pre-existing heart disease, high-output failure can occur in these conditions.

Symptoms and signs of pulmonary and systemic congestion are similar to those found in patients with low-output congestive heart failure. Because of the increased stroke volume, decreased peripheral vascular resistance, and increased rate of ejection, the pulses are bounding, with a rapid upstroke and a wide pulse pressure. Physical signs of the underlying process should be sought. Treatment involves the treatment of the etiological disorder.

REFERENCES

Chatterjee K, and Parmley WW: Vasodilator therapy for acute myocardial infarction and chronic congestive heart failure. J Am Coll Cardiol 1:133, 1983.

Goldenheim PD, and Kazemi H: Cardiopulmonary monitoring of critically ill patients. N Engl J Med 311:717, 776, 1984.

Gunnar RM, and Loeb HS: Shock in acute myocardial infarction: Evaluation of physiologic therapy. J Am Coll Cardiol 1:154, 1983.

Swan HJC, and Ganz W: Hemodynamic measurements in clinical practice: A decade in review. J Am Coll Cardiol 1:103, 1983

4 CONGENITAL HEART DISEASE

Congenital heart disease refers to cardiac lesions present at birth. Even though these abnormalities exist before birth, they often become clinically evident at the time of delivery, when profound physiological changes occur in the circulatory system, or months or years after birth. Congenital heart disease (excluding bicuspid aortic valve) occurs in approximately 0.8 per cent of live births and results from both genetic and environmental factors. Congenital heart disease may be familial in some instances, although a distinct pattern of inheritance is usually not recognized. It is more common in children of older mothers. Ventricular septal defect and patent ductus arteriosus are relatively common in premature infants. Environmental factors such as teratogens and maternal rubella are commonly recognized risk factors.

Congenital cardiac defects that are compatible with the fetal circulation (see Chapter 1) may produce symptoms once the child is born. The persistence of normal fetal structures in an infant, such as a patent ductus arteriosus allowing a left-to-right shunt, may be detrimental. However, an abnormal connection may be necessary for an infant to survive in the presence of another congen-

ital anomaly, such as transposition of the great arteries, which must have a connection between the two circuits (e.g., atrial septal defect, patent ductus arteriosus) to allow oxygenation of systemic blood and survival for any period of time after birth. Those at risk for developing endocarditis (see Chapter 10) should receive prophylactic antibiotics at appropriate times.

Congenital defects can be classified generally into acyanotic and cyanotic groups. The acyanotic congenital defects are those either without a shunt or with left-to-right shunts. Cyanosis occurs in the presence of a right-to-left shunt. In addition, it is important to identify whether malformations arise in the left or the right heart, the site of shunts if present, the status of the pulmonary blood flow (increased, normal, or decreased), and the presence of pulmonary hypertension (Tables 4–1, 4–2, and 4–3).

ACYANOTIC LESIONS

SITUS INVERSUS

Situs inversus involves a mirror image reversal of several organs, including the heart, the liver, and the gastrointestinal tract. These patients have normal longevity unless the disorder is associated with chronic sinusitis and bronchiectasis (Kartagener's syndrome). Situs inversus can be identified by physical examination and chest x-ray (cardiac apex and stomach bubble to the right, liver to the left). If the heart is in the right chest but the abdominal viscera are correctly located, dextroversion of the heart is present and, unlike situs inversus, is often associated with other congenital cardiac anomalies.

ATRIAL SEPTAL DEFECT

Atrial septal defects are classified according to their location in the atrial septum. Ostium secundum defects are in the region of the fossa ovalis, ostium primum in the low atrial septum, and sinus venosus in the upper septum near the junction of the vena cava and the right atrium. Ostium primum atrial septal defects are often associated with other endocardial cushion developmental defects, such as a cleft mitral valve or ventricular septal defect. Sinus venosus defects are almost always associated with partial anomolous pulmonary venous return (a pulmonary vein enters the right atrium or vena cava instead of the left atrium, adding to the left-to-right shunt).

In most atrial septal defects, the pressure equilibrates between the left and the right atrium, and the degree of left-to-right shunt depends not on a pressure gradient but instead on the relative compliance of the right ventricle and pulmonary arterial system compared to the left ventricle and systemic arterial system. Pulmonary vascular resistance and pulmonary arterial pressure tend to remain low, and thus pulmonary hypertension and right-to-left shunt (Eisenmenger's syndrome) do not occur commonly.

Atrial septal defects may go undetected in children because there are minimal or no symptoms and the ejection murmur across the pulmonic valve is thought to be functional. Survival into adulthood is expected but longevity is shortened, and death is usually due to cardiac failure. Occasionally, a young adult develops pulmonary hypertension. In addition to findings of congestive heart failure, atrial tachyarrhythmias become more frequent in patients over age 40 and may be the presenting symptom.

Patients with atrial septal defects generally appear normal. However, patients with the Holt-Oram syndrome have upper extremity skeletal abnormalities with a secundum defect, and patients with Down's syndrome have the typical features of mongolism and often a primum defect. The murmur is generated by the increased stroke volume flowing into a dilated pulmonary trunk; a murmur across the atrial septal defect is rare. Echocardiography reveals the dilated right ventricle and abnormal motion of the interventricular sepocardiography reveals the dilated right ventricle and abnormal motion of the interventricular septum; these findings are referred to as "right ventricular volume overload" and are also present in pulmonic regurgitation, tricuspid regurgitation, and Ebstein's anomaly. Ostium primum defects

and many ostium secundum defects can be visualized directly with two-dimensional echocardiography or indirectly after peripheral venous injection of echocardiographic contrast. However, cardiac catheterization may be required to determine the degree of shunt and evaluate for associated defects. Patients who have uncomplicated atrial septal defects without pulmonary hypertension and shunt ratios exceeding 1.5 should undergo repair electively, preferably during childhood.

VENTRICULAR SEPTAL DEFECT

Congenital ventricular septal defects are located most commonly in the region of the membranous interventricular septum. There is a tendency as a child grows for the relative size of the defect to diminish, and sometimes spontaneous closure occurs. The hemodynamic consequences of a ventricular septal defect depend on the size of the defect and on the extent of pulmonary vascular resistance. A small defect causes little problem, a moderate defect causes left-to-right shunting with minimal elevation of pulmonary arterial pressure, and a large defect may result in equalization of systolic pressures in the two ventricles with the result that the shunt flow depends on the relative resistance in the pulmonary versus the systemic circulations. As pulmonary vascular resistance increases secondary to the increased pulmonary pressure and flow, the left-to-right shunt may gradually decrease and even become right-to-left (Eisenmenger's complex). There is an increased incidence of aortic insufficiency in patients with large ventricular septal defects, in some patients due to primary aortic valve abnormality and in others due to herniation of a valve leaflet through the septal defect.

Echocardiography reveals left ventricular volume overload (hyperdynamic left ventricle). The defect usually cannot be directly visualized but may be indirectly visualized after a peripheral venous injection of echocardiographic contrast. Cardiac catheterization permits visualization and quantitation of the shunt and localizes it to the level of the ventricle. Associated defects are identified. Pulmonary artery pressure and pulmonary vascular resistance are determined.

Patients with small ventricular septal defects should be watched for gradual closure. Larger defects should be corrected surgically unless the pulmonary vascular resistance has become markedly elevated, at which time operative risk is high and results are poor because pulmonary vascular resistance fails to decrease significantly postoperatively.

PATENT DUCTUS ARTERIOSUS

A patent ductus arteriosus is common in premature infants and is more frequently seen in individuals born at high altitudes. In normal infants, the ductus functionally closes several hours after birth, and after four to eight weeks it closes anatomically. The pathophysiology of patent ductus

TABLE 4–1. COMMON CONGENITAL CARDIAC DEFECTS

TYPE	NATURAL HISTORY	PHYSICAL FINDINGS	ECG	X-RAY	ECHOCARDIOGRAM	THERAPY
Atrial septal defect	Congestive heart failure, atrial tachyarrhythmias in adulthood; occasionally pulmonary hypertension	Ejection murmur across pulmonic valve Hyperdynamic right ventricle Widely and fixed split S_2 Diastolic flow murmur across tricuspid valve	rSr^1 in V_1 (left axis with primum defect)	Large main pulmonary artery; increased pulmonary vascularity	Dilated RV, abnormal septal motion (right ventricular volume overload); direct or contrast visualization of defect	Surgical repair if shunt ratio exceeds 1.5
Ventricular septal defect	Spontaneous closure of small defects occurs; larger defects lead to heart failure or pulmonary hypertension with reversal of shunt (Eisenmenger's physiology)	Holosystolic left parasternal murmur, ± thrill Diastolic tricuspid flow murmur; occasionally murmur of associated aortic regurgitation Normal or widely split S_2 Findings of pulmonary hypertension if present (Table 4–3)	Biventricular hypertrophy	Increased pulmonary vasculature, large main pulmonary artery, dilation of both ventricles	Dilated hyperdynamic LV (left ventricular volume overload); direct or contrast visualization of defect	Larger defects repaired surgically unless pulmonary hypertension is present
Patent ductus arteriosus	Heart failure in infancy with larger shunts; eventual pulmonary hypertension	Wide aortic pulse pressure Hyperdynamic LV Continuous "machinery" murmur ± thrill Findings of pulmonary hypertension if present; "differential cyanosis" with right-to-left shunting (see text)	Left and/or right ventricular hypertrophy	Increased pulmonary vasculature; large main pulmonary artery; enlarged LA, LV aorta; occasionally a calcified ductus is visualized	Left ventricular volume overload, dilated LV, LA, and aorta	Usually requires surgery; may close spontaneously or with indomethacin in premature infants; recent catheter technique for closure
Pulmonic stenosis	May be asymptomatic for a long period of time; symptoms of RV failure when decompensation occurs	Large jugular a waves Pulmonic ejection sound RV lift Systolic ejection murmur ± thrill in second left intercostal space Widely split S_2 with soft (or absent) P_2	Right atrial enlargement Right axis QRS deviation RV hypertrophy	Normal pulmonary vascularity, post-stenotic pulmonary arterial dilation Enlarged RV	Differentiates valvular from nonvalvular	Valvulotomy if gradient > 50 mm Hg
Congenital aortic stenosis (valvular)	Exertional syncope, angina and heart failure depending on severity	Decreased pulse pressure and carotid pulse LV heave, palpable S_4, systolic ejection murmur ± thrill Aortic ejection click, preserved A_2 (non-	LV hypertrophy	Prominent LV Post-stenotic aortic dilation	Characteristic doming of aortic valve, LV hypertrophy	Aortic valvulotomy or replacement in symptomatic or severe cases

LV = left ventricle   LA = left atrium   RV = right ventricle   RA = right atrium

TABLE 4–2. CLASSIFICATION OF THE MORE COMMON CYANOTIC CONGENITAL CARDIAC DEFECTS

Increased pulmonary blood flow
    Transposition of the great arteries
    Truncus arteriosus
    Total anomalous pulmonary venous connection
Normal or decreased pulmonary blood flow
    I. Dominant left ventricle
        Tricuspid atresia
        Ebstein's anomaly of the tricuspid valve
    II. Dominant right ventricle
        a. Normal or low pulmonary arterial pressure
            Tetralogy of Fallot
        b. Elevated pulmonary arterial pressure
            Ventricular septal defect with reversed shunt (Eisenmenger's complex)

TABLE 4–1. *(continued)*

TYPE	NATURAL HISTORY	PHYSICAL FINDINGS	ECG	X-RAY	ECHOCARDIOGRAM	THERAPY
		calcified valve) with single or paradoxical splitting of S_2 S_4 gallop Concomitant aortic regurgitation common				
Coarctation of aorta	Most patients live to adulthood but eventually develop heart failure Aorta can dissect or rupture, cerebral hemorrhage occurs	Blood pressure in arms > legs Femoral pulses diminished or late, brisk upper extremity pulses Late systolic or continuous murmur LV lift S_4 gallop Evidence of associated bicuspid aortic valve	LV hypertrophy	Notching of inferior rib surfaces resulting from collateral flow through intercostal arteries Ascending aortic dilation; post-stenotic aortic dilation	Occasionally coarctation can be visualized	Surgical repair of all but mild cases
Ebstein's anomaly	Survival into adulthood but longevity decreased due to RV failure Arrhythmias from accessory bypass tracts	Acyanotic or cyanotic (right-to-left shunt due to increased RA pressure) Increased jugular venous pressure S_4 and/or S_3 gallops Systolic murmur of tricuspid regurgitation; large v waves do not occur due to the large compliant RA	RA enlargement Right bundle branch block PR prolongation Pre-excitation	Enlarged RA Pulmonary vasculature normal or decreased	Abnormal insertion and motion of tricuspid valve	Replace tricuspid valve when RV failure occurs
Tetralogy of Fallot	Usually depends on the degree of pulmonic stenosis: too much leads to right-to-left shunt and cyanosis, too little leads to left-to-right shunt and pulmonary hypertension Pulmonic stenosis tends to gradually increase	Most commonly cyanotic and clubbed but may be acyanotic; underdeveloped Loud pulmonic ejection murmur along left sternal border, softer with more severe stenosis No murmur across ventricular septal defect (equalization of pressure in LV and RV) Soft P_2 (mild stenosis) or absent P_2 (severe stenosis) Normal jugular venous pressure	RV hypertrophy	"Boot-shaped" heart due to RV hypertrophy, small LV, and small pulmonary artery	Pulmonic stenosis, ventricular septal defect, RV hypertrophy, overriding aorta all visualized	Complete surgical repair is usually treatment of choice

TABLE 4–3. PHYSICAL FINDINGS OF PULMONARY HYPERTENSION*

Cyanosis or clubbing from right-to-left shunt via congenital defect or propatent foramen ovale
Large jugular a wave (decreased right ventricular compliance)
Large jugular v wave if tricuspid regurgitation occurs
Left parasternal (right ventricular) lift
Palpable pulmonary arterial pulsations (second left intercostal space)
Pulmonic ejection murmur
Pulmonic ejection click
Loud P_2
Diastolic decrescendo murmur of pulmonic insufficiency (Graham Steell)
Holosystolic murmur of tricuspid regurgitation

*Not all manifestations are present in all patients.

arteriosus depends on the size of the ductus and the degree of pulmonary vascular resistance. After birth, as the pulmonary vascular resistance falls and the ductus fails to close, a left-to-right shunt occurs. When the ductus is small, pulmonary artery pressure is normal and there is little left-to-right shunting. If the defect is bigger, a large shunt results, and aortic pressure is transmitted to the pulmonary arterial tree. Pulmonary hypertension develops with a sizable left-to-right shunt, along with volume overload of the left heart and pressure overload of the right heart. Eventually, as pulmonary vascular resistance reflexly increases, left-to-right flow disappears, and in late stages the patient may develop a right-to-left shunt. The infant may fail to develop normally and, if the shunt is severe, demonstrates congestive heart failure. If right-to-left shunting occurs, "differential" cyanosis may be evident owing to nonoxygenated blood entering the aorta distal to the left subclavian artery via the patent ductus arteriosus, preferentially being shunted to the lower extremities and resulting in cyanotic toes but pink fingers.

Essentially all patients with persistent left-to-right shunt across a ductus should have surgical interruption; interruption also reduces the risk of bacterial endocarditis. Severely elevated pulmonary vascular resistance (Eisenmenger's syndrome) is not reversible and, if present, contraindicates surgery. The operation usually carries low risk, and cardiopulmonary bypass is not required. In older patients with a calcified ductus, ligation is slightly more risky although still indicated. Recently, insertion by catheter technique of an umbrella device into the ductus has been successful in occluding the ductus.

PULMONIC STENOSIS

Valvular pulmonic stenosis is more common than isolated subvalvular or supravalvular varieties. The murmur is present at birth, but survival into adulthood is common. Dyspnea and fatigue are the most frequent symptoms, but patients may remain asymptomatic for long periods as long as the right ventricle maintains a normal cardiac output via compensatory mechanisms (hypertrophy); if not, right ventricular failure ensues. Valvular pulmonic stenosis can cause hypertrophy of the right ventricular infundibulum, and secondary infundibular (subvalvular) stenosis can occur.

The longer the duration of the systolic murmur and the earlier the systolic ejection click, the higher the degree of stenosis. As the severity of pulmonic stenosis increases, widened splitting of S_2 occurs with a decrease and eventual disappearance of P_2.

Patients with mild pulmonic stenosis require no treatment other than endocarditis prophylaxis. Those with pulmonic valve gradients exceeding 50 mm Hg should have pulmonary valvulotomy. Balloon dilation techniques via cardiac catheterization are successful in some patients. Pulmonic regurgitation may occur postoperatively but is generally mild and functionally insignificant.

Secondary subpulmonic stenosis may require resection that complicates the procedure significantly.

AORTIC STENOSIS

Congenitally bicuspid aortic valves occur in up to 2 per cent of the population and are the most common congenital cardiac defect manifesting itself in the adult population. Bicuspid valves usually function normally throughout early and mid-life. However, progressive accelerated calcification of the valve can result in significant aortic stenosis during mid-adulthood. Occasionally bicuspid valves are incompetent, either inherently or secondary to damage from infective endocarditis. A short grade I-II/VI systolic murmur loudest at the second right intercostal space is typical and, if accompanied by an ejection sound or a soft murmur of aortic regurgitation, strongly suggests that the systolic murmur is pathological. Bicuspid aortic valve is predominantly a disease of males. The identification of a bicuspid valve can be suggested by echocardiography but is sometimes difficult to make.

In contrast to a bicuspid aortic valve, congenital aortic stenosis refers to an inherently stenotic left ventricular outflow tract. Congenital aortic stenosis is usually valvular but may be subvalvular or supravalvular. It is more common in males, with a ratio of approximately 4:1.

An ejection sound is present in valvular but not in nonvalvular aortic stenosis. It is generated by the sudden tensing upon opening of the abnormal aortic valve, implying good valve motion. In adults the abnormal valve gradually calcifies, and the ejection sound may disappear. In general, the longer and louder the murmur and the later its systolic peak, the greater the obstruction. The intensity of the murmur may decrease when the left ventricle fails, but it usually still peaks late in systole if stenosis is severe. An aortic regurgitation murmur may be present in valvular obstruction or, as the aortic cusps become distorted by the subvalvular jet, in subvalvular obstruction.

Cardiac catheterization is necessary to quantitate the degree of aortic stenosis. Aortic valvulotomy may be employed as a temporizing procedure in younger patients with significant aortic stenosis, but prosthetic aortic valves eventually are required in most severe cases.

Subvalvular stenosis is either dynamic (see Hypertrophic Cardiomyopathy in Chapter 9) or fixed. Two forms of fixed subaortic stenosis are the tunnel (fibromuscular) and the localized (fibromembranous) forms. These are unusual in adults. They can be identified with two-dimensional echocardiography. Surgical excision of an obstructing subvalvular membrane can be curative, but correction of a tunnel deformity is difficult. Supravalvular aortic stenosis often occurs in the presence of mental retardation and peculiar facies. The brachial and carotid arterial pressures may be reduced more on the left than on the right. Aortic regurgitation is rare (cf. subvalvular stenosis). The x-ray shows no post-stenotic dilatation of the ascending aorta, and the aorta is usually small.

COARCTATION OF THE AORTA

Coarctation refers to a narrowing of the aorta usually located immediately distal to the origin of the left subclavian artery and ligamentum arteriosum. It is associated with a bicuspid aortic valve in approximately 25 per cent of patients and occasionally a patent ductus arteriosus. Some patients have an associated aneurysm of the circle of Willis that may rupture. Other than coarctation associated with Turner's syndrome, males are more commonly affected than females. Most patients live to adulthood, but longevity is significantly decreased. Most patients are asymptomatic when the lesion is diagnosed. Discovery of upper extremity arterial hypertension is usually the initial finding. Patients develop one of four complications: congestive heart failure, rupture of the aorta or dissecting aneurysm, infective endarteritis or endocarditis, or cerebral hemorrhage. Endocarditis is more common on the bicuspid aortic valve than in the region of the coarctation.

Catheterization may be performed to assess the severity of the coarctation and to examine the collaterals. All but mild coarctations warrant surgical repair. In children the optimal age for elective correction is approximately the fifth year. Surgery becomes more difficult in adults.

MISCELLANEOUS NONCYANOTIC ABNORMALITIES

Congenital coronary arteriovenous (AV) fistulae, low resistance connections between the arterial and venous circulations without an intervening capillary bed, may steal blood flow away from a portion of the myocardium. Occasionally a coronary artery may originate from the pulmonary artery and cause myocardial ischemia. A coronary artery may arise from the wrong sinus of Valsalva, most commonly the left circumflex artery arising from the right sinus of Valsalva, and may be subject to compression, especially with exercise. In addition, the odd angle of takeoff from the abnormal ostium may limit flow. Congenital aneurysms of a sinus of Valsalva may occasionally rupture into the right atrium or right ventricle, resembling acute aortic regurgitation. Right ventricular dysplasia (Uhl's anomaly) involves a process whereby all or a portion of the right ventricular muscle is replaced with fat and fibrous tissue. It is often associated with ventricular tachycardia.

EBSTEIN'S ANOMALY OF THE TRICUSPID VALVE

In Ebstein's anomaly, the tricuspid valve leaflets are deformed and displaced into the right ventricular cavity, giving rise to a portion of the right ventricle that is functionally right atrium (atrial-ized right ventricle). Therefore, the pumping action of the right ventricle is decreased and the tricuspid valve is incompetent. Patients may be acyanotic, but a right-to-left shunt through a patent foramen ovale or an atrial septal defect due to elevated right atrial pressure can cause cyanosis. Ebstein's anomaly is compatible with survival into adulthood, but longevity is decreased. The anomaly is associated with right-sided accessory atrioventricular bypass tracts in approximately 10 per cent of cases (see Chapter 8). Patients can usually be managed medically. A tricuspid valve prosthesis is required when significant right ventricular failure occurs.

CYANOTIC LESIONS

TRANSPOSITION OF THE GREAT VESSELS

In complete transposition of the great arteries, the aorta and coronary arteries exit from the right ventricle while the pulmonary artery exits from the left ventricle. The left atrium empties into the left ventricle and the right atrium into the right ventricle. Therefore, the systemic and pulmonary circuits are arranged in parallel instead of in series. For the patient to survive, some means of exchange between the two parallel circuits must exist, for example, an atrial septal defect, ventricular septal defect, or patent ductus arteriosus. Transposition usually produces cyanosis and increased pulmonary blood flow. Bidirectional shunting must be present, and the greater the mixing between the two systems, the more likely the patient's survival. Diagnosis can be established by two-dimensional echocardiography. Palliation may be obtained by atrial septostomy via a balloon or surgery. Corrective surgery involves reversing the atrial input by inserting an atrial baffle that redirects the atrial flow to the opposite ventricle (Mustard procedure) or by transposing the pulmonary artery and aorta.

TOTAL ANOMALOUS PULMONARY VENOUS RETURN

In this condition, oxygenated blood returning from the lungs enters the right atrium instead of the left atrium, usually via a confluence of veins connected to the superior or inferior vena cava, the coronary sinus, or the right atrium directly. Blood from the right atrium enters the left atrium and left ventricle via an obligatory atrial septal defect, but because of the low pulmonary compliance most blood enters the right ventricle and pulmonary artery. Therefore, total anomalous pulmonary venous return is a cyanotic anomaly with increased pulmonary blood flow. Signs and symptoms are somewhat similar to those of atrial septal defect except that cyanosis and signs of pulmonary hypertension may exist. Echocardiography reveals findings similar to an atrial septal defect, but the confluence of veins can often be identified. Surgical correction involves an anastomosis of the confluence to the left atrium.

TRUNCUS ARTERIOSUS

In truncus arteriosus, one great artery with one semilunar valve exits the heart, receives blood from both ventricles, and gives rise to the coronary arteries, aorta, and pulmonary artery. Cyanosis and increased pulmonary blood flow are present. Most patients do not survive childhood. Surgical correction can be performed in which the ventricular septal defect is closed, with the left ventricle communicating with the truncus, and the pulmonary arteries are divided from the truncus and connected to the right ventricle by a valved conduit.

TETRALOGY OF FALLOT

Tetralogy of Fallot is the most common cyanotic congenital anomaly in adults. It includes a ventricular septal defect, pulmonic stenosis, an aorta overriding the ventricular septal defect, and right ventricular hypertrophy as a result of the first two defects. The ventricular septal defect is large and nonrestrictive. Right ventricular pressures are systemic. If the pulmonic stenosis is mild to moderate, the patient is acyanotic. If the pulmonic stenosis is severe, right-to-left shunting occurs across the ventricular septal defect and cyanosis results, the most common situation. Typically the pulmonic stenosis is infundibular, but it can be valvular or located elsewhere in the pulmonary outflow tract.

A large ventricular septal defect with mild pulmonic stenosis results in a left-to-right shunt and physiology similar to that of ventricular septal defect alone, i.e., increased pulmonary blood flow and left ventricular volume overload. With severe pulmonic stenosis, right ventricular pressure does not exceed systemic pressure because of the large ventricular septal defect; thus, right-to-left shunting occurs but right ventricular failure usually does not occur. Exercise increases right-to-left shunting and cyanosis by decreasing systemic vascular resistance. Patients typically have intermittent "spells" associated with hyperpnea, cyanosis, and lightheadedness or syncope thought to be due to an increase in right-to-left shunting. Children achieve relief from dyspnea by squatting, a maneuver that increases systemic vascular resistance and increases pulmonary blood flow. Infective endocarditis may occur, and there is a high incidence of brain abscess, presumably because the normal filtering mechanisms of the pulmonary vasculature are bypassed.

The natural history of tetralogy of Fallot is a gradual increase in severity of pulmonic stenosis so that cyanosis increases. Total surgical correction is the treatment of choice and can be performed even in infants; however, the creation of a systemic-to-pulmonary shunt (usually an anastomosis of the subclavian artery to the pulmonary artery, a Blalock-Taussig shunt) is still performed in very young cyanotic infants with complex lesions but adds to the risk of complete repair later. Right bundle branch block occurs after repair, and an increased incidence of ventricular arrhythmias, heart block, and sudden death have been reported years after surgery. Even with only moderate symptoms children should have a complete surgical correction by school age.

TRICUSPID ATRESIA

In tricuspid atresia no tricuspid valve is present, and the right atrium does not connect to the right ventricle. An interatrial connection allows blood to flow to the left heart, and a small ventricular septal defect usually allows some blood flow to the lungs via the rudimentary right ventricle. The patient is usually cyanotic with diminished pulmonary blood flow and has a dominant left ventricle. Transposition of the great arteries is often an associated defect. Systemic arterial to pulmonary arterial shunts and enlargement of the atrial septal defect by balloon septostomy are palliative. The insertion of a prosthetic conduit between the right atrium and pulmonary artery with closure of the atrial septal defect (Fontan procedure) may provide improvement.

GENERAL PROBLEMS DUE TO PROLONGED SURVIVAL

Because of cardiac surgery, more patients with congenital heart disease survive to become adults. Many patients have undergone complete repair of their defects and are asymptomatic. Others, however, may be symptomatic with residual defects or complications from surgery, and some patients may have merely had incomplete correction with palliative surgery. Pregnancy may be complicated in these patients. Infants of patients with cyanotic congenital heart disease tend to be small for their gestational age.

REFERENCES

Adams FH, and Emmanouilides GC: Moss' Heart Disease in Infants, Children, and Adolescents. 3rd ed. Baltimore, Williams & Wilkins, 1983.
Perloff JK: The Clinical Recognition of Congenital Heart Disease. 2nd ed. Philadelphia, WB Saunders Co, 1978.
Roberts WC: Congenital Heart Disease in Adults. 2nd ed. Philadelphia, FA Davis Co, 1984.

GENERAL CONSIDERATIONS

When an aortic or pulmonic valve is stenotic, the respective ventricle compensates by hypertrophying; that is, the mass of myocardium increases with little increase in the size of the ventricular cavity. Hypertrophy increases ventricular oxygen consumption and, because of the increased intramural pressure, decreases the diastolic flow of blood to the myocardium from the coronary arteries, resulting in an imbalance of myocardial oxygen demand and delivery. Aortic or pulmonic regurgitation places a diastolic volume overload on the respective ventricle and results in dilation with less hypertrophy. This increase in ventricular volume also leads to increased myocardial oxygen consumption via increased wall tension. Mitral or tricuspid regurgitation also places a diastolic volume overload on the ventricle although not as severe, since the ventricle empties into a lower pressure chamber and systolic pressures are not as high. Mitral regurgitation, therefore, is better tolerated than aortic regurgitation. Mitral and tricuspid stenosis do not overload the ventricle but instead the respective atrium dilates, and either pulmonary or systemic venous pressure may increase markedly. Ventricular myocardial dysfunction eventually occurs in both hypertrophy and dilation. An increase in venous pressure eventually may develop in any valvular lesion when cardiac decompensation occurs. The S_4 gallop correlates with left ventricular hypertrophy and decreased myocardial compliance, and the S_3 gallop correlates with increased blood volume filling the heart in early diastole and is common in volume overload states, usually with some degree of myocardial dysfunction. As left ventricular failure occurs and pulmonary venous pressures increase, right ventricular failure eventually may ensue.

Echocardiography may obviate the need for cardiac catheterization in certain lesions (for example, simple uncomplicated mitral stenosis). However, cardiac catheterization is the standard means to assess the severity or quantitate the degree of most valvular lesions in patients whose clinical status is thought possibly to warrant surgery. Catheterization may be needed to determine the relative severity of multivalvular lesions, to detect significant concomitant lesions, and to evaluate the status of the coronary circulation and to evaluate left ventricular function.

The decision of whether and when to replace an abnormal valve often is difficult, since the natural history of many valvular lesions is chronic and prolonged. In addition, prosthetic valves carry lifelong risks of endocarditis, emboli, and thrombosis, and the lifespan of many prosthetic valves is unknown. The natural history of each valvular lesion is different; some lesions (for example, aortic regurgitation) may be associated with irreversible myocardial damage before symptoms occur, whereas other lesions (for example, mitral stenosis) can await significant progression of symptoms before valve replacement is necessary, since the ventricle is protected by the stenotic valve. In addition, the patient's age, general medical status, and desire to return to previous levels of activity enter into the decision for valve replacement.

MITRAL STENOSIS
(Tables 5–1, 5–2, and 5–3)

Mitral stenosis almost always results from rheumatic fever and is rarely congenital in etiology. It

TABLE 5–1. ACQUIRED VALVULAR LESIONS: SYMPTOMS AND NATURAL HISTORY

LESION	MAJOR SYMPTOMS	NATURAL HISTORY
Mitral stenosis	Dyspnea, orthopnea, paroxysmal nocturnal dyspnea; later fatigue, wasting, hemoptysis, symptoms of right heart failure (Table 2–4) Systemic emboli not uncommon Acute decompensation with onset of atrial fibrillation	Onset of symptoms 10+ years after rheumatic fever; slowly progressive
Mitral regurgitation	Pulmonary congestion, fatigue; later right heart failure	Chronic: long asymptomatic phase despite moderately severe regurgitation Acute: if severe, rapid deterioration
Mitral valve prolapse	Chest pain atypical for angina pectoris; palpitations; rarely left heart failure from mitral regurgitation	Usually asymptomatic; endocarditis, rupture of chordae, progressive mitral regurgitation, and sudden death rarely occur
Aortic stenosis	Angina, LV failure; exertional syncope, presyncope	Rapid deterioration once symptoms appear; first manifestation in a rare patient is sudden death
Aortic regurgitation	LV failure Palpitations from arrhythmias or hyperdynamic circulation	Chronic: asymptomatic or minimally symptomatic stage may span years; irreversible myocardial damage may occur in the asymptomatic patient Acute: rapid deterioration
Tricuspid stenosis	Depends on associated mitral valve abnormalities Manifestations of right heart failure	Like mitral stenosis, gradually progressive with onset of symptoms in mid-adulthood
Tricuspid regurgitation	RV failure	Depends on underlying etiology; may improve if associated lesions are corrected

TABLE 5–2. ACQUIRED VALVULAR LESIONS: PHYSICAL AND LABORATORY EXAMINATION

LESION	PHYSICAL FINDINGS	ECG	X-RAY	ECHOCARDIOGRAM
Mitral stenosis	Decreased pulse pressure Loud S_1 Opening snap if mitral valve is pliable No S_3 or S_4 Diastolic rumble Concomitant murmur of mitral regurgitation or aortic involvement Late features include pulmonary hypertension (Table 4–3) and RV failure (Table 2–4)	Atrial fibrillation common Left atrial abnormality RV hypertrophy when pulmonary hypertension develops	Large LA: double density at right heart border, posterior displacement of esophagus, elevation of left mainstem bronchus, straightening of left heart border due to enlarged left atrial appendage Large pulmonary artery Pulmonary venous congestion	M-mode: thickened mitral leaflets, anterior movement of posterior leaflet during systole, decreased mid-diastolic mitral closure (decreased "E to F slope") Two-dimensional: mitral valve doming, visualization of decreased valve area
Mitral regurgitation	Hyperdynamic LV impulse displaced laterally Left parasternal lift from right ventricle or systolic LA expansion S_3, soft S_1, widely split S_2 (early A_2) S_4 absent in chronic, present in acute form Holosystolic murmur radiating to axilla; murmur may be atypical in acute mitral regurgitation, mitral valve prolapse, papillary muscle dysfunction Later features include pulmonary hypertension and RV failure	Atrial fibrillation less common than in mitral stenosis Left atrial enlargement LV hypertrophy	Enlarged LA and LV; pulmonary venous congestion	Large LV and LA with hyperdynamic LV motion (left ventricular volume overload) May reveal underlying cause of mitral regurgitation
Mitral valve prolapse	One or more systolic clicks, often followed by a late systolic murmur High incidence of bony chest abnormalities: straight back syndrome, pectus excavatum, thoracic scoliosis	Usually normal; occasionally ST depression and T wave inversion inferiorly Ventricular or supraventricular ectopy	Usually normal unless significant mitral regurgitation is present; bony abnormalities	Systolic bowing of anterior or posterior mitral leaflets into LA
Aortic stenosis	Pulsus parvus et tardus (may be absent in older patients or those with aortic insufficiency) Carotid "shudder" (thrill) Systolic ejection murmur in aortic area, usually with thrill, harsh quality, radiates to carotids, peaks late in systole if stenosis is severe Sustained, diffuse, but not displaced LV impulse (LV heave or lift) S_4 gallop, often palpable A_2 decreased, S_2 single or paradoxically split S_3 if LV failure is present Aortic ejection click in noncalcified congenital stenosis	LV hypertrophy Left bundle branch block and intraventricular conduction defects common Rare heart block from calcific involvement of the conduction system	LV predominance without dilation Post-stenotic aortic root dilation Calcification in region of aortic valve Cardiomegaly and pulmonary congestion with LV failure	Thick aortic valve leaflets with decreased excursion LV hypertrophy
Aortic regurgitation	Chronic: increased pulse pressure (head	LV hypertrophy often with "volume	LV and aortic dilation	Dilated LV and aorta Left ventricular volume

LESION	PHYSICAL FINDINGS	ECG	X-RAY	ECHOCARDIOGRAM
	bobbing), pistol-shot sounds over peripheral arteries, to-and-fro murmur over femoral arteries with light compression by stethoscope (Duroziez's sign), pulsatile blushing of nail beds (Quincke's sign), rapid upstroke with collapsing quality to pulse (water hammer pulse) Bifid pulse contour, especially if stenosis is also present Hyperkinetic, displaced apical impulse Diastolic decrescendo murmur, length correlates with severity Systolic flow murmur Systolic and/or diastolic thrill A$_2$ decreased or absent S$_3$ in early LV decompensation Austin Flint murmur *Acute:* apical impulse not displaced; pulse pressure increased much less Diastolic murmur shorter and softer (high LV diastolic pressure) S$_1$ decreased (because of early mitral valve closure) Severe LV failure	overload" pattern (narrow deep Q waves in left precordial leads)		overload Fluttering of anterior mitral valve leaflet Acute: premature diastolic closure of mitral valve
Tricuspid stenosis	Prominent a wave, attenuated v wave in jugular pulse Jugular venous distention, edema, hepatomegaly Tricuspid opening snap with diastolic rumble loudest in fourth left intercostal space, louder with inspiration	Atrial fibrillation common RA enlargement with RV hypertrophy	Associated valve lesions; large RA	Doming of tricuspid valve; associated lesions
Tricuspid regurgitation	Increased jugular venous pressure with large v waves Hepatomegaly with systolic pulsations Holosystolic murmur along left sternal border ± thrill, increases with inspiration Diastolic flow rumble Right ventricular S$_3$ (increases with inspiration loudest along left sternal border) Findings of pulmonary hypertension if tricuspid regurgitation is secondary	RV hypertrophy RA enlargement Atrial fibrillation is common	Enlarged RV and RA; other lesions may be evident	Underlying cause may be identified Contrast echo can establish the diagnosis

TABLE 5–3. ACQUIRED VALVULAR LESIONS: MEDICAL AND SURGICAL MANAGEMENT

LESION	MEDICAL MANAGEMENT	SURGICAL MANAGEMENT
Mitral stenosis	Rheumatic fever and endocarditis prophylaxis Diuretics, salt restriction Control of ventricular rate and anticoagulation in atrial fibrillation	*Indication:* Functional Class III despite medical therapy; severe pulmonary hypertension is not a surgical contraindication *Procedure:* Commissurotomy or valve replacement
Mitral regurgitation	Salt restriction, diuretics, digitalis, afterload-reduction Endocarditis prophylaxis	*Indication:* Functional Class III despite medical therapy; patients with lesser symptoms and evidence of myocardial dysfunction; acute severe mitral regurgitation *Procedure:* Mitral valve replacement
Mitral valve prolapse	Endocarditis prophylaxis Beta blockade for chest pain Beta blockade or other antiarrhythmic agents for arrhythmias	Mitral valve replacement for acute and/or severe mitral regurgitation
Aortic stenosis	Endocarditis prophylaxis Avoid strenuous exercise	*Indications:* Symptoms *Procedure:* Valve replacement
Aortic regurgitation	Endocarditis prophylaxis Salt restriction, diuretics, digitalis, afterload reduction	*Indication:* Controversial; greater than mild symptoms, evidence of early LV dysfunction in asymptomatic patients *Procedure:* Aortic valve replacement
Tricuspid stenosis	Endocarditis and rheumatic fever prophylaxis Depends on associated valvular lesions	*Indication:* Severe tricuspid stenosis, usually concomitant with mitral valve surgery *Procedure:* Tricuspid valve replacement
Tricuspid regurgitation	Endocarditis prophylaxis Treatment of associated lesions Diuretics, salt restriction, digitalis	*Indication:* Severe tricuspid regurgitation, often concomitant with mitral valve surgery *Procedure:* Tricuspid annuloplasty or valve replacement

is the most common lesion caused by rheumatic fever. Two thirds of patients with mitral stenosis are female. The valve leaflets become thickened, the commissures fused, and the chordae tendineae may fuse and shorten. Calcium may be deposited in the valve. This process of valve scarring progresses slowly and may take ten years or more after the episode of rheumatic fever to become hemodynamically significant. Because of the deformation of the mitral valve, mitral regurgitation also may be present. The left atrium enlarges, but the left ventricle remains normal in size unless mitral regurgitation also occurs. The elevated left atrial pressure determines the extent of pulmonary venous congestion that causes the major symptoms in mitral stenosis of dyspnea, orthopnea, and paroxysmal nocturnal dyspnea. Pulmonary arterial hypertension occurs not only secondary to the elevated pulmonary venous pressure but sometimes also secondary to a reactive increase in the pulmonary vascular resistance. Right ventricular failure and functional tricuspid regurgitation may result. Atrial fibrillation is common. Diastolic filling of the left ventricle is determined not only by the pressure gradient across the stenotic mitral valve but also by the amount of time spent in diastole during which the left ventricle can fill. Therefore, when the patient exercises and develops sinus tachycardia, or when atrial fibrillation occurs, the rapid ventricular rate diminishes the percentage of the cardiac cycle spent in diastole and ventricular filling is limited. A patient's first episode of pulmonary edema often occurs either with exercise or with the onset of atrial fibrillation.

Even though acute rheumatic fever may have occurred in childhood, the age at the onset of cardiac symptoms is usually between 25 and 45 years. There may be a relatively long period, 5 to 8 years, of mild to moderate pulmonary congestive symptoms before severe compromise occurs. Since reduction in cardiac output is a late finding, fatigue and physical wasting are also late manifestations. Occasionally, hemoptysis may occur due to leaking or rupture of pulmonary vessels. The occurrence of intermittent atrial fibrillation as the left atrium dilates may be associated with peripheral emboli. As pulmonary vascular resistance and reactive pulmonary arterial hypertension increase, flow from the right to left heart is limited, pulmonary venous hypertension stabilizes, and episodes of pulmonary edema may decrease; however, the complaint of fatigue becomes prominent. Findings of right heart failure with hepatomegaly, ascites, and peripheral edema may occur.

The first heart sound is loud because the mitral valve is maximally open at the onset of systole and the left ventricular pressure is rising rapidly when the valve closes because of the high left atrial pressure. An opening sound (snap) of the mitral valve, best heard at the lower left sternal border and apex, is present if the valve is pliable and not heavily calcified. More severe mitral stenosis shortens the interval between S_2 and the opening snap (the higher the left atrial pressure, the sooner the valve will open during isovolumic relaxation). A third heart sound rarely, if ever, occurs in mitral stenosis even with associated lesions. A diastolic, low-pitched, rumbling murmur located near the left ventricular apex immediately follows the opening snap. The rumble is loudest in early diastole during rapid ventricular filling and, if sinus rhythm is present, increases again with atrial contraction (presystolic accentuation). In mild mitral stenosis, as well as severe mitral stenosis with low cardiac output, the murmur may be difficult to hear and may be accentuated with the patient in the left lateral decubitus position, especially after exercise. In addition, a markedly enlarged right ventricle may displace the left ventricle posteriorly, making the murmur even harder to hear. Concomitant rheumatic involvement of the aortic valve may generate murmurs of aortic stenosis or regurgitation.

Echocardiography is diagnostic of mitral stenosis, revealing thickened mitral leaflets, anterior movement of the posterior leaflet during diastole, and decreased mid-diastolic mitral closure (decreased E to F slope). Characteristic "doming" of the valve is diagnostic on cross-sectional echocardiography. Cross-sectional echocardiography can be used to estimate accurately the valve orifice area in a high percentage of patients, possibly more accurately than the Gorlin formula at cardiac catheterization, since the presence of mitral regurgitation does not affect the valve area determined echocardiographically.

The patient with significant mitral stenosis has an elevated left atrial or pulmonary capillary wedge pressure with a pressure gradient between the left atrium and left ventricle during diastole. The Gorlin formula is used to calculate the valve area according to the equation:

$$\text{Valve Area} = \frac{\text{Transvalvular Flow}}{\text{constant} \times \sqrt{\text{Gradient}}}$$

Because the pressure gradient changes with the square of the flow, small increases in cardiac output are associated with relatively large elevations in left atrial pressure. Less severe cases of mitral stenosis have elevated pulmonary arterial pressures without a gradient between pulmonary arterial and venous pressures (passive pulmonary hypertension), whereas more severe cases have reactive pulmonary hypertension due to an increase in pulmonary vascular resistance. The area of a normal mitral valve is about 4 sq cm; severe mitral stenosis occurs when the valve area is less than 1 sq cm. Left ventricular function is generally normal unless complicating lesions are present.

Patients with mitral stenosis should receive both rheumatic fever and bacterial endocarditis prophylaxis. Since most symptoms in mild or moderate mitral stenosis are related to elevated left atrial pressures, diuretics may be used to decrease salt and water retention and decrease left atrial pressure. Control of the ventricular rate using digitalis in patients with atrial fibrillation decreases left atrial pressure. Patients with sinus rhythm experiencing exertional dyspnea may benefit from the administration of propranolol to prevent sinus tachycardia. Patients may be managed for many years medically. Patients who have had systemic emboli and probably patients with atrial fibrillation should receive anticoagulation therapy. Systemic embolization despite anticoagulation is an indication for surgery. Since systolic function of the ventricular myocardium is not impaired in uncomplicated mitral stenosis, the inotropic property of digitalis is not beneficial. When the patient experiences functional class III or IV symptoms despite medical therapy, surgery should be considered if cardiac catheterization or echocardiography shows severe mitral stenosis. Surgery is not contraindicated by severe pulmonary hypertension, since the increased pulmonary vascular resistance returns toward normal upon correction of the left atrial hypertension (cf. pulmonary hypertension in patients with left-to-right shunts, e.g., ventricular septal defect).

Mitral commissurotomy or valvuloplasty can be employed in patients with relatively pliable, noncalcified valves without mitral regurgitation. Commissurotomy spares the patient the risks of a prosthetic valve and anticoagulation for several years. A regurgitant valve is likely to become more regurgitant after commissurotomy, and valve replacement is therefore usually performed in patients with concomitant mitral regurgitation. The average patient experiences 8 to 12 years of symptomatic relief after commissurotomy, but progression of the disease occurs and usually valve replacement is necessary eventually. Perioperative mortality from open commissurotomy is approximately 2 per cent and with mitral valve replacement, about 5 per cent.

MITRAL REGURGITATION

The most common cause of mitral regurgitation is rheumatic fever, and it occurs more commonly in males. The murmur of mitral regurgitation may appear early after an episode of acute rheumatic fever. Concomitant aortic valve involvement suggests a rheumatic etiology. Other etiologies include congenital mitral regurgitation, which is sometimes associated with other lesions such as an ostium primum atrial septal defect. Mitral valve prolapse, mitral annular calcification, rupture of chordae tendineae from endocarditis, trauma, or degenerative diseases such as Marfan's syndrome may cause mitral regurgitation. Rupture of a papillary muscle after myocardial infarction results in severe, acute mitral regurgitation, while infarction of a papillary muscle can cause chronic papillary muscle dysfunction. Mitral regurgitation is common in patients with hypertrophic cardiomyopathy. It may occur secondary to left ventricular dilation; this "functional" mitral regurgitation probably occurs not so much from dilation of the mitral annulus as from distortion of the normal alignment of the papillary muscles.

Mitral regurgitation is holosystolic; that is, blood flows from the left ventricle to the low-pressure left atrium from the time the mitral valve closes to its opening after S_2. Left ventricular afterload is reduced. The v wave in the left atrial or pulmonary capillary wedge pressure tracing is often increased. However, large v waves can be seen in entities other than mitral regurgitation; if left atrial compliance is increased, v waves may not be present even in severe mitral regurgitation. Left ventricular diastolic volume increases in chronic mitral regurgitation. Because of the low pressure against which the left ventricle ejects blood (i.e., into the left atrium), the clinical course may extend over many years before decompensation occurs. However, as mitral regurgitation becomes severe and long-standing, left ventricular contractility may be irreversibly impaired. The left ventricular systolic as well as diastolic dimensions subsequently increase. Pulmonary hypertension, like that in mitral stenosis, may occur due to both increased pulmonary venous pressure and a reactive increase in pulmonary vascular resistance. In chronic mitral regurgitation, the increased volume of blood entering the left atrium is accommodated by dilation of the left atrium with a modest increase in left atrial pressure. However, in acute, severe mitral regurgitation (e.g., secondary to endocarditis or ruptured chordae tendineae), regurgitant blood enters a relatively small, noncompliant left atrium, and left atrial pressure may rise dramatically with very large v waves.

The severity of mitral regurgitation is estimated at catheterization by the amount of contrast regurgitated into the left atrium after injection into the left ventricle. A regurgitant fraction can be calculated but is fraught with error. There may be a pressure gradient across the mitral valve in early diastole in the absence of mitral stenosis because of the large volume of blood flowing across the valve. A normal ejection fraction may mask left ventricular dysfunction despite myocardial depression because of the marked afterload reduction afforded by the mitral regurgitation. Once the valve is replaced, however, the myocardial dysfunction may become evident.

Patients in functional Class III or IV despite medical therapy should be considered for surgery. Patients with lesser symptoms who display early evidence of myocardial dysfunction (e.g., increased systolic left ventricular diameter or decreasing ejection fraction) should be considered for surgery. Patients with severe myocardial dysfunction are poor surgical candidates because myocardial function usually does not improve after surgery. The mitral valve usually is replaced with a metal or bioprosthetic valve; valvuloplasty usually is not adequate. Metal valves in the mitral position require long-term anticoagulation; porcine mitral valves, if there is no history of previous embolus, left atrial clot, atrial fibrillation, or massively dilated left atrium, probably do not need chronic anticoagulation. When contemplating surgery, one must remember that patients may live for many years with symptoms well controlled with medications, and prosthetic valve replacement carries the immediate surgical risk plus the long-term risk of anticoagulation, thromboembolism, endocarditis, and valve malfunction. Acute severe mitral regurgitation generally is not well tolerated and requires emergency valve replacement. Potent afterload reduction, with intravenous nitroprusside, for example, may stabilize the patient until surgery can be performed.

MITRAL VALVE PROLAPSE

Mitral valve prolapse (floppy mitral valve, click murmur syndrome) is common and usually benign, reported to occur in 0.3 to 6 per cent of the population. It derives its clinical significance from its characteristic systolic click and late systolic murmur and the occasional patient who experiences significant mitral regurgitation, chordal rupture, endocarditis, arrhythmias, or sudden death. The severity of mitral regurgitation varies. The mitral valve leaflets are generally redundant, the chordae elongated, and pathology in more severe cases demonstrates myxomatous degeneration. Mitral regurgitation is occasionally progressive and severe and can occur acutely if a chordae ruptures because of myxomatous degeneration or endocarditis. The cause is unknown, although it is common in Marfan's syndrome and other connective tissue diseases. It has increased incidence in patients with ostium secundum atrial septal defect and hypertrophic cardiomyopathy. It is more common in females than males and occasionally will run in families.

Many symptoms have been attributed to mitral valve prolapse, but it is hard to definitely attribute symptoms to the syndrome, since it is so common. These patients commonly have chest pain that is atypical for angina pectoris; the pathogenesis of the chest pain is not clear but could be related to ischemia or tension on the papillary muscles. Patients may also have a variety of supraventricular or ventricular arrhythmias. Autonomic abnormalities such as orthostatic hypotension have been associated with mitral prolapse. However, the vast majority of patients with mitral valve prolapse are asymptomatic.

When the left ventricle contracts, the mitral valve initially closes normally; as ventricular volume decreases, however, the valve leaflets (anterior, posterior or both) abruptly prolapse into the atrium. This rapid motion generates the midsystolic click and subsequent mitral regurgitation creates the late systolic murmur. One or more high-pitched clicks, often followed by a systolic murmur, may occur at any time during systole. The murmur may be holosystolic in patients with early clicks and significant mitral regurgitation. Any maneuver that decreases the volume of the left ventricle causes the mitral valve to prolapse earlier during systole (for example, the Valsalva maneuver or standing), also causing the click and murmur to occur earlier in systole. The presence of clicks and the length and intensity of the murmur may vary from time to time in the same patient. There is no abnormality of the left ventricular impulse or jugular venous pressure as long as mitral regurgitation is absent or mild.

The classic features of mitral valve prolapse (posterior bowing of the posterior mitral leaflet into the left atrium during late systole) were first described with M-mode echocardiography. Two-dimensional echocardiography is the most sensitive technique for identifying mitral prolapse, diagnosed by bowing of either the anterior or posterior mitral leaflet beyond the plane of the mitral annulus into the left atrium during systole. There are a few patients who have the characteristic click and murmur on auscultation in whom no mitral valve prolapse is identified on echocardiography. Tricuspid valve prolapse is sometimes associated with mitral valve prolapse. Cardiac catheterization is not necessary unless severe mitral regurgitation has occurred.

The natural history of this syndrome is variable, and in most cases the syndrome is benign. Only a minority of patients develop severe mitral regurgitation. There is a risk of infective endocarditis, especially if a murmur is present. Sudden death is rare, and the risk of sudden death for any individual patient with mitral valve prolapse is very small unless ventricular tachycardia is demonstrated. Ventricular arrhythmias generally are not treated unless symptoms are present or ventricular tachycardia is demonstrated. These arrhythmias have been reported to respond to propranolol, but many cases are difficult to control with either propranolol or other antiarrhythmic agents. Chest pain often is treated effectively with beta-adrenergic blocking agents. If progressive or sudden mitral regurgitation occurs, mitral valve replacement may be necessary.

AORTIC STENOSIS

The most common cause of aortic stenosis is a congenitally bicuspid aortic valve (see Chapter 4) which, although usually not obstructive during childhood, gradually thickens, calcifies, and becomes stenotic by approximately the sixth decade of life. Tricuspid aortic valves may also thicken and calcify from wear and tear, causing aortic stenosis in a few patients. Rheumatic fever may cause aortic stenosis but is almost always accompanied by evidence of mitral valve involvement.

Aortic valve obstruction results in elevation of left ventricular systolic pressure, and the resultant left ventricular hypertrophy maintains cardiac output without dilation of the ventricular cavity. Therefore, the stroke volume is normal until the late stages of the disease. Forceful atrial contraction augments filling of the thick, noncompliant ventricle and generates a prominent S_4 gallop that elevates the left ventricular end-diastolic pressure. The mean left ventricular diastolic pressure is nearly normal unless myocardial decompensation occurs. Left ventricular hypertrophy and high intramyocardial wall tension account for the increased oxygen demand and, along with decreased diastolic coronary blood flow, account for the occurrence of angina pectoris even if coronary anatomy is normal. Compensatory mechanisms may be adequate for many years, although outflow obstruction is severe. However, once congestive heart failure, angina, or syncope occur the patient experiences a rapid clinical decline. The hypertrophied myocardium is not normal muscle, microscopically may contain myocardial fibrosis,

and eventually becomes unable to contract effectively. As the myocardium fails, mean left ventricular diastolic pressure increases and symptoms of pulmonary congestion ensue.

Aortic stenosis is three times more common in males than in females. Symptoms occur late, and many patients know of a murmur many years in advance of symptoms. Severe congenital aortic stenosis, however, may present in childhood. The three cardinal symptoms of aortic stenosis are angina, syncope, and left ventricular failure. In most cases, syncope is due to the inability of the left ventricle to maintain a normal cardiac output with exertion and peripheral vasodilation. A small percentage of patients (3 to 4 per cent) may have sudden death as their first symptom of aortic stenosis. The mechanism of sudden death is not known but is probably similar to that causing syncope or secondary to a ventricular arrhythmia. The onset of symptoms due to aortic stenosis is a grave prognostic sign and an indication for valve replacement.

An ejection murmur may occur across a deformed aortic valve owing to turbulence of flow without necessarily implying aortic stenosis. The murmur of significant aortic stenosis may diminish in the late stages of the disease when left ventricular failure occurs and flow across the stenotic orifice decreases.

Phonocardiography can be used to estimate noninvasively the severity of aortic stenosis by measuring the carotid pulse upstroke, the time of peaking of the ejection murmur, and the left ventricular ejection period (see Fig. 2–2). Echocardiography can detect thickening of the aortic valve leaflets with decreased systolic separation. However, because of the multiple echoes generated by the calcified valve, the severity of aortic stenosis often cannot be determined. In the adult the presence of thin, pliable aortic valve leaflets virtually excludes the diagnosis of aortic stenosis. However, in children and young adults the congenitally stenotic aortic valve may appear to move well on M-mode echocardiography, but two-dimensional echocardiography reveals the classic doming of the valve diagnostic of congenital aortic stenosis. Identification of a bicuspid valve with echocardiography is difficult. Echocardiographic degree of left ventricular hypertrophy correlates with the severity of aortic stenosis in children but not in adults. Measurement of aortic valve orifice by two-dimensional echocardiography is possible in a few patients but is not very reliable.

Cardiac catheterization is indicated in patients who have symptoms due to aortic stenosis and is the definitive test for determining the severity of stenosis. The gradient between the left ventricle and aorta is measured simultaneously with the cardiac output, and the valve area is calculated from the Gorlin equation. The pressure gradient alone often does not adequately define the severity of aortic stenosis, since the patient with an increased cardiac output may demonstrate an increased gradient across the aortic valve without necessarily having severe aortic stenosis, and a patient with severe aortic stenosis may demonstrate a decrease in the gradient as his ability to maintain cardiac output decreases. The normal valve area is approximately 2.5 sq cm, and no gradient is present normally. Aortic valvular area of less than 0.7 sq cm defines critical aortic stenosis and is usually associated with a gradient of 50 to 60 mm Hg or more. Right ventricular and pulmonary arterial pressures are normal unless left ventricular failure is present. Ventriculography is performed to assess left ventricular function, and most adult patients require coronary arteriography in case coronary revascularization is required along with aortic valve replacement.

Aortic stenosis can be complicated by the development of aortic insufficiency as the valve calcifies, stiffens, and fails to close properly or by the development of bacterial endocarditis. In younger patients, supravalvular or subvalvular aortic obstruction should be considered.

Patients with known significant aortic stenosis should not participate in strenuous physical exercise to avoid the risk of sudden death. The adult patient should undergo catheterization as soon as angina, syncope, or left ventricular failure appears. Surgical mortality is lowest in patients with good left ventricular function. In patients with poor ejection fraction who survive surgery, the ventricular function tends to improve considerably once the obstruction is relieved; therefore, poor left ventricular function does not contraindicate aortic valve replacement for aortic stenosis. Aortic valve replacement may be performed in children and young adults who have severe congenital aortic stenosis even in the absence of symptoms in order to lower the risk of sudden death. Operative mortality is approximately 3 to 6 per cent, but patients with severe left ventricular dysfunction may have an operative risk as high as 15 per cent. Once symptoms have appeared, survival is improved by surgery. Mechanical valves such as the Starr-Edwards are durable and reliable, but anticoagulation is required and thromboembolism occurs (approximately 2 to 3 per cent per year despite anticoagulation). Porcine aortic valves placed in the aortic position probably do not require chronic anticoagulation, although their life expectancy is somewhat less than that of the mechanical valves and emboli do occur.

AORTIC REGURGITATION

Rheumatic fever is the most common cause of aortic regurgitation. Isolated rheumatic aortic valve involvement without mitral valve involvement is unusual. Aortic regurgitation from rheumatic fever may occur with the aortic valvulitis at the time of the acute rheumatic fever or may occur late after the acute attack as the valve becomes thickened and the leaflets retract. Aortic stenosis and regurgitation often occur together in rheumatic heart disease as well as with bicuspid aortic valves. Aortic regurgitation may result from processes that either involve the valve directly or cause dilation of the aortic root. Aortic regurgitation can occur with discrete subvalvular stenosis or ventricular septal defects. Isolated congenital aortic regurgitation is unusual but may occur with a bicuspid aortic valve. Aortic regurgitation may occur after infective endocarditis. The aortic valve leaflets may be affected by rheumatoid arthritis. Conditions that may affect the ascending aorta and cause aortic regurgitation are syphilis, ankylosing spondylitis, Marfan's syndrome, systemic hypertension, aortic dissection, and aortic trauma.

Aortic regurgitation results in a volume overload of the left ventricle. The ventricle compensates by increasing its end-diastolic volume according to the Frank-Starling mechanism. Left ventricular end-diastolic pressure may not be elevated early in the course of the disease as the ventricle dilates and accommodates the increased volume. The amount of blood ejected with each contraction is abnormally increased, consisting of both the blood received from the left atrium and the regurgitant volume. As the ventricular volume increases beyond the capacity of the left ventricle to dilate, however, left ventricular end-diastolic and left atrial pressures may rise. Secondary mitral regurgitation may occur owing to the left ventricular dilation. The physiology of aortic regurgitation is somewhat similar to that of mitral regurgitation, except that the increased cardiac stroke volume is delivered into the high-pressure aorta instead of the low-pressure left atrium, tending to elevate left ventricular pressures instead of unloading the left ventricle. This, along with decreased aortic pressure during diastole when the majority of coronary flow occurs, may lead to greater oxygen demand than supply and angina may occur, even with normal coronary arteries. The systolic function of the left ventricle is normal in early chronic aortic regurgitation, but as dilation becomes severe, left ventricular function diminishes. Some patients experience an irreversible decrease in left ventricular function before any symptoms occur. The left ventricular dilation is thought to "overstretch" the myofibrils, leading to less actin-myosin interaction and decreased contractility. The mechanisms of compensation for chronic aortic regurgitation are very efficient, and patients with chronic severe aortic regurgitation may remain asymptomatic for years. However, the pathophysiology of acute, severe aortic regurgitation is different because the left ventricle has not had the opportunity to dilate, its compliance is relatively high, and the aortic regurgitation therefore leads to very high left ventricular end-diastolic pressures. The left atrium and pulmonary vasculature may be protected somewhat, since the elevated left ventricular end-diastolic pressure may cause the mitral valve to close early in diastole (mitral preclosure). However, if mitral regurgitation ensues, the elevated left ventricular diastolic pressure is reflected back to the pulmonary vasculature, and acute pulmonary edema may occur. Acute aortic regurgitation is caused most commonly by infective endocarditis, aortic dissection, and trauma. Acute aortic regurgitation results in a lower cardiac output, narrower aortic pulse pressure, and a smaller left ventricle than does chronic aortic regurgitation. Aortic diastolic pressure decreases in chronic aortic regurgitation because of both the regurgitation of blood into the left ventricle and a compensatory decrease in systemic vascular resistance to maintain forward cardiac flow to the periphery. In acute aortic regurgitation, however, left ventricular diastolic pressure is high, systemic vascular resistance is not low, and aortic diastolic pressure does not fall greatly.

Patients may have severe aortic regurgitation chronically for many years without the development of symptoms; once symptoms of left ventricular failure occur, they may be minimized with medical therapy. The time between the onset of symptoms and death in the natural history of the disease is relatively long compared to aortic stenosis. Palpitations may be related either to arrhythmias or to a sensation of the hyperdynamic circulatory system. Syncope from hemodynamic insufficiency is not common as in aortic stenosis, although sudden death does occur with severe aortic insufficiency. In patients with acute severe aortic regurgitation, left ventricular failure may be severe and intractable.

The increased pulse pressure in chronic aortic regurgitation is due to the large stroke volume, causing increased systolic and decreased diastolic pressure. This phenomenon determines many of the characteristic physical findings of aortic insufficiency (Table 5–2). Aortic regurgitation murmurs are heard best with the patient upright, leaning forward, and in end-expiration. The murmur of valvular aortic regurgitation is often loudest at the second left intercostal space, whereas the murmur of aortic regurgitation due to aortic dilation may be loudest in the second right intercostal space. Even if concomitant aortic stenosis is not present, a systolic ejection murmur reflecting a large stroke volume across a deformed valve is usually heard in the aortic area and may be transmitted to the carotids. In severe chronic aortic regurgitation, a diastolic low-pitched rumbling murmur may be heard at the apex (Austin Flint murmur), probably owing to flow across the mitral valve, which closes early because of the regurgitant jet from the aortic insufficiency and also the increased left ventricular diastolic pressure.

Echocardiography shows dilation of the left ventricle and sometimes aortic root. Wall motion is hyperdynamic if ventricular function is not impaired. Aortic regurgitation is characterized by diastolic fluttering of the anterior mitral valve leaflet caused by the regurgitant aortic jet striking the open mitral valve during diastole. Acute severe aortic regurgitation with marked elevation of left atrial pressures may result in closure of the mitral valve in diastole before ventricular systole has occurred (mitral preclosure). The cause of the aortic regurgitation may be identified, for example, aortic dissection or endocarditis. The presence of concomitant mitral valvular thickening or stenosis implies a rheumatic etiology.

During cardiac catheterization, supravalvular aortography defines aortic dimensions, and reflux of contrast into the left ventricle grossly quantitates the degree of aortic regurgitation. Left ventriculography is performed to evaluate left ventricular function, and reflux of contrast into the left atrium would reveal mitral regurgitation. Systolic left ventricular and aortic pressures are elevated, and aortic diastolic pressure is low. Left ventricular volume is increased. The left ventricular end-diastolic pressure is normal or only slightly increased until left ventricular failure ensues. Left ventricular dysfunction is demonstrated by decreased cardiac output, decreased ejection fraction, and increased left ventricular end-diastolic pressure. In severe aortic regurgitation, the normally functioning ventricle is hyperdynamic (increased ejection fraction), and even a normal ejection fraction may indicate decreased systolic function. The presence of left ventricular dysfunction markedly increases surgical complications and mortality, and left ventricular function may not be restored after surgery, in contrast to patients with pure aortic stenosis.

The timing of aortic valve replacement is difficult, since the natural history is prolonged and a long asymptomatic phase occurs. Early replacement of the aortic valve subjects the patient to the immediate surgical risk and the long-term risk created by prosthetic valves. However, if one waits to replace the aortic valve, irreversible left ventricular dysfunction may occur. Cardiac catheterization with consideration for valve replacement should be performed in patients with the onset of congestive heart failure. However, in some patients significant left ventricular dysfunction may occur in the absence of symptoms. Moderate depression of left ventricular function may reverse somewhat following surgery. In patients with no symptoms, evidence of progressive left ventricular systolic dysfunction may indicate surgery. (Suggested criteria include a left ventricular end-systolic diameter of 5.5 cm on M-mode echocardiography or a decrease in radionuclide left ventricular ejection fraction with exercise.) In patients with severe disease of the aortic root, replacement of a portion of the ascending aorta may be required in addition to the aortic valve replacement.

Patients who develop acute severe aortic regurgitation deteriorate rapidly, and aortic valve replacement must be performed emergently. Vasodilators such as nitroprusside can acutely reduce afterload and diminish aortic regurgitation to stabilize the patient for a short period of time until surgery can be performed. Intra-aortic balloon counterpulsation is not effective in the presence of aortic regurgitation.

TRICUSPID STENOSIS

Tricuspid stenosis is usually rheumatic in etiology and does not occur as an isolated lesion. Like mitral stenosis, it is gradually progressive, more common in women, and usually becomes symptomatic in mid-adulthood. Tricuspid stenosis can occasionally be caused by carcinoid, endomyocardial fibroelastosis, congenital valvular malformations, or right atrial myxoma.

Tricuspid stenosis results in increased right atrial pressures. Prominent a waves, reflecting atrial contraction against the stenotic valve, are present. The y descent (ventricular filling in early diastole) is attenuated. Because it is such a low-pressure system, relatively small gradients across the tricuspid valve (5 mm) may indicate significant tricuspid stenosis. Echocardiographic diagnosis is probably more accurate than catheterization because of the small gradient involved. Tricuspid stenosis can protect the patient with concomitant mitral stenosis from pulmonary congestion.

TRICUSPID REGURGITATION

Tricuspid regurgitation may occur as a result of rheumatic fever, often associated with tricuspid stenosis. Tricuspid regurgitation is most commonly a functional lesion secondary to right ventricular dilation and pulmonary hypertension, and as in patients with mitral regurgitation, the differentiation of functional from organic valvular regurgitation can be difficult. Functional tricuspid regurgitation can occur with forms of congenital heart disease associated with pulmonary hypertension and with severe pulmonary disease. Tricuspid regurgitation can occur with Ebstein's anomaly, carcinoid syndrome, intracardiac tumors, penetrating or nonpenetrating cardiac trauma, and endocarditis. Normal tricuspid valves may be affected by endocarditis, particularly in drug addicts.

Tricuspid regurgitation causes right ventricular volume overload. As tricuspid regurgitation becomes more severe, v waves become more prominent in the jugular venous pulse and mean venous pressure increases. Findings of pulmonary hypertension are present in patients with secondary tricuspid regurgitation.

Tricuspid regurgitation is not directly detectable by echocardiography, but the cause of tricuspid regurgitation (for example, tricuspid prolapse or tricuspid vegetation) may be evident. Contrast echocardiography using a contrast agent injected into a brachial vein may reveal tricuspid regurgitation by demonstrating regurgitation of contrast material into the inferior vena cava.

Functional tricuspid regurgitation may regress after associated lesions are corrected and pulmonary hypertension resolves. At times plication of the tricuspid annulus is required to improve functional tricuspid regurgitation. If annuloplasty is unsuccessful or if significant tricuspid stenosis is present, tricuspid valve replacement can be performed.

PULMONIC STENOSIS AND REGURGITATION

Pulmonic stenosis is usually congenital and is discussed in Chapter 4. It can occasionally occur in an acquired form with hypertrophic cardiomyopathy (due to bulging of the septum into the right ventricular outflow tract) or secondary to pericardial tumor involvement in the area.

Acquired pulmonary regurgitation is usually associated with pulmonary hypertension caused by left heart valvular disease (Graham Steell murmur) or pulmonary disease. The murmur sounds similar to that of aortic insufficiency and is heard best at the second left intercostal space. This murmur is high-pitched, early diastolic, and decrescendo in character. In distinction, isolated congenital pulmonic regurgitation results in a lower-pitched murmur that occurs later in diastole, is heard best at the third to fourth left intercostal space, and resembles more the murmur of tricuspid stenosis.

MULTIVALVULAR DISEASE

Combined valvular lesions are common, especially in rheumatic heart disease. In addition to organic lesions, development of mitral and tricuspid regurgitation or pulmonic regurgitation may occur secondary to the hemodynamic disturbance of other valvular lesions. In general, the manifestations of the more proximal valve lesion are the more prominent. For example, in patients with mitral and aortic valvular lesions of similar severity, mitral valve manifestations may predominate and the degree of aortic stenosis may be underestimated. Failure to correct all significant valvular lesions at the time of surgery may lead to an inadequate clinical result and illustrates the importance of excluding concomitant lesions at the time of catheterization. The surgical risk for double valve replacement is greater than that for single valve replacement.

RHEUMATIC FEVER

Rheumatic fever usually occurs in children 5 to 15 years of age. It is caused by group A beta hemolytic streptococcal pharyngitis that occurs one to three weeks prior to the clinical manifestations of rheumatic fever. It is believed that an immune response to the *Streptococcus* is responsible for the disease. Males and females are equally affected. It is more common in patients of lower socioeconomic level. The incidence of rheumatic fever in the United States has declined in recent years.

Aschoff nodules in the myocardium are the characteristic pathological feature of rheumatic fever. The most serious manifestation of rheumatic fever is a pancarditis that may involve the endocardium, myocardium, and pericardium. Usually the mitral valve, less frequently the aortic, and even less frequently the tricuspid valve are involved. Pulmonic valve involvement is extremely rare. Valvulitis is recognized by a new insufficiency murmur. Aortic and mitral stenosis murmurs are not heard acutely. Myocarditis may present with heart failure. Pericarditis may produce a friction rub, and the PR interval may prolong. Because of the difficulty in diagnosing rheumatic fever, guidelines (modified Jones criteria) for establishing the diagnosis were developed (Table 5–4).

Penicillin should be administered to eradicate streptococcal infection. Salicylates are effective rapidly for treating fever and arthritis but probably have no effect on carditis. The usefulness of steroids is unproven. Congestive heart failure is treated traditionally.

The relatively high recurrence rate of rheumatic fever after streptococcal infection continues for at least 5 to 10 years after the initial infection; therefore, rheumatic fever prophylaxis should be discontinued only in adults 5 to 10 years after the acute episode and only then if the risk of the streptococcal infection is low. Adults working with school-age children, those in the military service, those exposed to large numbers of people, and those in the medical or allied health professions should receive prophylaxis indefinitely. Patients who have a significant degree of rheumatic heart disease or a history of repeated occurrences should have prophylaxis indefinitely. The recommended regimen for prophylaxis is 1.2 million units of benzathine penicillin monthly. Oral penicillin, erythromycin, or sulfadiazine can be used but because of noncompliance are somewhat less effective than the parenteral regimen.

PROSTHETIC VALVES

Prosthetic valves may be either mechanical or bioprosthetic. The two basic designs of mechanical valves are the ball and cage and the tilting disk (like a toilet seat cover). Bioprosthetic valves are made from porcine valve tissue mounted on metal struts (Table 5–5).

All prosthetic valves are somewhat stenotic, and residual gradients over both aortic and mitral valves occur. Any prosthetic valve can develop a perivalvular leak, that is, a leak exterior to the valve sewing ring, resulting in aortic or mitral regurgitation. In addition to hemodynamic effects, the turbulence from a perivalvular leak can cause red cell hemolysis. Even normally functioning prosthetic valves can cause hemolysis in some patients. The mechanical portion of a prosthetic valve may clot or otherwise malfunction. The long-term durability of mechanical valves has been well documented, but the durability of bioprosthetic porcine valves is not established, and many appear to degenerate, especially in younger patients.

TABLE 5–4. JONES CRITERIA (REVISED)

MAJOR MANIFESTATIONS	MINOR MANIFESTATIONS
Carditis	Fever
Polyarthritis	Arthralgia
Chorea	Previous rheumatic fever or rheumatic heart disease
Erythema marginatum	Elevated erythrocyte sedimentation rate or positive C-reactive protein
Subcutaneous nodules	Prolonged PR interval

Plus supporting evidence of preceding streptococcal infection: history of recent scarlet fever; positive throat culture for group A streptococcus; increased ASO titer or other streptococcal antibodies.

Adapted from Jones Criteria (revised) for guidance in the diagnosis of rheumatic fever. Circulation 32:664, 1965. By permission of the American Heart Association, Inc.

All prosthetic valves carry a risk of thromboembolism. Valves in the aortic position are less likely to cause emboli than valves in the mitral position. Bioprosthetic valves are less likely to cause emboli than mechanical valves; however, a patient with a high embolic risk (for example, atrial fibrillation, markedly dilated left atrium, previous history of peripheral emboli, or documented intracardiac thrombus) requires chronic anticoagulation despite the presence of a porcine valve. All prosthetic valves are prone to developing endocarditis, and vigorous endocarditis prophylaxis should be administered prior to dental, GI, or GU surgery (see Chapter 10).

REFERENCES

Dalen JE, and Alpert JS (eds): Valvular Heart Disease. Boston, Little, Brown and Co, 1981.
Devereau RB, Perloff JK, Reicheck N, and Josephson ME: Mitral valve prolapse. Circulation 54:3, 1976.
Morganroth J, Perloff JK, Zeldis SM, and Dunkman WB: Acute severe aortic regurgitation. Ann Intern Med 87:223, 1977.
Rahimtoola SH: Valvular heart disease: A perspective. J Am Coll Cardiol 1:199, 1983.
Ross J: Left ventricular function and the timing of surgical treatment in valvular heart disease. Ann Intern Med 94:498, 1981.
Shulman ST, et al: Prevention of rheumatic fever. Circulation 70:1118A, 1984.

TABLE 5–5. PROSTHETIC VALVES

TYPE	EXAMPLES	ADVANTAGES	DISADVANTAGES
Ball and cage	Starr-Edwards	Good durability	Anticoagulation required; more hemolysis than other types
Tilting disc	Bjork-Shiley St. Jude	Most favorable hemodynamics (i.e., least residual stenosis for any given valve size); good durability	Anticoagulation required; most thrombogenic type
Bioprosthesis	Hancock, Carpentier-Edwards	Anticoagulation usually not required	Early degeneration, especially in younger patients

6 PULMONARY HEART DISEASE
(See also Chapter 21)

The normal pulmonary vasculature provides very low resistance to blood flow. However, when pulmonary hypertension occurs, right ventricular hypertrophy, dilation, and failure may develop. Pulmonary arterial hypertension results when there is increased flow in the pulmonary vasculature, when elevated pulmonary venous pressure is reflected back to the pulmonary arteries, or when the caliber of the pulmonary vasculature is decreased by either vasospasm or physical destruction. Pulmonary heart disease (cor pulmonale) occurs when pulmonary arterial pressure is elevated secondary to dysfunction of the lungs and its vasculature and produces right heart failure.

In primary pulmonary hypertension, intimal thickening of the pulmonary arteries and arterioles occurs with a characteristic "onion skin" vascular lesion. It occurs more frequently in women than in men. The pulmonary vascular resistance and pulmonary arterial pressure become markedly elevated. Left atrial and pulmonary capillary wedge pressures are normal, but right ventricular and right atrial pressures increase. The cardiac output may be normal or low, and the heart is unable to increase cardiac output with exercise. Functional tricuspid regurgitation may occur. Most patients become symptomatic late in the course of the disease. Fatigue and weakness are universal. Because of the low, fixed cardiac output, exertional syncope may result, which is an ominous sign; these patients may experience sudden cardiac death.

Secondary pulmonary hypertension can result from several etiologies. Pulmonary venous hypertension secondary to mitral stenosis often results in a "reactive" pulmonary arterial vasoconstriction, increasing pulmonary vascular resistance and causing pulmonary hypertension. The cause of this reactive pulmonary hypertension is unclear, but upon relief of the mitral stenosis and decline of the pulmonary venous pressure, it usually disappears. Various forms of congenital heart disease can result in pulmonary arterial hypertension, and many (for example, ventricular septal defect) are not reversible once present. Pulmonary parenchymal diseases such as chronic obstructive pulmonary disease, restrictive lung disease, pneumoconiosis, and sarcoidosis can lead to pulmonary heart disease. Pulmonary vascular diseases such as recurrent pulmonary embolism and scleroderma can result in pulmonary hypertension. In addition, patients with disorders of their chest wall and muscles of respiration that lead to hypoventilation, such as kyphoscoliosis or sleep apnea syndrome, can develop right heart failure.

Acute pulmonary edema can occur in apparently normal patients exposed to the hypoxia of high altitudes. The precise mechanism is unclear, but these patients tend to have an exaggerated vasoconstrictive response of the pulmonary arterioles to hypoxia. This syndrome responds very quickly to oxygen administration.

Chronic obstructive pulmonary disease (COPD) is the most common cause of pulmonary heart disease. Improvement of oxygenation is the best therapy for right heart failure associated with chronic lung disease. Aggressive treatment of the primary lung disorder with correction of hypoxia and acidosis decreases pulmonary vasoconstriction, and pulmonary hypertension improves.

Patients with pulmonary embolism may present with either dyspnea at rest, manifestations of pulmonary infarction including pleuritic pain, cough, and hemoptysis, circulatory collapse from massive pulmonary embolism, or unexplained exacerbation of known chronic heart failure. Large pulmonary emboli acutely elevate pulmonary arterial pressure and precipitate acute right heart failure.

7 CORONARY HEART DISEASE

Coronary artery disease is the leading cause of death in the United States and most of the industrialized Western world. In contrast, it is much less common in Asia, the Near East, Africa, and South and Central America. Inexplicably, death from coronary heart disease has declined in the United States since the late 1960's.

ATHEROSCLEROSIS

Atherosclerosis is a thickening and hardening of medium-size and larger arteries with narrowing of the arterial lumen by atherosclerotic plaques. Its cause is multifactorial. Preventable risk factors, genetic susceptibility, local arterial and hemodynamic factors, and sex influence the development of atherosclerosis.

The fatty streak, consisting of lipids and lipoid proteins, located in the intima of the vessel with the overlying endothelium intact, is the earliest form of atherosclerosis. This yellow fatty streak seen in childhood is not necessarily a precursor of adult atherosclerosis and occurs in populations in which atherosclerosis is uncommon; it is presumably reversible at this stage. Around age 25, in populations in which atherosclerosis is common, the fibrous plaque begins to develop. It is white, elevated, and may compromise the arterial lumen. Reversibility is questionable when fibrous tissue and intimal proliferation are present. In more advanced stages, deposition of fibrin and platelets and necrosis of tissue with growth of new vessels may occur. Cholesterol, calcification, and hemorrhage within the atherosclerotic plaque form complicated plaques. The intimal surface may ulcerate, thrombose, and occlude the vessel. Mechanical, chemical, or immunological injury that begins with the fatty streak may cause progression of the atherosclerotic lesion. Different arteries appear to have different degrees of susceptibility to atherosclerotic lesions; the coronary arteries are particularly susceptible, mostly within the first 6 cm of origin. Plaques tend to occur at arterial bifurcations, possibly due to the turbulent flow in these areas.

Atherosclerotic lesions in the coronary arteries may be detected during life by coronary arteriography (Fig. 7–1). When a radiopaque contrast agent is injected into a coronary artery, atherosclerotic plaques appear as narrowings in the column of contrast as it travels down the artery. Narrowing of vessels is described as a per cent diameter narrowing. Lesions >50 per cent are probably hemodynamically significant, causing approximately 75 per cent narrowing of cross-sectional area, while lesions > 75 per cent are definitely significant, producing 95 per cent cross-sectional narrowing. The gradation of obstruction at coronary angiography is approximate and often underestimates the actual degree of obstruction. Complete obstruction of a vessel at angiography is usually represented by a stump, the distal portion of the vessel often opacified via collateral circulation.

RISK FACTORS

Several risk factors for the development of coronary artery disease have been identified by epidemiological studies. The more risk factors present in any individual patient, the greater the likelihood that he will develop coronary artery disease. However, there is no absolute correlation between risk factors and incidence of coronary disease. Age, sex, and family history are strong risk factors for coronary artery disease that cannot be altered in any particular patient. Regardless of sex, the risk of developing symptomatic coronary artery disease increases with age. Mortality in males from coronary artery disease is much higher than in females, and females lag behind males in coronary artery disease deaths by approximately 10 years. Coronary disease mortality tends to equalize in men and women at age 50, possibly related to higher risk in women after menopause or the elimination of higher-risk males at an earlier age. The existence of coronary artery disease in a parent or sibling is a strong risk factor. Distinct differences, some of which may be due to genetic and environmental factors, are found in

the high incidence of coronary disease in white Western males and low incidence in Japanese males living in Japan.

Hypertension, hyperlipidemia, smoking, and glucose intolerance are potentially amenable risk factors that are independently associated with coronary risk. Hypertension is clearly associated with an increased risk of coronary and cerebral vascular disease. Treatment of even mild hypertension (diastolic pressure 90 to 104 mm Hg) reduces mortality from both stroke and myocardial infarction, implying not only an association but a causative role for hypertension. Both systolic and diastolic blood pressure elevation are associated with an increased risk. There is no distinct blood pressure value under which risk suddenly becomes low; that is, over a wide range of blood pressures, the higher the blood pressure, the higher the risk.

A strong relationship exists between total serum cholesterol and the development of coronary artery disease. The higher the serum cholesterol, the higher the risk of coronary disease, even

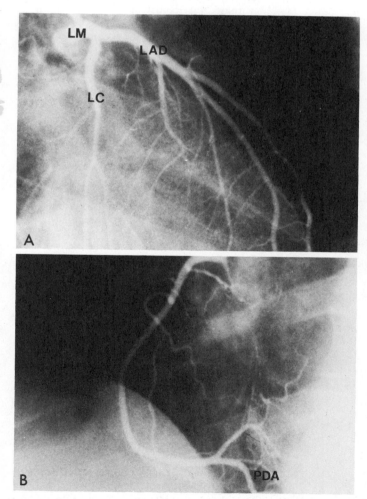

FIGURE 7–1. *A,* Normal left coronary arteriogram in the right anterior oblique projection. LM = Left main coronary artery; LAD = left anterior descending coronary artery; LC = left circumflex coronary artery. *B,* Normal right coronary arteriogram in the left anterior oblique projection. PDA = Posterior descending artery.

within the usually accepted "normal" cholesterol values of Americans. The low density lipoprotein (LDL) fraction of total cholesterol is directly associated with the risk of atherosclerosis, and the high density lipoprotein (HDL) fraction appears to be inversely related to the incidence of atherosclerosis. HDL levels are higher in women than in men at all age levels. They are increased by regular exercise and are reduced in diabetes mellitus. The serum triglyceride level is a weaker risk factor and may not be independent when adjusted for obesity or glucose intolerance. It is possible to lower serum cholesterol a small amount with diet and/or medications. Recent evidence implies that modifications in serum cholesterol may lead to a small improvement in risk. Many patients already have developed a manifestation of coronary artery disease when they consult a doctor, and "secondary prevention" (that is, prevention of more complications once one coronary event has already occurred) has been disappointing. However, dietary modification to lower serum cholesterol seems prudent in both asymptomatic patients with an elevated or high normal cholesterol (greater than 200 mg/dl) and in patients with known coronary artery disease. Drug treatment to effect marked reduction in serum cholesterol should probably be reserved for patients with well-defined hypercholesterolemia.

Cigarette smoking is a major independent risk for coronary artery disease that is proportional to the number of cigarettes smoked daily and applies equally to men and women. Those who stop smoking develop a lesser risk within a year or two of discontinuation, but the risk remains slightly higher than that of patients who never smoked. The risk of sudden death is sharply reduced after smoking is stopped.

Glucose intolerance is an independent risk factor for coronary artery disease that in women virtually eliminates the lower risk conferred by the female sex. Diabetes affects small as well as medium-sized vessels. There is currently no convincing evidence that rigid control of diabetes appreciably decreases the incidence of coronary atherosclerosis.

A variety of other risk factors have been described, but none of these factors has been shown to contribute independently to the development of atherosclerosis. Patients who are 20 per cent or more above ideal body weight have an increased risk of atherosclerosis, but this risk appears to be associated with the increased incidence of diabetes, hypertension, and hyperlipidemia. However, control of body weight is reasonable for both primary and secondary prevention. Likewise, the benefit of physical activity is controversial, and any protective aspect of physical activity may be secondary to the absence of other risk factors. "Type A" personality (aggressive, ambitious, and associated with a stressful environment) has been associated with coronary disease, but this personality is often associated with other adverse risk factors. There is little convincing evidence that modification of the type A personality is possible or alters risk.

The risk of atherosclerosis in women who use oral contraceptives and have other adverse factors (e.g., smoking) is elevated. Oral contraceptives may alter blood pressure, lipoproteins, and clotting mechanisms.

NONATHEROSCLEROTIC CAUSES OF CORONARY ARTERY OBSTRUCTION

Although uncommon, there are several nonatherosclerotic causes of coronary artery obstruction. Emboli to coronary arteries can occur in infective endocarditis, from mural thrombi in the left atrium or ventricle, from prosthetic valves, from cardiac myxomas, or associated with cardiopulmonary bypass or coronary arteriography. Trauma to coronary arteries can be associated with both penetrating and nonpenetrating injuries. Various forms of arteritis (syphilis, polyarteritis nodosa, Takayasu's disease, disseminated lupus erythematosus, and rheumatoid arthritis) can affect the coronary arteries. The mucocutaneous lymph node syndrome (Kawasaki's disease) presents as a febrile illness in a child usually below the age of 10. Multiple organ systems can develop vasculitis, but the most significant feature is a vasculitis involving intima, media, and adventitia of the coronary arteries that results in aneurysm and sometimes thrombus formation. Mortality is 1 to 2 per cent secondary to complications from coronary arterial involvement.

Dissection of the aorta involving the coronary arteries or dissection of the coronary arteries themselves may occur in patients with connective tissue abnormalities of the aorta (for example, Marfan's syndrome). In situ thrombosis may occur in certain rare disorders (for example, polycythemia vera, thrombocytosis, or disseminated intravascular coagulation). Spasm of the coronary artery (Prinzmetal's angina, discussed below) is another nonatherosclerotic cause of coronary obstruction.

NONOBSTRUCTIVE CAUSES OF ISCHEMIC HEART DISEASE

Situations associated with increased left ventricular pressure and wall tension, a decrease in diastolic perfusion pressure, and/or an increase in left ventricular mass (for example, aortic stenosis) may cause myocardial ischemia by altering the balance of oxygen supply and demand. In addition, conditions in which substrate delivery is decreased (for example, hypotension, anemia, and carbon monoxide poisoning) may cause myocardial ischemia, especially if preexisting coronary lesions are present.

A syndrome of myocardial infarction with angiographically normal coronary arteries exists. Approximately 2 per cent of patients with myocardial infarction demonstrate no obstructive lesions on coronary arteriography. These patients tend to be young, have a low incidence of coronary risk factors, and often have no history of angina pectoris prior to infarction. The prognosis for survival after the acute event is usually good. The cause is unknown, but possible etiologies include coronary emboli, coronary artery spasm, coronary artery disease in smaller vessels beyond the resolution of coronary arteriography, and coronary arterial thrombosis with recanalization.

PATHOPHYSIOLOGY OF ISCHEMIC HEART DISEASE

The manifestations of ischemic heart disease occur when the oxygen demand to the heart exceeds the oxygen supply. The most common cause of this imbalance is fixed obstruction within a coronary artery. Normally the arterioles regulate the blood flow to any particular area of the heart, and the more proximal epicardial "conductance" vessels, in the absence of a fixed or dynamic obstruction, do not restrict the flow. Once stenosis of 50 per cent or greater occurs in a conductance coronary artery, the vessel is unable to increase its flow sufficiently to maintain perfusion under conditions of increased demand despite the full dilation of the more distal arterioles. In addition to fixed obstruction, transient or "dynamic" obstruction of the conductance vessels may also occur. The caliber of these larger vessels can be altered by factors that are incompletely understood, and spasm of a localized area may decrease blood supply transiently to an area of the heart (variant or Prinzmetal's angina). Coronary artery spasm with or without the coexistent fixed coronary obstructive lesions may cause angina pectoris because of a temporary decrease in oxygen supply rather than any increase in oxygen demand.

Occasionally oxygen demand can exceed oxygen supply despite normal coronary arteries; the classic example is aortic stenosis when the hypertrophied muscle and increased wall tension increase oxygen demand, but increased intramural pressure and decreased aortic pressure decrease diastolic coronary artery flow and oxygen supply.

Ischemia affects the metabolism of cardiac cells, which can alter contractile and electrical functions. The inability to perform oxidative phosphorylation and generate high-energy compounds results in abnormal systolic myocardial contraction and also defects of diastolic compliance (relaxation). Dysfunction can be transient, for example, only after exercise-induced ischemia, or permanent, such as with myocardial infarction. Decreased compliance requires increased pressure to fill the heart to any given end-diastolic volume and accounts for the need to elevate somewhat the left ventricular filling pressure in order to maintain cardiac filling in patients with ischemic heart disease. The loss of cellular integrity allows release of enzymes (serum glutamine-ornithine transferase, lactate dehydrogenase, and creatine kinase) into the blood that are used clinically to detect the presence of myocardial infarction. Electrical changes occur owing to altered ion transport across the cell membrane. Serious arrhythmias, most frequently ventricular tachycardia and fibrillation, are common.

The time during which ischemia is reversible is clinically important, since interventions exist that may restore flow to myocardium distal to an acute occlusion. Reperfusion after complete occlusion of less than 15 to 20 minutes salvages most if not all of the ischemic tissue. However, longer periods of occlusion result in increased amounts of myocardium that remain irreversibly necrotic. After approximately four to six hours of occlusion, reperfusion salvages very little tissue.

In humans, collateral circulation (small vessels that course from a nonobstructed coronary system to the distal portion of an obstructed system) slowly develops as flow is gradually diminished by fixed coronary obstruction. Collateral flow does provide some perfusion to an ischemic vascular bed, but the adequacy of this perfusion is questionable, especially under periods of increased demand (for example, exercise). Collateral flow does not develop acutely after sudden obstruction of blood flow.

ANGINA PECTORIS

Angina pectoris is chest discomfort caused by transient myocardial ischemia without necrosis, usually resulting from the inability of atherosclerotic arteries to increase myocardial blood flow under conditions of increased demand. Coronary spasm may occur either alone or in the presence of fixed coronary obstruction and reduces flow without an increase in demand. Angina pectoris is considered stable when there exists a chronic course of predictable exertional chest pain and unstable if a change in chronic angina consisting of increased frequency, duration, or severity occurs. The onset of new angina, or angina occurring at rest or with minimal exertion, or angina awakening the patient from sleep is considered unstable. Unstable angina pectoris has also been termed preinfarction angina, crescendo angina, acute coronary insufficiency, and intermediate coronary syndrome and usually requires hospital admission to exclude an acute myocardial infarction (Table 7–1).

The patient's history is crucial in the diagnosis of angina pectoris (see Table 2–2). Even if coronary artery disease is known to exist anatomically, e.g., by arteriography, the functional significance of these lesions must be assessed from the patient's history of chest pain. The pattern of precipitation by exertion and disappearance with rest is one of the most characteristic features of angina pectoris. The pain or discomfort is often located in the left precordium or mid-chest directly under the sternum. It is sometimes not considered pain by the patient but described as pressure, burning, tightness, or fullness; the classic gesture is a clenched fist over the chest. The pain may appear over the period of a few seconds or minutes and disappears gradually in the same manner. It is usually not sharp or knifelike and does not occur suddenly at full intensity or leave abruptly. It lasts between one-half minute and approximately 20 minutes. Ischemic pain that lasts

TABLE 7–1. ANGINA PECTORIS

TYPE OF ANGINA	TYPICAL PATIENT CHARACTERISTICS	PATTERN	COMPLICATIONS	ECG	ANGIOGRAPHY	THERAPY
Stable	Older Male > Female Coronary risk factors	Stable, unchanging pattern of aggravation and relief; exertional, lasts <10 minutes	Usually none	Baseline ECG often demonstrates nonspecific ST-T changes or evidence of old MI but can be normal; ST depression or T wave inversion may occur with pain	Fixed obstructive coronary lesions	Nitrates Beta blockers Calcium blockers
Unstable	Same as above	Markedly increased frequency; prolonged, severe episodes; rest angina, nocturnal angina	Can lead to MI or ischemic arrhythmias	Same as stable angina; ST elevation occasionally occurs with pain	Fixed lesions (although coronary spasm can contribute)	Same as above Hospitalization Consider intra-aortic balloon pump, angiography, revascularization
Variant (atypical or Prinzmetal's)	Younger Male ≅ Female Lack of coronary risk factors	Typically severe pain at rest, can be provoked with exertion in a few cases; often early morning pattern	Syncope from tachyarrhythmias, heart block during pain; MI on rare occasions	Baseline ECG often normal; typically ST elevation with pain, although ST depression and T wave inversion also occur	Spontaneous or ergonovine-induced spasm in a normal vessel or at a region of a fixed but often nonstenotic lesion	Calcium blockers Nitrates Avoid beta blockers

longer suggests myocardial necrosis. Typical angina is relieved with nitroglycerin or rest over a period of 30 seconds to several minutes. Immediate relief (within a few seconds), incomplete relief, or relief 20 to 30 minutes after sublingual nitroglycerin is not typical of angina pectoris. The pain may radiate to the neck, jaw, epigastrium, shoulder, and the arms, most frequently the left arm. Pain localized to the left inframammary area is less characteristic. Chest wall tenderness is usually not present. Common precipitating factors are brisk walking, climbing stairs, using the hands above the head (for example, shaving, hair combing), emotional upset, exposure to cold, and a large meal. Redistribution of intravascular volume at night may cause angina decubitus, that is, angina occurring with the supine position. Existence of precipitating causes such as anemia, thyrotoxicosis, infection, aortic stenosis, arrhythmias, and hypertension should be excluded. Weakness, dyspnea, nausea, pallor, and diaphoresis may occur with the pain. Many patients misinterpret the sensation as "gas," and belching is not uncommon.

Findings on physical examination are nonspecific. An S_4 gallop is often present but may only be heard during an episode of acute ischemia (decreased diastolic compliance with ischemia). Likewise, a murmur of papillary muscle dysfunction may occur only with ischemia. When myocardial ischemia is not present at rest, exercise tests may unmask ECG evidence of ischemia (see Stress Testing in Chapter 2). Thallium perfusion scintigraphy or exercise radionuclide ventriculography increases the sensitivity and specificity of exercise testing, particularly in patients with abnormal baseline electrocardiograms because of digitalis, pre-existing nonspecific ST-T wave changes, or left bundle branch block. Exercise echocardiography has become practical with two-dimensional echo techniques and may reveal regional wall motion abnormality during or immediately after exercise. In addition to its diagnostic role, the treadmill exercise test is important to assess the functional capacity and prognosis of patients with known coronary artery disease.

If the patient presents with pain of unknown origin, exercise testing may be useful diagnostically, but only after rest and medication have relieved the pain and an acute myocardial infarction has been excluded. Patients with rest pain or particularly severe anginal syndromes should not undergo exercise testing but instead should proceed directly to coronary angiography after stabilization. Patients who present with unstable angina have a higher percentage of left main and severe three vessel disease than patients with chronic, stable angina.

The natural history of stable angina pectoris is variable, and several years may pass in some patients without the development of unstable angina or myocardial infarction. The most important factors to judge prognosis are measures of left ventricular function, the number of vessels containing significantly stenotic lesions, and exercise tolerance. Patients with significant left main coronary artery stenoses have a poor prognosis and are considered for surgery on the basis of their anatomy alone.

The indications for coronary angiography are relatively narrow (see Table 2–19). For patients in whom the differentiation of coronary artery disease from noncoronary causes of chest pain cannot be made despite a careful history and non-invasive evaluation, coronary arteriography may be the only means to exclude or establish the diagnosis of coronary artery disease. In addition, for patients in whom coronary artery spasm is suspected, the administration of ergonovine at cardiac catheterization may exclude or confirm that diagnosis. When ischemic pain is refractory to medical management, surgery very effectively eliminates pain (Table 7–2). Because specific subgroups of patients may demonstrate increased survival from coronary bypass surgery, some physicians recommend coronary angiography for any patient with known or suspected coronary artery disease in order to exclude left main or certain subsets of three-vessel coronary artery disease. Since this practice subjects many patients to the risk (albeit small) of coronary angiography, most physicians select patients for coronary angiography from subgroups at particularly high risk for having left main or three-vessel coronary artery disease, for example, patients with recurrent chest pain after myocardial infarction (especially sub-endocardial myocardial infarction), patients with poor exercise performance (positive test in first two stages or 6 minutes of exercise), and patients presenting with an unstable pattern of angina pectoris. Using these high-risk subgroups as a guide to selecting patients for catheterization, few patients with left main coronary artery stenosis would be missed. Many physicians also catheterize any young patient (below age 40) who presents with significant angina or myocardial infarction and any patient resuscitated from cardiac arrest. The ability of coronary artery bypass surgery to prolong life in many other subgroups of patients with coronary artery disease, particularly those patients with mild or moderate degrees of angina, is unproven.

Some patients, especially diabetics, may have "silent" ischemia, that is, episodes of ischemia,

TABLE 7–2. INDICATIONS FOR CORONARY REVASCULARIZATION

1. Relief of moderate to severe, significantly disabling stable angina in patients refractory or intolerant to medical management
2. Relief of unstable angina in patients refractory or intolerant to medical management; performed preferably after the patient is stable and pain-free, but can be done emergently if necessary
3. Improved survival in less symptomatic patients with left main coronary arterial stenosis and possibly certain subsets of three-vessel disease (for example, those with poor functional capacity or moderate left ventricular dysfunction)
4. Reperfusion during acute myocardial infarction to preserve myocardium (controversial; usually involves angioplasty rather than surgery)

well-documented by ECG, imaging, or echo techniques unassociated with chest discomfort. This lack of an anginal "warning system" may result from autonomic nervous system abnormalities and may be dangerous, since severe ischemia can occur without the patient's realizing that he needs to stop his activity. Some patients may manifest symptoms of ischemia as dyspnea rather than chest discomfort (angina-equivalent dyspnea).

MEDICAL MANAGEMENT OF ANGINA

Angina is treated by decreasing myocardial oxygen demand or increasing oxygen supply. Certain general measures may be helpful. Avoiding situations that may increase oxygen demand (for example, cold weather, particularly large meals,

TABLE 7–3. NITRATE PREPARATIONS FOR ANGINA

PREPARATION	INDICATION	ONSET*	DURATION*	USUAL DOSE	SIDE EFFECTS
Sublingual nitroglycerin	Acute anginal episodes; prophylaxis before specific activity	2 min	30 min	0.3-0.6 (usually 0.4) mg; can be repeated at 5-min intervals; if pain unrelieved after three doses patient is usually instructed to seek medical attention	Headache (tolerance may develop in 1-2 weeks) Flushing Tachycardia Dizziness Postural hypotension
Topical nitroglycerin 2% nitroglycerin ointment	Angina prophylaxis	15 min	4-6 hr (can be wiped off if side effects occur)	1-2 inches q6h; bedtime doses are useful	Same as above Messy
Sustained release transdermal		—	24 hr	q24h; dose depends on preparation	Variable drug levels and tolerance to nitrate effects have been reported; contact dermatitis
IV Nitroglycerin	Unstable, severe angina	Almost immediately	Effects gone 5-10 min after infusion is stopped	Continuous infusion; initially 10 µg/min, titrate upward at 5-min intervals to desired hemodynamic effect	Hypotension
Long-acting sublingual (e.g., isosorbide dinitrate)	Angina prophylaxis	5-10 min	1-3 hr	2.5-10 mg q2-3h	Same as above Ischemia may occur upon abrupt withdrawal
oral		15-20 min	4-6 hr	10-40 mg q3-6h (efficacy of long-acting nitrates administered q8-12h is questionable)	

*Varies widely

TABLE 7–4. BETA BLOCKING AGENTS

DRUG	USUAL DOSAGE	BETA-1 CARDIO-SELECTIVE	INTRINSIC AGONIST ACTIVITY	HYDRO-PHILIC
Propranolol	Oral: 40-480 mg/day in 2-4 doses; Intravenous: up to 0.10-0.15 mg/kg given as 1-mg increments at 3-5 minute intervals	–	–	low
Metoprolol	Oral: 50-100 mg twice a day	+	–	moderate
Nadolol	Oral: 40-160 mg once a day	–	–	high
Atenolol	Oral: 50-100 mg once a day	+	–	high
Timolol	Oral: 10-20 mg twice a day	–	–	moderate
Pindolol	Oral: 10-30 mg twice a day	–	+	moderate

+ = present
– = absent

and excessive exercise) may be effective. Control of hypertension and correction of other exacerbating conditions such as anemia, infection, hypoxia, and thyrotoxicosis is necessary. Cigarette smoking should be stopped. Treatment of congestive heart failure decreases oxygen consumption and improves oxygen delivery. After physical training under supervised programs the patient may be able to perform tasks with a lower heart rate–blood pressure product and less angina. Whether exercise increases collateral circulation and oxygen delivery is controversial.

The most time-honored antianginal medication is nitroglycerin (Table 7–3), a smooth muscle relaxant of both systemic arteries and veins, although it affects veins predominantly. A decrease in venous return to the heart decreases preload, decreases left ventricular volume, and subsequently reduces wall tension and afterload. These hemodynamic effects are also of value in treating congestive heart failure. In addition, nitroglycerin dilates the larger conductance coronary arteries and probably also the collateral vessels, thus directly increasing blood supply to ischemic myocardium. The reduction in ventricular diastolic pressure brought about by nitrates may lower resistance to coronary blood flow within the myocardium during diastole.

Beta-adrenergic receptor blockade (Tables 7–4

TABLE 7–5. SIDE EFFECTS OF BETA BLOCKERS

Beta-2 blocking effects:
 Bronchoconstriction
 Failure to initiate glycogenolysis in insulin-induced hypoglycemia
 Exacerbation of peripheral vascular disease
Other
 Exacerbation of congestive heart failure
 Bradycardia and heart block
 Ischemia upon abrupt withdrawal
 Fatigue, depression, impotence, nightmares

and 7–5) slows the resting heart rate, blunts the increase in heart rate with exercise, and decreases myocardial contractility, all of which decrease oxygen consumption. In addition, beta-blocking drugs are useful antihypertensive agents and may reduce cardiac afterload in such patients. Beta-adrenergic receptors can be divided into beta-1 and beta-2 subgroups. The beta-1 receptors mediate the cardiac actions of the sympathetic nervous system, whereas beta-2 receptors promote the glycogenolysis induced by catecholamines, vasodilation of peripheral blood vessels, and dilation of pulmonary bronchi. Therefore, beta blockers that have predominantly beta-1 rather than beta-2 sympathetic antagonism (e.g., atenolol and metoprolol) may be more useful in treating patients with bronchospastic pulmonary disease, chronic obstructive pulmonary disease, diabetes, and peripheral vascular disease. However, selective beta-1 blockade is only relative, and at higher doses (for example, above 100 mg a day of metoprolol) the selectivity may be lost. Hydrophilic beta blockers, for example atenolol and nadolol, have relatively long half-lives, can be administered once daily, and tend not to penetrate into the central nervous system, which may produce fewer neurological side effects such as mental depression and sleep disturbances. Thus, side effects attributed to one beta blocker may be eliminated by switching to another. Pindolol has mild intrinsic sympathomimetic activity in addition to its beta receptor–blocking activity; that is, it acts as a beta receptor agonist as well as antagonist. Theoretically, some of the effects at rest of beta-receptor blockade such as slow heart rate or peripheral vasoconstriction may be less prominent even though the sympathetic effects of exercise are blocked. Any clinical advantage to beta-receptor blockers with intrinsic sympathomimetic activity is not clear at present.

Calcium ions play critical roles in myocardial contraction, coronary vascular smooth muscle constriction, and the genesis of the cardiac action potential. Slow channel blocking agents are effective antianginal drugs when used either alone or in combination with beta-receptor adrenergic blockers or nitrates (Table 7–6). All three agents currently available in the United States (nifedipine, verapamil, and diltiazem) decrease myocardial contractility and relax coronary and peripheral vascular smooth muscle. Verapamil and diltiazem may decrease the sinus nodal discharge rate and prolong atrioventricular (AV) nodal conduction time. In clinically used doses, nifedipine is the most potent vasodilator of the three and exerts little action on myocardial contractility or on the sinus and AV nodes. Therefore, nifedipine decreases afterload via peripheral vasodilation and increases coronary blood flow via coronary vasodilation. The antianginal effect of verapamil may be related to both coronary artery vasodilation and decreased myocardial contractility, thus decreasing oxygen demand. The effects on contractility and sinus rate are minimized owing to reflex sympathetic stimulation in response to the peripheral vasodilation. Verapamil and the other

TABLE 7–6. CALCIUM ANTAGONISTS

	SINUS AND AV NODAL EFFECTS	NEGATIVE INOTROPIC EFFECTS	CORONARY AND PERIPHERAL VASODILATION	USUAL DOSE	SIDE EFFECTS
Nifedipine	0	0/+	+++	10-20 mg q6-8h	Hypotension Headache Dizziness Nausea Peripheral edema Reflex tachycardia with worsening of angina
Diltiazem	++	+	++	30-60 mg q6-8h	LV failure Bradycardia, AV block Hypotension Flushing
Verapamil	+++	++	++	80-120 mg q6-8h	LV failure Bradycardia, AV block Nausea Flushing Decreases excretion of digoxin by 30%

0 = none   ++ = moderate effect
+ = mild effect   +++ = strong effect

calcium antagonists enhance left ventricular diastolic filling (increase compliance); this is not an effect of simple beta blockade. In general, the effects of diltiazem are intermediate between those of verapamil and nifedipine.

Since the mechanisms of action of nitrates, beta-receptor blockers, and calcium antagonists differ, combination therapy of two or three of these drugs might be effective. Nitrates can cause reflex tachycardia that beta-receptor blockers can prevent. Therefore, in a patient with no contraindication to beta-receptor blockade, the combination of nitrates and a beta-receptor blocker may be beneficial antianginal therapy. In addition, the combination of beta blockers and calcium channel blockers is often useful if unwanted electrophysiological or inotropic side effects do not become manifest. Especially useful combinations may be a beta-receptor blocker plus nifedipine, or verapamil and a long-acting nitrate; these combinations would provide coronary arterial dilation along with decreased myocardial contractility and oxygen demand without subjecting the patient to two medications having similar side effects. Patients with particularly severe angina may require one drug from each of the three classes.

A patient experiencing a marked increase in the frequency or severity of angina, the new onset of angina at rest, or nocturnal angina should probably be admitted to an intensive care unit, placed at bed rest, and sedated if necessary. If not contraindicated, beta blockade should be instituted. Sublingual nitroglycerin, oral and/or cutaneous nitrates should be administered, and if pain recurs, intravenous nitroglycerin can be initiated. In addition, nifedipine may be useful in the patient with no hypotension or with congestive heart failure. Verapamil or diltiazem may be useful in the patient with no heart failure. Most patients having unstable angina experience relief of chest pain with this approach and further eval-

uation, probably including coronary arteriography, can be undertaken when the patient is stable and pain-free. If angina does not abate with aggressive medical therapy, the patient should be considered for early coronary arteriography and for angioplasty or bypass surgery. An intra-aortic balloon pump may be inserted before cardiac catheterization or surgery to improve diastolic filling of the coronary arteries and to decrease afterload. Many patients experience pain relief once balloon counterpulsation is initiated despite refractoriness to intensive medical antianginal therapy.

NONMEDICAL MANAGEMENT OF ANGINA PECTORIS

Coronary artery bypass surgery is useful to relieve angina unresponsive to medical therapy and, in certain subgroups, to prolong life. Coronary artery bypass surgery may be combined with aneurysmectomy in patients with refractory cardiac arrhythmias, congestive heart failure, or recurrent emboli due to a large ventricular aneurysm. Coronary artery bypass alone usually does not improve left ventricular function sufficiently to treat patients in whom congestive heart failure is the major manifestation of ischemic heart disease. Intractable, chronic ventricular arrhythmias also are not usually abolished by revascularization alone and require resection of the tachycardia focus.

Coronary artery bypass grafting most commonly involves harvesting saphenous veins from the legs to anastomose from the ascending aorta to the coronary artery at a site distal to the obstruction. The veins are reversed in direction to permit the flow of blood past the venous valves. As many major arterial branches as possible are grafted beyond significant obstructions. Internal mammary grafts demonstrate a superior long-term patency compared with saphenous grafts. Both the left and right internal mammary arteries may be dissected free and anastomosed to a coronary artery distal to its obstruction. The proximal take-off of the internal mammary artery remains intact from the subclavian artery. Internal mammary grafts are most commonly anastomosed to the left anterior descending coronary artery vessels. The distal coronary vessels must be at least 1 to 2 mm in diameter to accept a bypass graft, and the flow distal to the occlusion, determined at the time of coronary arteriography, should be sufficient to maintain flow in the grafts so that thrombosis is unlikely to occur. Left ventricular dysfunction increases the risk of surgery but does not necessarily contraindicate surgery if chest pain is refractory.

Perioperative mortality is approximately 0.7 per cent for those with normal left ventricular function and 1.8 per cent for those with abnormal ventricular function. Surgical mortality in patients with left main coronary artery disease is approximately 2.5 per cent, and if left ventricular function is abnormal, approaches 4 per cent. Surgical mortality increases with age, reaching 2 per cent in patients older than 65 years. The incidence of perioperative myocardial infarction is reported to be 5 to 10 per cent. Chest pain is completely relieved in approximately 65 per cent of patients, and significant improvement in pain occurs in an additional 25 per cent. The remaining patients are either not improved (5 per cent) or worse (5 per cent) after surgery. Approximately 2 to 4 per cent of patients per year have a recurrence of angina, due either to obstruction of the grafts or to progressive atherosclerosis in the native arteries. If angina recurs either early or late after surgery, repeat catheterization may be indicated if surgery or angioplasty is deemed necessary. Repeat operations carry a higher surgical risk and less successfully relieve pain. Patients with one- or two-vessel coronary artery disease have relatively good survival with medical or surgical therapy as long as their clinical status is stable, and they usually can be followed medically until refractory angina appears. The role of coronary artery bypass grafting in patients with three-vessel coronary artery disease is more controversial, but a recent study suggests that patients with three-vessel coronary artery disease who have either no symptoms or stable angina pectoris have no higher mortality with medicine than with surgery as their initial therapy. These patients, however, represent a select subgroup of relatively stable patients with three-vessel disease; patients with three-vessel disease and poor functional capacity, judged either on the treadmill or by their inability to perform as much daily activity as they would like, may benefit from bypass grafting. In addition, some studies demonstrate a tendency toward improved survival with surgery in patients with three-vessel disease and moderate ventricular dysfunction.

Percutaneous transluminal coronary angioplasty (PTCA) involves passing a balloon catheter into the coronary artery, positioning it across a stenotic lesion, and inflating the balloon with several atmospheres of pressure to dilate the stenosis. This procedure disrupts the intima, splits the atherosclerotic plaque, and often results in a small local dissection with relief of obstruction. Candidates for angioplasty have angina for which surgical revascularization would be recommended and discrete, relatively proximal stenoses in one or more coronary vessels. Studies demonstrate the feasibility of angioplasty on multiple lesions. Patients with left main coronary artery disease are not appropriate candidates for coronary angioplasty because a dissection in this vessel would jeopardize the majority of the myocardial blood flow. PTCA is successful (at least 25 to 50 per cent improvement in luminal diameter) in approximately 80 per cent of cases. In about 5 per cent of cases, coronary occlusion occurs and immediate coronary artery bypass grafting must be undertaken. Therefore, except under special circumstances, patients who are candidates for PTCA should also be candidates for operative intervention in case complications occur. Restenosis occurs in approximately 20 per cent of patients who initially have a good result, usually within the first six months. A second angioplasty is successful in some of these patients. The reported mortality from angioplasty ranges from 0.5 to 1 per cent. Long-term follow-up of patients after angioplasty is not yet available (Table 7–7).

Graft flow rates at the time of surgery can help predict graft closure. The average flow in a technically successful saphenous bypass graft is about 70 ml/min. Grafts in which the flow is less than 45 ml/min frequently occlude. Causes of poor graft flow include grafting to a vessel with a noncritical stenosis proximal to the graft anastomosis, a technically poor anastomosis, and poor distal run off secondary to distal vessel disease. Graft patency rates at 6 to 12 months are 75 to 87 per cent; since most patients receive more than one graft, 84 to 95 per cent of patients have at least one patent graft. Internal mammary grafts have a

TABLE 7–7. COMPARISON OF CORONARY ARTERY BYPASS GRAFTING (CABG) AND PERCUTANEOUS TRANSLUMINAL CORONARY ANGIOPLASTY (PTCA)

PTCA	CABG
Nonsurgical	Major surgery
Useful for proximal, discrete stenosis. Multiple vessels increase difficulty and risk. Lesions in some vessels (e.g., LAD) are more likely to be successfully dilated than others.	Useful for multiple, more distal and heavily calcified lesions as well as proximal, discrete lesions. Procedure of choice for left main stenosis
Risk of coronary artery dissection and emergency surgery	Risk of elective surgery
Patient should be a potential surgical candidate except under special circumstances.	Patient must be a surgical candidate
May be faster in an emergency situation (e.g., acute MI)	Associated defects (aneurysm, valve dysfunction) may be addressed
Long-term results unknown	Long-term results known

much higher patency rate than saphenous grafts, and over 95 per cent are patent after one year.

VARIANT ANGINA

In 1959 Prinzmetal described a syndrome of chest pain occurring unrelated to exertion and associated with ST segment elevation recorded on the ECG (see Table 7–1). The syndrome is often associated with cardiac arrhythmias, including ventricular fibrillation and heart block, and sudden death may occur. These episodes of angina more commonly occur between midnight and 8 a.m. Rarely, acute myocardial infarction results. Prinzmetal's angina appears to be due to spasm in the conductance portion of the coronary arteries, resulting in decreased oxygen delivery to the myocardium. Patients may have concomitant fixed obstructive lesions and therefore also experience angina with exertion. The classic electrocardiographic pattern of coronary spasm is localized ST elevation, although ST depression alone or T wave changes may occur. Coronary angiography during Prinzmetal's angina may reveal spasm at the site of a severe coronary atherosclerotic lesion, a mild atherosclerotic lesion, or a normal coronary artery. Patients with no or mild fixed coronary obstruction tend to have a more benign course than those with severe obstructions. The cause of coronary spasm is unknown. Provocative testing with ergonovine, an ergot alkaloid with alpha-adrenergic and serotoninergic effects, is a relatively sensitive and specific test for coronary artery spasm. Vessels prone to spasm appear to be supersensitive to its vasoconstrictive properties. When administered in incremental doses to a total of 0.05 to 0.4 mg intravenously, coronary artery spasm, chest pain, and ST elevation are provoked in susceptible individuals. Prolonged spasm with significant ischemia and serious arrhythmias is a potential hazard. Nitroglycerin may be injected directly into the coronary vasculature to quickly reverse the spasm if it is severe. Ergonovine testing generally is safe, especially if performed in the catheterization lab, but probably should not be done in patients who have flow-restricting coronary obstructions, and the drug should be administered in extremely low starting doses.

In patients with Prinzmetal's angina beta blockade may be detrimental by allowing unopposed alpha-adrenergic vasoconstriction. Calcium channel blockers are very effective in treating vasospastic angina, and their effects may be additive to that of nitrates, since the mechanism of action is different. Coronary artery bypass surgery is not helpful in patients with vasospasm and normal or nearly normal coronary arteries but may be useful in patients who have fixed significant stenoses.

ACUTE MYOCARDIAL INFARCTION

PATHOLOGY AND MECHANISM

Myocardial infarction refers to irreversible necrosis of myocardium. It usually results from atherosclerotic narrowing of a major coronary artery that creates an unfavorable balance of myocardial oxygen supply versus demand. Initially ischemia occurs and if severe and prolonged, myocardial infarction follows, the extent of which depends on the severity of the ischemia, the area of muscle supplied by the obstructed coronary artery, the extent of collateral blood flow, and the oxygen demands of the tissue supplied by the artery. Myocardial infarction may be transmural, that is, involving the full thickness of the left ventricular wall, or nontransmural, involving only the subendocardium and adjacent myocardium. The electrocardiographic findings of "transmural" versus "subendocardial" infarction do not correlate well with the pathological extent of infarction. No gross pathological changes occur in the myocardium until approximately six hours after myocardial infarction, and even light microscopic findings until that time are subtle. The myocardium initially appears pale and slightly edematous and over the next few days changes color as exudate and neutrophil infiltration occur. Eight to ten days after infarction the myocardium in the region of the infarction thins as debris is removed by mononuclear cells, and granulation tissue forms that by three to four weeks extends through the necrotic tissue. Subsequently, a thin scar develops that becomes firm over a six-week interval.

Ninety per cent of transmural myocardial infarctions are associated with complete obstruction of a coronary artery, consisting of fresh thrombus superimposed on a critically stenotic lesion. Nontransmural myocardial infarctions frequently occur distal to severely stenotic but still patent arteries. Mechanisms by which thrombosis occurs in the region of atherosclerotic plaques may include changes in the atherosclerotic intima promoting thrombosis, hemorrhage into the atherosclerotic plaque, ulceration of the plaque with activation of clotting factors, platelet thrombi, or coronary spasm at the site of a plaque causing sludging of blood flow and deposition of platelets and fibrin. Reperfusion can be achieved in many cases using intracoronary or intravenous fibrinolytic agents; however, residual high-grade atherosclerotic lesions are usually present at the site of occlusion after thrombi dissolution.

CLINICAL PRESENTATION

Signs and symptoms of acute myocardial infarction are summarized in Tables 7–8 and 2–2. The usual patient with myocardial infarction has severe chest pain that lasts until treated. Some patients are discovered to have suffered a myocardial infarction by electrocardiography or noninvasive evaluation of left ventricular function without any clinical history of infarction. In many of these patients, when a very careful history is obtained, an episode can be identified that probably represents the myocardial infarction. However, some people, especially diabetics, have true "silent" myocardial infarctions.

The electrocardiogram in acute myocardial in-

TABLE 7–8. SYMPTOMS AND SIGNS OF ACUTE MYOCARDIAL INFARCTION

Symptoms (see Table 2–2)
  Severe, prolonged chest pain, similar in quality to angina pectoris
  Nausea, vomiting
  Diaphoresis
  Shortness of breath
  Weakness
Signs
  Anxiety
  Elevated blood pressure (if shock not present)
  Tachycardia (may have bradycardia with inferior MI)
  Dyskinetic left ventricular impulse
  Small amplitude carotid pulses
  Soft heart sounds
  S_4 gallop
  Fixed or paradoxically split S_2
  Systolic murmur of papillary muscle dysfunction
  Loud systolic murmur with papillary muscle or ventricular septal
    rupture
  S_3 gallop and/or rales (congestive heart failure)
  Right ventricular S_3 gallop with jugular venous distention (right
    ventricular infarction)
  Signs of cardiogenic shock if > 40% of myocardium is infarcted
  Low-grade fever
  Pericardial friction rub (3rd-4th day, with transmural infarctions)
  Atrial or ventricular tachyarrhythmias, heart block

farction is discussed in Chapter 2 (see Tables 2–15 and 2–16 and Fig. 2–9). The diagnosis of subendocardial infarction may be suspected from electrocardiographic ST and T wave changes but must be confirmed by enzyme determinations. There are no chest x-ray findings characteristic of myocardial infarction. The white blood cell count rises the first day after a myocardial infarction and returns to normal within a week; it usually peaks between 12,000 and 15,000 cells/cu mm. Acute phase reactants, such as the erythrocyte sedimentation rate, may be elevated. Several cardiac enzymes released into the blood (Fig. 7–2) are used to diagnose myocardial infarction. Creatine kinase MB (the fraction characteristic of cardiac muscle) is the most sensitive and specific marker of myocardial necrosis, and an MB fraction exceeding 7 to 8 per cent is indicative of myocardial infarction even if the total CPK is not greater than normal. Injury to skeletal muscle causes the skeletal muscle fraction (MM) of CPK to rise. Other forms of injury to cardiac muscle, such as myocarditis, trauma, and cardiac surgery, may release significant amounts of creatine kinase MB fraction. Cardioversion and CPR usually do not elevate the MB function. Serum lactate dehydrogenase (LDH) may be fractionated into five isozymes. LDH_1 is principally from the heart, and if LDH_1 exceeds LDH_2, myocardial infarction is likely. LDH is sometimes useful in diagnosing myocardial infarction in a patient who presents several days after the event, when the creatine kinase has normalized. Hemolysis can raise LDH_1 activity, but LDH_2 also elevates and exceeds LDH_1. Liver and skeletal muscle contain mainly LDH_4 and LDH_5.

The use of infarct-avid scintigraphy has been discussed in Chapter 2. Echocardiography may demonstrate a segmental wall motion abnormality but cannot distinguish whether it is old or new.

GENERAL MANAGEMENT OF MYOCARDIAL INFARCTION

Since approximately 50 per cent of patients who die from myocardial infarction do so within the first four hours after the onset of chest pain, often before they ever arrive at the hospital, the prehospital management of myocardial infarction is important. Many large cities employ emergency medical technicians who can recognize the symptoms of myocardial infarction, initiate electrocardiographic monitoring, and treat ventricular tachyarrhythmias, terminating them with electrical defibrillation if necessary. Airway management, intravenous drug delivery, and cardiopulmonary resuscitation may be administered, if needed. Prehospital emergency cardiac care, especially the rapid treatment of life-threatening ventricular arrhythmias, improves both early and late survival from myocardial infarction.

The coronary intensive care unit allows continuous electrocardiographic and hemodynamic monitoring, delivery of intensive nursing care, and immediate treatment of arrhythmias or other problems. The advent of the coronary care unit has improved survival of patients with myocardial infarction mainly by reducing mortality from arrhythmias. Prevention of death from hemodynamic deterioration has been less successful and accounts for most of the mortality in coronary care units. Future progress in this area will probably come from thrombolysis of acute coronary obstructions.

Some general principles in treating patients with uncomplicated myocardial infarction include sedation if necessary, a calm, quiet coronary

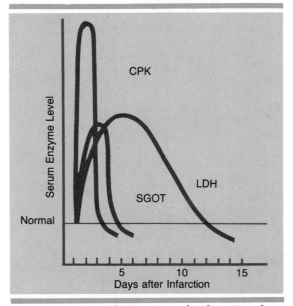

FIGURE 7–2. Typical time course for detection of enzymes released from the myocardium upon necrosis. CPK = Creatine phosphokinase; SGOT = serum glutamine ornithine transferase; LDH = lactic dehydrogenase.

care unit atmosphere, and control of pain to decrease patient anxiety, sympathetic drive, and myocardial oxygen demand. Morphine can be administered intravenously in doses of 2 to 8 mg repeated at intervals of 5 to 15 minutes until pain is relieved or drug side effects (e.g., hypotension, respiratory depression, nausea, vomiting, or vagal side effects such as bradycardia) appear. Small IV doses of atropine treat the vagomimetic side effects of morphine, and naloxone 0.4 mg IV at 5-minute intervals to a maximal dosage of 1.2 mg reverses respiratory depression if needed. After the acute severe pain is relieved, nitroglycerin can be used cautiously for recurrent angina, and chronic nitrate therapy may be initiated if angina persists. Oxygen can be omitted if the patient is not hypoxemic.

The patient with *uncomplicated* acute myocardial infarction should be confined to bed for the first 24 to 36 hours except for the use of a bedside commode. He should then be allowed to sit up out of bed for short periods of time and can be transferred out of the coronary care unit after three days, since life-threatening arrhythmias are uncommon after 36 to 48 hours. Ambulation is usually begun on the fourth to fifth day and is increased progressively so that at discharge the patient is able to walk up a flight of stairs. Early mobilization increases the patient's psychological well-being, prevents deconditioning, and decreases the incidence of thromboembolism. Many patients require stool softeners or laxatives to avoid constipation and straining at stool. Nausea and vomiting either from the infarction or drugs can be treated with a clear liquid diet. A gentle rectal examination in patients with acute myocardial infarction is not contraindicated.

The use of anticoagulation in acute myocardial infarction is controversial. If no contraindication exists, "minidose" heparin (5000 units subcutaneously every 8 to 12 hours) may decrease the incidence of deep vein thrombosis and possibly systemic embolization. In patients who have a high risk of embolization, such as those who have a ventricular aneurysm with thrombus, past or present thrombophlebitis, or previous systemic or pulmonary embolism, full systemic anticoagulation may be reasonable in the absence of contraindications. Systemic anticoagulation is contraindicated in patients with postinfarction pericarditis because of the risk of hemorrhage into the pericardium. Minidose heparin is stopped once the patient is ambulating, usually two to three days prior to hospital discharge. Continuation of systemic anticoagulation depends upon the original indication for therapy. Patients with left ventricular thrombi after myocardial infarction are at high risk of embolization, and this risk may be decreased by prophylactic systemic anticoagulation for about six months.

In patients with known or suspected acute myocardial infarction, lidocaine effectively prevents many ventricular tachyarrhthmias. If it is administered appropriately, side effects such as confusion, dizziness, and parasthesias can be minimized. Both the loading and maintenance doses of lidocaine should be decreased in elderly patients, patients with congestive heart failure, and patients with liver disease. Although ventricular fibrillation should be easily treatable in the coronary care unit, many physicians feel that, given the safety of lidocaine, it is advisable to attempt to prevent ventricular fibrillation rather than have to electrically defibrillate it should it occur. However, the prophylactic administration of lidocaine in this situation is still somewhat controversial. The dose of lidocaine should be increased if ventricular tachycardia occurs. Suppression of premature ventricular contractions (PVC's) is questionable, since their value (including "R on T" PVC's) as prognostic indicators or precipitators of the onset of more severe arrhythmias is questionable. Prophylactic lidocaine is continued for approximately 48 hours, after which the risk of ventricular tachyarrhythmias is reduced.

Patients with uncomplicated courses are usually discharged from the hospital between 7 and 12 days following infarction. The patient should gradually increase his activity but avoid isometric exercise (for example, lifting weights) and get adequate rest. He should be instructed in the use of sublingual nitroglycerin even if he requires no antianginal therapy on discharge. Many centers have formal rehabilitation programs in which the patient is supervised during activity and his electrocardiogram monitored. Exercise testing in patients after acute myocardial infarction helps determine what level of activity can be performed safely at home and is useful to identify those patients at high risk for recurrent events by finding a positive ST response and/or chest pain within the first two stages of exercise. Some physicians perform a limited treadmill test (the heart rate achieved is only 70 per cent of predicted maximum) just prior to hospital discharge, whereas others prefer a more normal stress test protocol six weeks after infarction. Patients who are considered at high risk on the basis of their clinical course and/or treadmill exercise test results may subsequently undergo coronary arteriography.

Large studies with timolol, propranolol, and metoprolol have shown that these agents reduce overall mortality, sudden death, and/or reinfarction if administered to patients after their first infarction. This outcome may be related to anti-ischemic effects, antianginal effects, or some other unknown effect of these drugs. Patients with contraindications to beta-adrenergic receptor blockers, especially heart failure, cannot receive these drugs; unfortunately, these patients are at the highest risk for a recurrent event. In addition, the mortality in the group of patients that can tolerate these drugs is relatively small, and thus even a 50 per cent reduction in sudden death or reinfarction does not represent a large proportion of the total patients. Despite these reservations, many physicians feel that it is advisable to administer beta-adrenergic receptor blocking drugs in doses sufficient to blunt the heart rate response to exercise in postinfarction patients who have no contraindication, and the drug should be continued for approximately two years.

FIGURE 7–3. Restoration of coronary blood flow after thrombolytic therapy with streptokinase. *A,* Completely obstructed vessel prior to administration of streptokinase. *B,* Restoration of flow after administration of intracoronary streptokinase. Note that a fixed atherosclerotic lesion is still present at the site of previous occlusion. *C,* Subsequent coronary angioplasty results in dilation of the fixed lesion. (Courtesy of James C. Dillon, M.D.)

Early ventricular tachyarrhythmias during acute myocardial infarction (i.e., first 24 to 48 hours) do not warrant chronic antiarrhythmic drug therapy. Patients with chronic complex ventricular ectopy, especially ventricular tachycardia, are at particularly high risk for sudden death in the first six months to a year after myocardial infarction. However, chronic antiarrhythmic therapy has not been shown to decrease mortality in patients with premature ventricular contractions (PVC's) or ventricular tachycardia after infarction. Therefore, at the present time there appears to be no compelling evidence to support treating patients with uniform or multiform PVC's or pairs of PVC's after infarction. In patients with episodes of nonsustained ventricular tachycardia after infarction, it seems prudent to treat with a type I antiarrhythmic agent (i.e., quinidine) to eliminate the spontaneous tachycardia, although there are no objective data to support this approach.

LIMITATION OF INFARCT SIZE

Any intervention to limit the size of an evolving infarction must be performed within the first four to six hours of infarction, before cells become irreversibly necrotic. The most promising techniques involve early reperfusion, i.e., fibrinolysis (e.g., streptokinase), coronary angioplasty, or surgery within the first four to six hours after infarction.

Most patients with acute transmural myocardial infarction have complete obstruction of a coronary artery due to thrombosis that can be documented safely with coronary arteriography within the first four hours of infarction. Administration of intracoronary streptokinase to lyse clots by activating plasminogen opens the coronary artery in 70 to 80 per cent of these patients (somewhat lower if intravenous streptokinase is employed) (Fig. 7–3). Electrocardiographic evidence of infarction usually still evolves. The time course of cardiac enzyme elevation is accelerated, thought to be evidence of washout of enzymes from the heart by reperfusion. Thus, even though this technique does not prevent infarction, it may salvage a portion of the myocardium in jeopardy. There is usually a high-grade stenosis in the area of thrombosis that can be dilated acutely with coronary angioplasty at the time of streptokinase infusion or approached with angioplasty or surgery at a later date to prevent reocclusion. Long-term results and potential complications (e.g., intramyocardial hemorrhage) are still being determined. Both intracoronary and intravenous streptokinase have profound systemic fibrinolytic effects, and massive bleeding may occur from arterial puncture sites or surgical wounds.

The role of angioplasty during acute myocardial infarction either with or without streptokinase administration is also under investigation. Even though early surgical revascularization is possible after myocardial infarction, it is logistically difficult to perform within the first four to six hours after the onset of chest pain and has not been demonstrated definitively to limit infarct size.

COMPLICATIONS OF MYOCARDIAL INFARCTION AND THEIR MANAGEMENT
(Table 7–9)

In patients who develop mild congestive heart failure with pulmonary congestion during acute myocardial infarction, administration of a diuretic may be sufficient therapy. Indications for hemodynamic monitoring are listed in Table 7–10. Hemodynamic monitoring allows measurement of left ventricular filling pressures (pulmonary capillary wedge pressure) and cardiac output, and the calculation of systemic vascular resistance. Patients with myocardial infarction may be grouped into subsets based on these measurements (Table 7–11). When the normal cardiac index (approximately 2.5 to 3.6 L/min/sq m) is reduced to 1.8 to 2.2 L/min/sq m, hypoperfusion occurs; shock occurs at levels less than 1.8 L/min/sq m. The normal pulmonary capillary wedge pressure is 10 to 12 mm Hg, but the optimum wedge pressure in a patient with acute myocardial infarction and a relatively noncompliant ventricle is usually 14 to 18 mm Hg.

Even if pharmacological therapy or intra-aortic balloon counterpulsation provides temporary improvement, patients with cardiogenic shock due to cardiac muscle destruction have a poor prognosis. However, patients who have cardiogenic shock secondary to surgically correctable mechanical factors, for example, acute mitral regurgitation or acquired ventricular septal defect, have a somewhat more favorable outlook. Myocardial revascularization improves an occasional patient with episodes of profound but reversible myocardial ischemia producing hypotension and shock.

Patients with right ventricular infarction may present with hypotension or shock (due to decreased cardiac output) and signs of right ventricular failure. The lungs are clear if left ventricular failure or pre-existing pulmonary disease is not present. Tricuspid insufficiency may occur. Fluid administration to raise right ventricular filling pressures and augment left ventricular filling reverses the shock and hypotension, even when jugular venous distention and other manifestations of systemic congestion exist. Right ventricular infarction is relatively common in patients with inferior myocardial infarction and is sometimes difficult to differentiate from cardiac tamponade. Most patients with right ventricular infarction do well, and their long-term prognosis depends on the extent of left ventricular infarction.

Approximately 20 per cent of patients extend their myocardial infarction within the first five days after infarction. The extension may be associated with recurrent chest pain that is sometimes difficult to distinguish from post–myocardial infarction pericarditis or recurrent angina. Continued angina and extension of myocardial infarction are usually unfavorable signs and may be indications for catheterization.

Many patients upon presentation with an acute myocardial infarction have mild to moderate hypertension because of pain, anxiety, and sometimes mild congestive heart failure. With relief of pain and treatment of heart failure, hypertension usually disappears within a few hours. However, sustained or severe blood pressure elevation should be treated vigorously to decrease myocardial oxygen consumption. Intravenous nitroprusside may be employed, and oral agents can be substituted as needed.

Rupture of an entire papillary muscle due to myocardial infarction is usually rapidly fatal owing to massive mitral regurgitation. However, rupture of one head of a papillary muscle may be tolerated for a period of time, allowing for diagnostic evaluation and surgical correction. Some form of papillary muscle rupture occurs in less than 5 per cent of patients with acute infarction. Papillary muscle dysfunction is more common than rupture and occurs when ischemia interferes with contraction of the papillary muscles and normal coaptation of the mitral valve leaflets. The degree of mitral regurgitation from papillary muscle dysfunction is usually less than that caused by papillary muscle rupture. Acute medical therapy for papillary muscle rupture may require inotropic agents, diuretics, vasodilators, or intra-aortic balloon counterpulsation. If the patient can be stabilized and weaned from balloon counterpulsation, surgical mitral valve replacement may be attempted four to six weeks after infarction when infarct scar formation is advanced. However, if hemodynamic stabilization cannot be obtained or requires intra-aortic balloon counterpulsation, early mitral valve replacement should be undertaken.

Rupture of the ventricular septum develops in about 1 per cent of myocardial infarctions and results in marked biventricular failure. It may occur with both inferior and anterior infarctions. It is associated with a holosystolic murmur along the left sternal border and is often difficult to differentiate from acute mitral insufficiency. A thrill is more common with ventricular septal defects than acute mitral regurgitation. Right heart (Swan-Ganz) catheterization may be necessary to distinguish acute ventricular septal rupture from mitral regurgitation by detecting an oxygen step-up between the right atrium and right ventricle. Increased pulmonary vascularity due to the left-to-right shunt may be seen on chest x-ray. Two-dimensional echocardiography can occasionally visualize the ventricular septal defect, but more often a septal aneurysm is demonstrated, with the ventricular septal defect presumably located in the apex of the aneurysm. Contrast echocardiography may define the defect. Surgical mortality is highest within the first month after infarction, but if ventricular failure is severe, surgery must be undertaken early.

A ventricular aneurysm is a localized area of thin, scarred myocardium that protrudes beyond and distorts the ventricular cavity (Fig. 7–4). Ventricular aneurysms may develop within days of myocardial infarction and gradually stretch, thin, and enlarge over weeks to months. The wall motion of an aneurysm on ventriculography may be

TABLE 7–9. COMPLICATIONS OF ACUTE MYOCARDIAL INFARCTION

COMPLICATION	CLINICAL PRESENTATION	PROGNOSIS/NATURAL HISTORY	THERAPY
Congestive heart failure	Symptoms and signs of heart failure (Table 2–4) or cardiogenic shock (Table 3–9)	Severe heart failure carries a poor prognosis unless a surgically correctable condition (e.g., ruptured ventricular septum or papillary muscle) is present.	See Table 3–7 See Table 3–10
Right ventricular infarction	Usually accompanies inferior MI; hypotension with clear lungs, distended jugular veins; cardiac output low, left ventricular filling pressure low; ST elevation in leads V_1 and V_{4R}	Depends on extent of LV infarction	Fluid administration
Extension of infarction	Recurrent chest pain after initial stabilization; further ECG changes and enzyme increases	Guarded prognosis	Pain relief Antianginal therapy Consider early catheterization and revascularization
Hypertension	Often related to pain or early heart failure May exacerbate angina	Usually responds to therapy	Pain relief Sedation Treat heart failure Antianginal vasodilators If BP elevation remains significant, may need to use IV nitroprusside
Papillary muscle rupture	Acute onset of congestive heart failure, usually 1-7 days after infarction; loud systolic murmur along left sternal border; echo may show flail mitral valve; Swan-Ganz shows no left-to-right shunt, often large v waves in wedge position	If patient can be stabilized, surgery can be postponed 4-6 weeks to allow healing of infarct; if not, early surgery may be life-saving although risky.	Afterload reduction Diuretics Digitalis Intra-aortic balloon pump Surgery
Ventricular septal rupture	Same presentation and murmur as above; contrast echo may demonstrate defect; Swan-Ganz shows left-to-right shunt.	Same as above	Same as above
Ventricular aneurysm	Often no symptoms, but may be associated with congestive heart failure, arrhythmias, or emboli; persistent ST elevation on ECG; visualized on two-dimensional echo	Does not rupture; prognosis depends on amount of remaining myocardium and complications (heart failure, arrhythmias, emboli)	Anticoagulation if mural thrombus is detected on echo or angiography Antiarrhythmic therapy as needed Treat heart failure Surgery if symptoms persist
Cardiac rupture	Acute onset of cardiogenic shock, usually within first week after infarction; occasional patient will wall off the rupture within the pericardial space (pseudoaneurysm) and survive; pseudoaneurysm detectable on echocardiography	Usually rapid death	Emergency surgery if possible
Deep venous thrombosis, pulmonary embolism	Warm, tender edematous extremity; with pulmonary embolus dyspnea, tachycardia, hypoxia, pleuritic chest pain, hemoptysis; cardiovascular collapse with massive pulmonary embolus; diagnosis via venogram, lung scan, and/or pulmonary angiogram	Recurrent emboli if therapy is not instituted	Anticoagulation with heparin, then warfarin

TABLE 7–9. COMPLICATIONS OF ACUTE MYOCARDIAL INFARCTION (*continued*)

COMPLICATION	CLINICAL PRESENTATION	PROGNOSIS/NATURAL HISTORY	THERAPY
Pericarditis early after MI	Chest pain sharper than that of infarction, usually located to the left of sternum toward the apex, not responsive to nitrates, better sitting up and leaning forward, occurs within a week after a transmural infarction; causes sinus tachycardia, diffuse ST elevation on ECG	Self-limited	Aspirin Nonsteroidal anti-inflammatory agents Avoid anticoagulation
Postinfarction (Dressler's) syndrome	Occurs 2 weeks to 9 months after MI; pericarditis, pericardial effusion, pleural effusion, pneumonitis, fever	Self-limited, but multiple recurrences may occur	Aspirin Nonsteroidal anti-inflammatory agents If above unsuccessful, short course of steroids
Arrhythmias (See also Chapter 8) a. Ventricular tachycardia or fibrillation	Syncope, cardiac arrest; dizziness, palpitations	Immediate prognosis depends on prompt termination; long-term prognosis depends on LV function and chronic recurrences	Cardioversion/defibrillation of sustained arrhythmias Lidocaine or other antiarrhythmic agent
b. Atrial fibrillation/flutter	Increased angina, heart failure, palpitations Associated with pericarditis, pulmonary embolus, and heart failure	Prognosis depends on underlying condition.	Digitalis ± quinidine Cardioversion
c. Heart block and conduction disturbances	Dizziness, syncope, increased angina, or heart failure if symptoms occur	Natural history depends on type of block present (see text); long-term prognosis depends on LV function	Indications for pacing in text

akinetic or dyskinetic. Large aneurysms may contribute to congestive heart failure by expanding during systole, decreasing the efficiency of blood expulsion. Most patients with ventricular aneurysms are asymptomatic. True ventricular aneurysms do not rupture. Mural thrombi commonly form in the ventricular aneurysms and appear less likely to embolize in patients who are systemically anticoagulated. Ventricular aneurysms often are associated with ventricular tachyarrhythmias originating from the edge of the aneurysm. Patients with ventricular aneurysms usually demonstrate electrocardiographic evidence of transmural myocardial infarction, and in many cases there is persistent ST segment elevation in the ECG leads with vectors pointing toward the aneurysm. Occasionally, the aneurysm can distort the cardiac silhouette enough to be visible on chest x-ray, appearing as a localized bulge on the surface of the left ventricle, sometimes with calcium in the wall. Two-dimensional echocardiography reliably delineates ventricular aneurysms. Refractory congestive heart failure or recurrent systemic emboli despite anticoagulation warrant aneurysmectomy. Aneurysmectomy alone is usually insufficient to control recurrent refractory ventricular tachyarrhythmias, which require combined aneurysmectomy with resection.

Rupture of the ventricular free wall is usually rapidly fatal. Rupture usually occurs within the first five days following transmural infarction. The patient's initial course may be uneventful until the abrupt occurrence of cardiogenic shock and rapid progression to death. Rare patients have survived after successful pericardiocentesis and emergency surgical repair. Occasionally, the course is less acute and blood is walled off within the pericardial space, giving rise to a pseudoaneurysm. In contrast to true aneurysms, pseudoaneurysms may rupture and require immediate intervention. The diagnosis of pseudoaneurysm is usually made by echocardiography, showing a narrow-based communication between the ventricular cavity and pseudoaneurysm, whereas the communication between a true aneurysm and the ventricular cavity is wide.

Early ambulation and the use of prophylactic subcutaneous minidose heparin have decreased the risk of venous thrombosis and pulmonary embolism after myocardial infarction. If deep vein thrombophlebitis or pulmonary embolism is doc-

TABLE 7–10. INDICATIONS FOR HEMODYNAMIC MONITORING IN ACUTE MYOCARDIAL INFARCTION

Hypotension unresponsive to simple measures such as treatment of bradycardia or fluid administration

Moderate or severe LV failure despite diuretic therapy, especially if blood pressure is unstable

Unexplained features such as persistent sinus tachycardia, cyanosis, hypoxia, or acidosis

Suspicion of ventricular septal defect, rupture of papillary muscle, or cardiac tamponade

TABLE 7–11. HEMODYNAMIC PARAMETERS IN ACUTE MYOCARDIAL INFARCTION

CLINICAL STATE	CARDIAC OUTPUT	PULMONIC CAPILLARY WEDGE	LIKELY CAUSE	THERAPY
No pulmonary congestion, normal systemic perfusion	normal	normal	Uncomplicated MI	None
Pulmonary congestion, normal perfusion	normal	↑	Mild to moderate heart failure	Diuretics, preload reduction
Hypoperfusion but no pulmonary congestion	↓	↓	Volume depletion RV infarction	Fluids
Hypoperfusion and pulmonary congestion	↓	↑	Severe heart failure, cardiogenic shock	Diuretics, preload and afterload reduction, inotropic agents, intra-aortic balloon pump

umented, intravenous heparin should be administered for at least seven days and followed by two to six months of oral warfarin. Patients who have systemic emboli also should be treated with intravenous heparin followed by two to six months of oral warfarin. Consideration should be given to removal of peripheral emboli by surgical embolectomy.

Pericarditis occurs in 7 to 15 per cent of patients within the first week after acute infarction, most frequently in those with transmural infarction of at least moderate size. If a pericardial friction rub is heard, the diagnosis is confirmed, but many patients do not have audible rubs. It is sometimes difficult to distinguish the pain of pericarditis from that of angina pectoris. Anticoagulation should be avoided in patients with active pericarditis because of the risk of developing hemorrhagic tamponade. Sinus tachycardia occurring with pericarditis must be differentiated from other causes of sinus tachycardia, for example, hemodynamic deterioration.

A small number of patients, probably less than 5 per cent, develop a late postinfarction syndrome (Dressler's syndrome) consisting of pericarditis, pericardial effusion, pleural effusion, and sometimes fever. The etiology is unknown but may be immunological. Multiple recurrences sometimes occur. If salicylates or nonsteroidal anti-inflammatory agents are not sufficient, short courses of high-dose corticosteroids provide relief.

FIGURE 7–4. Left ventriculogram in the right anterior oblique projection showing an anteroapical aneurysm. There is distortion of the ventricular contour in both systole (*A*) and diastole (*B*).

ARRHYTHMIAS IN ACUTE MYOCARDIAL INFARCTION

Arrhythmias occurring in patients with acute myocardial infarction should be treated if they cause hemodynamic compromise, augment myocardial oxygen requirements, or predispose to more malignant arrhythmias such as sustained ventricular tachycardia or fibrillation. Some rhythms not ordinarily deleterious may decrease cardiac output in patients who have stiff, noncompliant ventricles by the loss of atrioventricular synchrony. Reversible causes of ventricular ectopy, for example, digitalis excess or metabolic abnormalities, should be considered.

Ventricular premature complexes (PVC's) are very common following acute myocardial infarction. Unless very frequent, they usually cause no problem in themselves but may be forerunners of more serious sustained ventricular tachyarrhythmias. The danger of "R on T" PVC's (a ventricular premature complex occurring during the T wave of a previous complex) has probably been overestimated in the past and probably does not carry any worse prognosis than any other PVC. Even though PVC's are sometimes considered a warning arrhythmia for the subsequent development of ventricular tachycardia or fibrillation, many episodes of ventricular fibrillation occur without any warning arrhythmia. Approximately half of those patients who develop ventricular fibrillation have no warning PVC's, while half of those with warning PVC's do not develop a sustained ventricular tachyarrhythmia. If ventricular tachycardia is not suppressed by lidocaine, intravenous procainamide can be substituted or added to lidocaine. Intravenous bretylium may also be useful to prevent recurrence of sustained or symptomatic ventricular tachyarrhythmias. High-dose or multiple antiarrhythmic drug therapy in patients with simple ventricular ectopy is not warranted. If sustained ventricular tachycardia occurs, it should be cardioverted immediately if hemodynamic compromise occurs. If it is well-tolerated for a short period of time, a limited trial of lidocaine for termination may be tried. The patient with acute infarction should not be allowed to continue having sustained ventricular tachycardia for a prolonged period of time. Ventricular fibrillation occurs in 2 to 3 per cent of hospitalized patients with acute myocardial infarction and should be promptly defibrillated with 200 to 400 joules.

Ventricular tachycardia and fibrillation during the first 36 to 48 hours of acute myocardial infarction do not carry the same prognosis as when they occur later in the recovery period. These early ventricular arrhythmias appear to be due to acute ischemia and do not necessitate long-term, chronic antiarrhythmic therapy. On the other hand, ventricular tachycardia or fibrillation occurring more than 48 hours after infarction are probably due to different electrophysiological mechanisms and may be forerunners of severe, chronic arrhythmias.

Accelerated idioventricular rhythm with rates of 60 to 100 beats/minute occurs commonly during the acute infarction period. This arrhythmia probably does not increase the incidence of more rapid ventricular tachyarrhythmias. It usually does not cause hemodynamic deterioration unless cardiovascular compensation is tenuous and dependent upon normal atrioventricular synchrony. If the rhythm appears to be affecting hemodynamics adversely or increasing the incidence of ventricular ectopy, it can be treated by lidocaine or in some instances by accelerating the sinus rate slightly with atropine or atrial pacing.

Sinus tachycardia that persists in a patient with acute infarction after relief of pain and anxiety is often due to inability of the ventricle to maintain an adequate stroke volume. Not only is it a sign of hemodynamic impairment in some patients but also is detrimental by increasing oxygen demand. Pericarditis, pulmonary embolus, and fever commonly cause sinus tachycardia. The treatment of sinus tachycardia is directed at the underlying cause.

Sinus bradycardia often occurs early after acute inferior myocardial infarction and may be related to ischemia of the sinus node or abnormally elevated vagal tone. If asymptomatic and hemodynamically tolerated, it should not be treated. If it creates symptoms, atropine or temporary pacing may be required.

A rapid ventricular response caused by atrial flutter or fibrillation should be treated vigorously because of the increase in myocardial oxygen consumption. If the ventricular rate cannot be slowed pharmacologically, early electrical cardioversion should be considered. The treatment of atrial tachyarrhythmias is discussed in Chapter 8. Atrial tachyarrhythmias also may be features of pericarditis or pulmonary embolus.

First-degree AV block requires no therapy; if digitalis is thought to be the etiology, it should be discontinued. Second-degree AV block of the Mobitz type I (Wenckebach) type (see Chapter 8) is common in patients with inferior myocardial infarction due to increased vagal tone and/or ischemic involvement of the AV node. It is usually temporary and, if asymptomatic, requires no therapy. If hemodynamic compromise occurs, atropine is effective; if sustained improvement does not occur, temporary pacing may be needed. Type I AV block usually does not lead to high-degree AV block; if it does, the ventricular escape is junctional and usually reliable at reasonable rates (40 to 60/minute). Mobitz type II second-degree AV block is an indication for prophylactic pacing. Type I second-degree AV block is more common with inferior and type II more common with anterior myocardial infarctions.

A prophylactic temporary pacemaker is usually recommended for any patient who has developed complete heart block with an acute myocardial infarction, especially if the infarction is anterior and the site of the heart block likely to be in the His-Purkinje system. Complete AV block should be differentiated from AV dissociation, common

---

in inferior myocardial infarction due to sinus bradycardia with junctional escape or accelerated junctional rhythms (see Chapter 8).

The occurrence of new intraventricular conduction defects (left or right bundle branch block, or right bundle branch block with left anterior or posterior fascicular block) are associated with anterior more often than inferior infarction. The prognosis of these patients, as in those with Mobitz II second degree heart block, is poor, reflecting the extensive infarction rather than the conduction disturbance itself. Even though temporary pacing in these patients has not been shown definitely to increase survival, it is still reasonable to insert a temporary pacemaker if heart block is deemed likely. Therefore, temporary prophylactic pacing is indicated in patients who develop new bifascicular block. Temporary prophylactic pacing in patients who have a new right bundle branch block and a normal axis or a new left bundle branch block with a normal PR interval is more controversial. Patients who have pre-existing left or right bundle branch block with or without axis deviation probably do not require prophylactic pacing with acute infarction (see Table 8–5).

REFERENCES

CASS principal investigators and their associates: Coronary artery surgery study (CASS): A randomized trial of coronary artery bypass surgery. Survival data. Circulation 68:939, 1983.

Cohn PF: The role of noninvasive cardiac testing after an uncomplicated myocardial infarction. N Engl J Med 309:90, 1983.

Forrester JS, Diamond G, Chatterjee K, and Swan HJC: Medical therapy of acute myocardial infarction by application of hemodynamic subsets. N Engl J Med 295:1356, 1404, 1976.

Hillis LD, and Braunwald E: Coronary artery spasm. N Engl J Med 299:695, 1978.

Hillis LD, and Braunwald E: Myocardial ischemia. N Engl J Med 296:971, 1977.

Kannel WB, Castelli WP, and Gordon T: Cholesterol in the prediction of atherosclerotic disease. Ann Intern Med 90:85, 1979.

Koch-Weser J: β-adrenergic blockade for survivors of acute myocardial infarction. N Engl J Med 310:830, 1984.

Laffel GL, and Braunwald E: Thrombolytic therapy: A new strategy for the treatment of acute myocardial infarction. N Engl J Med 311:710, 770, 1984.

Lipid Research Clinics Program: The lipid research clinics coronary primary prevention trial results. I. Reduction in incidence of coronary heart disease. JAMA 251:351, 1984.

Rahimtoola SH: Coronary bypass surgery for chronic angina 1981. Circulation 65:225, 1982.

Ross R, and Glomset JA: The pathogenesis of atherosclerosis. N Engl J Med 295:369, 420, 1976.

Rude RE, Muller JE, and Braunwald E: Efforts to limit the size of myocardial infarcts. Ann Intern Med 95:736, 1981.

Silverman KJ, and Grossman W: Angina pectoris. Natural history and strategies for evaluation and management. N Engl J Med 310:1712, 1984.

8 ARRHYTHMIAS

MECHANISMS OF ARRHYTHMOGENESIS

The anatomy of the cardiac conduction system and basic electrophysiological principles are discussed in Chapter 1. The genesis of cardiac arrhythmias is divided into disorders of impulse formation, disorders of impulse conduction, and combinations of the two (Table 8–1). One cannot unequivocally determine the mechanism for most clinical arrhythmias, but each arrhythmia may be most consistent with or best explained by a particular electrophysiological mechanism. Disorders of impulse formation are defined as an inappropriate discharge rate of the normal pacemaker (the sinus node) or abnormal discharge from an ectopic pacemaker that usurps control of the atrial or ventricular rhythm. An appropriate discharge rate of a subsidiary pacemaker that takes control of the cardiac rhythm upon sinus slowing is termed an escape beat or rhythm, whereas an inappropriately rapid discharge rate of an ectopic pacemaker (abnormally increased automaticity) that usurps control of the cardiac rhythm from the normal sinus mechanism is termed a premature complex or, when they occur in a series, an ectopic tachycardia.

Parasystole may be due to abnormal automaticity and refers to an ectopic atrial or ventricular pacemaker that discharges regularly and appears to be protected from the dominate cardiac rhythm by entrance block into the area of abnormal automaticity. Therefore, it may depolarize the myocardium intermittently whenever the myocardium is excitable, but it is not discharged by the dominant rhythm. In addition, the abnormal focus may demonstrate variable degrees of exit block, and thus it may intermittently fail to depolarize the myocardium at a time when it would be expected. Characteristic features of ventricular parasystole are (1) premature ventricular parasystolic complexes that are a multiple of a common integer, (2) coupling of premature ventricular complexes to preceding normally conducted complexes that is not fixed, as it often is in patients with nonparasystolic premature ventricular complexes, and (3) periodic fusion complexes between the parasystolic and the normally conducted beat.

Disorders of impulse conduction include conduction delay and block that can result in brady-arrhythmias and provide the basis for re-entry, the most common mechanism responsible for arrhythmia development. Re-entry can occur at any level of the cardiac electrical system, including the sinus node, the atria, the AV node, the His-Purkinje system, and the ventricular myocardium. Normal cardiac tissue has relative homogeneity of conduction and refractoriness so that an impulse starts at the sinus node, travels through the atrium, the AV node, and the His-Purkinje system, and terminates with organized depolarization of ventricular muscle. Once all tissues are depolarized, the impulse is extinguished because there is no further tissue to activate. However, a re-entrant or reciprocating rhythm can occur within various tissues if certain criteria are met, giving rise to a continuous reactivation of tissue and generating a tachycardia. For re-entry to occur (Fig. 8–1) there must be two functionally dissociated pathways, permitting the impulse to travel in one direction down one pathway but blocking it in the other pathway. Thus, the pathway with longer refractoriness may block a premature impulse traveling antegradely. The first pathway, having shorter refractoriness but slower conduction, conducts the impulse to the distal common pathway with a delay that permits it to travel retrogradely up the second pathway and find the proximal tissue re-excitable. If this circus movement continues, a tachycardia occurs.

APPROACH TO THE PATIENT WITH SUSPECTED OR CONFIRMED ARRHYTHMIAS

History-taking in patients with suspected or confirmed rhythm abnormalities should be aimed at detecting the presence of cardiac or noncardiac disease that may be linked causally to the genesis of a rhythm abnormality. Common symptoms that prompt patients with rhythm disturbances to consult a physician are palpitations, syncope, presyncope, and congestive heart failure. The ability of a patient to sense an irregular, slow, or rapid heart rhythm varies greatly; some patients are completely unaware of a marked arrhythmia whereas others feel every premature impulse. In addition, some patients may complain of palpitations when they have no detectable rhythm disturbance or merely sinus tachycardia. Dizziness is a common complaint in people with tachy- or bradyarrhythmias but also may be due to nonarrhythmic causes. Syncope refers to complete but transient loss of consciousness and also has a variety of causes (see Table 8–9). Exacerbation of congestive heart failure may occur with arrhythmias. If a patient senses palpitations, the physician should determine whether the patient senses a slow heart beat, a rapid heart beat, a regular or irregular heart beat, its rate, and whether the onset and termination of the palpitations are sudden or gradual.

The physical examination is useful to detect evidence of underlying cardiac disease. In addition,

TABLE 8–1. GENESIS OF ARRHYTHMIAS

DISORDERS OF IMPULSE FORMATION	DISORDERS OF IMPULSE CONDUCTION
Atrial tachycardia with or without block	Heart block
Accelerated junctional rhythm	Reentry:
Nonparoxysmal AV junctional tachycardia	Paroxysmal supraventricular tachycardia
Accelerated idioventricular rhythm	Reciprocating tachycardia using an accessory pathway (Wolff-Parkinson-White syndrome)
Parasystole	Atrial flutter
	Atrial fibrillation
	Ventricular tachycardia
	Ventricular flutter
	Ventricular fibrillation

EITHER OR BOTH

Atrial, junctional, or ventricular extrasystoles
Flutter and fibrillation
Ventricular tachycardia

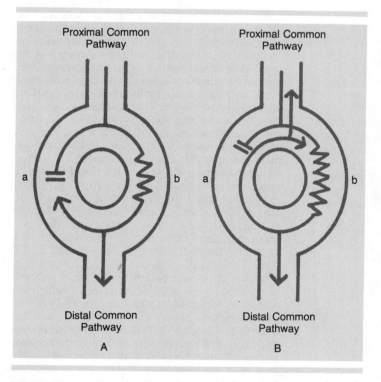

FIGURE 8–1. Mechanism of re-entry. Re-entry requires the presence of two separate pathways that join proximally and distally. Panel A illustrates a premature impulse that blocks antegrade in pathway a (double bars) but conducts down pathway b, albeit with a moderate conduction delay (serpentine arrow). The impulse attempts to return up pathway a but meets refractory tissue. In Panel B, a more premature impulse blocks earlier in pathway a and experiences more conduction delay in pathway b. This impulse finds pathway a recovered from its previous activation and returns retrogradely to the proximal common pathway. If able to again travel antegradely over pathway b, it would activate the distal common pathway prematurely. If this cycle were to continue, a circus movement or re-entrant tachycardia would result. For example, in AV nodal re-entrant tachycardia, the atrium represents the proximal common pathway and the His bundle represents the distal common pathway, with the re-entrant circuit located within the AV node.

abnormalities of the pulse may be noted, and clues regarding AV dissociation during an arrhythmia may be detected (for example, intermittent cannon a waves in the jugular venous pulse or varying intensity of S_1 during a regular tachyarrhythmia).

The resting electrocardiogram may reveal the specific arrhythmia responsible for symptoms or give clues regarding a tachyarrhythmia; for example, short episodes of nonsustained ventricular tachycardia may be recorded in a patient who has presented with syncope or cardiac arrest due to a sustained ventricular tachycardia. In addition, indirect evidence may be obtained from the electrocardiogram that may suggest the etiology of the arrhythmia; for example, the presence of a delta wave should alert the physician to the possibility that a tachycardia due to Wolff-Parkinson-White syndrome may be present. The electrocardiogram may also provide evidence as to the etiology of the arrhythmia, such as the presence of ischemic heart disease documented by ECG evidence of myocardial infarction.

Long-term ambulatory electrocardiography (Holter monitoring) is an important tool for evaluating patients with suspected arrhythmias. It permits quantitation of arrhythmia frequency and complexity, correlation with the patient's symptoms, potential diagnosis of an unknown arrhythmia, and evaluation of the effect of antiarrhythmic therapy. It can record arrhythmias while patients are engaged in their normal daily activities. It can also document alterations in the QRS, ST, and T waves and may be useful in documenting pacemaker function or malfunction. Certain arrhythmias are common during prolonged ECG monitoring in normal patients and may be of no clinical significance. In many patients symptoms are very infrequent and difficult to detect even with prolonged electrocardiographic monitoring. Exercise testing can be used to precipitate arrhythmias in some patients. Patients with no demonstrable structural heart disease may have an increase in premature ventricular or atrial complexes with exercise. However, patients who have ischemic heart disease are more likely to have ventricular ectopy at lower heart rates and in the early recovery period.

Invasive electrophysiological procedures are useful and involve introducing catheter electrodes into the heart to record electrical activity from the atria, ventricles, and the His bundle, and to stimulate the atria or ventricles electrically. Supraventricular or ventricular tachycardias may be induced by programmed electrical stimulation. The test may be used diagnostically to determine whether a particular rhythm disorder exists or to determine the mechanism of a known arrhythmia. The test may also be used therapeutically to terminate a tachycardia or to determine the efficacy of drug or other therapy. Electrophysiological testing is important in patients with resistant tachyarrhythmias undergoing either surgical resection or ablation of a tachycardia focus or accessory pathway. Patients considered candidates for antitachycardia pacemaker devices or implantable cardioverter-defibrillator devices require electrophysiological study to confirm the mechanism and origin of the arrhythmia and the efficacy and safety of this mode of therapy. Electrophysiological study may be helpful in identifying patients with sinus nodal dysfunction or atrioventricular block.

Esophageal electrocardiography is sometimes a useful noninvasive technique to diagnose arrhythmias. An electrode introduced approximately 40 cm from the patient's nares into the esophagus can record an atrial electrogram and often can be used to pace the atrium.

Autonomic and pharmacological manipulations sometimes aid in diagnosing arrhythmias. Most commonly, vagal maneuvers (e.g., carotid sinus massage), edrophonium, or administration of verapamil to slow AV nodal conduction are used. Carotid sinus massage is performed with the patient in the supine position. With the neck hyperextended and the head turned away from the side being tested, light pressure is applied to the carotid impulse at the angle of the jaw. If no change occurs, pressure is more firmly applied with a gentle rotating motion for approximately 5 seconds on one side and then on the other; both sides are not stimulated simultaneously. Prior to carotid sinus massage, the carotid artery should be auscultated; massage should not be performed in patients who have carotid bruits.

MANAGEMENT OF CARDIAC ARRHYTHMIAS

Before initiating antiarrhythmic therapy, one must determine whether the arrhythmia should be treated. Any arrhythmia that causes symptomatic hypotension or sudden death should be suppressed. However, the situation in which the arrhythmia occurs dictates whether chronic, long-term therapy is necessary. For example, an episode of ventricular fibrillation in a patient at the onset of an acute myocardial infarction does not necessarily require long-term drug therapy because of the low likelihood of recurrence. However, ventricular fibrillation in a patient without an acute myocardial infarction carries a high risk of recurrence. Some patients may have arrhythmias that, while not life-threatening, produce disabling symptoms of dizziness or palpitations and require therapy. Rhythms that are tolerated well in patients with structurally normal hearts (for example, paroxysms of supraventricular tachycardia) may not be tolerated in patients with diseased hearts (for example, ischemic heart disease or mitral stenosis) and may require therapy. The decision to treat a patient with an asymptomatic tachyarrhythmia is more difficult. Certain arrhythmias, such as short episodes of asymptomatic nonsustained ventricular tachycardia, are in themselves harmless but may be forerunners of more serious sustained ventricular tachyarrhythmias. The decision to treat is complicated by the side effects, occasionally life-threatening, of antiarrhythmic drugs, such as exacerbation of ventricular arrhythmias in 5 to 15 per cent of cases. Even though patients with premature ventricular complexes and complex ventricular ectopy after myocardial infarction are at increased risk of subsequent sudden death, it is not clear that antiarrhythmic treatment reduces the increased mortality.

Before beginning chronic antiarrhythmic therapy, factors contributing to the occurrence of the arrhythmia should be considered. These include digitalis excess, hypokalemia, hypomagnesemia, hypoxia, thyrotoxicosis, and other severe metabolic derangements. Congestive heart failure, anemia, or infection should be corrected. Smoking, excessive alcohol intake, caffeine- or theophylline-containing beverages or foods, fatigue, emotional upset, and some over-the-counter drugs (for example, nasal decongestants) may exacerbate arrhythmias.

DRUGS

"Therapeutic" serum concentrations of antiarrhythmic drugs are those that usually exert therapeutic effects without adverse effects in most patients. However, dosage and blood concentrations must be adjusted for any particular patient, and the measured serum concentration is of secondary importance if the response to the drug is appropriate and side effects absent. The therapeutic-to-toxic ratio of most antiarrhythmic drugs is relatively narrow, and knowledge of drug pharmacokinetics is important to avoid toxic peak and subtherapeutic trough concentrations. Most antiarrhythmic drugs can be administered at intervals equal to the elimination half-life of the drug after an initial loading dose. At a constant dosing interval without a loading dose, the time required to reach steady state is a function of the elimination half-life of the drug. Ninety-four per cent of steady-state level is achieved after four half-lives and 99 per cent after seven half-lives. The same principle applies to the decrease in drug levels after discontinuation of the drug. Therefore, a drug with a longer half-life takes longer to reach steady state and longer to be eliminated than does one with a shorter half-life. Drugs with shorter half-lives are inconvenient to administer orally because of more frequent dosing requirements. Some medications with relatively short half-lives can be given in long-acting forms that release the drug gradually and result in adequate blood concentrations for a longer period of time without a high peak level immediately upon administration of the drug. The pharmacokinetics of drug distribution and elimination are often important; for example, lidocaine blood concentrations may be high after an intravenous bolus but drop very quickly as the drug is redistributed throughout the body. Once this early redistribution phase occurs, blood concentrations fall much less precipitously during the elimination phase, at which time the lidocaine is metabolized by the liver. Therefore, to avoid very high serum concentrations within the first 10 minutes and a subtherapeutic nadir after redistribution has occurred, lidocaine therapy may be initiated in two or more boluses, 5 to 10 minutes apart instead of as one larger bolus.

TABLE 8–2. ANTIARRHYTHMIC DRUGS: DOSAGE AND PHARMACOKINETICS

DRUG	USUAL DOSE RANGES Intravenous (mg) Loading	Maintenance	Oral (mg) Loading	Maintenance	EFFECTIVE SERUM OR PLASMA CONCENTRATION (μg/ml)	ELIMINATION HALF-LIFE AFTER ORAL DOSE (hr)	MAJOR ROUTE OF ELIMINATION
Lidocaine	1 to 3 mg/kg at 20 to 50 mg/min	1 to 4 mg/min			1 to 5	1 to 2	Liver
Quinidine	6 to 10 mg/kg at 0.3 to 0.5 mg/kg/min		600 to 1000	300 to 600 q6h	3 to 6	5 to 9	Liver
Procainamide	6 to 13 mg/kg at 0.2 to 0.5 mg/kg/min	2 to 6 mg/min	500 to 1000	2000–6000 qd (q3-4h doses for procainamide, q6h doses for sustained-release form)	4 to 10	3 to 5	Kidneys
Disopyramide			300 to 400	100 to 400 q6-8h	2 to 5	8 to 9	Kidneys
Phenytoin	100 mg q5min for ≤ 1000 mg		1000	100 to 400 q12-24h	10 to 20	18 to 36	Liver
Propranolol	0.25 to 0.5 mg q5 min for ≤ 0.15 to 0.20 mg/kg			10 to 200 q6-8h		3 to 6	Liver
Bretylium	5 to 10 mg/kg at 1 to 2 mg/kg/min	1/2 to 2 mg/min			0.5 to 1.5	8 to 14	Kidneys
Verapamil	10 mg over 1 to 2 min	0.005 mg/kg/min		80 to 120 q6-8h	0.10 to 0.15	3 to 8	Liver
Amiodarone*	5 to 10 mg/kg		800 to 1200 qd for 1 to 4 weeks	200 to 800 qd	1 to 5	30 to 50 days	Liver
Tocainide			400 to 600	400 to 800 q8-12h	6 to 12	10 to 17	Liver

*Investigational
Results presented may vary according to doses, disease state, and IV or oral administration.

TABLE 8–3. ANTIARRHYTHMIC DRUGS: ELECTROCARDIOGRAPHIC EFFECTS

DRUG	SINUS RATE	PR	QRS	Q-T
Lidocaine	0	0	0	0
Quinidine	0 ↑	↓ 0 ↑	↑	↑
Procainamide	0	0 ↑	↑	↑
Disopyramide	0 ↑	0	0 ↑	0 ↑
Phenytoin	0	0	0	0 ↓
Propranolol	↓	0 ↑	0	0 ↓
Bretylium	0 ↓	0 ↑	0	0 ↑
Verapamil	0 ↓	↑	0	0
Amiodarone	↓	0 ↑	0	↑
Tocainide	0 ↓	0	0	0 ↓

The organ responsible for elimination of a particular drug, usually the kidneys or liver, must be known, and dosage adjustments must be made in patients with organ dysfunction. The per cent gastrointestinal absorption of some drugs is important to estimate intravenous versus oral dosages; for example, digoxin is only about 80 per cent ab-

TABLE 8–4. ANTIARRHYTHMIC DRUGS: SIDE EFFECTS

DRUG	MAJOR SIDE EFFECTS
Lidocaine	CNS: dizziness, paresthesias, confusion, delirium, stupor, coma, seizures
Quinidine	Hypotension GI: nausea, vomiting, diarrhea, anorexia, abdominal pain "Cinchonism": tinnitus, hearing loss, visual disturbances, confusion, psychosis Rash, fever, anemia, thrombocytopenia "Quinidine syncope"
Procainamide	Drug-induced lupus erythematosus Nausea, vomiting Hypotension Giddiness, psychosis
Disopyramide	Anticholinergic: urinary retention, constipation, blurred vision, closed-angle glaucoma Congestive heart failure
Phenytoin	CNS: nystagmus, ataxia, drowsiness, stupor Nausea, anorexia Rash, gingival hypertrophy, megaloblastic anemia, lymph node hyperplasia, peripheral neuropathy, hyperglycemia, hypocalcemia
Propranolol	See Table 7–5
Bretylium	Orthostatic hypotension Transient hypertension, tachycardia and worsening of arrhythmias (initial catecholamine release) Nausea, vomiting
Verapamil	See Table 7–6
Tocainide	CNS: dizziness, tremor, paresthesias, ataxia, confusion GI: nausea, vomiting
Amiodarone*	Pulmonary fibrosis, elevation of hepatic enzymes, corneal microdeposits, bluish-gray skin discoloration, hyper- or hypothyroidism, nausea, constipation, anorexia, bradycardia, exacerbation of heart failure; elevates plasma levels of digoxin, quinidine, procainamide; potentiates effects of warfarin

*Investigational

sorbed orally, compared to 100 per cent availability of an intravenous dose. Some drugs are metabolized to compounds that also demonstrate antiarrhythmic activity, such as N-acetyl procainamide, which is the active metabolite of procainamide. Drug interactions may necessitate dosage adjustments. For example, quinidine increases digoxin serum concentrations. Changes in pharmacokinetics may occur in some groups of patients, such as decreased lidocaine requirements in elderly patients or those with congestive heart failure. Disparity in drug absorption and metabolism may occur in different patients owing to genetically controlled enzyme systems that allow some patients to metabolize drugs such as procainamide quickly (rapid acetylators). The amount of drug bound to serum proteins affects the activity and metabolism of a drug and also may affect the interpretation of serum drug concentrations, since many assays measure both free and protein-bound drug.

Although in vitro electrophysiological properties are known for each drug and certain drugs are known to be more useful for one type of arrhythmia than another, much of antiarrhythmic drug therapy is trial and error. Even drugs grouped within the same class may vary in their clinical electrophysiological effects, and when one is unsuccessful in a particular patient, another drug from the same class may be effective. A common classification of antiarrhythmic drugs (Vaughn Williams) is as follows: class I drugs predominantly reduce the maximum velocity of the upstroke of the action potential (phase 0) and include quinidine, procainamide, and disopyramide (class IA); and lidocaine, phenytoin, and tocainide (class IB). Class II drugs inhibit sympathetic activity and include propranolol and other beta blockers. Class III drugs predominantly prolong action potential duration and include amiodarone and bretylium. Class IV drugs block the slow inward current and include verapamil. It is important to remember that this classification serves a useful communication purpose but cannot be applied rigidly for several reasons. All drugs assigned to a single group do not exhibit entirely similar actions, and some drugs have properties of more than one class. The classification is based on in vitro electrophysiological effects on normal Purkinje fibers; drug effects on diseased in vivo tissues may be different, or its mechanism of action may even have nothing to do with its direct electrophysiological actions. Tables 8–2, 8–3, and 8–4 summarize the currently available antiarrhythmic agents. It is important to remember that a potential adverse effect of any antiarrhythmic agent is arrhythmia exacerbation.

LIDOCAINE

Lidocaine has minimal effects on automaticity or conduction in vitro unless marked abnormalities are pre-existent. Lidocaine affects fast channel–dependent tissues (atrial and ventricular muscle and His-Purkinje tissue) but usually not slow channel–dependent tissues (sinus and AV nodes). It appears to be particularly potent at altering electrophysiological parameters in ischemic tissue. Lidocaine rarely causes clinically significant hemodynamic effects. It is used only parenterally because of extensive first-pass hepatic metabolism upon oral administration. Its metabolism is decreased in elderly patients and those with hepatic disease, heart failure, and shock. Maintenance doses should be reduced by one third to one half in patients with low cardiac output. Prolonged infusion of lidocaine can reduce its clearance, and dosage may have to be decreased after a day or so. Intramuscular administration has been advocated for use by emergency medical technicians when caring for a patient with an acute myocardial infarction before reaching the hospital, but lidocaine is usually administered intravenously. The ability to achieve rapid effective plasma concentrations and a fairly wide toxic-to-therapeutic ratio with a low incidence of hemodynamic complications makes lidocaine a very useful antiarrhythmic drug. It is effective against a variety of ventricular arrhythmias but is generally ineffective against supraventricular arrhythmias. The use of lidocaine prophylactically in patients with acute myocardial infarction is controversial (see Chapter 7). Lidocaine is usually the parenteral drug of first choice in patients with ventricular arrhythmias. Even though lidocaine may decrease ventricular response in some patients with Wolff-Parkinson-White syndrome and atrial fibrillation, it usually has no effect or can even accelerate the ventricular response in patients with rapid ventricular responses.

QUINIDINE

Quinidine is useful for long-term oral treatment of both atrial and ventricular arrhythmias. Quinidine has little effect on normal automaticity but depresses automaticity from abnormal cells. It prolongs conduction time and refractoriness in most cardiac tissues, and it increases the threshold of excitability in atrial and ventricular tissue. Although the direct effect of quinidine is to prolong conduction time in the AV node, its vagolytic actions may shorten conduction time, and the overall result is a balance between the two effects. Quinidine has alpha-adrenergic blocking effects that may cause significant hypotension, especially if vasodilators are administered concomitantly. If given slowly, quinidine may be administered intravenously. Intramuscular quinidine is incompletely absorbed and may cause tissue necrosis.

Quinidine prolongs the effective refractory period of atrial and ventricular muscle and accessory pathways. It may be effective in treating patients with AV nodal re-entry and tachycardias in Wolff-Parkinson-White syndrome. Quinidine may prevent supraventricular tachycardias not only by its effects on tissue refractoriness but also by preventing the atrial or ventricular premature complexes that may trigger the arrhythmia. Quinidine can terminate existing atrial flutter or fibrillation in about 10 to 20 per cent of patients,

especially if the arrhythmia is recent in onset and the atria are of normal size. Because quinidine slows the rate of atrial flutter and also exerts a vagolytic effect on AV nodal conduction, it may increase the ventricular response in patients with atrial flutter. Therefore, the patient should be treated with digitalis, propranolol, or verapamil to control the ventricular rate before administering quinidine. Prior to electrical cardioversion, quinidine may be administered to attempt chemical conversion of atrial fibrillation or atrial flutter and may also help maintain sinus rhythm once it is achieved, either chemically or electrically.

Quinidine may produce syncope in 0.5 to 2 per cent of patients, thought most often to result from a polymorphic ventricular tachyarrhythmia termed torsades de pointes when associated with a long QT interval. Many patients with quinidine syncope have significantly prolonged QT intervals and are also receiving digitalis. Treatment for quinidine syncope entails discontinuation of the drug and avoidance of similar antiarrhythmic agents. Drugs that do not prolong the QT interval, such as lidocaine, tocainide, or phenytoin, may be tried. Phenobarbital or phenytoin and related drugs that induce hepatic enzyme production shorten the duration of quinidine's action by increasing its elimination. Quinidine elevates serum digoxin and digitoxin concentrations.

PROCAINAMIDE

Electrophysiological effects of procainamide resemble those of quinidine. Procainamide exerts less intense anticholinergic effects than disopyramide and quinidine. It has a major metabolite, N-acetyl procainamide (NAPA), that exhibits much weaker electrophysiological effects than does procainamide. In patients with renal failure, NAPA levels increase more than procainamide levels and must be monitored to prevent toxicity. A sustained-release form is available that can be administered every 6 hours instead of every 3 to 4 hours; the total daily dose of both procainamide and the sustained release form of procainamide should be the same. Procainamide depresses myocardial contractility only in high doses. It may produce peripheral vasodilation, probably via a mild ganglionic blocking action. The clinical indications for procainamide are very similar to those for quinidine. Although the effects of both drugs are similar, an arrhythmia not suppressed by one drug may be suppressed by the other. Conduction disturbances and ventricular tachyarrhythmias similar to those caused by quinidine can occur.

Procainamide does not increase serum digoxin levels. A systemic lupus erythematosus–like syndrome including arthralgia, fever, pleuropericarditis, hepatomegaly, and hemorrhagic pericardial effusion with tamponade has been described. The brain and kidneys are usually spared and hematologic complications are unusual. Sixty to 70 per cent of patients who receive procainamide develop antinuclear antibodies, but clinical symptoms occur in 20 to 30 per cent and are reversible when the drug is stopped. A positive ANA is not necessarily a reason to stop procainamide therapy.

DISOPYRAMIDE

Disopyramide has electrophysiological actions similar to those of quinidine and procainamide but exerts greater anticholinergic effects than either, without antiadrenergic effects. Disopyramide has prominent negative inotropic effects, and patients who have evidence of abnormal ventricular function should receive the drug either not at all or only with extreme caution.

The role of disopyramide in the treatment of atrial and ventricular arrhythmias is similar to that of quinidine. Like quinidine, it can cause a 1:1 conduction during atrial flutter if the patient is not adequately digitalized. Disopyramide does not alter digitalis metabolism.

PHENYTOIN

Phenytoin is a potent medication to treat central nervous system seizures, but its antiarrhythmic actions are limited. It effectively abolishes abnormal automaticity caused by digitalis toxicity. Sinus nodal automaticity and AV conduction are only minimallly affected by phenytoin. Phenytoin's electrophysiological effects in vitro appear similar to those of lidocaine. It exerts minimal hemodynamic effects. Phenytoin may be successful in treating atrial and ventricular arrhythmias due to digitalis toxicity but is much less effective in treating arrhythmias of other etiologies.

TOCAINIDE

Tocainide is an analogue of lidocaine that undergoes negligible hepatic first-pass metabolism and therefore approaches 100 per cent oral bioavailability. It is effective for ventricular tachyarrhythmias, but its efficacy appears to be less than that of lidocaine. The effect of lidocaine on an arrhythmia may predict the efficacy of tocainide on that arrhythmia.

BETA BLOCKERS

Propranolol will be discussed as a prototype beta-adrenergic receptor blocker. Differences in the pharmacokinetics, beta-adrenergic receptor selectivity, and antagonist/agonist actions have been discussed in Chapter 7.

Propranolol slows the sinus nodal discharge rate and lengthens AV nodal conduction time (PR interval increases) and refractoriness. These effects may be marked if the heart rate or AV conduction is particularly dependent on sympathetic tone or if sinus or AV nodal dysfunction is present. There is no effect on refractoriness or conduction in the His-Purkinje system at usual doses, and the QRS complex and QT interval do not change. It appears that the beta-blocking activity of propranolol is responsible for its antiarrhythmic effects, since a local anesthetic (or quinidine-like) effect of propranolol is present only at doses ten times those causing the beta-blocking effect. There is variability in serum concentrations from patient to patient, and the appropriate dose is determined by the patient's physiological response, such as changes in resting heart rate or prevention of an increase in heart rate with exercise. If one beta blocker is ineffective against arrhythmias, the other beta blockers are usually also ineffective.

Propranolol is used most commonly to treat supraventricular tachyarrhythmias. Sinus tachycardia due to thyrotoxicosis, anxiety, and exercise may be slowed by propranolol. Propranolol does not usually terminate atrial flutter or fibrillation but may, by itself or combined with digitalis, control the ventricular response by prolonging AV nodal conduction time or refractoriness. Re-entrant supraventricular tachycardias using the AV node as one limb of the pathway (e.g., AV nodal re-entrant tachycardia and reciprocating tachycardias associated with the Wolff-Parkinson-White syndrome) may be prevented by propranolol alone or combined with other drugs. Propranolol is useful in treating ventricular arrhythmias associated with the prolonged QT syndrome and mitral valve prolapse. It usually does not prevent chronic recurrent ventricular tachycardia in patients with ischemic heart disease if the tachyarrhythmia occurs without acute ischemia.

BRETYLIUM TOSYLATE

Bretylium tosylate initially releases norepinephrine stores from adrenergic nerve terminals but subsequently prevents further norepinephrine release. This initial catecholamine release may aggravate some arrhythmias and produce transient hypertension. Although the chemical sympathectomy-like state may be antiarrhythmic, other electrophysiological properties may also contribute to the antiarrhythmic properties of bretylium. Bretylium does not depress myocardial contractility or affect vagal reflexes. After the initial increase in blood pressure, the drug may subsequently cause hypotension, usually orthostatic and controlled if the patient is supine. Bretylium is poorly absorbed orally and is commonly administered intravenously. Bretylium has been reported to induce spontaneous termination of ventricular fibrillation. Bretylium is indicated in patients with life-threatening ventricular arrhythmias that have not responded to lidocaine and possibly to other drugs.

VERAPAMIL

The calcium antagonists have been discussed in Chapter 7. Verapamil has the most potent antiarrhythmic actions. It does not affect cells with normal fast response characteristics (atrial and ventricular muscle, His-Purkinje system), but in fast channel–dependent cells rendered abnormal by disease, verapamil may suppress electrical activity. Slow channel–dependent tissue (sinus and AV nodes) exhibits an increase in conduction time and refractoriness after verapamil administration. Therefore, verapamil prolongs the AH interval without affecting His-Purkinje conduction or the QRS interval. Sinus rate may decrease, but in intact animals it often does not change significantly because of counteraction by sympathetic reflexes activated by peripheral vasodilation. Verapamil does not affect directly refractoriness of atrial or ventricular muscle or the accessory pathway. Combined therapy with propranolol and verapamil can be attempted in patients with normal cardiac contractility, but the patient should be observed for the development of heart failure and/or symptomatic bradycardias because the compensatory sympathetic response to slow channel blockade is blocked. Calcium infusion or isoproterenol may counteract some of the adverse effects of verapamil until temporary pacing can be initiated.

Intravenous verapamil is the drug of choice for terminating sustained paroxysmal supraventricular tachycardias that are not terminated by vagal maneuvers, such as those reciprocating tachycardias employing the AV node or SA node in the tachycardia circuit. Verapamil can decrease the ventricular response in patients with atrial fibrillation or flutter but converts only a small number of these rhythms to sinus rhythm. Verapamil may be used in patients with congestive heart failure and supraventricular tachycardia if it is thought that termination of the arrhythmia will relieve the heart failure. Verapamil may increase the ventricular response in patients with atrial fibrillation and Wolff-Parkinson-White syndrome, and the drug is relatively contraindicated in that situation. Verapamil is usually not effective in patients with recurrent ventricular tachyarrhythmias.

AMIODARONE

Amiodarone is an investigational antiarrhythmic agent initially introduced as an antianginal coronary vasodilator. It has a broad spectrum of antiarrhythmic efficacy against supraventricular and ventricular arrhythmias. Even though it prolongs the QT interval, it may suppress arrhythmias in patients with the long QT syndrome. It is effective in AV nodal reentry, reciprocating tachycardias associated with the Wolff-Parkinson-White syndrome, atrial flutter, and atrial fibrillation, as well as ventricular tachyarrhythmias. Antiarrhythmic efficacy develops after several days of oral administration but may occur earlier with intravenous administration. Amiodarone prolongs action potential duration and refractoriness in all cardiac tissues, slows sinus discharge, and prolongs AV nodal conduction time. Because of a variety of adverse effects, amiodarone should be administered to patients with highly symptomatic or life-threatening arrhythmias and only if conventional drug therapy has failed.

DC CARDIOVERSION AND DEFIBRILLATION

Direct current (DC) electrical cardioversion or defibrillation is the method of choice for terminating tachyarrhythmias that result in hemodynamic deterioration and those unresponsive to pharmacological termination. Cardioversion refers to the delivery of a DC shock, usually of relatively low energy, synchronized with the QRS complex of an organized tachyarrhythmia. QRS synchronization is important to avoid delivering a shock during ventricular repolarization (T wave) that may precipitate ventricular fibrillation. Defibrillation refers to an asynchronously delivered, relatively high energy shock to terminate ventricular fibrillation. Most supraventricular and ventricular tachyarrhythmias terminate with DC shock, although rhythms due to abnormally increased automaticity, especially if associated with digitalis intoxication, may not.

Prior to elective cardioversion the procedure should be explained to the patient and a physical examination, including palpation of all pulses, performed. Metabolic parameters (i.e., blood gases, electrolytes) should be normal, and ideally the patient should have fasted for 6 to 8 hours prior to the procedure. Digitalis should be withheld on the morning of cardioversion. Patients receiving digitalis without clinical evidence of toxicity are at very low risk for digitalis-induced complications. A short-acting barbiturate or diazepam can be used for anesthesia. Intravenous access should be available and resuscitation equipment at hand. Paddles should be lubricated with an electrolyte jelly and placed firmly to contact with the chest wall, either one paddle in the left infrascapular region and the other over the upper sternum at the third interspace, or one paddle to the right of the sternum at the first or second interspace and the other in the left midclavicular line at the fourth or fifth interspace. Shocks of 25 to 50 joules terminate most tachyarrhythmias except for atrial fibrillation that may require 100 to 200 joules and ventricular fibrillation that may require 100 to 400 joules. If the first low-energy shock fails to terminate the arrhythmia, the energy should be titrated upward.

Tachycardia that produces complications of hypotension, congestive heart failure, or angina and does not respond promptly to medical management should be terminated electrically. DC shock should be avoided if possible in patients with tachyarrhythmias caused by digitalis toxicity because of the risk of precipitating life-threatening refractory ventricular tachyarrhythmias. The administration of an antiarrhythmic drug prior to electrical termination of the arrhythmia may help maintain sinus rhythm after cardioversion. Many arrhythmias, especially chronic atrial fibrillation, commonly recur, and maintenance of sinus rhythm is sometimes a difficult problem.

Ventricular fibrillation due to an improperly synchronized or at times a properly synchronized shock is a complication of DC cardioversion. Immediate electrical defibrillation is mandatory. Systemic emboli occur, and patients with atrial fibrillation, especially those with a high risk for emboli (e.g., mitral stenosis, atrial fibrillation of recent onset, a history of emboli, a prosthetic mitral valve, enlarged left ventricle or left atrium, or

TABLE 8–5. INDICATIONS FOR TEMPORARY AND PERMANENT PACING

	DEFI-NITELY INDI-CATED	PROBA-BLY IN-DICATED	PROBA-BLY NOT INDI-CATED	DEFI-NITELY NOT IN-DICATED
Complete AV Block				
Congenital (AV nodal)				
Asymptomatic				X
Symptomatic	T,P			
Acquired (His-Pur-kinje)				
Asymptomatic		T,P		
Symptomatic	T,P			
Surgical (persistent)				
Asymptomatic	T	P		
Symptomatic	T,P			
Second-degree AV block				
Type I (AV nodal)				
Asymptomatic				X
Symptomatic	T,P			
Type II (His-Purkinje)				
Asymptomatic		T,P		
Symptomatic	T,P			
First-degree AV block				
AV Nodal				
Asymptomatic				X
Symptomatic			X	
His-Purkinje				
Asymptomatic				X
Symptomatic			X	
Bundle Branch Block				
Asymptomatic				X
Symptomatic		P†		
LBBB during right heart catheterization	T			
Acute Myocardial Infarction				
Newly acquired bifascicular BBB	T			
Preexisting BBB				X
Newly acquired BBB plus transient complete AV block	T	P		
Second-degree AV block				
Type I (asymptomatic)				X
Type II	T	P		
Complete AV block	T	P		
Atrial Fibrillation with Slow Ventricular Response				
Asymptomatic				X
Symptomatic	T,P			
Sick Sinus Syndrome (bradytachy syndrome)				
Asymptomatic			X	
Symptomatic	T,P			
Hypersensitive Carotid Sinus Syndrome				
Asymptomatic			X	
Symptomatic	T,P			

T = temporary
P = permanent
X = not indicated
† = no other cause found for symptoms

congestive heart failure) may require anticoagulation for two weeks before cardioversion to lower the risk of emboli. Anticoagulation should be continued for several weeks after cardioversion. Elevation of myocardial enzyme fractions after cardioversion is not common.

CARDIAC PACEMAKERS

Cardiac pacemakers are devices either implanted permanently or inserted temporarily, consisting of a pulse generator and an electrode that is either placed transvenously into the right ventricle and/or atrium or sutured directly into the epicardium at the time of surgery. Small electrical impulses, generated by the pulse generator and delivered via the electrode catheter, depolarize local cells to threshold potential and cause the entire chamber to depolarize. Pacemakers are widely used for treating bradyarrhythmias but can also be useful for treatment of some tachyarrhythmias. Indicators for temporary and permanent pacing are summarized in Table 8–5.

A five-position pacemaker code has been developed to describe the pacing modalities available in any particular pacemaker. The first three letters of the code are used commonly and the last two are optional. The first letter is the chamber paced (V=ventricle, A=atrium, and D=atrium and ventricle). The second letter is the chamber in which sensing occurs (V=ventricle, A=atrium, D=atrium and ventricle, and O=none). The third letter indicates the mode of response: sensed spontaneous activity inhibiting pacemaker output (I), trigger discharge into the refractory period (T), or trigger ventricular pacing in response to a sensed atrial event as well as inhibition of ventricular pacing during a sensed ventricular event (D). The fourth letter codes programmability of the pacemaker, and the fifth codes antitachyarrhythmia functions. Some examples are illustrated in Table 8–6. The main advantages of dual-chamber pacing modes are the preservation of AV synchrony and/or the ability to increase ventricular paced rate with an increase in atrial rate. Safeguards are built into the VDD and DDD modes so that the ventricular response cannot exceed a predetermined upper rate should an atrial tachyarrhythmia occur. A problem unique to dual-chamber pacing modes (DDD or VDD) that trigger ventricular depolarization from sensed atrial activity is pacemaker-mediated tachycardia. During pacemaker-mediated tachycardia, the pacemaker senses a retrograde P wave conducted after a paced ventricular beat or a premature ventricular complex and triggers a subsequent ventricular depolarization after the programmed AV delay. This paced ventricular complex can again conduct retrogradely to the atrium, creating a sensed P wave that generates another paced ventricular complex. If this continues, a sustained "reciprocating" tachycardia that utilizes the pacemaker as the antegrade limb may occur. Extensive programmability of the newer pacemaker models, particularly that of atrial re-

TABLE 8–6. COMMON PACEMAKERS

PACEMAKER TYPE	CODE	CHAMBER PACED	CHAMBER SENSED	MODE
Ventricular Asynchronous	VOO	V	None	Continuous pacing
Ventricular Demand	VVI	V	V	Ventricular pacing inhibited by spontaneous QRS
Atrial Demand	AAI	A	A	Atrial pacing inhibited by spontaneous P wave
Atrial Synchronous, Ventricular Inhibited	VDD	V	A,V	Ventricular pacing follows a sensed P wave after a preset AV delay; ventricular pacing inhibited by spontaneous QRS; no atrial pacing
AV Sequential	DVI	A,V	V	Ventricular pacing follows atrial pacing after a preset AV delay; ventricular and atrial pacing inhibited by spontaneous QRS; no P wave sensing
Optimal Sequential	DDD	A,V	A,V	Ventricular pacing follows sensed P waves or atrial pacing after a preset AV delay; ventricular pacing inhibited by spontaneous QRS, atrial pacing inhibited by spontaneous P wave

V = ventricle; A = atrium.

fractoriness, avoids pacemaker-mediated tachycardia in most cases.

For patients in whom a pacemaker is implanted only for an occasional symptomatic bradycardia or in whom optimal hemodynamic function is of no consequence, a simple VVI pacemaker may be sufficient. However, there are some patients in whom maintenance of physiological AV synchrony may be advantageous (Table 8–7). Pacemaker malfunction may be manifested by (1) failure to capture (activate myocardium), (2) abnormal sensing (oversensing or undersensing),

TABLE 8–7. INDICATIONS AND CONTRAINDICATIONS FOR PACING MODES

MODE	INDICATIONS	CONTRAINDICATIONS	ADVANTAGES	DISADVANTAGES
VOO	Obsolete			
AAI	SSS with normal AV conduction	Atrial inexcitability High atrial threshold Abnormal AV conduction	Simplest system providing properly timed sequential AV contraction; requires only one lead	Ventricle not paced should AV block develop
VVI	SSS without retrograde AV conduction SSS with no hemodynamic benefit of atrial pacing Chronic atrial fibrillation or flutter with AV block and a slow ventricular rate	Hemodynamic insufficiency due to loss of AV synchrony ("pacemaker syndrome")	Historical inertia Relative simplicity	Does not provide AV synchronous contraction Rate does not change in response to external demands
VDD	Normal sinus node function with impaired AV conduction	Inappropriate atrial tachycardia or bradycardia Retrograde atrial activation following ventricular stimulation or PVC's (relative contraindication) Extended periods of atrial fibrillation/flutter	Maintains atrial transport and normal sinus control of ventricular rate when atrial rate is within tracking limits of pacemaker	Does not maintain synchronous contractions during atrial bradycardia, since it does not pace the atria Requires two leads
DVI	Atrial bradyarrhythmias with or without impaired AV conduction	Retrograde atrial activation following ventricular stimulation or PVC's (relative contraindication) Extended periods of atrial fibrillation/flutter Frequent atrial tachycardias	Maintains sequential AV contraction during sinus bradycardia	Does not alter rate in response to physiological demands Does not maintain AV synchronous contractions during periods of normal sinus rhythm and AV block Competitive atrial pacing during normal sinus rhythm Requires two leads
DDD	Atrial bradyarrhythmias with or without impaired AV conduction Normal sinus node function with impaired AV conduction	Retrograde atrial activation following ventricular stimulation or PVC's (relative contraindication) Extended periods of atrial fibrillation/flutter Frequent atrial tachycardias	Maintains sequential AV contraction and sinus control of ventricular rate during normal sinus rhythm and during sinus bradycardia	Requires two leads

SSS = Sick sinus syndrome

TABLE 8—8. NONPHARMACOLOGICAL THERAPY OF TACHYARRHYTHMIAS

THERAPY	INDICATION	ADVANTAGES	DISADVANTAGES
Pacing	*Prevention* of drug-refractory tachyarrhythmias (for example, VT associated with bradycardia or prolonged QT syndrome)	Avoids drug side effects; may be the only effective therapy in some patients	Only effective for very narrow indications
	Termination of tachyarrhythmias (especially paroxysmal supraventricular tachycardia, atrial flutter)	Same as above	Requires electrophysiology study to determine efficacy Not effective for rapid VT or VF; may accelerate rather than terminate arrhythmia
Implantable cardioverter-defibrillator (investigational)	Ventricular tachycardia or fibrillation unresponsive to drug therapy	Failsafe to abort cardiac arrest or need for transthoracic DC shock	Does not prevent arrhythmia; drug therapy may still be required and syncope may occur before arrhythmia is terminated Can accelerate or precipitate arrhythmias Shock is uncomfortable Requires surgery, usually thoracotomy
Catheter ablation of arrhythmia focus or pathway (investigational)	Drug-resistant ventricular or supraventricular tachycardias in which the focus of origin of pathway can be located and is accessible to a catheter	Nonsurgical Avoids drug side effects	Only a minority of patients are candidates at present Safety and efficacy are unknown
Surgery	Cut accessory pathway in Wolff-Parkinson-White patients with markedly symptomatic or life-threatening arrhythmias; usually young or drug-refractory patients	Avoids drug side effects Definitive therapy	Surgical risk (small)
	Electrophysiologically guided aneurysmectomy for VT, usually drug-refractory	Avoids or decreases drug therapy Concomitant coronary bypass and aneurysmectomy	Surgical risk Not all patients are good candidates Not universally effective

or (3) abnormal discharge rate. Malfunction may be intermittent. Many pacemakers alter their discharge rate when the battery approaches depletion.

NONPHARMACOLOGICAL THERAPY OF TACHYARRHYTHMIAS

Electrical or surgical therapy may be useful in some patients with supraventricular or ventricular tachyarrhythmias (Table 8—8). Pacemakers activated by the patient or automatically when the pacemaker senses tachycardia can deliver timed single or multiple extrastimuli to the atrium, ventricle, or both chambers to interrupt the tachycardia circuit and terminate the arrhythmia. Before implantation, detailed electrophysiological evaluation should be performed to determine the pacing protocol that most safely and reliably terminates the tachycardia.

SPECIFIC ARRHYTHMIAS

SINUS NODAL RHYTHM DISTURBANCES
(Fig. 8—2)

Normal sinus rhythm refers to impulse formation beginning in the sinus node and, in adults, having a rate of between 60 and 100 beats per min-

ute. The P wave is upright in leads 1, 2, and aVF and negative in lead aVR. The rate of sinus nodal discharge is under autonomic control and increases with sympathetic and decreases with parasympathetic stimulation. Sinus tachycardia refers to a tachycardia of sinus origin with a rate exceeding 100 beats per minute. *Sinus tachycardia* occurs with stresses such as fever, hypotension, thyrotoxicosis, anemia, anxiety, exertion, hypovolemia, pulmonary emboli, myocardial ischemia, congestive heart failure, shock, drugs (e.g., atropine, catecholamines, thyroid, alcohol, caffeine), or inflammation. Therapy should be focused on the cause of the tachycardia. If the sinus tachycardia must be treated directly, propranolol may be used. *Sinus bradycardia* refers to sinus node discharge at a rate less than 60 beats per minute. The P wave contour is normal, but sinus arrhythmia is often present. Sinus bradycardia frequently occurs in young adults, especially well-trained athletes, and is common at night. Sinus bradycardia can be produced by a variety of conditions, including eye manipulation, increased intracranial pressure, myxedema, hypothermia, sepsis, fibrodegenerative changes, vagal stimulation, or vomiting, and the administration of parasympathomimetic drugs, beta-adrenergic blocking drugs, or amiodarone. It occurs commonly in the acute phase of myocardial infarction, especially inferior myocardial infarction. Treatment of asymptomatic sinus bradycardia is usually not necessary. If cardiac output is low or tachyarrhythmias occur owing to the slow heart rate, atropine or, if necessary, isoproterenol may be effective. There is no drug that effectively and safely increases the heart rate over a long period of time, and therefore electrical pacing is the treatment of choice chronically if symptomatic sinus bradycardia is present.

Sinus arrhythmia refers to phasic variation in the sinus cycle length by greater than 10 per cent. P wave morphology is normal. Respiratory sinus arrhythmia occurs when the PP interval shortens during inspiration as a result of reflex inhibition of vagal tone and lengthens during expiration. Nonrespiratory sinus arrhythmia refers to sinus arrhythmia not associated with the respiratory cycle. Symptoms are unusual and treatment not necessary.

In *sinus pause (sinus arrest)* and *sinoatrial exit block*, a sudden unexpected failure of a P wave occurs. In sinoatrial exit block, the PP interval surrounding the absent P wave is a multiple of the P to P intervals, implying that the sinus impulse was generated but did not propagate through the perinodal tissue to the atrium. If no such cycle relationship can be found, the term sinus pause

FIGURE 8–2. *A,* Sinus tachycardia (rate 150 beats/min) in a patient during acute myocardial ischemia; note ST segment depression. *B,* Sinus bradycardia (rate 46 beats/min) in a patient receiving propranolol. *C,* Respiratory sinus arrhythmia. The phasic variation in heart rate corresponds to a respiratory rate of approximately 12/min. *D,* Hypersensitive carotid sinus syndrome. Gentle left carotid sinus massage produced a prolonged period of asystole. *E,* Bradycardia-tachycardia syndrome. A fairly long period of asystole results before restoration of sinus rhythm upon termination of an episode of atrial fibrillation.

or sinus arrest is employed. Acute myocardial infarction, degenerative fibrotic changes, digitalis toxicity, or excessive vagal tone can produce sinus arrest or exit block. Therapy involves searching for the underlying etiology. Patients are not treated if they are asymptomatic. If they are symptomatic and the arrhythmia is not reversed by correcting the underlying etiologies, pacing is employed.

Wandering atrial pacemaker involves a transfer of the dominant pacemaker from the sinus node to latent pacemakers in other atrial sites or in the AV junction. The change from one pacemaker focus to another occurs gradually, associated with a change in the RR interval, PR interval, and P wave morphology. Treatment is usually not necessary except if symptoms occur from bradyarrhythmias.

The *hypersensitive carotid sinus syndrome* is characterized by cessation of atrial activity due to sinus arrest or sinoatrial exit block with light pressure over the carotid baroreceptors. In addition, AV block may be observed. Adequate junctional or ventricular escape complexes may not occur. Cardioinhibitory carotid sinus hypersensitivity is arbitrarily defined as ventricular asystole exceeding three seconds during carotid sinus stimulation. Vasodepressor carotid sinus hypersensitivity is defined as a fall in systolic blood pressure of 30 to 50 mm Hg without cardiac slowing, usually with reproduction of a patient's symptoms. The treatment in symptomatic patients is pacemaker implantation (to include at least a ventricular lead, since the sinus node slowing is usually also associated with AV block). Neither atropine nor pacing prevents the vasodepressor manifestations of carotid sinus hypersensitivity. Severe vasodepressor carotid sinus hypersensitivity occasionally requires denervation of the carotid sinus.

The *sick sinus syndrome* is applied to a variety of sinus nodal and AV nodal abnormalities that occur alone or in combination. They include (1) persistent spontaneous sinus bradycardia not caused by drugs and inappropriate to the physiological circumstances, (2) sinus arrest or exit block, (3) combinations of sinus and AV conduction disturbances, and (4) alternation of paroxysms of atrial tachyarrhythmias with periods of slow atrial and ventricular rates (bradycardia/tachycardia syndrome). The sick sinus syndrome may be associated with AV nodal or His-Purkinje conduction disturbances. If symptoms are present from bradyarrhythmias, pacemaker implantation is appropriate. Pacing for the symptomatic bradyarrhythmia combined with drug therapy for the tachyarrhythmia is often needed.

Sinus nodal re-entrant tachycardia accounts for 5 to 10 per cent of paroxysmal supraventricular tachycardias. Its mechanism is presumed to be re-entry within the sinus node and the perinodal tissues, giving rise to a tachycardia, usually with a rate of 130 to 140 beats per minute and containing P waves very similar to sinus P waves. AV block may occur without affecting the tachycardia. Vagal activation may slow and then abruptly terminate the tachycardia by its action on sinus nodal tissue. Tachycardia may be induced and terminated at electrophysiological study with premature atrial stimulation. Treatment with propranolol, verapamil, or digitalis is effective therapy.

ATRIAL RHYTHM DISTURBANCES (Fig. 8–3)

Premature atrial complexes (PAC's) are characterized by a premature P wave, usually of differing morphology from the sinus P wave. PAC's occurring very early in diastole may be followed by either aberrantly conducted QRS complexes or no QRS complexes (nonconducted PAC). In general, the shorter the interval from the last QRS to the P wave, the longer the PR interval after the PAC. PAC's are less likely to be followed by a fully compensatory pause than are PVC's (see discussion below). PAC's are common in normal people but may occur in a variety of situations, for example, infection, inflammation, myocardial ischemia, psychological stress, tobacco or alcohol use, or caffeine ingestion. PAC's can be the forerunner of a sustained supraventricular tachyarrhythmia. They do not require therapy unless they produce symptoms or precipitate tachyarrhythmias.

In *atrial flutter*, the atrial rate is usually 250 to 350 per minute. Ordinarily, the ventricular rate is half of the atrial rate. If AV block is greater than 2:1 in the absence of drugs, abnormal AV conduction is suggested. In children, patients with pre-excitation syndrome, or patients with hyperthyroidism, 1:1 AV conduction can occasionally occur. Drugs such as quinidine, procainamide, or disopyramide may reduce the atrial rate to the range of 200 per minute, raising the danger of 1:1 AV conduction. The atrial activity appears as regular sawtooth waves without an isoelectric interval between flutter waves. Flutter waves are commonly inverted in leads 2, 3, and aV_F. Ventricular response to atrial flutter may be irregular, generally of a Wenckebach nature, or regular. Chronic atrial flutter is usually associated with underlying heart disease, but paroxysmal atrial flutter may occur in patients without organic heart disease. Toxic and metabolic conditions such as thyrotoxicosis, alcoholism, or pericarditis may be associated with atrial flutter. There are fewer systemic emboli in patients with atrial flutter than in patients with atrial fibrillation, presumably because of the atrial contraction. Carotid sinus massage may decrease the ventricular response but does not terminate the arrhythmia. Cardioversion (less than 50 joules) usually restores sinus rhythm. If atrial fibrillation ensues, a second shock of higher energy may be necessary. Rapid atrial pacing also terminates atrial flutter, although some patients develop atrial fibrillation instead of sinus rhythm; however, atrial fibrillation is usually an easier arrhythmia in which to control the ventricular response.

Intravenous verapamil, beta blockers, or digitalis may slow the ventricular response to atrial flutter, and in a few patients may restore sinus

FIGURE 8—3. *A,* Premature atrial systoles with and without aberrancy. The first premature atrial systole (arrow) occurs at a shorter PR interval than does the second premature atrial systole (arrow) and conducts with a bundle branch block contour. The first premature atrial systole conducts with aberrancy, while the second does not because the first reaches the bundle branch system before complete recovery of repolarization. *B,* Atrial flutter. Flutter waves are indicated by arrows. The conduction ratio is 3:1, that is, three flutter waves to one QRS complex, and is a less common conduction ratio. *C,* Atrial fibrillation. Atrial activity is present as the undulating wavy base line seen in the midportion of the ECG strip. The premature ventricular complex would have to be differentiated from aberrant supraventricular conduction. *D,* Nonparoxysmal junctional tachycardia. *E,* Paroxysmal supraventricular tachycardia. Three sinus beats are interrupted by a premature atrial systole (arrow), which conducts with PR prolongation and initiates the supraventricular tachycardia. The most common mechanisms of this arrhythmia are AV nodal re-entry and atrioventricular re-entry using an accessory pathway as the retrograde limb.

rhythm. Type 1 antiarrhythmic drugs such as quinidine, procainamide, or disopyramide may terminate atrial flutter in some patients and are often useful to prevent recurrences. These drugs should not be administered unless AV nodal block has been previously achieved, since slowing the atrial flutter rate combined with the vagolytic effects of disopyramide or quinidine may lead to 1:1 AV conduction.

Atrial fibrillation is characterized by totally disorganized atrial activation without effective atrial contraction. The electrocardiogram shows small, irregular baseline undulations of variable amplitude. The ventricular response is irregularly irregular, usually between 100 and 160 beats per minute in the untreated patient with normal AV conduction. It is easier to slow the ventricular response with drugs in patients with atrial fibrillation than in patients with atrial flutter because of the greater number of atrial impulses reaching the AV node and decreasing the overall number of impulses that conduct to the ventricles. Chronic atrial fibrillation is usually associated with underlying heart disease, whereas paroxysmal atrial fibrillation may occur in apparently normal hearts. Atrial fibrillation commonly results from rheumatic heart disease (especially with mitral valve involvement), cardiomyopathy, hypertensive heart disease, pulmonary emboli, pericarditis, coronary heart disease, thyrotoxicosis, or heart failure from any cause. Episodes of atrial fibrillation may cause decompensation of patients with borderline cardiac function, especially those with mitral or aortic stenosis. Patients with chronic atrial fibrillation are at a greatly increased risk of developing systemic emboli, particularly if mitral valve disease is also present. Left atrial diameter tends to be smaller in patients with paroxysmal atrial fibrillation or in patients whose atrial fibrillation is easily terminated with cardioversion. Physical findings in patients with atrial fibrillation include a variation in the intensity of the first heart sound, absence of a waves in the jugular venous pulse, and an irregularly irregular ventricular rhythm. A pulse deficit may appear with faster ventricular rates; that is, the auscultated apical rate exceeds the palpable radial rate due to failure of many of the ventricular contractions to generate a palpable peripheral pulse. Although atrial fibrillation with a very rapid ventricular response can sometimes seem regular, it is always irregularly irregular upon careful measurement, and true regularization of the ventricular rhythm in patients with atrial fibrillation should suggest development of sinus rhythm, atrial flutter, junctional rhythm, or ventricular tachycardia (the latter two may be manifestations of digitalis intoxication).

It is important to correct any precipitating causes of atrial fibrillation such as thyrotoxicosis, mitral stenosis, pulmonary emboli, or pericarditis. If the onset of atrial fibrillation is associated with acute hemodynamic decompensation, DC cardioversion should be employed (usually requires 100 to 200 joules). In the absence of decompensation, the patient should be treated with digitalis to maintain a resting apical rate of 60 to 80 beats per minute that does not exceed 100 beats per minute after mild exercise. At times, the addition of a beta- or calcium-blocker may be useful to slow the ventricular rate. Quinidine or other type 1 antiarrhythmic drugs may be useful either to convert atrial fibrillation to sinus rhythm or to maintain sinus rhythm once it is restored with electrical cardioversion. Patients with atrial fibrillation of less than 12 months duration or without markedly enlarged left atria are more likely to remain in sinus rhythm after cardioversion. The role of anticoagulation is controversial, but anticoagulation prior to drug or electrical cardioversion is definitely indicated in patients at high risk of emboli, i.e., those with mitral stenosis, previous emboli, a prosthetic mitral valve, or cardiomegaly. Anticoagulation therapy should be administered two weeks prior to cardioversion and continued for about two weeks afterward. Rapid atrial pacing does not terminate atrial fibrillation.

In *atrial tachycardia with AV block*, the atrial rate is usually 150 to 200 beats per minute, and variable degrees of AV conduction are present. This rhythm is often associated with digitalis excess and occurs most commonly in patients with significant organic heart disease, such as coronary heart disease, cor pulmonale, and digitalis intoxication. Isoelectric intervals are present between P waves in contrast to atrial flutter. Carotid sinus massage should be performed with caution in patients suspected of having digitalis toxicity. If the patient is not receiving digitalis, the rhythm may be treated with digitalis to slow the ventricular response, and subsequently quinidine, disopyramide, or procainamide may be added. If atrial tachycardia occurs in a patient receiving digitalis, digitalis toxicity should be suspected. Usually the ventricular response is not rapid and withholding digitalis is sufficient therapy.

Chaotic or *multifocal atrial tachycardia* is characterized by atrial rates between 100 and 130 beats per minute with marked variation in P wave morphology and irregular PP intervals. It occurs commonly in patients with pulmonary disease and in diabetics or older patients who eventually may develop atrial fibrillation. Digitalis is usually not helpful in this arrhythmia. Therapy is directed toward the underlying disease.

AV JUNCTIONAL RHYTHM DISTURBANCES
(Fig. 8–3)

If suprajunctional pacemakers fail, a *junctional escape rhythm* may emerge at a rate of 35 to 60 beats per minute. The junctional escape rhythm is usually fairly regular, but the rate may increase gradually when the escape rhythm first begins (warm-up phenomenon). A junctional rhythm may be associated with retrograde P waves for each QRS complex, or AV dissociation may be present.

Premature junctional complexes arise from the AV junction. A retrograde P wave is usually present but may be prevented by a sinus P wave. They usually do not require therapy.

A regular junctional rhythm with a rate exceeding 60 beats per minute (usually between 70 and 130 per minute) is considered an accelerated junctional rhythm or *nonparoxysmal AV junctional tachycardia*. The gradual onset and termination account for the term nonparoxysmal and may imply that the mechanism of the tachycardia is increased automaticity. Retrograde activation of the atria or AV dissociation may be present. Nonparoxysmal AV junctional tachycardia occurs most commonly in patients with underlying heart disease, such as inferior myocardial infarction, myocarditis, and acute rheumatic fever, or after open heart surgery. The most common cause is digitalis excess. Therapy is directed toward the underlying etiological factor.

Paroxysmal supraventricular tachycardias (PSVT) are regular tachycardias that occur and terminate suddenly. They are due to a variety of mechanisms, the most common of which are atrioventricular (AV) nodal re-entry (approximately 60 per cent of cases) and AV re-entry using a concealed accessory bypass tract (approximately 30 per cent of cases). Sinus nodal re-entry, intra-atrial re-entry, and automatic atrial tachycardias account for the remaining PSVT's.

AV nodal re-entry is characterized by narrow QRS complexes (unless functional aberration has occurred), sudden onset and termination, and regular rates, usually between 150 and 250 beats per minute. Carotid sinus massage may slow the tachycardia slightly, and if termination occurs, it is abrupt. AV nodal re-entry commonly occurs in patients with no organic heart disease. Symptoms vary according to the rate of the tachycardia and the presence of organic heart disease. In some patients, rest, reassurance, and sedation may abort an attack. Vagal maneuvers including Valsalva, carotid sinus massage, and gagging may terminate the tachycardias and should be repeated after each pharmacological intervention. Intravenous verapamil, 5 to 10 mg, terminates AV nodal re-entry after about two minutes in over 90 per cent of cases and is the treatment of choice should vagal maneuvers fail. Edrophonium chloride, a short-acting cholinesterase inhibitor, may also terminate AV nodal re-entry and is administered in a total dose of 10 mg IV after a 1-mg test dose. Edrophonium should be used cautiously in patients who have hypotension or bronchospastic lung disease. Intravenous propranolol may be given (see Table 8–2) but must be used cautiously in patients with heart failure or chronic lung disease. Intravenous digoxin may also be used, but its onset of action is longer. If the patient is experiencing hemodynamic compromise, DC cardioversion with low energies is effective. Atrial or ventricular pacing also may restore sinus rhythm. In some patients, type I antiarrhythmic agents such as procainamide, quinidine, and disopyramide may be required to terminate AV nodal re-entry, but these drugs are used more often to prevent recurrences. Vasopressors (e.g., phenylephrine or metaraminol) may terminate AV nodal re-entry by inducing reflex vagal stimulation but are not commonly used. Digitalis is usually the initial drug choice for chronic therapy. If unsuccessful, verapamil, propranolol, or quinidine may be added. For some hard-to-control patients, antitachycardia pacemaker implantation or surgery may be considered.

PSVT may be caused by re-entry utilizing a retrograde concealed accessory pathway. The presence of the accessory pathway is not evident during sinus rhythm because antegrade conduction is not present, and therefore the ECG manifestations of the Wolff-Parkinson-White syndrome are not evident. However, the mechanism of tachycardia is the same as that in most patients with the Wolff-Parkinson-White syndrome, that is, antegrade conduction over the AV node and retrograde conduction over the accessory pathway. Since it takes a relatively long time for the impulse to travel through the ventricular tissue to the accessory pathway and back to the atrium, the retrograde P wave during this form of tachycardia occurs after completion of the QRS complex, usually in the ST segment or early T wave. In distinction, patients with AV nodal re-entrant tachycardias usually have their retrograde P wave inscribed during or just after the QRS complex, although longer retrograde conduction intervals can occur in AV nodal re-entry. Tachycardia rates tend to be somewhat faster than those in AV re-entry (≥200 per minute), but a great deal of overlap exists. Vagal maneuvers, verapamil, digitalis, and propranolol are acceptable choices for prompt termination. Chronic therapy often involves combinations of drugs that prolong accessory pathway conduction time and refractoriness (for example, quinidine, procainamide, and disopyramide) and drugs affecting AV nodal conduction.

PRE-EXCITATION SYNDROMES (Fig. 8–4)

Pre-excitation syndromes occur when ventricular activation occurs earlier than would be expected using the normal AV conduction system. There are several varieties of anomalous AV connections; the most common is the Wolff-Parkinson-White syndrome, in which an accessory atrioventricular pathway (Kent bundle) connects atrium with ventricle, short-circuiting the normal AV conduction system. A portion of the ventricle is activated via conduction over the accessory pathway before the remainder of the ventricle is activated via the normal AV conduction system, and the resultant QRS is a fusion of activation initiated by each of the two (normal and abnormal) AV pathways. Therefore, the PR interval is usually shortened (<0.12 sec) and the duration of the QRS is increased (>0.12 sec). The initial slurring of the QRS secondary to ventricular pre-excitation is referred to as the delta wave. Although the Wolff-Parkinson-White syndrome has been divided into Type A (positive delta wave in V_1 and V_6) and Type B (negative delta wave in V_1 and positive delta wave in V_6), this classification system is a gross oversimplification of the many ECG varieties produced by AV connections at different sites and is not very useful clinically. Accessory

FIGURE 8–4. Pre-excitation syndrome is apparent in the 12-lead ECG (short PR interval, wide QRS, delta wave). During atrial fibrillation the ventricular rate is extremely rapid, at times approaching 350 beats/min. The gross irregularity of the cycle lengths, wide QRS complexes interspersed with normal QRS complexes, and very rapid rate should suggest the diagnosis of atrial fibrillation and an atrioventricular bypass tract.

AV pathways may be located anywhere along the AV ring on either the left or right side or along the septum and are occasionally multiple.

The most common arrhythmia caused by an abnormal AV (Kent) connection is termed *orthodromic* reciprocating tachycardia: the antegrade limb of the re-entrant circuit is the AV node and the retrograde limb is the accessory pathway. *Antidromic* tachycardia utilizes the accessory pathway for the antegrade limb and the AV node as the retrograde limb. In the orthodromic variety, the QRS complexes either are normal or exhibit functional left or right bundle branch block. In the antidromic variety, the QRS complexes are totally pre-excited and consist of a wide, bizarre QRS. Similar pre-excited QRS complexes can occur when an atrial tachyarrhythmia (for example, atrial fibrillation) results in an extremely rapid ventricular response via the accessory AV connection. Arrhythmias involving the other types of anomalous connections are rare. Most adults with pre-excitation have normal hearts, although Ebstein's anomaly has an increased incidence of pre-excitation. Sudden death occurs rarely but may be a threat in patients with atrial fibrillation and rapid ventricular responses or in patients with associated congenital anomalies.

Patients who have frequent episodes of tachyarrhythmias and/or in whom the arrhythmias cause significant symptoms should receive therapy. Drugs that prolong refractoriness of the accessory pathway (e.g., quinidine, procainamide, and disopyramide) or the AV node (e.g., digitalis, verapamil, and propranolol) may be effective in treating the reciprocating tachycardia; long-term therapy may require one drug from each group. Drugs that prolong accessory pathway refractoriness are effective in slowing the ventricular rate during atrial flutter or atrial fibrillation. Because digitalis has been reported to shorten refractoriness in the accessory pathway and accelerate the ventricular response in some patients with atrial fibrillation, it is advisable not to use digitalis as a single drug in patients with the Wolff-Parkinson-White syndrome. Lidocaine and verapamil have also been reported to increase the ventricular response during atrial fibrillation in some patients with the Wolff-Parkinson-White syndrome. Termination of an acute episode of orthodromic reciprocating tachycardia may be approached as for AV nodal re-entry, but digitalis, verapamil, and lidocaine should be avoided in patients with atrial fibrillation or flutter. In patients with incomplete drug response or young patients who wish not to take drugs for the rest of their lives, antitachycardia pacing or surgical ablation of the accessory pathway is possible.

VENTRICULAR RHYTHM DISTURBANCES (Fig. 8–5)

Premature ventricular complexes (PVC's) are premature, bizarrely shaped QRS complexes of prolonged duration differing in contour from the dominant QRS complex. The T wave is large and oriented in the opposite direction from the major QRS deflection. The sinus node and atria are usually not activated prematurely by retrograde conduction from the PVC, and therefore a "compensatory pause" results; that is, the pause after the

PVC is sufficiently long that the interval between the two normally conducted QRS complexes flanking the PVC equals two sinus cycle lengths. A PVC that does not produce a pause is termed interpolated. Two successive premature PVC's are termed a pair or couplet, while three or more successive PVC's are arbitrarily termed ventricular tachycardia. If PVC's have different contours, they are called multifocal, multiform, polymorphic, or pleomorphic. If PVC's are not coupled to the previous QRS, parasystole should be considered; however, many nonparasystolic PVC's do not exhibit fixed coupling. The prevalence of PVC's increases with age. They are often asymptomatic but can give rise to palpitations, or if present in long runs of bigeminy, may produce hypotension, since they are premature and relatively ineffective at ejecting blood. The number of PVC's may increase during infection, ischemia, anesthesia, psychological stress, and excessive use of tobacco, caffeine, or alcohol. In the absence of underlying heart disease, the presence of PVC's probably has no significance regarding longevity or limitation of activity, and antiarrhythmic therapy is not indicated. The presence of PVC's identifies patients at an increased risk of cardiac death if they have coronary artery disease, hypertrophic cardiomyopathy, or mitral valve prolapse; however, treatment of PVC's has not been demonstrated to decrease sudden death. If drug therapy is indicated

FIGURE 8–5. A, Multiform premature ventricular systoles. Each sinus beat is followed by premature ventricular complexes that have two contours, one predominantly upright and the other predominantly negative. B, Accelerated idioventricular rhythm. The sinus rate slows slightly and allows the escape of an idioventricular rhythm. A fusion beat with a short PR interval results. Subsequently the sinus node once again regains control of the ventricular rhythm. C, Ventricular tachycardia. A regular wide complex tachycardia is present. Atrial activity is not readily apparent. The complexes marked C and F most likely represent capture and fusion complexes that confirm the ventricular origin of the arrhythmia. D, Ventricular flutter. Ventricular depolarization and repolarization appear as a sine wave with regular oscillations. The QRS complex cannot be distinguished from the ST segment or T wave. E, Ventricular fibrillation. The baseline is irregular and undulating without any electrical evidence of organized ventricular activity.

(usually only in patients with symptoms), lidocaine can be used acutely and procainamide, quinidine, or disopyramide may be considered for chronic therapy.

Ventricular tachycardia occurs when three or more consecutive PVC's occur with a rate exceeding 100 per minute. The QRS complexes usually have a prolonged duration and bizarre shape, with ST and T vectors opposite to the major QRS deflection. Atrial activity may be independent of ventricular activity (AV dissociation), or the atrium may be depolarized by the ventricles retrogradely (VA association). QRS contours may be unchanging (uniform) or may vary. The differentiation between sustained and nonsustained ventricular tachycardia is somewhat arbitrary but clinically useful; one guideline is that sustained ventricular tachycardia lasts at least 30 seconds or requires termination prior to 30 seconds because of hemodynamic decompensation.

The electrocardiographic distinction between supraventricular tachycardia with abnormal intraventricular conduction and ventricular tachycardia can be difficult. Supraventricular tachycardia may be associated with prolonged QRS complexes when pre-existing bundle branch block is present, functional aberration exists, or conduction over an accessory pathway is present. When fusion or capture QRS complexes occur during a wide-complex tachycardia (that is, early, narrow complexes that are either partially [fusion] or completely [capture] caused by activation from a supraventricular source), ventricular origin of the tachycardia can be assumed. The identification of AV dissociation, sometimes requiring esophageal or intracardiac recordings to determine atrial activity, is much more characteristic of ventricular than supraventricular tachycardia. However, only about 50 per cent of ventricular tachycardias demonstrate complete AV dissociation. In addition, the following characteristics favor a supraventricular origin: slowing or termination of the tachycardia by increased vagal tone, onset after a premature P wave; RP interval ≤ 100 msec, more atrial impulses than ventricular impulses (for example, 2:1 AV conduction), initiation of wide complexes after a long/short cycle sequence; and rsR' in V_1. With preceding normal QRS conduction, if left axis deviation or QRS duration of 140 msec or more is present during tachycardia, ventricular tachycardia is likely.

Ventricular tachycardia occurs in patients with ischemic heart disease, congestive and hypertrophic cardiomyopathy, mitral valve prolapse, valvular heart disease, and primary electrical disease (no identifiable structural heart disease). Even short runs of ventricular tachycardia may be important when detected in the late hospital phase of acute myocardial infarction, since the one-year mortality rate of this group appears to be much greater than for patients without tachycardia.

Deciding when to treat patients with ventricular tachycardia is sometimes difficult. Patients with chronic recurrent sustained ventricular tachycardia and those with symptomatic nonsustained ventricular tachycardia are treated. Treatment of patients with asymptomatic nonsustained ventricular tachycardia is controversial; we tend to treat those with structural heart disease, especially left ventricular dysfunction, and not treat those with no structural heart disease. Acute therapy of ventricular tachycardia is achieved with intravenous lidocaine; if unsuccessful, intravenous procainamide or bretylium may be used. If hypotension, shock, angina, congestive heart failure, or symptoms of cerebral hypoperfusion are present, the rhythm should be terminated promptly with DC cardioversion, beginning with very low energies (10 to 50 joules) synchronized with the QRS. DC cardioversion of digitalis-induced ventricular tachycardia may be hazardous but is sometimes necessary. If ventricular tachycardia is recurrent despite drug therapy, pacing may occasionally be useful for termination. Before embarking on chronic drug therapy, a search for reversible conditions contributing to the arrhythmia should be initiated; for example, metabolic abnormalities, hypoxia, digitalis excess, and congestive heart failure should be corrected. Effective drugs for chronic therapy include quinidine, procainamide, disopyramide, and tocainide. Phenytoin is usually not successful unless digitalis toxicity is present, and propranolol is usually unsuccessful unless the ventricular tachycardia is related to ischemia or catecholamine stimulation. Amiodarone (investigational) is very effective in patients in whom conventional agents have failed. Combinations of drugs are sometimes necessary. Surgery or implantable electrical devices may be considered in patients with ventricular tachycardia refractory to drug therapy.

Accelerated idioventricular rhythm refers to impulse formation originating in the ventricle with a rate of approximately 60 to 110 per minute. It often competes with the sinus node for control of the heart, and fusion and capture complexes occur commonly. The onset of the arrhythmia is often gradual (nonparoxysmal), and enhanced automaticity is presumed to be the mechanism. Precipitation of more rapid ventricular arrhythmias is not common. The arrhythmia usually occurs in patients with acute myocardial infarction or digitalis toxicity, and suppressive therapy is usually not necessary. If symptoms occur or if more malignant tachyarrhythmias result, therapy as noted above is indicated. Often simply increasing the sinus rate with atropine or atrial pacing suppresses the accelerated idioventricular rhythm.

The term *torsades de pointes* refers to a ventricular tachyarrhythmia characterized by QRS complexes of changing amplitude that appear to twist around the isoelectric line, occurring in the setting of a prolonged QT interval. Episodes of torsades de pointes often terminate spontaneously, but ventricular fibrillation may supervene. The syndrome may be either congenital or acquired. Acquired forms may be caused by any antiarrhythmic drug that prolongs the QT interval (for example, quinidine, procainamide, or disopyramide) or by psychoactive drugs such as phenothiazines and tricyclic antidepressants. In addition, potassium depletion, liquid protein diet, and other metabolic abnormalities may be associated with the long QT syndrome. Acute therapy involves withdrawing the offending drug and correcting metabolic abnormalities. Antiarrhythmic agents that prolong the QT interval may worsen the arrhythmia. Temporary ventricular or atrial pacing is the most effective therapy for suppressing the bursts of polymorphic tachycardia. Isoproterenol has been reported to be effective until pacing is instituted. Magnesium or bretylium therapy may be useful. If a polymorphic ventricular tachycardia resembling torsades de pointes is present but the QT interval is normal, standard antiarrhythmic drugs may be given.

Patients with congenital prolonged QT syndrome who are at increased risk for sudden death include those who have family members who died suddenly at an early age and those who have experienced syncope or torsades de pointes. Electrocardiograms should be obtained from all family members when a patient presents with suspected congenital long QT syndrome. Auditory stimuli, psychological stress, and exercise may provoke an arrhythmia in susceptible patients. For patients who have idiopathic long QT syndrome but no syncope, complex ventricular arrhythmias, or family history of sudden cardiac death, no therapy is recommended. In asymptomatic patients with long QT syndrome who have complex ventricular arrhythmias or a family history of premature sudden cardiac death, beta blockers at maximally tolerated doses are recommended. In patients with syncope, beta blockers at maximally tolerated doses, combined with phenytoin or phenobarbital if necessary, are suggested. For patients who continue to have syncope despite drug therapy, left-sided cervicothoracic sympathetic ganglionectomy has been effective, since sympathetic imbalance appears to be important in the pathogenesis of this syndrome.

Ventricular fibrillation generates little or no blood flow and is usually fatal within three to five minutes unless terminated. Ventricular fibrillation is recognized by the presence of irregular undulations of varying contour and amplitude without distinct QRS complexes, ST segments, or T waves. *Ventricular flutter* appears as a sine wave with regular, large oscillations occurring at a rate of 150 to 300 per minute. Ventricular fibrillation occurs in a variety of situations, including coronary artery disease, antiarrhythmic drug administration, hypoxia, ischemia, atrial fibrillation with rapid ventricular rates in the pre-excitation syndromes, accidental electrical shock, and poorly timed cardioversion. Most patients resuscitated from out-of-hospital cardiac arrest have ventricular fibrillation as their arrhythmia, often without acute myocardial infarction. Treatment is an immediate nonsynchronized DC shock using 200 to 400 joules. If ventricular fibrillation has been present for more than a few minutes, correction of metabolic abnormalities may aid in electrically converting the rhythm, although DC shock should not be delayed to await correction of hypoxia or acidosis. Once ventricular fibrilla-

tion has been terminated, medications to prevent recurrence of ventricular fibrillation should be initiated (e.g., lidocaine). Ventricular fibrillation rarely, if ever, terminates on its own and is lethal unless DC shock is applied.

HEART BLOCK (Fig. 8–6)

Heart block refers to a disturbance of impulse conduction and should be distinguished from interference, a normal phenomenon in which impulse conduction is blocked owing to physiological refractoriness in the wake of a preceding impulse. Heart block may occur anywhere in the heart but is commonly recognized electrocardiographically in the AV node, His bundle, or bundle branches. In *first-degree AV heart block*, AV conduction time is prolonged (PR interval ≥0.20 sec), but all impulses are conducted. *Second-degree heart block* occurs in two forms: *type I second-degree heart block (Wenckebach)* is characterized by a progressive lengthening of the PR interval until a P wave is not conducted. *Type II second-degree AV heart block* denotes occasional or repetitive sudden block of a P wave without prior measurable lengthening of the PR interval. Type II AV block often antedates the development of Stokes-Adams syncope and complete AV block, while type I AV block with a normal QRS complex is usually more benign and does not progress to advanced forms of AV conduction disturbances. In the patient with acute myocardial infarction, type I AV block usually accompanies inferior infarction, is transient, and does not require temporary pacing, whereas type II AV block usually accompanies anterior myocardial infarction, may require temporary or permanent pacing, and is associated with a high mortality, mostly due to pump failure. First-degree or type I second-degree AV block can occur in healthy young people, especially well-trained athletes. Any medication that affects AV nodal conduction (for example, digitalis, beta blockers, or verapamil) may cause first- or second-degree AV block.

Type I AV block with a normal QRS complex is usually at the level of the AV node proximal to the His bundle. Type II AV block usually occurs in association with a bundle branch block and is localized to the His-Purkinje system. Type I AV block in a patient with a bundle branch block may represent block in either the AV node or the His-Purkinje system. Type II AV block in a patient with a normal QRS complex may be due to intra-His block but is more likely to be type I AV nodal block that exhibits small increments in AV conduction time. Note that 2:1 AV block may represent either AV nodal or His-Purkinje block.

Complete AV block occurs when no atrial activity conducts to the ventricles. The atria and ventricles are controlled by independent pacemakers, and thus complete AV block is one cause of AV dissociation. The ventricular rhythm is usually regular. If the AV block is at the level of the AV node (for example, congenital AV block), the QRS complexes are normal in morphology and duration, with rates of 40 to 60 per minute, and

FIGURE 8–6. *A,* First-degree AV block. The PR interval is prolonged. *B,* Second-degree AV block (Type I, Wenckebach), characterized by progressive PR prolongation preceding the nonconducted P wave. In the setting of a normal QRS complex, Wenckebach almost always occurs at the level of the AV node. *C,* Second-degree AV block, Type II. Left bundle branch block is present in this recording of lead I. Sudden failure of AV conduction results, without antecedent PR prolongation. *D,* Acquired third-degree (complete) AV block. Complete AV dissociation is present owing to complete AV heart block. Atria and ventricles are under control of separate pacemakers, the sinus node and an idioventricular escape rhythm, respectively. *E,* Congenital third-degree (complete) AV block in a young adult at the level of the AV node. The QRS complex is normal.

respond to autonomic influences. If the AV block is in the His-Purkinje system (usually acquired), the escape rhythm originates within the ventricle, has a wide QRS and a slower rate, and is less reliable and under less autonomic influence. Causes of AV block include surgery, electrolyte disturbances, endocarditis, tumor, Chagas' disease, rheumatoid nodules, calcific aortic stenosis, myxedema, polymyositis, infiltrative processes such as amyloid, sarcoid, or scleroderma, drug toxicity, coronary disease, and degenerative processes. In children the most common cause of AV block is congenital and is usually asymptomatic; in some, however, symptoms eventually develop, requiring pacemaker implantation. The indications for pacemaker therapy in heart block are summarized in Table 8–5. Atropine (for AV nodal block) and isoproterenol (for heart block at any site) may be used transiently while preparations are made for ventricular pacing. Drugs cannot be relied on to increase the heart rate for more than several hours to a few days without producing significant side effects.

The term *AV dissociation* describes independent depolarization of the atria and ventricles. AV dissociation is not a primary disturbance of rhythm but is a "symptom" of an underlying rhythm disturbance produced by one or a combination of three causes that prevent the normal transmission of impulses from atrium to ventricle: (1) Slowing of the dominant pacemaker of the heart (usually the sinus node), allowing escape of a subsidiary or latent pacemaker. This is AV dissociation by default of the primary pacemaker and is often a normal phenomenon, e.g., sinus bradycardia and a junctional escape rhythm. (2) Acceleration of a latent pacemaker that usurps control of the ventricles. This abnormally enhanced discharge rate of a usually slower subsidiary pacemaker is pathological, e.g., junctional or ventricular tachycardia. (3) Block at the AV junction that prevents impulses formed at a normal rate in a dominant pacemaker from reaching the ventricles so that the ventricles beat under the control of a subsidiary pacemaker, e.g., complete AV block with a ventricular escape rhythm. It is important to remember that complete AV dissociation is not synonymous with complete AV block.

SYNCOPE

Syncope refers to sudden transient loss of consciousness, usually due to transient cerebral hypoperfusion. Presyncope is described as a light-headed spell that, if more prolonged, would cause loss of consciousness. Both may occur in the same patient and have similar etiologies. The causes of syncope are summarized in Table 8–9.

Cardiac syncope is due either to lesions that obstruct outflow of blood from the heart or to arrhythmias. In patients with severe aortic stenosis or other causes of obstructive syncope, when the systemic vascular resistance decreases upon exercise, the heart is unable to augment cardiac output sufficiently to maintain perfusion and syncope results. Both tachyarrhythmias and bradyarrhythmias that result in cerebral hypoperfusion can cause cardiac syncope. The hypersensitive carotid sinus syndrome, described above, is a well-recognized cause of syncope.

The history and physical examination are valuable in excluding many causes of syncope (Table 8–9). Even though the electrocardiogram may not reveal the actual arrhythmia causing syncope, electrocardiographic clues (for example, the presence of simple or complex ventricular ectopy, evidence of a previous myocardial infarction, or the delta wave of the Wolff-Parkinson-White syndrome) may suggest potential arrhythmic causes. Prolonged electrocardiographic (Holter) recording may be the cornerstone of diagnosis in arrhythmic syncope. On many occasions, more than 24 hours of recording are required to detect the responsible arrhythmia. Exercise testing is also valuable in some patients whose arrhythmias are exercise-induced. Patients with obstructive syncope such as aortic stenosis should not undergo exercise testing. In selected patients invasive electrophysiological studies may be useful to delineate the etiology of the syncope.

SUDDEN CARDIAC DEATH

The most commonly used definition of sudden death is unexpected, nontraumatic death occurring within an hour after the onset of symptoms; some studies have included death occurring within 24 hours of the onset of symptoms. Sudden cardiac death claims approximately 1200 lives daily in the United States and is the leading cause of death among men between the ages of 20 and 60. By far the most common cause of sudden death is cardiac, and within that group, the most common cause is ventricular tachyarrhythmias.

Nonarrhythmic causes of sudden death are listed in Table 8–10.

Ventricular tachyarrhythmias, generally related to ischemic heart disease, are the most common cause of sudden cardiac death. Although 75 per cent of patients resuscitated from ventricular fibrillation have extensive coronary artery disease, only 20 per cent have evidence of acute transmural myocardial infarction. Approximately 75 per cent of patients have a previous history of cardiac disease; sudden death is the first manifestation of cardiac disease in the remainder. The difference in recurrence of sudden death in patients with (2 per cent at one year) and without (22 per cent at one year) acute myocardial infarc-

TABLE 8–9.   CAUSES OF SYNCOPE

CAUSE	FEATURES
Peripheral Vascular or Circulatory Causes	
Vasovagal syncope	Prodrome of pallor, yawning, nausea, diaphoresis. Precipitated by stress or pain. Occurs when patient is upright, aborted by recumbency. Fall in blood pressure without appropriate rise in heart rate.
Micturition syncope	Syncope with urination (probably vagal)
Post-tussive syncope	Syncope after paroxysm of coughing
Hypersensitive carotid sinus syndrome	Vasodepressor and/or cardio-inhibitory responses with light carotid sinus massage (see text)
Drugs	Orthostasis
	Occurs with antihypertensive drugs, tricyclic antidepressants, phenothiazines
Volume depletion	Orthostasis
	Occurs with hemorrhage, excessive vomiting or diarrhea, Addison's disease
Autonomic dysfunction	Orthostasis
	Occurs in diabetes, alcoholism, Parkinson's disease, deconditioning after a prolonged illness
Central Nervous System	
Cerebrovascular	Transient ischemic attacks and strokes are unusual causes of syncope. Associated neurologic abnormalities are usually present.
Seizures	Warning aura sometimes present, jerking of extremities, tongue biting, urinary incontinence, postictal confusion
Metabolic	
Hypoglycemia	Confusion, tachycardia, jitteriness prior to syncope. Patient may be taking insulin.
Cardiac	
Obstructive	Syncope is often exertional. Physical findings consistent with aortic stenosis, hypertrophic obstructive cardiomyopathy, cardiac tamponade, atrial myxoma, prosthetic valve malfunction, Eisenmenger's syndrome, tetralogy of Fallot, primary pulmonary hypertension, pulmonic stenosis, massive pulmonary embolism
Arrhythmias	Syncope may be sudden; occurs in any position. Episodes of dizziness or palpitations. May be a history of heart disease. Brady- or tachyarrhythmias may be responsible; check for hypersensitive carotid sinus.

tion may be due to different arrhythmia mechanisms. Patients with ventricular fibrillation at the time of an acute myocardial infarction probably do not need long-term antiarrhythmic therapy unless chronic late ventricular tachycardia is documented. The risk of recurrent ventricular fibrillation is higher if there is evidence of left ventricular dysfunction or evidence of previous

TABLE 8–10. SELECTED CAUSES OF SUDDEN DEATH

Noncardiac
Central nervous system hemorrhage
Massive pulmonary embolus
Drug overdose
Hypoxia secondary to lung disease
Aortic dissection or rupture
Cardiac
Ventricular tachycardia
Bradyarrhythmias, sick sinus syndrome
Aortic stenosis
Tetralogy of Fallot
Pericardial tamponade
Cardiac tumors
Complications of infective endocarditis
Hypertrophic cardiomyopathy (arrhythmia or obstruction)
Myocardial ischemia
    Atherosclerosis
    Prinzmetal's angina
    Kawasaki's arteritis

myocardial infarction. Nonatherosclerotic etiologies of ventricular tachyarrhythmias associated with sudden death are mitral valve prolapse, hypertrophic or other cardiomyopathies, antiarrhythmic drugs, myocarditis, prolonged QT syndrome, and Wolff-Parkinson-White syndrome with rapid antegrade conduction over an accessory pathway.

The identification of patients at high risk for sudden cardiac death can be difficult. The occurrence of complex ventricular ectopy including multiform PVC's, pairs, and ventricular tachycardia in survivors of myocardial infarction is associated with a two- to three-fold increase in subsequent sudden death; however, suppression of ventricular ectopy with antiarrhythmic agents has not been proven to decrease the incidence of sudden death, and the necessity of suppressing less complex forms of ventricular ectopy is unclear. The risk of sudden cardiac death and the incidence of complex ectopy is greater in patients with poor left ventricular function.

The patient who has suffered sudden cardiac arrest in the absence of acute myocardial infarction and the patient with recurrent symptomatic ventricular tachyarrhythmias must be treated with antiarrhythmic therapy. The end point of antiarrhythmic therapy to be used to judge efficacy is often unclear. The mere attainment of "therapeutic" serum levels of an antiarrhythmic agent is not usually sufficient to guard against recurrent ventricular tachyarrhythmias. Prolonged electrocardiographic monitoring is noninvasive, simple, and widely available. However, many patients with sudden death demonstrate very little spontaneous ectopy between episodes; therefore, suppression of spontaneous ectopy cannot be used as an end point in these patients. In addition, even in patients with spontaneous ectopy, it is not clear whether an appropriate end point would be elimination of all ventricular tachycardia, all complex ectopy, or all PVC's. Drug evaluation using exercise testing and prolonged ambulatory recording to judge efficacy has been reported to decrease the incidence of recurrent malignant tachyarrhythmias but can only be used in patients with spontaneous high-grade ventricular ectopy between episodes of sustained tachyarrhythmia. Most investigators feel that patients experiencing sudden cardiac arrest in the absence of acute myocardial infarction should undergo serial electrophysiological testing to guide antiarrhythmic therapy. The suppression with a drug of ventricular tachycardia inducible by electrical stimulation appears to provide a better indicator of drug success than suppression of spontaneous ectopy and can be used in patients with little or no spontaneous ectopy. If arrhythmias cannot be controlled with drugs, the implantable cardioverter defibrillator and/or cardiac surgery are options. Coronary artery revascularization alone is usually not sufficient to prevent recurrent ventricular tachyarrhythmias.

Antiarrhythmic therapy in patients after myocardial infarction as prophylaxis for malignant cardiac arrhythmias has not been proven effective. However, in certain high-risk patients antiarrhythmic therapy may be warranted, for example, those with nonsustained ventricular tachycardia after infarction. Several large multicenter studies have demonstrated a decrease in the incidence of sudden death in patients treated with beta-adrenergic receptor blocking agents after myocardial infarction, and these drugs probably should be considered if no contraindication to their administration exists.

PRINCIPLES OF CARDIOPULMONARY RESUSCITATION

Cardiopulmonary resuscitation consists of basic and advanced life support. Upon evaluating a patient with suspected cardiac arrest, one should first quickly establish that the patient is truly unresponsive and not breathing. If a pulse is not present, a precordial thump to the midsternum may be tried. Subsequently, the "ABC's" of basic life support should be observed: Airway, Breathing, and Circulation. The mouth and pharynx should be examined to assure that no obstruction is present. The tongue should be removed from the posterior pharynx by tilting the head backward and hyperextending the neck. This maneuver can sometimes cause resumption of spontaneous respiration. If no breathing is noted, mouth-to-mouth or mouth-to-nose breathing should be initiated in four quick breaths. Time is often wasted trying to intubate a patient when adequate ventilation could be accomplished immediately via mouth or mask ventilation. One should check to see that the chest rises with each ventilation. If a carotid pulse is not present after the initial ventilations, external cardiac compression over the lower half of the sternum (not over the xiphoid process) should be initiated. The sternum should be depressed 3 to 5 cm, with the patient lying on a hard surface. Compressions should be approximately 60 per minute, with a ratio of 5 compressions to 1 ventilation if two rescuers are present. A single rescuer must give 15 chest compressions alternating with two ventilations every 15 seconds.

Advanced life support should be initiated while basic life support continues. Defibrillation should be applied if indicated as soon as possible and *is the single most definitive treatment available for most cardiac arrests.* Oxygen should be administered and an adequate intravenous access should be established. If circulation has not been restored quickly, sodium bicarbonate 1 mEq/kg IV is given to treat metabolic acidosis and is repeated after 10 minutes; further administration of sodium bicarbonate should be guided by blood gas and pH measurements once effective circulation is restored. Epinephrine (5 to 10 ml of a 1:10,000 solution administered via an intravenous, intracardiac, or endotracheal route every 5 minutes as needed) is useful in treating asystole and also in aiding defibrillation of fine (low-amplitude) ventricular fibrillation. Atropine (boluses of 0.5 mg IV at 5-minute intervals to a total dose of approximately 2 to 4 mg) can be administered for profound bradycardia. Isoproterenol given as a constant infusion (2 to 20 μg/min) and titrated according to response may be used to treat bradyarrhythmias if atropine is ineffective. Emergency cardiac pacing may be attempted for bradyarrhythmias if atropine and isoproterenol are unsuccessful.

Lidocaine, procainamide, or bretylium tosylate can be administered to help terminate ventricular tachyarrhythmias and prevent their recurrence. Intravenous furosemide and/or morphine may be used to relieve pulmonary edema. Calcium chloride (2.5 to 5 ml of a 10 per cent solution repeated if necessary in 10 minutes) is given to increase myocardial contractility, especially if electromechanical dissociation is present. Calcium should be used with caution in a patient with known digitalis excess. Calcium chloride will precipitate if given in the same intravenous line with sodium bicarbonate.

Electromechanical dissociation refers to the presence of cardiac electrical activity without appropriate mechanical activity. It may be caused by decreased filling of the heart (e.g., hypovolemia, cardiac tamponade, pulmonary embolus) or severe myocardial pump depression that may respond to calcium. Emergency pericardiocentesis may be attempted if cardiac tamponade is suspected.

The widespread application of cardiopulmonary resuscitation via education of the public and extensive emergency care systems in many cities has increased both the number of cardiac arrest victims who reach the hospital and the number who survive to be discharged. Survival critically depends on the time from arrest to the initiation of resuscitation and is best if basic life support can be initiated within 3 to 4 minutes and more definitive therapy (i.e., defibrillation) shortly thereafter.

REFERENCES

Bigger JT, Fleiss JL, Kleiger R, Miller JP, Rolnitzky L, et al: The relationships among ventricular arrhythmias, left ventricular dysfunction, and mortality in the 2 years after myocardial infarction. Circulation 69:250, 1984.

Cobb LA, Werner JA, and Trobaugh GB: Sudden cardiac death. I. A decade's experience with out-of-hospital resuscitation. II. Outcome of resuscitation; management, and future directions. Mod Concepts Cardiovasc Dis 19:31, 37, 1980.

Gallagher JJ, Pritchett ELC, Sealy WC, Kasell J, and Wallace AG: The preexcitation syndromes. Prog Cardiovasc Dis 20:285, 1978.

Health and Public Policy Committee, American College of Physicians: Diagnostic endocardial electrical recording and stimulation. Ann Intern Med 100:452, 1984.

Josephson ME, and Kastor JA: Supraventricular tachycardia: Mechanisms and management. Ann Intern Med 87:346, 1977.

Lown B: Sudden cardiac death: The major challenge confronting contemporary cardiology. Am J Cardiol 43:313, 1979.

Ludmer PL, and Goldschlager N: Cardiac pacing in the 1980's. N Engl J Med 311:1671, 1984.

Scheinman MM, and Morady F: Invasive cardiac electrophysiologic testing: The current state of the art. Circulation 67:1169, 1983.

Smith WM, and Gallagher JJ: "Les torsades de pointes": An unusual ventricular arrhythmia. Ann Intern Med 93:578, 1980.

Standards and guidelines for cardiopulmonary resuscitation (CPR) and emergency cardiac care (ECC). JAMA 244:453, 1980.

Zipes DP (ed): Symposium on Cardiac Arrhythmias I & II. Med Clin North Am, Vol 68, No 4 and 5 (July, September), 1984.

Zipes DP (ed): Arrhythmias I & II. Cardiol Clin, Vol 1, No 1 and 2 (February, May), 1983.

MYOCARDIAL AND PERICARDIAL DISEASE

9

MYOCARDIAL DISEASE

MYOCARDITIS

Acute myocardial inflammation is termed myocarditis and may be associated with fever, dyspnea, edema, fatigue, palpitations, and pleuro-pericardial pain. Myocarditis is frequently not clinically apparent and is suspected only on the basis of ST and T wave changes or a transient conduction defect on electrocardiography in a patient with a systemic illness. Physical examination may reveal signs of pericarditis or biventricular cardiac failure. Intraventricular or atrioventricular conduction disturbances or arrhythmias may occur.

Therapy is usually supportive. Congestive heart failure responds to routine management with digitalis, diuresis, and afterload reduction. Significant arrhythmias should be treated with antiarrhythmic agents. Steroids may be of benefit in acute rheumatic carditis but should be avoided in suspected infectious myocarditis. Immunosuppressive therapy may be helpful in selected patients.

Most patients recover completely. An unknown percentage of patients, probably small, develop a chronic process leading to a dilated cardiomyopathy after a varying latency period.

Infectious agents cause myocarditis by three basic mechanisms: (1) invasion of the myocardium, (2) production of a myocardial toxin, for example, diphtheria, and (3) autoimmunity, as in acute rheumatic fever. The infectious agents are multiple, most commonly thought to be viral, especially Coxsackie group B. Primary bacterial myocarditis is a rare but grave complication of bacterial endocarditis, most commonly caused by streptococci or staphylococci. *Mycoplasma pneumoniae* infections, toxoplasmosis, trichinosis, and rickettsial diseases such as Rocky Mountain spotted fever are associated with myocarditis. Protozoal myocarditis from trypanosomiasis (Chagas' disease) is common in Central and South America where it is a frequent cause of chronic congestive cardiomyopathy, heart block, and ventricular arrhythmias. Hypersensitivity reactions to various agents and radiation therapy can result in inflammation of the myocardium.

CARDIOMYOPATHY

Cardiomyopathy, a disease involving the heart muscle itself, is classified into three basic categories (Table 9–1). This classification is not rigid, and some cardiomyopathies may demonstrate characteristics that overlap among the three groups.

Dilated Cardiomyopathy

In dilated cardiomyopathy, ventricular enlargement occurs and systolic dysfunction results in symptoms of congestive heart failure. The cause of dilated cardiomyopathy is often not apparent but appears to be the end result of myocardial damage produced by a variety of toxic, metabolic, and infectious agents (Table 9–2). Clinical symptoms usually develop slowly, and patients may have ventricular dysfunction for some time before symptoms, usually of both left and right ventricular failure, appear. Q waves may be present on ECG without infarction when extensive left ventricular fibrosis has occurred. Echocardiography is important to exclude other causes of congestive

TABLE 9–1. CLASSIFICATION OF CARDIOMYOPATHY

TYPE	CHARACTERISTICS	SYMPTOMS AND SIGNS	LABORATORY DIAGNOSIS
Dilated (congestive)	Cardiac dilation, generalized hypocontractility	Left and right ventricular failure (see Table 2–4)	X-ray: cardiomegaly with pulmonary congestion ECG: sinus tachycardia, nonspecific ST-T changes, arrhythmias, conduction disturbances, Q waves Echo: dilated LV, generalized decreased wall motion, mitral valve motion consistent with low flow Catheterization: dilated hypocontractile ventricle; mitral regurgitation
Hypertrophic	Ventricular hypertrophy, especially the septum, with or without outflow tract obstruction Typically good systolic but poor diastolic (compliance) ventricular function	Dyspnea, angina, presyncope, syncope, palpitations Large jugular a wave, bifid carotid pulse, palpable S_4 gallop, prominent apical impulse; "dynamic" systolic murmur and thrill, mitral regurgitation murmur	X-ray: LV predominance, dilated left atrium ECG: left ventricular hypertrophy, Q waves, nonspecific ST-T waves; ventricular arrhythmias Echo: hypertrophy, usually asymmetric (septum > free wall); systolic anterior motion of mitral valve; midsystolic closure of aortic valve Catheterization: provokable outflow tract gradient; hypertrophy with vigorous systolic function and cavity obliteration; mitral regurgitation
Restrictive	Reduced diastolic compliance impeding ventricular filling; normal systolic function	Dyspnea, exercise intolerance, weakness Elevated jugular venous pressure, edema, hepatomegaly, ascites, S_4 & S_3 gallops, Kussmaul's sign	X-ray: mild cardiomegaly; pulmonary congestion ECG: low voltage, conduction disturbances, Q waves Echo: characteristic myocardial texture in amyloidosis with thickening of all cardiac structures Catheterization: square root sign; M-shaped atrial waveform, elevated left and right-sided filling pressures

909893

FIGURE 9–1. Typical electrocardiogram in pericarditis showing diffuse ST elevation.

heart failure. A pericardial effusion is sometimes present. Ventriculography shows enlargement of the left ventricle with diffuse wall motion reduction and sometimes left ventricular thrombi. Functional mitral regurgitation may be present, and occasionally it is difficult to distinguish from primary mitral regurgitation. The coronary arteries are normal or incidentally involved. Endomyocardial biopsy may sometimes be useful in diagnosing patients with cardiomyopathy.

Peripartum cardiomyopathy refers to congestive cardiomyopathy occurring in the last month of pregnancy or within five months of delivery in the absence of pre-existing heart disease. It occurs most frequently in multiparous blacks and is more common in older women and those with poor nutrition, poor prenatal care, or toxemia. Doxorubicin (Adriamycin) is an effective antitumor drug that commonly produces congestive cardiomyopathy. The risk of toxicity appears to be related to the cumulative dose, increasing as the dose increases but with a relatively abrupt increase in risk after approximately 450 to 550 mg/sq m. The prognosis after development of symptoms is extremely poor.

Hypertrophic Cardiomyopathy

Hypertrophic cardiomyopathy is characterized by myocardial hypertrophy, especially involving the interventricular septum. In many patients a dynamic pressure gradient can be detected in the subvalvular left ventricular outflow tract (hypertrophic obstructive cardiomyopathy or idiopathic hypertrophic subaortic stenosis). This gradient demonstrates wide fluctuations in severity and often is not present at rest, requiring physiological or pharmacological maneuvers to be precipitated. Even though much attention has been focused on

TABLE 9–2. CAUSES OF DILATED CARDIOMYOPATHY

Idiopathic
Infectious
  viral
  parasitic (e.g., Chagas' disease)
Toxins
  alcohol
  cobalt
  doxorubicin
Radiation
Systemic diseases
  connective tissue diseases (e.g., systemic lupus erythematosus)
  sarcoidosis
  hemochromatosis
Metabolic disorders
  thyrotoxicosis
  myxedema
  beriberi
  starvation
  glycogen storage diseases
  mucopolysaccharidoses
Neuromuscular disorders (e.g., certain muscular dystrophies)
Peripartum cardiomyopathy

the systolic gradient, the most characteristic pathophysiological abnormality in this syndrome is not systolic but rather diastolic dysfunction, characterized by abnormal stiffness of the left ventricle with impaired filling. Therefore, pulmonary venous pressures are elevated, and dyspnea is the most common symptom despite a typically hypercontractile left ventricle. In many patients the disease appears to be transmitted genetically as an autosomal dominant disorder with a high degree of penetrance, but sporadic cases do occur. Hypertrophy can involve predominantly the septum (asymmetric septal hypertrophy) or the septum and free wall equally (concentric left ventricular hypertrophy). Hypertrophied and bizarrely arranged myocardial cells are commonly but not always visualized pathologically, especially in the septum.

Signs and symptoms in hypertrophic cardiomyopathy are summarized in Table 9–1. A large jugular venous a wave may be present on physical examination owing to reduced compliance of the right ventricle. The carotid arterial upstroke is brisk and bifid in character with a rapid initial rise, a midsystolic dip, and a second late systolic rise characteristic of the dynamic outflow tract obstruction (see Fig. 2–2). The systolic outflow murmur typically is harsh, crescendo-decrescendo, often heard best between the apex and left sternal border, and radiates to the lower sternum, axilla, and base of the heart but often not into the neck. A murmur of concomitant mitral regurgitation is not uncommon. The systolic outflow murmur is said to be "dynamic" because its intensity varies inversely with the dimensions of the outflow tract. The outflow tract becomes larger with an increase in ventricular diastolic volume, an increase in systolic pressure against which the heart must pump, or a decrease in myocardial inotropic state. The outflow tract narrows with reversal of these factors (Table 9–3).

Left ventricular hypertrophy is common on ECG, and large Q waves, probably related to abnormal septal depolarization, may simulate septal myocardial infarction. Atrial fibrillation and other tachyarrhythmias are poorly tolerated owing to the hemodynamic abnormalities.

Echocardiography is the best technique for visualizing the hypertrophic myocardium and asymmetric septal hypertrophy. It is useful for screening family members of patients with hypertrophic cardiomyopathy. Narrowing of the left ventricular outflow tract by systolic anterior motion of the anterior leaflet of the mitral valve is characteristic of patients with obstructive cardiomyopathy, and the degree of systolic anterior motion appears to correlate with the degree of obstruction. The aortic valve may close partially in midsystole owing to the dynamic outflow obstruction; this finding, in addition to the systolic anterior motion, may be provoked with pharmacological manipulations (e.g., amyl nitrate, nitroglycerin, or isoproterenol). Mitral valve prolapse is sometimes observed along with evidence of a small left ventricular cavity and poor left ventricular compliance.

At cardiac catheterization, the systolic subvalvular gradient may or may not be present at rest, and provocative maneuvers such as nitroglycerin, amyl nitrate, isoproterenol infusion, and induced PVC's may provoke a gradient. The left ventricular end-diastolic pressure and a wave are elevated. Angiography demonstrates marked thickening of the ventricular septum and left ventricular free wall, with large papillary muscles distorting the ventricular shape and producing a characteristic hourglass configuration. The left ventricular cavity is usually small and systolic function vigorous, resulting in virtual obliteration of the ventricular cavity with systole. Mitral regurgitation is common.

The clinical course is variable, although symptoms may remain stable over a period of several years. Symptoms are often unrelated to the presence or severity of a gradient. Ventricular arrhythmias are common and sudden death may occur even in previously asymptomatic individuals. Any protective effect of medical therapy against arrhythmias is unproven.

Interventions that decrease ventricular contractility, increase ventricular volume, increase systemic arterial pressure, increase the dimensions of the outflow tract, or increase ventricular compliance decrease symptoms and vice versa. Digitalis should not be used unless atrial fibrillation with a rapid ventricular response or left ventricular dilation and dysfunction without a gradient occur. Diuretics should be used with caution as hypovolemia increases obstruction and symptoms. Beta-adrenergic receptor blockade can prevent the increase in outflow tract gradient that may occur with exercise; its efficacy at preventing sudden death has not been established. It also has antianginal effects. It can be used in large doses (propranolol ≥320 mg/day) if not limited by contraindications, but the overall efficacy of beta blockers is disappointing. Calcium channel blockers such as verapamil decrease myocardial contractility and probably decrease the outflow gradient. More importantly, both verapamil and nifedipine appear to improve the diastolic function (i.e., compliance) of the hypertrophic myocardium. Verapamil can exacerbate poor left ventricular contractility if present. Nifedipine has less negative inotropic effect but is a more potent vasodilator, which may be disadvantageous. Com-

TABLE 9–3. BEHAVIOR OF THE DYNAMIC OUTFLOW MURMUR IN HYPERTROPHIC OBSTRUCTIVE CARDIOMYOPATHY

MANEUVERS	PHYSIOLOGY	INTENSITY OF MURMUR
Valsalva Standing Amyl nitrate	Decrease LV cavity size	↑
Isoproterenol	Increase contractility	↑
Squatting Phenylephrine Elevation of legs Isometric exercise (handgrip)	Increase LV cavity size	↓

bined administration of a beta blocker and calcium antagonist may be effective in some patients. Patients with hypertrophic cardiomyopathy should receive endocarditis prophylaxis, since infection may occur on the aortic or mitral valves or on the endocardium at the site of septal contact of the anterior mitral leaflet. In the patient who is markedly symptomatic due to an outflow gradient and has not responded to medical management, septal myotomy-myectomy may be performed. This procedure usually relieves obstruction as well as mitral regurgitation.

Restrictive Cardiomyopathy

Restrictive cardiomyopathies are less common than the dilated and hypertrophic varieties. They are caused by a variety of infiltrative processes, including amyloidosis, hemochromatosis, sarcoidosis, endomyocardial fibrosis, Löfflers' endocarditis, and Fabry's disease. Restrictive cardiomyopathy is characterized by abnormal diastolic function that impedes ventricular filling. Contractile function is usually relatively normal. Restrictive cardiomyopathy is often difficult to distinguish from constrictive pericarditis, and endomyocardial biopsy may sometimes be necessary to make the distinction. Ventricular pressure recordings reveal a deep nadir in early diastole with a rapid rise to a plateau, termed the "square root" sign. The atrial pressure tracing demonstrates a corresponding prominent "y" descent with a rapid rise and plateau. The "x" descent and "a" wave are also often prominent, resulting in a characteristic M-shaped waveform. The left-sided filling pressures are often higher than the right-sided pressures, in distinction to the equalization of pressures in constrictive pericarditis.

Signs and symptoms are listed in Table 9–1. Kussmaul's sign (an inspiratory increase in central venous pressure) may be present. The apical impulse is usually palpable, in distinction to constrictive pericarditis.

Amyloidosis is characterized by deposition in many tissues of an amorphous, hyaline-like substance and is the most common cause of restrictive cardiomyopathy. In addition, it sometimes may cause systolic dysfunction and symptoms more typical of a dilated cardiomyopathy. Arrhythmias and conduction disturbances are common. The electrocardiogram in cardiac amyloidosis is usually abnormal and often demonstrates generalized decreased voltage. Q waves from myocardial infiltration may simulate myocardial infarction. Echocardiography reveals increased thickness of all cardiac structures, including the ventricular walls, the atrial septum, and the cardiac valves. A characteristic sparkling texture of the myocardium is typical on echocardiography. Diagnosis is made by biopsy of various tissues; if necessary, endomyocardial left or right ventricular biopsies may be performed. There is no treatment for the cardiac manifestations of amyloidosis, and the disease is slowly progressive. Digoxin must be used with caution because patients are particularly sensitive to its toxic effects.

Pacemaker implantation may be necessary in patients who develop atrioventricular block. Death from congestive heart failure as well as sudden death, presumably due to arrhythmias, occurs.

PERICARDIAL DISEASES

ACUTE PERICARDITIS

Inflammation of the pericardial lining around the heart from a variety of causes (Table 9–4) is termed acute pericarditis. Its typical manifestations include chest pain, a pericardial friction rub, and characteristic electrocardiographic changes. Chest pain, often localized substernally or to the left of the sternum, is usually worsened by lying down, coughing, and deep inspiration, and is relieved somewhat by sitting up and leaning forward. There is often adjacent pleural involvement. The pericardial friction rub, diagnostic of pericarditis, is a scratchy, high-pitched sound that has from one to three components corresponding to atrial systole, ventricular systole, and early diastolic ventricular filling. The ventricular systolic component is present most consistently. The rub is often transient; its absence does not exclude the diagnosis of pericarditis and its presence does not exclude the existence of a large pericardial effusion. The rub often is best heard with the diaphragm of the stethoscope as the patient sits forward at forced end-expiration. Single-component friction rubs must be differentiated from systolic cardiac murmurs, skin rubbing against the diaphragm of the stethoscope, and the crunching sound of mediastinal air.

The electrocardiogram may be diagnostic, especially if obtained serially, and reveals ST segment elevation with upright T waves at the onset of chest pain (Fig. 9–1). The ST elevation is characteristic in all leads except aV_R and V_1. The ST segments are often concave upward in distinction to those of acute myocardial infarction, but this distinction is often difficult or impossible to make. Reciprocal ST segment depression as in acute myocardial infarction generally does not occur. Several days later the ST segments characteristically return to normal, and the T waves begin to flatten. Subsequently, diffuse T wave inversion develops, usually after the ST segments return to normal, in contrast to the typical pattern of myocardial infarction. Weeks to months later the T waves usually return to normal but may remain abnormal indefinitely. The PR segment may be depressed, reflecting atrial injury. The ECG changes of acute pericarditis must be distinguished from early repolarization. Early repolarization is common in young patients, usually without PR segment depression, more often associated with sinus bradycardia than the sinus tachycardia of acute pericarditis, and without a characteristic evolution as described above for pericarditis. Atrial rhythm disturbances during pericarditis are common, especially intermittent atrial fibrillation; AV conduction disturbances and ventricular tachyarrhythmias are unusual and should suggest myocardial infarction. If a large

TABLE 9-4.   CAUSES OF PERICARDITIS

CAUSE	FEATURES
Idiopathic	Specific etiology not identified Common; symptoms and natural history resemble viral pericarditis
Viral Coxsackie B, echovirus, measles, mumps, influenza, infectious mononucleosis, poliomyelitis, varicella, hepatitis B, cytomegalovirus (*Mycoplasma pneumoniae*)	Prodromal syndrome resembling a "cold" Typical pericardial pain, rub, ECG changes Usually self-limited, lasts 1–3 weeks Associated myocarditis, recurrent pericarditis, tamponade, or later development of constrictive pericarditis occur infrequently Treatment: aspirin, nonsteroidal anti-inflammatory agents; short course of steroids if pain persists
Purulent Pericarditis Staphylococcus, streptococcus, pneumococcus	Associated with postoperative infection, endocarditis; hematogenous or contiguous spread High mortality; patients appear acutely ill: fever, chills, sweats, dyspnea; typical pericardial chest pain is unusual If suspected, pericardial fluid must be obtained immediately for examination Treatment: surgical drainage, antibiotics
Tuberculosis	Develops slowly; low grade fever, malaise, anorexia, weight loss, dyspnea; typical pericardial chest pain is unusual X-ray findings of tuberculosis are usually absent; tuberculin skin test is positive if patient not anergic Constrictive pericarditis common; pericardium may be calcified on x-ray Diagnostic yield is much higher if pericardial tissue as well as fluid is examined and cultured Treatment: antituberculous agents; pericardiectomy for constriction
Histoplasmosis	Usually occurs with a self-limited pulmonary infection Large pericardial effusions with

pericardial effusion is present, low QRS voltage and electrical alternans may occur.

The chest x-ray is of little value in the diagnosis of acute pericarditis, but an enlarged cardiac silhouette may be noted if a pericardial effusion is present. Calcification of the pericardium may be detected in patients with long-standing pericarditis, especially secondary to tuberculosis. The echocardiogram is extremely accurate for detection and quantitation of pericardial fluid and is also useful to evaluate suspected hemodynamic compromise (tamponade).

Nonspecific indicators of inflammation such as elevated erythrocyte sedimentation rate and leukocytosis are usually present. Cardiac isoenzymes are usually normal. Other laboratory tests that may exclude specific diagnoses include blood cultures, acute and convalescent viral serologies, fungal serology (e.g., histoplasmosis), ASO titer (rheumatic fever), cold agglutinins (mycoplasma),

heterophile test (mononucleosis), thyroid function tests (hypothyroidism), BUN and creatinine (uremia), and connective tissue disease screens such as ANA, rheumatoid factor, and complement.

Management of the patient with acute pericarditis involves treating its etiology. Patients are usually hospitalized to make sure that myocardial infarction is not present and to watch carefully for the occurrence of cardiac tamponade. Salicylates or nonsteroidal anti-inflammatory agents are often effective to relieve pain. Corticosteroids may be used if necessary, but long-term administration should be avoided. Anticoagulants should not be administered because of the risk of hemopericardium. In rare cases, pericardiectomy may be indicated to relieve recurrent symptoms. Most causes of pericarditis are self-limited, and inflammation abates after two to six weeks. Recurrent episodes of pericarditis occur in some pa-

TABLE 9–4. (*continued*)

CAUSE	FEATURES
	tamponade common; constriction uncommon
	Difficult to culture; serologic tests usually positive
	Hilar adenopathy common on x-ray
	Usually not treated with antifungal agents
Pericarditis after Myocardial Infarction (see Chapter 7)	Early form (usually 1-4 days after transmural infarction) probably due to local irritation and is self-limited
	Later form (>10 days after infarction, Dressler's syndrome) probably immunologic in etiology and tends to recur
Post-pericardiotomy Syndrome	Similar to Dressler's, usually occurs 1-4 weeks after cardiac surgery
Cardiac Trauma	Penetrating or nonpenetrating trauma
	Pericarditis can occur early due to direct pericardial injury or late analogous to Dressler's syndrome
Uremia	Large effusions with tamponade common
	May respond to vigorous dialysis but pericardiectomy is sometimes necessary
Neoplasm	Large effusions with tamponade common
	Most commonly due to metastatic lung and breast carcinoma, leukemia, lymphoma, and melanoma
	Tumor cells often detectable in pericardial fluid
	Treatment: needle or surgical drainage; systemic or local chemotherapy
Radiation	Usually doses >4000 rads to the heart
	May appear early or several months after radiation; constriction may eventually occur
Myxedema	Large pericardial effusions without tamponade are characteristic
Connective Tissue Diseases, Hypersensitivity Syndromes	For example, systemic lupus erythematosus, rheumatoid arthritis, scleroderma, polyarteritis nodosa, drug reactions (e.g., procainamide)

tients. Rarely, pericarditis eventually results in pericardial constriction or a combination of effusion and constriction (effusive-constrictive pericarditis).

PERICARDIAL EFFUSION

The hemodynamic effects of fluid in the pericardial cavity depend on the volume and rate of fluid accumulation. Because the pericardium is not compliant, an increase in pericardial effusion that occurs acutely may cause a rapid rise in intrapericardial pressure. If the accumulation of fluid is more gradual, the pericardium may accommodate, and the intrapericardial pressure increase is not as great for any given amount of pericardial fluid. Small increases in the volume of pericardial fluid may have little hemodynamic effect at first, but subsequent small increases may result in a rapid rise in intrapericardial pressure,

accounting for the rapid clinical deterioration of patients with stable pericardial effusion.

The patient with pericardial effusion and hemodynamic compromise has dyspnea, tachycardia, distended jugular veins, and a rapid thready pulse. Rales typical of pulmonary edema are absent. Dullness, increased fremitus, and bronchial breath sounds posteriorly below the angle of the left scapula due to compression of the left lower lung by the pericardium (Ewart's sign) may be present. The precordium often is quiet to auscultation, and the apical impulse frequently is not palpable. Kussmaul's sign, an increase in jugular venous pressure with inspiration, is unusual in pericardial effusion or tamponade. When cardiac tamponade results, pulsus paradoxus, characterized by a decrease in the systolic blood pressure of more than 10 mm Hg with normal inspiration, frequently is present. The paradoxical pulse often can be noted by marked weakening or disappearance of a peripheral pulse during inspiration. Paradoxical pulse is not diagnostic of pericardial tamponade and can occur in chronic lung disease, acute asthma, and severe congestive heart failure.

Any cause of acute pericarditis can lead to pericardial effusion. The electrocardiogram may be normal, may demonstrate low voltage, or may reveal ST and T wave changes typical of pericarditis. Electrical alternans, a variation in voltage of P, QRS, and T waves in alternate beats, may occur in patients with large effusions. The chest x-ray may show an enlarged "water bottle" cardiac silhouette, but if the pericardial effusion has developed rapidly, the chest x-ray may show a normal heart size. Definitive diagnosis of pericardial effusion is usually obtained by echocardiography. Cardiac catheterization shows pulsus paradoxus, equalization of diastolic pressures throughout the heart, elevated systemic venous pressure, and normal or reduced cardiac output with reduced stroke volume.

The management of pericardial effusion without tamponade is similar to that of acute pericarditis. Patients with acute significant pericardial effusions should be hospitalized to monitor for impending tamponade. If tamponade occurs, the pericardium should be drained by pericardiocentesis or surgery. Patients with cardiac tamponade and hypotension should receive intravenous volume (and possibly isoproterenol) to optimize cardiac performance until pericardial drainage can be performed. Diuresis is contraindicated.

The pericardial fluid should be examined microscopically for bacteria, cells, cytology, culture, glucose, and protein content. An indwelling catheter or drain is sometimes left in place for subsequent drainage of pericardial fluid or chemotherapy instillation.

CONSTRICTIVE PERICARDITIS

Constrictive pericarditis results from pericardial thickening and fibrosis occurring long after acute episodes of pericarditis. It is less common since the advent of antituberculous therapy but can occur after bacterial, fungal, viral, neoplastic, or uremic pericarditis. The fundamental hemodynamic abnormality is abnormal diastolic filling. Eventually the underlying myocardial tissue may atrophy and decreased systolic function may result. Pericardial effusion and constriction may occur together (effusive-constrictive pericarditis), in which case pericardiocentesis may only partially relieve the symptoms. Occasionally constriction can be localized to only certain chambers of the heart.

Symptoms of dyspnea, peripheral edema, abdominal swelling, and fatigue usually develop gradually. On physical examination, the jugular veins are distended with a prominent y descent (corresponding to early rapid ventricular filling). Tachycardia, hepatomegaly, ascites, and peripheral edema are common. Splenomegaly may occur. The pulse pressure is usually normal, and pulsus paradoxus is usually not present. Kussmaul's sign may be present. The apical impulse

sometimes is not palpable or may retract with systole. An early diastolic apical sound termed a pericardial knock is often present and can be confused with an S_3 gallop.

Electrocardiographic findings include low voltage and nonspecific T wave changes. The chest x-ray reveals clear lungs and normal or only slightly increased heart size. Pericardial calcification is most common in tuberculous constriction. Echocardiography sometimes can suggest constrictive pericarditis but is usually not diagnostic. At cardiac catheterization the right and left ventricular pressures may demonstrate an early diastolic dip with a subsequent rise termed a square root sign. The right atrial pressure tracings may show sharp x and y descents, generating a typical M-shaped contour. There is equalization of end diastolic pressures in all four chambers and the pulmonary artery. Occasionally these findings become evident only after an infusion of saline (occult constriction).

It is sometimes difficult to distinguish constrictive pericarditis from restrictive cardiomyopathy. Left ventricular ejection fraction is more likely to be decreased in patients with restrictive cardiomyopathy than constrictive pericarditis. Comerized tomography is the procedure of choice to demonstrate the thickened pericardium. Endocardial biopsy or even surgical exploration is sometimes necessary.

Constrictive pericarditis is slowly progressive. Patients may be managed conservatively with mild sodium restriction and diuretics; however, the mortality and morbidity of pericardiectomy is less when performed early than after progressive calcification and fibrosis have occurred. Therefore, pericardiectomy should probably not be performed in patients with very mild, early disease or elderly patients with severe disease and a fibrotic, calcified pericardium. Improvement occurs in about 75 per cent of patients who survive the operation but may be delayed for several weeks or months postoperatively. Cardiac function may not normalize after pericardiectomy either because of inability to completely remove the pericardium or fibrosis and atrophy of the underlying myocardium.

REFERENCES

Fowles RE, and Mason JW: Endomyocardial biopsy. Ann Intern Med 97:885, 1982.

Fuster V, Gersh BJ, Giuliani ER, Tajik AJ, Brandenberg RO, and Frye RL: The natural history of idiopathic dilated cardiomyopathy. Am J Cardiol 47:525, 1981.

Maron BJ, and Epstein SE: Hypertrophic cardiomyopathy. Recent observations regarding the specificity of three hallmarks of the disease: Asymmetric septal hypertrophy, septal disorganization, and systolic anterior motion of the anterior mitral leaflet. Am J Cardiol 45:141, 1980.

Shabetai R: Cardiomyopathy: How far have we come in 25 years, how far yet to go? J Am Coll Cardiol 1:252, 1983.

Spodick DH: The normal and diseased pericardium: Current concepts of pericardial physiology, diagnosis, and treatment. J Am Coll Cardiol 1:240, 1983.

INFECTIVE ENDOCARDITIS

10

Infection of the endocardium, usually involving diseased cardiac valves, is termed infective endocarditis. It is most frequently caused by bacteria but can also be caused by fungi. It is classified as acute or subacute depending on the clinical course of the disease. More virulent organisms (e.g., staphylococci, group A beta-hemolytic streptococci, and pneumococci) tend to produce the acute form of the disease with rapid progression and death within a few weeks if untreated. *Streptococcus viridans* (alpha-hemolytic streptococci) causes approximately 50 per cent of all cases of endocarditis and usually follows a subacute course, also eventually fatal if untreated but lasting several months. It is commonly preceded by dental surgery. Other bacteria that cause endocarditis relatively commonly include the enterococci, gonococci, and *Streptococcus bovis* (a group D nonenterococcal streptococcus). Gram-negative organisms uncommonly cause infective endocarditis. Enterococcal and *Streptococcus bovis* endocarditis may occur after genitourinary or gastrointestinal surgery. The incidence of *Streptococcus bovis* endocarditis is increased in patients with carcinoma of the colon. Staphylococcal endocarditis, common in narcotic addicts, may follow wound infections or prosthetic cardiac valve surgery. *Staphylococcus aureus* usually results in acute endocarditis, whereas *Staphylococcus epidermidis* endocarditis is usually subacute. Fungal endocarditis, rare but increasing in frequency, probably owing to more patients with valvular prostheses and drug addiction, is usually due to *Candida albicans*, *Histoplasma capsulatum*, or *Aspergillus*. A variety of other organisms can rarely cause endocarditis.

Endocarditis is characterized by vegetations, consisting of infecting organisms embedded in platelet-fibrin thrombi with an inflammatory reaction mainly of mononuclear cells, usually located on the valvular leaflets. The valve tissue beneath the vegetation undergoes destruction. Endocarditis occurs in the left more commonly than the right heart. The mitral valve is involved most frequently, followed by the aortic and tricuspid valves. Right-sided lesions such as on apparently normal tricuspid valves have become more common recently due to intravenous drug addiction.

The infection may cause rupture of the valve tissue itself or of its chordal structures, leading to either gradual or acute valvular regurgitation. Some virulent bacterial (for example, *Staphylococcus aureus*) or fungal vegetations may become large enough to obstruct the valve orifice or create a large embolus. Aneurysms of a sinus of Valsalva may occur and can rupture into the pericardial space. The infection may invade the interventricular septum, causing intramyocardial abscesses or septal rupture that can involve the conduction system of the heart. Peripheral septic emboli may occur with left-sided and septic pulmonary emboli with right-sided endocarditis.

Patients with pre-existing valvular heart disease are at particular risk for developing endocarditis. Rheumatic heart disease, congenital heart disease, hypertrophic obstructive cardiomyopathy, mitral valve prolapse, degenerative changes in valves, and prosthetic valves are predisposing features. All these lesions are characterized by the production of turbulent flow. Once endothelium has been damaged and bacteremia has occurred, a vegetation may be established, usually on the valve surface toward the chamber of lower pressure (for example, on the atrial surface of an abnormal mitral valve). Infective endocarditis in a patient with a patent ductus arteriosus occurs on the low pressure pulmonic side where more turbulence and eddying of blood occur. Atrial septal defects do not predispose to infective endocarditis because little turbulent flow is created from this defect. Dental, gastrointestinal, and genitourinary manipulations are the most frequent sources of bacteremia causing endocarditis. This transient bacteremia, in the presence of pre-existing valvular lesions, is the most common predisposing factor to endocarditis, followed by intravenous drug addiction and cardiac surgery. In acute infective endocarditis, previously normal valves may be involved in up to half of cases. Only a small number of these highly invasive bacteria appear to be required to initiate infection. On the other hand, in the subacute infection, sterile platelet-fibrin thrombi caused by the trauma of the jet from the turbulent hemodynamics are thought to precede and subsequently become infected from the transient bacteremia.

Males are affected more commonly than females. Patients with subacute endocarditis are often minimally symptomatic, most commonly having nonspecific symptoms that may be overlooked such as fever, chills, sweats, malaise, anorexia, or weight loss. Acute endocarditis presents with a more dramatic illness and may include acute congestive heart failure or manifestations of pulmonary or systemic emboli (e.g., renal, splenic, retinal, coronary, or cerebral infarction). Mycotic (infected) aneurysms can occur, especially in the cerebral circulation, giving rise to subarachnoid hemorrhages.

Heart murmur and fever are the two major findings and are present in about 95 per cent of patients. The heart murmurs are regurgitant, systolic if due to mitral or tricuspid infection, and diastolic if due to aortic regurgitation. Rarely obstructive murmurs result. A murmur varying in duration and intensity over time suggests endocarditis. The murmurs of the underlying cardiac disease may be present and sometimes confuse the diagnosis. In patients with tricuspid endocarditis, a heart murmur may be absent. In addition, patients with acute endocarditis of the left heart may develop a murmur only during the course of therapy after the diagnosis has been made from positive blood cultures or a peripheral embolic phenom-

TABLE 10–1. MANIFESTATIONS OF ENDOCARDITIS

Clinical
Fever
Pallor
Wasting
Clubbing
Splenomegaly
"Peripheral stigmata"
  Petechiae
  Splinter hemorrhages under fingernails
  Osler's nodes (tender red nodules on fingers or toes)
  Janeway's lesions (nontender flat lesion on palms and soles)
  Roth spots (retinal fundal hemorrhages with a white central area)
  Scleral or conjunctival hemorrhages
Murmur (valvular regurgitant)
Symptoms and signs of congestive heart failure
Peripheral emboli
  Gangrene of extremities
  Flank tenderness from renal or splenic infarction
Neurologic abnormalities
  Cerebral embolism
  Ruptured mycotic aneurysm
  Meningitis
Laboratory
Elevated erythrocyte sedimentation rate
Anemia
Positive test for rheumatoid factor (subacute form)
Urinalysis
  Proteinuria
  Hematuria
  Red blood cell casts (glomerulonephritis)
Positive blood cultures

TABLE 10–2. ENDOCARDITIS PROPHYLAXIS IN SPECIFIC CARDIAC CONDITIONS*

Endocarditis Prophylaxis Recommended
  Prosthetic cardiac valves (including biosynthetic valves)
  Most congenital cardiac malformations
  Surgically constructed systemic-pulmonary shunts
  Rheumatic and other acquired valvular dysfunction
  Idiopathic hypertrophic subaortic stenosis (IHSS)
  Previous history of bacterial endocarditis
  Mitral valve prolapse with insufficiency†
Endocarditis Prophylaxis Not Recommended
  Isolated secundum atrial septal defect
  Secundum atrial septal defect repaired without a patch six or more months earlier
  Patent ductus arteriosus ligated and divided six or more months earlier
  Postoperative coronary artery bypass graft (CABG) surgery

* This table lists common conditions but is not meant to be all-inclusive.
† Definitive data to provide guidance in management of patients with mitral valve prolapse are particularly limited. It is clear that in general such patients are at low risk of development of endocarditis, but the risk-benefit ratio of prophylaxis in mitral valve prolapse is uncertain.

Adapted from Shulman ST, et al: Prevention of bacterial endocarditis. Circulation 70:1123A, 1984. By permission of the American Heart Association, Inc.

enon. A murmur usually appears at some time during the course or treatment of acute endocarditis.

Clinical and laboratory manifestations of endocarditis are summarized in Table 10–1. Peripheral stigmata are much less frequent than in the pre-antibiotic era and are thought to be caused by septic, embolic, and immunologic consequences of the infection. Chest x-ray findings are nonspecific and show evidence of any pre-existing cardiac disease in addition to signs of progressive ventricular failure from the endocarditis. Multiple pulmonary infiltrates may be a manifestation of septic pulmonary infarctions from right-sided endocarditis.

The most important laboratory evaluation is the blood culture. Three to six cultures should be obtained over a period of several hours. A small number of patients may have persistently negative blood cultures secondary either to infection with an organism difficult to culture (for example, fungal endocarditis) or to previous antibiotic therapy. Aerobic and anaerobic cultures should be obtained. If previous antibiotic therapy has been administered, cultures should be obtained over several days if possible.

Echocardiography may establish any underlying valvular abnormality predisposing the patient to endocarditis, or the complications of endocarditis such as flail mitral valve leaflet, intramyocardial abscess, or hemodynamic abnormalities. Vegetations may be identified directly if they exceed approximately 3 mm in diameter. Smaller vegetations may not be noted, and therefore failure to visualize vegetations does not exclude endocarditis. Echocardiography can identify fungal vegetations most frequently because these vegetations are generally large. In many patients the diagnosis is clear, and cardiac surgery may be performed without cardiac catheterization. If catheterization is done, one must be cautious not to dislodge a vegetation.

The differential diagnosis of infective endocarditis is broad and includes viral syndromes, acute rheumatic fever, atrial myxoma, connective tissue diseases such as lupus erythematosus, neurologic disorders, and occult neoplasms. Definitive diagnosis usually relies on blood culture results. When cultures are negative, the diagnosis must be made indirectly by echocardiography and peripheral stigmata. It is sometimes difficult to determine in an elderly patient with a systolic murmur whether positive blood cultures represent endocarditis or bacterial seeding of the blood from another source; at times, empirical treatment for endocarditis without confirmation of the diagnosis may be required.

Endocarditis on a prosthetic valve usually presents similarly to native valve endocarditis. The organisms causing prosthetic valve endocarditis in the early postoperative period are usually those involved in infected surgical wounds (e.g., staphylococci) and in pulmonary and urinary tract infections. Endocarditis in the late postoperative period commonly involves organisms that occur in bacteremia related with dental, gastrointestinal, or genitourinary procedures as does native endocarditis.

The natural history of untreated endocarditis is universally fatal, although the time course for acute and subacute forms is different. Despite the availability of antibiotic and surgical therapy, the mortality and morbidity are still high. Patients who are older, have more virulent organisms, have a longer duration of illness before the institution of therapy, have extensive valvular damage, congestive heart failure, renal involvement, or other complications such as myocarditis, myocardial abscess, mycotic aneurysms, or embolization are more likely to have an unfavorable outcome.

Bactericidal antibiotics that have been demonstrated to be effective toward the specific organism isolated should be employed. Dosage should be followed by measuring the antibacterial activity of the patient's serum against the organism, and dilutions of at least 1:8 of the patient's serum should inhibit bacterial growth. The duration of therapy is controversial but is usually recommended to be six weeks for most infecting organisms. Initial treatment can be delayed until identification of the infecting organism in patients with subacute endocarditis but must be instituted empirically immediately *after* obtaining cultures in patients with acute endocarditis. Antibiotics are usually administered intravenously. *Streptococcus viridans* responds to penicillin G; streptomycin or gentamicin is sometimes added to the regimen because of in vitro synergy. Vancomycin can be substituted in individuals allergic to penicillin. Enterococcal endocarditis must be treated with penicillin or vancomycin, plus an aminoglycoside. *Streptococcus bovis* is sensitive to penicillin, and therapy is the same as for viridans streptococci. Staphylococci are treated with penicillin G if they are non–penicillinase-producing or with semisynthetic penicillins such as nafcillin, oxacillin, or methicillin if they produce penicillinase or if that fact is unknown. Methicillin-resistant strains have been identified for which vancomycin must be used. Therapy for gram-negative bacteria should be guided by antibiotic sensitivity testing and may include drugs such as carbenicillin and/or aminoglycosides. Fungal endocarditis is treated with amphotericin B, sometimes with flucytosine added. Fungal endocarditis usually requires surgical intervention.

Heart failure is treated conventionally with digitalis, diuretics, and afterload reduction. Regurgitant mitral or aortic valve lesions may respond to afterload therapy with intravenous nitroprusside as a temporizing measure. Severe heart failure must be treated with valve replacement, waiting until the infection has been effectively treated if possible, but in the presence of active infection with concomitant antibiotic therapy if necessary. Indications for surgery in infective endocarditis include heart failure not responding to medical management; recurrent infection despite apparently adequate medical therapy; infections on most prosthetic valves, especially if prosthetic valve malfunction is present; infections with or-

ganisms not usually responsive to medical therapy, such as fungi; repeated embolic episodes; presence of a septal abscess or aneurysms of the sinus of Valsalva.

Patients with cardiac lesions predisposing to infective endocarditis should have antibacterial prophylaxis when dental or surgical instrumentation is likely to produce transient bacteremia (Tables 10–2 and 10–3). Patients with prosthetic

TABLE 10–3. PROCEDURES FOR WHICH ENDOCARDITIS PROPHYLAXIS IS INDICATED

All dental procedures likely to induce gingival bleeding
Tonsillectomy and/or adenoidectomy
Surgical procedures or biopsy involving respiratory mucosa
Bronchoscopy, especially with a rigid bronchoscope
Incision and drainage of infected tissue
Genitourinary and gastrointestinal procedures
  Cystoscopy
  Prostatic and urinary tract surgery
  Urethral catheterization (especially in the presence of infection)
  Vaginal hysterectomy
  Gallbladder or colonic surgery
  Colonoscopy
  Upper GI endoscopic or proctosigmoidoscopic biopsy
  Other GI/GU procedures in patients at especially high risk for endocarditis (e.g., prosthetic valves)

Adapted from Shulman ST, et al: Prevention of bacterial endocarditis. Circulation 70:1123A, 1984. By permission of the American Heart Association, Inc.

TABLE 10–4. SUMMARY OF RECOMMENDED ANTIBIOTIC REGIMENS FOR DENTAL/RESPIRATORY TRACT PROCEDURES

STANDARD REGIMEN	
For dental prodecures that cause gingival bleeding, and oral/respiratory tract surgery	Penicillin V 2.0 grams orally 1 hour before, then 1.0 gram 6 hours later. For patients unable to take oral medications, 2 million units of aqueous penicillin G IV or IM 30-60 minutes before a procedure and 1 million units 6 hours later may be substituted.
SPECIAL REGIMENS	
Parenteral regimen for use when maximal protection is desired, e.g., for patients with prosthetic valves	Ampicillin 1.0-2.0 grams IM or IV plus gentamicin 1.5 mg/kg IM or IV ½ hour before procedure, followed by 1.0 gram oral pencillin V 6 hours later. Alternatively, the parenteral regimen may be repeated once eight hours later.
Oral regimen for penicillin-allergic patients	Erythromycin 1.0 gram orally 1 hour before, then 500 mg 6 hours later.
Parenteral regimen for penicillin-allergic patients	Vancomycin 1.0 gram IV slowly over 1 hour, starting 1 hour before. No repeat dose is necessary.

Adapted from Shulman ST, et al: Prevention of bacterial endocarditis. Circulation 70:1123A, 1984. By permission of the American Heart Association, Inc.

TABLE 10–5. SUMMARY OF RECOMMENDED REGIMENS FOR GASTROINTESTINAL GENITOURINARY PROCEDURES

STANDARD REGIMEN

For genitourinary/gastrointestinal tract procedures	Ampicillin 2.0 grams IM or IV plus gentamicin 1.5 mg/kg IM or IV, given ½ to 1 hour before procedure. One follow-up dose may be given 8 hours later.

SPECIAL REGIMENS

Oral regimen for minor or repetitive procedures in low-risk patients	Amoxicillin 3.0 grams orally 1 hour before procedure and 1.5 grams 6 hours later.
Penicillin-allergic patients	Vancomycin 1.0 gram IV slowly over 1 hour, plus gentamicin 1.5 mg/kg IM or IV given 1 hour before procedure. May be repeated once 8-12 hours later.

Adapted from Shulman ST, et al: Prevention of bacterial endocarditis. Circulation 70:1123A, 1984. By permission of the American Heart Association, Inc.

heart valves are at particularly high risk. Alpha-hemolytic (viridans) streptococci are the most common causes of endocarditis following dental procedures, and antibiotic prophylaxis should be directed at these organisms, whereas prophylaxis after gastrointestinal/genitourinary procedures must include antibiotics to treat enterococcal infections. Antibiotic regimens are described in Tables 10–4 and 10–5.

REFERENCES

Brandenburg RO, Giuliani ER, Wilson WR, and Geraci JE: Infective endocarditis—a 25 year overview of diagnosis and therapy. J Am Coll Cardiol 1:280, 1983.
Dinubile MJ: Surgery in active endocarditis. Ann Intern Med 96:650, 1982.
Shulman ST, et al: Prevention of bacterial endocarditis. Circulation 70:1123A, 1984.

11 CARDIAC TUMORS

Tumors involving the heart may be primary or metastatic; both are rare. Although a variety of metastatic tumors has been described in the heart, the most common are malignant melanomas, leukemia, and lymphomas. The treatment of metastatic tumors is treatment of the primary malignancy.

Primary cardiac tumors may be benign or malignant. Myxoma is the most common primary tumor of the heart and is usually benign. Almost all malignant cardiac tumors are sarcomas, angiosarcoma and rhabdomyosarcoma being the most frequent. It is impossible prior to histologic examination to distinguish benign from malignant tumors, but malignant tumors are more likely to present with evidence of metastases, invasion, or rapid growth. Tumor type may be identified occasionally from tissue at the time of peripheral embolectomy. Malignant primary tumors of the heart have a very poor prognosis.

Myxomas may arise from the endocardial surface of any cardiac chamber, but the majority arise from the left atrium, most commonly in the region of the fossa ovalis. They are usually pedunculated. As a general rule, 10 per cent of cardiac myxomas manifest malignant characteristics and 10 per cent arise in locations other than the left atrium. Occasionally they can be bilateral and usually present in one of three general ways: (1) progressive interference with mitral valve function that causes decreased exercise tolerance, dyspnea on exertion, and pulmonary edema; syncope or presyncope may occur; (2) stroke or occlusion of a major systemic artery due to an embolus; (3) systemic manifestations that include fever, wasting, arthralgias, malaise, anemia, or Raynaud's phenomenon.

If the left atrial myxoma interferes with mitral valve function, a regurgitant valvular murmur may occur. A murmur resembling mitral stenosis may be present owing to obstruction of the valve orifice during diastole. The intensity of the murmur may change with changes in body position. An early diastolic sound termed a "tumor plop" may occur secondary to movement of the tumor toward the left ventricle in early diastole. The erythrocyte sedimentation rate, gamma globulins, and white blood cell count may be elevated. The cause of the systemic manifestations is not clear but may result from products secreted by the tumor, necrotic tumor debris, or an immunologic reaction.

Cardiac myxoma is usually diagnosed by echocardiography. Two-dimensional echocardiography shows the tumor location and movement with the cardiac cycle. Cardiac catheterization with angiocardiography usually is not necessary when the diagnosis has been established noninvasively and is associated with risk of tumor embolus.

Cardiac myxomas should be excised surgically once identified. A recurrent or second myxoma occurs following resection in a small number of patients. Atrial myxoma occasionally may behave as a malignant tumor and demonstrate metastases.

REFERENCES

Peters MN, Hall RJ, Cooley DA, Leachman RD, and Garcia E: The clinical syndrome of atrial myxoma. JAMA 230:695, 1974.
Sutton M, Mercier L, Guiliani E, and Lie J: Atrial myxomas. A review of clinical experience in 40 patients. Mayo Clin Proc 55:371, 1980.

CARDIAC TRAUMA

12

Penetrating or nonpenetrating (blunt) chest trauma can injure any cardiac structure, most seriously producing exsanguinating hemorrhage and cardiac tamponade, and can be overlooked in patients who have obvious injuries elsewhere.

NONPENETRATING TRAUMA

Blunt chest trauma is especially common after steering wheel impact from an automobile accident. It may produce myocardial contusion, resulting in myocardial hemorrhage and at times some degree of necrosis. Often there is little or no residual myocardial scar once healing is complete. Large contusions may lead to myocardial scars, cardiac or septal rupture, congestive heart failure, or formation of true or false aneurysms. Necrosis or hemorrhage involving the cardiac conduction system can produce intraventricular or atrioventricular block. Coronary artery laceration, valvular damage, or pericardial tears may occasionally occur after blunt trauma. The chest pain of myocardial contusion is similar to that of myocardial infarction and is often confused with musculoskeletal pain from the chest trauma. The electrocardiogram at the time of injury may show a diffuse injury pattern similar to that of pericarditis. Later, the electrocardiogram may reveal serial development of Q waves similar to that of acute myocardial infarction if significant necrosis has occurred. Bradyarrhythmias and tachyarrhythmias are common. Contractile abnormalities are usually not severe unless concomitant injury to a valve or the septum has occurred. The MB fraction of creatine kinase is elevated. Myocardial contusion is usually treated similarly to myocardial infarction with initial monitoring and subsequent progressive ambulation. Anticoagulants should not be administered to patients with myocardial contusion. If the patient survives the acute episode, his long-term prognosis is usually good, although late complications such as ventricular arrhythmias occasionally occur.

Rupture of the aorta is a common consequence of blunt trauma. It most commonly occurs just distal to the take-off of the left subclavian artery. The patient may complain of pain in the back or chest similar to that of aortic dissection. The chest x-ray usually reveals widening of the mediastinum. Many patients demonstrate increased arterial pressure in the upper extremities and decreased arterial presure and pulse pressure in the lower extremities. Signs of decreased renal or spinal cord perfusion may become evident. The diagnosis is usually confirmed by aortography, and the treatment is surgical.

PENETRATING TRAUMA

Penetrating cardiac injuries may be due to external objects such as bullets or knives and also bony fragments occurring from chest injury. Because of its anterior location, the right ventricle is most commonly involved. Iatrogenic causes of cardiac penetrating injury include perforation of the heart during catheterization or cardiac trauma from cardiopulmonary resuscitation.

Penetrating injury to the heart may present as exsanguinating hemorrhage with hemothorax or cardiac tamponade if hemorrhage has been limited to within the pericardial sac. Immediate pericardiocentesis and administration of large volumes of fluids may be performed as preparations are being made for emergency surgery. A "post-pericardiotomy" type of pericarditis, infection, arrhythmias, aneurysm formation, and ventricular septal defects are late complications of penetrating cardiac injury. The risk of bacterial endocarditis, infection from a retained foreign body, and foreign body embolus are complications peculiar to penetrating as opposed to nonpenetrating injuries.

REFERENCE

Symbas PN: Trauma to the Heart and Great Vessels. New York, Grune & Stratton, 1978.

AORTIC DISEASE

13

AORTIC ANEURYSMS

Aortic aneurysms, localized areas of increased aortic diameter, may occur in the ascending aorta, aortic arch, descending thoracic aorta, or abdominal aorta, depending on the etiology. For example, aneurysms of the sinuses of Valsalva may occur in Marfan's syndrome, syphilis, as a complication of infective endocarditis, or as a congenital lesion, while aneurysms of the ascending aorta or aortic arch occur in syphilis, aortic dissection, or cystic medial necrosis with or without Marfan's syndrome. Aneurysms of the descending thoracic aorta occur from syphilis, atherosclerosis, or dissection. Aneurysms just distal to the take-off of the left subclavian artery are commonly due to trauma. Abdominal aortic aneurysms are usually atherosclerotic but can be secondary to syphilis or extension of a dissection from above. Connective tissue diseases such as Takayasu's aortitis can lead to aneurysm formation anywhere in the aorta, most commonly the proximal portion.

Arteriosclerotic aneurysms usually occur in the abdominal aorta, most often between the renal arteries and the aortic bifurcation, and are most common in males older than 50 years. Abdominal aortic aneurysms may cause back or epigastric pain but usually produce no symptoms. Their first manifestion may be rupture with severe pain and exsanguinating hemorrhage. Impending rupture of an aneurysm is often heralded by increasing abdominal or back pain, usually constant, "gnawing" in quality, and not affected by movement. Aneurysms may be tender to palpation. Some patients seek medical attention because of fullness or abnormal pulsations in their abdomen. A prominent abdominal aortic pulsation may be felt in normally thin people and be mistakenly diagnosed as an abdominal aortic aneurysm; on the other hand, an abdominal aortic aneurysm may not be palpable in patients who are obese or who have muscular abdominal walls. On occasion, manifestations of peripheral emboli secondary to debris from the aneurysm may be noted in the feet and toes. Bruits may be heard over the aneurysm, and associated occlusive peripheral vascular disease is often present. Aneurysms may rupture into the inferior vena cava producing an arteriovenous fistula, into the duodenum with acute massive gastrointestinal hemorrhage, into the retroperitoneal space manifested by flank or groin hematomas, or into the abdominal cavity causing abdominal distention.

The size of the aneurysm can be estimated from physical examination, routine chest x-ray if calcification of the aortic wall is present, abdominal ultrasound, CT scan, and aortography. The normal aorta is no more than 2 cm in diameter. Physical examination is the least accurate method for estimating abdominal aortic size; abdominal ultrasound is simple and very accurate. Angiography may be less accurate because mural clot may cause the lumen to appear smaller than it really is. If surgery is contemplated, however, aortography is necessary to assess the extent of aortic involvement and the status of the aortic branches.

Half of all aneurysms exceeding a 6-cm diameter rupture within one year, and surgical resection with prosthetic graft replacement is usually recommended. Aneurysms less than 6 cm also may rupture. In patients with relatively high surgical risk, aneurysms of 4 to 6 cm should be followed closely and surgery undertaken upon signs of expansion or impending rupture.

Three-fourths of atherosclerotic aneurysms are confined to the abdominal aorta. One-fourth also involve the thoracic aorta, most commonly the descending aorta. Thoracic aortic aneurysms may cause tracheal deviation with pulmonary complications, hoarseness due to recurrent laryngeal nerve compression, dysphagia from obstruction of the esophagus, Horner's syndrome from compression of the sympathetic chain, or superior vena caval obstruction. Steady, gnawing pain may occur, and occasionally a visible aneurysmal pulsation can be noted in the sternum or in the suprasternal notch. Rupture of the aneurysm is associated with severe chest or back pain. Thoracic aortic aneurysms are usually visible on chest x-ray and must be differentiated from other mediastinal masses. The aneurysms can be identified by CT scan, but aortography usually is necessary before surgery. Larger thoracic aortic aneurysms, especially those exceeding 6 to 7 cm in diameter and those showing evidence of expansion or causing symptoms, should be resected and replaced with a vascular prosthesis if possible. Aortic valve surgery may be required if the aneurysm involves the ascending aorta, and reimplantation of the great vessels or coronary arteries is sometimes necessary. In patients who are poor surgical risks or in whom an extensive aneurysm obviates surgery, reduction of blood pressure and force of ventricular ejection with beta blockade is reasonable.

A dissecting aneurysm is caused by a tear of the aortic intima with formation of a false channel within the aortic media. Blood in the false channel may re-enter the true aortic channel via a second intimal tear or rupture through the adventitia into the periaortic tissues. Aortic dissections, probably not related to atherosclerosis of the aorta, tend to occur in middle-aged men with hypertension, Marfan's syndrome, cystic medial necrosis, and coarctation of the aorta. They are also somewhat more common during pregnancy. They may be caused by trauma and may be a complication of aortic angiography. If the dissection travels retrogradely toward the aortic valve, severe aortic valvular regurgitation may occur. Involvement of the coronary, carotid, or spinal cord arteries may produce myocardial infarction, stroke, or paraplegia, respectively. Dissections can rupture into the pericardium and cause cardiac tamponade or renal impairment if the dissection extends to the renal arteries.

Most dissections arise either in the ascending aorta within several centimeters of the aortic valve or in the descending thoracic aorta just beyond the origin of the left subclavian artery in the region of the ligamentum arteriosum. Dissections have been classified into three types: type I begins in the proximal ascending aorta and extends to the descending aorta, type II is confined to the ascending aorta, and type III begins in the descending aorta and extends distally. Patients with proximal dissections tend to be younger and have a higher incidence of Marfan's syndrome and cystic medial necrosis; distal dissections more commonly involve older patients with hypertension.

Dissecting aortic aneurysms are usually associated with chest pain radiating into the abdomen or the back. The pain is usually severe, sudden, maximal in intensity at its onset, and described as sharp or tearing. An occasional patient presents with aortic insufficiency and heart failure without the history of an acute painful episode. Physical examination may reveal hypertension. Pulses are often but not always asymmetrical. Abnormal pulsations may be felt in the region of the sternoclavicular joints. The electrocardiogram is usually nonspecific but may show evidence of complicating pericarditis or myocardial infarction. The chest x-ray often but not always reveals widening of the mediastinum.

CT scan with contrast injection is very accurate in diagnosing both ascending and descending dissecting aortic aneurysms. Echocardiography can sometimes demonstrate ascending aortic involvement. Angiography is necessary to identify the site of the intimal tear, to determine the full extent of aortic involvement, to evaluate the competency of the aortic valve, and to determine the relationship of the dissection to the aortic branches.

The prognosis is usually poor. Surgical therapy should be undertaken when a dissection involves the ascending aorta or arch, or the distal aorta when there is evidence of leaking or retrograde extension, impairment of cerebral or other vital circulations, inability to control pain or blood pressure, and when hypertension is absent and thought not to be the etiology of the dissection. Patients with distal dissections tend to be older, have more generalized atherosclerosis, and have more cardiopulmonary disease. Thus, surgery generally is indicated in type I and type II, while medical therapy may be the treatment of choice for uncomplicated distal dissection (type III). Medical therapy must be administered to surgical patients both during the preoperative stabilization period and chronically postoperatively to prevent the risk of progression or repeat dissection. Medical management involves control of hypertension and lessening the force of ventricular contraction. Potent antihypertensive agents such as intravenous sodium nitroprusside or trimethaphan may be used. Trimethaphan has the advantage of also decreasing the force of myocardial ejection but exhibits both unpleasant side effects and tachyphylaxis. Therefore, sodium nitroprusside, combined with beta blockade to lessen the force of contraction, is usually the medical treatment of choice.

AORTIC ARTERITIS

Aortitis is an inflammatory process of the aortic wall that may be caused by several disease processes. When it involves the origin of various aortic branches (e.g., the innominate artery, the left common carotid artery, and the left subclavian artery), it is termed the "aortic arch syndrome" and is characteristically produced by Takayasu's syndrome but also by syphilis, arteriosclerosis, or dissecting aneurysm. Takayasu's arteritis or pulseless disease appears to be most common in Japanese females and is an aortic panarteritis that leads to eventual luminal obliteration from the thickened walls and superimposed thrombus. Localized aneurysm formation may occur. The process may involve the coronary ostia or any of the branches of the aortic arch. Tertiary syphilis causes an aortic arteritis that may lead to an as-

cending aortic aneurysm, aortic valvulitis with insufficiency, and/or coronary ostial stenosis. It is a late manifestation of syphilis, usually occurring 10 to 30 years after the primary infection. Routine serological tests may be negative, but the *Treponema pallidum* immobilization or the fluorescent Treponemal antibody absorption test are almost always positive. The media of the aorta is destroyed from necrosis of smooth muscle and elastic tissue. The intima assumes a wrinkled appearance referred to as "tree barking." Involvement is much more prominent in the aortic root than in the distal aorta, in contrast to atherosclerotic aortic aneurysms. This whole process is often asymptomatic and detected by egg shell calcification of the ascending aorta on chest x-ray.

MISCELLANEOUS AORTIC DISEASE

Large peripheral arterial emboli may obstruct the abdominal aortic bifurcation, resulting in so-called saddle emboli. These usually originate from the left heart but rarely may originate from the aorta itself in the area of an atherosclerotic lesion. Other rarer causes are "paradoxical emboli" (from the right heart or venous system in patients with right-to-left shunts), atrial myxomas, or infective endocarditis (very large emboli can occur in acute endocarditis and fungal endocarditis). Obstruction at the aortic bifurcation is characterized by the sudden onset of severe pain in both legs, peripheral neurological abnormalities, and evidence of decreased perfusion bilaterally. It must be differentiated from acute atherosclerotic aortic thrombosis and dissecting aneurysm. The diagnosis is confirmed by angiography. Surgical removal of the clot with subsequent anticoagulation and/or treatment of the underlying etiology is necessary.

Infected aortic aneurysms are rare. The most common congenital aortic anomaly is coarctation of the aorta (see Chapter 4). Congenital aortic aneurysms of the sinus of Valsalva may rupture into the right atrium or ventricle, producing a continuous murmur. Sinus of Valsalva aneurysms can occasionally produce coronary occlusion, conduction disturbances, or valvular malfunction.

REFERENCES

Roberts W: Aortic dissection: Anatomy, consequences, and causes. Am Heart J 101:195, 1981.
Sabiston DC (ed): Textbook of Surgery. 12th ed, Philadelphia, WB Saunders Co, 1981, pp 1855–2018.
Schwartz SI, Shives GT, Spencer FC, and Storer EH (eds): Principles of Surgery. 4th ed, New York, McGraw-Hill Book Co, 1984, pp 873–1002.

14 PERIPHERAL VASCULAR DISEASE

ARTERIOSCLEROSIS OBLITERANS

Arteriosclerosis obliterans refers to atherosclerotic narrowing of large and medium-sized arteries. It most commonly involves arteries supplying the lower extremities, mostly the superficial femoral artery, the aortoiliac area, and the popliteal artery. It is the leading cause of obstructive peripheral arterial disease in patients after the age of 30 and more common in males and in diabetics. The process is often segmental, and there may be areas of normal or nearly normal vessel between areas of severe involvement. Symptoms may occur at rest but are usual with exertion and are due to decreased perfusion of the tissues distal to the obstruction.

Intermittent claudication is most common and is characterized by cramping, pain, and fatigue in muscles upon exercise, relieved promptly with rest. It often occurs in the calf muscles in patients with femoral artery disease, but the site of claudication may be higher, for example, in the low back, buttocks, or thigh in patients with more proximal arterial obstruction. Rest pain is a sign of severe vascular compromise; it usually has a stocking-like distribution and is often worse at night. The patient also may complain of coldness, numbness, and paresthesias. Diminished or absent pulses help localize the obstruction. Bruits can often be heard over the aorta and iliac or femoral arteries. Signs of limb ischemia include coolness, pallor, cyanosis, shiny dry skin with absence of hair, nail changes, and prolonged venous filling time when an elevated extremity becomes dependent. Localized ulcerations and gangrene may occur. Aortoiliac obstruction may produce a syndrome of intermittent claudication of the low back, buttocks, or thighs along with atrophy of the lower extremities, hypertension of the upper extremities, and sometimes impotence (Leriche's syndrome). The symptoms of claudication may remain stable over a very long time period. Many of these patients eventually die from other complications of atherosclerosis. Obstruction at the origin of the subclavian artery can cause "subclavian steal," i.e., reversal of flow in the ipsilateral vertebral artery with arm exertion.

The patient with intermittent claudication but normal appearance of his extremity should be treated without surgery. Exercise is advised (but to be discontinued once pain occurs) and may gradually increase the patient's exercise duration. The patient should avoid tobacco and drugs that decrease peripheral blood flow (for example, beta blockers). The patients should protect their extremities from cold temperature and trauma, and the skin should be cared for carefully with special attention to any apparently minor infections or ulcers. Toenail trimming must be done carefully. Surgery is indicated in patients with progressive claudication that interferes with their lifestyle or with the development of ischemic signs or symptoms at rest. Doppler examination can localize and quantitate obstruction fairly reliably. Arteriography is necessary if surgical intervention is contemplated. Surgery usually involves a saphenous bypass graft across the area of stenosis. Percutaneous transluminal balloon angioplasty of discrete lesions is feasible and appears to be associated with favorable long-term patency. Vasodilating drugs have little or no efficacy in the treatment of arteriosclerosis obliterans and may even decrease blood flow to ischemic areas. Amputation of the affected limb may be necessary in patients in whom gangrene occurs.

THROMBOANGIITIS OBLITERANS

Thromboangiitis obliterans or Buerger's disease is an inflammatory process causing obliteration of peripheral arteries and veins. Men are affected much more frequently than women, and it usually occurs before age 30. Its etiology is not fully understood, but a relationship to cigarette smoking is suspected. Like arteriosclerosis obliterans, the lesions are often segmental, but smaller arteries are involved. The pathology consists of intimal proliferation and thrombi in small to medium-sized vessels with inflammatory infiltrates. The process may alternate between periods of activity and quiescence, and peripheral ischemia develops gradually over the course of a few years. In its later stages, it may be difficult to differentiate from arteriosclerosis obliterans. The lower extremities are commonly affected, but involvement of the upper extremities is more common than in arteriosclerosis obliterans. The patient is often a cigarette smoker who complains of cold extremities and may manifest digital ulcers and Raynaud's phenomenon. Up to half of the patients have a history of migratory thrombophlebitis. Involvement of the lower extremity may produce claudication, gangrene, ulcers, and rest pain similar to arteriosclerosis obliterans, but obstruction is usually more distal (instep or hand claudication is characteristic). Occasionally the coronary, cerebral, mesenteric, or renal arteries are involved. The diagnosis can be suspected by the characteristic clinical findings in a young male and is proven by biopsy of an involved artery.

Patients may do well for long periods of time, but the need for amputation of distal extremities is common if patients continue to smoke. No medication has been shown to be helpful. Sympathectomy to prevent vasospasm may be effective if conservative therapy fails.

ARTERIAL EMBOLISM

Peripheral arterial emboli usually originate from thrombi in either the left atrium or left ventricle or, uncommonly, from atheromatous emboli located in atherosclerotic plaques in the aorta. A "paradoxical embolus" refers to an embolus originating from the venous system, passing through a right-to-left intracardiac shunt, and lodging in the systemic arterial tree. Septic emboli may occur with endocarditis and tumor emboli with cardiac myxoma, diagnosed by pathologic examination of the embolus upon removal. Emboli tend to lodge at arterial bifurcations and areas already narrowed by atherosclerosis; for example, a common site is in the femoral artery at the origin of the deep femoral artery. A very large embolus may lodge at the bifurcation of the aorta and is referred to as a "saddle embolus." Embolic occlusion of an artery usually is followed by propagation of thrombus distal and often proximal to the embolus.

Some patients present with the sudden onset of a severely painful extremity, but others manifest a more slowly developing course of numbness and paresthesias over a period of several hours. Pain is usually present eventually and is often severe. The extremity, pale and cold distal to the embolus, is demarcated from more normal circulation proximally. Pulses are absent below the site of embolization. The extremity may demonstrate decreased reflexes or weakness. If some collateral circulation is present, the clinical presentation may not be as striking, and gangrene formation is not as likely.

Acute thrombosis of a vessel is sometimes difficult to distinguish from embolism but should be suspected if no source for emboli is present and if concomitant severe atherosclerotic disease is present. Surgical therapy is indicated, especially when larger vessels are involved (e.g., aortic bifurcation or femoral or popliteal arteries). Surgical embolectomy should be performed as soon as possible, and results are less favorable if surgery is delayed for greater than about eight hours. Conservative medical management is sometimes successful with small distal emboli, especially if good collateral circulation is present. The limb should be kept warm to prevent vasospasm. Heparin should be administered immediately to prevent recurrent emboli and to prevent thombus propagation distal to the embolus even if surgery is to be performed. Streptokinase administration may dissolve the embolus in some patients and should be followed with anticoagulation; surgical embolectomy is usually preferred, however. If gangrene is already present, amputation is usually required. Chronic anticoagulation may be necessary to prevent recurrent emboli, and the source of embolization should be eliminated if possible. Anticoagulation probably does not prevent atheromatous emboli, for example, from an atherosclerotic abdominal aorta. Residual symptoms of claudication may develop. Mortality is relatively high because of the high incidence of associated diseases and advanced age.

RAYNAUD'S PHENOMENON

Raynaud's phenomenon involves bilateral paroxysmal ischemia of fingers or toes, usually precipitated by cold and relieved by heat. The entire hand or foot is usually not affected. Raynaud's phenomenon may be secondary to a variety of underlying diseases, including arterial occlusive diseases (e.g., arteriosclerosis obliterans or thromboangiitis obliterans), connective tissue diseases (e.g., scleroderma, rheumatoid disease, systemic lupus erythematosus, or polyarteritis nodosa), trauma (e.g., air hammer operators or typists), various neurologic diseases (e.g., multiple sclerosis or peripheral neuropathy), ingestion of certain drugs (e.g., ergotamine, methysergide, or beta-adrenergic blocking drugs), nerve compression syndromes (e.g., thoracic outlet or carpal tunnel syndrome), hematologic abnormalities (e.g., cryoglobulinemia or cold agglutinins), and late after-cold injuries (e.g., frostbite or trench foot). The phenomenon probably occurs secondary to abnormalities of the sympathetic nerves, abnormal reactivity of the blood vessels, and/or sludging of blood cells in the capillaries. If no underlying disease can be found, the patient is said to have Raynaud's disease. Raynaud's disease affects women more frequently than men, most commonly between the ages of puberty and 40.

At the time of an attack, the affected digit initially turns white and subsequently becomes cyanotic. Upon resumption of circulation, it may appear hyperemic because of vasodilation. These changes are usually precipitated by exposure to cold but may also occur with emotional upset. In Raynaud's disease the changes are usually bilateral. Between attacks, normal pulses are present, and the digits usually appear normal. In more severe cases "trophic" changes in the fingers or toes may occur consisting of smooth, shiny, tightly stretched skin over the digits (sclerodactyly) and nail changes. Small painful areas of gangrene may appear on the tips of digits and leave scars upon healing. Amputations of digits in patients with Raynaud's disease are rare.

Mild cases should be treated by limitation of cold exposure. Smoking should be avoided. In more severe cases, vasodilating agents such as calcium-channel blocking agents may be used. Some patients may respond to regional sympathectomy. In Raynaud's phenomenon treatment should be aimed at the underlying cause.

ENVIRONMENTAL DAMAGE OF THE EXTREMITIES

Both freezing (frostbite) and nonfreezing injuries may damage the extremities. The presence of dampness or peripheral vascular disease enhances the tissue loss for any given temperature reduction or duration of exposure. Tissue damage is probably due to a combination of direct freezing and marked vasoconstriction. Cold produces numbness in tissues that may allow freezing without warning, so that the first indication of frostbite may be a prickling feeling. The affected area initially looks pale or waxy yellow and may be anesthetic. In severe frostbite, edema and bullae formation occur with thawing, and gangrene may result. Frostbite should be treated immediately by rewarming, but excessive warming, massage, and exercise should be avoided. Infection is the greatest danger and the affected areas must be handled with aseptic technique.

Prolonged immersion of extremities in water leads to a syndrome known as immersion foot or trench foot. Wetness plus cold produces the most serious form of the syndrome. It does not necessarily require freezing temperatures and is due in part to direct and reflex vasoconstriction.

PERIPHERAL ANEURYSMS AND FISTULAE

Occasionally true or false aneurysms may occur in peripheral vessels. True aneurysms are usually secondary to atherosclerosis; false aneurysms (i.e., a tear in the arterial wall allowing accumulation of blood in the perivascular tissues) may be associated with trauma or rupture of a true aneurysm. True aneurysms of peripheral vessels are located most commonly in the popliteal artery but can occur in the femoral artery, iliac artery, arteries of the upper extremities, and occasionally visceral arteries such as renal or splenic arteries. Aneurysms of the popliteal and femoral arteries are often palpable. Aneurysms may occasionally be infected (mycotic). Symptoms result from arterial occlusion, rupture, distal embolization, or local pressure on adjacent structures such as nerves or veins. Surgery for renal or splenic artery aneurysms is usually recommended in patients who are pregnant (increased incidence of rupture) or whose aneurysm is symptomatic, enlarging, or more than 1.5 to 2.0 cm in diameter. Femoral and popliteal aneurysms should be treated surgically if the patient's condition allows.

Arteriovenous fistulae are acquired or congenital abnormal communications between arteries and veins without an intervening capillary network. Acquired fistulae may be created to facilitate hemodialysis or may occur after trauma such as a gunshot or stab wound. Increased blood flow leads to venous dilation and makes the region of the fistula abnormally warm; the area distal to the fistula may be cool. If the fistula is large, a high cardiac output state may occur and may produce heart failure. Because of the low resistance pathway, diastolic blood pressure tends to decrease, and systolic blood pressure and pulse pressure increase. A bruit and thrill may be present over the fistula. If the artery serving the fistula is compressed, shunting via the low resistance circuit is prevented, and a prompt decrease in the pulse rate may occur (Branham's sign). Acquired fistulae are best treated surgically. Congenital AV fistulae are usually multiple, small, and often accompanied by cutaneous birthmarks. Enlargement of the entire involved limb may occur, since the fistulae are present during the period of rapid bone growth. Bruits and pulsatile masses are uncommon, since the fistulae are small and multiple. Treatment is less satisfactory than that of large acquired AV fistulae.

ARTERIAL TRAUMA

Arterial trauma is usually a surgical emergency. It occurs with penetrating or blunt trauma, including fractures and dislocations. Swelling within a compartment of an extremity after blunt trauma can cause both arterial and neurological damage and responds to decompression of that compartment. Direct arterial injury from trauma requires acute surgical repair. Arterial injury may be iatrogenic from catheterization of brachial or femoral arteries. Loss of local pulse after a catheterization procedure should be approached surgically with early thrombectomy and/or repair, since waiting may necessitate more complicated procedures.

PERIPHERAL VENOUS DISEASE

The most common disorder involving the peripheral veins is venous thrombosis and thrombophlebitis. Thrombophlebitis refers to inflammation of the vein, usually from thrombus but occasionally from trauma or infection. Predisposing factors to thrombophlebitis are venous stasis, local venous injury, and hypercoagulable states. Particular risk factors for thrombophlebitis include oral contraceptives, trauma or fractures of the extremities, pregnancy, major surgery, prolonged immobilization, heart disease, varicose veins, and myeloproliferative syndromes. Local thrombophlebitis may occur from administration of irritating drugs such as chemotherapeutic agents or from indwelling intravenous catheters, especially if infection has supervened (septic phlebitis). Patients with malignancies appear to be prone to migrating, recurrent thrombophlebitis. Thrombophlebitis can occur with thromboangiitis obliterans or processes causing extrinsic obstruction of venous flow. In some patients no predisposing factors can be found. Low-dose subcutaneous heparin appears to be effective prophylaxis against deep vein thrombosis in patients with a variety of medical or surgical conditions.

Symptoms and signs of venous thrombosis and thrombophlebitis in the leg vary. The onset may be inapparent until pulmonary embolism occurs. Warmth and edema may occur, and the affected leg may become larger than the other. Tenderness over the deep vein upon palpation or inflation of a blood pressure cuff may be noted. Pain upon dorsiflexion of the foot (Homans' sign) is neither sensitive nor specific. Skin changes such as mottling or cyanosis may be present. A palpable venous "cord" occurs in only about 20 per cent of patients. When thrombophlebitis is superficial, red, tender, indurated areas occur just beneath the skin, often corresponding to the distribution of the superficial veins. The distinction, usually requiring laboratory evaluation, between deep and superficial thrombophlebitis is critical because the former is prone to embolization whereas the latter is not.

The clinical presentation of iliofemoral thrombosis is characterized by unilateral leg swelling, and the diagnosis usually can be confirmed by Doppler examination. The main differential diagnosis of this syndrome is extrinsic venous obstruction by tumor or adenopathy. Deep venous thrombosis in calf veins is more difficult to diagnose clinically. Doppler studies and impedance plethysmography may be helpful, but a venogram is usually necessary. Venograms are usually reliable diagnostically; however, inadequate opacification of the deep venous system may occur, and areas of previous thrombophlebitis may be difficult to distinguish from new thrombophlebitis. Phlebitis may occur as a complication of venography in a small number of patients.

Management of deep venous thombosis includes heat, elevation of the extremity, and administration of anti-inflammatory agents. Anticoagulation is required to prevent additional thrombus formation and pulmonary embolism. Heparin should be used for immediate anticoagulation to keep the activated partial thromboplastin time 2 to 2.5 times normal. Heparin is continued for seven to ten days. Warfarin should be given for several days before heparin is discontinued, and its effect may be estimated using the prothrombin time. Bed rest is necessary for several days until pain and swelling have improved. Upon ambulation, an elastic support stocking should be worn. The duration of anticoagulation therapy is controversial but is usually between six weeks and six months. If risk factors for thrombophlebitis cannot be corrected or if recurrent thrombophlebitis occurs, chronic anticoagulation may be necessary. In patients with deep vein thrombosis who have contraindications to anticoagulation or in whom pulmonary embolism recurs despite anticoagulation, surgical plication of the inferior vena cava or insertion of an inferior vena caval umbrella is indicated to prevent pulmonary embolism. Fibrinolytic agents such as urokinase or streptokinase may be useful to treat deep venous thrombosis but should be used only in patients with serious iliofemoral thrombophlebitis.

Superficial thrombophlebitis caused by intravenous indwelling catheters is treated by removal of the catheter and warm heat. Because of this potential complication, IV's should not be inserted in the leg. If infection is present, appropriate antibiotics should be given. Anticoagulation is not used unless lower extremity deep venous involvement is present. Heat and elevation should be applied. Ambulation with elastic stockings is possible. Anti-inflammatory drugs may aid in alleviating the symptoms.

Varicose veins (distended, tortuous superficial veins with incompetent valves) can result from thrombophlebitis but may also occur congenitally or in conditions associated with increased venous pressure such as pregnancy, prolonged standing, and ascites. In most people the edema resolves overnight. Many people complain of aching discomfort from the superficial varicosities, relieved by elastic stockings and leg elevation. Occasionally stripping or sclerosing of the saphenous veins may be necessary. Chronic deep venous insufficiency is more serious and gives rise to more edema, darkening and induration of the skin and sometimes indolent skin ulcers (stasis dermatitis). Arterial pulses are normal. The post-phlebitic syndrome refers to chronic swelling and skin changes in extremities due to chronic venous insufficiency, often caused by a previous episode of thrombophlebitis.

Swelling of an extremity can also occur from obstruction of the lymphatic outflow (lymphedema). Lymphedema may be idiopathic (primary) or more commonly secondary (for example, due to lymphangitis, neoplasms, adenopathy, or surgical removal of lymph nodes). Venous distention, stasis dermatitis, and ulcers are usually not present, but lymphangiography and/or venography may be necessary to differentiate lymphedema from venous obstruction.

REFERENCES

Coffman JD, and Davies WT: Vasospastic diseases: A review. Prog Cardiovasc Dis 18:123, 1975.

Coffman JD: Intermittent claudication and rest pain; physiologic concepts and therapeutic approaches. Prog Cardiovasc Dis 22:53, 1979.

Moser KM, and Fedullo PF: Venous thromboembolism. Three simple decisions. Chest 83:117, 256, 1983.

SURGERY AND CARDIAC DISEASE   15

GENERAL PRINCIPLES OF CARDIAC SURGERY

Surgical results are excellent in simple abnormalities such as uncomplicated atrial septal defects, but the mortality and morbidity are higher for repair of more complex lesions such as tetrology of Fallot. Results also depend on whether the surgery is corrective or palliative; i.e., lesions that are incompletely corrected at the time of surgery inherently have less favorable outcome. Overall ventricular function is one of the most important determinations of cardiac surgical risk.

The prognosis for postoperative recovery of left ventricular function differs depending on the underlying disease. For example, left ventricular function may not improve postoperatively in a patient with a large myocardial scar from previous infarction, whereas the patient with left ventricular dysfunction secondary to aortic stenosis is likely to show improvement in left ventricular function upon correction of the aortic stenosis.

The general medical status of the patient may affect cardiac surgical results. For example, abnormal pulmonary function is a common cause of complications after cardiac surgery. In addition to pre-existing primary lung diseases such as chronic obstructive pulmonary disease, pulmonary hypertension secondary to heart disease may increase the risk of surgery. Severe irreversible pulmonary hypertension from left-to-right shunts (for example, ventricular septal defect) is a contraindication to surgery, but pulmonary hypertension and increased pulmonary vascular resistance secondary to mitral stenosis usually resolves after surgical correction. The pre-existence of chronic renal failure increases the risk of acute renal failure in the postoperative period. Even mild hepatic disease may be exacerbated after cardiac surgery, increasing the risk of acute hepatic failure. Pre-existing neurological defects may be exacerbated by cardiopulmonary bypass but usually eventually return to baseline. In patients with serious carotid artery obstruction, care must be taken to maintain flow during cardiopulmonary bypass to minimize the risk of neurological injury.

All noncardiac medical conditions should be investigated and treated before cardiac surgery. Most medications required for optimal medical management should be administered up until the evening before or day of surgery, including beta blockers and antihypertensive medication. Continuous monitoring of the electrocardiogram, arterial pressure, central venous pressure, and pulmonary arterial and wedge pressures is usually initiated prior to induction of anesthesia to obtain baseline values. An intra-aortic balloon counterpulsation device may be inserted preoperatively in selected high-risk patients.

Complications of cardiopulmonary bypass involve those related to the cannulation and the technical institution of bypass and those related to the secondary effects of extracorporeal circulation on various organ systems. An example of the first category is a dissection of the aorta while introducing the aortic cannula. Pulmonary, renal, or neurological dysfunction is common following cardiopulmonary bypass, especially if disease is pre-existent.

Convalescence after cardiac surgery depends on the extent of pre-existing cardiac and noncardiac disease, the direct trauma of the operation, and the response to cardiopulmonary bypass. The thermodilution cardiac output should be periodically monitored in the early postoperative hours. The adequacy of arterial pressure, peripheral pulses, skin temperature, urinary output, arterial blood gases, and mixed venous oxygenation is periodically assessed. Arterial pressure may be a poor indicator of adequate output after surgery because peripheral arterial resistance may be markedly elevated. If cardiac output is insufficient, the patient may require fluids, afterload reduction, inotropic drugs and/or improvement in oxygenation. Measurement of left ventricular filling pressure is important to assess adequacy of fluid volume. If bradycardia is present, pacing via surgically implanted temporary wires (preferably atrial or AV sequential pacing) may optimize cardiac output. If pharmacological manipulation does not improve cardiac output, intra-aortic balloon counterpulsation may be required and may be of more value than inotropic agents if ischemia or arrhythmias are a particular problem. Tachyarrhythmias must be treated vigorously. Exacerbating factors such as hypoxia, anemia, or electrolyte abnormalities should be corrected. The pacing wires can be used to terminate atrial tachyarrhythmias such as atrial flutter. Complex ventricular arrhythmias are treated with lidocaine as the drug of first choice. Atrial tachyarrhythmias may require treatment with digoxin, beta blockers, or in some cases membrane-active agents such as procainamide.

Ventilation with positive end-expiratory pressure should be employed but used cautiously in patients with chronic obstructive pulmonary disease. Patients are usually extubated within four to eight hours after surgery but sometimes not until the next morning.

If bleeding occurs postoperatively, examination of hematological parameters such as fibrinogen, platelets, and coagulation times should be obtained. Blood and blood products should be administered as indicated. Drainage from pleural and pericardial tubes should be monitored, and if excessive the patient may need to be returned to surgery for exploration. Cardiac tamponade is an occasional complication requiring early reoperation.

GENERAL SURGERY IN THE PATIENT WITH HEART DISEASE

Noncardiac surgery is particularly stressful in patients with pre-existing heart disease. The burdens of anesthesia, surgical trauma, wound healing, infection, hemorrhage, and pulmonary insufficiency may overwhelm the diseased heart. The internist is often asked to assess cardiovascular risk in patients undergoing noncardiac surgery and to aid in their preoperative and postoperative management.

General anesthetics reduce myocardial contactility and also have autonomic nervous system effects that may cause either hypotension or hypertension. Regional, spinal, or epidural anesthesia minimizes myocardial depression, but sympathetic blockade and hypotension still may result. In general, there appears to be no difference in risk between general anesthesia and spinal anesthesia in cardiac patients. The anesthesiologist must maintain adequate ventilation, oxygenation, and blood pH throughout the procedure. The ECG is routinely monitored throughout surgery. If cardiac disease is significant, arterial blood pressure, central venous pressure and/or pulmonary arterial wedge pressure may need to be monitored throughout the procedure. Cardiac arrhythmias are particularly likely in patients with heart disease and occur most commonly during induction of anesthesia and intubation. Excessive vagal tone can cause bradyarrhythmias and usually responds to adjusting the depth of anesthesia or administering atropine. Antiarrhythmic agents may be administered if needed.

Some patients have life-threatening indications for surgery, and cardiac risk does not affect whether or not the surgery should be performed. In elective surgery, however, the timing of the operation or even whether the operation should be done may depend upon a preoperative estimation of surgical risk. Cardiac risk is strongly associated with the type of surgical procedure. Herniorrhaphy and transurethral resection of the prostate carry relatively low risk, whereas chest, abdominal, and retroperitoneal surgery have a relatively high risk. Emergency surgery is associated with greater risk than nonemergent surgery because there is no time to optimize the patient's cardiac status.

Ischemic heart disease is one of the major determinants of cardiac risk. The incidence of perioperative myocardial infarction is 4 to 8 per cent in patients who have had remote prior infarctions. In addition, the mortality from perioperative myocardial infarction is two to three times greater in patients with previous infarction as compared to those without previous infarction. Particularly high risk of reinfarction occurs if surgery is performed early after infarction, but levels off if surgery is delayed until six months after infarction. The surgical risk in patients with stable angina pectoris is about the same as that in patients with remote myocardial infarction. Patients with unstable angina pectoris should not have elective surgery until the angina is stabilized and possibly invasive evaluation of the coronary arteries obtained.

Decompensated congestive heart failure is another major operative risk factor and should be treated vigorously prior to noncardiac surgery. Patients with congestive heart failure or atrial tachy-arrhythmias should probably receive digitalis prior to surgery.

Patients with symptomatic heart block may need prophylactic pacing prior to surgery. Patients with chronic bifascicular block or asymptomatic type I second-degree AV block probably do not require prophylactic pacemaker placement prior to anesthesia. Patients with frequent or symptomatic atrial or ventricular tachyarrhythmias should be treated prior to surgery.

Patients with valvular heart disease tend to tolerate the operation according to their pre-existing functional status. Patients with critical aortic or mitral stenosis are at particularly high risk. Treatment of heart failure should be optimized preoperatively, and those with severe valvular lesions should be considered for corrective surgery prior to elective noncardiac operation. In patients with valvular disease or prosthetic heart valves, endocarditis prophylaxis should be administered if appropriate (see Chapter 10). In patients with prosthetic heart valves, anticoagulation can usually be stopped temporarily immediately preoperatively and in the early postoperative period in order to prevent bleeding complications.

Mild to moderate hypertension does not alter surgical risk. Severe hypertension should be controlled prior to surgery, as should heart failure or angina associated with it.

Patients with congenital heart disease are at increased risk according to their functional disability. Patients with cyanotic congenital heart disease and polycythemia have an increased risk of hemorrhage due to coagulation defects and thrombocytopenia, and they may tolerate hypotension and hypoxia poorly. Appropriate endocarditis prophylaxis should be administered. Patients with right-to-left shunts are at risk for paradoxical emboli.

In addition to evaluating and optimizing the patient's cardiac status, the general medical status should also be optimized. Pulmonary function is especially important; cessation of smoking and treatment of chronic bronchitis may improve risk.

REFERENCE

Goldman L: Cardiac risks and complications of noncardiac surgery. Ann Intern Med 98:504, 1983.

HEART DISEASE AND PREGNANCY 16

Marked changes in normal circulatory physiology occur during pregnancy. The cardiac output rises by the end of the first trimester, peaking at a level (30 to 50 per cent rise) in the twentieth to twenty-fourth week that is maintained until after delivery. Increases in stroke volume, heart rate (10 beats per minute) and blood volume (40 to 50 per cent) and decreases in systolic blood pressure and the systemic and pulmonary vascular resistances result. Oxygen consumption and minute ventilation increase. Easy fatigability, decreased exercise tolerance, dyspnea, peripheral edema, a third heart sound, and a midsystolic murmur may be normal in pregnancy. The mechanical pressure of a gravid uterus on the inferior vena cava may decrease venous return and reduce cardiac output. The hemodynamic stresses of pregnancy can exacerbate any pre-existing cardiac abnormality.

Most rheumatic valvular disease in young women involves mitral stenosis. Mitral stenosis is aggravated by the increased cardiac output and heart rate required during pregnancy. The incidence of heart failure increases as pregnancy progresses. These patients have an increased risk of complications from atrial fibrillation, emboli, or endocarditis during pregnancy. Nevertheless, most of these patients can be managed carefully through a relatively uneventful pregnancy. Right ventricular failure may increase the peripheral edema, venous stasis, and risk of pulmonary embolism.

Women with significant mitral or aortic valvular disease who desire children may require surgical correction of the lesion before conception. Cardiac surgical intervention during pregnancy carries an increased risk for both mother and fetus. If a valve is inserted, one should consider a porcine valve so that anticoagulation may be avoided. Warfarin crosses the placenta but heparin does not. Warfarin may produce fetal developmental abnormalities if administered in the first trimester. The use of heparin versus warfarin during various stages of pregnancy is controversial, but it is clear that warfarin should be replaced by heparin during the last two to three weeks of pregnancy. Heparin is discontinued and if necessary protamine administered upon the onset of labor. Patients given warfarin should not breast feed, since it is excreted in breast milk. Patients with prosthetic valves probably should receive peripartum endocarditis prophylaxis.

Survival to reproductive age in patients with congenital heart disease has become more common since the advent of surgical intervention. The risk of pregnancy in patients after surgical correction of congenital heart lesions depends on the completeness of their repair and residual defects such as left ventricular dysfunction or pulmonary hypertension. Patients with uncomplicated cardiac lesions such as ostium secundum atrial septal defects usually tolerate pregnancy without any problem. Patients with uncorrected cyanotic heart disease such as tetralogy of Fallot may have difficulty carrying a pregnancy to term. The infants often have low birth weights. Adverse hemodynamics may result in increased right-to-left shunt and increasing maternal cyanosis, increasing the risk to both mother and child. In patients with severe pulmonary vascular obstruction (for example, Eisenmenger's syndrome), the fixed resistance allows little circulatory reserve, and fluctuations in systemic vascular resistance, cardiac output, and blood volume are very poorly tolerated, especially during labor and the puerperium. Severe aortic stenosis also limits cardiac reserve, and the risk of exertional syncope may increase during pregnancy. Patients with Marfan's syndrome are at markedly increased risk of aortic dissection during pregnancy. Women with coarctation of the aorta also have an increased risk of aortic dissection during pregnancy. Women with persistent cardiomegaly following peripartum cardiomyopathy are at high risk during subsequent pregnancies.

Maternal and fetal complications and mortality are directly related to functional class, and therapy should be optimized throughout pregnancy. Heart failure should be treated by decreased activity, decreased salt intake, and administration of digitalis and diuretics. If heart failure is refractory to medical therapy, termination of pregnancy should be considered. Patients with heart failure may need to be hospitalized during the final weeks of pregnancy. Serious arrhythmias are managed with conventional therapy. Chest x-rays and cardiac catheterization should be avoided if possible because of the radiation risks to the fetus. Factors that may exacerbate heart failure should be eliminated. Most women with heart disease should undergo a spontaneous term vaginal delivery, although Caesarean section may be necessary in selected seriously ill patients.

REFERENCE

Ueland K: Pregnancy and cardiovascular disease. Med Clin North Am 61:17, 1977.

GENERAL REFERENCES

Braunwald E (ed): Heart Disease. A Textbook of Cardiovascular Medicine. 2nd ed. Philadelphia, WB Saunders Co, 1984.

Hurst JW (ed): The Heart. Arteries and Veins. 5th ed. New York, McGraw-Hill Book Co, 1982.

Wallace AG (ed): Cardiovascular diseases. In Wyngaarden JB, and Smith LH (eds): Cecil Textbook of Medicine. 17th ed. Philadelphia, WB Saunders Co, 1985.

SECTION

II

RESPIRATORY DISEASES

17 ANATOMICAL AND PHYSIOLOGICAL CONSIDERATIONS

The major function of the lung is to deliver to the tissues sufficient oxygen (O_2) to meet their energy demands and to remove the carbon dioxide (CO_2) formed as a byproduct of metabolism. This demand varies dramatically from basal requirements of 3 to 4 ml of $O_2 \cdot kg^{-1} \cdot min^{-1}$ to as much as 60 ml of $O_2 \cdot kg^{-1} \cdot min^{-1}$. To accomplish this, sufficient blood and gas must be brought together at a sufficiently large surface area to allow for rapid and adequate gas exchange.

THE AIRWAY

STRUCTURE

The inspired air travels through a complex pathway on its way to the alveoli. Most people (85 per cent) breathe through the nose, although the mouth is an additional route of air passage when ventilatory requirements are high (in excess of 35 to 40 L/min). The nose and pharynx serve to heat, humidify, and filter the air. Air then passes through the larynx, a complex group of muscles and cartilages, which remains patent during inspiration and closes during swallowing and maneuvers that require an increase in intrathoracic pressure, such as defecation and vomiting.

Beyond the larynx is the trachea, a 10- to 12-cm tube supported by U-shaped cartilages and a fibrous posterior membrane. The trachea divides into two mainstem bronchi at the carina. The right mainstem bronchus is a more direct continuation of the trachea, and thus aspirated foreign bodies tend to lodge on the right side. Moving further out, the airways branch in an irregular dichotomous pattern. In the smaller airways, the cartilage becomes less complete and disappears when the airways are 1 to 2 mm in diameter. The first 19 branches, ending at the terminal bronchioles, provide a rapid and enormous expansion of the total airway cross-sectional area, increasing from 2.5 sq cm in the trachea to approximately 900 sq cm (Fig. 17–1). Beyond this are three generations of respiratory bronchioles with their walls made up of increasing proportions of alveoli. This progresses into the alveolar ducts and culminates in the alveolar sacs. At this point, the cross-sectional area of the alveolar capillary membrane has increased to an incredible 50 to 100 sq meters.

The epithelial surface of the alveolar capillary membrane, the site of gas exchange, consists of Type I and Type II pneumocytes, the latter thought to be the progenitor of the former. The Type II cell is responsible for the production of

	CROSS-SECTIONAL AREA (cm²)	RESISTANCE (cm H₂O · L⁻¹ · sec)
LARYNX		0.5
TRACHEA	2.5	0.5
BRONCHI	2.0	
BRONCHIOLES	5.0	0.2
	1.8×10^2	
	9.4×10^2	
ALVEOLAR DUCTS	5.8×10^3	
ALVEOLI	5.6×10^7	

FIGURE 17–1. The subdivision of the airways and their nomenclature. The cross-sectional area increases dramatically as we reach the peripheral, small airways. (Adapted from Weibel ER: Morphometry of the Human Lung. Berlin, Springer, 1963.)

surfactant and possibly for other metabolic activities within the lung. Following a significant injury to the alveolar-capillary membrane, this cell proliferates and is probably responsible for the repair.

VENTILATION

During inspiration air enters the lung consequent to the negative airway pressure generated by the increase in intrathoracic volume secondary to inspiratory muscle contraction. Expiration is passive, as the intrinsic elasticity of the lung and chest wall return the volume of the system back to its resting position. With increased ventilatory requirements, the expiratory muscles may be enlisted to assist in lung emptying.

The respiratory muscles include the diaphragm, the intercostal and accessory muscles, and the abdominal muscles. The diaphragm, the major muscle of inspiration, arises from the lower ribs and inserts into the central tendon under the heart. When the diaphragm contracts, it pushes down against the abdominal contents, causing the thoracic cage to expand by moving the chest wall in a cephalad direction. The increase in abdominal pressure causes an outward motion of the abdominal wall, the clinical hallmark of diaphragmatic contraction. The external and internal intercostal muscles serve inspiratory and expiratory functions, respectively. The accessory muscles, primarily the sternocleidomastoid and the scalene muscles, facilitate inspiration by directly elevating the chest wall. The abdominal muscles increase abdominal pressure and drive the relaxed diaphragm upward during expiration and other situations requiring increases in intrathoracic pressure, such as coughing. As expiration is passive, abdominal muscle activity does not normally commence until minute ventilation increases to 40 L/min.

The respiratory muscles are much like other skeletal muscles in terms of their physiological behavior. If stressed they may fatigue, and proper training can induce a small but significant increase in their strength and endurance. The typical relationship between resting length and the amount of tension developed also exists. For the respiratory muscles, length can be translated into lung volume, and when increased, as in emphysema, inspiratory muscle efficiency is decreased (Fig. 17–2).

The major work of the respiratory muscles is expended in overcoming the elastic and resistive forces encountered in breathing. If the lungs of a normal individual were removed from the chest, they would collapse until the airways close (minimal volume). Concurrently the elastic forces of the chest wall would increase the thoracic volume to about 80 per cent of the total capacity of the thoracic space. Thus, when combined, the lungs and chest wall pull in opposite directions, with the resting volume of the system, the functional residual capacity (FRC), occurring at the volume at which the outward pull of the chest wall equals the inward pull of the lungs, which is normally less than 50 per cent of total lung capacity (TLC).

Changes in elasticity are commonly considered in terms of its inverse: compliance (C) = change in volume/change in pressure. In normal lungs, near FRC, it takes an average of 1 cm H_2O to inflate the lungs by 200 ml (Fig. 17–3); i.e., compliance at this volume is 200 ml/cm H_2O. However, near TLC the lung and chest wall get stiffer, requiring greater inflationary pressure. Compliance decreases with pulmonary fibrosis or pulmonary edema and increases with emphysema. The normal compliance of the chest wall is also 200 ml/cm H_2O, and this may be decreased by skeletal abnormalities such as scoliosis or increased by the

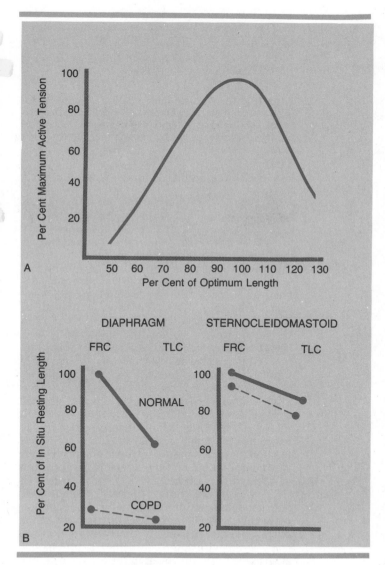

FIGURE 17–2. A, The length-tension curve for the diaphragm. At lengths above or below the optimal in situ resting length, the amount of tension generated decreases. B, The change in the length of the diaphragm and sternocleidomastoid muscles at functional residual capacity (FRC) and total lung capacity (TLC) in a normal subject and a patient with chronic obstructive lung disease (COPD) and hyperinflation. Increased FRC shortens the resting length of the diaphragm so that contraction during inspiration becomes inefficient. Consequently, rib cage expansion becomes more dependent on accessory muscle contraction. (From Druz et al: Am Rev Disp Dis 119:145, 1979.)

FIGURE 17–3. The compliance curves for normal subjects and patients with emphysema and pulmonary fibrosis. An increase in the transpulmonary pressure required to achieve a given lung volume increases the work of breathing.

loss of respiratory muscle tone in neuromuscular disease.

The second force that must be overcome during breathing is airways resistance, defined as the driving pressure divided by air flow, normally 1 to 2 cm $H_2O \cdot L^{-1} \cdot sec^{-1}$. It is greatly dependent on the total cross-sectional area of the airways and thus, even though the individual peripheral airways are narrow, the overall airway resistance decreases because of the increase in total cross-sectional area (Fig. 17–1). Because of their small contribution to overall resistance, early disease in the small airways is often difficult to detect; thus, the airways are called the silent zone. Many factors influence airway resistance, most commonly lung volume, as an increase in lung volume decreases resistance because of the tethering effect of the alveoli on the airways. Thus, resistance should be referenced to the lung volume at which it is measured. Other factors that influence airway resistance include bronchial smooth muscle contraction (bronchospasm), intrinsic or extrinsic airway compression, and the dynamic compression of a forced expiration.

The work of breathing is the product of the pressure generated and the change in volume. In normal subjects, this represents a tiny fraction of the overall energy utilized by the body (4 to 5 per cent), even with high ventilatory requirements, such as exercise. However, in the presence of lung disease, as the work of breathing increases, the O_2 requirements of the respiratory muscles can become inordinant (greater than 25 per cent of total), so that any improvement in gas exchange is offset, or even exceeded, by the increased O_2 consumption and CO_2 production.

Gas entering the lungs is divided into that entering the gas exchanging regions of the lung, the alveolar volume (V_A), and that remaining in the conducting airways, the dead space (V_D). At end expiration, V_D is filled with gas that has already equilibrated with pulmonary capillary blood, and thus on the subsequent inspiration the amount of fresh gas reaching the alveoli is equal to the tidal volume (V_T) minus V_D. Measurement of V_D as a fraction of V_T is quantitated from the Bohr equation:

$$V_D/V_T = \frac{P_aCO_2 - P_ECO_2}{P_aCO_2}$$

where P_aCO_2 and P_ECO_2 are the arterial and mixed expired PCO_2, respectively. In normal subjects, V_D is 20 to 40 per cent of V_T and made up almost entirely of the anatomic volume of the airways. In patients with lung disease there is an additional component of alveolar deadspace due to the presence of ventilation-perfusion (V_A/Q) inequality. The combination of anatomic and alveolar dead space is termed physiologic dead space.

Distribution of V_A within the lung depends on the regional pleural pressure. Normally, pleural pressure is most negative at the apex of the lung and becomes less negative as we move toward the lung base. This gradient is caused by a combination of gravity due to the weight of the lung and the different stresses imposed by the shape of the lung and chest wall. As a result of this gradient, the lung bases are better ventilated than the apices, since during tidal breathing they are on a steeper portion of the compliance curve.

THE BLOOD VESSELS

STRUCTURE

The lung receives its blood supply from two vascular systems—the bronchial and pulmonary circulations. The nutritive blood flow to all but the alveolar structures comes from the bronchial circulation. About one third of the venous effluent drains into the systemic veins and back to the right ventricle. The remainder drains into the pulmonary veins and, along with the Thebesian veins in the heart, represents a component of the 1 to 2 per cent right-to-left shunt found in normal subjects.

The pulmonary arterial system runs alongside the airways from the hila to the periphery. The arteries down to the level of the subsegmental airways (2 mm diameter) are thin-walled, predominantly elastic vessels. Beyond this, the arteries become muscularized until they reach diameters of 30 μm, where the muscular coat disappears. Most of the arterial pressure drop takes place in these small muscular arteries, which are responsible for the active control of blood flow distribution in the lung. The pulmonary arterioles empty into an extensive capillary network and drain into thin-walled pulmonary veins, which eventually join with the arteries and bronchi at the hilum and exit the lung to enter the left atrium.

PERFUSION

The pulmonary vascular bed serves as a source of nutritive blood to the alveolar membrane, but its most important role is in pulmonary gas exchange. It delivers the entire venous return to the pulmonary capillary bed, where exchange of O_2 and CO_2 occurs. While it receives the same blood flow per minute as the systemic circulation, there are many differences between the vascular beds. First, since the pulmonary vascular resistance calculated as

$$\frac{\text{pulmonary artery pressure} - \text{left arterial pressure}}{\text{cardiac output}}$$

is also only about one tenth of systemic vascular resistance, the pressure in the pulmonary vascular bed is consequently only one tenth of that in the systemic circulation. Second, all structures within the thorax, including the pulmonary vascular bed, the heart, and the great vessels, are exposed to the surrounding pressures, both pleural and alveolar, which vary during respiration.

Many factors affect the pressure-flow relationships in the pulmonary circulation. When blood flow increases in upright man, as during exercise, pulmonary vascular pressure increases, but pulmonary vascular resistance actually falls owing to the ability to recruit new vessels and distend the ones already open. This allows large increases in blood flow with lesser increases in pressure, thus preventing the transudation of fluid into the lungs due to a higher microvascular pressure. Pulmonary vascular resistance is also affected by lung volume and is lowest at FRC.

In addition to these passive influences, a number of factors actively affect pulmonary vascular tone. The most important is alveolar hypoxia, which results in constriction of the perfusing artery by as-yet-unknown mechanisms. This may be a conservative mechanism when alveolar hypoxia is localized, since reduction in perfusion to poorly ventilated alveoli reduces the abnormality of gas exchange, which is otherwise inevitable. During generalized hypoxia, its beneficial nature is not always apparent, as in sojourners at high altitude, in whom it may be a major cause of pulmonary edema. Acidosis causes a vasoconstrictor response of lesser magnitude. Other vasoactive compounds produced in the body, such as prostaglandins and adrenergic substances, may also alter pulmonary vascular tone.

Blood entering the lung at the hilum must either be pumped upward toward the lung apex or flow down with the help of gravity toward the base. Thus pulmonary arterial pressures display great variation from the apex to the lung base, whereas the alveolar pressure is the same throughout the lung. The blood flow through any alveolus and therefore the distribution of blood in the lung depend on the interaction of the vascular pressure across the capillary bed (arterial-venous difference) and the surrounding alveolar pressure (Fig. 17–4). At the apex, pulmonary artery pressure is usually just able to overcome alveolar pressure. However, a fall in arterial pressure or any rise in alveolar pressure (positive pressure breathing) may cause alveolar pressure to exceed arterial

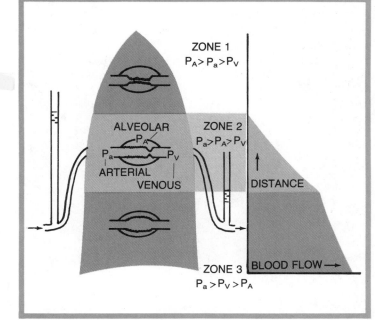

FIGURE 17–4. The zonal model of blood flow in the lung. Because of the interrelationship of vascular and alveolar pressures, the lung base receives the most flow (see text for explanation). (From West et al: J Appl Physiol 19:713, 1964.)

pressure, with cessation of flow. This is known as Zone 1 conditions. Below this lies Zone 2, where the alveolar pressure is less than arterial pressure but greater than venous pressure. Thus, blood flow depends on the difference between arterial pressure and the surrounding alveolar pressure. Blood flow continues to increase with increasing arterial pressure and eventually reaches a point, Zone 3, where venous pressure exceeds alveolar pressure and flow becomes dependent on arterial-venous pressure difference.

GAS TRANSFER

CO_2 and O_2 are transported between the environment and the tissues by convection and diffusion (Fig. 17–5). In the blood, O_2 combines with hemoglobin, and the resulting O_2 saturation is determined by the oxyhemoglobin dissociation curve (Fig. 17–6A). More than 98 per cent of the O_2 in the blood travels combined with hemoglobin; the remainder is dissolved in the plasma. Above a P_aO_2 of 150 mm Hg, hemoglobin is totally saturated and carries 1.34 ml O_2/gm hemoglobin; further rises in P_aO_2 increase only the amount of O_2 dissolved in the plasma at the rate of 0.003 ml O_2/100 ml blood/mm Hg PO_2. CO_2 is carried in the blood in three forms: bicarbonate (90 per cent), dissolved in plasma, or combined with protein, predominantly hemoglobin. The relationship between the PCO_2 and the CO_2 content is represented by the carboxyhemoglobin dissociation curve (Fig. 17–6B), which is steeper and more linear than the oxyhemoglobin dissociation curve.

A number of factors influence the relationship

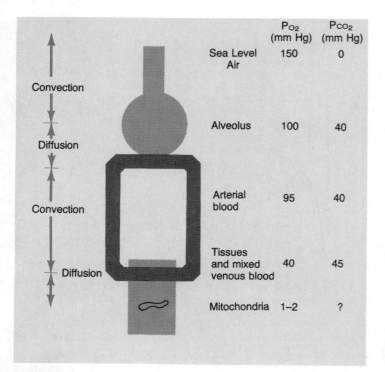

		P_{O_2} (mm Hg)	P_{CO_2} (mm Hg)
Convection	Sea Level Air	150	0
Diffusion	Alveolus	100	40
Convection	Arterial blood	95	40
Diffusion	Tissues and mixed venous blood	40	45
	Mitochondria	1–2	?

FIGURE 17–5. The transfer of O_2 and CO_2 from the atmosphere to the mitochondria.

ment system, the alveolar $P_{CO_2}(P_{A_{CO_2}})$ and thus the arterial $P_{CO_2}(P_{a_{CO_2}})$ depend on the alveolar ventilation ($\dot{V}_A$) and $\dot{V}_{CO_2}$, as

$$P_{A_{CO_2}} = \frac{\dot{V}_{CO_2}}{\dot{V}_A} \times k$$

where k is constant. Any decrease in ventilation will lead to a concomitant rise in $P_{A_{CO_2}}$, provided $\dot{V}_{CO_2}$ remains unchanged. The effect of this on alveolar $P_{O_2}(P_{A_{O_2}})$ can be appreciated using the alveolar air equation

$$P_{A_{O_2}} = (P_B - P_{H_2O}) \cdot F_{I_{O_2}} - \frac{P_{a_{CO_2}}}{R}$$

FIGURE 17–6. *A*, The oxyhemoglobin dissociation curve. The bulk of the O_2 is carried combined with hemoglobin. The various factors that shift the curve, either increasing or decreasing the hemoglobin O_2 affinity, are shown. *B*, The carboxyhemoglobin dissociation curve. It is more linear than the oxyhemoglobin curve throughout the physiological range. Increased P_{O_2} shifts the curve to the right, which decreases CO_2 content for any given P_{CO_2} and thus facilitates CO_2 off-loading in the lungs. The shift to the left at a lower P_{O_2} facilitates CO_2 on-loading at the tissues.

between P_{O_2} and P_{CO_2} and their contents, which can be described as changes in the shape or position of the respective dissociation curves. Increased P_{CO_2} and temperature and decreased pH shift the oxyhemoglobin dissociation curve to the right, decreasing affinity of hemoglobin for O_2 and expediting its release to the tissues. Converse changes in the above factors have the opposite effect. Increased levels of 2,3-DPG, produced during chronic hypoxemia or anemia, also shift the curve to the right, while carbon monoxide shifts it to the left. The most important influence on the carboxyhemoglobin dissociation curve is P_{O_2}; increased P_{O_2} shifts the curve to the right, thus reducing the CO_2 content for any given P_{CO_2} and assisting in the unloading of CO_2 in the lungs.

PULMONARY GAS EXCHANGE

The arterial blood gas values are determined by the gas composition in the alveoli and its successful equilibration with the blood in the pulmonary capillaries. The P_{O_2} and P_{CO_2} in the alveoli, in turn, are determined by the inspired gas tensions, the mixed venous P_{O_2} and P_{CO_2}, the total ventilation and blood flow, and most importantly the success with which the lung is able to match ventilation and blood flow. Abnormality of any of these factors leads to hypoxemia and/or hypercapnia. For convenience they are grouped into four basic mechanisms.

HYPOVENTILATION. Hypoventilation is characterized by a minute ventilation insufficient to maintain a normal $P_{a_{CO_2}}$ for the level of metabolic activity, as measured by CO_2 production ($\dot{V}_{CO_2}$). If the lung is considered as a simple one-compartwhere P_{AO_2} is alveolar P_{O_2}, P_B is atmospheric pressure (usually 760 mm Hg), P_{H_2O} is the partial pressure of water vapor (47 mm Hg), F_{IO_2} is the fractional concentration of inspired O_2, and R is the respiratory exchange ratio (which can be estimated at 0.8). We see that any rise in P_{aCO_2} leads to a concomitant fall in P_{AO_2} and thus in P_{aO_2}. The presence of hypoventilation should direct attention to abnormalities of the chest wall, respiratory muscles, or respiratory center drive.

ABNORMAL DIFFUSION. Under normal conditions, blood spends about 0.75 second in the pulmonary capillaries. Since it ordinarily takes only about one third of this time for the blood to equilibrate with alveolar gas, there is a wide safety margin before abnormal pathology would result in nonequilibration, i.e., a diffusion impairment. It has been estimated that the diffusing capacity of the lung must fall to less than 10 per cent of normal before it affects P_{aO_2} at rest. Three factors may stress the system sufficiently to interfere with complete equilibration: increased diffusion distance due to a thickening of the alveolar capillary membrane; increased rate of blood flow or a reduction in the number of open capillaries, decreasing the time the blood spends in the process of equilibration; and reduced driving pressure from alveolus to blood, as seen at extreme altitudes. Diffusion impairment almost never plays a role in the hypoxemia of disease unless at least two of the above factors are in force. Even when abnormal diffusion is present, it usually accounts for only a minimal amount of the observed disturbance in gas exchange.

VENTILATION-PERFUSION INEQUALITY. The proper matching of ventilation and blood flow within the lung is necessary for the adequate uptake of O_2 and elimination of CO_2. While the lung is sometimes regarded as a single gas-exchanging unit, it really contains units that differ in their relative amounts of blood flow and ventilation. In normals, the span of $\dot{V}_A/\dot{Q}$ ratios is very small, varying from about 0.5 to 3.0, with an average of 0.8. As lung disease develops, the range increasingly widens, with some units receiving very little ventilation relative to perfusion while others are excessively ventilated. If $\dot{V}_A/\dot{Q}$ inequality is imposed on a lung, the arterial P_{O_2} will fall and the P_{CO_2} will rise (Fig. 17–7). In patients with normal chemosensitivity and without severe limitation in ventilatory capacity, the increasing P_{CO_2} leads to a progressive increase in ventilation. This increase in ventilation is capable of bringing the P_{CO_2} back toward normal but only minimally attenuates the fall in the P_{O_2} because of the different shapes of the oxy- and carboxyhemoglobin dissociation curves. The oxyhemoglobin dissociation curve plateaus at a high P_{O_2}, and thus the increased P_{O_2} in alveoli receiving increased ventilation fails to increase the O_2 content of blood leaving that unit. The carboxyhemoglobin dissociation curve, on the other hand, is linear through the physiological range, and any decrease in P_{CO_2} is accompanied by a fall in CO_2 content, compensating for the failure of poorly ventilated lung units to eliminate CO_2. As $\dot{V}_A/\dot{Q}$ inequality wors-

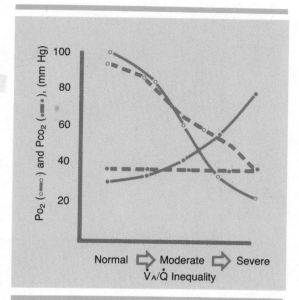

FIGURE 17–7. The effect of increasing ventilation-perfusion ($\dot{V}_A/\dot{Q}$) inequality on arterial P_{O_2} and P_{CO_2}. The solid lines show the change in gas tensions when cardiac output and minute ventilation are held constant. The change in gas tensions when ventilation is allowed to increase to maintain arterial P_{CO_2} at 40 mm Hg is shown by the dotted lines. (From Dantzker DR: Gas exchange abnormalities. *In* Montenegro H (ed): Chronic Obstructive Pulmonary Disease. New York, Churchill Livingstone, 1984, pp 141–160.)

ens with progression of the underlying disease, further increases in ventilation eventually become impossible, and both hypoxemia and hypercapnia result. $\dot{V}_A/\dot{Q}$ inequality is the characteristic abnormality of gas exchange in chronic obstructive and restrictive lung diseases.

SHUNT. Intrapulmonary or intracardiac shunt, where blood bypasses ventilated lung units, is a most potent source of hypoxemia, but hypercapnia is not seen (Fig. 17–8). In fact, as the hypoxemia progresses, hypocapnia is usually found owing to the stimulatory effects of the low P_{aO_2} on ventilatory drive. Shunt is the major mechanism of hypoxemia in pulmonary edema, pneumonia, and atelectasis.

NONPULMONARY FACTORS

Abnormalities other than alterations in lung function may influence the P_{aO_2} through their effect on the mixed venous $P_{O_2}(P_{\bar{v}O_2})$. The $P_{\bar{v}O_2}$ is decreased when cardiac output is inappropriately low, when O_2 consumption ($\dot{V}_{O_2}$) is increased (as with exercise or fever), or when the hemoglobin concentration or O_2 saturation is low. For any lung unit, the resultant end-capillary P_{O_2} is influenced by the $P_{\bar{v}O_2}$, although the magnitude of this effect on the arterial O_2 content will be greatest in lungs with $\dot{V}_A/\dot{Q}$ inequality or shunt (Fig. 17–9). The importance of this phenomenon is the recognition that a fall in P_{aO_2} in a patient with lung disease may be due to one of these nonpulmonary

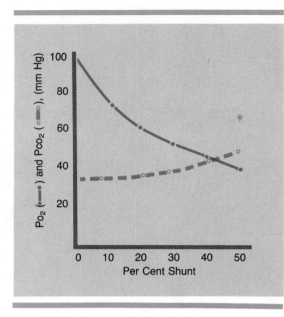

FIGURE 17–8. The effect of increasing shunt on the arterial P_{O_2} and P_{CO_2}. The minute ventilation has been held constant in this example. Under normal circumstances, the hypoxemia would lead to an increased minute ventilation and a fall in the P_{CO_2} as the shunt increases. (From Dantzker DR: Gas exchange abnormalities. *In* Montenegro H (ed): Chronic Obstructive Pulmonary Disease. New York, Churchill Livingstone, 1984, pp 141–160.)

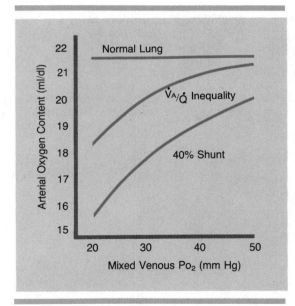

FIGURE 17–9. The effect of altering mixed venous $P_{O_2}(P_vO_2)$ on the arterial oxygen content under three assumed conditions: a normal lung, severe ventilation-perfusion (V_A/Q) inequality, and the presence of a 40 per cent shunt. For each situation the patient is breathing 50 per cent O_2 and the P_vO_2 is altered, keeping all other variables constant. (From Dantzker DR: Gas exchange in the adult respiratory distress syndrome. Clin Chest Med 3:57, 1982.)

factors rather than a deterioration in lung function, thus requiring a very different intervention.

ASSESSING THE EFFICIENCY OF PULMONARY GAS EXCHANGE

A number of indices are used to assess the efficiency of pulmonary gas exchange. The simplest are the arterial blood gases. While extremely useful in patient management, they are neither sensitive nor specific to changes in the efficiency of gas exchange because they are influenced not only by changes in overall minute ventilation but also by nonpulmonary factors that alter the mixed venous P_{O_2} and P_{CO_2}. When breathing enriched O_2 mixtures, arterial blood gases become an even less accurate guide to impairment of gas exchange. With normal lungs, or in patients with small shunts or minor degrees of V_A/Q inequality, P_aO_2 increases almost linearly as F_{IO_2} is increased. However, with progressive lung disease, the response is less predictable.

The alveolar-arterial O_2 difference (A-a D_{O_2}) is a derived measure of gas exchange efficiency that is not influenced by changes in overall minute ventilation. The ideal P_{AO_2} is calculated from the alveolar gas equation. If gas exchange is optimal, then calculated P_{AO_2} should be close to measured P_aO_2. Any factor making gas exchange less efficient will widen the A-a D_{O_2}. In normals, this is usually less than 10 mm Hg, increasing as high as 20 mm Hg in older normal subjects. When hypoxemia is due to hypoventilation, the A-a D_{O_2} remains normal, since the fall in P_{O_2} is due to the rise in P_{CO_2} and the calculated P_{AO_2} should fall to the same degree as the P_aO_2. Thus, the A-a D_{O_2} is a practical way of differentiating hypoventilation from the other causes of hypoxemia.

The second derived index of gas exchange efficiency is the calculation of venous admixture (Q_S/Q_T). The model on which this index is based assumes that the lung has two compartments: one is a shunt, and so blood flowing through this compartment (Q_S) has a P_{O_2} equal to that of mixed venous blood ($P_{\bar{v}}O_2$); the second is well-ventilated and receives the remainder of the cardiac output (Q_T) (i.e., $\dot{Q}_T - \dot{Q}_S$) and has a P_{O_2} equal to that of alveolar gas (P_{AO_2}). Thus, O_2 content of systemic arterial blood (C_aO_2) is the weighted contribution of blood from these compartments:

$$\dot{Q}_T \times C_aO_2 = \dot{Q}_S \times C_vO_2 + \dot{Q}(T - s) \times C_cO_2$$

and solving for venous admixture

$$\dot{Q}_S/\dot{Q}_T = (C_cO_2 - C_aO_2)/(C_cO_2 - C_{\bar{v}}O_2)$$

The C_aO_2 and the $C_{\bar{v}}O_2$ are calculated from measurements of partial pressures and saturations of the arterial and mixed venous blood. The O_2 content of end-capillary blood (C_cO_2) cannot be measured and is derived from the calculated P_{AO_2}, assuming that P_cO_2 equals P_{AO_2}. If P_{AO_2} is greater than 150 mm Hg, then the saturation of end-capillary blood can be assumed to be 100 per cent. If $P_{A_{O_2}}$ is lower, then the saturation must be calculated from one of the many algorithms for the oxyhemoglobin dissociation curve. Modifications of the shunt equation have been suggested in order to make the calculations easier, but should be avoided. They assume either a standard arterial–mixed venous O_2 difference or that both the $P_{a_{O_2}}$ and $P_{c_{O_2}}$ are fully saturated, an unlikely situation in patients with lung disease. An increased Q_S/Q_T in a patient breathing room air is usually due to V_A/Q inequality or shunt. When the patient is breathing 100 per cent O_2, the Q_S/Q_T quantitates the amount of the shunt that is present, as the contribution of V_A/Q inequality is abolished at an $F_{I_{O_2}}$ of 1.0.

NONRESPIRATORY FUNCTIONS OF THE LUNG

In addition to its central role in gas exchange, the lung is active in both the metabolism and the degradation of many substances. Surfactant production by the alveolar Type II cell is an important metabolic function of the lungs. This phospholipid minimizes surface tension and thus confers stability on the alveoli and small airways, preventing atelectasis and decreasing the work of breathing. The failure of the immature lung to produce sufficient surfactant leads to the respiratory distress syndrome (RDS) of the newborn. The lung is also involved in the biosynthesis of arachidonic acid into products of both the lipoxygenase and cyclo-oxygenase pathways. While a myriad of physiological functions have been ascribed to these agents, a clear relationship to pulmonary function is still lacking. Additionally, the lung is capable of removing or inactivating a large number of biologically active substances, including serotonin, bradykinin, and prostaglandins. It is also the principal site of the conversion of angiotensin I to angiotensin II.

REFERENCES

Murray JF: The Normal Lung. Philadelphia, WB Saunders Co, 1976.

West JB: Respiratory Physiology—The Essentials, 2nd ed. Baltimore, Williams and Wilkins, 1979.

CLINICAL MANIFESTATIONS AND DIAGNOSTIC PROCEDURES

18

The correct diagnosis of respiratory illness requires careful attention to both the history and physical examination, as well as to the use of carefully chosen diagnostic studies.

COMMON PRESENTING COMPLAINTS

Cough is "the watchdog of the lungs." It is provoked by mechanical or chemical stimulation of the airways. The cough is preceded by a deep breath followed by glottic closure. Then active compression causes a rapid rise in intrathoracic pressure until sudden opening of the glottis allows rapid decompression. The high flow velocity achieved serves to clear the airway of secretions or foreign bodies. Cough may be caused by the presence of secretions, viral infection of the airway epithelium, or stimulation of parenchymal receptors by pulmonary edema or fibrotic lung disease or may be the sole manifestation of bronchospasm. Chronic cough at night can often be ascribed to the presence of postnasal drip, reflux esophagitis, or aspiration. Recent alteration in the character of a chronic cough may be due to bronchial carcinoma. The cause of chronic isolated cough can usually be elucidated without recourse to invasive measures.

Hemoptysis requires immediate evaluation. A bleeding site in the upper airway should be excluded. Blood-streaked sputum is commonly seen in bronchitis, bronchiectasis, pneumonia, and tuberculosis, but in the absence of infection, persistent or intermittent hemoptysis usually indicates the presence of tumor. Massive hemoptysis is a medical emergency and unless promptly treated the patient may asphyxiate. Unexplained hemoptysis requires a complete evaluation, including a chest x-ray, and fiberoptic bronchoscopy may eventually be required.

Breathing is an automatic, unconscious act. Dyspnea indicates an awareness of increased difficulty in breathing. Its pathophysiology is unclear but may be due to a disproportion between the perceptive demand for ventilation and that achieved. This may result from a change in the relationship between respiratory center drive and minute ventilation or the work of breathing. Clarification of the predisposing factors is important in the diagnosis of its origin. Episodic dyspnea associated with wheezing at rest or following exercise may indicate bronchospasm. Dyspnea causing arousal from sleep may be due to nocturnal asthma, pulmonary edema, sleep apnea syndrome, or aspiration. Dyspnea on exertion may be cardiac or pulmonary in origin, and differentiation often requires exercise testing.

Chest pain originates in the chest wall, the parietal pleura, the large airways, and the structures located within the mediastinum, as the lung parenchyma and visceral pleura are insensitive to painful stimuli. Pleuritic pain is distinctive, being sharp and knifelike and exacerbated by breathing and coughing. It must be differentiated from pericardial pain, involvement of the intercostal nerves by herpes zoster, and inflammation of the costochondral junctions (Tietze's syndrome). Disease involvement of the diaphragmatic pleura may cause referred pain to the shoulder, because the phrenic nerve supply arises from the cervical roots (C3, 4, 5).

Careful review of the remainder of the history is important. Prior episodes of respiratory infection may indicate acquired or congenital abnormalities of pulmonary clearance mechanisms. Similar findings in family members may suggest an inherited disorder such as immotile cilia syndrome. Attention should be paid to occupation, travel, habits (smoking), and hobbies (pets).

PHYSICAL EXAMINATION

The physical examination of the chest remains a cornerstone of the diagnostic process, and it is wise to follow a set system to avoid inadvertently neglecting some aspects of the examination (Table 18–1). Unobtrusive observation of the patient as he breathes quietly is important. A respiratory rate above 22 breaths per minute suggests underlying lung disease. Normally the ribcage and ab-

domen move synchronously on respiration, both moving out on inspiration and in on expiration. Inward motion of the abdomen during inspiration suggests paralysis or dysfunction of the diaphragm, while chaotic in and out movements of the abdominal wall during inspiration may be an early sign of impending respiratory muscle fatigue. Retraction of the intercostal, supraclavicular, and suprasternal spaces reflects the generation of increased negative intrathoracic pressure in the presence of lung disease. Downward pull of the trachea—tracheal tug—is commonly observed in obstructive lung disease. The distance between the cricoid cartilage and the sternal notch is less than the usual three to four finger breadths in patients with hyperinflation.

Cyanosis is a bluish discoloration of the skin, generally indicating an O_2 saturation of 80 per cent or less, representing about 3g/dl, rather than the usually stated 5 g/dl, of reduced hemoglobin. Accuracy diminishes in the presence of inadequate capillary blood flow or anemia. Finger clubbing is recognized by loss of the angle between the nail and the nail bed. It may be associated with painless swelling of tissues of the terminal phalanx and/or arthralgias of the wrist and ankles (hypertrophic pulmonary osteoarthropathy). Common causes include chronic suppurative diseases, chronic interstitial lung disease, pulmonary malignancy, cyanotic congenital heart disease, endocarditis, chronic liver and bowel disease, as well as a congenital idiopathic form.

Contraction of the sternomastoid muscles during resting breathing is an important indicator of respiratory distress. Patients with obstructive lung disease often derive symptomatic benefit from pursed-lip breathing, but the mechanism of this improvement is unknown. A "barrel-shaped" chest wall is seen in emphysema, while deformity of the chest wall may explain a restrictive pattern on pulmonary function testing.

Reduction in movement of one side of the chest on palpation indicates the presence of ipsilateral lung disease. Deviation of the trachea from the midline may reflect a shift in the mediastinum and is helpful in the diagnosis of a pneumothorax (Table 18–2). Vocal fremitus is the palpable vibration associated with transmission of the spoken word to the chest wall. It is increased with consolidation and decreased if fluid or air is present in the pleural space. Its absence helps to differentiate pleural effusion from dense parenchymal infiltrates seen on x-ray.

Percussion helps in detecting the interface between the aerated lung and solid structures (liver, pleural fluid, or consolidation). Determination of heart and mediastinal size and probably also the extent of diaphragmatic movement is better done radiographically.

During auscultation, the observer needs to compare the two sides of the chest at equidistant points from the midline and *while* listening answer only two questions: (1) what is the character of the breath sounds? and (2) are added sounds present, and if so what is their nature?

TABLE 18–1. SYSTEMATIC APPROACH TO PHYSICAL EXAMINATION OF THE CHEST

I. **Inspection**
   Initial impression—distress, wheeze, malnourished, etc.
   Respiratory rate, depth, and pattern
   Asynchronous motion of the ribcage and abdomen
   Recession of the intercostal, supraclavicular, or suprasternal spaces
   Tracheal tug
   Cyanosis
   Finger clubbing or nicotine stains
   Accessory muscle employment
   Pursed-lip breathing
   Chest wall shape and deformity
II. **Palpation**
   Tracheal deviation
   Chest expansion (globally/locally)
   Vocal fremitus
   Pleural rub
   Lymphadenopathy
   Subcutaneous emphysema
III. **Percussion**
   Normal, dull, or increased
IV. **Auscultation**
   Breath sounds—can only be normal, reduced, or bronchial (latter associated with increased vocal resonance, whispering pectoriloquy, and egophony)
   Added sounds—can only be absent, wheezes, crackles, or pleural rub

TABLE 18–2. PHYSICAL FINDINGS IN COMMON PULMONARY DISORDERS

DISORDER	MEDIASTINAL DISPLACEMENT	CHEST WALL MOVEMENT	VOCAL FREMITUS	PERCUSSION NOTE	BREATH SOUNDS	ADDED SOUNDS	VOICE SOUNDS
Pleural effusion	Heart displaced to opposite side	Reduced over affected area	Absent or markedly decreased	Stony dull	Absent over fluid; bronchial at upper border	Absent; pleural rub may be found above effusion	Absent over effusion; increased with egophony at upper border
Consolidation	None	Reduced over affected area	Increased	Dull	Bronchial	Crackles	Increased with egophony and whispering pectoriloquy
Pneumothorax	Tracheal deviation to opposite side if under tension	Decreased over affected area	Absent	Resonant	Absent	Absent	Absent
Atelectasis	Ipsilateral shift	Decreased over affected area	Absent	Dull	Absent or diminished	Absent	Absent
Bronchospasm	None	Decreased symmetrically	Normal or decreased	Normal or decreased	Normal	Wheeze	Normal or decreased
Interstitial fibrosis	None	Decreased symmetrically	Normal or increased	Normal	Normal	Coarse crackles unaffected by cough or posture	Normal

Breath sounds are caused by turbulent air flow, with the intensity depending on the flow rate. They are produced almost entirely in the trachea and large airways and transmitted to the chest wall initially by the smaller airways and finally through the lung parenchyma. The passage through the lung filters out the high frequencies and accounts for the differences in normal breath sounds heard at different places.

Bronchial breath sounds are essentially unaltered, and both inspiration and expiration are clearly heard. These are heard normally over the trachea and the central airways in the back. As we move away from the central airways to the periphery of the lung, the filtering effect serves to diminish the inspiration and almost eliminate the expiratory noise. This is the normal vesicular breath sound.

The breath sounds can only be normal, decreased, or increased. Decreased intensity of the breath sounds is due to either (1) impaired movement of air that normally generates the breath sounds, such as in emphysema, diaphragmatic paralysis, or bronchial obstruction, or (2) impaired transmission from the lung to the chest wall due to pneumothorax or pleural effusion or thickening. An increased transmission of the breath sounds is characterized by the finding of bronchial breath sounds (similar to the sound normally heard over the trachea) over the peripheral lung fields. Bronchial breathing is most commonly found with consolidation but can also occur at the interface with a pleural effusion where the lung is compressed. Upon completion of initial auscultation, the examiner can verify the presence of bronchial breathing by demonstrating the presence of the associated features: increased vocal resonance, whispering pectoriloquy (whispered sounds are heard more clearly), and egophony (the phonated e is heard as a).

Added sounds can be of only three types: wheezes, crackles, and pleural sounds. Wheezes are continuous, musical sounds thought to occur as air passes through a narrowed airway, setting up oscillations in the walls. They are more common during expiration, since dynamic compression exaggerates the constriction. Wheezes may be diffuse in asthma or chronic bronchitis, or localized in the case of a partially obstructed bronchus (tumor, secretions, or foreign body).

Crackles, formerly called râles or crepitations, are short sequences of discontinuous sounds that may be heard during inspiration or expiration. Very coarse crackles heard over the large airways are thought to result from air moving through secretions. However, most crackles are generated further out in the lung as a result of the popping open of small airways that were closed during the previous expiration owing to low lung volumes, alterations in lung compliance, or increases in interstitial pressure. These factors are magnified in the bases, and they are more common there even if the underlying process is diffuse. When fine, the sound is mimicked by rubbing hair close to the ear between the thumb and finger, while the coarse crackle is like the sound of a Velcro fastener opening. The finding of crackles is a nonspecific indicator of pulmonary parenchymal disease, and the crackles of congestive failure cannot be differentiated from those of pulmonary infection.

Pleural sounds may be a rub, like the creaking of leather, found with pleural inflammation or the mediastinal crunching sound synchronous with systole found with a pneumomediastinum and likened to the sound created while walking through snow.

The typical physical findings in the major pulmonary disorders are outlined in Table 18–2.

DIAGNOSTIC TECHNIQUES AND THEIR INDICATIONS

IMAGING PROCEDURES

The standard chest roentgenogram complements the history and physical exam as the starting point for the diagnosis of pulmonary disorders. The chest x-ray may demonstrate a density that only physical exam can differentiate between consolidation and loculated pleural fluid. Conversely, the chest x-ray may show dramatic involvement of the lung by tuberculosis while the physical exam is not remarkable. Standard views include the posteroanterior and the left lateral projections; they reduce disproportionate magnification of the heart and anterior mediastinal structures. These films allow visualization of the air-containing lung, vascular markings, heart and mediastinal structures, pleura, lymph nodes, ribs, spine, and soft tissues of the thorax. Correct interpretation requires that the film be taken as close to total lung capacity as possible. A correctly ex-posed film allows the vertebral bodies to be barely visible behind the heart. A number of specialized views and procedures can be added to the standard PA and lateral films (Table 18–3).

Significant improvement in visualization of chest structures has resulted with computed tomography (CT), which provides excellent visibility of areas previously difficult to see and has ten times the contrast resolution of conventional radiography. Excellent evaluation of the mediastinum makes it valuable in the work-up of bronchogenic neoplasms. Differentiating pleural from parenchymal densities, a common problem on the routine film, has been improved. Computed tomography has virtually replaced the standard radiographs for evaluating the presence of early metastatic spread to the lung parenchyma; unfortunately, specificity is low, and 20 to 60 per cent of nodules visualized on CT scan but not on x-ray are benign. In addition, CT is useful for detecting calcification in pulmonary nodules.

Ultrasound is useful in helping to differentiate pleural opacities into solids or fluid and to localize loculated pleural effusions. Other imaging methods such as nuclear magnetic resonance and digital subtraction angiography are not generally available, and their superiority over available methods has yet to be proven.

PULMONARY FUNCTION EVALUATION

In the pulmonary function laboratory, routine studies can be grouped into four categories: lung volumes, air flow, diffusing capacity, and maximal pressures. Additional studies such as measurements of lung compliance rarely provide additional information to that obtained by more easily performed measurements.

The lung is conveniently divided into four volumes and three capacities, as shown in Figure 18–1. The components of the vital capacity can be obtained with routine spirometry. The residual

TABLE 18–3. SPECIALIZED RADIOGRAPHIC TECHNIQUES

STUDY OR VIEW	INDICATION	COMMENT
Oblique	Visualization of hilum and pleural plaques. Contralateral oblique is best view for apical disease.	Better done with CT
Lordotic	Right middle lobe and lingular disease	
Lateral decubitus	Identification of pleural effusions, air-fluid levels, and fungus balls	Both left and right should always be done
Upright-supine	Differentiation of pleural from parenchymal disease in critically ill patients requiring portable radiography	
Inspiratory-expiratory	Obstruction of bronchus or air-trapping in enclosed pleural or lung spaces	
Tomograms	Visualization of lesions obscured by overlying tissue; visualization of bronchi, pulmonary vessels, and hili; demonstration of parenchymal calcifications	Better done with CT
Bronchograms	Diagnosis of bronchiectasis	Only indicated in the rare situation when surgery is contemplated; can now be diagnosed by CT
Pulmonary angiogram	Detection of congenital anomalies of the pulmonary vasculature. Diagnosis of pulmonary emboli	
Fluoroscopy	Diaphragmatic movement. Differentiation between chest wall lesions and lung parenchymal lesions	

volume (RV), however, must be measured indirectly, since it represents the air left in the lungs at completion of a full expiration. In fact, we actually measure functional residual capacity (FRC) rather than RV, since the former, i.e., the volume at the end of a normal expiration, is a more reproducible point. The expiratory reserve volume (ERV) is then subtracted from FRC to obtain the residual volume.

Three techniques are commonly used to measure FRC: nitrogen washout, helium dilution, and body plethysmography. The first two techniques are limited by the ability of the test gas to either wash out or equilibrate completely with all portions of the lung. In the presence of significant airways obstruction this will not occur and the FRC will be significantly underestimated. Body plethysmography eliminates this problem and measures the total thoracic gas volume, whether it is located in a bulla or in direct communication with the airway, and thus provides a more accurate reflection of the FRC.

The dynamics of airflow can be evaluated during a forced expiratory maneuver by recording the change in volume against time to calculate flow rate or by directly measuring volume and flow (Figs. 18–2 and 18–3). The flow-volume loop is particularly useful in demonstrating the presence of upper airway obstruction, which by affecting primarily the peak inspiratory and expiratory flows gives a characteristic loop (Fig. 18–3). An estimate of total airway resistance can be determined by the body plethysmograph.

The measurement of the diffusing capacity for carbon monoxide ($D_{L}CO$) is an indicator of the adequacy of the alveolar-capillary membrane and so is reduced when the latter is decreased, as in pulmonary fibrosis, emphysema, and pulmonary vascular disease. In patients with a restrictive physiological defect, diffusing capacity helps to differentiate chest bellows ($D_{L}CO$ normal) from pa-

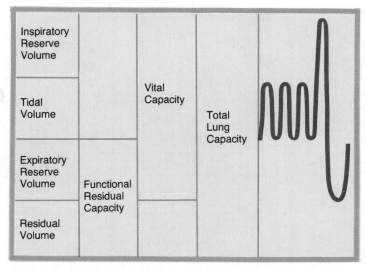

FIGURE 18–1. Lung volumes and capacities. While vital capacity and its subdivision can be measured by spirometry, calculation of residual volume requires measurement of functional residual capacity by body plethysmography, helium dilution technique, or nitrogen washout.

renchymal disease ($D_{L}CO$ decreased). While it provides little insight into the mechanism of abnormal lung function, it is useful as a marker of improvement or deterioration of the existing disease process.

Measurement of maximal static respiratory pressures is probably the most sensitive and specific method of diagnosing respiratory dysfunction in patients with neuromuscular disease. Maximal inspiratory pressure is obtained by recording mouth pressure during a maximal inspiratory effort from residual volume, and maximal expiratory pressure is recorded during a maximum expiratory effort from total lung capacity.

Interpretation of pulmonary function studies requires consideration of the technical quality of

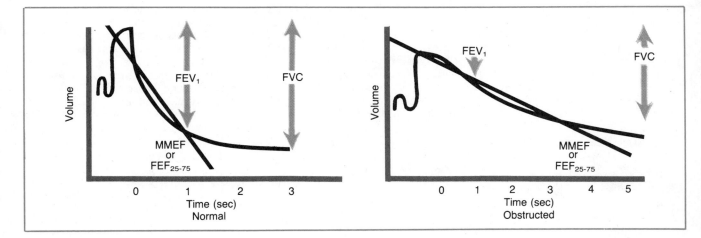

FIGURE 18–2. Spirometry in a normal subject and a patient with obstructive lung disease. FEV_1 represents the forced expired volume in 1 sec and FVC represents the forced vital capacity. The slope of the line connecting the points at 25 per cent and 75 per cent of the FVC represents the forced expired flow, FEF_{25-75}, or maximum mid-expiratory flow (MMEF). The FEF_{25-75} is less reproducible and less specific than the FEV_1.

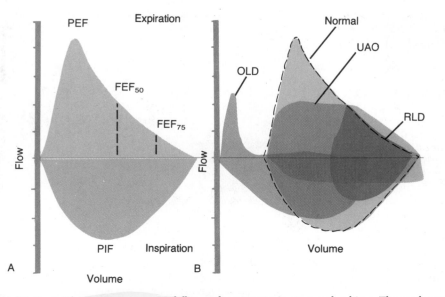

FIGURE 18–3. *A,* The maximum expired flow-volume curve in a normal subject. The peak expiratory flow (PEF) and forced expiratory flows at 50 per cent and 75 per cent of the exhaled vital capacity are indicated. *B,* In obstructive lung disease (OLD) hyperinflation pushes the position of the curve to the left, and there is characteristic scalloping on expiration. In restrictive lung disease (RLD), lung volumes are reduced but flow for any one point in volume is normal. In upper airway obstruction (UAO), the flow-volume curve shows a reduction in the peak flow rates.

the tracings and a knowledge of the degree of variation for a particular index. Small deviations in vital capacity may be abnormal, whereas larger deviations in D_{LCO} are required to confidently diagnose abnormality. Fixed percentages of a normal value should not be considered to indicate disease.

Measurement of lung volumes and flow rates after certain challenges such as methacholine, exercise, cold air, or exposure to organic or inorganic substances helps in the diagnosis of bronchospasm. Acute reversibility is determined by their repetition after bronchodilator administration. However, failure of flow to improve following a single dose of a bronchodilator does not necessarily indicate irreversible disease and does not exclude the possibility of a clinical response to bronchodilator treatment.

More complex testing is occasionally required to answer specific questions. Exercise studies are valuable in judging the degree of disability as well as elucidating the cause of dyspnea on exertion. Expired gas, minute ventilation, heart rate, and arterial oxygenation are measured during increased workloads. The degree of limitation and the relative contribution of ventilatory and cardiovascular factors can be assessed. Polysomnography is an essential tool in the diagnosis of sleep apnea (see Chapter 25).

ARTERIAL BLOOD GASES

The arterial partial pressures of oxygen and carbon dioxide (P_aO_2 and P_aCO_2) and pH as well as parameters derived from these values such as the alveolar-arterial O_2 difference (A-a Do_2) and venous admixture ($\dot{Q}_S/\dot{Q}_T$) are the most commonly evaluated parameters of lung function (see Chapter 17). When measured while breathing room air and 100 percent O_2, they can often diagnose the mechanism of abnormal pulmonary gas exchange (Table 18–4). Measurement of these parameters requires arterial puncture, which is uncomfortable for the patient and occasionally difficult or dangerous to perform. When multiple samples are required over a relatively short period of time, an indwelling arterial catheter may be useful.

INVASIVE DIAGNOSTIC TECHNIQUES

Bronchoscopy. This is used to visualize the airways, to sample secretions, and to perform forceps biopsy. The rigid scope remains the instrument of choice when a wide channel is required, such as in massive hemoptysis and removal of large foreign bodies. Otherwise the flexible scope is preferable because it is easy to maneuver. It is invaluable in the evaluation and biopsy of endobronchial lesions and in localizing the site of hemoptysis, since it allows visual access out to

TABLE 18–4. DIFFERENTIAL DIAGNOSIS OF HYPOXEMIA

	P_aO_2	P_aCO_2	A-a Do_2		$\dot{Q}_S/\dot{Q}_T$	
			RA	100% O_2	RA	100% O_2
Hypoventilation	D	I	N	N	N	N
Abnormal diffusion	D	N	I	N	I	N
Shunt	D	N or D	I	I	I	I
$\dot{V}_A/\dot{Q}$ inequality	D	N or I	I	N	I	N

Abbreviations: RA = room air; D = decreased; I = increased; N = normal; $\dot{V}_A/\dot{Q}$ = ventilation–perfusion.

the segmental airways. It can be used together with fluoroscopy to biopsy peripheral lung lesions. In the immunocompromised host it is the standard technique in the diagnosis of fungal or pneumocystic pneumonia. It is also effective in the diagnosis of tuberculosis in a patient not producing sputum. Its indication in the diagnosis of common bacterial infections is less clear, although the development of special protective brushes has reduced the problem of contamination with upper airway flora. In most patients requiring bronchial toilet and drainage, physical therapy is sufficient, but when that fails, especially in patients on mechanical ventilation, bronchoscopy may be effective in re-expanding atelectatic areas.

While generally a benign procedure, bronchoscopy has a number of complications. Worsening of hypoxemia is almost inevitable, and supplemental O_2 should be used in hypoxemic patients. Laryngospasm, bronchospasm, fever, and new pulmonary infiltrates may occur. Significant bleeding and pneumothorax infrequently follow lung biopsy.

Transthoracic Needle Aspiration. Aspiration of lung tissue through a skinny needle inserted percutaneously is most useful with peripheral lesions, with which the bronchoscope has its least success. It provides material for cytologic examination or microbial studies rather than histologic examinations. The major complication is pneumothorax, occurring in 20 to 30 per cent, although chest tube drainage is required in only 1 to 15 per cent. Hemoptysis may occur but is rarely of clinical significance.

Thoracocentesis and Pleural Biopsy. Pleural fluid examination and interpretation are covered in Chapter 26. Parietal pleural biopsy can be ac-complished if sufficient fluid separates the lung from the chest wall. Histologic examination reveals granulomas in greater than 60 per cent of cases of suspected tuberculosis effusion, and when histology is combined with culture of the tissue sample the yield may be 90 per cent. Biopsy is positive in 39 to 75 per cent of cases of suspected malignancy, which is less than with cytologic examination of the fluid. Thoracoscopy with biopsy of pleural lesions under direct vision can be performed when the pleural effusion remains undiagnosed after thoracocentesis and biopsy.

Mediastinoscopy. A small tube is passed into the mediastinum through an incision in the sternal notch. Lymph nodes in the anterior mediastinum and the right paratracheal region can be biopsied.

Open Lung Biopsy. When the above procedures are negative, an open lung biopsy may be indicated. In the immunocompromised host, it has a greater diagnostic yield than transbronchial biopsy using a fiberoptic bronchoscopy, but still a proportion of patients display nonspecific findings. Despite the critical nature of the patients' illness, the mortality in large series of open lung biopsy is less than 0.5 per cent, with a complication rate of 11 per cent.

REFERENCES

Fraser RG, and Pare JAP: Diagnosis of Diseases of the Chest. 2nd ed. Philadelphia, WB Saunders Co, 1977.

Intermountain Thoracic Society: Clinical Pulmonary Function Testing: A Manual of Uniform Laboratory Procedures. 2nd ed. Salt Lake City, 1984.

Sackner MA : Diagnostic Techniques in Pulmonary Disease, Parts I and II. New York, Marcel-Dekker, 1981.

OBSTRUCTIVE LUNG DISEASE 19

The obstructive lung diseases are characterized by reduction of expiratory flow rates and include asthma, emphysema, chronic bronchitis, bronchiectasis and cystic fibrosis. However controversy and confusion reign over the definition of these individual disorders because of the marked overlap of clinical and pathophysiological features. Some have even suggested the abandonment of the traditional names and the substitution of groupings based on signs and symptoms. Chronic mucus hypersecretion, with or without obstruction, and chronic airways obstruction, reversible or nonreversible, are probably more useful designations than debating whether a patient has chronic bronchitis or asthma. However, because these are not in general use, we will try to define each of the diseases as currently understood, pointing out overlap when it exists (Table 19–1).

PATHOPHYSIOLOGY OF AIRWAY OBSTRUCTION

The mechanism of the airway obstruction in these disorders is always multifactorial, although in any individual patient one mechanism may play a dominant role. Air flow in the lungs is directly proportional to the driving pressure and inversely related to the airway resistance. During most of a forced expiration, the effective driving pressure is the elastic recoil pressure of the lung.

TABLE 19–1. OBSTRUCTIVE LUNG DISEASES

DISORDER	MAJOR CLINICAL CRITERIA	DISTINCTIVE LABORATORY FINDINGS
Emphysema	Hyperinflation, little or no sputum production, cachexia	Well preserved ABG's, low carbon monoxide diffusing capacity, and increased lung compliance
Chronic bronchitis		
Simple	Cough and sputum production, history of chronic irritant exposure (i.e., tobacco, industry)	No significant physiological impairment
Obstructed	Cough and sputum production, congestive heart failure common	Hypoxemic ± hypercapnia
Asthma	Episodic dyspnea, may be associated with clear-cut allergy	Marked airways reactivity
Bronchiectasis	Large volume sputum production, clubbing	Chest x-ray finding of thickened bronchial walls
Immotile cilia syndrome	Associated with situs inversus or dextrocardia, sinusitis, and infertility	Abnormal sperm anatomy
Hypogammaglobulinemia		Abnormal decrease in one or more immunoglobulins
Cystic fibrosis	Bronchiectasis associated with GI disease, sinusitis, and infertility	Increased sweat Cl and Na, abnormal pancreatic function

Thus, reduction in elasticity, as in emphysema, decreases the maximum expiratory flow. Decreased elasticity also increases airway resistance, since the elastic recoil pressure exerts radial traction on the airways, which limits their dynamic compression during expiration.

A second cause of increased airway resistance is bronchoconstriction. The airways are lined by smooth muscle that is innervated by both adrenergic (bronchodilating) and cholinergic (bronchoconstricting) pathways. Cholinergic control is mediated by a vagal reflex, via irritant receptors lying just beneath the mucosa of the large airways, trachea, and upper respiratory tract. Stimulation of these receptors by inhaled irritants or inflammation produces bronchoconstriction. In addition, endogenous mediators such as histamine and prostaglandins may dilate or constrict bronchial smooth muscle directly or reflexly by exciting the irritant receptors. Such mechanisms function to protect the lungs of normal subjects from noxious agents, but hyperreactivity of these pathways exists in patients with obstructive lung disease.

A third cause of increased airway resistance is chronic inflammation. In response to irritation in the form of external pollutants, recurrent infection, or chronic immunological stimulation, there is hyperplasia and hypertrophy of the bronchial glands, inflammatory narrowing of the airways, and the production of excessive, thick secretions. If this process is allowed to continue it often results in the loss of ciliated epithelium, squamous metaplasia, and eventual peribronchial fibrosis.

Airway obstruction leads to characteristic changes in lung volumes, with an increase in residual volume (RV) and functional residual capacity (FRC) and a normal or increased total lung capacity (TLC). The vital capacity (VC) is decreased as the RV takes up more and more of the thoracic gas volume. The mechanism of the increase in RV and FRC is not completely under-

stood, although several factors are likely to contribute to a variable degree depending on the specific etiology involved. Decrease in the elastic recoil of the lungs moves the FRC closer to the relaxed volume of the chest wall (about two thirds of TLC). A second factor is the greater tendency for abnormal airways, particularly at the lung base, to collapse during expiration, trapping air behind the closed airways. Finally, certain patients with asthma have persistent activity of the inspiratory muscles during expiration, which actively maintains a high FRC.

There are three major consequences of these changes in lung volume. Because of the nonlinear nature of the pressure-volume relationship of the lung, breathing at high lung volumes along the flat portion of the curve requires a greater pressure for the same change in volume (see Fig. 17–3), further increasing the work of breathing, which is already high owing to the abnormal airway resistance. In addition, the higher the resting lung volume, the shorter the inspiratory muscles are at the beginning of the breath (see Fig. 17–2). This places them at a disadvantageous position on their length-tension curve and predisposes them to fatigue. Hyperinflation, however, has one beneficial effect. Owing to the tethering effect of the lung parenchyma on the airways, there is an inverse relationship between lung volume and airway resistance. Thus, hyperinflation is the one strategy immediately available in asthmatics to minimize sudden changes in airway caliber.

Abnormal pulmonary gas exchange is an inevitable consequence of obstructive lung disease. Airway obstruction and the breakdown of alveolar walls produce ventilation-perfusion mismatch, which interferes with the efficient transfer of both O_2 and CO_2. Up to a certain point, patients with obstructive lung disease can increase their minute ventilation sufficiently to prevent the development of hypercapnia despite worsening hypoxemia (see Fig. 17–9). However, with continued progression of the disease a point is reached beyond which further increase in ventilation is impractical because of either the high energy requirements or the development of muscle fatigue. At that point, it is more efficient, physiologically, to allow P_aCO_2 to rise, thus eliminating it at both a lower minute ventilation and metabolic cost but at a higher concentration. The onset of hypercapnia is not always clearly related to the degree of mechanical impairment, and it appears that some patients prefer to work harder to maintain normocapnia, while others with the same degree of impairment are satisfied to breathe less and allow worse gas exchange (see Chapter 25).

Acute exacerbations of the chronic process brought on by infection or congestive heart failure may lead to the development of intrapulmonary shunt and further worsen gas exchange. During sleep, gas exchange is also usually worse owing to a characteristic reduction in minute ventilation. A patient with adequate arterial blood gases during the day may develop significant hypercapnia and arterial desaturation at night.

EMPHYSEMA

Emphysema is characterized by two features. Anatomically, it is defined as an abnormal enlargement of the airspaces distal to the terminal bronchioles, accompanied by destructive changes in the alveolar walls. Physiologically, it is characterized by a loss of elastic recoil and thus an increased lung compliance. The correlation between the anatomic and physiological criteria is good but not invariable.

The pathogenesis of emphysema has yet to be determined with certainty, although most workers favor an imbalance of proteases and antiproteases in the lung, with resultant lung destruction. This theory is based on the discovery of a small number of patients with an inherited deficiency of $alpha_1$-antitrypsin, the major antiprotease, who develop emphysema at a young age even without other risk factors. Cigarette smoke, the major etiologic factor in the development of emphysema, has been shown to increase the numbers of alveolar macrophages and neutrophils in the lung, enhance protease release, and impair the activity of antiproteases. However, other factors must determine susceptibility to emphysema, as less than 10 to 15 per cent of smokers develop clinical evidence of airway obstruction. Patients with emphysema usually present with dyspnea, exercise intolerance, and in its purest form minimal cough and sputum production. On physical examination they have hyperinflation, decreased breath sounds, and prominent use of accessory muscles. They are usually thin, even cachectic looking, and rarely have evidence of congestive heart failure. Despite severe obstructive lung disease, they usually preserve their arterial oxygen saturation and are generally normocapnic.

In the absence of pathological material, the diagnosis of emphysema is inferred from the clinical and laboratory findings. Chest roentgenograms demonstrate hyperinflation with depressed diaphragms, increased anteroposterior diameter, and widened retrosternal airspace. These findings, however, are seen whenever hyperinflation is present, and more specific features in emphysema include attenuation of the pulmonary vasculature and the presence of bullous lines. The routine pulmonary function studies are also nonspecific, showing a decrease in the VC and increased RV, FRC, and TLC, along with decreased forced expired volume in 1 sec (FEV_1) and flow rates. While flow rates may increase with bronchodilator administration, the improvement is less than that observed in asthma. The one finding that correlates well with the anatomical presence of emphysema is a reduction in diffusing capacity because of the loss of alveolar capillary surface area.

CHRONIC BRONCHITIS

Chronic bronchitis is defined as a persistent cough resulting in sputum production for more than three months in each year over the previous three years. Diagnosis requires exclusion of other conditions associated with cough and sputum production, such as bronchiectasis. As with emphysema, cigarette smoke is the major etiologic factor, although exposure to other pollutants such as dusts may play a role by causing chronic irritation. The airway obstruction seen in the setting of chronic bronchitis is due to associated emphysema, bronchospasm, and obstruction of the peripheral airways.

The findings on physical examination, pulmonary function assessment, and x-ray depend on the degree of associated airway obstruction. They range from normal to the pattern observed in emphysema, with the exception that diffusing capacity remains normal. Gas exchange is worse than in patients with predominant emphysema, with hypoxemia and eventual hypercapnia increasing as the degree of air flow obstruction worsens. The marked hypoxemia leads to hypoxic pulmonary vasoconstriction and is responsible for the presence of pulmonary hypertension and the subsequent right-sided heart failure (cor pulmonale) often found in these patients. It also may result in significant polycythemia.

Chronic bronchitis and emphysema are marked by intermittent exacerbations that may precipitate acute respiratory failure. The underlying causes of these exacerbations include acute pulmonary infection, development of heart failure, and poor patient compliance. Until recently, an episode of acute respiratory failure in these patients was associated with a poor prognosis following discharge (only 30 per cent survived five years), but with modern management such an episode does not appear to alter overall prognosis.

ASTHMA

Asthma has been defined as a disease in which there is an increased responsiveness of the airways to various stimuli, causing widespread narrowing of the airways which varies over time. The stimulus may be immunologic in origin, as in clas-

TABLE 19–2. TYPES OF ASTHMA

CLASSIFICATION	INITIATING FACTORS
Extrinsic	IgE-mediated external allergens
Intrinsic	?
Adult onset	?
Exercise induced	Alteration in airway temperature and humidity; mediator release
Aspirin sensitive (associated with nasal polyps)	Aspirin and other nonsteroidal anti-inflammatory drugs
Allergic bronchopulmonary aspergillosis	Hypersensitivity to *Aspergillus* species (not infection)
Occupational	Metal salts (platinum, chrome, and nickel)
	Antibiotic powder (penicillin, sulfathiazole, tetracycline)
	Toluene diisocyanate (TDI)
	Flour
	Wood dusts
	Cotton dust (byssinosis)
	Animal proteins

sic extrinsic asthma, in which mast cells, sensitized by IgE antibodies, degranulate and release bronchoactive mediators following exposure to a specific antigen. The cause may also be unclear, as in adult-onset asthma, in which the patients frequently show no evidence of allergy. The airway obstruction may be due to bronchoconstriction alone or may involve mucosal inflammation and excessive mucus production. Symptoms may be intermittent, or they may gradually become persistent. The recognized categories of asthma are listed in Table 19–2. Clinical differentiation is important only in situations in which there are

TABLE 19–3. DIAGNOSTIC STUDIES IN ASTHMA

1.	Routine pulmonary function test	Decreased FEV_1; hyperinflation; improvement with bronchodilator
2.	Special pulmonary function test	
	a. methacholine, histamine or cold-air challenge	Indicate the presence of nonspecific bronchial hyper-reactivity; bronchoconstriction occurs at lower dose in asthma
	b. challenge with specific agents: occupational, drugs, etc.	Occasionally performed
	c. portable peak flow measurements	Helpful in diagnosis of occupational asthma and managment of brittle asthmatic
3.	Chest x-ray	Fleeting infiltrates and central bronchiectasis in ABPA
4.	Skin tests	Demonstrate atopy; little value except prick test to *Aspergillus fumigatus* positive in ABPA
5.	Blood tests	Eosinophils and IgE usually increased in atopy; levels may be very high in ABPA. *Aspergillus* precipitins increased in many but not all patients with ABPA

Abbreviation: ABPA = allergic bronchopulmonary aspergillosis.

clear-cut, easily identifiable, and avoidable extrinsic factors, such as drugs or industrial substances.

The diagnosis of asthma is based on the presence of episodic dyspnea associated with wheezing. Intermittent cough, probably due to stimulation of the irritant receptors, is the sole presenting symptom in some patients. Typically, symptoms are worse at night, following exercise, after going out in the cold, while exposed to irritating gases, etc.

Laboratory studies may be required to determine the presence of specific types of asthma (Table 19–3). The chest x-ray demonstrates hyperinflation in the symptomatic patient, while in patients with allergic bronchopulmonary aspergillosis, serial films may show infiltrates that change location or features suggestive of central bronchiectasis. Pulmonary function studies show the findings of obstruction, which improve significantly following the acute administration of bronchodilators. During the asymptomatic phase, the diagnosis can often be made by producing obstruction by the inhalation of histamine, methacholine, or cold air.

Acute severe asthma (status asthmaticus) refers to an attack of increased severity that is unresponsive to routine therapy. While the attack is sometimes prolonged, fatal episodes may occur unexpectedly with overwhelming suddenness. A history of increasing bronchodilator use with little benefit is expected, but clinical signs, including pulsus paradoxus, are extremely unreliable in judging the severity. The degree of physiological disturbance can best be appreciated by a measure of expiratory flow rates. In the emergency room management of these patients such indices are very helpful in assessing the response to therapy, as they provide immediate quantitative information and can be obtained at frequent intervals without discomfort. Complementary information can be obtained by measurement of arterial blood gases, and this may be the only measurement possible in the critically ill asthmatic. Hypoxemia is usually, but not invariably, present, and P_aCO_2 is typically reduced early in an attack. With increasing severity, P_aO_2 falls and P_aCO_2 returns to normal and then rises, accompanied by a mixed respiratory and metabolic acidosis, such that intubation and mechanical ventilation may become necessary. Hypercapnia at presentation is not an indication for intubation, as most patients improve, but careful monitoring is essential. In general, arterial blood gas measurements are less sensitive and specific than assessment of airway obstruction in judging the response to therapy.

BRONCHIECTASIS

Bronchiectasis is an abnormal and persistent dilatation of the bronchi due to destructive changes in the elastic and muscular layers of the walls. It may be widespread or localized to a single lung segment. It is usually a consequence of a severe necrotizing lung infection. In the past it was often seen as a sequela of measles or pertussis pneumonia, whereas today it is more likely to be a residual from a gram-negative infection. Immune deficiency states such as hypogammaglobulinemia predispose to frequent respiratory tract infections and the development of bronchiectasis. Exposure to corrosive gases is an additional inflammatory injury that may result in permanent airway damage. Interference with the normal clearance mechanisms may also cause chronic inflammation and bronchiectasis. An unusual congenital cause of decreased lung clearance and bronchiectasis is the immotile cilia syndrome due to structural abnormalities in the microtubular system. This is often associated with sinusitis, situs inversus or dextrocardia, and infertility.

The diagnosis in general is made by a history of long-standing chronic cough and the production of large quantities of foul sputum, occasionally blood tinged, and physical findings of persistent crackles over the affected lung regions. With severe, long-standing disease, clubbing and cor pulmonale are frequent and massive hemoptysis may occasionally occur. The chest x-ray may be normal or may display minor nonspecific features, such as increased markings or linear atelectasis. On occasion, the x-ray is very suggestive of bronchiectasis, demonstrating thickening of the bronchial walls well out to the lung periphery and even cystic lesions. Definitive diagnosis usually requires contrast bronchography, but this is rarely indicated. More recently CT scanning has been able to resolve the presence of bronchiectasis with a high degree of sensitivity. Pulmonary function studies invariably show obstruction and occasionally significant hyperinflation, although with severe disease restricted lung volumes may be present.

CYSTIC FIBROSIS

Cystic fibrosis is a common generalized disorder of exocrine gland function, which impairs clearance of secretions in a variety of organs (Table 19–4). This autosomal recessive disorder occurs in about 1 in every 2000 white births. The underlying defect is unknown, but the pulmonary pathophysiology is similar to other causes of bronchiectasis, with tenacious mucus and impaired ciliary function resulting in recurrent infections, chronic inflammation, and bronchial wall destruction.

The disease is usually manifest in childhood, often with gastrointestinal symptoms, particularly steatorrhea and bowel obstruction (Table 19–4). However, the pulmonary features pose the biggest problem. Classically, *Staphylococcus aureus* in childhood and the mucoid strain of *Pseudomonas aeruginosa* in later years cause recurrent respiratory infections that are particularly difficult to treat because of chronic colonization of the airways. Definitive diagnosis requires the finding of an elevated concentration of sodium or chloride in the sweat. When correctly collected and analyzed, levels above 60 mEq/L in children or 80 mEq/L in adults are diagnostic in the proper clin-

TABLE 19–4. CYSTIC FIBROSIS—ORGAN INVOLVEMENT

I. **Pulmonary**
 Cough and sputum production
 Recurrent pneumonias
 Bronchial hyper-reactivity
 Hemoptysis
 Pneumothorax
 Marked digital clubbing
 Cor pulmonale
II. **Upper Respiratory Tract**
 Nasal polyps
 Chronic sinusitis
III. **Gastrointestinal**
 Meconium ileus in the neonate
 Meconium ileus equivalent (childhood, adult)
 Rectal prolapse
 Hernias
 Chronic pancreatic dysfunction causing steatorrhea, malnutrition, and vitamin deficiency
 Acute pancreatitis (rare)
 Diabetes mellitus
 Cirrhosis and portal hypertension
 Salivary gland inflammation
IV. **Genitourinary**
 Sterility in men
 Low fertility rate in women

ical setting. The course is usually one of gradual but progressive respiratory failure. Some patients with milder disease escape diagnosis until their late teens or even early 20's. These patients usually have minimal extrapulmonary problems and have been carried for years with a diagnosis of asthma or even just recurrent bronchitis. The true diagnosis is usually made when the disease worsens or problems with another organ system, such as the discovery of infertility, lead to a more complete evaluation. Recent improvements in antibiotics, nutritional therapy, and supportive care, however, have improved the prognosis such that the median survival has increased from less than two years in the 1940's up to more than 20 years today.

TREATMENT

Our current rudimentary knowledge of the etiology of the various obstructive lung diseases prevents specific therapy aimed at basic pathophysiological mechanisms. Thus, the treatment of all forms of obstructive lung disease is symptomatic and directed toward the reduction of abnormal airway tone and specific complications such as infection, excessive bronchial secretions, hypoxemia, and cor pulmonale.

BRONCHODILATORS

Drugs directed toward reducing airway tone can be divided into four groups (Table 19–5). The sympathomimetics are the most potent bronchodilators. Subcutaneous epinephrine and nebulized isoproterenol have a relatively short duration of action and act on both beta-1 and beta-2 receptors, whereas epinephrine has additional,

TABLE 19–5. BRONCHODILATORS

Sympathomimetics
  Epinephrine
  Isoproterenol
  Beta-2–specific agents—metaproterenol,
    terbutaline, albuterol
Xanthines
  Theophylline
  Aminophylline
Anticholinergics
  Atropine
  Ipratropium bromide
Corticosteroids
  Hydrocortisone
  Prednisone
  Beclomethasone

undesirable alpha effects. The development of noncatecholamine, beta-2–specific agents has improved the specificity of the sympathomimetic agents for the adrenergic receptor found in airway smooth muscle, but more importantly has increased the duration of action from 60 to 90 minutes to more than 4 hours and permits oral administration. Aerosol therapy is the preferred route of administration, because the lower total dose reduces side effects. Oral use often leads to muscle twitching, and parenteral administration appears to markedly reduce their apparent beta-2 specificity.

When sympathomimetic agents are insufficient, the addition of a methylxanthine, such as theophylline, is quite useful. Effectiveness appears to be dose related, but the incidence of cardiac, gastrointestinal, and neurologic toxicity is unacceptable at serum levels above 20 μg/ml. It is most effective when a stable blood level is maintained. Factors that alter theophylline levels are shown in Table 19–6.

Anticholinergic agents were the first clinically available bronchodilators, but their usage declined because of concerns about their side effects, specifically the purported inhibition of lower airway secretions, which is no longer considered to be a problem. As the importance of vagally mediated mechanisms of bronchospasm have been elucidated, these agents have received renewed interest. They are particularly effective in patients with chronic airway obstruction, and newer agents with fewer extrapulmonary effects are being developed.

Corticosteroids are invaluable, although they do not work acutely to relieve airway obstruction. Their usage early and in sufficient doses in the treatment of acute asthma or the acute exacerbation of chronic airflow obstruction has been shown to lessen the degree of airway obstruction (over 12 to 24 hours), to decrease the total time of hospitalization, and to reduce recurrence. The complications of chronic administration limit their usefulness, although the introduction of potent, inhaled agents (beclomethasone) has significantly reduced this problem. Unfortunately, an alternate-day regimen, to minimize steroid complications, is usually ineffective in patients with bronchospastic lung disease.

Inhaled sodium cromolyn prevents bronchospasm and is not helpful in the management of an acute asthmatic attack. While stabilization of the mast cell membrane and the prevention of mediator release are the major proposed mechanisms of action, it is also effective in forms of asthma without an atopic association. In asthmatics who are difficult to control, it is a useful drug to try before turning to chronic oral steroid therapy. The drug has a slow onset of action and should be used for three to four weeks before deciding on its efficacy. It may also be used intranasally to relieve the symptoms of allergic rhinitis.

A suggested scheme for the administration of the bronchodilators is shown in Figure 19–1.

OXYGEN

The hypoxemia seen in obstructive lung disease has two major deleterious consequences: decreased O_2 delivery to the tissues and hypoxic pulmonary vasoconstriction with resultant cor pulmonale. Oxygen therapy is thus an intergral part of the treatment of patients with obstructive lung disease and should be used whenever the arterial saturation falls below 90 per cent. In some patients O_2 may be required only with acute exacerbations, but in those with chronic disease it may be needed during sleep, with exercise, or continuously, depending on when desaturation occurs. Because of the mechanism of the hypoxemia, namely ventilation-perfusion inequality, the desaturation can be corrected by small increases in the inspired fractional O_2 concentrations, achieved with less than 4 L/min of nasal flow. It has been clearly demonstrated in patients with chronic obstructive lung disease with a resting P_aO_2 below 55 torr that long-term O_2 therapy markedly improves survival, and maximal benefit is achieved when it is delivered throughout the 24 hours of the day.

ANTIBIOTICS

Many exacerbations of airway obstruction are secondary to acute infections. In patients with

TABLE 19–6. FACTORS AFFECTING THEOPHYLLINE CLEARANCE

Clearance increased by	Cigarette smoking
	Marijuana smoking
	Charcoal-broiled meat
	Phenobarbital
Clearance decreased	Erythromycin
by 25%	Propranolol
	Allopurinol
	Oral contraceptives
by 50%	Cimetidine
	Phenytoin
	Influenza vaccine
	Infection
by 100% or more	Heart failure
	Hepatic cirrhosis

bronchiectasis, the specific organism responsible, usually *S. aureus* or *Pseudomonas*, is easily identifiable. However, in patients with bronchitis or asthma, a specific agent associated with periodic increases in cough and sputum is not usually isolated. In the first case, the appropriate antibiotic can be chosen, while in the latter case it is often more cost-efficient to administer a broad-spectrum antibiotic such as ampicillin, trimethoprim-sulfamethoxazole, or tetracycline. The route of administration depends on the specific agent and the acuteness of the process.

IPPB AND NEBULIZATION THERAPY

Intermittent positive-pressure breathing (IPPB) has recently been shown to have no specific value in the managment of patients with airway obstruction. Powered nebulizers can be used to deliver bronchodilators but have no clear advantages over metered dose canisters except in the patient unable to synchronize canister actuation with inhalation. Their major value is in acute airway obstruction. Thinning of secretions is a controversial topic. While a normal state of hydration is probably important to maintain normal bronchial secretions, there is no evidence that additional fluids have any effect. Neither is there evidence for the efficacy of nebulized saline, mucolytics, enzymes, detergents, or iodides, and side effects may be significant. Probably the most important steps to improve airway secretions are to control the primary irritants by eliminating smoking, maximizing bronchodilation, and utilizing antibiotics when indicated.

SMOKING CESSATION

One of the most important factors in the management of patients with COPD is the cessation of cigarette smoking. Susceptible smokers who develop COPD have an increased rate of decline in lung function measured as FEV_1 (80 ml/yr) compared to nonsusceptible smokers and nonsmokers (30 ml/yr) (Fig. 19–2). Following cessation of smoking, the rate of decline in the susceptible smoker is reduced to that in the nonsmoker (30 ml/yr).

PHYSICAL THERAPY AND REHABILITATION

Chest physiotherapy (percussion and postural drainage) is employed on the assumption that sputum retention has undesirable consequences. While this is a reasonable although unproved assumption and while physiotherapy increases the immediate volume of sputum cleared, there is no evidence that it affects the natural history of any disease. Similarly, breathing training and exercise rehabilitation lack a clear scientific basis. However, patients with pulmonary disease of sufficient severity to prevent normal daily living commonly demonstrate an improved quality of life

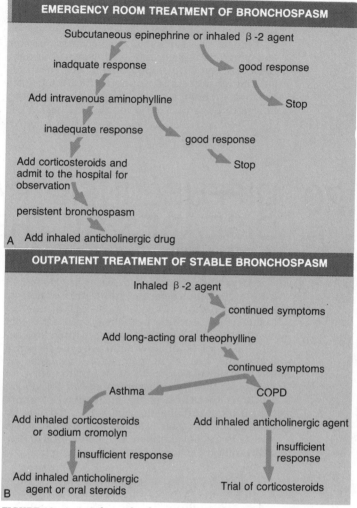

FIGURE 19–1. *A*, Scheme for the treatment of bronchospasm in the emergency room. In patients presenting with severe asthma, all three agents—sympathomimetics, aminophylline, and corticosteroids—will be combined in the initial therapy. *B*, Scheme for the management of bronchospasm in outpatients.

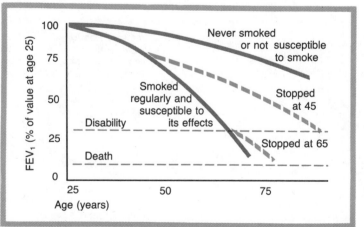

FIGURE 19–2. Pattern of decline in FEV_1, with risk of morbidity and mortality from respiratory disease in a susceptible smoker compared to a normal subject or nonsusceptible smoker. While cessation of smoking does not replenish the lung function already lost in a susceptible smoker, it decreases the further rate of decline. (Adapted from Fletcher and Peto: Br Med J 1:1645, 1977.)

when enrolled in a properly run rehabilitation program. Finally, nutritional needs in these patients must be addressed. This is important in cystic fibrosis, as supplemental pancreatic enzymes and vitamins are necessary. However, the debilitated patient with emphysema must also be considered for nutritional support, since poor nutrition may render him susceptible to respiratory failure through decreased muscle strength.

REFERENCES

Clark THJ, and Godfrey S: Asthma. 2nd ed, London, Chapman and Hall, 1983.
Paterson JW, Woolcock AJ, and Shenfield GM: Bronchodilator drugs, state of the art. Am Rev Respir Dis 120:1149–1188, 1979.
Snider GL: Emphysema. Clin Chest Med, Vol 4, 1983.
Wood RE, Boat TF, and Doershuk CF: Cystic fibrosis, state of the art. Am Rev Respir Dis 113:275–320, 1976.

20 DIFFUSE INFILTRATIVE DISEASES OF THE LUNG

A large number of lung diseases are characterized by the replacement or infiltration of normal lung by abnormal tissue (Fig. 20–1). On rare occasions, the insulting agent may be well recognized, as in silicosis, although more often the causative process is unknown and only the response is obvious. The insult may cause lung injury by direct toxicity, as a result of an inflammatory response, or through an immunologically mediated reaction. Regardless of the mechanism of injury the influx of inflammatory cells into the lung interstitium, perivascular space, and alveolar space results in the development of an alveolitis or vasculitis and if carried to completion, lung fibrosis.

CLINICAL MANIFESTATIONS

The spectrum of clinical presentation in this group of disorders is as varied as the conditions themselves. The majority of patients present with an insidious onset of dyspnea, exercise limitation, and a dry, nonproductive cough. Certain histori-

cal features may suggest a specific diagnosis as detailed in the discussion of each entity. Examination of the chest characteristically reveals mid to late inspiratory crackles and tachypnea. Physical findings of pulmonary hypertension, cor pulmonale, and cyanosis are usually late findings. Evidence of extrathoracic disease is valuable in suggesting a specific diagnosis, such as the skin lesions of sarcoidosis or the arthritis of a collagen-vascular disease. The chest x-ray may confirm the presence of diffuse infiltrative disease but is rarely diagnostic on its own.

The physiological consequences depend on the proportion of lung involved and the speed with which the infiltration develops. As fibrosis replaces normal lung structures, there is a decrease in all lung volumes, a fall in lung compliance, and a decline in the diffusing capacity. The loss of alveolar space and airway abnormalities produce ventilation-perfusion inequality, but hypoxemia is usually mild until the disease progresses to a significant degree and hypercapnia is uncommon.

FIGURE 20–1. Pathophysiology and outcome of diffuse infiltrative lung disease.

A specific diagnosis, when not clear from the presentation, depends on lung biopsy findings. In certain diseases, such as sarcoidosis, sufficient tissue can be obtained using a fiberoptic bronchoscope and a transbronchial biopsy, but this may be insufficient in others, such as idiopathic pulmonary fibrosis, and an open lung biopsy may be required.

SPECIFIC ENTITIES

DISEASES WITH KNOWN ETIOLOGIES

Pneumoconioses

Pneumoconioses are lung diseases produced by the inhalation of inorganic dust. These dusts may be fibrous minerals, such as asbestos, or nonfibrous minerals, like silica or metals. The clinical spectrum varies widely according to the nature of the inhaled substance and the type of response it evokes in the lung. Some substances such as asbestos lead to progressive fibrosis, while others such as iron dust produce little or no reaction even when deposited in large amounts. The common organic dusts are listed in Table 20–1 and are divided according to their structure and fibrogenic potential.

Among the fibrous minerals, asbestos is the most important health hazard (Table 20–2). The pulmonary fibrosis (asbestosis) is dose-dependent, while diseases in the pleural space do not seem to be related to the intensity of exposure. In addition to pulmonary fibrosis and benign pleural disease, there is a five-fold increase in the rate of bronchogenic carcinoma among nonsmoking asbestos workers when compared to a nonsmoking control population. Among smoking asbestos workers the risk is 60- to 90-fold. Malignant mesotheliomas of the pleura and peritoneum are also associated with asbestos exposure but bear no apparent relationship to smoking. There is a prolonged latency period between the exposure and the development of the tumors, usually at least 20 years and sometimes as long as 30 to 40 years.

Deposition of coal dust around the first- and second-order respiratory bronchioles causes coal workers' pneumoconiosis or "black lung." This may be accompanied by minimal inflammation but is insufficiently severe to cause symptoms or measurable physiological derangement in most workers. Simple pneumoconiosis consisting of a fine, diffuse reticulonodular pattern seen on chest roentgenogram and a productive cough develop in 5 per cent of coal workers. Physiological impairment when present is slight. In a smaller number of miners, perhaps 0.4 per cent, nodular densities of 1 cm or greater may be present on chest x-ray, representing dense collagenous nodules (complicated coal workers' pneumoconiosis). Unlike the simple form, this can eventually result in progressive massive fibrosis and restrictive lung disease.

The pulmonary response to a more fibrogenic dust, such as silica, is dramatically magnified. Silica exposure occurs in most mining operations,

sandblasting, pottery working, brick making, and foundries. In most cases, silicosis develops after at least 20 years of exposure, although it can develop in 5 years or less with intense exposure to a high concentration of dust. Roentgenographic gradation of disease ranges from small diffuse nodules with minimal hilar node enlargement to large nodules, predominantly in the upper lobes, that vary from about 1 cm to conglomerate masses occupying most of a lobe (progressive massive fibrosis). Eggshell calcification of the hilar nodes is characteristic. The chest x-ray findings do not correlate well with the symptomatology and physiological impairment in silicosis. The course of the disease may be modified by other factors such as coexisting smoke or superinfection with mycobacterial disease, either M. tuberculosis, M. intracellulare, or M. kansasii. The more acute the silicosis, the more likely it will be complicated by tuberculosis.

No specific treatment exists for any pneumoconiosis, and only removal from the offending environment may modify the eventual progression

TABLE 20–1. PNEUMOCONIOSES

SUBSTANCE	FIBROGENICITY	OCCUPATION
I. Fibrous minerals		
Asbestos	High	Asbestos mining, shipyard and boiler workers, insulators
Talc	High	Talc mining and milling
Fiberglass	Low	Insulation
II. Non-fibrous minerals		
Silica	High	Mining, sandblasting, etc.
Coal	Low	Mining
III. Metals		
Iron	Low	Mining, refining, and fabricating
Aluminum	Uncertain	Mining, refining, and fabricating
Beryllium	High	Mining and fabricating

TABLE 20–2. ASBESTOS-RELATED RESPIRATORY DISEASE

FORM	COMMENT
1. Asbestosis	Interstitial fibrosis; long latent period; clubbing; crackles
2. Pleural thickening	Calcified plaques; intensity proportional to exposure; only significant in that it indicates prior exposure
3. Benign effusions	Hemorrhagic; asymptomatic; spontaneous remission and recurrence
4. Pleural mesothelioma	Latent interval 20 to 40 years; not dose-related; probably unrelated to smoking; median survival 12 months
5. Bronchogenic carcinoma	Five-fold increased risk in exposed nonsmoker and 60- to 90-fold risk in exposed smoker

TABLE 20–3. HYPERSENSITIVITY PNEUMONITIS

ANTIGEN	SOURCE	DISEASE EXAMPLES
Thermophilic bacteria	Moldy hay and other organic material, heated humidifiers	Farmer's lung, bagassosis, humidifier's lung
Other bacteria, particularly *Bacillus subtilis*	Water	Detergent worker's and humidifer's lung
Fungi	Moldy organic material, water	Maple bark–stripper's lung, suberosis, sequoiosis
Animal protein	Bird droppings, animal dander	Pigeon breeder's lung, rodent handler's disease
Amoeba	Water	Humidifier's lung

to respiratory failure. A careful and repeated search for mycobacterial disease is mandatory in silicosis, especially with sudden worsening of the condition. Cessation of smoking, aggressive treatment of routine bacterial infections, and the use of oxygen to treat complicating cor pulmonale may improve function and prolong life.

Hypersensitivity Pneumonitis

Hypersensitivity pneumonitis or extrinsic allergic alveolitis occurs in individuals who have developed an abnormal sensitivity to some organic agent. Four to six hours following exposure in a sensitized subject there is the onset of cough, dyspnea, fever, and malaise; wheezing is usually absent. Diffuse crackles are heard on auscultation

and the x-ray reveals nodular or reticulonodular infiltrates with relative sparing of the apices. In most cases there is gradual resolution of these symptoms, which recur on subsequent exposure. The duration of symptoms may gradually increase with repeated exposure and eventually result in the development of pulmonary fibrosis and restrictive lung disease.

A vast array of substances can cause this disorder (Table 20–3), the prototype being farmer's lung, a hypersensitivity to thermophilic actinomycetes, fungus-like organisms found in moldy hay. Patients with these disorders have serum precipitins to specific proteins, although the presence of precipitins does not, by itself, define the disease, since 50 per cent of similarly exposed subjects develop precipitins but remain asymptomatic.

The treatment is to remove or avoid the offending agent. Occasionally in the acute situation corticosteroids are required. The efficacy of corticosteroids in the chronic phase, once fibrosis has set in, however, is less clear, although a trial in symptomatic patients is usually worthwhile.

Other Clearly Extrinsic Causes of Diffuse Infiltrative Lung Disease

External radiation in doses in excess of 5000 rads over a 4- to 6-week period frequently produces radiation pneumonitis and the response usually occurs within the first 6 months following exposure and almost always by 13 months. Many drugs cause diffuse lung disease (Table 20–4). Some cancer chemotherapeutic agents such as chlorambucil result in dose-related toxicity while others, like methotrexate, produce hypersensitivity reactions. Both phenomena occur with bleomycin, an acute syndrome and a chronic illness almost inevitable when greater than 400 to 500 units are used. Synergism with other causes of lung injury such as radiation and high concentrations of oxygen is suspected. Antibiotics, especially nitrofurantoin and sulfonamides, may cause hypersensitivity lung disease, while a number of sedatives and hypnotics have been implicated in noncardiogenic pulmonary edema, especially with intravenous abuse. Exposure to noxious gases such as chlorine, ammonia, phosgene, ozone, hydrogen sulfide, and nitrogen dioxide can cause severe lung injury. The nature of the injury depends upon the reactivity of the gas, its concentration, and the length of exposure and ranges from tracheobronchitis to adult respiratory distress syndrome.

DIFFUSE LUNG DISEASE OF UNKNOWN ETIOLOGY

Collagen-Vascular Diseases

Rheumatoid arthritis is associated with five different pulmonary manifestations present in a high percentage of seropositive cases: exudative pleural effusion characterized by a very low glucose concentration; pulmonary nodules varying from a few millimeters to greater than 5 cm in diameter; rheumatoid nodules in association with

TABLE 20–4. COMMON DRUG-INDUCED LUNG DISEASES

DRUG	DOSE RELATION	PATHOLOGICAL AND CLINICAL APPEARANCE
I. Cancer chemotherapeutic agents		
Bleomycin	Both acute and dose-dependent	Pulmonary fibrosis
Busulfan	Greater than 600 mg	Pulmonary fibrosis
Chlorambucil	Greater than 2 g	Pulmonary fibrosis
Methotrexate	None	Pneumonitis
II. Analgesics and hypnotics		
Aspirin	Serum level greater than 45 mg/dl	Pulmonary edema
Ethchlorvynol, propoxyphene hydrochloride, heroin	Overdose	Pulmonary edema
Opiates and other psychotropic drugs	Chronic intravenous abuse	Pulmonary fibrosis and vasculitis
III. Antibiotics		
Nitrofurantoin	Acute	Hypersensitivity pneumonitis
Sulfonamides	Chronic	Pulmonary fibrosis, Löffler's syndrome

coal workers' pneumoconiosis (Caplan's syndrome); diffuse interstitial fibrosis; and pulmonary vasculitis. With the exception of the nodules and the low glucose in the pleural fluid, patients with systemic lupus erythematosus (SLE) may have many of the same manifestations. Pleuritis and pneumonitis have also been described in Sjögren's syndrome, polymyositis, and dermatomyositis. The lung is commonly involved in scleroderma presenting as pulmonary fibrosis and/or pulmonary hypertension.

Pulmonary Vasculitis

Pulmonary vasculitis may occur as a part of one of the aforementioned connective tissue disorders or in the course of a systemic granulomatous or hypersensitivity vasculitis.

The granulomatous vasculitides include classic Wegener's granulomatosis, limited Wegener's, and lymphomatoid granulomatosis. Classic Wegener's is a necrotizing vasculitis initially described as involving three organ systems: the lung, the upper respiratory tract, and the kidneys. However, many other organs in the body may be affected. Lung involvement usually takes the form of single or multiple nodular lesions that have a propensity to cavitate. The limited form of Wegener's granulomatosis refers to patients with similar pathology but free of renal disease. Both diseases respond well to cyclophosphamide. Lymphomatoid granulomatosis resembles Wegener's but differs in three important features: there is frequent central nervous system involvement, more than 15 per cent develop malignant lymphoma, and although cyclophosphamide may achieve remission, relapses are very common.

In hypersensitivity vasculitis, pulmonary involvement is a less prominent part of a systemic disease. The disorders in which this is most commonly seen are anaphylactoid purpura, essential mixed cryoglobulinemia, and the vasculitis associated with malignancy, infection, or drugs.

Pulmonary Infiltrates with Eosinophilia (PIE)

The combination of pulmonary infiltrates and peripheral eosinophilia occurs in five relatively well-characterized disorders. *Löffler's syndrome* is a benign condition characterized by fleeting pulmonary infiltrates and eosinophilia, probably related to an immune response to some external agent. It is often asymptomatic, but fever and cough may occur. Although recurrent, it usually clears within 4 to 6 weeks, and it also displays a rapid response to steroids. *Chronic eosinophilic pneumonia* is a more symptomatic form of PIE, often persistent or recurrent in nature. Because of its tendency to involve the periphery of the lung, its roentgenographic appearance is called the inverse of pulmonary edema. Despite a rapid response to corticosteroids, relapse may occur once treatment is discontinued, so that therapy may be required for a year or more. PIE in *asthma* is most commonly due to allergic bronchopulmonary aspergillosis, which may result in a central destructive bronchiectasis. *Tropical eosinophilia* consists of symptoms of wheeze, fever, and a diffuse reticulonodular pattern on the x-ray that is thought to result from an infestation with microfilaria of *Wuchereria bancrofti*. Finally, it may be associated with a *collagen-vascular disease*, in which case the underlying disorder determines the overall presentation.

Sarcoidosis

Sarcoidosis is a systemic disease of unknown etiology characterized by abnormal T cell function and noncaseating granulomas found diffusely throughout the body. It occurs most commonly in the third and fourth decades, is slightly more likely in women, and is approximately ten times more frequent in black people in the United States.

Most of the dysfunction associated with sarcoidosis results from the physical presence of the granulomas in the tissues, although systemic signs of inflammation may also be present. Organs commonly involved include the lungs, skin, lymph nodes, liver, spleen, eyes, joints, central nervous system, and muscle (Table 20–5). The presenting symptoms are quite variable, although in the United States 50 per cent of patients will present with pulmonary disease, 25 per cent with constitutional symptoms, and 7 per cent with extrapulmonary involvement, and the remainder are asymptomatic and disease is discovered during routine examination.

Diagnosis depends on the finding of noncaseating granulomata in the setting of a characteristic clinical picture with typical radiographic findings, in the absence of another specific cause of granulomatous disease, such as tuberculosis, fungal disease, carcinoma, and lymphoma. Histological confirmation is most commonly obtained by a transbronchial biopsy during bronchoscopy. Conventional chest x-ray staging is as

TABLE 20–5. CLINICAL MANIFESTATIONS OF SARCOIDOSIS

Pulmonary
Asymptomatic with abnormal chest x-ray
Gradually progressive cough and shortness of breath
Pulmonary fibrosis with pulmonary insufficiency
Laryngeal and endobronchial obstruction

Extrapulmonary
Lofgren's syndrome—fever, arthralgias, bilateral hilar adenopathy, erythema nodosum
Heerfordt's syndrome (uveoparotid fever)—fever, swelling of parotid gland and uveal tracts, VII nerve palsy
Skin—lupus pernio or skin plaques
Central nervous system—cranial nerve palsies, subacute meningitis, diabetes insipidus
Joints—polyarticular and monoarticular arthritis
Erythema nodosum
Punched-out cystic lesions in phalangeal and metacarpal bones
Peripheral lymphadenopathy and/or splenomegaly
Heart—paroxysmal arrythmias, conduction disturbances
Eye—chorioretinitis, anterior uveitis, keratoconjunctivitis
Hypercalcemia with nephrocalcinosis or nephrolithiasis
Granulomatous hepatitis

follows; stage O, normal film; stage 1, bilateral hilar adenopathy; stage 2, adenopathy plus pulmonary infiltrates; and, stage 3, pulmonary infiltrates alone. There is no evidence that staging has any relationship to the natural progression of disease. Rarely, the x-ray may show multiple nodules similar to those seen with a metastatic tumor or a pleural effusion. Nonspecific laboratory abnormalities include hypercalcemia, anemia, hypergammaglobulinemia, and an elevated angiotensin-converting enzyme level. Skin test anergy is usually present in association with lymphopenia and decreased number and function of peripheral blood T cells.

The disorder is usually self-limited, with complete resolution of symptoms and chest x-ray changes within a year or two. A minority have a persistent mild abnormality with some fibrotic changes on chest x-ray. Approximately 10 per cent develop severe progressive disease with progressive pulmonary fibrosis or significant extrapulmonary involvement.

Because of the self-limiting nature of the disease, treatment is usually reserved for patients with significant symptomatic abnormalities of pulmonary function and with granulomas in the eye or central nervous system, where scarring will lead to significant problems. Corticosteroids are quite effective in ameliorating the acute granulomatous inflammation, but their efficacy in altering the long-term prognosis is unproven.

Pulmonary Hemorrhagic Disorders

The combination of hemoptysis, anemia, and diffuse pulmonary infiltrates along with the development of glomerulonephritis is known as Goodpasture's syndrome. This is predominantly a disease of young white males. The etiology is unknown, but the presence of antiglomerular basement membrane antibodies lining both the glomerulus and the alveolus suggests an autoimmune mechanism. While the lung disease may be intermittent, the kidney disease rapidly progresses to renal failure. On occasion, hemoptysis by itself may be life-threatening. Bilateral nephrectomy results in cessation of hemoptysis, but present therapy is directed at the presumed immunological basis for the disease. Plasmapheresis is used to remove the antibodies, immunosuppressive drugs are administered to decrease their production, and steroids are given empirically to decrease the pulmonary hemorrhage. Untreated patients usually die within two years.

Idiopathic pulmonary hemosiderosis can present similarly to Goodpasture's syndrome, although it predominantly affects young girls and does not involve the kidneys. The etiology is unknown and there are no clear-cut immunological markers. Despite this, treatment similar to that for Goodpasture's syndrome is usually attempted, although the efficacy in this disease is much less clear, and average survival is about two to three years.

Finally, pulmonary hemorrhage, with or without renal disease, may accompany one of the collagen-vascular diseases, particularly SLE and periarteritis nodosa. It may also be seen with systemic vasculitis, in particular Wegener's granulomatosis, hypersensitivity vasculitis, mixed cryoglobulinemia, and Behçet's syndrome.

Miscellaneous

Pulmonary histiocytosis X, or eosinophilic granuloma of the lung, is a relatively benign disease presenting with dyspnea and x-ray evidence of diffuse nodular or reticulonodular infiltrates with relative sparing of the lung bases. It should be suspected in patients in the third and fourth decades presenting with diffusely abnormal chest x-rays. It is easy to confuse with sarcoidosis, although pneumothorax or honeycombing on the chest x-ray and the rarity of hilar adenopathy favor histiocytosis X. Diagnosis is made pathologically, treatment is uncertain, and spontaneous remissions are common.

The lymphocytic infiltrative disorders include lymphocytic interstitial pneumonia and immunoblastic lymphadenopathy, among other specific entities. They differ from other interstitial lung diseases by their common association with dysproteinemia and frequent progression to lymphoid malignancy.

Pulmonary alveolar proteinosis is a rare, idiopathic disease in which the alveoli become filled with a proteinaceous material rich in lipids. Most patients recover spontaneously, but total lung lavage is necessary when diffuse involvement causes severe hypoxemia. These patients are particularly prone to infection with *Nocardia*, and less so to *Aspergillus* and *Cryptococcus*.

Idiopathic Pulmonary Fibrosis

A large number of patients with diffuse interstitial lung disease will not fit into any of the previously mentioned categories. These patients, usually middle aged with no sex predominance, present with dyspnea and x-ray evidence of interstitial disease. Rarely, the disease progresses very rapidly to death from respiratory failure within six months of the onset of symptoms (Hamman-Rich syndrome). When the disease is more slowly progressive, it is termed idiopathic pulmonary fibrosis or cryptogenic fibrosing alveolitis.

TREATMENT

While the treatment of these disorders depends on the particular one being discussed, certain general statements can be made. The most rational decisions can be made only if a clear diagnosis has been obtained. If the offending substance is identified, as in the pneumoconioses and the hypersensitivity pneumonitides, avoidance is the best solution. When there is an active alveolitis component, corticosteroids may be of benefit. Dosage should be high (60 to 100 mg prednisone) initially and then reduced to the lowest possible dose that successfully suppresses the inflammatory response. Immunosuppressive agents are added to effect remission in certain vasculitides, such as Wegener's granulomatosis, but are of questionable value in Goodpasture's syndrome and have little efficacy in idiopathic pulmonary fibrosis. Plasmapheresis should be reserved for illnesses in which circulating antibody is known to be the etiological factor, as in Goodpasture's syndrome.

The decision to initiate therapy with one of these relatively high-risk agents and how long to maintain treatment depend on the ability to evaluate the presence of active alveolitis and to judge the effect of the therapeutic regimen. The chest roentgenogram does not ordinarily determine the acuteness of the process, although a diffuse honeycomb pattern usually suggests severe fibrosis. It is useful, however, to follow the course of the disease, although in itself it may not accurately predict the course or response to therapy. Like the chest x-ray, the pulmonary function studies give an indication of the degree of involvement, but they are not reliable in separating reversible phases of inflammation from far-advanced fibro-

sis. They are used predominantly to follow the course of the disease and the response to therapy. Depending on the initial abnormalities, any of a number of studies may be used, including the measurement of lung volumes, diffusing capacity, arterial blood gases at rest or during exercise, and maximum exercise tolerance. Gallium lung scanning and bronchoalveolar lavage are providing interesting insights into the mechanism of these disorders but have no proven clinical utility.

REFERENCES

Crystal RG, Bitterman PB, Rennard SE, Hance AJ, and Keogh BA: Interstitial lung diseases of unknown cause. N Engl J Med 310:154–166, 235–244, 1984.

Fulmer JD: Symposium on interstitial lung diseases. Clin Chest Med 1982, Vol 3.

Hunninghake GW, and Fauci AS: Pulmonary involvement in the collagen-vascular diseases, state of the art. Am Rev Respir Dis 119:417–501, 1979.

Morgan WKC, and Seaton A: Occupational Lung Disease. 2nd ed. Philadelphia, WB Saunders Co, 1984.

PULMONARY VASCULAR DISEASES

21

The pulmonary vascular bed is a low-pressure, low-resistance system through which the entire cardiac output passes. A number of disorders can affect this system, leading to an increase in these pressures and resistance, with significant consequences on cardiorespiratory function.

PHYSIOLOGICAL EFFECTS OF PULMONARY HYPERTENSION ON CARDIAC FUNCTION

The right and left sides of the heart are functionally integrated by their anatomical contiguity. There is continuity between their free walls, they share a common wall (the intraventricular septum), and they are covered by the pericardium. When pulmonary vascular resistance is normal, the right ventricle serves as a capacitance chamber, performing only minimal contractile work. It compensates ineffectually for acute rises in pulmonary artery pressure, and acutely it can only generate a mean pressure of 40 mm Hg. Acute elevations of right ventricular pressures also interfere with left ventricular performance, presumably owing to a shift in the intraventricular septum to the left. Chronic elevations of pulmonary artery pressure cause gradual hypertrophy of the right ventricle, which eventually allows it to

generate pressures equal to those in the left ventricle.

EFFECTS OF PULMONARY HYPERTENSION ON PULMONARY FUNCTION

Abnormalities of pulmonary function in patients with pulmonary vascular disease are usually a consequence of the underlying lung disease rather than an intrinsic effect of the pulmonary vascular disease. An exception is the decreased diffusing capacity due to capillary obliteration. In addition, pulmonary vascular occlusion and obliteration cause shunt and ventilation-perfusion inequality by undefined mechanisms. The resulting hypoxemia is further exaggerated by the associated reduction of cardiac output and low mixed venous P_{O_2}.

CLINICAL FEATURES OF PULMONARY HYPERTENSION

Clinical onset may be acute or chronic, depending on the cause. Acute pulmonary hypertension is usually due to thromboembolism, and patients may complain of sudden dyspnea with

TABLE 21–1. PULMONARY HYPERTENSION

1. Hyperkinetic Pulmonary Hypertension
     Atrial and ventricular septal defects
     Patent ductus arteriosus
     Peripheral arteriovenus shunts
2. Postcapillary Pulmonary Hypertension
     Left ventricular failure
     Mitral valve disease
     Left atrial myxoma
3. Obliterative or Obstructive Hypertension
     Embolic
     Parenchymal lung disease
     Arteritis
     Pulmonary artery stenosis
     Primary
4. Reactive Hypertension
     High altitude
     Chronic obstructive lung disease
     Persistent or intermittent hypoventilation
        Neuromuscular disease
        Sleep apnea syndrome

or without hemoptysis and pleuritic chest pain. Physical examination is frequently normal or may reveal tachypnea, a loud P_2, a right ventricular heave, and a pleural rub or effusion. Gradually progressive dyspnea is the major symptom of chronic pulmonary hypertension and in addition to a loud P_2 and right ventricular heave, features of right heart failure—i.e., elevated jugular venous pressure, tender hepatomegaly, and pedal edema—may be found.

CAUSES OF PULMONARY HYPERTENSION

These disorders are classified by the proposed major mechanism for increased pulmonary vascular resistance, although the etiology is usually multifactorial (Table 21–1).

HYPERKINETIC PULMONARY HYPERTENSION

Since pulmonary artery pressure is the product of pulmonary vascular resistance and cardiac output, any increase in pulmonary blood flow is invariably associated with an increase in pulmonary artery pressure. If the increased flow is sustained,

TABLE 21–2. SOURCES OF EMBOLIC MATERIAL

Present with symptoms due to vascular obstruction
     Thromboemboli
     Sepsis
     Tumor
     Parasites
     Foreign material
     Sickled red cells
Present with symptoms due to development of ARDS
     Fat
     Amniotic fluid
     Air

as in intracardiac shunts, anatomical changes occur in the pulmonary vessels (vascular remodeling) which increase vascular resistance and further increase pulmonary artery pressure, causing the pulmonary hypertension to persist even after the initial stimulus is corrected. Remodeling consists initially of the muscularization and hypertrophy of previously unmuscularized small arteries, followed by medial hypertrophy and intimal proliferation in the larger pulmonary arteries. Both of these changes are reversible if the pulmonary hypertension is reduced. However, persistently high pressures produce permanent obstructive changes such as necrotizing arteritis and complex dilatations known as plexiform lesions.

POSTCAPILLARY PULMONARY HYPERTENSION

This results from the passive effects of an elevated left atrial pressure due to mitral valve disease or prolonged left ventricular failure. If it persists, pulmonary artery pressure gradually increases above that explained by passive transmission of the elevated outflow pressure. Initially this increase is due to reflex vasoconstriction, but eventually vascular remodeling occurs. This additional contribution to pulmonary hypertension can be quantified by the increasing gradient between the pulmonary diastolic pressure and the left atrial pressure.

OBLITERATIVE OR OBSTRUCTIVE PULMONARY HYPERTENSION

The largest group of disorders that affect the pulmonary vascular bed are those in which its cross-sectional area is decreased, obstructed, or obliterated.

EMBOLIC DISEASE

Thromboemboli directly or indirectly cause 200,000 deaths per year. Common and uncommon sources of emboli are listed in Table 21–2. Clinical presentation results from physiological abnormalities caused by increases in pulmonary vascular resistance. Significant alterations occur only after more than 50 per cent of the pulmonary vascular bed has been occluded. Embolization of substances such as fat, amniotic fluid, or air, however, markedly alter alveolar capillary membrane integrity and present as the adult respiratory distress syndrome (ARDS) (see Chapter 22). The most frequently embolized material is blood clot, an extremely common cause of hospital morbidity and mortality.

Most thromboemboli (> 85 per cent) originate in the ileofemoral deep veins. Less common sources include pelvic veins, upper extremities, and mural thrombi in the right side of the heart. Stasis and intimal injury are important factors in the development of thrombosis. The clinical diagnosis of deep venous thrombosis is highly inaccurate, as physical examination is often misleading and specialized diagnostic techniques should be utilized whenever it is suspected (Table 21–3).

The diagnosis of pulmonary embolism is often missed in sick hospitalized patients, while in the healthy outpatient population it is overdiagnosed. Predisposing situations are listed in Table 21–4. Clinical findings suggestive of pulmonary embolism are nonspecific and are often more commonly indicative of other acute cardiopulmonary disorders. Typical symptoms include dyspnea, pleuritic chest pain, and hemoptysis (20 to 30 per cent). Physical findings include tachypnea (invariable), obvious thrombophlebitis (unusual), acute right ventricular strain (right ventricular heave, increased P_2, gallop) in less than 40 per cent of cases, and occasionally rubs, crackles, or wheezing. A normal chest examination is not unusual. Cardiac output is decreased in severe cases. Excluding a diagnosis of pneumonia or pleurisy is difficult, as all may be associated with pyrexia and leukocytosis, although persistent high fever and marked leukocytosis are unusual in embolic disease.

Abnormal chest x-ray findings are common but nonspecific: atelectasis, infiltrates, pleural effusions, and an elevated diaphragm. Clear-cut hypovascularity is difficult to detect. The electrocardiograph (EKG) helps to exclude myocardial infarction and may show right ventricular strain, but nonspecific ST and T wave changes are more common and sinus tachycardia is usually the only abnormality. Hypoxemia and hypocapnia are typical, but arterial Po_2 is greater than 80 mm Hg in 13 per cent of patients. In summary, the clinical presentation and routine laboratory studies may suggest the diagnosis, but confirmation requires specific investigations.

Absence of activity on the perfusion lung scan, which visualizes the gross distribution of blood flow in the lung, may be due to anatomical blockage of the vessels or to vasoconstriction. A normal scan excludes pulmonary embolism. Lobar or multiple segmental defects that do not correspond to abnormalities on chest x-ray are considered high-probability scans consistent with pulmonary emboli. A ventilation scan helps to differentiate anatomical from functional blockage of blood flow. Inhalation of radioactive gas defines the distribution of ventilation, and delayed clearance during washout of the gas suggests that airway disease may have caused the decreased perfusion secondary to hypoxic vasoconstriction. A normal ventilation scan with a high-probability perfusion scan is highly successful at diagnosing pulmonary embolism. A normal perfusion scan excludes pulmonary emboli, but anything other than a high-probability perfusion scan with a normal ventilation scan is nondiagnostic and cannot confirm or exclude pulmonary embolism.

When the lung scan is not diagnostic, the anatomy of the pulmonary vessels must be visualized by angiography. With a markedly abnormal chest x-ray or severe cardiopulmonary disease, the lung scan is not likely to be useful, and immediate angiography is logical. Angiography has a sufficiently low risk to make it practical in routine di-

TABLE 21–3. METHODS OF DIAGNOSING DEEP VENOUS THROMBOSIS

METHOD	USEFULNESS
1. Contrast venography	The "gold standard"; low incidence of post-study phlebitis.
2. Impedance plethysmography (IPG)	Most sensitive noninvasive technique for detecting thrombi above the knee. Detects only 30% of thrombi confined to calf veins.
3. Doppler ultrasound	May add to diagnostic accuracy of IPG.
4. Radioiodine fibrinogen scanning	Most sensitive of all but not as specific as IPG; better for calf and low thigh thrombosis.
5. Nuclide venography	Functional study; high incidence of false positive studies.

agnosis, and it is almost always positive within 10 to 14 days of the embolic event. Definitive diagnosis of pulmonary emboli is vital, as both missed diagnosis and unwarranted anticoagulation have high morbidity and mortality rates. A diagnostic decision tree is shown in Figure 21–1.

Treatment consists of anticoagulation with heparin, by continuous infusion, for 7 to 10 days at a dosage to prolong clotting (PTT 1.5 or 2 times control). Recommendations for oral anticoagulation (warfarin) range from six weeks to three months, or longer if a predisposing factor clearly exists. Rarely additional therapy may be required (Table 21–5), but it should be undertaken only when clear indications are present because of significant added risks. Preventive therapy is valuable and includes early ambulation and subcutaneous heparin, 5000 units every 8 to 12 hours. Most emboli completely resolve, and chronic persistent pulmonary hypertension develops in less than 2 per cent of patients.

PRIMARY PULMONARY HYPERTENSION

Primary pulmonary hypertension occurs predominantly in young children and between the ages of 20 and 40 years. In children, there is no apparent sexual predominance, but there is a marked predilection for females in the older pa-

TABLE 21–4. FACTORS PREDISPOSING TO PULMONARY THROMBOEMBOLI

Prolonged immobilization—bed rest, travel, limb casts
Lower extremity trauma or surgery
Abdominal surgery
Underlying malignancy
Congestive heart failure
Pregnancy
Abnormal clotting—thrombocytosis, anti-thrombin III deficiency
Obesity?
Oral contraceptives?

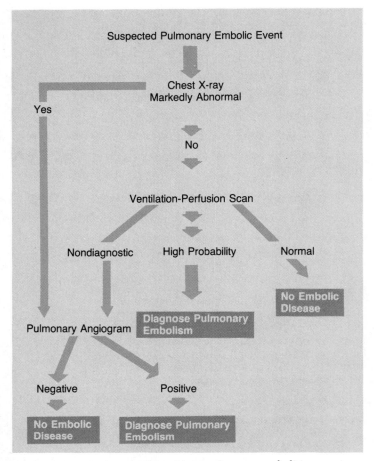

FIGURE 21–1. Diagnostic approach to pulmonary embolism.

tients. The etiology is unknown but is possibly related to increased vasoconstrictors or a vascular bed abnormally responsive to vasoconstrictor substances. Occasional clinical associations include chronic portal hypertension, ingestions of an appetite suppressant (aminorex), and a family history.

TABLE 21–5. TREATMENT OF PULMONARY EMBOLI

TREATMENT	INDICATION
Anticoagulation	All patients with pulmonary emboli unless risk of bleeding is unacceptable
Fibrinolytic drugs—streptokinase and urokinase	Patients with massive emboli and hemodynamic instability
Vena caval interruption—vena cava filters or surgical approach	When anticoagulants are contraindicated or have failed
Acute embolectomy	Rarely, if ever, useful because of high mortality

Patients present with progressive dyspnea and marked exercise limitation. With time features of cor pulmonale or syncopal episodes on exertion (decreased left ventricular output) develop. Physical examination may be normal or may reveal evidence of pulmonary hypertension. The chest x-ray shows an enlarged right ventricle and main pulmonary arteries with oligemia in the outer lung fields. EKG evidence of right ventricular hypertrophy is invariable when the mean pulmonary artery pressures are chronically elevated above 40 mm Hg. Pulmonary function studies are often normal except for a small reduction in diffusing capacity. Diagnosis is made by catheterization and by excluding other causes of pulmonary hypertension. Prognosis is dreadful, with only 20 per cent surviving three years.

Drug therapy is actively being investigated. Nitroglycerine, hydralazine, and calcium blockers, among other agents, reduce pulmonary vascular resistance in 30 to 50 per cent of patients, but it is not known if they alter the natural course of the disease.

A number of other conditions may lead to obliterative pulmonary hypertension. Severe parenchymal lung disease, usually pulmonary fibrosis, may destroy enough vessels to cause elevations in pulmonary artery pressure. The pulmonary vessels may also be involved by a systemic vasculitis, most commonly scleroderma. Congenital pulmonary artery stenosis and fibrosing mediastinitis are rare causes of pulmonary hypertension.

REACTIVE PULMONARY HYPERTENSION

Alveolar hypoxia, which normally modulates pulmonary vascular tone, may by itself cause pulmonary hypertension or amplify the response of the pulmonary vascular bed to other insults. Significant vasoconstriction occurs at an alveolar P_{O_2} below 60 mm Hg. Increases in P_{CO_2} may also cause vasoconstriction, although its physiological importance is much less. Hypoxic vasoconstriction is the major initiating factor in the pulmonary hypertension associated with chronic obstructive lung disease and along with subsequent vascular remodeling is responsible for the development of cor pulmonale in those patients (see Chapter 19).

REFERENCES

Harris P, and Heath D: The Human Pulmonary Circulation. 2nd ed. Edinburgh, Churchill Livingstone, 1977.

Hyers TM: Pulmonary embolism and hypertension. Clin Chest Med, 1984, Vol 5.

Rubin LJ: Pulmonary Heart Disease. Boston, Martinus Nijhoff, 1984.

Weir EK, and Reeves JT: Pulmonary Hypertension. Mount Kisco, NY, Futura Publishing Co, 1984.

THE ADULT RESPIRATORY DISTRESS SYNDROME

22

In 1967 a syndrome of acute respiratory failure characterized by severe hypoxemia, bilateral pulmonary infiltrates, and decreased lung compliance, usually occurring without preceding lung disease, was dubbed the adult respiratory distress syndrome (ARDS). Since that time, its incidence has increased as improvements in intensive care allow more patients to survive the catastrophic illnesses that act as the initiating events, but its mortality rate remains unacceptably high.

PATHOPHYSIOLOGY

The physiological abnormalities in ARDS, regardless of the predisposing event, are associated with an increase in extravascular lung water. Water movement in the lung is governed by vascular permeability and the balance of the hydrostatic and oncotic pressures across the capillary endothelium as described in the Starling equation (Fig. 22–1). Hydrostatic forces favor fluid filtration, while oncotic pressure promotes reabsorption. Normally, filtration forces dominate and fluid continuously moves from the vascular space into the interstitium. Despite this, extravascular water does not accumulate because the lung lymphatics effectively remove the filtered fluid and return it to the circulation. However, the capacity of the lymphatic system is limited and if the rate

of fluid filtration exceeds its functional capabilities water accumulates. Initially, it accumulates in the loose interstitial tissues around the airways, pulmonary arteries, and later the alveolar walls (interstitial edema). This causes increased lung stiffness and dyspnea due to stimulation of lung receptors but rarely produces significant abnormalities in the arterial blood gases. If the process continues the excess fluid pours into the alveolar space with two consequences: alveolar surface forces are altered, leading to a further reduction in compliance and a decreased lung volume, and the flooded alveoli can no longer be ventilated, thus converting their blood supply into intrapulmonary shunt. Shunt is the major cause of the severe hypoxemia characteristic of ARDS (see Chapter 17).

Two major alterations of the Starling equation are seen clinically. The commonest is an increase in hydrostatic pressure as with cardiogenic pulmonary edema and fluid overload. Edema fluid in this setting has a low protein content and is essentially an ultrafiltrate of plasma. In ARDS, fluid accumulation is due to an alteration in alveolar-capillary membrane permeability, which may result from either endothelial or epithelial cell injury (Fig. 22–2). The etiology of the injury is occasionally clear-cut, as in gastric aspiration or viral pneumonia, but is more commonly elusive and ascribed to complex immunologic or bio-

FIGURE 22–1. Factors affecting fluid filtration in the lung. The net filtration is from the pulmonary microcirculation into the interstitium of the lung. Normally excessive accumulation of fluid is prevented by the capacity of the lymphatics to drain it back into the systemic circulation.

$$\text{Fluid Flux} = K_w [(P_{mv} - P_{is}) - \sigma_s (\pi_{mv} - \pi_{is})]$$

where

K_w = Filtration coefficient of water ("leakiness" to water)
P_{mv} = Hydrostatic pressure of the microcirculation
P_{is} = Hydrostatic pressure of the interstitium
π_{mv} = Oncotic pressure of the microcirculation
π_{is} = Oncotic pressure of the interstitium
σ_s = Reflection coefficient of the membrane ("leakiness" to solutes)

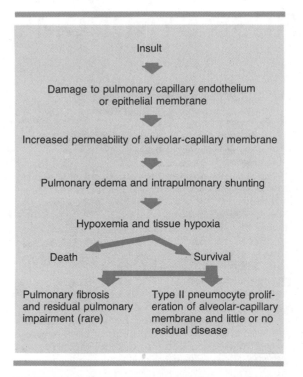

FIGURE 22—2. Pathogenesis and outcome of the adult respiratory distress syndrome.

chemical events involving complement activation, arachidonic acid metabolites, leukocyte trapping in the lung, and O_2 radical release. The resulting edema has a high protein content similar to that of plasma. While alterations in oncotic pressure are unusual as the sole cause of pul-

TABLE 22—1. DIAGNOSIS OF ARDS

1. Proper clinical setting (Table 22–2) and the exclusion of left ventricular failure or chronic lung disease
2. Diffuse pulmonary infiltrates on chest x-ray
3. $P_aO_2 < 50$ mm Hg on $F_IO_2 > 0.60$
4. Decreased respiratory compliance <50 ml/cm H_2O

TABLE 22—2. CONDITIONS ASSOCIATED WITH ARDS

Inhalant injuries
  aspiration
  smoke and toxic gases
  near drowning
  oxygen toxicity
Infections
  gram-negative sepsis
  viral, bacterial, and *Pneumocystis carinii* pneumonia
  miliary tuberculosis
Drug overdose—heroin, methadone, propoxyphene, aspirin
Disseminated intravascular coagulopathy
Burns
Pancreatitis
Multiple transfusions
Trauma—lung contusion, fat emboli
Uremia
Head injury
Amniotic fluid and air emboli

monary edema, the presence of low intravascular oncotic pressure increases the rate of fluid transudation in both low- and high-pressure pulmonary edema. Similarly, any increase in microvascular hydrostatic pressure in the setting of increased capillary permeability dramatically increases the rate of fluid filtration.

CLINICAL PRESENTATION AND DIAGNOSIS

As with any clinically defined syndrome, the diagnosis of ARDS is made by finding the appropriate signs and symptoms (Table 22–1) in the proper clinical setting (Table 22–2). Some predisposing conditions are more likely to result in ARDS than others, such as lung injury secondary to aspiration of gastric contents, pneumonias and sepsis requiring admission to the intensive care unit, and disseminated intravascular coagulopathy.

Clinical presentation is relatively uniform regardless of etiology. Initially signs and symptoms are limited to those of the primary disorder. However, within the first 12 to 24 hours early accumulation of lung water causes dyspnea, hyperventilation, and the appearance of a fine diffuse reticular infiltrate on chest x-ray. Unless the underlying disease can be rapidly reversed, as in sepsis, the patient quickly progresses to the full-blown syndrome with the development of progressive bilateral pulmonary infiltrates, severe hypoxemia, and a dramatic fall in lung compliance. Most patients manifest respiratory failure within 24 hours of the onset of the predisposing event, and almost 90 per cent of those who eventually develop ARDS will do so by 72 hours. Treatment is generally supportive and directed at maintaining an adequate delivery of O_2 to the tissues while minimizing iatrogenic complications. Therapy directed at the predisposing condition, when known, is imperative, since its continued presence leads to the persistence of the ARDS.

OXYGEN THERAPY AND MECHANICAL VENTILATION

Correction of the severe hypoxemia by increasing the fractional concentration of the inspired O_2 (F_IO_2) is useful early in the disease. However, because the hypoxemia is due to shunt this is less effective than in patients with obstructive or restrictive lung disease in which ventilation-perfusion inequality is the major underlying mechanism. Figure 22–3 plots the relationship between the F_IO_2 and arterial PO_2 (P_aO_2) and O_2 content for different levels of shunt. Increasing the F_IO_2 may significantly increase O_2 content and thus the O_2 delivery despite the negligible increase in P_aO_2. While O_2 content can be increased substantially, a high F_IO_2 by itself is toxic to the lung, and thus this strategy has distinct limitations. O_2 toxicity depends on a number of factors, including F_IO_2,

FIGURE 22–3. The effect of changing the inspired oxygen concentration on the arterial P_{O_2} and O_2 content for lungs having shunts of 10 to 50 per cent. When the shunt is small, as may be seen early in the course of ARDS, increasing the inspired oxygen to 40 to 50 per cent will effectively increase the P_aO_2. As the shunt increases and approaches 30 to 50 per cent, the levels commonly seen in ARDS, only small increases in arterial P_{O_2} will be achieved even when 100 per cent O_2 is administered. Although P_{O_2} increases very little (*left panel*), this occurs at a steep portion of the O_2 dissociation curve so that O_2 saturation increases disproportionately, resulting in a considerable increase in O_2 content (*right panel*). (From Dantzker D. Gas exchange in the adult respiratory distress syndrome. Clin Chest Med 3:57–67, 1982.)

duration of treatment, and the underlying condition of the lung. The F_IO_2 likely to induce toxicity in man is unknown, although it is probable that a continuum rather than a threshold exists. As a general rule, an F_IO_2 above 0.60 can be tolerated for short periods such as 24 hours, but after 72 hours O_2 toxicity may contribute to further lung damage.

When adequate oxygenation cannot be maintained by O_2 therapy alone, or if hypercapnia develops, mechanical ventilation is essential. The positive pressure generated by the ventilator increases mean airway pressure, which in turn increases lung volume. This results in an increase in alveolar size, spreading the fluid that is present over a greater surface area and allowing gas exchange to take place. Mechanical ventilation also reduces the O_2 demands on the body caused by increased O_2 consumption by the respiratory muscles as patients try to cope with the increased work of breathing.

An oral or nasal endotracheal tube is necessary for mechanical ventilation. While nasal tubes often seem to be more comfortable to the patient, they usually are smaller in diameter than an oral tube and tend to cause difficulties in suctioning and to increase the work of breathing during the weaning period. In addition, a tube in the nasopharynx may lead to the development of a purulent otitis media, as it interferes with eustachian

tube drainage. With proper care, low compliance cuffed tubes can be left in place for at least three to four weeks. The major complication from endotracheal tubes is damage to the larynx resulting from tube motion as the patient moves about, which can be minimized by adequate fixation of the tube at the mouth or nose. The decision to proceed to a tracheostomy should not be made on the basis of any arbitrary time limit. Tracheostomy has its own complications, e.g., tracheal stenosis, which may exceed the morbidity associated with endotracheal tubes. Thus a tracheostomy should be performed only if it is necessary for adequate care or if it is clear that continued mechanical ventilation will be required for a prolonged time.

Mechanical ventilators are classified on the basis of what terminates inspiratory flow. Pressure-cycled ventilators terminate flow when a preset pressure is reached in the airway. Consequently, tidal volumes and minute ventilation vary with changes in airways resistance and lung compliance, which makes them unsuitable for use in patients with ARDS. Volume-cycled ventilators provide a preset volume to the patient over a range of airway pressures. A pressure limit is set to prevent the development of trauma to the lung in the event of a sudden change in pulmonary mechanics when airway pressure increases in an attempt to achieve the required tidal volume. Although the precise volume delivered to the patient may vary somewhat with changes in lung mechanics and compliance of the ventilator circuit, volume-cycled ventilators allow greater control of the patient's ventilation.

Mechanical ventilators can be set to operate in a variety of modes (Fig. 22–4). Controlled ventilation, in which both tidal volume and rate are determined by the machine, are used only when the patient is unable to initiate a spontaneous breath, e.g., drug overdose, severe neuromuscular disease, muscle relaxants, or excessive sedation. The modes most commonly used in the treatment of ARDS are intermittent mandatory ventilation (IMV) and assist-control ventilation (AC). While controversy exists as to which of these modes is more effective, no good comparison has been made, and for most patients it probably makes very little difference as long as sufficient support is provided.

The goal of increased lung volume is achieved by two strategies regardless of the ventilatory mode: (1) high tidal volume, such as 10 or even 15 ml/kg rather than the normal 6 ml/kg; (2) positive end-expiratory pressure (PEEP), which prevents the airway pressure from falling back to atmospheric at end-expiration. While these strategies allow inspired gas to enter previously unventilated alveoli, there is no convincing evidence that increasing lung volume alters the primary pathological process or reverses the transudation of fluid from the blood vessels into the lung. Thus, these ventilatory techniques should be used only to the degree that they may help in achieving an adequate O_2 saturation (90 per cent) at a relatively nontoxic F_IO_2 (0.60). However, improvement in arterial oxygenation by itself is an insufficient guide to ventilatory therapy, as the increase in airway pressure may cause a fall in cardiac output with an overall reduction in O_2 delivery to the tissues. Pulmonary barotrauma, manifested as subcutaneous emphysema, pneumomomediastinum, and pneumothorax, is an additional serious complication.

The mechanism by which high intrathoracic pressure interferes with cardiac output is complex, with a reduction in venous return to the heart playing a major role. With small increases in intrathoracic pressure (5 to 10 cm of PEEP) impairment of cardiac output may be minimal as long as cardiac filling pressures are adequate. With higher levels of PEEP, cardiac output is invariably reduced unless filling pressures are increased above normal. This reduction in cardiac output results in a decrease in O_2 delivery to the tissues despite a concomitant increase in P_aO_2. The increase in filling pressure required to maintain cardiac output in the face of large increases in PEEP is likely to increase the accumulation of extravascular lung water. To monitor these important variables, especially in patients with a questionable cardiovascular status or those in whom high levels of PEEP are required, a flow-directed pulmonary artery catheter is often useful. The catheter is inserted at the bedside, preferably through an internal jugular vein, and is carried by the flow of blood through the right heart until its balloon occludes a pulmonary artery. In this position both pulmonary artery and occlusion pressure (an index of left arterial pressure) can be monitored as well as cardiac output measured by thermodilution. In addition to evaluating the adequacy of cardiac filling pressure, the catheter is often required to distinguish between ARDS and congestive heart failure, a distinction that is difficult by physical examination alone in many sick patients. The insertion and maintenance of the pulmonary artery catheter must be accomplished with great care to limit the risk of complications, including pneumothorax, myocardial or vascular perforation, bleeding, air embolism, arrhythmias, valve trauma or endocarditis, sepsis, and pulmonary infarction.

Care must be taken in interpreting readings obtained from the pulmonary artery catheters in patients on mechanical ventilation, since a variable amount of the positive pressure applied to the lungs is transmitted to the heart. This leads to an apparent rise in vascular pressures during inspi-

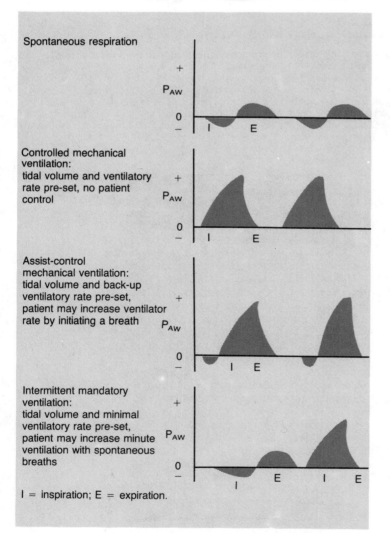

Spontaneous respiration

Controlled mechanical ventilation: tidal volume and ventilatory rate pre-set, no patient control

Assist-control mechanical ventilation: tidal volume and back-up ventilatory rate pre-set, patient may increase ventilator rate by initiating a breath

Intermittent mandatory ventilation: tidal volume and minimal ventilatory rate pre-set, patient may increase minute ventilation with spontaneous breaths

I = inspiration; E = expiration.

FIGURE 22–4. Changes in airway pressure during spontaneous respiration and various modes of mechanical ventilation.

ration. The amount of the pressure transmitted depends on a number of complex factors, including the compliance of the lungs and the cardiovascular system and the intravascular volume. The vascular pressures should be read at the same point in the breathing cycle, preferably at end-expiration. This requires reading the pressures from a continuous recording, since digital displays record mean pressures throughout the respiratory cycle.

Since hypoxemia in ARDS is due to shunting of systemic venous blood through the lung, any alteration in mixed venous P_{O_2} ($P_{\bar{v}O_2}$) proportionally alters the $P_{a}O_2$ resulting from a given amount of shunt. Increase in the O_2 consumption, decrease in cardiac output, and fall in the hemoglobin concentration may all necessitate increased O_2 extraction by the tissues and thus decrease $P_{\bar{v}O_2}$. Unless this is kept in mind, it is possible that a fall in $P_{a}O_2$ due to one of these factors may be misinterpreted as a worsening of ARDS and corrective therapy aimed in the wrong direction.

Assessing the adequacy of O_2 and ventilatory therapy in these complex conditions is a major challenge. Clearly, $P_{a}O_2$ is an inadequate index, since it reflects only one facet of O_2 delivery (O_2 Del), which is defined as:

$$O_2 \text{ Del} = \text{cardiac output} \times \text{arterial } O_2 \text{ content}$$

Thus, O_2 Del also includes a convection term, cardiac output, and a capacitance term, O_2 content, which, in addition to $P_{a}O_2$, includes O_2 saturation and hemoglobin concentration. All components must be adequate to ensure sufficient peripheral delivery of O_2. In addition to O_2 Del, tissue oxygenation depends on the distribution of blood flow within various tissues, about which little is known.

Is there a useful parameter to monitor which will reflect the adequacy of O_2 Del? The $P_{\bar{v}O_2}$ has been suggested, but this represents the weighted mean from all the tissues and thus is markedly influenced by the distribution of blood flow. For example, in septic shock, because blood flow is redistributed to tissues with a low O_2 extraction, the $P_{\bar{v}O_2}$ may actually rise pari passu with the development of systemic acidosis. In this instance, $P_{\bar{v}O_2}$ misrepresents the true status of O_2 delivery. Lactic acidosis is a sure sign of inadequate tissue O_2 Del, but since lactic acid is rapidly cleared by a well-perfused and functioning liver while its washout is delayed from poorly perfused tissues, the appearance of lactic acidosis is a late indicator of O_2 deficiency. The best current indicators are the performance of the end-organs (heart, kidney, and liver).

OTHER THERAPEUTIC MODALITIES

The development of pharmacological agents to treat or, more importantly, prevent ARDS would represent a major advancement. Early administration of high-dose corticosteriods over a brief period is of questionable value in gram-negative sepsis and has no proven efficacy in ARDS due to other etiologies. Antiprostaglandin agents, e.g., ibuprofen, affect the course of experimental disease leading to ARDS, but extension to the bedside is premature.

Antibiotics are the most important group of agents, as correct treatment of infection may be lifesaving while the failure to recognize infection ensures the continuation of the pulmonary capillary leak. As far as possible, antibiotics should be selected on the basis of reliable microbial studies, but until the results are known empiric therapy is not only appropriate but necessary. Continued sepsis in the face of appropriate antibiotics raises the spectre of an abscess and should lead to an aggressive diagnostic search, as this is a common cause of persistent ARDS and a fatal outcome. The lungs and the peritoneal cavity are the commonest sites of undiagnosed infection.

Appropriate fluid management is important to ensure adequate cardiac output and thus O_2 delivery. Fluid loading to maintain adequate cardiac filling pressures in the face of the high intrathoracic pressures generated during mechanical ventilation must be balanced against the resultant increase in microvascular pressure and its tendency to increase the extravascular lung water accumulation. The controversy over the use of colloid vs. crystalloid therapy is moot in the presence of such marked alterations in microvascular permeability. Until more is known concerning the dynamics of fluid movement in this disease, a good rule of thumb is to maintain filling pressures in a normal range (pulmonary artery wedge pressures of about 10 cm H_2O).

PROGNOSIS

The mortality rate in ARDS is 50 to 80 per cent. In any particular patient this is strongly influenced by the presence of other acute or chronic disorders. The cause of death is often unclear. Infection, particularly when associated with bacteremia of unknown origin, is a major determinant of mortality. Inadequate tissue oxygenation and organ failure are also likely to play significant roles.

Of those patients who survive the acute event, the prognosis depends primarily on the presence of other underlying disease. For most patients who began with normal lungs, pulmonary function returns slowly toward normal. A small number of patients will be left with residual fibrosis, rarely of a severe nature.

REFERENCES

Bone RC: Symposium on adult respiratory distress syndrome. Clin Chest Med, Vol 3, 1982.

Bone RC: Critical Care, a Comprehensive Approach. Chicago, American College of Chest Physicians, 1984.

Fowler AA, Hamman RF, Good JT, et al: Adult respiratory distress syndrome: Risk with common predispositions. Ann Intern Med 98:593–597, 1983.

O'Quinn R, and Marini JJ: Pulmonary artery occlusion pressure: Clinical physiology, measurements, and interpretation. Am Rev Respir Dis 128:319–326, 1983.

23 INFECTIOUS DISEASES OF THE RESPIRATORY TRACT

Medical science has made considerable advances in our understanding of the pathogenesis of respiratory tract infections in the hundred years that have elapsed since the identification of the *Pneumococcus*. In particular, the discovery of penicillin and other antibiotics has revolutionized management of pneumonia so that it is no longer "the captain of the men of death," as characterized by Osler. For a time, antibiotics may have lulled physicians into a false sense of security, but in recent years pulmonary infections have taken on a new importance with the emergence of antibiotic-resistant organisms, the increased numbers of immunocompromised hosts, and the entrance of hitherto undiscovered organisms (such as *Legionella*) and disease states (such as the acquired immunodeficiency syndrome, AIDS).

PATHOGENESIS OF RESPIRATORY TRACT INFECTION

Development of pulmonary infection reflects a victory for microbial load and virulence over the lung's defense system found throughout the airways from the nose to the alveoli. An understanding of the various abnormalities of lung defense expected in different clinical situations often helps point toward the correct etiological agent (Table 23–1). Organisms may enter the lung by direct extension from an adjacent infected site, hematogenous transfer, inhalation of aerosolized particles, or, most commonly, aspiration of oropharyngeal secretions following colonization of the upper airways. The factors determining microbial adherence to the buccal mucosa remain unclear, but it is known that colonization with gram-negative bacilli (GNB) is seen only in 2 to 18 per cent of healthy subjects, whereas it is universally observed in some patients in intensive care units (ICU).

When an organism breaches the anatomic and cough defenses, the mucociliary system aids in its removal by trapping it in the mucous layer and the cilia propel it cephalad. Abnormalities of mucociliary clearance may be aquired as a result of viral infections that denude the epithelium or may be inherited, as with defects in ciliary microtubular structure (immotile cilia syndrome) and cystic fibrosis, in which tenacious airway secretions impair ciliary beating.

In the distal respiratory tract, organisms encounter a dual phagocytic system, pulmonary alveolar macrophages and polymorphonuclear neutrophils. The macrophages are vital for protection against intracellular organisms such as mycobacteria and some other bacteria, fungi, and viruses. Macrophage function may be disrupted by viral infection or immunosuppressive therapy. Neutrophilic recruitment may be the most important component of the host's defense once the inflammatory response has commenced and, in conjunction with antibodies and complement, provides important protection against pyogenic bacterial infection. In addition, neutrophils protect against invasive and systemic infection with opportunistic fungi such as *Candida*, *Aspergillus*, and *Mucor*, which rarely, if ever, produce infection in healthy subjects.

Humoral and cellular responses depend on the host's previous exposure to the organism. Antibody in secretions interferes with local spread of

---

TABLE 23–1.   HOST DEFENSE SYSTEM

COMPONENT	ABNORMAL IN	CONSEQUENCES	PATHOGENS
Cough reflex/laryngeal barrier	Neuromuscular disease, drug overdose, intubation	Aspiration	Anaerobes, gram-positive and gram-negative organisms
Mucociliary clearance	Immotile cilia syndrome, cystic fibrosis, viral infection	Bronchiectasis	Gram-positive and gram-negative organisms
Secretory IgA	Congenital deficiency	Increased bacterial adherence and colonization	Viruses and bacteria
Pulmonary alveolar macrophage	Viral infection, immunosuppressive agents	Impaired phagocytosis and inactivation of organisms	*Pneumocystis carinii*, *Legionella*, and mycobacteria
Polymorphonuclear granulocyte	Neutropenia	Impaired phagocytosis and parenchymal inflammatory response	Gram-negative bacilli, *S. aureus*, *Aspergillus*, *Mucor*, fungi
Humoral antibody	Congenital or acquired hypogammaglobulinemia	Impaired opsonization causing inefficient phagocytosis	*S. pneumoniae*, *H. influenzae*
Cellular immunity	Lymphoreticular disease, immunosuppressive agents, organ transplantation, AIDS	Impaired attraction and activation of pulmonary alveolar macrophages	Herpesvirus group, *P. carinii*, *Cryptococcus*, *Nocardia*, mycobacteria, *Legionella*
Complement	Genetic deficiencies	Impaired opsonization and inefficient phagocytosis	Pyogenic bacterial infection

organisms, while circulating antibody helps in preventing spread to distant sites by maximizing phagocytosis (opsonization). Antibody also causes direct bacterial killing in conjunction with complement. Actively sensitized T lymphocytes release lymphokines that attract and activate macrophages to enhance their phagocytic function. This cell-mediated immunity is particularly important in protection against viruses, facultative intracellular bacteria such as mycobacteria, *Legionella*, *Brucella*, and *Listeria*, and most systemic fungi. Both the classic and alternate pathways of complement activation help with opsonization and direct microbial killing and lysis.

CLINICAL PRESENTATION

If the infectious process overwhelms the host defenses but is restricted to the large airways, a tracheobronchitis results, whereas involvement of the lung parenchyma represents pneumonia. Pneumonia may occur in four major settings: community-acquired, hospital-acquired, immunocompromised host, and following aspiration, each varying in etiology, presentation, diagnostic approach, and therapy.

Community-Acquired Pneumonia

A specific etiological diagnosis is often difficult or impossible to make in community-acquired pneumonia. Given this, the true incidence of each microbial etiology is unknown. In an otherwise healthy host, probably 95 to 99 per cent of community-acquired pneumonias are due to viral, mycoplasma, pneumococcal (*Streptococcus pneumoniae*) or *Legionella* infections, and some authors estimate that viruses and mycoplasma account for more than half. In patients with underlying disease, other organisms may be found

which fortunately tend to follow a certain predictable pattern: *Streptococcus pneumoniae*, *Staphylococcus aureus*, and *Haemophilus influenzae* are commonly responsible for bacterial pneumonia following influenza; *S. pneumoniae* and *H. influenzae* in patients with chronic bronchitis; and anaerobes in patients with pneumonia following aspiration of oropharyngeal contents. Highly resistant gram-negative bacilli are very rarely responsible for community-acquired pneumonia.

If pneumonia is suspected, a physical examination is essential; however, even in the absence of abnormal physical signs, such as crackles or evidence of consolidation, pneumonia may be present. A chest x-ray is required to differentiate pneumonia (infiltrate expected) from bronchitis. While certain radiological patterns have been associated with different organisms, such associations are of a nonspecific nature and are of little value in an individual patient. Serology may be obtained if viral, mycoplasma, or *Legionella* infection is suspected but does not aid immediate clinical decisions because a delay is incurred in demonstrating a rising titer (up to five weeks). Sputum cultures are also of limited value. Sensitivity is only 50 per cent for pneumococci, and other fastidious organisms are difficult to culture or are overgrown by oral flora. If positive, cultures of blood or pleural fluid provide a precise etiological diagnosis, but negative results are much more common. Sputum Gram's stain remains the time-honored approach, but some patients are unable to expectorate, and even when sputum is obtained, it is usually of poor quality and contaminated by oral flora 75 per cent of the time. When an optimal specimen is obtained with extreme care, there is still a 38 per cent false-negative rate for pneumococcal pneumonia. Invasive techniques to obtain selective cultures are rarely required in community-acquired pneumonia.

FIGURE 23–1. Empirical approach to the treatment of community-acquired pneumonia.

Therapy is commonly instituted on an empirical basis because of the limited information provided by the above diagnostic approaches. One suggested approach is depicted in Figure 23–1. In the normal host, a viral etiology is suggested by the presence of a dry cough and systemic illness in a young person. A bacterial infection is commoner in adult patients, who often present suddenly with rigors, productive cough, chest pain, and a high white cell count. Patients with *Legionella* infection have features of both. Erythromycin is the most practical empirical agent, as it is the drug of choice for mycoplasma and *Legionella* infection and is also useful in pneumococcal pneumonia. The antibiotic selected for an abnormal host depends on the specific circumstances (Fig. 23–1). The decision of whether to hospitalize the patient is often based on the patient's underlying disease status.

Nosocomial Pneumonia

Lung infection in a hospitalized patient is termed nosocomial pneumonia. It occurs in 1 to 5 per cent of all hospitalized patients and is responsible for 15 per cent of hospital deaths. Up to 60 per cent of ICU patients may develop pneumonia, and up to half of these die. More than 60 per cent of nosocomial pneumonias are due to gram-negative bacilli (GNB), and the main source of organisms is the patient's own oropharynx. Subsequent entry into the lung is probably achieved by aspiration. In mechanically ventilated patients, direct entry is further facilitated by the presence of an endotracheal or tracheostomy tube. Organisms reach the oropharynx by a number of routes, including fecal contamination of the hands of the patient or attendant, or more commonly by retrograde movement from the stomach to the oropharynx. A less frequent source is the surrounding environment, such as sinks, food, and flowers. Antibiotics reduce the normal inhibitory flora and predispose to GNB colonization. There is a marked difference in the rate of oropharyngeal colonization with GNB in healthy subjects (2 to 18 per cent) compared to medical ICU patients (50 per cent) and ICU patients with a primary respiratory diagnosis (100 per cent), possibly related to the increased adherence of bacilli to the regional epithelium in seriously ill patients. Colonization also confounds the etiological diagnosis, because expectorated or aspirated tracheobronchial secretions are usually contaminated by the colonizing upper airway organisms. In this setting, precise bacteriological diagnosis is particularly perplexing, and culture of secretions, with the inevitable recovery of a diverse array of potential pathogens, is likely to be misleading and to result in patient mismanagement. Differentiation of colonization from infection should be based on an overall evaluation of the patient, taking into account fever, leukocytosis, the presence of purulent secretions, and a new or progressive infiltrate on chest x-ray, although the value of these findings is lessened in patients with underlying lung disease. Blood cultures, when positive (which is rare), are helpful. If a precise etiological diagnosis is desired, invasive measures are usually required, such as transtracheal aspiration, transthoracic aspiration, or fiberoptic bronchoscopy employing a plugged telescoping catheter brush technique. In patients receiving multiple antibiotics even this is often misleading. Commonly, antibiotic therapy, including coverage for gram-positive and gram-negative organisms, is instituted on an empirical basis.

Pneumonia in the Immunocompromised Host

Increased susceptibility to infection is axiomatic to the immunocompromised host, and infections involving the lung have the greatest impact on patient morbidity and mortality. Development of a fever and pulmonary infiltrate in these patients is associated with a mortality rate of up to 50 per cent and thus poses a grave situation requiring prompt assessment and management. The potential causes of such an infiltrate are sundry and include not only the common viruses and bacteria but a galaxy of unusual organisms and a host of noninfectious conditions. While precise etiological diagnosis is extremely difficult in this setting, careful clinical assessment helps to narrow the differential diagnosis (Table 23–2). Knowledge of the particular defect in host defenses provides a valuable clue to the spectrum of possible pathogens (see Table 23–1). A complete examination of the patient is a prerequisite. Cardiac failure may masquerade as a pneumonia and must be carefully excluded. While the radiographic pattern may offer some guidance, it is

TABLE 23–2. DIAGNOSTIC APPROACH TO PNEUMONIA IN IMMUNOCOMPROMISED PATIENTS

PHENOMENON	COMMENT
History	
Nature of underlying condition	see Table 23–1
Time of onset	
CMV pneumonia following renal transplant	Between 1 and 4 months
Radiation pneumonitis	Usually latent interval of 8 weeks
Leukoagglutinin reaction	Minutes to hours
Rate of progression	
Rapid	*P. carinii*, cytomegalovirus, bacteria, tuberculosis, *Cryptococcus*
Slow	Nocardia
Intermediate	Cytomegalovirus, *Aspergillus*, *Mucor*
Physical Examination	
Skin lesions	Bacteremia, *Cryptococcus*, *Nocardia*
Eye lesions	*Candida*, cytomegalovirus, *Aspergillus*, *Toxoplasma*
Nasal necrosis	*Mucor*, less so gram-negative bacilli, *Aspergillus*
CNS—meningitis	*Cryptococcus*, tuberculosis, neoplasia
—encephalitis	Herpes simplex, *Toxoplasma*
—mass lesion effect	*Nocardia*, *Mucor*, neoplasia

rarely specific for any organism. Skin tests or serology do not provide information with sufficient accuracy or speed to be helpful in immediate management. Staining of respiratory secretions provides immediate information: cryptococci may be identified by an India ink preparation, methenamine silver nitrate may reveal *Pneumocystis*, and direct fluorescent antibody may demonstrate *Legionella*. Sputum cultures are commonly contaminated by upper airway colonizing organisms, but the presence of certain organisms, such as *Aspergillus*, *Cryptococcus*, and *Nocardia* (but not *Candida*) in the immunocompromised patient should suggest the possibility of infection even though these may be saprophytes in a normal host. Invasive techniques such as bronchoscopy, to obtain bronchial washings or brushings, or lung biopsy, to derive material for histological examination, are generally necessary to make a firm diagnosis. While empirical therapy may be instituted in the absence of an etiological diagnosis, definitive diagnostic studies should be undertaken in all but the most unstable patients.

Aspiration Pneumonia and Lung Abscess

Aspiration pneumonia may be due to inhalation of gastric juice or oropharyngeal contents, foreign body aspiration, and the spontaneous intrabronchial drainage of purulent material from a diseased lung to the contralateral healthy lung. Impairment of the airway's protective mechanisms, especially cough and glottic closure, is the major predisposing factor and is most often seen in patients with neurological disorders or acute loss of consciousness, especially in the presence of poor dentition. Pulmonary injury includes chemical pneumonitis, necrotizing pneumonia, lung abscess, and empyema. Anaerobic bacteria are the major pathogens in community-acquired aspiration pneumonia, while aerobic organisms such as S. aureus, S. pyogenes, and various GNB are less commonly responsible but predominate in hospitalized patients. Onset of disease is insidious, beginning as an acute pneumonic process with the development of an abscess or empyema after one to two weeks. Dependent areas of the lung are particularly involved. The sputum and discharges are usually putrid and foul-smelling, but this is not invariable. Diagnosis of bacterial etiology should not be based on sputum examination because of the frequency of contamination by upper airway organisms. If a specific bacteriological diagnosis is desired, invasive techniques such as transtracheal aspiration, transthoracic aspiration, or bronchoscopy are required. Since S. aureus and GNB are so easily recovered from mixed culture samples, their absence in a purulent specimen usually excludes their presence in the lower respiratory tract. The converse cannot be said, however, and their growth should not be taken as an indication of their involvement. Treatment is usually empirical and consists of penicillin G, which is effective even against organisms such as B. fragilis that display *in vitro* resistance. Clindamycin is a

reasonable alternative agent. Surgical resection of the abscess cavity or decortication of the pleural peel is rarely required.

SPECIFIC PATHOGENIC ORGANISMS

Viral Agents. Viral infection is usually limited to the upper respiratory tract, and only a small proportion of infected patients develop pneumonia. In children, viruses are the commonest cause of pneumonia, and respiratory syncytial virus is the most frequent organism. In adults, viruses are estimated to account for less than 10 per cent of pneumonias, and influenza is the commonest organism. Patients at increased risk of influenzal pneumonia include the aged, patients with chronic disease of the heart, lung, or kidney, and women in the last trimester of pregnancy. Cytomegalovirus has developed prominence as a cause of pneumonia in immunosuppressed patients, particularly in AIDS and the post-transplantation state, in which it has a mortality rate of about 50 per cent. When varicella occurs in adults some 10 to 20 per cent develop pneumonia, which commonly leaves a pattern of diffuse punctate calcification on chest x-ray. Measles is occasionally complicated by a typical viral pneumonia. Viral pneumonias typically occur in community epidemics and usually develop 1 to 2 days after the onset of "flu-like" symptoms. Major features include a dry cough, dyspnea, generalized discomfort, unremarkable physical examination, and an interstitial pattern on chest x-ray. A presumptive diagnosis may be made on the basis of the clinical presentation and the epidemiologic setting. Viral isolation or serology is required for confirmation but is rarely of clinical value.

Streptococcus pneumoniae. The pneumococcus is still the commonest bacterial cause of pneumonia in the community and in hospital. The organism is carried in the nose in up to 25 per cent of healthy adults. An increased predisposition to pneumococcal pneumonia is observed in sickle-cell disease, prior splenectomy, chronic lung disease, hematologic malignancy, diabetes mellitus, and renal failure. Clinical features include fever, rigors, chills, cough, respiratory distress, signs of pulmonary consolidation, confusion, and herpes labialis. Chest x-ray typically shows lobar consolidation with air bronchograms, but a patchy bronchopneumonic pattern may also be found. Abscess or cavitation almost never occurs. Sterile pleural effusions occur in up to 25 per cent and empyema in 1 per cent. Typically, a leukocytosis of 15,000 to 30,000 cells/cu mm with neutrophilia is found, but leukopenia may be observed with fulminant infection. While demonstration of gram-positive diplococci is valuable, it should be remembered that 75 per cent of sputum samples are of poor quality and contaminated by organisms colonizing the upper airways, and even with an ideal sample there is a 38 per cent false-negative rate. Sputum culture is positive in only half of the patients with pneumococcal pneumonia. Positive blood cultures are found in 20 to 25 per cent of patients. Penicillin G remains the treatment of choice, although recently resistant forms have been described which are sensitive only to vancomycin.

Staphylococcus aureus. This accounts for 2 to 5 per cent of community-acquired pneumonia, 11 per cent of hospital-acquired pneumonia, and 26 per cent of pneumonia following a viral infection. Persistent nasal colonization is observed in 15 to 30 per cent of adults, and 90 per cent display intermittent colonization. Presentation is similar to that of pneumococcal pneumonia, but contrasting features include the development of parenchymal necrosis and abscess formation in up to 25 per cent, empyema in 10 per cent, and a hematogenous source of infection, particularly septic thrombophlebitis, infective endocarditis, or an infected intravascular device. If the pneumonia is hematogenous in origin, blood cultures are usually positive and associated skin lesions occur in 40 per cent. Sputum Gram's stain may reveal grapelike clusters of gram-positive cocci. *S. aureus* is recovered very easily from mixed culture samples so that its absence in a purulent specimen usually excludes it as a cause of the pneumonia. Treatment requires a penicillinase-resistant agent such as nafcillin.

Streptococcus pyogenes. This is now a rare cause of pneumonia, probably accounting for less than 1 per cent of all cases. Carriage rate in the pharynx, about 3 per cent in adults, is less than with the other gram-positive cocci. Presentation is similar to that observed with *S. pneumoniae* and *S. aureus*, except that empyema is found in 30 to 40 per cent of cases. Gram's stain reveals gram-positive cocci in pairs or chains. Penicillin G is the treatment of choice.

Gram-Negative Bacilli. GNB have emerged as pathogens of major importance with the introduction of potent antibiotics and the proliferation of ICU's. They are frequently encountered in patients with debilitating diseases such as chronic alcoholism, cystic fibrosis, neutropenia, diabetes mellitus, malignancy, and chronic diseases of the lungs, heart, or kidney. They are ubiquitous throughout the hospital, contaminating equipment and instruments, and are the major source of nosocomial pneumonia. Specific organisms are associated with certain situations; e.g., *Klebsiella pneumonia* is particularly common in chronic alcoholics, *Escherichia coli* pneumonia is associated with bacteremias arising from the intestinal or urinary tracts, and *Pseudomonas aeruginosa* is almost universal in cystic fibrosis. Precise etiological diagnosis is confounded by the frequency with which these organisms colonize the upper airways in predisposed patients. Treatment in this situation generally includes the use of a penicillinase-resistant penicillin or a cephalosporin and an aminoglycoside. *Haemophilus influenzae* is a gram-negative coccobacillus almost universally present in the upper respiratory tract; thus its identification in sputum samples carries no sig-

nificance. Diagnosis depends on isolating the organism in the blood, pleural fluid, or lung tissue. Pneumonia is complicated by a high incidence of pleural reactions. Ampicillin is the treatment of choice, but 20 per cent show resistance due to beta-lactamase production.

Mycoplasma pneumoniae. This is not only a common cause of pneumonia in young adults, but it also produces a wide range of extrapulmonary features that may be the only findings. Less than 10 per cent of infected patients develop symptoms of lower respiratory tract infection. Respiratory findings resemble those of viral pneumonia. Nonpulmonary features include myalgias, arthralgias, skin lesions (rashes, erythema nodosum and multiforme, Stevens-Johnson syndrome) and neurological complications (meningitis, encephalitis, transverse myelitis, neuropathy). Definitive diagnosis is delayed by technological limitations. Isolation and serology take several weeks for positive results. Cold agglutinins are found in 50 per cent of patients but take 7 to 14 days of infection before becoming positive, and they are also elevated in other respiratory infections. Tetracycline and erythromycin decrease the duration of symptoms and hasten radiographic resolution but do not eradicate the organism from the respiratory tract.

Pneumocystis carinii. This protozoan parasite exists as a cyst, 5 μm in diameter, containing oval bodies or sporozoites. Severe clinical infection is probably secondary to reactivation of latent infection due to immunosuppression, particularly affecting cell-mediated immunity. Corticosteroids seem to be more important than cytotoxic therapy in predisposing to infection. Currently, this is the major pulmonary infection in patients with AIDS. Patients usually present with dyspnea, dry cough, and diffuse patchy infiltrates. Diagnosis requires bronchoscopy, with bronchoalveolar lavage and transbronchial biopsy, or open-lung biopsy. Gomori methenamine silver nitrate usually stains the cyst wall black or brown. Definitive etiological diagnosis rather than employment of empirical therapy is desirable, as *P. carinii* accounts for no more than one third of diffuse pulmonary infiltrates in immunocompromised patients. Treatment of choice is trimethoprim-sulfamethoxazole, or pentamidine if the patient is allergic to the former agent.

Legionella species. These are fastidious GNB that were responsible for respiratory infections long before the outbreak of Legionnaires' disease in 1976. They are distributed widely in water, and outbreaks have been related to their presence in cooling towers, condensers, potable water, and even hospital shower heads. Infection may occur sporadically or in outbreaks. While healthy subjects are affected, there is an increased risk in patients with chronic diseases of the heart, lungs, or kidneys, malignancy, and impairment of cell-mediated immunity. After an incubation period of two to ten days the illness usually gradually begins with a dry cough, respiratory distress, fever, rigors, malaise, weakness, headache, confusion, and gastrointestinal disturbance. The chest x-ray shows alveolar shadowing that may have a lobar or patchy distribution, with or without pleural effusions. The diagnosis is clinically suggested by the combination of a nonconsolidating pneumonia, dry cough, multiorgan involvement, and failure to respond to antibiotics other than erythromycin (although the latter should not be necessary to arouse suspicion).

Diagnosis can be made by four methods. (1) Indirect fluorescent antibody testing is positive in 75 per cent of patients, but up to eight weeks is required for seroconversion. (2) Direct fluorescent antibody of respiratory secretions is the most rapid method of establishing the diagnosis and has a specificity of 95 per cent. (3) Fresh fluids and tissues should be subjected to the Gimenez stain, which is more sensitive and specific than the previously employed Dieterle silver stain. (4) The organism can be cultured on charcoal yeast extract medium, but up to ten days is required for growth.

Erythromycin is the treatment of choice and appears to result in a four-fold reduction in mortality. Patients usually respond within 12 to 48 hours, and it is very unusual for fever, leukocytosis, and confusion to persist after four days of therapy. In the untreated situation, the recorded mortality rate is 20 to 30 per cent in a previously healthy host and 80 per cent in immunocompromised patients.

Tuberculosis. Mycobacterium tuberculosis is transmitted in aerosolized droplets, and the majority of infected patients develop an asymptomatic, self-limited pneumonia that heals by granuloma formation with eventual scarring and calcification. Sensitization develops two to ten weeks after infection, evidence of which can be obtained by demonstrating reactivity on skin testing with an extract of the tuberculous bacillus (purified protein derivative, PPD). Less than 15 per cent of infected patients ever develop active disease. The onset of symptoms may follow directly after infection or may occur many years later owing to the breakdown of a previously healed focus of disease. The risk of progressing to disease is increased in certain situations such as immunocompromise, diabetes mellitus, malnutrition, silicosis, and maintenance hemodialysis. Active disease may involve any organ system. In the lung it may proliferate locally, producing caseation and necrosis, or it may rupture into a bronchus and result in pneumonia. On the chest x-ray the apical and posterior segments of the upper lobes are most commonly involved, and the appearance may be that of a single nodule, segmental infiltrate, or diffuse acinar shadow, with or without calcification and cavitation. Other sites include the pleural space, genitourinary tract, bone, pericardium, meninges, and peritoneum. Invasion of a blood vessel with hematogenous spread may result in miliary tuberculosis, so termed because of the appearance of millet-seed type shadows on the chest x-ray. With a characteristic x-ray, diagnosis is easy, but the features of miliary tuberculosis may be subtle and it may present as a fever of unknown origin without obvious pulmonary involvement.

Isolation of the organism is required for diagnosis. Ziehl-Neelsen stain of the sputum demonstrates the acid-fast organisms but must be differentiated from atypical mycobacteria or nocardia. Fluorescent microscopy is more sensitive but less specific. Culture takes three to eight weeks before yielding positive results. Single morning sputum samples are the preferred source of material. If no sputum can be obtained, gastric aspirates or bronchial washings should be obtained. A negative sputum smear in the presence of cavitary disease places the diagnosis in doubt. Most patients with active disease demonstrate sensitivity on skin testing when 0.1 ml of standard PPD (intermediate strength) is injected intradermally. Induration of at least 10 mm in diameter is deemed significant, but this varies with the prevalence in the community. Interpretation is complicated by the fact that some patients with active disease are anergic.

Currently the recommended treatment is isoniazid (300 mg/day) and rifampin (600 mg/day) for nine months, which results in treatment failures and relapses in only 1 per cent of patients. The addition of a third agent (such as ethambutol or

TABLE 23–3. FUNGAL INFECTION IN THE NORMAL HOST

ORGANISM	PULMONARY FINDINGS	SEROLOGY	DIAGNOSIS	TREATMENT
Histoplasma capsulatum	Acute pneumonia, multiple nodules or chronic fibronodular infiltrate	Rising titer signifies infection	Sputum or biopsy: smear and culture; exposure to bird or bat droppings or residence in river valleys of eastern to central North America	Not required in most cases of acute disease; amphotericin B for chronic disease or dissemination
Coccidioides immitis	Acute flulike illness, pneumonia, nodules, and cavities	High titers indicate dissemination	Sputum or biopsy: smear and culture; residence in southwestern United States	Not required unless disseminated or present in immunosuppressed host; then amphotericin B
Blastomyces dermatitidis	Pneumonia; pulmonary nodule; chronic fibronodules; or cavitation; hilar adenopathy uncommon	Not helpful	Residence in southeast or central United States; genitourinary and skin involvement common	Treatment of progressive pulmonary disease, dissemination; or immunosuppressed host with amphotericin B

TABLE 23–4. OPPORTUNISTIC FUNGAL PNEUMONIAS

ORGANISM	PULMONARY FINDINGS	DIAGNOSIS	TREATMENT
Aspergillus	(a) Aspergilloma: mass in lung cavity surrounded by crescent of air	Serum percipitins to aspergillus in almost 100%	Observation or surgery if significant hemoptysis
	(b) Allergic bronchopulmonary aspergillosis: hypersensitivity to fungus causing sputum plugs and fleeting chest x-ray shadows in an asthmatic. Not an infection; rather an infestation	Intradermal prick test, sputum and blood eosinophilia, elevated IgE	Corticosteroids
	(c) Invasive aspergillosis: parenchymal consolidation containing a rim of air	Sputum culture, lung aspirate or biopsy	Amphotericin B
Mucor	Chronic infection resembles aspergilloma; acute infection resembles invasive aspergillosis associated with rhinocerebral involvement	Sputum, blood cultures almost always negative; lung aspirate or biopsy required	Amphotericin B
Candida	Rarely a cause of primary pneumonia; no typical radiological pattern	Growth in sputum is of no value; serology unreliable; lung biopsy required	Amphotericin B
Cryptococcus neoformans	Single or multiple nodules without hilar involvement; associated neurological involvement	Sputum culture may be unreliable; serology less frequently positive in the absence of CNS involvement; lung biopsy required	Close observation or amphotericin B and flucytosine

streptomycin) does not improve the rate of sputum conversion but may increase toxicity.

Mycobacteria other than M. tuberculosis are frequent causes of chronic pulmonary infection, particularly in patients with chronic lung diseases such as COPD and silicosis. Fifteen per cent of mycobacterial infections are estimated to be due to such agents. The most common organisms are M. kansasii and M. avium-intracellulare. Disease is usually confined to the lung and while possible, extrapulmonary involvement is rare. The exception to this is in patients with AIDS, in whom disseminated M. avium-intracellulare is becoming an increasingly common problem. This organism displays marked antibiotic resistance.

Fungi. Although an uncommon cause of pneumonia, the lungs are frequently involved in systemic fungal infections. The responsible organisms can be divided into two groups: those associated with impaired host defenses (*Aspergillus, Mucor,* and *Candida*) and those occurring in normal subjects (*Histoplasma capsulatum, Coccidioides immitis,* and *Blastomyces dermatitidis*). *Cryptococcus neoformans* may infect both normal and immunocompromised hosts. These are discussed briefly in Tables 23–3 and 23–4.

REFERENCES

Dixon RE: Symposium on nosocomial infections (Parts I, II and III). Am J Med 70:379–473,631–744,899–986, 1981.

Green GM, Daniel TM, and Ball WC: Koch Centennial Memorial. Am Rev Resp Dis 125:1–31 (Suppl), 1982.

Pennington JE: Respiratory Infections: Diagnosis and Management. New York, Raven Press, 1983.

24 NEOPLASTIC DISEASES OF THE LUNG

Lung cancer causes over 120,000 deaths per year in the United States and has long been the leading cause of cancer deaths in men and recently has become more common than breast carcinoma in women. Carcinoma of the lung is most common in the fifth and sixth decades and is rarely seen before the age of 35.

Cigarette smoking is the most important causative factor, with lung cancer being 10 to 30 times more common among smokers; approximately 4 per cent of those who have smoked for 40 years develop lung cancer. All cell types except bronchoalveolar carcinoma are associated with smoking. Of the other causative agents, asbestos is the most important, especially when combined with cigarette smoking, and up to 14 per cent of smokers with asbestosis develop lung cancer. Other industrial risks include uranium, arsenic, chromium, chloromethyl, methylethers, polycyclic aromatic hydrocarbons, nickel, and possibly beryllium. Lung cancer may rarely develop in preexisting scars due to old granulomatous disease, diffuse interstitial fibrosis, or scleroderma.

PATHOLOGY

Benign tumors, composing 5 per cent of the total, are usually diagnosed on routine chest x-rays, and symptoms, if present, are usually related to bronchial obstruction. The commonest central tumor is the bronchial adenoma, which usually appears benign but is potentially malignant and rarely produces features of the carcinoid syndrome. The most common peripheral tumor is the pulmonary hamartoma, which has a characteristic "popcorn" pattern of calcification.

Primary malignant neoplasms of the lung can be classified on the basis of their cell type, as summarized in Table 24–1. The relative incidence of each cell type varies from study to study. Currently, squamous cell carcinoma and adenocarcinoma each represent one third of the cases, with the remainder made up of large cell and small cell tumors. Bronchoalveolar carcinoma is considered a variant of adenocarcinoma. Small cell undifferentiated carcinoma or oat cell carcinoma has the greatest propensity to metastasize early in its course, leading most clinicians to assume disseminated disease at diagnosis even without objective evidence.

Starting as a single malignant cell (10 μ size), 30 volume doublings are required to produce a tumor of 1 cm diameter, the smallest size detectable on a chest x-ray (Table 24–1). Ten further doublings produce a tumor 10 cm in diameter, but most patients die before the tumor reaches this size. Small cell carcinoma has the fastest doubling time and the worst prognosis. While adenocarcinoma has the longest doubling time, it has a worse prognosis than squamous cancers because of early extrathoracic spread.

Metastatic spread of neoplasms to the lung is common, involving the parenchyma, endobronchial mucosa, chest wall, pleural space, or mediastinum. Direct extension is the least common mode of spread, occurring with breast, liver, and pancreatic tumors. Hematogenous spread is common with renal, thyroid, and testicular tumors and bone sarcomas and presents with asymptomatic discrete nodules on chest x-ray. Lymphangitic spread presents as an infiltrate or diffuse reticulonodular pattern on chest x-ray and causes severe dyspnea, usually out of proportion to the x-ray findings. This pattern is typical of spread from adenocarcinoma of the breast, stomach, pancreas, ovary, prostate, and lung.

CLINICAL PRESENTATION

Clinical presentation may be related to tumor location within the chest, metastatic spread, or extrapulmonary paraneoplastic manifestations. Most patients present with weight loss and symptoms related to local involvement such as cough (75 per cent) that has changed in character, hemoptysis (50 per cent) that is rarely life-threatening, dyspnea (60 per cent), chest pain (40 per cent), and a marked increase in sputum production with bronchoalveolar carcinoma. Pancoast's syndrome refers to apical tumors that involve the brachial plexus and often leads to Horner's syndrome resulting from invasion of the inferior cervical ganglion. Compression and obstruction of the superior vena cava, usually by oat cell tumor, causes facial and upper extremity edema, dyspnea, stridor, and symptoms related to increased intracranial pressure. Partial obstruction of a bronchus may lead to unilateral, persistent wheezing, whereas complete obstruction causes postobstructive pneumonia. Recurrent laryngeal nerve involvement, typical of a left hilar mass, causes hoarseness. Phrenic nerve entrapment by a mediastinal mass causes diaphragmatic paralysis. Finally, direct spread of the tumor to the pleural or pericardial space will result in effusions. Bronchogenic carcinoma is frequently discovered only after it metastasizes to other organs. The brain, liver, bone, and lymph nodes are common sites,

TABLE 24–1. FEATURES OF MALIGNANT NEOPLASMS

CELL TYPE	PATHOLOGICAL FEATURES	COMMON CHEST X-RAY FINDING	VOLUME DOUBLING TIME (DAYS)
Squamous cell carcinoma	Keratin production, intercellular bridges	Central lesion with hilar involvement, cavitation not infrequent	90
Adenocarcinoma	Gland formation, mucin production	Peripheral lesion, cavitation may occur	180
Bronchoalveolar carcinoma	Distinction from adenocarcinoma imprecise	Usually peripheral lesion, pneumonic-like infiltrate, occasionally multifocal	
Large cell carcinoma	Probably represents poorly differentiated adenocarcinoma	Usually peripheral lesion, larger than adenocarcinoma with tendency to cavitate	90
Small cell carcinoma	Involvement by cells twice the size of lymphocytes	Central lesion, hilar mass common, early mediastinal involvement, no cavitation	30

TABLE 24–2. COMMON PARANEOPLASTIC SYNDROMES ASSOCIATED WITH BRONCHOGENIC CARCINOMA

SYNDROME	CELL TYPE USUALLY IMPLICATED	MECHANISM
Hypertrophic pulmonary osteoarthropathy	All types except small cell	Unknown
Gynecomastia	Large cell	Chronic gonadotrophin production
Syndrome of inappropriate ADH (SIADH) secretion	Usually small cell (may be associated with any cell type)	Inappropriate ADH release
Hypercalcemia	Usually squamous cell	Direct involvement of bone, prostaglandins, osteoclast-activating factor, PTH-like action
Cushing's syndrome	Usually small cell	Ectopic ACTH production
Eaton-Lambert myasthenic syndrome	Usually small cell	Unknown
Other neuromyopathic disorders (see appropriate chapter)	Frequently small cell but reported with most types	Unknown
Thrombophlebitis	All types	Unknown

and the evaluation of tumor found in these locations, in a smoker, should include a search for a primary lung neoplasm. In 10 to 50 per cent of patients, bronchogenic carcinoma produces one or more paraneoplastic syndromes. These may manifest themselves as neuromuscular, skeletal, endocrine, hematologic, cutaneous, or cardiovascular abnormalities (Table 24–2).

DIAGNOSIS AND EVALUATION

A careful history and physical examination are crucial in patient evaluation, and availability of a previous chest x-ray is of tremendous value. Certain generalizations regarding the relationship of the chest x-ray to the tissue type can be made: (1) A hilar mass as the only abnormal finding is most common in small cell carcinoma and almost never seen in adenocarcinoma. (2) A peripheral mass 4 cm or less in diameter is most likely an adenocarcinoma, while one greater than 4 cm may be any of the cell types except small cell carcinoma. (3) Multiple masses are very rare in primary lung cancer. (4) Apical tumors are usually squamous cell carcinoma. (5) Atelectasis strongly suggests squamous cell carcinoma. (6) Consolidation is a rare finding in all cell types. (7) Cavitation is most common in squamous cell, is less common with large cell and adenocarcinoma, and is never seen in small cell carcinoma. (8) Mediastinal widening usually signifies spread from small cell carcinoma (after Fraser and Paré).

Routine laboratory studies are rarely helpful in the diagnosis of bronchogenic carcinoma but can be invaluable in evaluating extrathoracic spread of the disease, especially liver function studies and serum calcium and alkaline phosphatase, which screen for bone metastases.

Therapeutic decisions are based on a correct tissue diagnosis. Cytological examination of expectorated sputum is the easiest and least invasive approach. False-positive results are rare, but false-negative results are relatively common (40 to 50 per cent), especially with peripheral lesions. When cytological examination of expectorated sputum is negative, bronchoscopy should be the next procedure in patients with central lesions, lung infiltrates, hoarseness, or hemoptysis. Positive yield ranges from 90 per cent for central endobronchially visible tumors to 50 per cent for peripheral lesions. Small peripheral lung nodules should probably be approached by percutaneous needle aspiration performed under fluoroscopic guidance, which provides material for cytological examination. Diagnostic accuracy is greater than 80 per cent for malignant disease but is disturbingly less accurate with benign lesions.

Once bronchogenic carcinoma is diagnosed, therapeutic decisions depend on both physiological and anatomical considerations (Fig. 24–1). Since successful surgery offers the only chance of cure, clinical evaluation is directed toward determining suitability for resection. Spirometric measurement of the forced expired volume in one second (FEV_1) is sufficient for screening. As a rule of thumb, an FEV_1 of less than 2.0 liters preoperatively may result in an FEV_1 of 0.8 liter or less after pneumonectomy, a value generally considered to preclude surgery. When the clinical evaluation of the patient differs markedly from the findings on spirometry, a useful estimate of the relative contribution of each lung to overall function can be obtained using a nuclear perfusion scan.

Determination of anatomical operability is the next step. Endobronchial lesions within 2 cm of the carina on bronchoscopy are inoperable. Intrathoracic spread to the lungs and to the hilar or mediastinal lymph nodes can often be determined from the plain radiograph, but computed tomography (CT) may be required. In situations of doubt, biopsy through the mediastinoscope (false negative rate of 20 per cent) or an anterior mediastinotomy may be required.

Once intrathoracic spread is excluded, a negative history and physical examination combined with a normal routine laboratory evaluation is usually adequate to exclude metastatic spread. Multiple imaging techniques in the absence of symptoms or signs suggesting specific organ involvement are cost-inefficient and are frequently misleading.

SOLITARY PULMONARY NODULE

A solitary pulmonary nodule is defined as a rounded lesion with well-demarcated margins. Between 5 and 40 per cent are malignant. Benign lesions are usually smaller (less than 2 cm), have sharp borders and no satellite lesions, and are present in younger people (less than 40 years). Three characteristics help to separate benign from malignant nodules. Nodules with doubling times

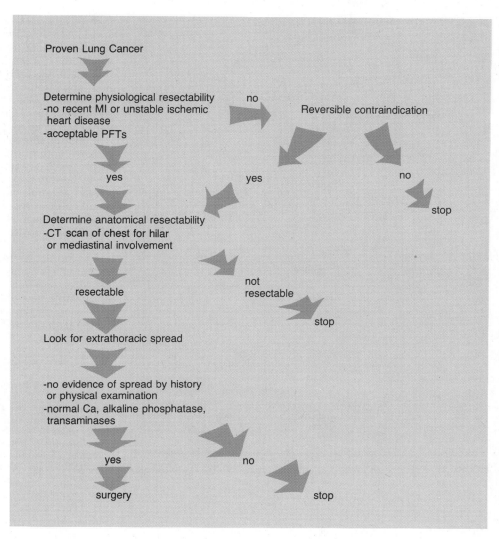

FIGURE 24—1. Decision tree for management of a solitary pulmonary nodule.

of less than 10 to 20 or more than 450 days are most likely benign. The presence of calcification with a central, speckled, diffuse, laminar, or "popcorn" pattern, but not eccentric calcification, is also evidence of its benign nature. On rare occasions the clinical picture is clearly benign, e.g., a patient with a previously normal chest x-ray who develops well-documented histoplasmosis that resolves leaving a single histoplasmoma. A suggested decision tree for the approach to the solitary nodule is shown in Figure 24–2.

TREATMENT AND PROGNOSIS

Surgery is the therapy of choice for patients with non–small cell carcinoma who meet both physiological and anatomical criteria and have no evidence of extrathoracic spread. There is no evidence that postoperative radiation therapy or chemotherapy improves survival.

For those patients with small cell carcinoma or nonoperable non–small cell tumors, radiation

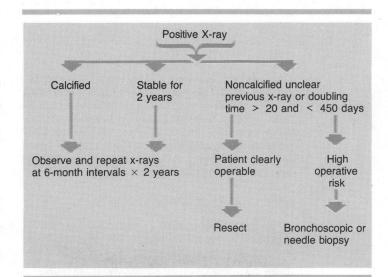

FIGURE 24—2. Decision regarding operability in the presence of proven lung cancer.

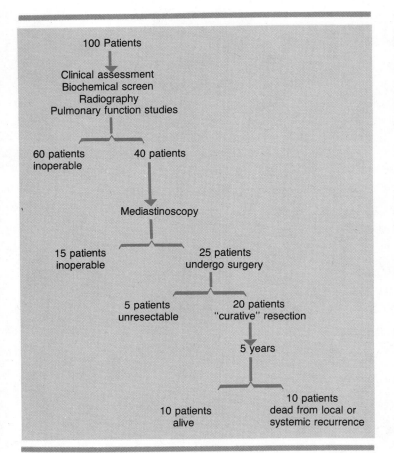

FIGURE 24–3. Outcome in 100 patients with non–small cell carcinoma.

therapy and chemotherapy are the only other modalities. Chemotherapy in various combinations has improved the median survival of patients with small cell carcinoma limited to the thorax from the 3 months, untreated, to 16 to 17 months. For non–small cell carcinoma, chemotherapy has not significantly altered the outcome and because of the significant toxicity involved, it should not be used except in controlled experimental settings.

Radiation therapy is often used in small cell carcinoma, both to treat the primary lung lesion and as prophylaxis against cerebral metastases. However, there is no evidence that this prolongs survival. Radiation therapy is not beneficial in non–small cell carcinoma and is limited to the palliative management of pain, recurrent hemoptysis, effusions, or obstruction of airways or the superior vena cava.

The prognosis for patients with bronchogenic carcinoma is poor and has improved only slightly over the past few years despite the introduction of multiple new chemotherapeutic agents. Figure 24–3 depicts the expected outcome of 100 unselected patients with non–small cell carcinoma.

REFERENCES

Fraser RG, and Paré JAP: Diagnosis of Diseases of the Chest. 2nd ed. Philadelphia, WB Saunders Co, 1977.

Hande KR, and Des Prez RM: Current perspectives in small cell lung cancer. Chest 85:669–677, 1984.

Rohwedder JJ: Neoplastic disease and mediastinal disorders. In: Guenter CA, and Welch MH (eds): Pulmonary Medicine. 2nd ed. Philadelphia, JB Lippincott, 1982, pp 795–929.

25 CONTROL OF BREATHING

Arterial P_{O_2} and P_{CO_2} are remarkably stable despite up to 20-fold increases in O_2 consumption and CO_2 production. This precise adjustment is performed by balancing tidal volume and respiratory frequency through the integrative function of the three components of the respiratory control system: respiratory control centers, respiratory sensors, and respiratory effectors (Figure 25–1).

RESPIRATORY CONTROL CENTERS

The neurons controlling respiration are located at several levels in the brain stem. The most important network resides in the medulla oblongata, where respiratory rhythm originates. The pons contains an apneustic center, uninhibited activity of which results in sustained inspiratory spasm (apneusis) and a pneumotactic center, which regulates respiratory timing, thus determining the relative duration of inspiration and expiration. While these brain stem centers are responsible for the automatic control of ventilation, the cerebral cortex can override them during wakefulness to permit speech and other actions requiring voluntary control of ventilation.

RESPIRATORY SENSORS

The respiratory sensors consist of the central and peripheral chemoreceptors and the chest wall and intrapulmonary sensory receptors. The central chemoreceptors, located on the ventral surface of the medulla oblongata, rapidly respond to any increase in CO_2 or hydrogen ion concentration by increasing ventilation (Fig. 25–2A). Under normal circumstances these receptors are very sensitive, keeping the $P_{a CO_2}$ constant despite marked variability in CO_2 production. In contrast,

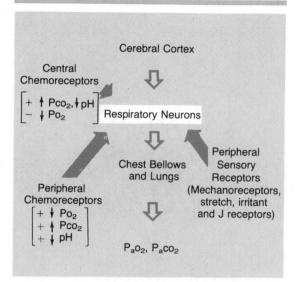

FIGURE 25–1. Schematic representation of the respiratory control system. The respiratory neurons in the brain stem receive information from the chemoreceptors, peripheral sensory receptors, and cerebral cortex. This information is integrated, and the resulting neural output is transmitted to the chest bellows and lungs.

hypoxia does not act as a central respiratory stimulant but instead depresses the central chemoreceptors. Conversely, the peripheral chemoreceptors, located at the bifurcation of the carotid arteries and along the aortic arch, are activated mainly by hypoxia and less so by CO_2 and hydrogen ion. They are also sensitive to a fall in blood pressure, which may partly account for hyperventilation seen in shock. Unlike the central response to P_{CO_2}, the peripheral chemoreceptors cause little increase in ventilation until there is significant hypoxemia (P_{O_2} less than 60 mm Hg) (Fig. 25–2B). Mechanoreceptors in the chest wall respond to stretch of the intercostal muscles and reflexly modulate the rate and depth of breathing. Tidal volume and respiratory frequency may also be reflexly affected by stimuli arising in (1) airway irritant receptors, which respond to physical or chemical stimulation, (2) pulmonary stretch receptors, which respond to marked increases in lung volume (Hering-Breuer reflex), or (3) J receptors found in the juxtacapillary junctions, which respond to vascular engorgement and congestion.

EFFECTORS OF THE RESPIRATORY SYSTEM

Signals are transmitted from the respiratory center to the chest bellows apparatus by (1) the phrenic nerves, which supply the diaphragm, (2) the intercostal nerves, which innervate the intercostal and abdominal muscles, (3) the accessory cranial nerves, which supply the sternomastoid muscles, and (4) the lower cervical nerves, which supply the scalene muscles. In addition, a variety of muscles acting on the soft palate, tongue, and hyoid bone maintain upper airway patency and offset the collapsing effect of the negative pressures generated by the respiratory muscles. During wakefulness, both the upper airway and chest wall muscles display rhythmic inspiratory activity. During sleep, upper airway muscle activity wanes, whereas diaphragmatic activation changes little.

CLINICAL ASSESSMENT OF THE REGULATION OF VENTILATION

Clinical assessment is currently limited to the chemical control of ventilation, as the precise role of sensory receptor influences is unknown and satisfactory techniques for their assessment do not exist. Depressed chemosensitivity should be suspected when one of the conditions listed in Table

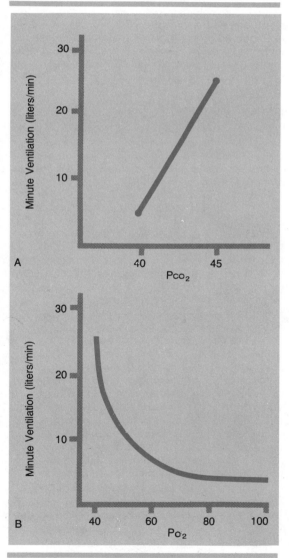

FIGURE 25–2. Minute ventilation increases linearly with rising P_{CO_2} (A) and increases exponentially with falling P_{O_2} (B).

TABLE 25–1. SUSPECT IMPAIRED CHEMOSENSITIVITY IN THE PRESENCE OF HYPERCAPNIA AND THE FOLLOWING

1. Disproportionately small reduction in FEV_1
2. Normal alveolar-arterial Po_2 gradient
3. Ability to achieve normocapnia with voluntary hyperventilation
4. Ability to generate a negative inspiratory pressure of at least minus 30 torr, which eliminates muscle weakness as a cause of hypercapnia

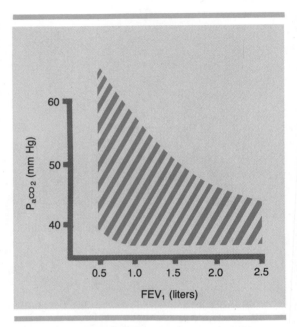

FIGURE 25–3. The increase in $Paco_2$ as airway obstruction becomes more severe, as reflected by decreasing FEV_1. Note the large scatter of Pco_2 values for any level of obstruction.

25–1 is present, and formal assessment of respiratory center function should be considered.

The rebreathing test is the commonest clinical method of assessing CO_2 sensitivity. Normally minute ventilation increases by an average of 2 L/min/mm Hg CO_2 (range 1 to 8 L/min/mm Hg CO_2) (Figure 25–2A). Blunting of the CO_2 response occurs in idiopathic hypoventilation, obesity-hypoventilation syndrome, narcotic or sedative ingestion, hypothyroidism, metabolic alkalosis, and primary neurological disorders. The reduced response in patients with COPD and CO_2 retention is discussed later. Chemosensitivity to hypoxia is technically more difficult to measure, and generally there is a good relationship between reduced chemosensitivity to O_2 and CO_2.

CONTROL OF BREATHING IN DISEASE STATES

Disordered respiratory control usually accompanies other states and rarely in itself constitutes an independent clinical disorder.

Chronic Obstructive Pulmonary Disease (COPD). Patients with physiologically significant COPD have a reduced ventilatory response to hypoxia and hypercapnia. While this was formerly thought to be entirely due to decreased chemosensitivity of the respiratory centers, most of these patients display an *increased* resting respiratory center drive. In hypercapnic patients this heightened respiratory drive fails to translate into a sufficiently increased minute ventilation to maintain a normal Pco_2 owing to the increased work of breathing and marked ventilation-perfusion mismatch. The level of hypercapnia is related in general to the degree of obstruction, although lung mechanics, resting respiratory drive, and the pattern of breathing are often similar in patients with and without CO_2 retention (Fig. 25–3). Development of hypercapnia depends on poorly understood interactions of inherited respiratory drive, peripheral sensory receptor stimulation, associated hypoxemia, degree of ventilation-perfusion mismatching, and the metabolic milieu.

Asthma. Patients with acute asthma display hyperventilation and hypocapnia, presumably due to stimulation of lung sensory receptors. CO_2 retention is a late finding in the progression of a severe asthmatic attack. Indeed, eucapnia, rather than the expected hypocapnia, is a warning sign of impending deterioration.

Other disorders in which abnormal peripheral sensory receptor stimulation is thought to result in an increased respiratory drive with resultant dyspnea, tachypnea, and hypocapnia include restrictive lung disease, pulmonary vascular disease, and abnormalities of the chest wall.

Central Hypoventilation. This may occur secondary to brain stem involvement by tumor, ischemia, or inflammatory disease; a primary, idiopathic form has also been described. Patients display decreased chemosensitivity, often with resting hypercapnia and cor pulmonale. Rarely the impairment of chemosensitivity may be so severe that the patient breathes adequately only when stimulated by wakefulness but hypoventilates and becomes apneic during sleep, when rostral neural influences are removed.

Obesity-Hypoventilation Syndrome. Some patients with obesity display chronic hypoventilation with hypoxia, hypercapnia, reduced chemosensitivity, and cor pulmonale. The hypoventilation may partly reflect the response to the increased load of fatty tissue on the chest wall, although hypoventilation is not directly related to the degree of obesity. Independent neural factors, yet undefined, are probably important. A subgroup called pickwickian have obesity, daytime hypoventilation, hypersomnolence, polycythemia, and cor pulmonale. All patients with the pickwickian syndrome probably have sleep apnea.

Breathing Pattern Abnormalities Associated with Neurological Disease. Central neurogenic hyperventilation has been considered a characteristic feature of lower brain stem and upper pontine disease. Rarely is it an isolated finding, as most patients display associated pulmonary complications that could reflexly stimulate the respiratory center through hypoxia or activation of intrapulmonary sensory receptors. Apneustic breathing consists of sustained inspiratory pauses, localizing damage to the mid pons, most commonly due to a basilar artery infarct. Biot's or ataxic breathing, a haphazard random distribution of deep and shallow breaths, is caused by disruption of the respiratory rhythm generator in the medulla.

Cheyne-Stokes respiration is characterized by regular cycles of crescendo-decrescendo changes in tidal volume separated by apneic or hypopneic pauses. Many affected patients have evidence of cardiac or neurological disease. In patients with cardiac disease the disturbance arises because of prolongation of the circulation time, which delays transmission of information concerning arterial Po_2 and Pco_2 to the respiratory centers, thus leading to system instability with resulting oscillations in tidal volume. It has no localizing value in patients with neurological disease but has generally been considered to be an ominous sign. While this is sometimes the case, many patients display subtle evidence of Cheyne-Stokes respiration, especially during sleep, without serious consequences, and it is not an uncommon finding in otherwise normal elderly subjects.

Neuromuscular Disease. Respiratory center function is poorly defined in neuromuscular disease. Decreased ventilatory capacity may result from impaired neural output or poor translation of this neural output into respiratory muscle contraction. Typically, the patients display an increased respiratory rate and inability to take deep breaths, with consequent susceptibility to atelectasis. Paradoxical motion of the rib cage and abdomen is commonly observed. Typical causes include inflammatory polyneuropathy, amyotrophic lateral sclerosis, myasthenia gravis, and poliomyelitis. The features of diaphragmatic paralysis are discussed in Chapter 26.

THE SLEEP APNEA SYNDROME

The sleep apnea syndrome is characterized by daytime hypersomnolence in patients who display at least 30 apneic episodes of 10 seconds or longer during six hours of nocturnal sleep. The apneic episodes are of two types: (1) central apnea due to decreased respiratory center output and manifested by cessation of breathing efforts (Fig. 25–4A) and (2) obstructive apnea due to upper airway obstruction and characterized by continued respiratory efforts, indicated by paradoxical motion of the rib cage and abdomen, during the period of absent airflow (Fig. 25–4B). Commonly both types combine to give mixed apnea. The less common central type usually causes little physiological disturbance, whereas the obstructive variety is accompanied by severe O_2 desaturation with occasional values below 50 per cent (Po_2, 27 torr). Arrhythmias are common and may rarely result in sudden death.

The prevalence of this syndrome is unknown, but it probably affects more than 1 per cent of the general population. The major predisposing con-

FIGURE 25–4. *A,* Central sleep apnea. There is absence of abdominal (ABD) and rib cage (RC) movement, and their sum (V_T), during central apnea associated with a small fall of arterial oxygen saturation (O_2 Sat %) measured by ear oximetry. *B,* Obstructive sleep apnea. This depicts obstructive apnea terminated by deep breaths. Apnea in midportion of recording is marked by absence of sum movements (V_T) despite respiratory efforts indicated by paradoxical movement of rib cage (RC) (movement downward) and abdominal (ABD) (movement upward) compartments that is associated with marked fall in arterial oxygen saturation (O_2 Sat %) measured by ear oximetry. (Reproduced with permission from Tobin MJ, et al.: Breathing abnormalities during sleep. Arch Intern Med 143:1221, 1983.)

ditions can be grouped as (1) neurological states associated with impaired respiratory drive (previously discussed) and (2) conditions associated with upper airway obstruction such as enlarged tonsils and adenoids, retrognathia, fat deposition in obesity, macroglossia associated with acromegaly, myxedema, and Down's syndrome, and nasal packing for nosebleeds or nasal surgery.

Characteristically, these patients have a long history of loud, sonorous snoring, often combined with thrashing movements of the limbs. Repetitive arousals produce sleep deprivation and lead to excessive daytime sleepiness. Many patients are obese, but this is not invariable, and only a small fraction can be classified as pickwickian. Other features of the sleep apnea syndrome include hypertension, morning headache, intellectual deterioration, and reduced libido.

Polysomnography, including the monitoring of the electroencephalogram (EEG), electro-oculogram, motion of the rib cage and abdomen, and arterial O_2 saturation, is required to make a definite diagnosis.

Treatment may include respiratory stimulants, especially medroxyprogesterone, the application of continuous positive airway pressure (CPAP) to the nose, or tracheostomy to bypass the site of upper airway occlusion. In some obese patients, marked weight loss has led to an improvement in the obstruction.

REFERENCES

Hornbein TF: Regulation of Breathing, Parts I and II. New York, Marcel Dekker, Inc., 1981.
Tobin, MJ, Cohn MA, and Sackner MA: Breathing abnormalities during sleep. Arch Intern Med 143:1221–1228, 1983.

26 DISORDERS OF THE PLEURAL SPACE, MEDIASTINUM, AND CHEST WALL

PLEURAL DISEASE

The pleural spaces are defined by the visceral pleura of the lungs and the parietal pleura of the rib cage, diaphragm, and mediastinum. The spaces themselves are potential rather than real,

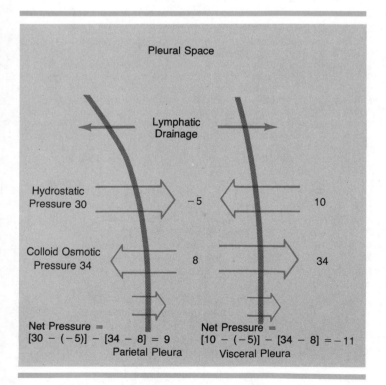

FIGURE 26–1. Factors affecting fluid and solute movement in the pleural space. The blood supply of the parietal pleura is from the intercostal arteries (branches of the systemic circulation), while the visceral pleura is predominantly supplied by the pulmonary circulation, a low-pressure system. Taking into account the osmotic pressure in the parietal and visceral vessels, which are roughly equal, and the changes in intrapleural pressure, fluid flows from the parietal surface into the pleural space and is subsequently reabsorbed by the visceral pleura (indicated pressures are in cm H$_2$0).

since the visceral and parietal pleura are normally separated by only a thin film of fluid.

The lung's elastic recoil pulls the visceral pleura inward, and the chest wall's recoil pulls the parietal pleura outward. The net pressure in the pleural space at functional residual capacity is below atmospheric pressure. In the pleural space fluid flows from the parietal surface into the pleural space, with subsequent reabsorption by the capillaries of the visceral pleura (Fig. 26–1). This system is remarkably well-balanced and ordinarily prevents the collection of significant amounts of fluid despite the formation and absorption of 5 to 10 liters of pleural fluid each day. In addition, fluid and leakage of protein are drained by lymphatics, which can increase their absorptive capacity several-fold.

Fluid accumulates with abnormalities in hydrostatic and osmotic pressure, increased permeability of the capillaries, or lymphatic dysfunction. Pleural inflammation, either infectious or noninfectious, increases permeability and results in the collection of a high-protein pleural fluid. Alterations in the systemic and pulmonary venous pressures, as in heart failure, increase fluid transudation from the parietal capillaries and decrease reabsorption on the visceral side. Decreasing the osmotic pressure (hypoalbuminemia) may also result in more rapid fluid transudation. Finally, lymphatic dysfunction due to anatomical or functional obstruction also facilitates the accumulation of pleural fluid.

PLEURAL EFFUSIONS

Causes of pleural effusions are best considered in terms of the underlying pathophysiology: transudates due to abnormalities of hydrostatic or osmotic pressures, and exudates resulting from increased permeability or trauma (Table 26–1).

Patients present with dyspnea, nonspecific discomfort, or pleuritic chest pain—a sharp, stabbing pain exacerbated by coughing or breathing. Such pain must be carefully differentiated from pericardial or musculoskeletal pain. Rarely, the effusion will be asymptomatic and discovered only on chest x-ray.

Physical examination reveals decreased vocal fremitus, dullness on percussion, and decreased breath sounds over the effusion, with bronchial breathing and egophony at its upper limit. Greater than 250 ml of fluid can be seen on the upright chest x-ray as blunting of the costophrenic angle. Increasing amounts cause dense opacification of the lung fields with a concave meniscus. In certain situations the initial x-ray is misleading and further studies are required: (1) a subpulmonic effusion presenting as an elevated hemidiaphragm can be confirmed on lateral decubitus x-ray; (2) a hazy diffuse density on the supine film in a seriously ill patient will disappear on an upright x-ray; and (3) a loculated effusion, especially with coexisting parenchymal disease, may require ultrasound or CT scan for diagnosis.

Thoracentesis is essential in the differential diagnosis. The gross appearance of the fluid is rarely helpful except when frank blood or the milky fluid of a chylous effusion is encountered. Criteria for the separation of the fluid into transudate and exudate (Table 26–2) are not infallible, and an effusion due to congestive heart failure may occasionally be exudative, while a transudate may occur with malignancy. Pleural fluid glucose concentrations less than 10 to 20 mg/dl are usually diagnostic of rheumatoid arthritis but may be seen in cancer and infection. Pleural fluid amylase is about twice normal in effusions due to pancreatitis and esophageal perforation, while smaller elevations may be seen with malignancy. The presence of a high rheumatoid factor or LE cells in the fluid is strong evidence that the effusion is due to rheumatoid arthritis and systemic lupus erythematosus, respectively. Measurement of pleural fluid pH is usually of little value in the diagnosis and management of empyema.

Surprisingly few red blood cells are required to impart a red color to the fluid, and a hemothorax should be diagnosed only when the pleural fluid hematocrit is greater than 20 per cent. Bloody fluid should arouse suspicion of malignancy, trauma, or pulmonary embolus but may also occur with other disease entities. The number of polymorphonuclear neutrophils is of little or no specific diagnostic value. A high eosinophil count is usually due to air or blood in the pleural space. There is a high probability that an exudate is due to tuberculosis or malignancy if small lymphocytes constitute more than 50 per cent of the white cells. Cytological examinations for malignant cells is positive in about 60 per cent of patients on first thoracentesis, rising to about 80 per cent if three separate samples are obtained. Gram's stain and routine culture should always be done and special stains and cultures added when tuberculosis or fungal disease is suspected. Transcutaneous needle biopsy at the bedside with subsequent histology and culture is positive in over 90 per cent of tuberculous effusions, whereas fluid culture is positive in only 25 per

cent. Although less frequently positive (40 per cent) than cytological examination, biopsy occasionally makes a diagnosis of malignant effusion when cytology is negative.

Treatment depends on the underlying etiology and the degree of physiological impairment. Specific therapy to control the underlying etiology is the only successful approach. Although removal of fluid results in symptomatic improvement, lung volumes and gas exchange improve very little. Parapneumonic effusions resolve with antibiotic therapy (90 per cent), but empyemas, i.e., fluid with positive smear or culture, should be drained by repeated aspirations or tube thoracostomy; otherwise the fluid may spontaneously drain through the chest wall (*empyema necessitans*) or lead to subpleural lung necrosis with resultant bronchopleural fistula and endobronchial spread of infection. Palliative therapy should be considered for a malignant effusion only if the patient is symptomatic and displays benefit from thoracentesis. Repeated thoracentesis should be avoided, as significant protein loss results and the fluid reaccumulates within one to three days. Chemical pleurodesis using intrapleural tetracycline obliterates the pleural space and is helpful in about 80 per cent of malignant effusions.

TABLE 26–1. PLEURAL EFFUSIONS

Transudates
  Congestive heart failure
  Hypoalbuminemia—nephrotic syndrome, starvation, cirrhosis
  Abdominal fluid collection—ascites, peritoneal dialysis
Exudates
  Infection
    Empyema
    Bacterial—Gram-positive and negative, *Actinomyces*, *Mycobacterium tuberculosis*
    Viral—Coxsackie virus, *Mycoplasma*
    Fungal—*Nocardia*, *Coccidioides* (rarely)
    Parasitic—*Amoeba*, *Echinococcus*
    Parapneumonic
  Malignancy—bronchogenic Ca, mesothelioma, lymphoma
        metastatic Ca—breast, ovary, kidney, pancreas, GI tract
  Pulmonary embolism and infarction
  Collagen vascular disease—systemic lupus erythematosus, rheumatoid arthritis
  Intra-abdominal processes—pancreatitis, subphrenic abscess, Meig's syndrome, postabdominal surgery
  Trauma—hemothorax, chylothorax, ruptured esophagus
  Miscellaneous—myxedema, uremia, asbestosis, lymphedema (yellow nail syndrome), drug sensitivity, Dressler's syndrome

TABLE 26–2. DIFFERENTIATION OF EXUDATIVE AND TRANSUDATIVE PLEURAL EFFUSION

	EXUDATE	TRANSUDATE
Protein	>3 g/dl	<3 g/dl
Pleural/serum protein	>0.5	<0.5
LDH	>200 IU/L	<200 IU/L
Pleural/serum LDH	>0.6	<0.6

PNEUMOTHORAX

The most common causes of air in the pleural space are listed in Table 26–3. Idiopathic spontaneous pneumothorax typically causes dyspnea, chest pain, and few abnormalities on physical examination. On chest x-ray, the one-dimensional view grossly underestimates its true volume. Without surgery, 50 per cent develop a recurrence, usually within two years. Unlike the low mortality with idiopathic pneumothorax, that due to underlying lung disease has a 15 per cent mortality rate. Under certain circumstances, particularly in patients on mechanical ventilators, the rent in the pleura forms a one-way valve that permits air to enter but not escape and positive pressure builds up in the chest (tension pneumothorax).

Treatment depends on the amount of air and the underlying status of the patient. Spontaneous pneumothorax in a healthy asymptomatic patient may require no treatment, whereas treatment is required for the same size pneumothorax in a patient with cardiopulmonary insufficiency. Treatment is almost always required for pneumothoraces greater than 50 per cent in size and for a pneumothorax of any size in patients on mechanical ventilation or with diffuse lung disease. Drainage by tube thoracostomy is successful in most instances, and instillation of tetracycline to produce pleurodesis may prevent recurrences. Sometimes open thoracotomy with partial pleurectomy and oversewing of apical blebs or abrasion of the pleural surface is required.

TUMORS OF THE PLEURAL SPACE

Mesotheliomas may be localized, benign growths curable by surgical resection or aggressive, untreatable malignancies spreading extensively in the pleural space and beyond. Malignant mesotheliomas are almost always associated with asbestos exposure. More commonly, neoplasms of the pleural space are due to adjacent spread (bronchogenic carcinoma) or metastatic disease (carcinoma of the breast, ovary, and kidney and lymphoma). These produce bloody pleural effusions, although chylous effusions resulting from lymphatic obstruction are also seen.

TABLE 26–3. CAUSES OF PNEUMOTHORAX

Spontaneous
  Idiopathic
  Emphysema
  Interstitial lung disease
  Eosinophilic granuloma/histiocytosis X
  Cystic fibrosis
  Asthma
  Malignancy
Traumatic
  Penetrating and nonpenetrating chest trauma
  Transbronchoscopic or transthoracic lung biopsy
  Thoracentesis
  Mechanical ventilation
  Esophageal perforation

MEDIASTINAL DISEASE

The mediastinum is bounded by the thoracic outlet, the diaphragm, the sternum, the vertebral column, and the medial borders of the lungs. It contains the heart, esophagus, trachea, lymphatics, thymus gland, and a large number of nerves and blood vessels. Generally, benign mediastinal masses grow slowly, displace surrounding structures, and are painless, whereas malignant lesions invade and compress the important mediastinal structures, giving rise to earlier symptoms such as pain, dysphagia, hoarseness, stridor, cough, and dyspnea and features of Horner's and superior vena cava syndromes. Myasthenia gravis is associated with thymomas, while neurogenic tumors cause spinal cord or nerve compression.

The chest x-ray localizes the process and often suggests the correct diagnosis. CT is invaluable, as it separates vascular from nonvascular lesions and cystic from solid structures and identifies local invasion. Definitive diagnosis often depends on obtaining tissue.

MEDIASTINITIS

Acute mediastinitis is usually due to esophageal perforation or to traumatic rupture of the airway, or rarely to spread of infection from the neck or abdomen. Features are usually typical of mediastinal disease, along with fever, leukocytosis, pneumomediastinum, pneumothorax, and often a pleural effusion. Distinctive features include a high pleural fluid amylase with esophageal perforation and fracture of the first three ribs seen with bronchial rupture. Treatment includes antibiotics, surgical drainage, and closure of the perforated viscus.

Chronic mediastinitis is usually caused by a granulomatous process, most often histoplasmosis, and less frequently by other fungal infections, tuberculosis, and syphilis. Noninfectious causes include sarcoidosis and, in the past, the use of methysergide. An idiopathic cause should be considered only when specific disorders are ruled out. Treatment other than that specifically directed at the underlying disorder, such as surgery, is usually unsuccessful.

MEDIASTINAL MASSES

These are mostly tumors, but also include glandular lesions, vascular abnormalities, and esophageal disease. They are conveniently divided by anatomical location (Fig. 26–2).

CHEST WALL DISEASE

Adequate ventilation depends on efficient movement of the chest wall in response to neural stimulation. Interference with this may result in increased work of breathing, restricted lung volumes, exercise limitation, and gradual progres-

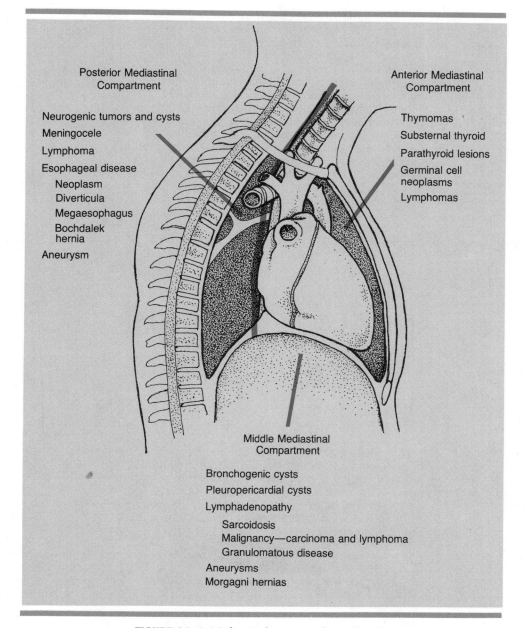

Posterior Mediastinal
Compartment

Neurogenic tumors and cysts
Meningocele
Lymphoma
Esophageal disease
  Neoplasm
  Diverticula
  Megaesophagus
  Bochdalek
  hernia
Aneurysm

Anterior Mediastinal
Compartment

Thymomas
Substernal thyroid
Parathyroid lesions
Germinal cell
neoplasms
Lymphomas

Middle Mediastinal
Compartment

Bronchogenic cysts
Pleuropericardial cysts
Lymphadenopathy

  Sarcoidosis
  Malignancy—carcinoma and lymphoma
  Granulomatous disease
Aneurysms
Morgagni hernias

FIGURE 26–2. Mediastinal masses indicated by their anatomical location.

sion to respiratory failure. Total lung capacity and vital capacity are decreased, but unlike parenchymal restrictive lung disease the residual volume is usually normal or even increased. Hypoventilation is the predominant mechanism of abnormal gas exchange, and thus hypercapnia is found at much higher levels of arterial Po_2 than in parenchymal lung disease. In addition, progressive ventilation-perfusion inequality resulting from basilar atelectasis causes gradual widening of the alveolar-arterial gradient. Continued, prolonged hypoxemia eventually causes cor pulmonale.

Kyphoscoliosis. Kyphoscoliosis is usually idiopathic but may be associated with Marfan's syndrome or poliomyelitis. Most patients are asymp-

tomatic, but respiratory disturbance develops in 1 in 10,000. Surgical correction of the deformity in adults does not influence the incidence of respiratory complications.

Ankylosing Spondylitis. Respiratory failure in the absence of additional parenchymal lung disease is extremely rare. Apical fibrocavity disease develops in rare instances.

Obesity. Patients have a small expiratory reserve volume (ERV) and thus breathe close to residual volume. This leads to decreased ventilation of the lung bases and hypoxemia. This is magnified in the supine posture, which further decreases ERV. These abnormalities may be further complicated by disorders of ventilatory control and upper airway obstruction (see Chapter 25).

Diaphragmatic Paralysis. Causes of unilateral diaphragmatic paralysis include phrenic nerve involvement by tumor, trauma, or herpes zoster, but many are idiopathic in origin. Patients are asymptomatic, with an elevated hemidiaphragm on chest x-ray, a 25 per cent reduction in lung volume, and evidence of hypoxemia on recumbency. Fluoroscopic examination shows paradoxical upward motion of the diaphragm during sniffing. Bilateral diaphragmatic paralysis is rare and may be due to chest trauma, cervical surgery, neuromuscular disease, or phrenic nerve injury during topical cardiac hypothermia employed in cardiopulmonary bypass. Severe orthopnea combined with paradoxical inward motion of the abdomen during inspiration are the clinical hallmarks. Assumption of the supine posture is associated with hypoxemia and a 50 per cent fall in vital capacity, and the ERV may become undetectable.

TREATMENT

Treatment is directed at reversible abnormalities and at minimizing the development of parenchymal lung disease. Respiratory failure develops in some patients, and mechanical ventilation is required. Initially this is particularly valuable during sleep at night, but eventually mechanical ventilation may be required on a continuous basis.

REFERENCES

Bergofsky EH: Respiratory failure in disorders of the thoracic cage: State of the art. Am Rev Respir Dis 119:643–669, 1979.
Heitzman ER: The Mediastinum: Radiologic Correlations with Anatomy and Pathology. St Louis, The C V Mosby Co., 1977.
Light RW: Pleural Diseases. Philadelphia, Lea and Febiger, 1983.

27 INHALATIONAL INJURY

DROWNING AND NEAR-DROWNING

The pathophysiology of near-drowning in both freshwater and saltwater is similar. Survival depends on the pulmonary insult, the amount of hypoxemic brain damage, and the degree of acidosis. A drowning victim responds initially by closing his glottis, and 10 per cent of drowned victims aspirate no fluid but die from asphyxia. The remainder aspirate fluid, develop pulmonary edema and intrapulmonary shunt, and may progress to profound hypoxemia accompanied by a clinical picture identical to the adult respiratory distress syndrome (ARDS). The quantity of aspirated fluid is rarely sufficient to produce a significant change in blood volume. Occasionally, however, near-drowning in hypotonic freshwater can cause transient hypervolemia, whereas hypovolemia may follow hypertonic saltwater aspiration. Alterations in hematocrit or serum electrolytes are rarely life-threatening and not different with either salt- or freshwater near-drowning. Metabolic acidosis develops in 70 per cent of victims. Renal function remains normal in most, but some develop hemoglobinuria, albuminuria, or oliguria and acute tubular necrosis. The cardiovascular system displays remarkable stability, and alterations are primarily a consequence of hypoxemia or acidosis. The likelihood of neurological impairment depends on the duration of immersion and possibly the temperature of the water. Recovery has been reported after submersion in very cold water for up to 40 minutes. This may be due partly to the diving reflex, which is initiated by facial immersion in cold water (<20°C) and re-

sults in severe bradycardia and the shunting of blood to the heart and brain in an attempt to limit hypoxic damage. Additionally, hypothermia lowers O_2 requirements and prolongs the tolerance of the brain and heart to severe hypoxemia.

The most decisive factor in the management of near-drowning victims is resumption of ventilation using mouth-to-mouth resuscitation. Even in victims with evident aspiration of fluid, time should not be wasted in attempting to drain liquid from the lungs, as large volumes are rarely aspirated. In the absence of an effective pulse, closed-chest cardiac resuscitation is required. Admission to hospital is imperative for all surviving victims because the patient's clinical status may belie life-threatening hypoxemia, and supplemental O_2 should be continued until the measurement of $P_{a}O_2$ indicates a satisfactory level. Intubation, mechanical ventilation, and hemodynamic monitoring (as described in Chapter 22) will be required in patients who subsequently develop ARDS. Bronchodilators counteract bronchospasm, and bicarbonate administration is usually necessary to correct metabolic acidosis. Electrolyte disturbances, hemolysis, and renal failure should be treated appropriately. Prophylactic steroid or antibiotic therapy is not indicated. Prognosis is good in patients who are alert or who have a blunted level of consciousness on admission to the emergency room, but poor in those in coma.

SMOKE INHALATION

Pulmonary injury due to inhalation of the thermal, gaseous, or particulate products of combustion is the commonest cause of death in fire injury victims. Two major types of lung injury are observed: thermal injury of the airways, and inhalation of gaseous or particulate matter.

Thermal injury is usually limited to structures above the vocal cords because the airways possess a very efficient cooling system. Combustion (flame) and pyrolysis (smolder) of materials release a complex array of organic acids, aldehydes, and gases that may induce a chemical injury of the airway mucosa with resultant peribronchial edema and bronchoconstriction. Asphyxia may also occur, as the ambient F_IO_2 in the area of a fire usually falls to about 0.10 because combustion uses O_2. Impairment of mucociliary and phagocytic function predisposes to subsequent lung infection. Alveolar damage may result in ARDS but this is uncommon, possibly because the degree of exposure required for ARDS is likely to result in fatal carbon monoxide poisoning. Carbon monoxide is an odorless, tasteless, and colorless gas that does not produce lung injury but has a dual effect on tissue oxygenation. Its marked affinity for hemoglobin (210 times that of O_2) limits the O_2-carrying capacity of blood. In addition, it shifts the O_2 dissociation curve to the left, which impairs O_2 release to the tissues.

Clinical presentation depends on the predominant form of injury. Facial burns and singed nasal hairs should arouse suspicion of lung injury, although pulmonary involvement occurs in only a small proportion of such patients. Thermal injury may produce upper airway obstruction with stridor, hoarseness, and phonation difficulties, necessitating further evaluation (with possible bronchoscopy) and intubation to maintain a patent airway. Lower airway involvement may be associated with the production of carbonaceous sputum, wheezes, and crackles. The chest x-ray is insensitive in the early stages, although pulmonary infiltrates or edema may subsequently develop. Features associated with carbon monoxide intoxication include headache, nausea, fatigue, behavioral change, ataxia, and hypoxic damage to the heart or brain. Cherry red coloration of the lips is usually absent unless the carboxyhemoglobin (COHb) concentration is above 40 per cent. An intoxicated patient displays a normal P_aO_2 and *calculated* O_2 saturation, but there is a severe reduction in O_2 saturation when it is measured. Despite the severe O_2 desaturation, minute ventilation is not increased in carbon monoxide intoxication, as the cartoid body responds to P_aO_2. Confirmation is made by measurement of blood COHb: below 2 per cent in healthy subjects, 5 to 10 per cent in cigarette smokers, and 30 to 50 per cent in fire injury victims.

Management includes removing the victim from exposure, checking vital signs, and establishing a patent airway. Administration of supplemental O_2 relieves hypoxemia and enhances the dissociation of carbon monoxide from hemoglobin, decreasing the half-time for elimination from 300 minutes on room air to 60 minutes with an F_IO_2 of 1.0. In order to achieve an adequate F_IO_2, intubation and mechanical ventilation may be required. The use of hyperbaric O_2 has been suggested for patients with severe CO intoxication, although its advantage over breathing 100 per cent O_2 is unproven. Bronchospasm usually responds to bronchodilators, but corticosteroids may be required if it is severe and unresponsive or severe upper airway obstruction is present. Antibiotics should be prescribed only if there is evidence of infection. In the rare cases in which ARDS supervenes, the management is identical to that described in Chapter 22. Patients surviving the acute clinical course usually recover completely. Long-term complications of tracheal stenosis, bronchiolitis obliterans, or bronchiectasis are rare.

NOXIOUS GASES AND FUMES

Exposure to toxic gases and fumes is an increasing problem in modern industrial society and may cause harm by four basic mechanisms (Table 27–1). Asphyxia occurs when the O_2 in inspired air is displaced by another gas. The commonest mechanism of injury is local irritation, the form and extent of which depend on the concentration, solubility, and duration of exposure to the toxic gas. Highly soluble gases, such as *ammonia*, rapidly injure the mucous membranes of the eye and upper airway, causing an intense burning pain in the eyes, nose, and throat, with lacrimation, rhinorrhea, and a sense of suffocation. This, combined with the strong pungent odor of ammonia, causes the victim to flee from the site of exposure. Lower airway injury is not observed unless the victim is trapped or a massive spill occurs, in

TABLE 27–1. TOXIC GASES AND FUMES

MECHANISM OF INJURY	AGENT	OCCUPATIONAL EXPOSURE
Asphyxia	Carbon dioxide	Mining, foundry work
	Nitrogen	Mining, underwater work
	Carbon monoxide	Mining, petroleum refining, air pollution
	Methane	Mining
Local irritation	Ammonia	Fertilizer, refrigerator, cleaning agents
	Nitrogen dioxide	Farming (silo), fertilizer, welding
	Chlorine	Bleaching, disinfectant
	Sulfur dioxide	Smelting, air pollution
Toxic absorption	Carbon monoxide	Mining, petroleum refining
	Cyanide	Electroplating, fumigants
	"Metal fume fever" (metal oxides)	Welding, galvanizing, smelting
Allergy	Isocyanates	Plastics, paint
	Platinum	Electroplating, photography
	Formalin	Insulation, textiles, chemical manufacturing

which case laryngeal or pulmonary edema may ensue. In contrast, insoluble gases, such as nitrogen dioxide, are distributed to the peripheral airways and usually cause a diffuse lung injury. Exposure to *nitrogen dioxide* is classically encountered in farmers, as large quantities of this gas are formed by fermentation during the first week after filling a silo pit. The victim typically presents with cough, dyspnea, bronchospasm, and weakness, with little evidence of ocular or upper airway irritation. After a lag of one or more hours there may be progression to frank pulmonary edema. Following recovery from the acute illness the patient may develop bronchiolitis obliterans, characterized by progressive dyspnea. Absorption of a toxic gas with systemic consequences is best characterized by carbon monoxide, as discussed under smoke inhalation. Exposure to isocyanate, platinum compounds, or formalin vapors may cause asthma, either immediate or delayed in onset, and is more fully discussed in Chapter 19.

Management of exposure to a toxic gas is generally supportive in nature. The victim should be removed from the source of exposure, and a patent airway with adequate ventilation should be ensured. Correction of hypoxemia may be possible with supplemental O_2, or intubation and mechanical ventilation may be necessary. The patient should be carefully monitored for a delayed reaction to the agent. Additional measures that may be required include bronchodilators and correction of acid-base disturbance and shock. The role of prophylactic antibiotics and steroids remains undetermined, although a trial of steroids is usually employed in patients with bronchiolitis obliterans.

REFERENCES

Fein A, Leff A, and Hopewell PC: Pathophysiology and management of the complications resulting from fire and the inhaled products of combustion: Review of the literature. Crit Care Med 8:94–98, 1980.

Modell JH: Biology of drowning. Ann Rev Med 29:1–8, 1978.

Morgan WKC, and Seaton A: Occupational Lung Diseases. 2nd ed. Philadelphia, WB Saunders Co., 1984.

SECTION III

RENAL DISEASE

28 ESSENTIALS OF NORMAL RENAL FUNCTION

The kidney has one major function: to maintain nearly constant the volume and composition of body fluids. The renal contribution to the homeostasis of body fluids involves a number of individual, specialized renal functions; these include the excretion of metabolic end products and toxins, the regulation of body fluid volume and solute composition, and a number of metabolic and hormonal functions. The kidney thus permits fluctuations in the volume and composition of daily intake as well as safe habitation in a wide range of external environments, all the while maintaining nearly invariant the internal fluid environment of the individual.

Body fluids are confined to discrete "compartments" that are separated by semipermeable barriers. The volume of these individual fluid compartments can be approximated by considering that two thirds of body weight is water, that two thirds of body water is intracellular fluid (ICF), and that the remaining extracellular fluid (ECF) has two thirds of its volume in the interstitium and only one third in the vascular space. Thus, a 70-kg individual has about 46 L of body water, of which about 15 L is in the ECF. The vascular fluid volume, a subcompartment of the ECF, is about 5 L.

The vascular volume is confined by the vascular endothelium, which is permeable to water and small solutes but not to proteins or cells. The intra- and extracellular compartments are separated by cell membranes, which are, with few exceptions, freely permeable to water but impermeable to most solutes. The kidney operates directly on the fluid of the vascular compartment of the ECF to alter its volume and composition. The appropriate movement of water and/or solutes across the compartmental barriers maintains equilibrium among body fluid compartments and allows the kidney to regulate the volume, content, and composition of *all* body fluids.

The major renal functions are conducted by two serial processes: glomerular ultrafiltration and tubular resorption/secretion. The cooperative actions of glomerular filtration and tubular resorption/secretion cause the kidney to process up to 12 times the volume of the extracellular fluid each day in order to excrete a small volume (1 to 2 L) of urine in which wastes and excess solutes are concentrated 100- to 200-fold above the concentrations normally present in plasma water. Both processes are regulated by feedback loops that work through sensors and signals that are both intrinsic to and extrinsic to the kidney.

This chapter will first consider the elements and operation of the functional renal unit, the nephron, which carries out the two processes noted above. It will next describe the individual homeostatic functions maintained by the integrated operation of nephron units.

THE NEPHRON

The nephron is the basic functional unit of the kidney and consists of a specialized capillary vascular bed (the glomerulus) connected to a continuum of specialized epithelial segments (the tubule). Each human kidney has about one million individual nephrons. The glomerular capillary bed is enclosed in a capsule of urinary epithelium that is continuous with the epithelium of the tubule. The tubule has three functional divisions, each of which is composed of a number of discrete anatomical segments. The divisions (Fig. 28–1) are the proximal tubule, divided into a convoluted and a straight portion; the loop of Henle, consisting of thin descending, thin ascending, and thick ascending limbs; and the distal nephron, containing the distal convolutions and the cortical, medullary, and papillary collecting ducts. Nephrons display heterogeneity based on the level in the renal cortex at which the glomerulus lies. Juxtamedullary nephrons have larger glomeruli and their loops of Henle descend deep into the renal papillae. Superficial nephrons have smaller glomeruli and shorter loops of Henle with a more shallow medullary penetration.

The juxtaglomerular apparatus (JGA) is a distinctive region of the nephron composed of both tubular and vascular elements. The macula densa is a cluster of specialized epithelial cells that marks the beginning of the distal tubule and represents the tubular component of the JGA. The macula densa of each nephron makes contact with the vascular pole of its glomerulus. Cells of the afferent and efferent arterioles and distinctive extraglomerular mesangial cells comprise the remainder of the JGA. Adrenergic nerve fibers make contact with the vascular elements of the JGA.

The JGA is the site of renin synthesis and secretion within the kidney. Three sets of stimuli may contribute to renin release by the JGA. The sodium or chloride content of tubular fluid passing the macula densa may determine some part of renin release. The degree of volume- or pressure-mediated stretch of the vascular elements of the JGA may also influence renin secretion. Finally, direct adrenergic stimulation may be a regulatory factor in renin secretion.

The work of the nephron can be considered in relation to the functional anatomy of the nephron. The glomerulus, by delivering a pure ultrafiltrate of plasma to the tubule, supplies the substrate for urine formation. The proximal tubule reclaims the bulk, about two thirds, of the volume of the ultrafiltrate by a process that does not alter the tonicity of the intratubular fluid but does change its composition. The loop of Henle absorbs less than one fifth of the ultrafiltrate volume but does so by separating the absorption of salt from water.

This differential absorption sets the stage for urinary dilution and concentration. Finally, the distal tubule, which handles less than 15 per cent of the ultrafiltrate volume, performs the final adjustments to urine composition and volume.

The Glomerulus

Blood flow enters the kidney by a single renal artery which, after several divisions, supplies the arcuate arteries that lie at the junction of the renal cortex and medulla. From this vascular arc, non-anastomosing interlobular arteries radiate into the cortex and directly supply the glomerular capillaries through afferent arterioles. The glomerular capillary bed is drained by a second muscular vessel, the efferent arteriole. This unique suspension of a capillary network between two resistance vessels, as opposed to the arteriole-capillary-venule arrangement of other tissues, makes possible the fine regulation of blood flow and maintenance of high intracapillary hydrostatic pressures that drive ultrafiltration across the glomerular capillary wall.

Renal blood flow is maintained nearly constant over a wide range of mean aortic pressure. Renal autoregulation of blood flow preserves glomerular blood flow in hypotensive states and protects the glomerulus from pressure injury and hyperfiltration in most hypertensive states. Part of this autoregulatory response includes the action of the intrinsic renal vasoconstrictor angiotensin II (AII); the effect of opposing vasodilating renal prostaglandins, PGE_2 and PGI_2; and the contractile response of the glomerular mesangium.

Glomerular ultrafiltration occurs as a result of an outwardly directed net pressure that moves fluid across the semipermeable capillary wall. Net ultrafiltration pressure (P_{UF}) is the sum of Starling forces across the capillary wall and can be expressed as:

$$P_{UF} = (P_{GC} + \pi_{US}) - (\pi_{GC} + P_{US}).$$

Glomerular capillary hydrostatic pressure ($P_{GC} \sim 45$ mm Hg) plus the colloid osmotic (oncotic) pressure (π_{US}) of the urinary space favors fluid movement from capillary to urinary space. Since negligible quantities of protein enter the urinary space, π_{US} is normally zero. The hydrostatic pressure of the urinary space ($P_{US}, \sim 10$ mm Hg) plus the mean glomerular capillary oncotic pressure (π_{GC}) opposes ultrafiltration. The values for P_{GC} and P_{US} are relatively constant along the length of the capillary bed, while the value of π_{GC} rises progressively as protein-free fluid exits, causing capillary protein concentrations to rise. As a consequence of ultrafiltration, the value of π_{GC} rises from about 20 mm Hg at the afferent end of the glomerular capillary to nearly 35 mm Hg at the efferent end.

The glomerular filtration rate (GFR) can then be expressed as:

$$GFR = K_f(\Delta P - \pi_{GC}),$$

where ΔP is the net hydrostatic pressure that favors ultrafiltration ($P_{GC} - P_{US}$) and π_{GC} is the

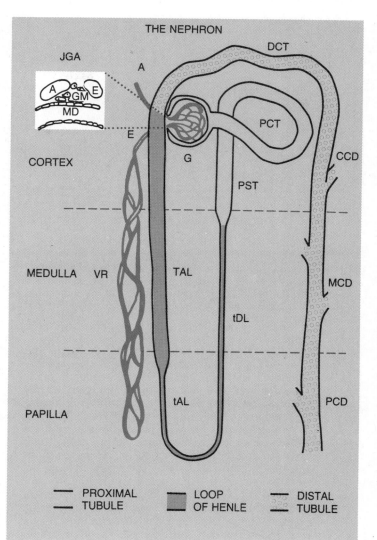

FIGURE 28–1. Functional and anatomical divisions of the nephron. PCT, Proximal convoluted tubule; PST, proximal straight tubule; tDL, thin descending limb; tAL, thin ascending limb; TAL, thick ascending limb; DCT, distal convoluted tubule; CCD/M CD/PCD, cortical/medullary/papillary collecting ducts; JGA, juxtaglomerular apparatus; A, afferent arteriole; E, efferent arteriole; G, glomerulus; GM, extraglomerular matrix; MD, macula densa; VR, vasa recta.

mean oncotic pressure in the glomerular capillary that retards ultrafiltration. K_f is a factor that expresses the permeability of the glomerular ultrafiltration barrier and the surface area of the capillary bed available for ultrafiltration.

Clinically important alterations in GFR may result from changes in the hydrostatic pressure gradient (ΔP), which result from changes in the tone in the afferent and/or efferent arterioles or from changes in hydrostatic pressure in the tubule lumen. Afferent and efferent arteriolar tone is regulated, in part, by the opposing influences of vasoconstrictors (AII) and vasodilators (PGE_2, PGI_2). GFR can also be altered by changes in the rate of rise of the glomerular capillary protein concentration. Finally, changes in the permeability or surface area of the glomerular capillary bed will affect the GFR.

GLOMERULAR FILTRATION BARRIER

US
EPI
GBM
ENDO
H₂O   PROTEIN   UREA   NaCl
CAPILLARY LUMEN

FIGURE 28–2. Elements of the glomerular capillary wall, showing filtration paths of water and small solute and rejection of protein. EPI, urinary epithelial cell; GBM, glomerular basement membrane; ENDO, capillary endothelial cell; US, urinary space: ɪɪɪɪɪɪɪɪ. polyanion coating; ⊠. GBM anionic clusters.

The *glomerular capillary filtration barrier* has three main components (Fig. 28–2): the capillary endothelial cell, the capillary basement membrane, and the urinary epithelial cell. During ultrafiltration, water and small solutes in plasma water move freely into the urinary space. The concentration of any small solute in the urinary space is equal to its free concentration in plasma water (PW); i.e., $[NaCl]_{PW} = [NaCl]_{US}$. By contrast, all cells and most macromolecules (proteins) are totally excluded from passage into the urinary space. The basis for this discriminatory nature of glomerular ultrafiltration is in the unique structural arrangement and chemical composition of the ultrafiltration barrier.

The glomerular basement membrane (GBM) appears to be the structure that limits passage of solute into the urinary space based on the molecular radius of the solute. The GBM is a hydrated gel of intertwined collagenous fibers and can be pictured as containing water-filled channels of 2 to 4 nm radius. Passage of solutes with molecular radii of 2 to 4 nm is progressively restricted, and molecules of greater than 4.0 to 4.2 nm radius do not appear in the glomerular ultrafiltrate. Owing to clusters of anion-rich macromolecules both within the GBM and lining the epithelial and endothelial cell margins, a further restriction to filtration is placed on macromolecules that carry a net negative charge. The negative charge of the filtration barrier provides an explanation for the fact that anionic albumin, which has a molecular radius (3.6 nm) less than the limiting pore size of 4.0 to 4.2 nm, does not normally enter the urinary space.

The Proximal Tubule

The primary function of the proximal tubule is bulk isosmotic reabsorption of ultrafiltrate. Under normal, euvolemic conditions, about two thirds of ultrafiltrate volume is absorbed in the proximal tubule. A major feature of this absorptive process is its adaptability to changes in extracellular fluid volume. When ECF volume is reduced, with no change in GFR, the percentage of ultrafiltrate absorbed in the proximal tubule increases, sometimes up to 80 per cent. Conversely, ECF volume expansion leads to a fall in fractional absorption in the proximal tubule so that only 40 per cent of the ultrafiltrate may be absorbed. Alterations in the rate of absorption in the proximal tubule result in delivery of greater or lesser volumes of isotonic fluid to the loop of Henle, where solute and water absorption are separated. The relation between proximal tubular fluid absorption and distal delivery of ultrafiltrate is useful in understanding the renal response to certain systemic diseases and in managing certain types of renal dysfunction.

A number of solutes undergo nearly complete reabsorption in the proximal tubule. Active H^+ secretion leads to reclamation of the vast majority of the filtered bicarbonate (Fig. 28–3). By a mechanism coupled to active sodium absorption, glucose, amino acids, and other organic solutes are completely resorbed in this segment. The proximal tubule is responsible for the bulk of phosphate reabsorption. Calcium is absorbed in parallel with sodium in the proximal tubule. In the more distal, straight portion of the proximal tubule, secretion of organic acids, including uric acid and drugs such as penicillins, occurs.

The Loop of Henle

The loop of Henle begins at the corticomedullary junction with the thin descending limb, continues around a hairpin turn as the thin ascending limb, and becomes the thick ascending limb in the outer medulla. The segment ends in the macula densa at the level of the glomerulus from which it originated. Each segment of the loop has different permeabilities to sodium chloride and water, so that about 15 per cent of the volume of the isosmotic ultrafiltrate is absorbed but about 25 per cent of the sodium chloride is absorbed. This differential absorption converts the isotonic fluid entering from the proximal tubule into a dilute (hypotonic to plasma) fluid delivered to the distal tubule. This dilution of tubular fluid occurs regardless of the final concentration of the urine. The net salt abstraction is important in establishing the medullary interstitial hypertonicity required for urinary concentration. In addition, a major portion of calcium absorption occurs in the loop of Henle.

Salt and water movement across the thin limbs is passive, driven by osmotic gradients that change from the corticomedullary junction to the papillary tip (Fig. 28–3). The thin descending limb is water-permeable but has a low permeability to sodium chloride. The tubular fluid reaches osmotic equilibrium with the surrounding hypertonic interstitium by passive water movement out of the tubule. The thin ascending limb is impermeable to water but has a high permeability to sodium chloride. As fluid rounds

SEGMENTAL NEPHRON FUNCTION

FIGURE 28–3. Major transport functions of each nephron segment, including representative osmolalities (color) in vasa recta, interstitium, and tubule at different levels within kidney. Glu, Glucose; OA, organic acid.

the bend of the loop, salt diffuses passively into the interstitium while water remains inside the tubular lumen. As the fluid ascends inside the thin ascending limb, it remains in osmotic equilibrium with the interstitium and becomes more dilute as salt is abstracted.

The thick ascending limb absorbs sodium chloride by an active, energy-dependent process. Since the thick ascending limb is also impermeable to water, the luminal fluid leaving the thick ascending limb is made hypotonic with respect to plasma by active salt absorption. In addition, the transfer of sodium chloride from the tubule lumen to the interstitium is the primary step that allows a multiplication process to build and maintain interstitial hypertonicity. Since a high solute concentration in the medullary interstitium is necessary to absorb water from the terminal nephron, this portion of salt absorption is critical in determining maximum urinary concentrating ability.

The hairpin arrangement of the loop, with flow in descending and ascending limbs directed in opposite directions, minimizes the work needed to maintain a papillary osmolality of 1200 mOsm/kg H_2O compared to the 300 mOsm/kg H_2O osmolality of the cortex. In addition, the vasa recta, capillaries that branch from juxtamedullary glomerular efferent arterioles, has a similar counter-

current flow into and out of the papillae. The parallel flow of blood and tubular fluid allows sodium chloride absorbed from the loop of Henle and urea absorbed from the papillary collecting duct to be trapped within the interstitium at increasing concentrations. The anatomic arrangement and orderly regulation of vasa recta blood flow are essential to the concentrating ability of the kidney.

The Distal Nephron

Two distinct functional segments make up the distal portion of the nephron. The distal convoluted tubule is a water-impermeable cortical structure that continues the dilution of luminal fluid through active sodium chloride absorption. Since the cortical interstitium remains isotonic to plasma, salt absorption from cortical portions of the thick ascending limb or the distal convoluted tubule affects only urinary dilution but not urinary concentration. Potassium secretion and H^+ secretion are also seen in the distal convolution. Calcium absorption continues in this nephron segment.

The collecting ducts (cortical, medullary, and papillary) are the primary sites of antidiuretic hormone (ADH) action (Fig. 28–3). They are virtually impermeable to water in the absence of ADH and, in that circumstance, can deliver the hypotonic (50 to 100 mOsm/kg H_2O) fluid issuing from the distal convoluted tubule unchanged into the urine. When ADH is present, water passes across the tubule wall readily and the luminal fluid tonicity approaches that of the interstitium at any level. Thus, a fluid of 100 mOsm/kg H_2O entering the cortical collecting duct reaches 300 mOsm/kg H_2O (the cortical interstitial tonicity) by the beginning of the medullary collecting duct. Likewise, fluid in the papillary collecting duct will approach the tonicity of the interstitium at the papillary tip. The effect of ADH on collecting ducts is modulated by intrinsic renal prostaglandins. PGE_2 reduces the ADH-induced increase in collecting duct water permeability.

Distal nephron segments reabsorb sodium and secrete protons (H^+) and potassium. All three processes are stimulated by aldosterone. Active sodium absorption increases the lumen-negative voltage of the distal convoluted tubule and collecting ducts. In states of volume depletion and maximal aldosterone production, the urine can be rendered virtually free of sodium. Parathyroid hormone increases calcium absorption in the distal nephron. At this point, sodium and calcium resorption are independently mediated by different hormones.

Potassium secretion begins in the late distal convoluted tubule and continues through the collecting ducts. Potassium is concentrated within tubule cells by the energy-consuming (Na^+ + K^+)-ATPase located on basolateral membranes. The activity of this enzyme "pump" is increased by potassium loading and by aldosterone. Potassium secretion proceeds by diffusion of the intracellular cation down both concentration and electrical gradients into the tubule lumen. Increases in the flow rate of fluid in the distal nephron increase potassium secretion by keeping the concentration gradient from cell to tubule lumen at a maximum. Both an increase in the delivery of sodium to the distal nephron and an increase in aldosterone activity increase the rate of sodium absorption and thereby increase the lumen-negative voltage that favors potassium diffusion from tubule cells. The presence in the distal nephron of poorly absorbed anions (sulfate, penicillins) also increases the lumen-negative voltage and increases potassium secretion.

Proton (H^+) secretion in the distal nephron allows absorption of any bicarbonate present in this segment, thereby completing reclamation of filtered bicarbonate. The major contribution of the distal nephron to acid-base homeostasis is the generation of new bicarbonate. Within tubule cells, the reaction

$$CO_2 + H_2O \rightleftarrows H_2CO_3 \rightleftarrows H^+ + HCO_3^-$$

takes place. The protons (H^+) are secreted into the tubular fluid and are buffered by phosphate ($Na_2HPO_4 + H^+ \rightarrow NaH_2PO_4 + Na^+$) or ammonia ($NH_3 + H^+ \rightarrow NH_4^+$). In addition, the collecting duct can maintain an intraluminal free H^+ concentration 1000 times that of blood, i.e., urine pH 4.4 versus plasma pH 7.4. The bicarbonate generated within the cell diffuses into the blood to replenish the bicarbonate consumed during buffering of nonvolatile acids. The quantity of new bicarbonate added to body fluids amounts to about 1 mEq HCO_3^- per kg of body weight per day under usual conditions of dietary intake and metabolism.

Summary

The kidney regulates the volume and composition of the extracellular fluids by modifying an ultrafiltrate of plasma water. The majority of this ultrafiltrate is returned to the circulation by selective tubular reabsorption. A very small portion of the ultrafiltrate is excreted as urine, carrying with it the undesirable or excess solutes that threaten the homeostatic balance of body fluids.

The proximal tubule absorbs the bulk of the ultrafiltrate volume, and almost all of the filtered glucose, amino acids, and bicarbonate, by a process that leaves the tubular fluid isotonic to plasma. The volume of proximal tubular absorption is influenced by changes in GFR and ECF volume. The loop of Henle, through its unique structure, separates the absorption of salt and water and sets the conditions for urinary dilution or concentration. The distal nephron is regulated by specific hormones and establishes the final composition of the urine. ADH activity determines the osmotic concentration of urine by governing H_2O absorption in the collecting ducts. Aldosterone regulates sodium, potassium, and hydrogen concentrations in the urine.

RENAL HOMEOSTATIC FUNCTIONS

The contribution of the kidney to maintaining a constant internal environment can be categorized in a number of ways. Table 28–1 presents one such list. It is evident that a given renal function may overlap these homeostatic categories. For instance, salt and water absorption contribute to both volume and blood pressure regulation. This section will describe these homeostatic functions.

Renal homeostasis operates to maintain each component of body fluid composition within a narrow range of values. In order to achieve this end, the kidney must match urinary output of any substance to total intake, regardless of the rate of glomerular filtration. Figure 28–4A demonstrates

TABLE 28–1. HOMEOSTATIC FUNCTIONS OF THE KIDNEY

Waste/toxin excretion
Extracellular fluid volume regulation
Body fluid osmolar regulation
Blood pressure regulation
Acid-base regulation
Mineral regulation
Metabolic and hormonal regulation

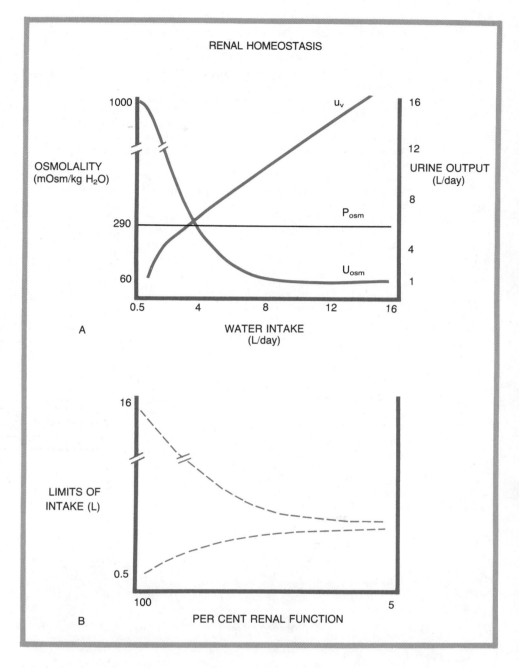

FIGURE 28–4. *A*, Maintenance of nearly constant body water balance (P_{osm}, black line) by increasing renal excretion of solute-free water (U_v and U_{osm}, blue lines) as water intake (abscissa) increases. *B*, Decreasing tolerance of range of water intake (ordinate) as range of urinary water excretion (dotted lines) converges on a fixed value during progressive decrease in renal function (abscissa).

this principle applied to body water homeostasis, which is estimated via the plasma osmolality. The plasma osmolality is maintained nearly invariant (<2 per cent variation) by the excretion of a small volume of highly concentrated urine when water intake is curtailed, or the excretion of large volumes of maximally dilute urine when water intake is great. The kidney rapidly adjusts renal water excretion so that the volume of solute-free water in urine is equal to the volume of water ingested over any short time period.

A second important facet of renal homeostasis is illustrated in Figure 28–4*B*. Again, water balance is used as an example. When renal function (GFR plus tubular function) is totally normal, the kidney can maintain homeostasis despite a wide

range of intake. For the case of water regulation, the kidney accommodates ingestion of as much as 16 to 18 L daily or as little as 0.5 L daily without perturbation of total body water balance (Fig. 28–4*A*). However, as renal function decreases, the kidney's ability to excrete excess ingested water or to conserve water when intake is reduced is diminished. Thus, the *range* of tolerable intake is progressively narrowed and approaches a fixed value. At minimally tolerable levels of renal function, body homeostasis is maintained only by regulating intake at some nearly invariant level.

Waste/Toxin Excretion

One of the most obvious functions of the kidney is to eliminate endogenous end products of metabolism as well as exogenous toxins and drugs from the circulation. Two nitrogenous metabolic products—urea, derived from protein/amino acid catabolism, and creatinine, derived from muscle creatine metabolism—are used as the major clinical markers of intact renal excretory function.

As indicated above, glomerular filtration is the first step in the elimination of most substances by the kidney. Since homeostatic requirements necessitate the maintenance of low concentrations of most metabolic end products and toxins within the circulation, very large volumes of ultrafiltrate formation are needed to deliver into the urine the absolute quantity of material requiring excretion. The production of up to 180 L/24 hr of glomerular ultrafiltrate makes possible the mass elimination of a compound normally present in a low concentration in plasma. Once in the ultrafiltrate, the tubule need only not reabsorb the compound while the majority of ultrafiltrate volume (99 to 99.5 per cent) is reclaimed. By this means, a daily urine output of 900 to 1800 ml can contain waste products concentrated 100- to 200-fold above their concentration in plasma.

A second means of solute entry into the urine is via tubular secretion. Organic acids (such as urate, citrate, and lactate) and organic bases (such as creatinine) can be taken up by proximal tubular cells from capillary blood and secreted directly into the tubular fluid. A large number of drugs, including antibiotics and diuretics, are also eliminated via these transport processes. In most cases, the secretory process and the filtration process work in concert to clear the blood of the particular substance. However, for substances that are protein-bound and have a low free-solution concentration for ultrafiltration, the secretory process may be the major means of elimination.

Extracellular Fluid Volume Regulation

About 60 per cent of body weight, or about 42 liters in a 70-kg individual, is water. Approximately one third of that volume is contained in the extracellular (blood vessels plus interstitium) fluid (ECF) compartment. Since sodium salts account for almost 90 per cent of the solute in this compartment, the ECF volume can be considered, for practical purposes, to be composed of isotonic saline. Operationally, the kidney regulates NaCl absorption as the primary adjustment to ECF volume. The requisite water absorption needed to maintain an isotonic state is controlled by osmotic regulatory influences.

Renal NaCl absorption is controlled by the volume regulatory scheme depicted in Figure 28–5. Both extrarenal and intrarenal systems act to regulate salt absorption from proximal and distal nephron sites.

Baroreceptors in the atria, pulmonary vessels, aortic arch, and carotid bifurcations sense volume changes in the vascular compartment of the ECF. Sending signals to the CNS via cranial nerves IX and X, these receptors influence peripheral sympathetic nerve activity. Sympathetic tone, in turn, regulates renal perfusion pressure, renal vascular tone, glomerular blood flow, and proximal tubular fluid absorption. In addition to changes in sympathetic nerve activity, systemic vasoactive hormones such as vasopressin and angiotensin II are released into the circulation. ECF volume contraction, operating through the above hemodynamic and direct tubular influences, causes an increase in fractional volume absorption in the proximal nephron with little or no change in GFR.

Through increased sympathetic tone, the direct influence of efferent arteriolar pressure, and the

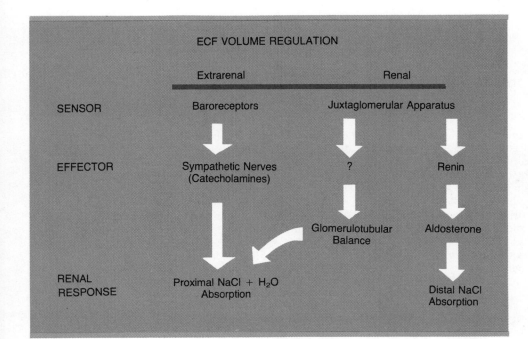

FIGURE 28–5. Scheme of renal regulation of extracellular fluid volume.

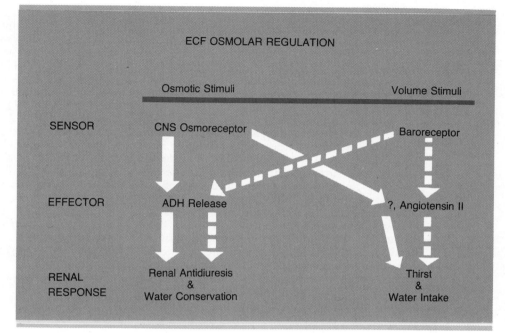

FIGURE 28–6. Scheme of renal regulation of extracellular fluid osmolality.

composition of tubular fluid leaving the loop of Henle, the juxtaglomerular apparatus (JGA) is stimulated to increase the rate of renin secretion. Intrarenal angiotensin II (AII) further regulates renal and glomerular hemodynamics. In addition, AII stimulates aldosterone secretion by the adrenal gland. Under the influence of aldosterone, it is possible for sodium to be reclaimed almost completely from the distal tubular fluid.

In conditions in which the intake of sodium is negligible or in the repair of ECF volume losses (hemorrhage, emesis), the renal excretion of sodium is nearly zero and the defense of ECF volume maximal. This is accomplished by an increase in NaCl and water absorption by the proximal tubule, resulting in delivery of a reduced volume to the distal nephron. This decreased distal delivery, coupled to the aldosterone-dependent increase in distal nephron sodium avidity, makes possible the complete recovery of sodium from the urine.

When ECF volume is expanded, proximal tubular absorption of sodium and water is decreased and aldosterone secretion is suppressed. In addition, a polypeptide natriuretic factor that originates from the right atrium may augment renal sodium excretion in certain volume-expanded and hypertensive states. The predominant mode of action of atrial natriuretic factor appears to be an alteration of renal hemodynamics that leads to an increase in the filtered load of NaCl. In this case, a greater delivery of NaCl to the distal nephron is coupled to a hormonal environment that does not favor sodium absorption. As a result, more sodium is lost in the urine and the excess ECF volume is eliminated.

Body Fluid Osmolar Regulation

Body fluid osmolality, the ratio of solute to water in all fluid compartments, is maintained within a very narrow range. Unlike volume regulation, which is keyed to renal handling of sodium, osmolar balance depends on close renal regulation of ECF water. Since water moves freely across most cell membranes, the osmolality of intracellular fluid is dictated by water balance in extracellular fluids. Therefore, the kidney is able to regulate the osmolality of all body fluids via adjustments of water balance in the ECF.

ECF osmolality is regulated by dual pathways in the water repletion reaction, as shown in Figure 28–6. The primary sensing element in this system is the CNS osmoreceptor, located along the wall of the third ventricle. Osmoreceptor cells sense as little as 1 to 2 per cent change in the osmolality of blood in the internal carotid circulation. Neuronal signals from osmoreceptors stimulate the release of ADH from the posterior pituitary gland and simultaneously stimulate the sensation of thirst. The former action, ADH release, causes water conservation in the kidney by increasing water permeability and water absorption in collecting ducts. The latter response, thirst, leads to an increase in water intake. An excess of body water has the opposite effect. ADH release and thirst are suppressed, dilute fluid from the loop of Henle passes through the collecting ducts unchanged, and the excess water is excreted. Because of the high sensitivity of the osmotic regulation of renal water absorption, the sodium chloride absorbed in operation of the ECF volume regulatory scheme is accompanied by a volume of water sufficient to maintain isotonicity of the extracellular fluid.

When the ECF volume is reduced by about 10 per cent (Fig. 28–6), however, water repletion is activated as a means of replenishing ECF volume irrespective of ECF osmolality. In this case, baroreceptors in the venous and arterial circulations stimulate ADH release through neuronal pathways. This nonosmotic stimulation of ADH release occurs independently of osmoreceptor function. Thirst is also stimulated, probably by increased generation of angiotensin II. The volume stimulus to ADH secretion can override osmoregulation via osmoreceptors, and water will be resorbed by the kidney even in the face of continuing dilution of body fluids.

Successful osmoregulation depends on the normal function of nephron segments proximal to the collecting ducts, regardless of the level of circulating ADH. Adequate volumes of filtrate must be delivered to the loop of Henle to form the quantity of solute-free water needed for excretion in states of body water excess. Excessive filtrate delivery may hinder the ability of the loop of Henle to dilute the tubular fluid. The loop of Henle itself must be intact to dilute the luminal fluid maximally when water excretion is required or to set medullary hypertonicity at a maximum when water resorption is needed. The highly ordered medullary structure of countercurrent tubular fluid and blood flow must also be intact in order to maintain medullary hypertonicity.

Blood Pressure Regulation

The two major renal inputs into the complex scheme of blood pressure regulation are through control of ECF volume and generation of vasoactive compounds. Because virtually all types of hypertension are ultimately responsive to changes in ECF volume, there must be some degree of impairment in the renal regulation of the ECF volume in many types of hypertension. In these cases, the maintenance of salt balance appears to depend on a "resetting" of the mean arterial pressure to a higher level. The role of the kidney in setting total systemic vascular resistance through the control of vasoactive substances, particularly angiotensin II, is well-documented in some forms of hypertension.

The renal response to hypotension, sensed either at central vascular baroreceptors or at the renal efferent arteriole, is the generation and release of renin. Renin enzymatically converts plasma angiotensinogen into angiotensin I, which is converted into the potent vasoconstrictor angiotensin II (AII). The latter (AII) increases systemic vascular resistance and blood pressure. Angiotensin II stimulation of aldosterone secretion ultimately complements the vasoconstrictor effect through aldosterone-dependent augmentation of sodium absorption and an increase in ECF volume. Restoration of blood pressure may allow relaxation of this response, or maintenance of blood pressure may become dependent on its continuation.

The role of the kidney in decreasing systemic vascular tone is far less certain. Two potent vasodepressor substances, prostaglandins and kinins, are produced in the kidney. These compounds, however, probably act only as intrarenal vasodilators and have little or no systemic effect.

Acid-Base Regulation

The kidney contributes to acid-base homeostasis by the reclamation in the proximal tubule of the bulk of the filtered load of bicarbonate, and by the generation in the distal tubule of new bicarbonate, which replenishes the body buffer stores. Both bicarbonate reclamation and generation depend on the active secretion of hydrogen ion by the respective tubule segments (Fig. 28–7).

The filtered load of bicarbonate buffer amounts

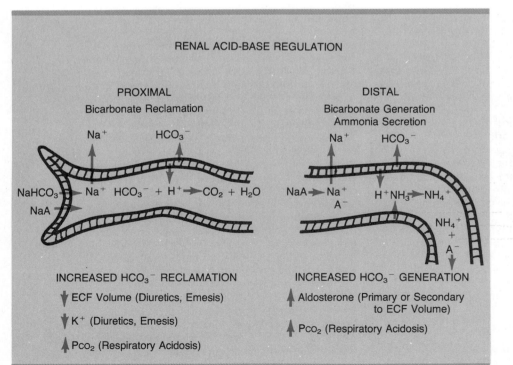

FIGURE 28–7. Scheme of renal acid-base regulation with representative reactions in both proximal and distal tubules.

to about 4500 mEq daily. The proximal tubule has an apparent maximal reabsorptive rate for bicarbonate that can be increased by ECF volume depletion. Rates of bicarbonate reabsorption in the proximal tubule are also increased by an increase in P_{CO_2}, as occurs in chronic respiratory acidosis, or by hypokalemia. Conversely, ECF volume expansion or a lowering of P_{CO_2}, as seen in respiratory alkalosis, lowers the proximal tubular resorptive rate for bicarbonate. ECF volume contraction, an elevation of P_{CO_2}, and hypokalemia permit the maintenance of an increase in serum bicarbonate concentrations by increasing the rate of proximal tubular bicarbonate absorption. In contrast, ECF volume expansion and a lowered P_{CO_2} permit a reduction in serum bicarbonate concentrations.

As nonvolatile acid is formed from metabolic processes, bicarbonate is consumed in buffering the acid in the ECF. The acid anion is filtered at the glomerulus as a sodium salt. In the distal nephron, H^+ is secreted in an amount equal to the amount of filtered acid anion. This H^+ is excreted in phosphate or ammonium buffer, or as free proton. Simultaneously, an equivalent amount of bicarbonate is made available for addition to blood, thereby replenishing the bicarbonate consumed in the original buffering reaction. About 50 to 70 mEq of acid is processed daily in this manner. Factors that increase H^+ secretion in the distal nephron, such as aldosterone or an elevated P_{CO_2}, may lead to the addition of an amount of bicarbonate to blood that is in excess of the amount consumed in buffering metabolic acids.

Mineral Regulation

The kidney maintains the composition of the ECF with respect to a number of minerals. This section will consider the three most important of these: potassium, calcium, and magnesium. Potassium, the major intracellular cation, is freely filtered at the glomerulus and undergoes resorption along the length of the proximal nephron. In the distal nephron, potassium is secreted under the control of several influences. As noted above, aldosterone promotes potassium secretion in association with sodium absorption. Two other factors are also important determinants of the rate of potassium secretion. Distal nephron potassium secretion increases as the rate of fluid flow through the distal nephron increases and as the absolute amount of sodium delivered to the distal tubule increases. Thus, it is not surprising that the administration of diuretics that inhibit the absorption of sodium in the loop of Henle is associated with an increase in potassium secretion.

Conservation of potassium is less well-regulated. While sodium can be virtually eliminated from the urine when aldosterone is present, the minimum urinary concentration of K^+ is seldom less than 10 to 12 mEq/L. Only when body and cellular potassium stores are severely depleted does the renal conservation of potassium become maximal.

Since about 40 per cent of total serum calcium is protein-bound, the concentration of calcium in glomerular ultrafiltrate equals only about 60 per cent that of total serum calcium. The bulk of calcium, about 60 per cent, is absorbed in the proximal tubule in parallel with sodium. Factors that change fractional proximal tubular reabsorption greatly influence calcium excretion. The separation of calcium and sodium absorption occurs in the distal nephron. Parathyroid hormone (PTH) governs the rate of calcium absorption in this nephron segment.

While PTH-dependent calcium absorption acts efficiently to correct hypocalcemia, the renal response to hypercalcemia is less satisfactory. If PTH is suppressed, the only way to augment calcium excretion is by increasing sodium excretion. However, hypovolemia, which often is associated with hypercalcemic states, may trigger renal sodium conservation and further increase the tubular reabsorption of calcium. In addition, elevations of serum calcium to 12 to 15 mg/dl may suppress GFR and further limit the urinary excretion of calcium.

Magnesium is absorbed in the proximal tubule at a rate less than that of sodium absorption. The loop of Henle accounts for the majority of magnesium absorption. Both decreases in fractional proximal tubular absorption (ECF volume expansion) and decreases in loop of Henle NaCl absorption (diuretics) increase the excretion of magnesium. Renal loss of magnesium is a common cause of hypomagnesemia, and hypermagnesemia is almost always the result of severe decreases in GFR.

Renal Metabolic and Hormonal Regulation

The kidney contributes to the metabolic degradation of a number of peptide hormones, including most pituitary hormones, glucagon, and insulin. Decreased renal catabolism of insulin in diabetics with renal insufficiency may be manifest as a prolongation of the effect of exogenous insulin.

Aside from regulation of calcium excretion, the kidney plays a major role in total calcium metabolism. Vitamin D, cholecalciferol, requires two *in vivo* hydroxylations to become the potent hormone that regulates intestinal calcium absorption. The first hydroxylation occurs in the liver at position 25 of the molecule, while the second hydroxylation occurs in the kidney. Depending on the state of calcium balance, PTH levels, and intracellular phosphorus levels, renal proximal tubule cells may add a second hydroxyl ion at the 1-position of the molecule. This hydroxylation yields 1,25-dihydroxycholecalciferol, the potent hormonal form of the vitamin. Renal hydroxylation at all other sites on the molecule yields other metabolites whose biological activities are less well-defined.

The kidney is the major site for production of an erythrocyte-promoting factor, erythropoietin. Erythropoietin production increases in states of decreased tissue O_2 delivery. This may occur as a result of chronic hypoxemia, as is seen in patients living in high altitudes or with lung disease; decreased O_2-carrying capacity of blood, as is seen in anemic individuals; or decreased blood flow to the kidney, as is seen in chronic renal insufficiency.

SUMMARY

This chapter has introduced the individual elements of renal function performed by the specialized renal unit, the nephron. A segmental functional anatomy of the nephron can be used to describe its work. Bulk glomerular ultrafiltration allows large quantities of a solute to enter the urine while maintaining a low serum concentration of that solute. The proximal tubule resorbs the bulk of the ultrafiltrate. The loop of Henle sets the mechanism for urinary concentration or dilution. Finally, the distal nephron, working on a greatly reduced volume of filtrate, determines the final volume and composition of excreted urine.

The combined and closely regulated operation of these segmental functions provides both for maintenance of the volume and composition of body fluids within narrow limits and for the elimination of waste products. The kidney acts as a target organ for a number of regulatory hormones and either produces or metabolizes a number of vital hormones. These renal contributions to homeostasis of the internal fluid environment allow great latitude in the interaction of an individual with the external environment.

REFERENCES

Bricker NS, Schultze RG, and Licht A: Renal function: General concepts. In Maxwell MH, and Kleeman CR (eds): Clinical Disorders of Fluid and Electrolyte Metabolism. 3rd ed. New York, McGraw-Hill Book Co, 1980, pp 233–268.
Fried TA, and Stein JH: Glomerular dynamics. Arch Intern Med 143:787–791, 1983.
Knepper M, and Burg M: Organization of nephron function. Am J Physiol 244:F579–F589, 1983.

29 ELECTROLYTE AND VOLUME DISORDERS

This chapter considers common disorders of volume status and electrolyte abnormalities encountered in clinical medicine. The volume and composition of the body fluid compartments normally remain constant despite wide daily variations in solute and water intake, or in the face of significant environmental fluctuations. When the volume or composition of body fluids varies beyond acceptable limits, sensor elements trigger afferent stimuli, which activate homeostatic responses. Negative feedback systems set the limits of these responses by deactivating the effectors.

VOLUME DISORDERS

Body water comprises approximately 60 per cent of body weight: the intracellular compartment (ICF) contains two thirds of body water, or 40 per cent of body weight; and the extracellular compartment (ECF) contains the remaining one third of total body water. The total blood volume, that is, plasma plus formed elements, constitutes one third of the total ECF.

Protection of the ECF volume, and more specifically of the effective circulating volume, is the most fundamental characteristic of fluid homeostasis. The details of the mechanisms regulating extracellular fluid volume have been presented in Chapter 28. When considered in an overall context, two features are noteworthy. First, redundant mechanisms protect effective circulating volume. For example, angiotensin II release and catecholamine release produce overlapping results: each agent affects both the peripheral vasculature and renal sodium conservation. Second, the magnitude of the volume repletion reaction varies with the degree of volume contraction.

VOLUME DEPLETION

Volume contraction may be the result of renal or extrarenal losses (Table 29–1). The cardinal hormones regulating renal water and sodium conservation are ADH and aldosterone, respectively. In diabetes insipidus, a large fraction of hypotonic distal tubular fluid escapes collecting duct reabsorption and appears in the urine. Impaired aldosterone production, either in Addison's disease or in interstitial renal disease, leads to renal sodium wasting. Renal tubular deficits in sodium or water conservation may be grouped into three classes: specific tubular nephropathies; osmotic diuresis, which overwhelms renal tubular reabsorptive capacity for water and salt; and chronic renal failure.

The major extrarenal volume losses occur in hemorrhage, excessive sweating, burns, and vomiting or diarrhea. Excessive sweating is characterized by loss of water in excess of salt, so that body water osmolality rises. Burns allow the loss of large amounts of plasma and interstitial fluid through affected areas and therefore lead to profound ECF losses. Finally, gastrointestinal volume losses from either vomiting or diarrhea result in a loss of a fraction of the 8 to 10 liters of normal daily gastrointestinal secretions.

Clinical Manifestations

The clinical findings in volume contraction are referable to underfilling of the arterial tree and to the renal and hemodynamic responses to this underfilling. Mild volume contraction is characterized by mild postural giddiness and tachycardia. In more advanced volume depletion, particularly when acute, there is recumbent hypotension, tachycardia, and a reduced urine volume. Finally, when volume contraction is severe, the combination of fluid loss and increased sympathetic activity produces vasoconstricted circulatory collapse: extreme hypotension, recumbent tachycardia, cold extremities, and oliguria.

The clinical manifestations of volume contraction vary directly with the volume and rate of fluid loss. The kind of fluid lost also affects findings in volume contraction. The acute loss of one liter of predominantly solute-free water, as in diabetes insipidus, produces only a 2.5 per cent reduction in blood volume. The acute loss of one liter of predominantly extracellular fluid, as in a burn, produces a 6.6 per cent reduction in blood volume, since sodium is confined to the ECF. Lastly, an acute hemorrhage of one liter of blood reduces blood volume by 20 per cent.

Diagnosis and Treatment

The physical examination provides an initial assessment of circulatory dynamics. In critically ill patients who are hemodynamically unstable, monitoring of the pulmonary capillary wedge pressure with a flow-directed catheter may be required. However, even the pulmonary capillary wedge pressure may remain within normal limits when blood volume has been reduced by 5 to 10 per cent. Consequently, a fluid challenge may be useful in evaluating volume status. A convenient protocol is to administer 500 ml of normal saline over one to three hours and to measure the change in the pulmonary capillary wedge pressure or the cardiac output.

The renal response to volume contraction is sodium avidity. As indicated in Chapter 28, the urinary sodium concentration and the fraction of filtered sodium excreted in the urine, denoted as Fe_{Na}, are clinically useful indices of renal sodium avidity. These indices are not reliable when there is obligatory renal sodium wasting.

The treatment of volume contraction is to expand circulating volume by replacing fluid deficits. The degree to which a given solution expands blood volume depends on composition. One liter of 5 per cent dextrose in water expands the blood volume by 75 to 100 ml, that is, by about 2 per cent. One liter of a normal saline solution will increase blood volume by about 300 ml, or about

TABLE 29–1. MAJOR CAUSES OF VOLUME DEPLETION

RENAL LOSSES	EXTRA-RENAL LOSSES
Hormone Deficit	**Hemorrhage**
Pituitary diabetes insipidus	**Cutaneous Losses**
Aldosterone insufficiency	*Sweating*
Addison's disease	*Burns*
Interstitial nephritis	**Gastrointestinal Losses**
Renal Deficit	*Vomiting*
Tubular nephropathies	*Diarrhea*
Renal tubular acidosis	*Gastrointestinal fistulae*
Bartter's syndrome	
Nephrogenic diabetes insipidus	
Diuretic abuse	
Post-obstructive diuresis	
Osmotic diuresis	
Chronic renal failure	

Adapted from Andreoli TE: Disorders of fluid volume, electrolyte, and acid-base balance. In Wyngaarden JB, and Smith LH Jr (eds): Cecil Textbook of Medicine. 17th ed. Philadelphia, WB Saunders Co, 1985, p 518.

6 per cent; the remaining portion is distributed in the interstitial compartment. Colloid-containing solutions, such as iso-oncotic albumin solutions, plasma, and blood, are mainly restricted to the intravascular space.

CIRCULATORY COMPROMISE WITHOUT VOLUME CONTRACTION

These disorders include illnesses in which inadequate arterial filling occurs in the absence of external fluid losses. Table 29–2 lists three commonly encountered classes of derangements that may present with signs of circulatory collapse in the absence of external volume losses.

With an *impaired cardiac output*, the heart fails to translocate blood adequately from venous to arterial beds. Circulatory collapse also occurs when there is a sudden increase in *venous capacitance*, as in sepsis, and is characterized by the combined occurrence of warm extremities, hypotension, and oliguria. Finally, circulatory collapse occurs when there is a rapid *fluid translocation* from vascular to interstitial compartments, as in acute pancreatitis and rhabdomyolysis.

TABLE 29–2. CIRCULATORY COMPROMISE WITHOUT EXTERNAL FLUID LOSSES

Impaired Cardiac Output
Acute myocardial infarction
Pericardial tamponade
Increased Vascular Capacitance
Septic shock
Vascular → Interstitial Fluid Shifts
Acute pancreatitis
Bowel infarction
Rhabdomyolysis
Noncardiogenic pulmonary edema

From Andreoli TE: Disorders of fluid volume, electrolyte, and acid-base balance. In Wyngaarden JB, and Smith LH Jr (eds): Cecil Textbook of Medicine. 17th ed. Philadelphia, WB Saunders Co, 1985, p 521.

TABLE 29–3. VOLUME-EXPANDED STATES

Disturbed Starling Forces: Edema States
  Systemic venous pressure increases
    Right heart failure
    Constrictive pericarditis
  Local venous pressure increases
    Left heart failure
    Portal vein obstruction
  Reduced oncotic pressure
    Nephrotic syndrome
  Combined disorders
    Cirrhosis
Primary Hormone Excess: Nonedematous States
  Primary aldosteronism
  Cushing's syndrome
  SIADH
Primary Renal Sodium Retention
  Acute glomerulonephritis

Adapted from Andreoli TE: Disorders of fluid volume, electrolyte, and acid-base balance. In Wyngaarden JB, and Smith LH Jr (eds): Cecil Textbook of Medicine. 17th ed. Philadelphia, WB Saunders Co, 1985, p 522.

VOLUME-EXPANDED DISORDERS

Table 29–3 presents a format for classifying disorders having an increase in total body sodium and water. The first group of disorders is characterized by an *abnormality in Starling forces*, which tends to result in renal Na$^+$ avidity, edema formation, and a reduced effective circulating volume. The plasma renin activity and aldosterone concentrations in these disorders tend to be elevated, although the results are variable.

The major *hormonal disturbances* leading to volume excess are those in which there is unregulated production of mineralocorticoids or of ADH. Mineralocorticoid excess produces sodium retention, preferential expansion of the ECF, a normal serum sodium, and hypertension. The syndrome of inappropriate ADH production (SIADH) produces water retention and dilutional hyponatremia. Edema is not characteristic of either disorder. Finally, acute glomerulonephritis is an example of *primary renal salt retention*: salt retention, hypertension, and edema formation occur without excesses in aldosterone production or reductions in filtration rate or circulating volume.

DIURETICS

Table 29–4 provides a summary of the properties of common diuretics. Acetazolamide is a carbonic anhydrase inhibitor that blocks proximal reabsorption of sodium bicarbonate. The prolonged use of acetazolamide may lead to hyperchloremic acidosis. Metolazone is a congener of the thiazide diuretics that blocks sodium chloride absorption in at least two nephron sites: the proximal tubule and the early distal tubule.

Loop diuretics, such as ethacrynic acid and furosemide, inhibit sodium chloride absorption in the thick ascending limb of Henle: early distal tubule diuretics, such as chlorothiazide, block sodium absorption in early segments of the distal convoluted tubule. Hypokalemia and metabolic alkalosis may complicate therapy with loop diuretics and early distal tubular diuretics, because these agents increase salt delivery to the late distal nephron and therefore enhance rates of late distal proton and potassium secretion.

Finally, agents such as amiloride, triamterene, and spironolactone inhibit sodium absorption in terminal regions of the distal tubule. Prolonged use of these agents can lead to hyperkalemia and hyperchloremic metabolic acidosis.

OSMOLALITY DISTURBANCES

Normally, the serum osmolality is virtually constant. The mechanisms that adjust water balance are determined by changes in cell volume that result from variations in effective ECF osmolality. If the ECF osmolality is increased by sol-

TABLE 29–4. DIURETICS

	PRIMARY EFFECT	SECONDARY EFFECT	COMPLICATIONS
Proximal Diuretics			
Acetazolamide	↓ Na$^+$/H$^+$ exchange	↑ K$^+$ loss, ↑ HCO$_3^-$ loss	hypokalemic, hyperchloremic acidosis
Metolazone	↓ Na$^+$ absorption	↑ K$^+$ loss, ↑ Cl$^-$ loss	hypokalemic alkalosis
Loop Diuretics			
Furosemide / Ethacrynic acid	↓ Na$^+$:K$^+$:2Cl$^-$ absorption	↑ K$^+$ loss, ↑ H$^+$ secretion	hypokalemic alkalosis
Early Distal Diuretics			
Thiazide / Metolazone	↓ Na$^+$ absorption	↑ K$^+$ loss, ↑ H$^+$ secretion	hypokalemic alkalosis
Late Distal Diuretics			
Aldosterone antagonists Spironolactone	↓ Na$^+$ absorption	↓ K$^+$ loss, ↓ H$^+$ secretion	hyperkalemic acidosis
Nonaldosterone antagonists Triamterene Amiloride	↓ Na$^+$ absorption	↓ K$^+$ loss, ↓ H$^+$ secretion	hyperkalemic acidosis

Adapted from Andreoli TE: Disorders of fluid volume, electrolyte, and acid-base balance. In Wyngaarden JB, and Smith LH Jr (eds): Cecil Textbook of Medicine. 17th ed. Philadelphia, WB Saunders Co, 1985, p 522.

utes that penetrate cell membranes readily, such as urea, acute cell shrinkage does not occur.

The osmolalities of intracellular and extracellular fluids are virtually identical. Two factors are responsible for this: cell membranes are freely permeable to water, and cell membrane-bound $(Na^+ + K^+)$-ATPase maintains the sum of cation concentrations in intracellular fluids equal to the sum of cation concentrations in extracellular fluids.

In *acute hypotonic* disorders, the primary event mediating osmotic equilibration between the ICF and ECF is cellular water gain. Thus cerebral edema is the most ominous consequence of acute water intoxication. In *chronic hypotonic* disorders, cell swelling is offset by solute loss from cells, particularly in the central nervous system. Thus in chronic hyponatremia, brain volume may be normal while brain solute content is reduced.

The most lethal consequence of *acute hypertonic* disorders is water loss from the central nervous system and brain shrinkage. In *chronic hypertonic* disorders, brain shrinkage is minimized by the accumulation of additional solutes within brain cells. These latter solutes are often called "idogenic osmoles."

HYPOTONIC DISORDERS

A hypotonic disorder is one in which the serum osmolality and serum sodium are both reduced in parallel. True hypotonicity must be distinguished from disorders in which the *measured* serum sodium is low while the *measured* serum osmolality is either normal or increased. The latter generally occurs because of an increased concentration of a nonsodium solute such as glucose in the ECF.

The regulatory mechanism for ECF osmolality shown in Figure 28-6 provides a convenient frame of reference for classifying hypotonic syndromes. Hyponatremia can be due to an absolute increase in water intake that exceeds the ability of a normal kidney to excrete free water, for example, in primary polydipsia. However, profound hyponatremia is rare because the ability to excrete a maximally dilute urine is not impaired.

Clinically significant hyponatremia is most often due to an inability to excrete a maximally dilute urine. This diluting impairment may occur (1) because of reductions in the amount of salt absorbed by the thick ascending limb of Henle; (2) because of sustained nonosmotic ADH release; and (3) because of a combination of these factors. Table 29-5 summarizes these disorders.

A *reduced sodium* intake impairs the maximal rate of dilute urine formation. Since the minimum urinary osmolality is usually 50 mOsm/kg H_2O, the excretion of 15 L of highly dilute urine requires the excretion of 750 mOsm of solute. If urinary solute excretion falls, the maximal daily rate of dilute urine formation is also reduced.

The prototypes of *primary ADH excess* include the syndrome of inappropriate ADH production (SIADH) and drug-induced ADH release. SIADH is a disorder in which hyponatremia occurs as a result of sustained endogenous production and release of ADH or ADH-like substances. The disorder occurs most commonly in pulmonary diseases; in cranial disorders; and in a number of neoplasms, particularly bronchogenic carcinoma. Patients with SIADH retain ingested water, become hyponatremic and modestly volume-expanded, and generally increase body weight by 5 to 10 per cent. The volume expansion generally results in a natriuresis, so that edema is uncommon, and in a reduced serum concentration of uric acid. The glomerular filtration rate is normal, as is adrenal and thyroid function. The urine osmolality in patients with SIADH need not be hypertonic to plasma, but only inappropriately high for the level of serum osmolality.

Finally, hyponatremia occurs commonly in *mixed disorders*, in which nonosmotic ADH release and reductions in the rate of urinary sodium excretion blunt urinary diluting capacity. This phenomenon occurs in advanced volume contraction, in intractable heart failure, and in advanced hepatic cirrhosis with ascites.

Diagnosis

The clinical manifestations of hyponatremia are produced by brain swelling and usually occur when the serum sodium concentration falls to 120 mEq/L or less. An early symptom of lethargy can proceed rapidly to seizures and coma, so that acute water intoxication is a medical emergency. In chronic hyponatremia, central nervous system manifestations are far less common, because the loss of brain solutes minimizes brain cell swelling.

The most difficult differential diagnosis among hyponatremic disorders involves the distinction between patients who are modestly volume contracted and those who have SIADH. In volume contraction due to extrarenal causes, the urinary sodium concentration is less than 10 to 15 mEq/L and the Fe_{Na} is generally less than 1 per cent. In patients with SIADH, the urinary sodium con-

TABLE 29-5. HYPONATREMIA DUE TO IMPAIRED RENAL WATER EXCRETION

Reduced Sodium Delivery to the Diluting Segment
  Starvation
  Beer potomania
  ? Myxedema
Primary Excess of ADH
  SIADH
  Drug-induced ADH production
  Drug potentiation of ADH action
  Trauma
  Potassium depletion
  ? Myxedema
  ? Acute intermittent porphyria
Mixed Disorders
  Volume contraction (Addison's disease)
  Advanced edema states (congestive heart failure, constrictive
    pericarditis, and cirrhosis)

Adapted from Andreoli TE: Disorders of fluid volume, electrolyte, and acid-base balance. In Wyngaarden JB, and Smith LH Jr (eds): Cecil Textbook of Medicine. 17th ed. Philadelphia, WB Saunders Co, 1985, p 525.

centration usually exceeds 30 mEq/L, the Fe_{Na} is greater than 1 per cent, and the serum uric acid is reduced. Tests of adrenal function are normal. Patients with SIADH exhibit a characteristic response to water restriction: a 2- to 3-kg weight loss is accompanied by correction of hyponatremia and cessation of salt wasting, usually over a period of two to three days.

Treatment

The goal of treatment in hyponatremia is to correct body water osmolality and restore cell volume by raising the ratio of sodium to water in extracellular fluid. Acute hyponatremia associated with a serum sodium concentration below 120 to 125 mEq/L and central nervous system manifestations requires immediate therapy. In volume-contracted states, the serum sodium can be raised to 125 mEq/L by administering hypertonic 3 to 5 per cent saline.

Hypertonic saline solutions are hazardous in volume-expanded states such as congestive heart failure. Hypertonic saline may be ineffective in correcting hyponatremia in SIADH because the administered salt is excreted promptly. In such circumstances, one may use normal saline solutions in combination with furosemide administration. During furosemide therapy, urinary concentrating ability is blunted and the urinary sodium concentration is lower than that in plasma. Consequently, the combination of intravenous normal saline, coupled with a furosemide diuresis, provides an effective way of raising the serum sodium concentration.

Chronic hyponatremia in SIADH may be corrected by restricting water intake. An alternative approach involves the use of agents such as lithium or demethylchlortetracycline, which interfere with the renal tubular effects of ADH. Finally, oral salt loading in combination with oral furosemide therapy will also correct chronic hyponatremia.

The rapid elevation of serum sodium concentrations to levels greater than 125 mEq/L is hazardous, either in acute or chronic hyponatremia, since the ECF may become hypertonic to brain cells partially solute-depleted during hyponatremia. Consequently, raising the serum sodium rapidly can result in acute brain shrinkage.

HYPERTONIC DISORDERS

The most common reasons for clinically significant hypernatremia (Table 29–6) include three pathogenic mechanisms: impaired thirst; solute, or osmotic, diuresis; and excessive losses of water, either via the kidneys or extrarenally.

Inadequate water intake occurs in patients who are either comatose or unable to communicate thirst. The increased rates of urinary solute excretion in *osmotic diuresis* produce renal water losses in excess of sodium losses, and therefore hypertonicity. The serum sodium is generally reduced in the early stages of osmotic diuresis and raised in later stages. *Excess water losses* in pituitary or nephrogenic diabetes insipidus can lead to profound water deficits and hypernatremia. Striking water losses may also occur with excessive sweating.

Clinical Findings and Treatment

The clinical manifestations of hypernatremia or hyperglycemia are referable to circulatory collapse and to brain shrinkage due to water loss. In acute hypertonicity, confusion and somnolence generally appear when the effective ECF osmolality exceeds 350 mOsm/kg H_2O. Chronic hypertonicity produces fewer central nervous system manifestations because brain cells accumulate solutes that minimize the tendency to brain shrinkage.

The treatment of acute hypernatremia requires intravenous fluids. An isotonic saline solution has particular advantages in acute hypernatremia. It provides fluid resuscitation in impending cardiovascular collapse. The isotonic salt solution, which is hypotonic with respect to the hypertonic patient, also avoids unnecessarily rapid falls in the serum sodium. Since solute accumulation by brain cells occurs in hypertonic disorders, a rapid reduction in serum osmolality may produce cerebral edema.

TABLE 29–6. MAJOR CAUSES OF HYPERNATREMIA

Impaired Thirst
  Coma
  Essential hypernatremia
Solute Diuresis
  Osmotic diuresis: diabetic ketoacidosis, nonketotic
                 hyperosmolar coma, mannitol administration
Excessive Water Losses
  Renal
    Pituitary diabetes insipidus
    Nephrogenic diabetes insipidus
  Extrarenal
    Sweating
Combined Disorders
  Coma plus hypertonic nasogastric feeding

From Andreoli TE: Disorders of fluid volume, electrolyte, and acid-base balance. In Wyngaarden JB, and Smith LH Jr (eds): Cecil Textbook of Medicine. 17th ed. Philadelphia, WB Saunders Co, 1985, p 528.

POTASSIUM DERANGEMENTS

The body contains approximately 3500 mEq of potassium, 60 mEq of which are extracellular. The cardinal transport process regulating K^+ distribution between ICF and ECF is cell membrane–bound $(Na^+ + K^+)$-ATPase, which actively transports potassium into cells and counterbalances the passive leak of potassium from cells into interstitial fluid. Insulin and beta-adrenergic agents promote cellular uptake of potassium by stimulating $(Na^+ + K^+)$-ATPase.

A number of passive mechanisms also regulate the partition of potassium between the ICF and ECF. A 0.1 unit change in arterial pH produces a 0.6 mEq inverse change in the serum K^+. Second, cellular shrinkage raises the intracellular potassium concentration and thereby increases the rate of passive potassium leakage from the ICF to the ECF.

The renal handling of potassium is discussed in Chapter 28. Stated briefly, virtually all dietary potassium appears in the urine because of tubular secretion of potassium in distal tubular segments. The major elements that regulate distal potassium secretion include the rate of distal tubular sodium delivery; dietary potassium intake; and aldosterone. Impermeant anions such as carbenicillin produce greater distal luminal electronegativity and also enhance K^+ secretion.

The clinical consequences of hypokalemia and hyperkalemia are referable to changes in the characteristics of excitable tissues. At rest, excitable tissues are far more permeable to potassium than to sodium, and the cell interior is electronegative. During deplorization, there is a profound increase in membrane permeability to sodium, which accounts for the initial spike of the action potential.

If an excitable cell is partially depolarized in the resting state by hyperkalemia, the increase in sodium permeability that accompanies the action potential is reduced, and the rate of phase zero cardiac depolarization is therefore slowed. The net effect of progressive hyperkalemia, therefore, is to make the heart refractory to excitation.

The effects of hypokalemia on excitable tissues are more complex. Because the K_i/K_o ratio rises in hypokalemia, excitable cells are initially hyperpolarized. Eventually, resting depolarization follows, because the high K_i/K_o ratio by itself reduces potassium permeability. The net effect is to increase the likelihood of arrhythmia formation.

HYPOKALEMIA

Chronic hypokalemia indicates a reduction in total body potassium; a 1-mEq reduction in serum potassium indicates a net loss of 100 to 200 mEq of potassium. An acute reduction in serum potassium occurs when potassium is shifted from extracellular to intracellular compartments.

The four major causes for hypokalemia are given in Table 29–7. A *reduced intake* may result in potassium depletion and hypokalemia, because maximal renal conservation of potassium requires 7 to 10 days. During this interval, the net renal potassium loss may be as much as 250 to 300 mEq.

Excessive renal losses of potassium are common in states of mineralocorticoid excess and with diuretic excess. In chronic metabolic alkalosis associated with volume contraction, secondary hyperaldosteronism results in renal potassium losses. In fact, the hypokalemia associated with vomiting is primarily due to renal potassium losses. Upper gastrointestinal tract losses are small, since upper gastrointestinal tract fluid contains only about 10 mEq/L of potassium.

Gastrointestinal losses due to diarrhea also produce significant potassium losses, since diarrheal fluid contains 30 mEq/L of potassium. The most striking diarrheal potassium losses occur in secretory diarrheas.

Finally, acute hypokalemia with a normal total

TABLE 29–7. MAJOR CAUSES OF HYPOKALEMIA

Inadequate Intake
Excess Renal Loss
  Mineralocorticoid excess
  Bartter's syndrome
  Diuresis
    Diuretics with a pre-late distal locus osmotic diuresis
  Chronic metabolic alkalosis
  Impermeant anion antibiotics
    Carbenicillin
  Renal tubular acidosis
Gastrointestinal Losses
  Vomiting
  Diarrhea, particularly secretory diarrheas
  Villous adenoma
ECF → ICF Shifts
  Acute alkalosis
  Hypokalemic periodic paralysis
  Insulin therapy
  Vitamin B_{12} therapy

Adapted from Andreoli TE: Disorders of fluid volume, electrolyte, and acid-base balance. In Wyngaarden JB, and Smith LH Jr (eds): Cecil Textbook of Medicine. 17th ed. Philadelphia, WB Saunders Co, 1985, p 532.

body potasssium may occur because of *potassium shifts* from the ECF to the ICF. Such shifts occur in hypokalemic periodic paralysis and in association with insulin therapy.

Manifestations and Treatment

The most serious disturbances in potassium deficiencies are those affecting excitable tissues. At serum potassium concentrations in the range of 2 to 2.5 mEq/L, muscular weakness and arrhythmias are likely to occur; with more severe hypokalemia, areflexic paralysis may occur. The electrocardiographic abnormalities of potassium depletion include sagging of the ST segment, depression of the T wave, and elevation of the U wave.

The treatment of hypokalemia involves replacement therapy. Except in extreme circumstances, oral therapy with organic potassium salts rather than parenteral potassium replacement is prudent. When parenteral therapy is indicated, potassium chloride can be added to intravenous solutions and given at rates of 10 to 20 mEq per hour. Parenteral potassium therapy should be avoided in azotemic patients.

HYPERKALEMIA

Acute or chronic hyperkalemia occurs most commonly either because of diminished renal excretion or because there is a sudden transcellular shift of potassium from the ICF to the ECF. The major causes for hyperkalemia are listed in Table 29–8.

Hyperkalemia due to *diminished renal excretion* may occur whenever the glomerular filtration rate has been reduced. Hyperkalemia also occurs with modest reductions in the glomerular filtration rate if there is impairment of potassium secretion by the distal nephron.

Hyperkalemia also occurs in situations in

TABLE 29–8. HYPERKALEMIC SYNDROMES

Diminished Renal Excretion
  Reduced GFR
    Acute oliguric renal failure
    Chronic renal failure
  Reduced tubular secretion
    Addison's disease
    Hyporeninemic hypoaldosteronism
    Potassium-sparing diuretics
Transcellular Shifts
  Acidosis
  Cell destruction
    Trauma, burns
    Rhabdomyolysis
    Hemolysis
    Tumor lysis
  Hyperkalemic periodic paralysis
  Diabetic hyperglycemia
    Insulin dependence plus aldosterone lack
  Depolarizing muscle paralysis
    Succinylcholine

Adapted from Andreoli TE: Disorders of fluid volume, electrolyte, and acid-base balance. In Wyngaarden JB, and Smith LH Jr (eds): Cecil Textbook of Medicine. 17th ed. Philadelphia, WB Saunders Co, 1985, p 534.

which there is a *potassium shift* from the ICF to the ECF. This occurs in acidosis or in circumstances that result in cell destruction; the latter occurs commonly with tissue trauma, burns, rhabdomyolysis or hemolysis, and with lysis of large masses of tumor cells. Paradoxical hyperkalemia occurs when sudden hyperglycemia develops in insulin-dependent diabetics who also have interstitial renal disease and associated hyporeninemic hypoaldosteronism.

Pseudohyperkalemia may occur in thrombocytosis or leukocytosis, because clotting of blood promotes potassium release from these cells. Pseudohyperkalemia is identified by noting that the serum potassium is elevated while the plasma potassium is normal.

Manifestations and Treatment

The most important clinical manifestations of hyperkalemia relate to alterations in cardiac excitability. The earliest electrocardiographic manifestation of hyperkalemia is the development of peaked T waves, usually when the serum potassium exceeds 6.5 mEq/L. Higher potassium levels produce prolongation of the PR interval followed by a loss of P waves and widening of the QRS complex. The latter, known as a sine wave electrocardiogram, is followed by cardiac arrest.

Three kinds of maneuvers are used in the treatment of hyperkalemia. First, insulin promotes potassium entry into cells; glucose is administered with insulin to prevent hypoglycemia. Alkalinization also drives potassium into cells. Second, gastrointestinal potassium losses may be produced by the use of cation exchange resins such as sodium polystyrene sulfonate (Kayexalate). Hemodialysis is also an effective means for potassium removal.

Finally, calcium salts do not alter the serum potassium concentration. However, the calcium re-

stores cardiac excitability and antagonizes the cardiotoxic effects of hyperkalemia and is therefore useful in hyperkalemic cardiotoxicity.

ACID-BASE DISORDERS

The arterial pH normally ranges between 7.35 and 7.45; the widest range of pH values compatible with life is 6.8 to 7.8, or an interval of one pH unit. The major buffer system in extracellular fluid is the bicarbonate–carbonic acid pair. While proton shifts between the ECF and ICF help stabilize the plasma pH against acute fluctuations, the ultimate maintenance of pH balance requires that input of acid or base into the body be matched by output of acid or base.

Acid Handling. The largest source of endogenous acid production is from combustion of glucose and fatty acids to carbon dioxide and water, or in other words, to a volatile acid. The rate of volatile acid production amounts to about 22,000 mEq of hydrogen ion daily.

The prime factors regulating alterations in the rate of minute ventilation are subtle changes in cerebrospinal fluid (CSF) pH or arterial pH. On an average, a 1 mEq/L reduction in plasma bicarbonate produced by metabolic acidosis will increase ventilation and produce a 1.2 mm Hg fall in the P_aCO_2. Conversely, a 3 mEq/L rise in bicarbonate due to metabolic alkalosis produces a 1 mm Hg rise in P_aCO_2.

In addition to volatile acids, cellular metabolism also results in the formation of a number of nonvolatile acids; the major source for the latter is metabolism of sulfur-containing amino acids. The daily rate of nonvolatile acid production under normal conditions is about 1 mEq/kg of body weight. The details of the renal secretory mechanisms for eliminating these nonvolatile acids have been discussed in Chapter 28.

The kidneys also filter large quantities of bicarbonate daily, virtually all of which is absorbed together with sodium by the proximal tubule. The rate of proximal bicarbonate reabsorption is increased by three major factors: a fall in effective circulating volume, a rise in P_aCO_2, and hypokalemia.

The Anion Gap. A convenient formula for calculating the anion gap is:

$$\text{anion gap} = Na - (Cl + HCO_3)$$

where Na, Cl, and HCO_3 are the serum sodium, chloride, and bicarbonate concentrations, respectively. The anion gap includes phosphate and sulfate, lactate and ketoacids, and albumin.

An *increased* anion gap generally indicates the presence of metabolic acidosis. The anion gap will be *reduced* if the sodium concentration falls while the chloride and bicarbonate concentrations are unchanged; this may occur in severe multiple myeloma of the IgG variety, since the myeloma proteins are cationic at pH 7.4. Lithium intoxication, hypermagnesemia, and hypercalcemia rarely raise the nonsodium cation concentrations sufficiently high to reduce the anion gap.

METABOLIC ACIDOSIS

A convenient way to consider the metabolic acidoses is to divide them into those having a normal anion gap and those having an increased anion gap. Table 29–9 presents a classification of metabolic acidosis according to this format.

Normal Anion Gap Metabolic Acidosis

The metabolic acidoses having a normal anion gap occur for three classes of reasons: (1) The kidneys fail to reabsorb or regenerate bicarbonate because of specific tubular deficits. Renal tubular acidosis is described in Chapter 34. (2) There are extrarenal losses of bicarbonate, generally due to diarrhea. (3) Excessive amounts of substances yielding hydrochloric acid (see Table 29–9) have been administered. The presence of a normal anion gap implies that the glomerular filtration rate is sufficient to excrete sulfates and phosphates, that there is no endogenous overproduction of organic acids, and that there has not been ingestion of substances that lead to organic acid accumulation.

Increased Anion Gap Metabolic Acidosis

Metabolic acidoses characterized by an increased anion gap occur either because the kidneys fail to excrete inorganic acids or because there is net accumulation of organic acids. *Retention* of sulfates and phosphates occurs in acute or chronic renal failure. In chronic renal failure, metabolic acidosis occurs because the net amount of ammonium excreted daily falls as functional renal mass diminishes. The plasma bicarbonate concentration in most patients with acute or chronic renal failure ranges between 16 and 20 mEq/L.

Organic acid accumulation represents the second major cause for metabolic acidosis with an increased anion gap. Normally, the complete combustion of carbohydrates and fatty acids to carbon dioxide and water equals the production of approximately 22,000 mEq of hydrogen ion per day. Processes that impair cellular respiration, and therefore result in nonvolatile rather than volatile acid production, can lead to profound metabolic acidosis.

The syndrome of lactic acidosis results from impaired cellular respiration. Lactic acid is produced in muscle, red blood cells, and other tissues as a consequence of anaerobic glycolysis. When lactic acid oxidation is limited because of impaired cellular respiration, the lactate-to-pyruvate ratio (L/P) rises. Lactic acidosis occurs most commonly in disorders characterized by inadequate oxygen delivery to tissues, such as shock, septicemia, and profound hypoxemia; with phenformin or isoniazid toxicity; and in leukemia and diabetes mellitus.

Accelerated rates of organic acid production

TABLE 29–9. MAJOR CAUSES OF METABOLIC ACIDOSIS

NORMAL ANION GAP	INCREASED ANION GAP
Bicarbonate Loss Proximal renal tubular acidosis Diarrheal states Small bowel drainage Ureterosigmoidostomy	**Reduced Excretion of Inorganic Acids** Renal failure
Failure of Bicarbonate Regeneration Distal, gradient-limited renal tubular acidosis Hyporeninemic hypoaldosteronism Diuretics: triamterene, spironolactone	**Accumulation of Organic Acids** Lactic acidosis Ketoacidosis: alcoholic, diabetic, starvation Ingestion: salicylates, paraldehyde, methanol, ethylene glycol
Acidifying Salts Ammonium chloride Lysine hydrochloride Arginine hydrochloride Hyperalimentation	

Adapted from Andreoli TE: Disorders of fluid volume, electrolyte, and acid-base balance. In Wyngaarden JB, and Smith LH Jr (eds): Cecil Textbook of Medicine. 17th ed. Philadelphia, WB Saunders Co, 1985, p 539.

also result in an anion gap acidosis. Alcoholic ketoacidosis occurs in alcoholic patients with recent binge drinking and depends on accelerated lipolysis because of reduced insulin secretion secondary to starvation. Diabetic ketoacidosis with an increased anion gap occurs because of increased rates of ketogenesis due to insulin lack. Starvation produces metabolic acidosis by a similar mechanism. Thus alcoholic ketoacidosis, diabetic ketoacidosis, and starvation share a common feature: accelerated lipolysis and ketogenesis due at least in part to insulin lack.

Finally, *ingested substances* can also result in severe metabolic acidosis with a large anion gap. The most common of these are listed in Table 29–9

DIAGNOSIS AND TREATMENT

The diagnosis of metabolic acidosis requires analysis of serum electrolytes and, when indicated, measurement of arterial pH and $P_{a}CO_2$. A cardinal clinical manifestation of metabolic acidosis is hyperventilation, usually as Kussmaul respiration. Severe metabolic acidosis exerts a negative inotropic effect on the heart, since acidosis diminishes tissue responsiveness to catecholamines. Acidosis also tends to reduce red blood cell 2,3-DPG; this may offset partially the compensatory Bohr effect and therefore aggravate inadequate tissue oxygenation in acidosis.

The treatment of metabolic acidosis involves correction of the underlying disorder and, where appropriate, alkali therapy with sodium bicarbonate. In chronic renal failure and in distal renal tubular acidosis, relatively modest amounts of bicarbonate—in the range of 30 to 60 mEq daily—are adequate. In proximal renal tubular acidosis, bicarbonate therapy is not helpful because of renal bicarbonate wasting. Rather, attempts to minimize renal bicarbonate wasting by salt restriction are more helpful.

The treatment of acidoses due to accumulation of organic acids varies with the disorder. In lactic acidosis, therapy should be directed toward improving tissue perfusion. Large amounts of sodium bicarbonate may be required to avoid the development of lethal acidosis.

The treatment of alcoholic ketoacidosis generally requires only the administration of saline solutions and glucose. Alkali therapy is not needed unless the metabolic acidosis is in the lethal range. The same considerations apply to starvation ketosis. In diabetic ketoacidosis, insulin therapy promotes glucose utilization and consequently complete oxidation of ketoacids; simultaneously, ketogenesis is reduced. Therefore alkali therapy is ordinarily not required, except when profound reductions in the arterial pH, to values less than 7.0, impair cardiac contractility.

METABOLIC ALKALOSIS

While metabolic alkalosis may be initiated by the loss of hydrogen ion from the body, for example during gastric drainage, maintenance of metabolic alkalosis requires that the rate of renal bicarbonate reabsorption be greater than normal. Table 29–10 lists the major clinical causes of metabolic alkalosis.

Volume contraction can sustain metabolic alkalosis because of an increase in the apparent rate of bicarbonate reabsorption by the proximal tubule. The most common cause for initiating this kind of alkalosis is hydrochloric acid loss because of vomiting or gastric suction. *Potassium depletion*, when sufficiently severe, can sustain metabolic alkalosis by raising the rate of renal bicarbonate reabsorption. When serum potassium concentrations are reduced to about 2 mEq/L, metabolic alkalosis due to gastric fluid loss becomes saline-resistant but responsive to potassium chloride administration.

Situations in which there occurs *enhanced delivery of sodium chloride* to terminal nephron segments lead to metabolic alkalosis by increasing the rate of renal bicarbonate generation. This effect occurs with loop diuretics (see Table 29–4) like furosemide. The alkalosis of *mineralocorticoid excess* occurs because of increased genera-

TABLE 29–10. MAJOR MECHANISMS FOR METABOLIC ALKALOSIS

ECF volume contraction
Potassium depletion
Increased distal salt delivery
Mineralocorticoid excess
Liddle's syndrome
Bicarbonate loading (post-hypercapneic alkalosis)
Delayed conversion of administered organic acids

From Andreoli TE: Disorders of fluid volume, electrolyte, and acid-base balance. In Wyngaarden JB, and Smith LH Jr: Cecil Textbook of Medicine. 17th ed. Philadelphia, WB Saunders Co, 1985, p 542.

tion of bicarbonate by terminal nephron segments and is accentuated by potassium depletion.

Post-hypercapneic alkalosis occurs in patients with chronic hypercapnia, who have a compensatory increase in serum bicarbonate and in whom the arterial P_aCO_2 is lowered abruptly by assisted ventilation. Delayed conversion of *accumulated organic acids* is a second mechanism for producing transient metabolic alkalosis. This may occur after insulin therapy for diabetic ketoacidosis, during the recovery phase of lactic acidosis, and following high-efficiency hemodialysis.

MANIFESTATIONS AND TREATMENT

Metabolic alkalosis can result in cardiac arrhythmias, and severe metabolic alkalosis can also result in severe hypoventilation. The diagnosis is inferred by routine measurements of serum electrolytes and confirmed by arterial blood gas analysis. Hypokalemia is generally present. The urinary chloride concentration is useful in distinguishing metabolic alkalosis due to volume contraction from that due to primary mineralocorticoid excess.

Metabolic alkalosis associated with hypokalemia and volume contraction is treated by volume expansion and potassium replacement. If the metabolic alkalosis is sufficiently severe that significant hypoventilation is present, dilute hydrochloric acid or acidifying salts may be required.

RESPIRATORY ACIDOSIS

Respiratory acidosis occurs when there is impairment in the rate of alveolar ventilation. *Acute respiratory acidosis* occurs with sudden depressions of the medullary respiratory center, with paralysis of respiratory muscles, with airway obstruction, and with trauma that impedes ventilation. *Chronic respiratory acidosis* generally occurs in individuals with emphysema, in patients with extreme kyphoscoliosis, and in individuals with extreme obesity (Pickwickian syndrome).

The arterial pH and plasma bicarbonate concentrations differ in acute and chronic respiratory acidosis. The compensatory response to carbon dioxide retention is to increase the plasma bicarbonate concentration by approximately 0.3 mEq for every millimeter of mercury increase in the P_aCO_2. This compensatory increase in plasma bicarbonate concentration generally requires two to three days. Consequently, the plasma bicarbonate is generally increased in chronic but not acute respiratory acidosis.

MANIFESTATIONS AND TREATMENT

Acute increases in P_aCO_2 values result in somnolence, confusion, and ultimately CO_2 narcosis. Asterixis may also be present. The only practical treatment for acute respiratory acidosis involves treatment of the underlying disorder and ventilatory support. Naloxone (Narcan) therapy should be considered in comatose patients with no apparent cause for respiratory depression.

Oxygen therapy in patients with chronic hypercapnia should be instituted with caution, since hypoxemia may be the primary stimulus to respiration in this setting. Alkalinizing salts have no place in the management of chronic respiratory acidosis.

RESPIRATORY ALKALOSIS

Acute respiratory alkalosis is most commonly the result of the hyperventilation syndrome. Acute hyperventilation may also occur because of damage to the respiratory centers; in acute salicylism; and in association with pneumonia, pulmonary emboli, or congestive heart failure. The disorder may also be produced iatrogenically by injudicious mechanical ventilatory support. Chronic hyperventilation occurs in the acclimation response to exposure to high altitudes (a low ambient oxygen tension), in advanced hepatic insufficiency, and in pregnancy.

MANIFESTATIONS AND TREATMENT

Acute hyperventilation syndrome is characterized by lightheadedness, paresthesias, circumoral numbness, and tingling of the extremities. Tetany occurs in severe cases.

The treatment of acute respiratory alkalosis involves correction of underlying disorders. When anxiety produces hyperventilation, air rebreathing generally terminates the attack.

REFERENCES

Andreoli TE: Disorders of fluid volume, electrolyte, and acid-base balance. In Wyngaarden JB, and Smith HL Jr (eds): Cecil Textbook of Medicine. 17th ed. Philadelphia, W B Saunders Co, 1985, pp 515–544.

Cohen JJ: Disorders of potassium balance. Hosp Pract 14:119–128, 1979.

Gabow PA, Kaehny WD, Fennessey PV, Goodman SI, Gross PA, and Schrier RW: Diagnostic importance of an increased serum anion gap. N Engl J Med 303:854–858, 1980.

Kreisberg RA: Lactate homeostasis and lactic acidosis. Ann Intern Med 92:227–327, 1980.

Miller M, Dalakos T, Moses AM, Fellerman H, and Streeten DHP: Recognition of partial defects in antidiuretic hormone secretion. Ann Intern Med 73:721–729, 1970.

Miller M, and Moses AM: Drug-induced states of impaired water excretion. Kidney Int 10:96–103, 1976.

Thier SO: The kidney. Diuretics. In Smith LH, and Thier SO (eds): Pathophysiology. 2nd ed. Philadelphia, WB Saunders Co, 1985, pp 715–722.

Weitzman RE, and Kleeman CR: The clinical physiology of water metabolism. Part III: The water depletion (hyperosmolar) and water excess (hyposmolar) syndromes. West J Med 132:16–38, 1980.

ARTERIAL HYPERTENSION 30

Elevation of the systemic arterial blood pressure is one of the most common problems in clinical medicine. Approximately 20 to 25 million Americans have hypertension. Although many of these individuals are asymptomatic, chronic elevation of the systemic arterial blood pressure may lead to significant morbid complications, including congestive heart failure, myocardial infarction, cerebrovascular accident, and/or renal insufficiency. Because effective therapy is available for the patient with hypertension, many of these sequelae can be prevented if the disease is diagnosed and treated properly.

DEFINITION AND EPIDEMIOLOGY

There is no strict definition of hypertension because the precise dividing line between normal and elevated blood pressure is not clear-cut. However, a blood pressure of greater than 140/90 is usually considered abnormally high, particularly if it can be reproduced on more than two occasions. Hypertension is commonly classified as mild, moderate, or severe depending on the level of the diastolic blood pressure (Table 30–1). However, isolated systolic hypertension may occur and is defined as a systolic blood pressure greater than or equal to 160 mm Hg associated with a normal diastolic value. Prospective studies indicate that morbidity and mortality increase in direct proportion to the level of blood pressure beginning at levels well *below* 140/90.

In the United States, approximately 15 per cent of the adult white population and 25 per cent of

TABLE 30–1. CLASSIFICATION OF HYPERTENSION

RANGE (mm Hg)	CLASSIFICATION
DIASTOLIC	
<85	normal
85–89	high normal
90–104	mild hypertension
105–114	moderate hypertension
>115	severe hypertension
SYSTOLIC (when diastolic <90)	
<140	normal
140–159	borderline systolic hypertension
>160	isolated systolic hypertension

the adult black population can be considered hypertensive. The blood pressure in healthy children and pregnant women is typically lower, so that values in excess of 120/80 should be viewed with suspicion. Many factors affect the risk of an individual's developing hypertension. The incidence of the disease clearly increases with age. Heredity plays a strong role, with approximately 80 per cent of hypertensive patients displaying a positive family history of the disease. Obesity and the dietary intake of sodium are two other variables that increase the risk of hypertension in susceptible individuals. Whereas heredity and age cannot be controlled, factors such as body weight and diet can be modified.

THE PATHOPHYSIOLOGY OF HYPERTENSION

A review of the physiological determinants of normal blood pressure provides a way of introducing the factors that play a role in the development of hypertension. The blood pressure is generated by cardiac contraction, which produces its maximal pressure, the *systolic blood pressure*, during ejection. This is followed by cardiac relaxation, which results in a fall in blood pressure to its nadir level, the *diastolic blood pressure*. The *mean arterial blood pressure* lies between the systolic and diastolic pressures and can be defined as a function of cardiac output and systemic vascular resistance (Table 30–2). The mean arterial pressure is tightly regulated within a range that maintains tissue perfusion but minimizes vascu-

TABLE 30–2. DETERMINANTS OF BLOOD PRESSURE

MAP	= mean arterial pressure
DBP	= diastolic blood pressure
SBP	= systolic blood pressure
CO	= cardiac output
SVR	= systemic vascular resistance
HR	= heart rate
SV	= stroke volume
MAP	= DBP + (SBP − DBP)/3
MAP	= CO × SVR, and since CO = HR × SV,
MAP	= HR × SV × SVR

lar trauma. Three major mechanisms maintain the blood pressure within these limits.

The first of these is the *baroreceptor reflex*, a virtually instantaneous response that regulates the blood pressure by controlling autonomic discharge from the brain stem. Specialized receptors in the carotid sinus detect fluctuations in the mean arterial blood pressure and transmit this to the brain stem. From here, changes in the adrenergic outflow from the brain stem directly modify heart rate, cardiac contractility, and systemic vascular resistance in order to restore the blood pressure toward its prior set-point.

The second mechanism centers on the *renin-angiotensin system* (Fig. 30–1). The kidney produces *renin*, an enzyme that acts on a plasma protein, termed renin substrate, to form *angiotensin I*, which is subsequently converted, primarily in the lungs, to *angiotensin II*. Angiotensin II is a potent vasoconstricting hormone that raises systemic vascular resistance. Angiotensin II also stimulates the adrenal gland to synthesize *aldosterone*, a mineralocorticoid hormone that promotes reabsorption of salt and water by the kidney. Multiple factors affect the release of renin from the juxtaglomerular cells of the kidney, including changes in renal perfusion pressure, changes in the sodium content of the distal renal tubule, beta-adrenergic stimuli, and the influence of locally produced prostaglandins.

Third, because plasma volume directly affects blood pressure, it must be closely regulated within a range that will maintain adequate tissue perfusion. The kidneys play an important role in preserving plasma volume in states of extracellular fluid depletion by the avid reabsorption of salt and water from the renal tubules. Conversely, if the blood pressure rises because of an increased plasma volume, the kidney undergoes a natriuresis in order to return plasma volume to its baseline.

CLINICAL ASPECTS OF HYPERTENSION

The vast majority of patients with hypertension (90 to 95 per cent) will not have a definable cause

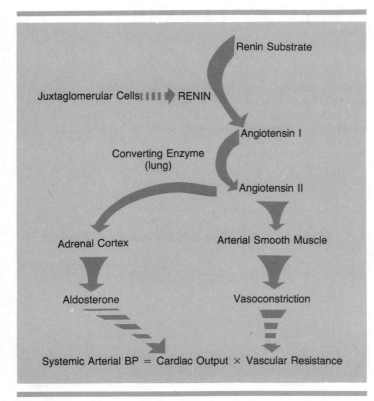

FIGURE 30–1. The renin-angiotensin-aldosterone system.

for their disease and are given the diagnosis of primary or *essential hypertension*. Instead of being a discrete entity, essential hypertension appears to be a heterogeneous syndrome in which multiple factors contribute to the elevated blood pressure through an effect on cardiac output, systemic vascular resistance, and/or salt balance.

Although there may be an increase in cardiac output and/or systemic vascular resistance in the initial phase of hypertension, established hypertension is most often maintained by an elevated systemic vascular resistance as cardiac output returns to normal. The kidney probably plays an important role in the maintenance of hypertension as well by the upward "resetting" of the pressure level at which natriuresis occurs. Furthermore, the enhanced vascular tone in hypertensive patients may be the result of the influence of angiotensin II, sympathetic nervous system discharge, arteriolar hyperplasia, and other factors.

Although essential hypertension is usually detected during middle age, the disease probably begins during the early teenage years. It is typically of insidious onset and asymptomatic for many years. If the hypertensive patient remains undetected or is inadequately treated, morbidity and mortality may be significant. Although elevated blood pressure in itself can lead to vascular injury and end-organ damage, a second major mediator of disease in the hypertensive patient is accelerated atherosclerosis. The most commonly involved target organs are the brain, heart, kidney, and major blood vessels (Table 30–3). The main causes of death in the hypertensive patient are the result of these pathological processes. Myocardial infarction and cerebrovascular accident lead the list. These sequelae can largely be prevented if effective treatment is instituted before the development of irreversible end-organ damage.

The approach to the patient with hypertension begins with an evaluation of the severity of the disease as assessed by its effects on target organs. Although many patients have asymptomatic elevations of blood pressure, neurological or cardiovascular complaints are often elicted. A detailed examination of the optic fundus provides an excellent chance to view the vascular effects of hypertension directly and, when combined with a careful physical examination, can be used to assess the damage incurred by elevated blood pressure. Routine laboratory studies in a newly diagnosed hypertensive patient should include an electrocardiogram, complete blood count, urinalysis, and blood chemistries such as serum electrolytes, creatinine, glucose, triglycerides, cholesterol, and uric acid.

A subset of patients with hypertension may develop rapidly progressive, aggressive disease that is termed *accelerated* or *malignant hypertension*. It is characterized by a severe elevation of blood pressure (diastolic values usually in excess of 120 mm Hg and as high as 150 mm Hg) and widespread end-organ dysfunction. If untreated, it leads to irreversible tissue damage and death. Widespread fibrinoid necrosis of arterioles is the major pathological finding. The patient most often

TABLE 30–3. HYPERTENSIVE COMPLICATIONS

TARGET ORGAN	HYPERTENSIVE	ATHEROSCLEROTIC
Brain/Eye	Intracerebral hemorrhage	Thrombotic stroke
	Lacunar infarcts	TIA
	Encephalopathy	
	Fundal hemorrhages, exudates, papilledema	
Heart	Congestive failure	Myocardial infarct
	Ventricular hypertrophy	Angina
Kidney	Nephrosclerosis	Renal artery stenosis
Vessels	Aortic dissection	Diffuse atheromata

appears ill and may have complaints of headache, blurred vision, and dyspnea. The typical retinal findings include papilledema, fundal hemorrhages, and infarctions (cotton wool spots). Encephalopathy and congestive cardiac failure may also occur. Microangiopathic hemolytic anemia is common, and renal function is often significantly impaired.

REMEDIABLE CAUSES OF HYPERTENSION

Only about 5 to 10 per cent of patients with hypertension are found to have a secondary cause for their elevated blood pressure. However, because the management of hypertension in these patients is significantly different and because the disease is potentially curable, it is important to consider these conditions. A detailed evaluation designed to exclude all causes of secondary hypertension is not warranted in most patients. However, a more thorough investigation should be pursued in the young patient with severe hypertension, the individual whose blood pressure is poorly controlled on antihypertensive therapy, or the person whose initial screening evaluation is suspicious for the presence of a secondary cause (Table 30–4).

A brief description of the major causes of secondary hypertension and the approach to diagnosis are as follows.

Renovascular Hypertension. In this condition one or both renal arteries are affected by a stenotic lesion that causes renal ischemia and subsequent stimulation of the renin-angiotensin system. The stenotic lesions are of two varieties. The first, termed fibromuscular hyperplasia, is characterized by proliferation of the vascular media and is more commonly seen in young, otherwise healthy women. The second type is an atheromatous lesion that affects the proximal renal artery and is usually seen in older men who have evidence of widespread atherosclerotic disease. The diagnosis usually requires a renal arteriogram to assess the vascular anatomy and selective renal vein renin levels to confirm the role of renin-angiotensin in the hypertension. Unilateral renal artery stenosis is characterized by a high venous renin level on the affected side and a suppressed level on the

TABLE 30–4. SECONDARY CAUSES OF HYPERTENSION

CAUSE	SYMPTOMS/SIGNS	ASSOCIATIONS	CONFIRMATION
Renovascular	Flank bruit, diffuse atherosclerosis	$\downarrow K^+$, $\uparrow$ Creatinine	Arteriogram, $\uparrow$ Renal vein, renin level
Renal disease	Edema	Acute/chronic renal disease	$\uparrow$ Creatinine, $\uparrow$ BUN
Pheochromocytoma	Paroxysmal sweating, palpitations, flushing, headache, weight loss, episodic hypertension, tachycardia, orthostatic hypotension	$\uparrow$ Urine VMA, metanephrines, catecholamines	CAT scan, arteriography
Mineralocorticoid excess	Weakness, muscle cramps	Hypokalemia, alkalosis, $\downarrow$ renin	$\uparrow$ Aldosterone level, CAT scan
Aortic coarctation	$\uparrow$ BP in arms, $\downarrow$ BP in legs	Rib notching on chest x-ray	Arteriography

unaffected side. Treatment of renovascular hypertension should be individualized; surgical revascularization is possible in some patients, whereas in others medical treatment with angiotensin-converting enzyme inhibitors and/or other antihypertensive drugs is the better choice.

Parenchymal Renal Disease. Hypertension is a common finding in many acute and chronic renal diseases. The mechanism is most often the result of hypervolemia, although in some patients the renin-angiotensin system mediates the hypertension. Although most chronic renal diseases cannot be reversed, treatment of the associated hypertension may slow the progression of the renal disease and reduce the risk of other morbid complications.

Pheochromocytoma. Hypertension is the hallmark of pheochromocytoma, a rare tumor of chromaffin cells that secretes norepinephrine and epinephrine. These tumors are most often located within the adrenal medulla but may occur along the sympathetic ganglia in the abdomen and chest. Patients typically describe symptoms of paroxysmal sweating, flushing, palpitations, and orthostasis associated with the finding of intermittent hypertension. However, not all patients present with these classic findings and may simply have sustained hypertension. The diagnosis is made by detecting elevated urinary excretion of catecholamines or the metabolites, vanillylmandelic acid (VMA) and metanephrine. The tumor can usually be localized by computed tomography. Surgical removal of the tumor is the preferred treatment for pheochromocytoma, but preoperative control of the blood pressure and extracellular fluid volume is critically important.

Mineralocorticoid Excess. The most common cause of mineralocorticoid excess is primary hyperaldosteronism. A solitary adrenal adenoma, usually benign, or bilateral adrenal hyperplasia is responsible for excess production of aldosterone in this disease. Hypertension is initiated by volume expansion, a direct consequence of aldosterone-mediated sodium reabsorption in the distal nephron. The major symptoms in these patients are referable to the hypokalemia that is almost universally present because of enhanced distal tubule secretion of potassium. Metabolic alkalosis may occur because of augmented hydrogen ion secretion. The diagnosis is confirmed by the detection of a high level of aldosterone and a suppressed level of renin in the plasma. If an adrenal adenoma can be detected, surgical removal should be considered. The use of an aldosterone antagonist such as spironolactone may be helpful in the treatment of hypertension and hypokalemia in patients who are not considered surgical candidates.

Coarctation of the Aorta. Coarctation of the aorta is most often a congenital disorder in which the aorta is narrowed, usually just distal to the left subclavian artery. Mechanical impairment of blood flow to the kidneys leading to stimulation of the renin-angiotensin axis is the probable initiating mechanism in the hypertension of aortic coarctation. The hallmark on physical examination is an elevated blood pressure in the arms associated with a lower blood pressure in the legs. The disease is most commonly diagnosed during childhood, and the treatment is surgical repair of the vascular narrowing.

TREATMENT OF HYPERTENSION

The goal of treatment in the hypertensive patient is to reduce the risk of morbid sequelae and death due to cerebrovascular, cardiovascular, and renal disease. Individuals with diastolic blood pressures consistently greater than 95 mm Hg benefit from treatment directed at lowering blood pressure. For individuals with diastolic blood pressures between 90 and 95 mm Hg, the approach should be individualized. If other risk factors such as diabetes mellitus or hyperlipidemia are coexistent, treatment should be strongly considered. Antihypertensive therapy should be designed to maintain diastolic blood pressure below 90 mm Hg or at the lowest level consistent with patient tolerance.

Antihypertensive therapy involves nonpharmacological intervention as well as specific drug treatments. The former approach includes such recommendations as dietary sodium restriction, exercise, weight loss, behavior modification, and the limitation of heavy alcohol or tobacco consumption. These interventions may be all that is required in the patient with mild hypertension (diastolic BP 90 to 95 mm Hg). Antihypertensive

TABLE 30–5.   COMMONLY PRESCRIBED ORAL ANTIHYPERTENSIVE DRUGS

CLASSIFICATION	EXAMPLE	MECHANISM	SIDE EFFECTS	PRECAUTIONS/ CONSIDERATIONS
Diuretics	Thiazide, Furosemide	Salt/water diuresis	Hypokalemia, hyperuricemia, hyperglycemia	Furosemide is more useful in chronic renal insufficiency
	Spironolactone	Aldosterone antagonist	Hyperkalemia	Should be avoided in renal insufficiency
Beta-adrenergic blockers	Propranolol	↓ Cardiac contractility and heart rate, may ↓ renin release	Bradycardia, fatigue, insomnia	Avoid in patients with obstructive airway disease, congestive heart failure, heart block
Central adrenergic inhibitors	Clonidine, Methyldopa	Decreased CNS sympathetic outflow	Drowsiness, dry mouth, fatigue, sexual dysfunction	Rapid clonidine withdrawal may lead to rebound hypertension
Peripheral adrenergic inhibitors	Guanethidine	Vasodilation	Orthostatic hypotension, sexual dysfunction	Use with caution in the elderly
Alpha-1–adrenergic blocker	Prazosin	Vasodilation	"First dose" hypotension, orthostatic hypotension, tachycardia	Tachyphylaxis to drug effect often noted
Combined alpha/beta blocker	Labetolol	↓ Cardiac contractility and heart rate vasodilation	Dizziness, fatigue, headache	Avoid in patients with obstructive airway disease, congestive heart failure, heart block
Vasodilators	Hydralazine, Minoxidil	Vasodilation	Tachycardia, fluid retention	Positive antinuclear antibody, lupus syndrome with hydralazine, hypertrichosis with minoxidil
Calcium channel blockers	Nifedipine	Vasodilation	Tachycardia, fluid retention	Usually combined with beta blockers; useful in patients with hypertension and heart failure
Angiotensin-converting enzyme inhibitor	Captopril	Inhibition of angiotensin II production	Skin rash, neutropenia	May cause worsening of renal function, proteinuria in patients with renal disease

drugs are almost always necessary in the management of most other patients but should be prescribed in conjunction with nonpharmacological therapy.

The majority of patients with hypertension can be managed effectively in an outpatient setting as long as the response to antihypertensive therapy is followed closely and the potential adverse side effects of the drug(s) are recognized (Table 30–5). One of the most effective antihypertensive drug regimens is termed the "stepped-care" approach, outlined in Table 30–6. Initial therapy begins with a low dose of a single drug, such as a thiazide diuretic or beta-adrenergic blocker. The dose is then increased to full strength as necessary. If the blood pressure remains elevated, additional drugs are added or substituted until an acceptable blood pressure is achieved. Synergistic effects of antihypertensive drugs will often permit smaller doses of individual drugs. The majority (70 to 80 per cent) of patients will achieve acceptable blood pressure control by step 1 or 2.

Malignant hypertension is a medical emergency that demands a more aggressive approach than that outlined for the stable hypertensive patient. Intensive treatment in a hospital setting is indicated in order to avoid permanent damage to target organs, particularly the kidney. Renal function may deteriorate rapidly during a hypertensive crisis, and deterioration is often not reversible. Equally disturbing is the occasional continued deterioration of kidney function even when the blood pressure is brought under control. Parenterally administered antihypertensive drugs such as sodium nitroprusside, hydralazine, or diazoxide are usually required for optimal management of these critically ill patients.

TABLE 30–6.   "STEPPED CARE" APPROACH TO HYPERTENSION

Step 1	BEGIN	a diuretic or beta-adrenergic blocker
Step 2	ADD	a centrally acting adrenergic blocker* OR a diuretic or beta blocker (if not used in step 1) OR a peripheral alpha blocker†
Step 3	ADD	a vasodilator‡ OR a converting enzyme inhibitor§ OR calcium channel blocker**
Step 4	ADD	guanethidine or minoxidil

Examples:
* clonidine, methyldopa
† prazosin
‡ hydralazine, prazosin
§ captopril
** nifedipine

REFERENCES

Dollery CT: Arterial hypertension. In Wyngaarden JB, and Smith LH Jr (eds): Cecil Textbook of Medicine. 17th ed. Philadelphia, W B Saunders Co, 1985, pp 266–280.

The 1984 Report of the Joint National Committee on Detection, Evaluation, and Treatment of High Blood Pressure. Arch Intern Med 144:1045–1057, 1984.

Wallace AG, and Waugh RA: Hypertension. In Smith LH Jr, and Thier SO (eds): Pathophysiology. 2nd ed. Philadelphia, W B Saunders Co, 1985, pp 915–922.

31 APPROACH TO THE PATIENT WITH RENAL DISEASE

The patient with renal disease often comes to the attention of a physician because of mild, nonspecific signs and symptoms but may also present with severe, life-threatening manifestations of renal dysfunction. Certain signs and symptoms should alert the physician to the possibility that renal disease is present. Complaints of flank pain, dysuria, gross hematuria, or the passage of a renal stone are directly referable to the urinary tract. Other findings such as hypertension, edema, congestive heart failure, or constitutional symptoms of lethargy, anorexia, or pruritus are nonspecific but may reflect the impact of reduced renal function on other organ systems. The approach to the patient with suspected renal disease begins with a careful history and physical examination. Table 31–1 outlines some of the important features of the history and physical examination that should not be overlooked. A particular renal syndrome such as chronic renal failure, glomerulonephritis, urinary tract infection, or urinary tract obstruction is often suggested by the constellation of presenting signs and symptoms. This initial impression can then be used in the formulation of a differential diagnosis and in the design of a diagnostic evaluation.

ASSESSMENT OF RENAL FUNCTION AND STRUCTURE

Specific laboratory tests and renal imaging studies are often indicated in the evaluation of the patient with suspected renal disease. These studies are particularly useful in defining the renal disease, the extent of functional and anatomical impairment, and the rate of progression.

Urinalysis

A complete analysis of the urine is a simple, noninvasive, and inexpensive means of detecting renal pathology. A first morning voided urine specimen obtained by a clean catch technique yields the most information. The urine should be examined promptly by both chemical and microscopic means.

Normal urine ranges from almost colorless to deep yellow, depending on the concentration of urochrome pigment. Abnormal urine colors may be a sign of disease or may indicate the presence of a pigmented drug or dye (Table 31–2). The presence of red blood cells in the urine or large amounts of free hemoglobin or myoglobin will often result in red or smoke-colored urine. Cloudy urine may occur with a heavy white blood cell content (pyuria) or with the precipitation of amorphous phosphate in alkaline urine.

Chemical assessment of the urine is performed with the "dipstick," a chemically impregnated plastic strip that will detect the presence of protein, occult blood, glucose, and ketones in the urine. When the dipstick is placed in urine, the color changes in the various reagent strips provide an approximate quantitation of the amount of substance present. The dipstick method for the detection of urinary protein is very sensitive to albumin but will not detect immunoglobulins or tubular proteins (Tamm-Horsfall mucoprotein). The urine sulfosalicylic acid test will detect all proteins by a process of precipitation and can be used as an alternative means of detecting urinary protein. A very concentrated urine may show trace to 1+ protein (10 to 30 mg/dl) in a normal individual. The finding of occult blood in the urine

---

TABLE 31–1. IMPORTANT FEATURES OF THE HISTORY AND PHYSICAL EXAMINATION IN THE PATIENT WITH RENAL DISEASE

Historical Data
  Familial Renal Disease—polycystic kidney disease, hereditary nephritis, renal calculi
  Systemic Disease—systemic lupus erythematosus, diabetes mellitus, hypertension, sickle cell anemia
  Toxic Exposure—heavy metals, radiographic contrast material, drugs: analgesics, antibiotics, nonsteroidal anti-inflammatory agents
  Associated Symptoms
    General: fever, weight loss, fatigue, skin rash, pruritis, sore throat
    Cardiovascular: dyspnea, chest pain, edema
    Gastrointestinal: anorexia, nausea, vomiting
    Genitourinary: polyuria, dysuria, flank pain, hematuria, passage of a renal stone
Physical Examination
  Cardiovascular: hypertension, cardiac failure, pericardial rub, edema
  Genitourinary: palpable kidneys or bladder, prostatic enlargement
  Neurological: peripheral neuropathy, asterixis, encephalopathy
  Funduscopic: signs of diabetes, systemic lupus erythematosus, hypertension

is abnormal and signifies the presence of either intact red blood cells or free hemoglobin or myoglobin molecules.

Microscopic examination of the urine sediment may reveal the presence of cellular elements, casts, crystals, or micro-organisms (Table 31–3). Microscopic hematuria is defined as more than two red blood cells per high-power field on a centrifuged urine specimen in the absence of contamination by menstrual blood. Pyuria is defined as the presence of more than four white blood cells per high-power field. Epithelial cells are commonly found in the urinary sediment and may derive from any point along the urinary tract from the renal parenchyma to the urethra. Renal tubular cells that contain absorbed lipids are termed oval fat bodies. Free fat droplets composed primarily of cholesterol esters may also be observed in the urine, particularly in association with heavy proteinuria. Both the oval fat body and free fat droplets have doubly refractile characteristics under the polarizing microscope and share the characteristic "Maltese cross" appearance. Urinary casts are cylindrical elements derived from the intratubular precipitation of mucoprotein and cellular debris. Hyaline casts, composed of mucoprotein, are a common finding in concentrated urine. Casts composed of cellular elements in addition to protein are named according to the predominant cell type. The presence of red or white blood cell casts is strong evidence of inflammatory parenchymal renal disease. Granular, waxy, or broad casts represent successive stages in the degeneration of cellular casts.

Crystals of calcium oxalate (envelope-shaped) and uric acid (rhomboid) are often identified in acid urine depending on the degree of supersaturation but are usually of little clinical significance. Cystine crystals provide a clue to the rare disease cystinuria. Triple phosphate crystals ("coffin lid"–shaped) may be identified in alkaline urine. Bacteria in the urine are almost always recognized in a centrifuged specimen but do not necessarily imply significant bacteriuria. The presence of bacteria in an unspun specimen, however, is significant and provides presumptive evidence for a urinary tract infection.

Renal Function Tests

Specific tests of renal function are used to assess both the glomerular and tubular functional capacity of the kidney. The glomerular filtration rate is most accurately determined by measurement of the clearance of a marker that is completely filtered by the glomerulus and neither reabsorbed, secreted, nor metabolized by the renal tubule. The sugar inulin is an ideal marker for such a study. Because inulin is not an endogenous substance, performance of an inulin clearance study is not practical in the routine clinical setting. Determination of the clearance of endogenous creatinine is a more convenient test and provides a reasonable estimate of the glomerular filtration rate. Because roughly 10 per cent of creatinine is excreted by the process of tubular se-

cretion, the creatinine clearance will overestimate the true glomerular filtration rate. The creatinine clearance (C_{cr}) is calculated as $C = U_{cr}V/P_{cr}$. P_{cr} is the plasma creatinine in mg/dl, U_{cr} is the urine creatinine in mg/dl, and V is the volume of urine excreted over a specific time interval in ml/min. Normal values of C_{cr} range from 75 to 160 ml/min or 95 to 105 ml/min/1.73 sq m when normalized to body surface area (Table 31–4). The creatinine clearance is normally increased 30 to 50 per cent

TABLE 31–2. URINE COLORS

COLOR	ASSOCIATION
colorless	dilute urine, diabetes mellitus, diabetes insipidus
yellow	normal, riboflavin, quinacrine
amber	concentrated urine, Pyridium, sulfasalizine
blue, blue-green	biliverdin, methylene blue, amitriptyline, triamterene
red	hematuria, hemoglobinuria, myoglobinuria, phenytoin, phenolphthalein, rifampin, adriamycin, anthrocyanin (pigment in beets and blackberries)
red-brown	porphyria, urobilinogen, bilirubin, nitrofurantoin, primaquine, chloroquine, metronidazole
brown-black	acidification of hemoglobin pigment, melanin, alkaptonuria, senna, cascara, rhubarb
milky white	chyluria, pyuria

TABLE 31–3. MICROSCOPIC EXAMINATION OF THE URINE

	FINDING	ASSOCIATIONS
Casts	Red blood cell	glomerulonephritis, vasculitis
	White blood cell	interstitial nephritis, pyelonephritis
	Epithelial cell	acute tubular necrosis, interstitial nephritis, glomerulonephritis
	Granular	renal parenchymal disease (nonspecific)
	Waxy, broad	advanced renal failure
	Hyaline	normal finding in concentrated urine
	Fatty	heavy proteinuria
Cells	Red blood cell	urinary tract infection, urinary tract inflammation
	White blood cell	urinary tract infection, urinary tract inflammation
	Eosinophil	drug-induced interstitial nephritis
	(Squamous) epithelial cell	contaminants
Crystals	Uric acid	acid urine, acute uric acid nephropathy, hyperuricosuria
	Calcium phosphate	alkaline urine
	Calcium oxalate	acid urine, hyperoxaluria, ethylene glycol poisoning
	Cystine	Cystinuria
	Sulfur	Sulfadiazine antibiotics

TABLE 31–4. CALCULATION OF THE CREATININE CLEARANCE

$$C_{cr} = U_{creat} \times V/P_{creat}$$

C_{cr} = clearance of creatinine (ml/min)
U_{creat} = urine creatinine (mg/dl)
V = volume of urine (ml/min) (for 24 hour volume: divide by 1440)
P_{creat} = plasma creatinine (mg/dl)
Normal range: 95 to 105 ml/min/1.73 sq m

over baseline values in pregnancy because of the increase in renal plasma flow during gestation. Protein loading is also associated with an incremental rise in creatinine clearance on the basis of similar intrarenal hemodynamic changes and can be used as a measure of the functional reserve capacity of the kidney.

An approximate assessment of glomerular filtration is easily obtained by the measurement of the concentration of creatinine and urea nitrogen in the serum. Creatinine is a metabolite of creatine, a major muscle constituent. In a given individual, the daily rate of production of creatinine is constant and determined by the mass of skeletal muscle. Because body creatinine is disposed almost entirely by glomerular filtration, its steady-state concentration in the serum has been used as a marker of glomerular function. The "normal" range for serum creatinine is 0.5 to 1.5 mg/dl. In any individual, however, a value in this range does not necessarily imply normal renal function. A more accurate assessment of renal function is obtained by determining the creatinine clearance. However, once the relationship between the serum creatinine and the creatinine clearance is established for a given patient, the serum creatinine can be followed as a reliable indicator of renal function.

The urea nitrogen concentration in the serum (BUN) is often used in conjunction with the serum creatinine as a measure of renal function. Urea is the major end product of protein metabolism, and its production reflects the dietary intake of protein as well as the protein catabolic rate. Urea is excreted by glomerular filtration but significant amounts of urea are reabsorbed along the renal tubule, particularly when the kidney is salt- and water-avid, as in extracellular volume contraction. Consequently, the BUN may vary in relation to the extracellular fluid volume, whereas the serum concentration of creatinine does not. The usual ratio of urea nitrogen to creatinine concentration in the serum is 10:1. This ratio is altered in a number of clinical settings and may suggest a specific diagnosis (Table 31–5).

Renal tubular function is evaluated by tests that examine the ability of the kidney to maintain salt and water balance as well as acid-base homeostasis. Maximal urinary concentrating ability is assessed by restriction of water intake until three consecutive urine specimens show no increase in urine osmolality or until the subject has lost a maximum of 5 per cent of body weight. The normal individual is able to concentrate the urine to

between 800 and 1200 mOsm/kg H_2O. A further increase in the osmolality is not observed following the administration of aqueous vasopressin.

The fractional excretion of various solutes provides useful information about the handling of a solute relative to its glomerular filtration. This is carried out by measuring the urinary excretion of the solute in question relative to the excretion of creatinine. The fractional excretion is calculated as the clearance of the solute divided by the clearance of creatinine $\times$ 100 and is expressed as a per cent. The fractional excretion of sodium, for example, is the fraction of sodium filtered at the glomerulus that is ultimately excreted in the urine (Table 31–6). Determination of the fractional excretion of sodium is most useful in the differential diagnosis of a patient with acute renal insufficiency. Determination of the fractional excretion of calcium, phosphate, uric acid, and amino acids is useful in the evaluation of patients with suspected disorders of renal tubular function or in the evaluation of renal stone disease. Acidification of the urine is an important tubular function that can be assessed by the measurement of the urine pH. In the presence of systemic acidosis, the urine pH should be 5.3 or less.

A timed urine collection for determination of the rate of protein excretion is an important study in the evaluation of glomerular and tubular diseases of the kidney. In normal individuals, urinary protein excretion is less than 150 mg/24 hr. In patients with various glomerular or tubular disorders, the renal excretion of protein may be increased significantly. In glomerular disease, the urinary excretion of protein is usually in excess of 2 to 3 grams per day. Because the daily urinary excretion of creatinine is relatively constant and

TABLE 31–5. CAUSES OF ALTERED UREA NITROGEN–TO–CREATININE RATIO

Increased Ratio (>10:1)
  Increased urea input
    Increased dietary protein intake
    Gastrointestinal hemorrhage
    Hemolysis
    Sepsis/catabolic states
    Drugs that inhibit anabolism
      Corticosteroids
      Tetracyclines
  Decreased effective circulating volume
    Volume depletion
    Congestive heart failure
    Cirrhosis/ascites
    Nephrotic syndrome
  Obstructive uropathy
Decreased Ratio (<10:1)
  Decreased urea input
    Starvation
    Liver disease
  Increased creatinine production
    Rhabdomyolysis
  Volume expansion
    SIADH
    Iatrogenic
  Chronic renal failure with dialysis

averages 10 to 20 mg/kg in women and 15 to 25 mg/kg in men, the rate of creatinine excretion in any timed urine collection should be determined to verify that the collection was complete. If the creatinine excretion deviates significantly from these guidelines, the collection should be repeated.

Anatomical Imaging of the Urinary Tract

The plain film of the abdomen, or KUB, is a simple way of determining renal size and shape. The normal kidney shadow will approximate the length of three and one-half vertebral bodies or about 12 cm. Bilaterally small kidneys in a patient with renal insufficiency implies a chronic, irreversible process, whereas the presence of enlarged kidneys suggests obstructive, inflammatory, infiltrative, or cystic disease. Radiopaque renal calculi composed of calcium, magnesium ammonium phosphate (struvite), or cystine are often apparent on a plain film of the abdomen. Renal ultrasonography is another noninvasive method of obtaining an anatomical image of the kidney and the collecting system. Renal ultrasonography is particularly useful in the detection of renal masses, renal cysts, and dilation of portions of the urinary tract (hydronephrosis). An accurate determination of renal size and shape can also be discerned from the sonogram.

The radioisotopic renal scan provides information about renal blood flow and tubular function. The test involves the intravenous administration of radiolabeled compounds that are excreted by the kidney. An external scintillation camera provides an image of the kidneys and calculates the rate of uptake and excretion of the labeled compound. Technetium-99 DPTA is the compound used to assess renal vascular perfusion qualitatively. Impaired renal perfusion, as in the setting of unilateral renal artery stenosis or renal infarction, is characterized by asymmetric uptake of technetium. Generalized renal hypoperfusion, as in the setting of acute glomerulonephritis or renal transplant rejection, can be recognized also. An evaluation of renal tubular function may be obtained by the use of hippuran ^{131}I, a compound eliminated by tubular secretion. Impaired hippuran excretion in the face of a normal technetium perfusion is commonly observed with acute tubular necrosis or chronic renal disease.

The intravenous pyelogram involves the intravenous injection of iodinated radiographic contrast medium that is excreted by glomerular filtration. The contrast medium is concentrated in the renal tubules as water is reabsorbed, and this produces a nephrogram image within the first few minutes after injection. As the medium passes into the collecting system, the calyces, renal pelvis, ureters, and bladder are visualized. This study is useful in the identification of lesions such as renal calculi, pyelonephritic scars, cysts, or renal tumors. The computerized axial tomograph (CAT) scan of the kidney provides similar information about renal anatomy but, in contrast to the intra-

TABLE 31–6. CALCULATION OF THE FRACTIONAL EXCRETION OF SODIUM

Fractional excretion of sodium ($FeNa^+$) = fraction of sodium filtered at the glomerulus that is ultimately excreted in the urine

$$FeNa^+ = \frac{\text{amount } Na^+ \text{ excreted/volume}}{\text{amount } Na^+ \text{ filtered/volume}} = \frac{U_{Na} \times V}{P_{Na} \times GFR}$$

$$GFR = C_{cr} = \frac{U_{cr} \times V}{P_{cr}}$$

$$FeNa^+ = \frac{U_{Na} \times V}{P_{Na}} \times \frac{1}{U_{cr} \times V/P_{cr}} = \frac{U_{Na} \times P_{cr}}{U_{cr} \times P_{Na}} \times 100$$

P_{Na} = plasma sodium (mEq/L)

P_{cr} = plasma creatinine (mg/dl)

U_{Na} = urine sodium (mEq/L)

U_{cr} = urine creatinine (mg/dl)

venous pyelogram, provides more precise differentiation of solid from cystic lesions. In both studies, the uptake and excretion of contrast by the kidney is prolonged in patients with renal insufficiency. In these patients, useful information can still be obtained from these tests by examining radiographs taken 24 to 48 hours after the injection of contrast medium. The risk of contrast medium–induced nephrotoxicity is the major limiting factor to these tests and for this reason they should be used with caution in high-risk patients. Individuals with underlying renal dysfunction, multiple myeloma, or diabetes mellitus should be well-hydrated to reduce this risk.

Retrograde pyelography is performed by the injection of radiocontrast material directly into the ureters at the time of cystoscopy. It is useful in the definition of obstructing lesions within the ureter or renal pelvis, particularly in the setting of a nonvisualizing kidney on intravenous pyelography. If an obstruction is identified, it can often be removed or bypassed by the placement of a ureteral catheter at the time of the procedure. Cystoscopy is often indicated in the evaluation of unexplained hematuria when bladder lesions are suspected.

Renal arteriography involves the direct injection of radiographic contrast medium into the aorta and renal arteries and is used to define the renal vasculature. Renal arteriography is particularly useful in the evaluation of patients with suspected renal artery stenosis or thrombosis and in those with a renal mass. Because renal arteriography is a more invasive test, its use should be limited to those situations in which a strong clinical indication exists and the patient is considered a candidate for surgical intervention. Renal venography is used to confirm the diagnosis of renal vein thrombosis.

Renal Biopsy

A renal biopsy should be considered in a patient with parenchymal renal disease when the diagnosis or the extent of disease cannot be ascertained by the studies outlined earlier. Most renal biopsies are performed when a glomerular lesion is suspected. It is often clinically important that the disease be diagnosed before commencing treatment with potent drugs such as corticosteroids or immunosuppressive agents. The percutaneous biopsy is the most commonly employed technique and is a relatively safe procedure. An open renal biopsy is considered in the patient with a solitary functioning kidney or a bleeding diathesis when adequate hemostasis is critical to prevent loss of the kidney. The biopsy specimen should be submitted for light, immunofluorescent, and electron microscopy. Potential complications of a renal biopsy include hematuria, renal hematoma, vascular laceration with the development of arteriovenous fistulas, or the inadvertent biopsy of liver, spleen, or bowel.

SPECIFIC MANIFESTATIONS OF RENAL DISEASE

This section reviews the approach to the patient with specific manifestations of renal disease such as proteinuria, hematuria, pyuria, or azotemia. The evaluation of all such patients includes a detailed history and physical examination, a urinalysis, and determination of the serum concentration of creatinine, urea nitrogen, and electrolytes. A timed collection of urine for calculation of the creatinine clearance and rate of protein excretion is often helpful. Other studies, including anatomical imaging of the urinary tract or renal biopsy, may be indicated.

Proteinuria

In a normal individual, less than 150 mg of low molecular weight tubular protein is excreted in the urine per day. The glomerular basement membrane acts as an effective barrier to the passage of high molecular weight proteins, such as albumin, and the renal tubules function to reabsorb the small amount of protein that is filtered. Proteinuria may occur as a transient phenomenon in individuals with febrile illnesses or congestive heart failure or after vigorous exercise. Persistent proteinuria, however, is almost always indicative of renal disease.

Nephrotic range proteinuria (>3.5 grams/24 hr) is indicative of glomerular disease. Lesser amounts of protein may be excreted in various tubulointerstitial diseases or in some cases of acute or chronic renal failure. When proteinuria is associated with red blood cell casts, glomerulonephritis should be suspected. Tubulointerstitial pathology is suggested by the association of proteinuria with alterations in tubular function such as concentrating or acidifying defects. Proteinuria is often asymptomatic, although nephrotic range proteinuria will often result in hypoalbuminemia and resultant edema formation.

The laboratory evaluation of the patient with proteinuria begins with a quantitation of protein excretion in a 24-hour urine specimen. A urine protein electrophoresis should be obtained to identify the major urinary proteins. Diseases of the glomerulus are characterized by predominant albuminuria, whereas tubulointerstitial disease results in the excretion of low molecular weight proteins. Detection of a monoclonal immunoglobulin spike in the urine is suggestive of multiple myeloma or amyloidosis. A renal biopsy should be considered when the cause of heavy proteinuria is not apparent from the initial evaluation.

Hematuria

The presence of red blood cells in the urine, either microscopic or macroscopic, should be regarded as a significant finding. Hematuria is a sign of genitourinary tract inflammation and occurs in a number of disorders, including glomerulonephritis, acute and chronic renal failure, urinary tract infection, urinary tract obstruction, and neoplasia. Although the source of bleeding cannot be defined on the basis of the presenting signs and symptoms or the urinalysis, certain specific findings are helpful. The presence of red blood cell casts and associated proteinuria is good evidence for a glomerular inflammatory lesion. Smoke-colored urine is also considered a sign of glomerular bleeding, since the contact time of the red blood cells with the urine is prolonged and allows for the formation of methemoglobin. The passage of gross clots in the urine is suggestive of bleeding distal to the renal tubule.

The evaluation of the patient with hematuria will often require anatomical imaging of the urinary tract to exclude a neoplastic lesion or renal stone. Cystoscopy may be indicated to exclude an inflammatory lesion of the bladder. A urine culture should be obtained to rule out the possibility of hemorrhagic bacterial cystitis. If the bleeding is of glomerular or tubular origin and a specific diagnosis cannot be made by other means, a renal biopsy may be helpful.

Pyuria

The finding of more than four white blood cells per high-power field on a urine specimen is suggestive of urinary tract inflammation, although as with hematuria, the precise site is not identified. Pyuria as an isolated finding is most commonly associated with bacterial urinary tract infection. When associated with hematuria or proteinuria, pyuria is suggestive of parenchymal renal disease such as glomerulonephritis or interstitial nephritis.

The presence of pyuria should initiate a search for urinary tract infection, particularly when the patient complains of dysuria, flank pain, or fever. Renal imaging studies are often indicated to exclude the presence of renal parenchymal scarring, obstruction, or abscess formation, particularly when accompanied by signs of renal dysfunction such as azotemia. Sterile pyuria may be a sign of occult renal tuberculosis. A Wright's stain of the urine for eosinophils is often helpful in the patient suspected of having acute allergic interstitial nephritis.

Azotemia

The patient with azotemia often comes to the attention of a physician because of signs or symptoms referable to impaired renal function. Occasionally, an elevation of the plasma concentration of urea nitrogen or creatinine is an incidental finding on a screening laboratory profile in an asymptomatic patient. In either case, the major clinical questions are (1) is the renal dysfunction acute or chronic? and (2) what is the rate of progression of the renal disease?

The history of the patient and prior blood chemistry determinations, if available, provide important information in distinguishing acute from chronic renal disease. The presence of small kidneys assessed by renal imaging studies is most suggestive of chronic disease. The presence of normal-sized or enlarged kidneys, however, does not exclude the diagnosis of chronic renal insufficiency. Patients with chronic renal failure as compared to those with acute renal failure tend to be more anemic and to have higher plasma concentrations of phosphate. Neither of these determinations, however, is sufficiently discriminating to differentiate acute from chronic disease. The patient must be evaluated for the presence of any potentially reversible coexisting insults to the kidney, such as hydronephrosis or drug-induced renal insufficiency.

Evaluation of the rate of progression of renal insufficiency is important, as it provides an estimate of when a patient will require renal replacement therapy. Most patients with uncomplicated chronic renal failure have a slow progressive deterioration in renal function. Secondary insults such as disturbances in the volume or composition of the extracellular fluid volume, obstruction to urine flow, urinary tract infection, exposure to nephrotoxins, or uncontrolled severe hypertension may accelerate the rate of deterioration in renal function in a patient with underlying chronic renal disease. A valuable method of evaluating such individuals is to graph the reciprocal of the serum creatinine concentration (1/Cr) versus time (Fig. 31–1). Such a graph describes a straight line with a negative slope in patients with progressive renal failure. Secondary insults would be indicated by a relatively abrupt increase in the slope of the relationship. In addition, such

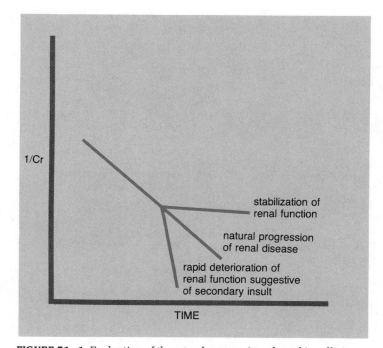

FIGURE 31–1. Evaluation of the rate of progression of renal insufficiency by graphing the reciprocal of the serum creatinine concentration (1/Cr) versus time.

a graph can be used to evaluate the response to therapy in a patient with renal disease. A decrease in the slope of 1/Cr versus time indicates a slowing in the rate of deterioration of renal function. A graph of 1/Cr versus time is also of value in predicting when a given patient will require dialysis treatment or consideration for renal transplantation.

REFERENCES

Abuelo JG: Proteinuria: Diagnostic principles and procedures. Ann Intern Med 98:186, 1983.
Race GJ, and White MG: Basic Urinalysis. Hagerstown, MD, Harper and Row, 1979.
Steiner RW: Interpreting the fractional excretion of sodium. Am J Med 77:699, 1984.

ACUTE RENAL INSUFFICIENCY 32

Acute or subacute declines in the glomerular filtration rate and/or in tubular function (acute renal insufficiency) can occur in a variety of clinical settings and as a consequence of different types of insults to the kidney (Table 32–1). Decreases in the effective circulating blood volume or renal blood flow may result in a decline in the glomerular filtration rate with relatively intact tubular function. Such conditions are termed *prerenal azotemia*. Obstruction to urine flow results in an acute decrease in renal function and the development of *obstructive nephropathy*. Renal parenchymal inflammatory diseases such as glomerulonephritis and interstitial nephritis can also

TABLE 32–1. ETIOLOGIES OF ACUTE RENAL INSUFFICIENCY

TYPE	EXAMPLES
Prerenal Azotemia	External losses of fluid and electrolytes—vomiting, diarrhea, diuretic administration, burns
	Internal sequestrations of extracellular fluid—peritonitis, pancreatitis
	Decreased effective circulating volume—congestive heart failure, liver disease with ascites
Diseases of the Renal Arteries or Veins	Direct trauma to renal vasculature, dissecting aortic aneurysm
Intrinsic Renal Disease	
Glomerulonephritis	Postinfectious glomerulonephritis, antibasement membrane antibody disease, collagen vascular diseases
Acute interstitial nephritis	Drug associated acute interstitial nephritis
Acute tubular necrosis	Vasomotor nephropathy, toxic nephropathy
Intratubular obstruction	Rhabdomyolysis, multiple myeloma, uric acid–induced acute renal failure (tumor lysis syndrome)
Obstruction of Collecting System	Bladder outlet obstruction, bilateral ureteral obstruction (rare), ureteral obstruction in a solitary kidney

result in acute changes in kidney function. The term *acute tubular necrosis* (ATN) is generally taken to describe a clinical syndrome in which there is a simultaneous and progressive deterioration of both glomerular and tubular function in the absence of documented glomerular or interstitial nephritis, vascular disease, or obstruction of the collecting system. It is to be noted that the term acute tubular necrosis is not a valid histological description of this syndrome (see page 215). Nonetheless, this terminology is widely used and will be employed in this chapter. Synonyms for acute tubular necrosis include vasomotor nephropathy, toxic nephropathy, and the acute renal failure syndrome. Acute tubular necrosis usually refers to rapid changes in renal function consequent to a severe reduction in the effective circulating extracellular fluid volume and/or the ingestion, administration, or generation of substances that are directly toxic to the renal tubular cells. In the clinical setting, the diagnosis of ATN is often suggested from the history and physical examination of the patient but is, in fact, a diagnosis of exclusion. Said in another way, it is necessary to carefully exclude the other defined renal syndromes before concluding that ATN is present. In the first part of the present chapter, the general approach to a patient with an acute decline in renal function is considered. The second part of this chapter deals more specifically with the ATN syndrome.

CLINICAL PRESENTATION

Renal insufficiency results in signs and symptoms that reflect loss of the regulatory, excretory, and endocrine functions of the kidney. The inability to regulate the volume of body fluid compartments may be expressed as edema, hypertension, or congestive heart failure. The loss of ability to regulate the composition of the body fluids is evidenced by the development of hyperkalemia, metabolic acidosis, and hyperphosphatemia.

The loss of excretory ability of the kidney is expressed by a rise in the plasma concentration of specific substances normally excreted by the kidney. The most widely monitored indices are the blood urea nitrogen (BUN) and concentration of creatinine in the serum. The rate of rise of BUN and creatinine reflects the impairment in the filtration function of the kidney and the rate of generation of urea nitrogen and creatinine. Creatinine generation is proportional to muscle mass. Accordingly, a patient with acute renal failure and a large mass of muscle may have an increase in the serum concentration of creatinine of several milligrams per deciliter per day. A patient with smaller initial muscle mass but with the same degree of renal filtration failure may have a slower rate of rise. Urea nitrogen derives from the catabolism of protein. In a catabolic patient, blood urea nitrogen may increase by over 40 mg/dl/day. In a patient who is not catabolic and in whom the dietary intake of protein is low, the rate of urea nitrogen generation will be less and the blood level will increase at a slower rate. Thus, while increases in the serum concentration of urea nitrogen and creatinine indicate the presence of renal disease, the absolute blood concentrations obtained and the rate of change are related to both the degree of renal injury and the rate of generation. A thin, elderly individual can be severely and symptomatically uremic despite the fact that the serum concentration of creatinine is only 2 mg/dl. Conversely, such a value would be only modestly abnormal in a young, muscular, athletic person.

DIAGNOSTIC WORK-UP OF THE PATIENT WITH ACUTE RENAL INSUFFICIENCY (TABLE 32–2)

History and Physical

A history and physical examination provide useful diagnostic information. Careful review of medical records, if available, and medications should be performed. Certain signs and symptoms may provide clues to specific disease entities. The presence of red blood cell casts would indicate glomerulonephritis; the presence of swelling and edema of muscle might indicate rhabdomyolysis. The findings of abdominal or flank pain could be the result of renal infarctions, obstruction to urine flow, or acute inflammation of the kidney. The signs and symptoms of specific disease entities are discussed more completely in other chapters. It is important to note that virtually all renal injuries may result in the development of acute renal insufficiency.

Blood Chemistries

Routine, and where appropriate special blood chemistries, a hemogram, and a urinalysis should be obtained. The choice of special laboratory tests depends upon the clinical circumstances. If a collagen vascular or immune complex disease is suspected, the serum complement should be measured. Determination of the titer of antinuclear antibodies is indicated in patients suspected to have systemic lupus erythematosus. In patients with a clinical picture consistent with rapidly progressive glomerulonephritis or Goodpasture's syndrome, the serum should be checked for the presence of anti–glomerular basement membrane antibodies. Serum and urine protein electrophoresis is indicated in patients in whom the diagnosis of multiple myeloma is suggested.

Urinalysis, Renal Tubular Function, and Urine Flow Rate

A careful *urinalysis* should be performed to determine the presence or absence of red blood cell casts. The presence of red blood cell casts indicates inflammation of the glomerulus. The presence of red blood cells but not red blood cell casts is less diagnostic and may indicate disease in the kidney itself or in the collecting system. White blood cell casts reflect inflammation (but not necessarily infection) of the renal parenchyma. Polymorphonuclear leukocytes may derive from the kidney and/or the collecting system. The presence of lymphocytes and/or eosinophils may suggest the diagnosis of acute interstitial nephritis. The urinalysis of a patient with obstruction to flow in the collecting system is variable. An important diagnostic point is that the presence of azotemia in the face of a totally normal appearing urinalysis is highly suggestive of obstruction. The presence of red or white blood cells, however, does not rule out the diagnosis of obstruction. The urine of patients with acute tubular necrosis usually contains protein and, on microscopic examination, granular casts. Glucose may be detected in the urine in the absence of hyperglycemia, a finding that reflects the tubular damage. In acute tubular necrosis, the urinalysis is almost always abnormal but nondiagnostic. It is, however, an important test to rule out other etiologies of acute renal insufficiency.

An important diagnostic issue is the determination of *tubular function*. The most widely used and convenient tests are measurements of the concentration of electrolytes and osmolality of the urine and the calculation of the fractional excretion of sodium. To be of optimal clinical value, such measurements must be obtained prior to the administration of diuretics and considered in concert with other assessments of the state of hydration of the individual. The utility of these urinary indices is highest in patients with oliguria and azotemia. The urine indices are not diagnostic in and of themselves. In general, the acute tubular necrosis is characterized by defects in tubular absorptive function as expressed by the findings of a urine concentration of sodium of greater than 40

TABLE 32–2. DIAGNOSTIC APPROACH TO A PATIENT WITH ACUTE RENAL INSUFFICIENCY

1. History and physical examination and review of medications
2. Routine and special laboratory tests
3. Examination of the urine, measurement of renal tubular function, and determination of the urine flow rate
4. Determination of the anatomy of the kidney and, when indicated, the renal blood flow
5. Other diagnostic tests when indicated

mEq/L on a spot sample, a fractional excretion of sodium of greater than 1 per cent, and a urine osmolality that approaches that of the serum.

Prerenal azotemia is characterized by a decrease in the glomerular filtration rate as manifest by a rise in the BUN and creatinine and by normal tubular function as evidenced by a low urine concentration of sodium, a high urine osmolality, and a fractional excretion of sodium of less than 1 per cent. Patients with acute renal insufficiency secondary to acute glomerulonephritis may also have well-preserved renal tubular function early in the course of their disease, as may patients with the acute onset of partial urinary tract obstruction.

The major value of determining the urine concentration of sodium and the fractional excretion of sodium is in formulating a differential diagnosis in a patient with decreased renal function. Interpretations of these tests, however, must be made in conjunction with other assessments of the patient. While patients with renal tubular disease frequently have high urine concentrations and fractional excretions of sodium and patients with prerenal disease manifest sodium avidity, there are clinically important exceptions to these generalizations. Certain types of ATN such as radiographic dye–induced renal injury may present with all the clinical characteristics of ATN, but with fractional excretions of sodium of less than 1 per cent. Conversely, a patient with depletion of the extracellular fluid volume may have a high urine concentration and fractional excretion of sodium if diuretics have been administered, during the generation phase of metabolic alkalosis, and when there was pre-existing renal tubular disease with renal salt wasting. In these latter conditions, the urinary excretion of sodium does not reflect the state of hydration of the patient.

Determination of the *urine flow rate* is not helpful in formulating a differential diagnosis of the etiology of the acute renal insufficiency but is important in clinical management. Oliguria is considered to be present when the urine volume is less than 500 ml/day. Patients with acute tubular necrosis may be oliguric or polyuric. The distinction between these two forms may reflect differences in the etiology and/or the severity of the insult. Acute partial obstruction to urine flow may be associated with a decreased or variable urine output. However, the presence of a normal urine volume does not exclude the diagnosis. Obstruction of modest duration may result in loss of concentrating ability by the kidney and, as a consequence, the excretion of an apparently normal volume of urine.

The presence of total anuria provides an important diagnostic clue in the evaluation of a patient with acute renal insufficiency and somewhat reduces the differential diagnostic list. Acute arterial or venous catastrophes, total urinary tract obstruction, severe cortical necrosis, severe acute glomerulonephritis and, occasionally, severe acute tubular necrosis may present with anuria.

Determination of Kidney Anatomy and Renal Blood Flow

Sonography provides a good noninvasive method of obtaining an estimate of the size of the kidney, of detecting cysts and masses in or near the kidney, and of determining the presence or absence of dilatation of the ureter. It is therefore an important and safe screening test to rule out obstruction and to differentiate between acute and chronic disease. Large kidneys may indicate inflammatory disease or infiltrative disease of the kidneys. Further delineation of the anatomy of the kidney may require radiocontrast dyes. In patients with renal insufficiency, the quality of the x-rays obtained with the use of radiocontrast agents may be suboptimal, and the radiocontrast dyes themselves may be nephrotoxic.

Radionuclide methods are available to assess renal blood flow. These studies can easily discriminate between the presence or absence of renal blood flow and the symmetry of flow to the two kidneys but are less accurate in quantitating the absolute rates of flow. In a patient who presents with anuria or who develops renal failure after abdominal trauma or retroperitoneal surgery, in an elderly individual in whom the etiology of the acute renal insufficiency is obscure, and in patients with abdominal, flank, or back pain, it is prudent to determine that blood is flowing to the kidney. Angiography is required if equivocal results are obtained by nuclide scanning, in a patient suspected of acute renal venous disease, or when time does not permit a lengthy evaluation such as in a patient with suspected dissecting aortic aneurysm.

Renal blood flow as assessed by nuclide scanning is normal or only slightly decreased in a patient with established ATN. Renal blood flow is clearly decreased in patients with glomerulonephritis or transplant rejection. Assessment of renal blood flow may be of particular value in differentiating between renal transplant ATN and rejection.

Renal Biopsy and Other Diagnostic Tests

A percutaneous or open *renal biopsy* may be indicated in patients suspected of having glomerulonephritis or acute interstitial nephritis. The value of a renal biopsy is to confirm the diagnosis and predict outcome prior to the use of steroids and other potent immunosuppressive agents and before instituting difficult therapeutic procedures such as plasmapheresis. Other diagnostic tests may be indicated depending upon the clinical circumstances.

DIAGNOSTIC QUESTIONS IN THE PATIENT WITH ACUTE RENAL INSUFFICIENCY (TABLE 32–3)

Evaluation of a patient with presumed renal disease should proceed in an organized fashion. The patient may present only with biochemical abnormalities (azotemia) or with both biochemical abnormalities and symptomatic manifestations (uremia). In the initial evaluation of the patient who has significant renal insufficiency, several considerations must be addressed:

1. Etiology of acute renal insufficiency (see Table 32–1).

2. Acute versus chronic disease: If no prior history or laboratory tests are available, it may be difficult, in an individual case, to determine if the renal insufficiency is of long duration or of acute onset. The presence of shrunken, scarred, or calcified kidneys as determined by radiographic or sonographic methods usually indicates chronic, long-standing disease. These tests are also useful to evaluate for obstruction to urine flow. The presence of normal-size kidneys, however, does not necessarily indicate acute onset of disease, since several chronic forms of renal disease may be characterized by normal-sized or enlarged kidneys. Anemia and hyperphosphatemia are usually present in patients with advanced chronic disease but are not sufficiently specific findings to differentiate acute from chronic disease.

3. Systemic disease with renal involvement versus primary renal disease: Several systemic diseases may present with acute renal insufficiency alone or in conjunction with other manifestations. For example, patients with systemic lupus erythematosus or Goodpasture's syndrome may have, as part of the disease process, acute renal injury. The distinction between systemic disease with renal involvement and primary renal

TABLE 32–3. DIAGNOSTIC QUESTIONS IN PATIENTS WITH ACUTE RENAL INSUFFICIENCY

QUESTION	EVALUATION
Etiology of acute renal insufficiency	See Table 32–1
Acute versus chronic disease	Clinical history, prior laboratory tests, determination of kidney size
Systemic disease versus primary renal disease	Rule out systemic lupus erythematosus, Goodpasture's syndrome, etc.
Acute disease in a patient with underlying chronic disease	Graph 1/Cr versus time (see Chapter 31); evaluate fluid and electrolyte status; rule out obstruction, exposure to toxins, and infections

disease, particularly acute tubular necrosis, is important in planning the diagnostic work-up and therapy of the patient as well as in predicting the probability for recovery.

4. Acute disease in a patient with underlying chronic renal failure: If a patient with previously documented impairment in renal function is found on re-evaluation to have more advanced disease, it is necessary to determine if the deterioration in renal function is the result of the natural progression of the disease or the consequence of other secondary insults to the kidney. Secondary insults may include exposure to nephrotoxic drugs, alterations in the extracellular fluid volume, the development of hypercalcemia or other electrolyte abnormalities, infections in the kidney, or obstruction to urine flow. The presence of these secondary insults may indicate the possibility of partial reversal of the functional impairment. Often, clinical findings and the history of the patient will provide information as to the possibility of secondary insults to the kidney. If the data are available, a graph of 1/Cr versus time may be of considerable value in determining if the observed level of renal function represents the progression of chronic disease or the imposition of an acute insult on the chronic renal failure (see Chapter 30).

ACUTE TUBULAR NECROSIS (ATN)

Clinical Course, Pathogenesis, and Anatomy of Acute Tubular Necrosis

ATN syndrome is characterized by an acute and usually progressive loss of tubular and glomerular function. The vast majority of patients with ATN have as their initiating event either a decrease in renal plasma flow or exposure to a nephrotoxic agent. The vasomotor nephropathy variant of ATN occurs in a patient in whom there is a decrease in blood pressure and/or in the effective circulating volume. The pathophysiological events in the generation of vasomotor nephropathy are not known with certainty (Stein et al., 1978). An initial decrease in renal blood flow appears to be a requisite for the development of ATN. However, blood flow returns nearly to normal within 24 to 48 hours after the initial insult. Despite adequate renal blood flow, tubular dysfunction persists and the glomerular filtration rate remains depressed. The factor or factors that sustain the renal functional impairment after the primary insult depend upon the the nature of the original insult. Leakage of glomerular ultrafiltrate from the tubular lumen into the interstitium across the damaged renal tubular cells, obstruction to flow due to debris or crystals in the lumen of the tubules, loss of high-energy intermediates in renal tubular cells, and a decrease in the glomerular capillary ultrafiltration coefficient (K_f) have all been proposed to play a pathophysiological role in sustaining the clinical picture of ATN.

The toxic nephropathy variant of ATN occurs in clinical circumstances in which the patient has been exposed to a nephrotoxic agent. These agents impair tubular function and cause a secondary decrease in filtration. Many drugs have been implicated in causing toxic nephropathy. Antibiotics, particularly the aminoglycoside antibiotics, and specific cancer chemotherapeutic agents are two classes of drugs commonly associated with ATN. Specific forms of toxic nephropathy are discussed in Chapter 35.

Histologically, the kidney may appear nearly normal. The brush border membranes of the proximal convoluted tubule may be absent and cellular debris may be observed in the tubule lumens. In patients with rhabdomyolysis and ATN, myoglobin-stained casts may be observed on histological examination of the kidney. Cellular infiltrates are not usually prominent unless there is an associated interstitial nephritis. There is, however, edema of the interstitium. Aminoglycoside antibiotic toxicity may be suggested by the presence of lipid whorls in the cytoplasm of the renal tubular cells. It is to be stressed that in the vast majority of patients with ATN, the histological picture is nondiagnostic. Despite the common use of the term acute tubular necrosis, necrosis of the tubules is rarely observed. The glomeruli appear normal by light microscopy. The functional abnormalities of ATN are not expressed in the histology of the kidney.

Differential Diagnosis and Evaluation of the Patient (Fig. 32–1 and Table 32–4)

A careful history for exposure to nephrotoxic drugs and a physical examination with a particular emphasis on the evaluation of the circulating volume are required in any patient with suspected ATN. Routine blood and urine chemistries and a urinalysis should be performed. A sonogram of the kidney should be obtained, and where indicated, renal blood flow should be determined. More invasive tests such as angiography and/or renal biopsy are required in special circumstances. ATN is a diagnosis of exclusion. The clinical history and the determination of the functional status of the kidney remain the cornerstone of the differential diagnosis.

Prerenal azotemia is a clinical condition in which there is a rise in the plasma concentration of BUN and creatinine consequent to a reduced or ineffective circulating fluid volume and renal plasma flow. Prerenal azotemia differs from ATN by virtue of the fact that it is reversible when the circulating volume is restored and by the presence of normal tubular function. A patient with prerenal azotemia will be characterized by an elevated BUN-to-creatinine ratio in the blood (greater than 20:1) if the patient has a source of nitrogen intake, a low concentration of sodium and chloride in the urine on a spot sample (less than 20 mEq/L), a fractional excretion of sodium of less than 1 per cent, and a urine osmolality higher than that of plasma. These determinations must be obtained

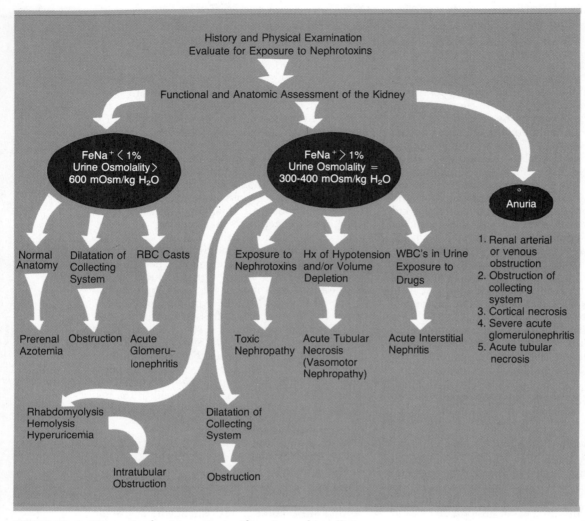

FIGURE 32—1. Diagnostic plan in a patient with acute renal insufficiency.

prior to the administration of diuretics. The above findings would indicate the normal renal response to conserve salt and water in the face of a decrease in the real or effective circulating blood volume. The patient may manifest other clinical signs of depletion of the extracellular fluid volume. Central hemodynamic monitoring may be necessary when clinical estimates of the circulating volume are unreliable, such as in the elderly, in patients with heart or liver disease, and in patients receiving vasoactive drugs.

Acute partial bilateral obstruction to urine flow may also be associated with an elevated BUN-to-creatinine ratio in blood, a low urine concentration of sodium, and a low fractional excretion of sodium. Thus, partial obstruction to urine flow may mimic the findings of depletion of the extracellular fluid volume. In both extracellular fluid volume depletion and partial obstruction, the urinalysis may be nearly normal, a feature differentiating it from ATN. With obstruction of longer duration, tubular injury occurs, the excretion of sodium increases, and the urine osmolality decreases. The sonogram of the kidneys will usually detect the presence of dilatation of the urinary collecting system.

The diagnosis of ATN is suggested in a patient with a BUN-to-creatinine ratio of less than 20:1, a urinary excretion of sodium and fractional excretion of sodium that is high (greater than 40 mEq/L and 1 per cent, respectively), and a urine osmolality between 250 and 400 mOsm/kg H_2O. The urinalysis reveals the presence of protein and granular casts.

Management

The general principles of management of acutely ill patients have been discussed elsewhere. There are absolute and relative indications for dialysis. Dialytic therapy should be instituted for uremic symptoms such as encephalopathy or pericarditis. Other indications for dialysis include severe fluid overload, hyperkalemia, metabolic acidosis, and life-threatening abnormalities in serum concentrations of electrolytes that cannot be effectively managed by conservative means. In a patient who is asymptomatic and without the above clinical and laboratory find-

TABLE 32–4. DIFFERENTIAL DIAGNOSIS OF ACUTE RENAL INSUFFICIENCY

DIAGNOSIS	SERUM BUN:Cr	URINALYSIS	URINE SODIUM (mEq/L)	FeNa (%)	URINE OSMOLALITY (mOsm/kg H_2O	COMMENTS
Prerenal Azotemia	>20:1	Hyaline casts; may be nearly normal	<20	<1%	>600	Clinical signs of volume depletion. Hx of vomiting, diarrhea, or sweating. Hx of diuretic administration.
Acute Arterial or Venous Disease	<20:1	May present with anuria	—	—	—	Arterial: Hx of abdominal trauma or manipulation of aorta or renal arteries. Venous: Hx of nephrotic syndrome, trauma, or severe dehydration (in children). Renal arteriography or venography may be indicated.
Intrinsic Renal Disease Acute glomerulonephritis	>20:1	RBC's, RBC casts, proteinuria	<20	<1%	>600	Hx of sore throat, pyoderma, or other infections. Renal biopsy may be indicated.
Acute interstitial nephritis	<20:1	WBC's, WBC casts, eosinophiluria	Variable	Variable	Variable	Hx of exposure to drugs that cause interstitial nephritis. Eosinophilia.
Acute tubular necrosis	<20:1	Granular casts, proteinuria, ± RBC's, ± WBC's	>20	>1%	~250–300	Vasomotor nephropathy: Hx of volume depletion or decrease in blood pressure. Toxic nephropathy: Hx of exposure to nephrotoxic drugs or radiocontrast dyes.
Intratubular obstruction	>20:1	Variable	Variable	Variable	Variable	Signs, symptoms, and laboratory findings of rhabdomyolysis or multiple myeloma. Hx of lymphoma or leukemia with hyperuricemia.
Obstruction of collecting system	>20:1	Variable, may be normal	Variable; may be <20	Variable; may be <1%	Variable	Hx of fluctuating urine volume. Sonogram of kidney showing bilateral dilatation of ureters.

ings, a trial of conservative nondialytic management may be attempted. In a patient who is catabolic with increases of BUN of greater than 20 mg/dl/day, it is reasonable to institute dialysis prior to the development of severe clinical symptoms. Moreover, sustained serum concentrations of BUN greater than 70 mg/dl are associated with platelet dysfunction, poor function of white blood cells, poor wound healing, and possibly a higher rate of mortality and morbidity. If instituted, dialysis (hemodialysis or peritoneal dialysis)

should be performed as often as is required to obtain the therapeutic goal.

The principles and techniques involved in hemodialysis and peritoneal dialysis are discussed in Chapter 33. The following considerations relate to the use of hemodialysis or peritoneal dialysis in the acute clinical situation. Hemodialysis requires the use of heparin to prevent the clotting of blood during its extracorporeal circulation. Hemodialysis is absolutely or relatively contraindicated in patients with acute intracerebral hemorrhage or active gastrointestinal bleeding and in the immediate postoperative period. Hemodialysis must also be used with caution in patients with pericarditis and/or pericardial effusions, acute myocardial infarctions, and underlying bleeding disorders. In the above clinical circumstances, peritoneal dialysis may be the preferred type of dialytic therapy.

The relative inefficiency of peritoneal dialysis may render this form of dialysis suboptimal in the acute treatment of very catabolic patients, in patients with marked hyperkalemia, and in patients with severe metabolic acidosis. Peritoneal dialysis is also not the preferred treatment option when dialysis is being performed for drug overdoses. Whether or not dialysis is instituted, there are several distinct clinical problems unique to the patient with ATN.

Sodium and Water Balance. The dietary or intravenous administration of sodium and water should be matched to the urine output and nonurinary losses of the patient once a nearly normal state of hydration is achieved. Diuretic administration may be attempted to increase the urine output if the above measures are not effective and the extracellular fluid volume is expanded (see below). If diuretics are unsuccessful in preventing expansion of the extracellular fluid volume, dialysis is required. In patients who require large amounts of intravenously infused fluids, such as patients receiving intravenous alimentation, dialysis may be required on a daily basis. When dialysis is instituted, the removal of sodium and water by dialysis must be considered in the calculation of the net water and sodium balance of the patient.

Potassium Homeostasis. Hyperkalemia is a life-threatening complication of ATN, and dialysis is required if severe hyperkalemia is present. In these patients, the electrocardiogram will reflect the severity of the hyperkalemia. Resins that bind potassium in the gut may be used as adjunctive therapy in a hyperkalemic individual or as sole therapy in a patient who does not have an urgent requirement for dialysis.

Acid-Base Abnormalities. Most patients with ATN are acidotic. An occasional ATN patient with vomiting or nasogastric suction may develop alkalosis if the rate of hydrogen ion loss exceeds the rate of production. Acidosis can be treated by administration of bicarbonate or bicarbonate equivalents. Dialysis is required for severe acidosis. Alkalosis can be treated by the oral or intravenous administration of acid or by employing dialysis baths with reduced concentrations of base.

Phosphate Balance. Hyperphosphatemia is treated by limiting the dietary absorption of phosphate by phosphate-binding antacids. If the patient is not eating, hyperphosphatemia can effectively be managed by dialysis.

Diet. A source of protein is required in patients with ATN, since the underlying disease process as well as the presence of renal insufficiency results in increased catabolism and decreased anabolism of protein. On the other hand, protein contributes to the generation of urea nitrogen and perhaps other products thought to be involved in the genesis of the "uremic syndrome." In a patient who is not severely catabolic and not requiring dialysis, protein intake should be limited to 40 grams/day and protein should contain a high content of essential amino acids (high biological value protein). Carbohydrates should be administered to provide sufficient calories. If the patient is severely catabolic, as evidenced by a rise in the urea nitrogen concentration of over 20 mg/dl/day, higher intakes of protein are often required to maintain nitrogen balance. In this circumstance, dialysis is almost always indicated.

Adjustment in Drug-Dosing Regimens. Drug-induced renal failure is a common clinical problem. In addition, renal failure is associated with abnormalities in the metabolism of a number of commonly used drugs. The relationship between drugs and renal disease is discussed more fully in Chapter 35. It is critical, however, to carefully review the indications for and the dose of all drugs administered to patients with ATN. A question that often arises relates to the administration of potentially nephrotoxic drugs to a patient with ATN due to some other cause. For example, a patient with ATN may require an aminoglycoside antibiotic for life-threatening sepsis. In this clinical circumstance, the following points need to be considered. If there is an equally effective drug that has less or no renal toxicity, it should be employed. If no alternative is available, the drug should be administered in amounts required to achieve the desired therapeutic effect. The amount of drug to be administered and the dosing intervals, however, need to be carefully considered. For drugs that are removed by dialysis, the pharmacokinetics of the drug are even more complex. Monitoring of blood concentrations is an important adjunct to effective treatment. The critical point is that potentially life-saving but nephrotoxic drugs should not be withheld in a patient with ATN. The same general considerations apply to the requirement for radiographic studies involving potentially nephrotoxic radiocontrast dyes. If indicated for the effective management of a patient with ATN, the tests should be performed. Dialysis is effective in removing the water-soluble x-ray contrast agents.

Other. Vitamins are often administered to patients with ATN. Since the water-soluble vitamins and folate are removed by dialysis, they should be provided routinely in patients requiring dialysis. Blood transfusions may be required in some patients with ATN. Because of the potential for overexpansion of the extracellular fluid volume and hyperkalemia consequent to infusion of large amounts of blood to a patient with ATN, elective or semielective blood transfusions are often given during dialysis.

The Use of Diuretics. It has been established that pretreatment of the subject with vigorous hydration, osmotic diuretics, or loop diuretics protects the kidney from some forms of renal injury.

Accordingly, patients who will be exposed to potentially injurious stimuli such as radiocontrast dyes, vascular surgery, or nephrotoxic drugs should be maintained with high rates of urine flow and replete extracellular fluid volumes. The value of diuretics when administered after the injurious insult is controversial. Most studies indicate that diuretics do not alter the severity or the duration of ATN. Loop-acting diuretics, however, may convert oliguric ATN into a polyuric form. Some clinicians therefore advocate administration of a bolus dose of a loop-acting diuretic once the diagnosis is established. If the diuretic fails to induce a diuretic response, it is discontinued. Although the diuretics do not alter the course of ATN, it is generally easier to manage the polyuric as compared to the oliguric form of ATN.

Outcome and Prognosis

The outcome of patients who develop ATN is quite variable and dependent upon the nature of the underlying disease. With the availability of dialysis, death is rarely due to renal failure directly. In modern acute-care hospitals, mortality rates may be in excess of 50 per cent, a figure that reflects the advanced age, severity of disease, and number of coexisting illnesses in this patient population. Outcome is considerably more favorable in younger patients with fewer coexisting diseases. As a generalization, patients with antibiotic-induced acute renal failure appear to have a more favorable outcome than those with vasomotor nephropathy. The same generalization is true of patients presenting with nonoliguric as compared to oliguric ATN.

In a patient with established ATN who is not exposed to additional insults to the kidney, renal function may recover. The onset of recovery averages 7 to 10 days, although shorter and longer periods of renal dysfunction are not uncommon. In patients who are oliguric, recovery is heralded by an increase in urine output. Generally, in a patient not undergoing dialysis, the urine output doubles every 24 to 48 hours until an output of 3000 to 4000 ml/day is attained. The serum concentration of urea nitrogen and creatinine decreases 48 to 72 hours after the onset of the increase in urine output. The progressive increase in urine output should be carefully monitored. A patient with oliguric ATN who begins to manifest an increase in urine output usually demonstrates complete progression to urine output of 3000 ml or more per day. If a patient fails to reach this value or if urine output decreases after an initial increase, the possibility of an additional renal insult should be carefully considered.

REFERENCES

Epstein M, Schneider NS, and Befler B: Effect of intrarenal furosemide on renal function and intrarenal hemodynamics in acute renal failure. Am J Med 58:510–516, 1975.

Miller TR, Anderson RJ, Linas SL, Henrich WL, Berns AS, Gabow PA, and Schrier RW: Urinary diagnostic indices in acute renal failure. Ann Intern Med 89:47–50, 1978.

Stein JH, Lifschitz MD, and Barnes LD: Current concepts on the pathophysiology of acute renal failure. Am J Physiol 234:F171–F181, 1978.

CHRONIC RENAL FAILURE 33

The term chronic renal failure describes the existence of irreversibly advanced and usually progressive renal insufficiency. End-stage renal disease (ESRD) is that stage of chronic renal failure at which renal function is no longer sufficient to sustain life. The incidence of newly diagnosed end-stage renal failure is approximately 50 to 100 new cases per million population. There are approximately 80,000 patients currently maintained on chronic dialysis in the United States.

Specific Etiologies (Table 33–1)

The outcome from any specific form of renal injury and the progression to end-stage renal disease have been reviewed in Chapter 32. The most common etiologies of renal disease in patients being considered for dialysis and transplantation are chronic glomerulonephritis, hypertensive nephrosclerosis, chronic interstitial nephritis, polycystic kidney disease, and diabetes mellitus. The inclusion of diabetes mellitus in such a list reflects recent improvement in the care and management of this patient population such that greater numbers survive the intercurrent devastations of this illness to manifest ESRD.

TABLE 33–1. COMMON CAUSES OF END-STAGE RENAL DISEASE

Chronic glomerulonephritis
Hypertensive nephrosclerosis
Chronic interstitial nephritis
Chronic diabetic glomerulosclerosis
Polycystic kidney disease

ADAPTATION TO NEPHRON LOSS

The kidney has great functional reserve and is able to compensate for progressive loss of functioning nephrons. The homeostatic, excretory and, in part, endocrine functions of the kidney are

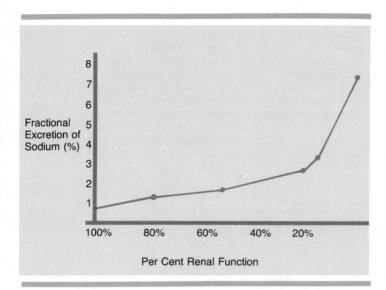

FIGURE 33—1. Changes in the fractional excretion of sodium required to maintain homeostatic balance in a patient ingesting a diet containing 100 mEq of sodium and undergoing progressive loss of renal function.

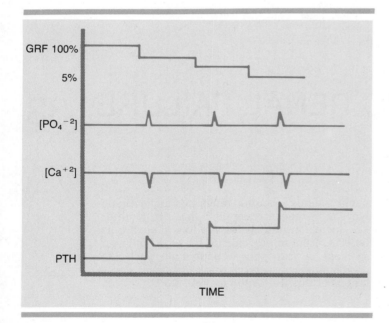

FIGURE 33—2. Schematized representation of the changes in the serum concentrations of calcium (Ca^{+2}), phosphate (PO_4^{-2}), and parathyroid hormone (PTH) in a patient undergoing a stepwise reduction in renal function. The dietary intake of phosphate is constant throughout the time period. The changes in the plasma concentration of calcium and phosphate are not observable clinically owing to the rapid adjustments mediated by PTH. (Adapted from Bricker NS, Slatopolsky E, Reiss E, and Avioli LV: Calcium, phosphorus and bone in renal disease and transplantation. Arch Intern Med 123:543–553, 1969.

maintained even when function of the kidney is only 10 per cent of normal. Further degrees of nephron loss usually result in clinical sequelae.

The adaptation to nephron loss can be illustrated for a single solute such as sodium (Fig. 33–1). In an individual with a glomerular filtration rate of 100 ml/min and ingesting 100 mEq of sodium per day, the urinary excretion of sodium must be 100 mEq/day in order to maintain constant body weight and composition of body fluid compartments. In such an individual, 25,000 mEq of sodium are filtered at the glomerulus per day. Since only 100 of the 25,000 mEq of sodium that are filtered at the glomerulus are excreted, the fractional rate of excretion is 0.4 per cent. If the filtration rate were to be reduced by 50 per cent, the filtered load of sodium would be reduced proportionately. In order to maintain overall balance, 100 mEq of sodium would still have to be excreted. Under these circumstances, the fractional excretion of the filtered load of sodium by the kidney would be increased to 0.8 per cent. In the face of progressive reductions in the rates of filtration, the constancy of the composition and volume of body fluid compartments is maintained by progressive increases in the fractional rates of excretion of filtered sodium such that intake and output are matched. As renal function decreases, however, there is a narrowing of the range of intake that can be tolerated (see Chapter 28). In general, renal adjustments in the rate of excretion are adequate to accommodate normal rates of intake down to rates of filtration of 10 to 20 per cent of normal.

The above example highlights several important points in the adaptation to nephron loss. The nephrons that remain functional in the presence of a decrease in total number of functioning units are not damaged units. Rather, they behave in a normal or supernormal manner and respond appropriately to physiological stimuli. The above defines the concept of the "intact nephron hypothesis." Said in another way, in a kidney that has sustained loss of nephrons, the remaining nephrons display a high degree of organization and respond appropriately to the needs of the organism.

The adaptive changes in nephron function are mediated by stimuli generated both outside the kidney and within the kidney itself. The nature of the stimuli is not known for all solutes but has been well studied in the adaptation of calcium and phosphate metabolism to progressive renal disease (Fig. 33–2). In the presence of a constant intake of phosphate and progressive loss of nephrons, the following sequence of events ensues. With each decrease in the glomerular filtration rate, the dietary intake of phosphate results in a transient increase in serum phosphate and, as a consequence, a decrease in the serum concentration of ionized calcium. The decrease in ionized calcium causes release of parathyroid hormone. Parathyroid hormone, in turn, causes an increase in the urinary excretion of phosphate and a normalization of the serum concentrations of calcium and phosphate. The intact nephrons respond appropriately to parathyroid hormone. In this example, normal plasma concentrations of calcium and phosphate are maintained, but there is a progressive rise in the concentration of parathyroid hormone. Thus, the intact nephron hypothesis has been extended to include the "trade-off hypothesis." In this circumstance, normal calcium and phosphate homeostasis is maintained at the expense of development of secondary hyperparathyroidism. The negative aspect of this trade-off is hyperparathyroid-associated disease of bone and dysfunction of other organ systems. The trade-offs for maintenance of balance of other solutes aside from phosphate have not been elucidated clearly, but it is likely that the general thesis applies to multiple regulatory functions of the kidney.

When renal failure is far advanced, the adaptive response of the kidney to changes in the dietary intake of solute is severely compromised and the urinary excretion rates tend to become fixed. This loss of regulatory capacity of the kidney provides an explanation for the findings that in patients with advanced renal failure, alterations in dietary intake can be associated with states of depletion or excess. For example, ingestion of amounts of sodium in excess of the excretory capacity of the kidney results in expansion of the extracellular fluid volume. Conversely, ingestion of amounts of sodium that are less than the fixed rate of urinary excretion results in depletion of the extracellular fluid volume.

FACTORS AFFECTING THE RATE OF LOSS OF NEPHRONS

It has been appreciated for some time that many patients have a slow, steady decline in renal function over a period of months to years (see Fig. 31–1). A number of pathogenetic mechanisms have been implicated in the slow decline in renal function.

Continuing Primary Insult. It is often suggested that the disease initially causing the renal injury is still active and results in progressive damage. Frequently, despite the progressive loss of renal function, it is not possible to identify continued activity of the primary disease or exposure to toxins.

Secondary Renal Insults. In some circumstances, there may be development of secondary insults to the kidney, and these secondary processes could account for the progression of renal insufficiency. Congestive heart failure, hypercalcemia, infection, obstruction to urine flow, exposure to nephrotoxic drugs, or alterations in the extracellular fluid volume may result in further decreases in renal function.

Alterations in Glomerular Hemodynamics, Parathyroid Hormone Metabolism, and Systemic Arterial Blood Pressure.

Alterations in Glomerular Hemodynamics in Renal Disease. The nephrons that remain functional in the presence of renal injury are, as noted earlier, not damaged but rather supernormal. Morphologically and functionally, these nephrons are larger and have higher than normal rates of glomerular plasma flow and filtration. The reason for the increase in the glomerular plasma flow and the rate of filtration is not known with certainty but is related, at least in part, to the dietary intake of protein. Protein or its peptide fragments cause renal vasodilation, an increase in glomerular plasma flow, and an increase in the glomerular hydrostatic pressure. It has been proposed that in renal insufficiency, the superperfusion and hyperfiltration of remaining nephrons, in and of itself, results in glomerulosclerosis and further loss of nephrons. Administration of a low-protein diet containing proteins of high biological value (proteins with a high content of essential amino acids) may result in a reduction in glomerular blood flow, glomerular hydrostatic pressure, and hyperfiltration and thus slow the progression of the renal disease.

The Role of Parathyroid Hormone. In adapting to a constant intake of phosphate, calcium and phosphate homeostasis are maintained at the expense of development of hyperparathyroidism. Parathyroid hormone, however, has several actions that may be detrimental to the kidney. PTH may contribute to injury of renal cells by facilitating deposition of calcium in the renal parenchyma or by translocating calcium into the cells and the mitochondria. The net effect of parathyroid hormone would be further loss of nephrons and increasing degrees of hyperparathyroidism.

The Role of Blood Pressure. Regardless of the nature of the primary renal insult, the codevelopment of elevation of the blood pressure results in a significant acceleration in the rate of nephron loss. It has been suggested that aggressive and early treatment of blood pressure elevations, even elevations in the range in which therapy is of questionable value in patients without renal disease, is indicated.

In the evaluation of a patient with progressive renal injury, the clinician must carefully determine if there is evidence of continued activity of primary disease and/or exposure to nephrotoxins. The patient should be carefully evaluated for the existence of secondary forms of renal injury and, if such is present, treated appropriately. If there is neither evidence for active primary disease nor secondary insults, a low-protein diet containing proteins of high biological value should be instituted. In addition, correction of the phosphate-calcium-parathyroid hormone interactions should be considered. Finally, the institution of blood pressure control is of critical therapeutic importance.

CLINICAL MANIFESTATIONS OF END-STAGE RENAL DISEASE

The clinical manifestations of ESRD are protean. The initial clinical presentation is also extremely varied. Clinical signs and symptoms may arise as a direct consequence of organ dysfunction secondary to the "uremic state" or as an indirect consequence of primary dysfunction of another system. There is not one single compound or pathophysiological event that explains the multiple organ and systems abnormalities in uremia. Urea, monitored as the blood urea nitrogen concentration (BUN), is not, in and of itself, the "uremic toxin." Much discussion has focused on the possible role of the so-called middle molecules, molecules of molecular weight of 500 to 2000 (Navarro et al., 1982). These middle molecules are retained in patients with renal disease, but their exact pathophysiological role remains to be defined. It has also been proposed that PTH may be an important factor in the genesis of some of the clinical manifestations of ESRD.

Table 33–2 lists the major clinical manifestation of ESRD and divides them into those that are life-threatening, those that are common but not an immediate threat to existence, and those that occur with variable clinical frequency and expression. This division, however, is arbitrary and in any given patient, one organ system dysfunction may be the major threat to life or rehabilitation. The major causes of death in patients with ESRD are cardiovascular catastrophes and infections. The major morbid complications are the development of uremic bone disease (uremic osteodystrophy) and neuropathy.

Blood Chemistries

Analysis of serum chemistries reveals a variety of abnormalities in patients with ESRD. The BUN and creatinine are increased to a variable degree.

Since the blood level attained reflects not only the impairment in filtration function of the kidney but also the rate of generation of these substances, the development of "uremic" symptoms may not correlate directly with blood values. Metabolic acidosis is commonly observed and is usually a hyperchloremic acidosis. In far-advanced renal failure, the acidosis may be associated with an increased anion gap. Hyperkalemia is observed when renal failure is far-advanced or in patients with coexisting deficiency or tubular insensitivity to aldosterone. Patients with ESRD are "potassium adapted" and tolerate mild degrees of hyperkalemia ($K^+ = 5.5$ mEq/L) with no clinical sequelae. In far-advanced renal failure, the serum concentration of phosphate is increased. Bone-derived alkaline phosphatase increases over time in the ESRD patient and can be used to follow the development of uremic osteodystrophy. Serum concentrations of uric acid and magnesium are often elevated.

Cardiovascular

Cardiovascular disease is one of the most common causes of death in patients with ESRD. The incidence of coronary artery disease in ESRD patients is significant and may be related to the presence of hypertension, glucose intolerance, and/or the abnormalities in lipid metabolism. Renal disease may also result in accelerated arterosclerotic disease and a form of cardiomyopathy. Ingestion of sodium and water in excess of the excretory capacity of the kidney can result in expansion of the extracellular fluid volume. Tolerance to expansion of the extracellular fluid volume is dependent, in part, on cardiac function. The clinical manifestations of expansion of the extracellular

TABLE 33–2. MANIFESTATIONS OF END-STAGE RENAL DISEASE

	LIFE-THREATENING	COMMON	UNCOMMON OR VARIABLE FREQUENCY
Blood chemistries	Acidosis, ↑ K^+	↑ BUN/creatinine, ↑ PO_4^{-2}, ↑ alkaline phosphatase, ↑ urate, ↑ Mg^{+2}	↑ Amylase, ↓ SGOT
Cardiovascular system	Pulmonary edema, cardiac tamponade	↑ Blood pressure, coronary artery disease, arrhythmias, congestive heart failure, pericarditis	Pericarditis ± pericardial effusion
Uremic osteodystrophy		↑ Alkaline phosphatase, ↑ PTH, ↓ 1,25 $(OH)_2$ Vit D	Bone pain, fractures
Nervous system	Encephalopathy	Peripheral neuropathy	
Hematopoietic system		Anemia, ↓ platelet function, ↓ WBC function, ↓ immune responsivity, coagulopathy	
Gastrointestinal system	Gastrointestinal hemorrhage	Gastroenteritis, colitis, hepatitis	Ascites
Skin and conjunctiva		Pruritus	Darkening of skin, conjunctivitis
Endocrine system		Glucose intolerance, ↑ blood levels of peptide hormones, ↓ erythropoietin	Gonadal dysfunction, abnormal thyroid function tests
Muscular and articular system			Proximal myopathy, arthritis (pseudogout)
Genitourinary system		Urinary tract infections, cystic degeneration of the kidney, carcinoma of the kidney	
Pulmonary system		Pulmonary congestion, infections	Poor gas exchange, pleural effusions

fluid volume include hypertension, congestive heart failure, and peripheral edema.

Involvement of the pericardium is common in ESRD patients. Clinical manifestations may include pericarditis with pain, fever, and a pericardial friction rub, or pericardial effusion with or without clinically apparent pericarditis. Pericardial tamponade and constrictive pericarditis are less common manifestations but are more life-threatening. Pericarditis occurs in two distinct clinical situations. In the newly diagnosed uremic patient or in patients who have been inadequately dialyzed, institution of regular dialytic treatment results in resolution of the pericarditis. Pericarditis can also arise in patients who are already established on dialysis and who appear to be well-dialyzed. In this circumstance, increasing the number or duration of dialytic treatments does not hasten the resolution of the pericarditis. Cardiac tamponade requires immediate drainage of the pericardial fluid. Constrictive pericarditis requires surgical intervention.

Uremic Osteodystrophy (Fig. 33–3)

The development of bone disease is universal in patients with renal disease. Clinical manifestation varies widely, ranging from only laboratory abnormalities (elevated alkaline phosphatase) or radiographic findings to severe and disabling bone pain and fractures. Three distinctive metabolic bone diseases occur in association with ESRD. Although all are present to a variable degree, one subtype may dominate the clinical picture. Hyperparathyroidism is universal in ESRD; the bone manifestations are the development of osteitis fibrosa cystica. In advanced renal disease, there is a failure to convert vitamin D to its active metabolite, $1,25(OH)_2$ vitamin D and, as a consequence, rickets or osteomalacia develops. In addition, recent evidence indicates that the accumulation of aluminum metabolites in bone results in a form of vitamin D–resistant rickets. Owing to a variety of factors, including sustained acidosis and poor nutrition, osteoporosis is common.

Neurologic Manifestations

Central nervous system manifestations of ESRD may range from mild changes in mentation to coma, convulsions, and death. The more severe clinical manifestations occur in patients with advanced uremia and are alleviated by the institution of dialysis. In a patient with severe uremic central nervous system manifestations, the initial dialysis treatments should be brief so as to avoid the development of a disequilibrium syndrome, manifested by cerebral edema and worsening neurologic findings. Usually after a few dialytic treatments, the patient becomes adapted and no longer manifests this dialysis disequilibrium condition. A rare but severe neurologic syndrome may occur in patients maintained on dialysis,

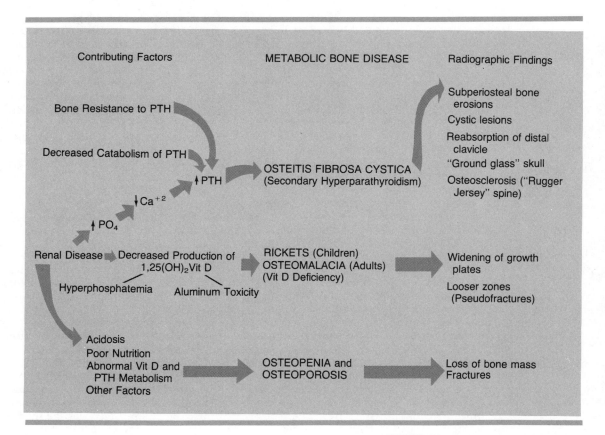

FIGURE 33–3. Uremic osteodystrophy.

called "dialysis dementia." This dementing syndrome is also associated with a movement disorder and has a fatal outcome in the majority of patients. Finally, the presence of arteriosclerosis and hypertension makes the ESRD patient vulnerable to the development of cerebrovascular disease.

The peripheral nervous system is frequently involved in advanced renal disease and is manifest by a glove-stocking peripheral neuropathy. In some patients, the neuropathy may be quite severe and precludes successful rehabilitation. The institution of dialysis may stabilize the neuropathy, but only rarely is a severe neuropathy reversed. In some patients, the neuropathy may progress despite seemingly adequate dialysis.

The development of ESRD may also result in dysfunction of the autonomic nervous system. Clinical manifestations may include abnormalities in motility of the gastrointestinal tract with the findings of gastroparesis and/or diarrhea, labile blood pressure, and intolerance to dialysis. Dialysis generally does not reverse the overt manifestations of the autonomic neuropathy.

Hematopoietic System

Anemia is a nearly universal finding in patients with advanced renal disease. The etiology of the anemia is multifactorial. Red blood cell production is decreased owing to the lack of erythropoietin production by the kidney, the presence of products retained in uremia which inhibit erythropoiesis, and fibrosis of the bone marrow. Red blood cell loss may be accelerated owing to the presence of uremic gastroenteritis and the disordered function of platelets. The anemia may be exacerbated by associated dietary limitations or malabsorption of essential foodstuffs required for red cell production, such as folic acid and iron.

Total white blood cell counts are normal to low in ESRD. Some patients manifest poor polymorphonuclear leukocyte chemotaxis. Although not present in all ESRD patients, blunted production of antibodies and/or cellular immune responsivity is present in a significant number of such patients. The nature of the defects in white blood cell function are not known with certainty but appear to include both an inherent defect in the cells themselves and a response to a circulating factor. These defects in white blood cell function, in conjunction with other factors, may provide an explanation for the findings that infections are a common cause of death in ESRD patients.

Platelet counts are normal in patients with advanced renal disease, but qualitative defects in platelet function have been well-documented. Abnormalities in activity of clotting factors and in factors mediating the bleeding time have been described in ESRD patients. The abnormalities of hemostasis are not totally reversed by dialysis and may contribute to the frequent findings of gastrointestinal blood loss and subcutaneous hematomas in patients with ESRD. The defects in hemostasis are also important considerations in the evaluation of an ESRD patient who requires surgery.

Gastrointestinal Tract

In untreated uremic patients, gastroenteritis and/or colitis is frequently reported. Patients may present with anorexia, nausea, vomiting, or gastrointestinal bleeding. These symptoms may improve when dialysis is instituted. In addition, there are abnormalities in the motility of the gastrointestinal tract in some patients as well as abnormalities in the absorptive functions of the gut.

Particularly in patients on dialysis, hepatitis is common owing to exposure to blood and blood products. Transaminase activity in serum, however, may be only minimally elevated in patients with significant liver disease because of suppression in transaminase activity in uremic serum.

Skin and Conjunctiva

Itching and conjunctivitis are common manifestations of end-stage renal disease and appear to represent the clinical sequelae of microcrystallization of calcium. In addition, PTH itself may cause pruritus. As a consequence of poor nutrition and the defects in platelet function, poor skin texture and bruising are common. In long-standing ESRD patients, there is darkening of the skin, perhaps related to retention of substances that stimulate melanin production.

Endocrine Systems

The kidney is the organ that produces erythropoietin and $1,25(OH)_2$ vitamin D, the active metabolite of vitamin D. Renal disease is associated with low or absent levels of both these hormones. The kidney is also the organ of catabolism of several peptide hormones such as insulin, glucagon, parathyroid hormone, and gonadotropic hormones. Glucose intolerance is common in patients with ESRD due, in part, to the abnormal circulating levels of hormones, to alterations in hormone-receptor interactions, and to changes in post–hormone-receptor events in given cells. Abnormalities in gonadal function are common in patients with advanced renal insufficiency. Pregnancies and term deliveries are rare in females with ESRD. Menstrual periods also tend to be irregular.

Muscular and Articular System

Generalized malaise, muscle fatigue, weakness, and twitching may be seen in patients with ESRD. A proximal myopathy, perhaps related to hyperparathyroidism, may occur. The fasciculation and twitching of muscles may be related to depolarization of muscle cells secondary to uremia.

Articular symptoms, including overt arthritis, occur in uremic individuals. Although any form of arthritis may occur, pseudogout due to the deposition of calcium pyrophosphate seems to occur with increased frequency in patients with renal disease. Interestingly, despite the presence of hyperuricemia, overt attacks of gout are rare.

Genitourinary System

Urinary tract infection is common in patients with ESRD and may be related to stasis in the collecting system due to low rates of urine flow. In patients maintained on chronic dialysis for a period of time, there is a significant incidence of cystic degeneration of the kidney. There is also a significant increase in the incidence of carcinoma of the kidney.

Pulmonary System

Infections of the lung occur more commonly in renal disease patients and may be the consequence of poor clearing of secretions and impaired host defenses. Calcium may be deposited in the lung parenchyma and contribute to poor exchange of gases seen in some uremic individuals. Pulmonary congestion secondary to overexpansion of the extracellular fluid volume and/or congestive heart failure is a common clinical problem. Patients with uremia may also develop pleural effusions not due to other recognizable causes.

TREATMENT OPTIONS

CONSERVATIVE MANAGEMENT

Conservative management of patients with advanced renal disease is feasible in most (but not all) patients even when the glomerular filtration rate is as low as 10 ml/min. Some patients with even lower levels of function can be managed conservatively over short periods of time while awaiting evaluation and preparation for longer-term management.

Regulation of Fluids and Electrolytes

The cardinal pathophysiological abnormality of fluid and electrolyte homeostasis in advanced renal failure is the inability of the kidney to adjust the rates of excretion to widely varying rates of intake. The urinary excretion of *water* and *solutes* tends to be fixed over a narrow range. Thus, when the rate of intake exceeds the rate of output, a state of retention will result. Rates of intake that are less than output will result in states of depletion. A patient with advanced renal failure is simultaneously a waster and a retainer of solute and water, depending upon intake. Management of such individuals therefore requires matching of dietary intake to output. Practically, this involves ingestion of enough sodium and water to maintain the extracellular fluid volume at normal levels. *Potassium* intake usually requires careful monitoring. Once a dietary regimen is instituted, serial measurements of body weights, blood pressure, and blood electrolytes are required to ensure that the patient has achieved the steady-state balance felt to be optimal clinically. Diuretics may be of value in patients unable to restrict their intake of sodium. Oral potassium-binding resins, which allow elimination of potassium by the gut, can be used in patients exhibiting frequent and life-threatening hyperkalemia. *Bicarbonate* or bicarbonate equivalents are used to partially correct systemic acidosis. *Antihypertensive* agents are indicated if hypertension is still evident after control of the fluid and electrolyte status of the patient. In patients who are unable to adjust sodium and water balance by diet, with or without the use of diuretics, and/or those who are persistently hyperkalemic or acidotic, dialysis therapy is usually indicated.

The dietary intake of *phosphate* is intimately involved in the genesis of secondary hyperparathyroidism. It is not feasible to severely restrict the dietary intake of phosphate, since such diets are unpalatable. Aluminum-based antacids bind phosphate in the gastrointestinal tract and prevent its absorption. These antacids can aid in control of the plasma concentration of phosphate and in the correction of the abnormalities in the metabolism of calcium and parathyroid hormone. If the plasma concentration of phosphate can be controlled, it may be possible to administer calcium and/or analogues of vitamin D to increase calcium absorption in the gut and further suppress the stimulation of parathyroid hormone release. The net effect of the use of phosphate-binding antacids, calcium, and vitamin D analogues is to restore serum concentrations of calcium and phosphate to values as close to normal as possible.

While the above regimen is widely used, certain precautions need to be considered. Aluminum toxicity may be involved in the development of some types of uremic osteodystrophy and play a role in the generation of a dementing syndrome reported in dialysis patients. Second, the administration of calcium and/or vitamin D analogues must be carefully monitored so as to avoid elevation of the product of the serum concentration of calcium and phosphate. Deposition of calcium in body tissues may be involved in some of the systemic manifestations of renal failure.

Despite therapeutic maneuvers designed to control the abnormalities in calcium, phosphate, and parathyroid hormone metabolism, progressive hyperparathyroidism may develop. A parathyroidectomy may be indicated in patients with progressive hyperparathyroidism as manifested by overt hypercalcemia, a markedly elevated alkaline phosphatase, bone pain and/or fractures, and x-ray evidence of advanced and progressive changes (Fig. 33–3). If bone disease continues to progress despite optimal medical management and adequate dialysis, renal transplantation may be the preferred treatment option.

Elimination of Waste Products of Metabolism and Drugs

As noted earlier, there is no consensus on the nature of the uremic toxins. Nonetheless, the dietary intake of protein contributes to the genesis of uremic symptoms. While urea is not a toxic product in and of itself, the BUN concentration does correlate both with the dietary intake of protein and with the systemic manifestations of end-stage renal disease. It is generally believed that BUN reflects the accumulation of other products of protein catabolism, some of which may contribute to clinical symptoms. Restriction of dietary intake of protein can lead to symptomatic improvement in the nausea, vomiting, malaise, and encephalopathy of end-stage renal disease. Such improvements are usually associated with a decrease in BUN. On the other hand, uremic patients have a decreased protein anabolic rate and an increased rate of protein catabolism. Marked restrictions in protein intake, therefore, can result in protein malnutrition. A patient with end-stage renal disease can usually be maintained in nitrogen balance by restriction of the dietary intake of protein to 40 grams per day. Moreover, proteins providing essential amino acids (high biological value proteins) are indicated to stimulate the reincorporation of urea nitrogen into new protein synthesis and prevent accumulation of nitrogen metabolites that are not essential. Additional calories need to be provided when protein intake is restricted. The use of a low-protein diet containing proteins of high biological value can lead to symptomatic improvement and prolong the time until a patient must have dialytic therapy or transplantation.

The kidney is a major route of excretion of drugs. Moreover, renal failure is associated with alterations in the binding of drugs by plasma proteins and in the overall metabolism and distribution of drugs within the body. These considerations are reviewed in Chapter 35.

Endocrine and Other Considerations

The relationship between calcium, phosphate, and parathyroid hormone has already been considered. Glucose intolerance is common in patients with end-stage renal disease. A patient with pre-existing diabetes mellitus may experience marked changes in insulin and carbohydrate requirements as renal function deteriorates. If anorexia limits the intake of carbohydrates, hypoglycemia may ensue if the insulin dose is not adjusted. In addition, some uremic patients have impaired gluconeogenesis. On the other hand, the following factors may result in hyperglycemia. Uremic patients have defects in the tissue uptake and metabolism of glucose and in the number and action of insulin receptors. Carbohydrate intake as a percentage of total calories is increased by the dietary regimen. The plasma concentration of glucagon is also elevated in patients with renal failure. Finally, advanced renal disease limits the urinary excretion of glucose when hyperglycemia is present. In the diabetic patient with advanced renal failure, frequent monitoring of blood sugar concentrations, adjustments in the doses of insulin, and alterations in the diet are required. There is no clinical method to assess the relative influence of all of the multiple factors that affect glucose metabolism in the ESRD patient. Measurements of glycosylated hemoglobin concentra-

tions as an index of glucose control are not valid in patients with advanced renal disease.

Administration of androgens may be of value as a stimulus to the production of red blood cells in men. In females, anabolic steroids with low androgenic activity are used for stimulation of the bone marrow. A variety of abnormalities in thyroid function tests have been described in patients with advanced renal failure. These tests need to be carefully correlated with the clinical assessment of the patient prior to administration of thyroid hormone replacement. Despite laboratory tests that, if considered by themselves, might suggest hypothyroidism, the incidence of hypothyroidism is probably not significantly increased in patients with end-stage renal disease.

Anemia is very common in patients with ESRD, and the average patient on dialysis has hematocrit readings of 20 to 30 per cent. Folate is provided to all patients on dialysis, since it is removed by dialysis. Iron supplements are given if iron deficiency is documented. Iron should not routinely be provided, since excess iron administration may result in the development of hemochromatosis. Blood transfusions may be indicated in patients who are unable to maintain their red cell mass and are symptomatic from the anemia. Transfusions are also given prior to surgery to improve tolerance to the stress of anesthesia and surgical manipulations. Treatable causes of gastrointestinal bleeding should also be addressed.

Vitamin supplements are indicated in most ESRD patients. Water-soluble vitamins are removed by dialysis and supplements are clearly indicated in patients on dialysis.

DIALYTIC THERAPY

Principles and Technology of Dialysis

The principles underlying the use of dialysis are those of diffusion and convection (Fig. 33–4). Blood is separated from a dialysis solution by a semipermeable membrane. For hemodialysis, blood is pumped into a dialyzer containing an artificial semipermeable membrane. The dialysis solution bathes the opposite side of the membrane. In peritoneal dialysis, the capillaries of the peritoneal membrane serve as the semipermeable membrane, dialysis solution being instilled into the peritoneal cavity.

The physical separation of blood from the dialysis solution by a semipermeable membrane sets conditions favorable for net transfer of solutes and water from one compartment to the other. If a concentration gradient for a substance can be established, passive diffusion of that substance across the membrane can occur. The rate of transfer depends on the concentration gradient of the substance in question and its permeability across the semipermeable membrane. For example, urea in blood will diffuse from blood into the dialysis bath, which initially contains no urea. In this example, urea removed from the body is associated with a decrease in the blood concentration of urea.

Another example is the removal of potassium from plasma by using dialysis baths with concentrations of potassium lower than that of the plasma. By imposing the appropriate gradients, substances can be made to diffuse into or out of the blood. For other substances, such as sodium, it is not advisable to markedly alter the plasma concentration. Net removal of these substances, however, can be accomplished by inducing a flow of water across the membrane. In hemodialysis, water flow is accomplished by imposing a hydrostatic pressure gradient across the membrane. In peritoneal dialysis, water flow is induced by imposing an osmotic gradient across the membrane. In either mode, the membrane behaves as if pierced with large, water-filled channels that offer little resistance to flow of solutes dissolved in water. Thus, if the dialysis bath contains sodium in a concentration that approximates that of plasma, this convective pathway will permit net sodium removal from the body without inducing a change in the plasma concentration of sodium.

The vascular access required for chronic hemodialysis is created by forming an arteriovenous fistula by direct anastomosis of native vessels, or by the use of artificial grafts. Blood is pumped into the dialyzer and flows along one side of the artificial membrane. The dialysis solution is pumped in a counterflow direction across the other side of the membrane. The effluent blood is then returned to the patient. Dialysis machines permit regulation of the rate of blood flow and dialysate flow and the hydrostatic pressure gradient across the membrane. Peritoneal dialysis is accomplished by placement of a soft catheter through the abdominal wall into the peritoneal cavity. The external end of the catheter is attached in a closed system to a bag containing dialysis solution. Dialysis solution is instilled into the peritoneal cavity, permitted to dwell for varying periods of time, and then drained from the peritoneal cavity. These fill-dwell-drain cycles may be performed intermittently or continuously. The osmolality of the dialysis solution is adjusted by varying the concentration of glucose. The hypertonic dialysate creates an osmotic gradient for water removal equivalent to the hydrostatic pressure gradient of hemodialysis.

Indications for Dialysis and Adequacy of Dialysis

The major goals of dialysis (hemodialysis or peritoneal dialysis) are to maintain fluid and electrolyte balance and to rid the body of waste products. Dialysis is indicated in patients with severe abnormalities in fluid and electrolyte balance such as fluid overload, volume-dependent hypertension, acidosis, or hyperkalemia; in patients with "uremic" symptoms such as pericarditis or encephalopathy; and in patients whose renal function is 5 per cent or less of normal regardless of symptoms. The adequacy of dialysis has not been clearly defined in quantitative terms. Adequacy, however, may be defined clinically by the

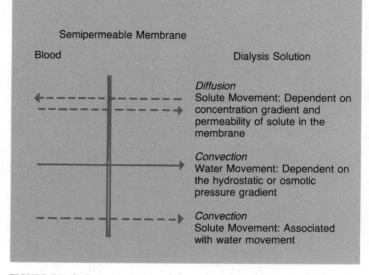

FIGURE 33–4. Representation of the principles of dialysis. Solutes that are permeable in the semipermeable membrane will diffuse along their concentration gradient. Additional solutes may be transferred associated with bulk water flow. Water movement is dependent upon the prevailing hydrostatic and/or osmotic pressure gradient across the semipermeable membrane.

well-being of the patient and correction of the regulatory and excretory defects of the kidney. Dialysis is not total renal replacement therapy. The endocrine abnormalities are not corrected by dialysis. Uremic bone disease and neuropathy may persist and accelerate despite seemingly adequate dialysis. Diet and medication must be carefully monitored as discussed earlier. Owing to the time required for dialysis, the psychological adjustments to the presence of organ failure, and the dependence on machines to sustain life, the impact of end-stage renal disease requiring chronic dialytic therapy on the life-style of an individual is significant. Management of dialysis patients therefore requires input not only from physicians, but also from individuals in nursing, dietary, social work, and psychology services.

Complications of Dialysis

Clotting or infection of the vascular access is a common problem in patients maintained on hemodialysis. In addition, the hemodialysis machine functions as a low-resistance arteriovenous fistula, requiring that cardiac output and/or peripheral vascular resistance increase so as to maintain systemic arterial blood pressure. In patients with significant heart disease or autonomic neuropathy (particularly diabetics) or those receiving drugs that inhibit the normal response of the autonomic nervous system, failure to manifest the appropriate cardiovascular response may result in intolerance to hemodialysis. The changes in extracellular fluid volume and in the composition of blood following hemodialysis may also contribute to the patient's intolerance to hemodialysis. Peritonitis is the most common complication of peritoneal dialysis and occurs following the inadvertent introduction of bacteria into the peritoneal space through the peritoneal dialysis catheter. Infections may also occur along the intra-abdominal tract of the catheter. In patients on peritoneal dialysis for extended periods (years), there may be a progressive loss in the efficiency of dialysis.

Factors Involved in the Choice of Type of Dialysis

Chronic hemodialysis can be performed in the home, if the patient has a dialysis partner, or in an outpatient dialysis facility. Chronic peritoneal dialysis is usually a home-based, rather than a facility-based, treatment. The morbidity and mortality of ESRD patients treated with either hemodialysis or peritoneal dialysis are approximately the same. The choice of one modality versus the other, therefore, is often predicated on nonmedical considerations, such as the patient's desire to directly participate in his or her care, the home and work situation of the patient, and the proximity of the patient to a kidney treatment center. In certain acute and chronic circumstances, however, one modality may be the preferred treatment option.

1. Cardiovascular instability is more common in patients treated with hemodialysis than in those treated with peritoneal dialysis. Peritoneal dialysis does not require an extracorporeal low-resistance blood circuit. In addition, by virtue of the fact that peritoneal dialysis is a less efficient modality on a per minute basis, the changes in blood chemistries and in the extracellular fluid volume occur more slowly. In a patient who is experiencing instability or intolerance to hemodialysis, peritoneal dialysis may be the preferred treatment option.

2. In the patient with diabetes mellitus, peritoneal dialysis is the preferred choice of dialytic therapy. Peritoneal dialysis avoids the requirement for heparin, with the attendant risk of blindness in the diabetic patient with retinopathy. There is a significant increase in the incidence of blindness in diabetic patients treated with chronic hemodialysis. In addition, patients with diabetes mellitus who reach ESRD have a high incidence of associated cardiac disease and autonomic neuropathy and, as a consequence, are less tolerant of hemodialysis.

3. The presence of intra-abdominal adhesions, communications between the pleural and peritoneal spaces, or abdominal wall hernias is a contraindication to institution or continuation of peritoneal dialysis. Obesity and abnormalities in serum lipids may be exacerbated by the glucose absorbed from the peritoneal dialysis fluid. The presence or worsening of these conditions is a relative contraindication to peritoneal dialysis.

Outcomes of Dialysis

Death rates in patients on chronic dialysis average 10 to 15 per cent per year but are quite variable. In recent years, the age of patients who are maintained on chronic dialysis has increased, as have the number and severity of coexisting illnesses. The major causes of mortality and morbidity are infections and cardiovascular events. Patients can be maintained on dialysis while awaiting renal transplantation, and patients who have undergone unsuccessful attempts at renal transplantation can be returned to chronic dialysis therapy.

TRANSPLANTATION

In suitable individuals, renal transplantation is a valid option for treatment of patients with end-stage renal disease. Although patient survival is approximately equal in patients receiving a renal transplantation and those treated by dialysis, there are significant differences between these forms of replacement therapy. A successful transplant more closely approximates the function of the normal kidney than does dialysis. Dietary restrictions are considerably less and the patient is no longer obligated to the time required to perform dialysis. The advantages of transplantation are partially offset by the requirement for immunosuppressive drugs, with the consequent results of infections and neoplasms and the risks associated with immunological rejection of the transplanted kidney.

The success of a renal transplant is dependent upon a number of factors. Perhaps the most important factor is the immune tolerance of the recipient. In general, the better the match of tissue antigens between donor and recipient, the better the outcome. Organ donation by a living relative therefore has a better renal outcome than does donation from a cadaveric source. The inherent immune responsivity of the recipient also determines the tolerance to a transplanted organ. Finally, the ability of drugs to modify the immune response is a factor in the overall success rate of renal transplantation. Tissue typing and measurements of reactivity of the recipient to the donor are determined by clinical laboratory methods. The use of these tests has improved the outcome from transplantation by providing a closer match between donor and recipient and avoiding transplantation in patients with unfavorable immunological parameters. In addition, considerable progress has been made in modulating the immune response of the recipient by the use of immunosuppressive drugs, including corticosteroids, azathioprine, cyclophosphamide, and cyclosporine, and by the use of other immunomodulating agents, such as antilymphocyte globulins, monoclonal antibodies, and pretransplant blood transfusions. It is likely that continued development of better matching techniques and the ability to modulate the immune response with drugs and agents with acceptable toxicities will improve the success rate of renal transplants.

SUMMARY

End-stage renal disease can result directly from many types of renal injury or may be a secondary consequence of processes that are initiated by the original insult. Such factors as hyperfiltration, hyperparathyroidism, and hypertension may be amenable to therapy. Careful conservative management, therefore, may not only slow the progression of disease but may also relieve some of the clinical consequences of renal disease. Dialysis and transplantation provide renal replacement therapy that can sustain life and allow for medical and social rehabilitation of the patient.

REFERENCES

Brenner BM, Meyer TW, and Hostetter TH: Dietary protein intake and the progressive nature of kidney disease: The role of hemodynamically mediated glomerular injury in the pathogenesis of progressive glomerular sclerosis in aging, renal ablation, and intrinsic renal disease. N Engl J Med 307:652–659, 1982.
Bricker NS: On the meaning of the intact nephron hypothesis. Am J Med 46:1–11, 1969.
Bricker NS: On the pathogenesis of the uremic state: An exposition of the "Trade-off hypothesis." N Engl J Med 286:1093–1099, 1972.
Bricker NS, Slatopolsky E, Reiss E, and Avioli LV: Calcium, phosphorus and bone in renal disease and transplantation. Arch Intern Med 123:543–553, 1969.
Fisher JW: Mechanism of the anemia of chronic renal failure. Nephron 25:106–111, 1980.
Massry SG, and Goldstein DA: Role of parathyroid hormone in uremic toxicity. Kidney Int 13 (Suppl 8):S39–42, 1978.
Mooradian AD, and Morley JE: Endocrine dysfunction in chronic renal failure. Arch Intern Med 144:351–353, 1984.
Navarro J, Contreas P, Touraine JL, Freyria AM, Later R, and Traeger J: Are "middle molecules" responsible for toxic phenomena in chronic renal failure? Nephron 32:301–307, 1982.
Raskin NH, and Fishman RA: Neurologic disorders in renal failure. N Engl J Med 294:143–148, 204–210, 1976.
Renfrew R, Buselmeier TJ, and Kjellstrand CM: Pericarditis and renal failure. Annu Rev Med 31:345–360, 1980.

RENAL PARENCHYMAL DISEASE 34

Individual syndromes of altered renal function can be grouped according to the structural element of the kidney affected by the disorder. These elements include the major vessels, arteries, and veins of the kidney; the glomerulus; the renal tubules and interstitium; and the conduits for urine flow from the renal calyces through the urethra. Specific diseases involving each of the structures will be discussed in this chapter. In addition, certain diseases and conditions of systemic origin may affect one or more of these renal structures and present with renal manifestations.

Glomerular disease rarely causes local symptoms; it is more likely detected by the presence of either edema or hypertension, the cardiovascular complications of this disorder. Smoky or bloody urine may be evident. Disordered glomerular function—either proteinuria consequent to an altered glomerular filtration barrier or a reduced glomerular filtration rate (GFR) secondary to altered glomerular ultrafiltration dynamics—characterizes these diseases. *Tubulointerstitial diseases* are usually asymptomatic until renal damage is far advanced. These disorders characteristically present as abnormalities of urine composition, i.e., failure of urinary concentrating ability, saltwasting, failure of urinary acidification, or failure of complete resorption of organic solutes such as glucose. A decrease in GFR is a late manifestation of these diseases. *Vascular disease* of the kidney may be associated with flank or abdominal pain and causes alteration of both glomerular and tubular function. *Obstruction* of the urinary drainage system usually causes alterations in patterns of urination (oliguria, anuria, nocturia) and may also present with localized pain. Both glomerular and tubular function are disrupted.

GLOMERULAR DISEASE

CLINICAL PRESENTATION

Proteinuria in excess of 0.5 to 1 gm/24 hr is the hallmark of glomerular disease and indicates a functional impairment in the sieving ability of the glomerular capillary with respect to serum macromolecules (proteins). The second common sign of glomerular disease consists of cellular elements, red and white blood cells, and cellular casts in the urinary sediment. Sterile pyuria and hematuria with red blood cell (RBC) casts are indicators of inflammatory processes. Regardless of the etiology of the glomerular injury, the clinical presentation and course of glomerular diseases converge on the following general patterns.

Nephrosis is a presentation of glomerular injury characterized predominantly by proteinuria with minimal or no cellular sediment in the urine. Nephrosis is expressed clinically in edema formation, normal to reduced blood pressure, and normal or slowly decreasing rates of glomerular filtration (GFR). The *nephrotic syndrome* is a clinical syndrome in which heavy proteinuria (usually >3 gm/24 hr) leads to a reduction in the serum albumin (usually <3.0 gm/dl) and is associated with edema formation. Renal salt retention in nephrotic glomerulopathies results in expansion of the interstitial compartment of the extracellular fluid volume. Hyperlipidemia and lipiduria are frequent findings in the syndrome.

Nephritis describes a presentation of glomerular injury in which hematuria or a prominent cellular urinary sediment occurs along with slight to moderate proteinuria. Hypertension and/or heart failure occur regularly in nephritic glomerulopathies because salt retained by the diseased kidneys results primarily in expansion of the intravascular volume. A reduced GFR is usually seen at an early stage in the course of nephritic diseases. Focal glomerulonephritis, which affects portions of some glomeruli, may present only with hematuria and proteinuria; the GFR and systemic hemodynamic functions may be little affected. Diffuse glomerulonephritis, which affects the entirety of most glomeruli, more often presents with clinical signs of ECF volume excess and azotemia in addition to hematuria and proteinuria.

Mechanism of Injury

In most glomerular diseases, in which the kidney is the primary focus of the disease process, injury is believed to occur through immunological processes. The primary indicator of this association comes from the regular finding by immunofluorescent staining of immune reactants (IgG, IgM, IgA, C_3, or C_4) within the glomeruli (Fig. 34–1).

Complement can be activated through the binding of antigen by specific antibody (IgG or IgM). Three modes of antigen-antibody interaction have been described for the activation of complement within the glomerulus. *Circulating immune complexes* (CIC) form within the circulation and may be trapped in the glomerular capillary wall during ultrafiltration. *In situ immune complex* formation takes place when circulating free antigen lodges within the glomerulus and antibody subsequently binds to the trapped antigen. Finally, *antirenal antibody* (specifically, anti–glomerular basement membrane antibody) may form, bind to an element of the glomerulus, and activate injury pathways.

Complement activation via the classic pathway is inferred from the presence of IgG or IgM plus C_4 and C_3 within glomeruli. The presence of C_3, sometimes with properdin, but the absence of C_4 and IgG or IgM indicates alternate pathway complement activation within glomeruli.

Attraction of polymorphonuclear leukocytes (PMN's) appears to be the most direct consequence of immune complex complement activation. However, injury does occur in a number of glomerular diseases associated with immune deposits in which PMN infiltration is minimal or absent. Moreover, in some common human glomerulopathies, immune reactants are absent. The mode of glomerular injury and/or dysfunction in these instances is uncertain. Glomerular injury in diseases such as diabetes mellitus and amyloidosis likely proceeds from a metabolic etiology. Finally, hemodynamic insults to the glomerular capillary bed may lead to glomerular necrosis, as in the case of severe hypertension, or sclerosis, as with sustained glomerular hyperfiltration.

Mechanism of Proteinuria

The serum proteins, which carry a net negative charge, are excluded from the urine on the basis of both their size and their net charge. The latter causes them to be repelled by the fixed negative charge of the glomerular capillary wall. Albumin, with a molecular radius of about 3.6 nm, is almost totally excluded from passage into the urine, but a neutral molecule of equal size would appear in urine at a concentration of approximately 20 per cent that in the blood.

Proteinuria in glomerular disease most likely represents a loss of the functional, negatively charged barrier of the glomerulus rather than a disruption in the structural integrity of the capillary wall by "holes." Proteinuria of glomerular disease does not represent either a failure by the tubules to reabsorb normally filtered proteins or an increase in the tubular secretion of serum proteins.

FIGURE 34–1. Patterns of immune deposits in glomeruli. *A*, Normal capillary loop (see Fig. 28–2). *B*, Subendothelial deposits. *C*, Intramembranous deposits. *D*, Subepithelial "humps." *E*, Fine, epimembranous deposits. *F*, Linear glomerular basement membrane deposits. *G*, Mesangial deposits.

Sodium Retention

Renal salt retention, expressed clinically either as edema formation or as volume overload and hypertension, is another common feature of glomerular disease. A reduction in GFR may account for some of the decreased ability to excrete salt, but other factors are usually present. Alterations in glomerular hemodynamics may independently compromise the ability of the kidney to excrete sodium. In this case, a change in glomerulotubular balance leads to increased salt and volume absorption in the proximal nephron. A decrease in the effective circulating blood volume due to a reduction in oncotic pressure may stimulate the renin-aldosterone axis and lead to hormone-dependent renal sodium retention in nephrotic patients. Renin and aldosterone secretion may also be increased in cases of nephritis in which renal blood flow is significantly reduced.

Reduction in GFR

As noted in Chapter 28, the rate of glomerular filtration may fall as a result of a decrease in capillary hydrostatic pressure, a change in the rate of rise of capillary oncotic pressure, or a decrease in the permeability of the capillary wall. Endothelial cell swelling, capillary occlusion or sclerosis, and glomerular scarring all decrease glomerular capillary pressure and blood flow. In other cases, glomerular architecture is little affected. In animals, a reduction in the permeability (K_f) of the glomerular capillary has been found in similar circumstances.

Even when glomerular permeability is reduced, GFR can be maintained near normal by raising the hydrostatic pressure and/or blood flow within the glomerular capillary bed. This may be accomplished by relaxation of the tone of the afferent arteriole relative to the efferent arteriole. Vasoactive agents of renal origin appear to participate in this response. In some glomerular diseases, a progressive fall in GFR is seen, continuing long after any evidence for immunological injury can be found. In such cases, these adaptive hemodynamic changes in the glomerulus lead to physical, nonimmunological injury of the glomerular capillaries and result in progressive glomerular sclerosis.

CLASSIFICATION OF GLOMERULAR DISEASES

The classification of glomerulopathies is very confusing, because groupings can be made according to the histological pattern of injury, the etiology of injury, or the mode of clinical presentation. In addition, the nomenclature includes a bewildering mixture of clinical, etiological, and pathological descriptive terms with many synonyms for the same disorder. This section will first divide glomerular diseases by their chief pattern of clinical presentation (nephrosis, nephritis, or mixed) and then order the individual entities by the dominant renal histopathological pattern.

TABLE 34–1. GLOMERULOPATHIES ASSOCIATED WITH THE NEPHROTIC SYNDROME

Minimal Change Nephropathy (Nil Lesion, Lipoid Nephrosis)
  Idiopathic
  Secondary: Hodgkin's lymphoma
Membranous Glomerulopathy (Epimembranous or Perimembranous Nephropathy)
  Idiopathic
  Secondary: Infections—hepatitis B, syphilis
             Neoplasms—carcinoma of lung, stomach, breast
             Drugs—gold, D-penicillamine
             Systemic lupus erythematosus
Focal Glomerular Sclerosis (Focal and Segmental Glomerulosclerosis, Focal Sclerosing Glomerulopathy)
  Idiopathic
  Secondary: Heroin abuse
             Chronic vesicoureteral reflux
Diabetic Glomerulosclerosis (Kimmelstiel-Wilson Glomerulosclerosis)
Amyloidosis
Idiopathic amyloid
Secondary amyloid: Multiple myeloma
                      Chronic infection—osteomyelitis, tuberculosis
                      Familial Mediterranean fever
Essential Cryoglobulinemia
Membranoproliferative Glomerulonephritis
Mesangioproliferative Glomerulonephritis

NEPHROTIC GLOMERULOPATHIES

The nephrotic syndrome may occur in the course of a number of glomerulopathies, each having a distinctive pattern of renal histopathology. Table 34–1 lists the more common renal lesions that present clinically with nephrotic-range proteinuria. The entries listed in boldface type present almost solely as the nephrotic syndrome and will be discussed in this section. Each of these histopathological patterns may occur as a primary (idiopathic) renal lesion, in which no contributory disease process has been identified, or secondary to a known disease process. Clinical entities are listed but are not discussed separately in this section. Entries in blue type may have manifestations other than the nephrotic syndrome and are discussed in subsequent sections.

Minimal Change Nephropathy

This glomerulopathy is the most common cause of childhood nephrotic syndrome, is most prevalent in children aged 2 to 6 years, and displays a 3:1 male predominance. Up to 25 per cent of cases of adult nephrotic syndrome may be minimal change. Edema in an otherwise healthy individual is the mode of clinical presentation in over 75 per cent of cases. Up to one third of childhood cases appear to follow an upper respiratory infection.

Proteinuria over 50 mg/kg/day with a serum albumin <2.0 gm/dl and a serum cholesterol >300 mg/dl are typical findings. The proteinuria is highly selective in children, being mostly albuminuria, but is less selective in adults. Lipiduria, seen as lipid droplets or "Maltese crosses" under polarized light, is characteristic. Microscopic hematuria occurs in a minority of patients. Serum complement levels are normal. IgG levels may be severely depressed, especially in patients with heavy proteinuria.

Renal insufficiency and azotemia do not occur unless caused by severe vascular volume contraction. Postural hypotension and circulatory collapse may occur in the face of severe reductions of serum oncotic pressure. An increased susceptibility to infection by encapsulated organisms (*Pneumococcus, Haemophilus, Klebsiella*) is notable when proteinuria is great and may relate to an acquired IgG deficiency. Thrombosis of renal and peripheral veins, associated with a hypercoagulable state, is not uncommon.

The term minimal change or nil lesion refers to the fact that the glomeruli appear normal on light microscopy (Fig. 34–1A). There is no significant or consistent staining for immune reactants. Electron microscopy reveals nothing more than the "fusion" of epithelial cell foot processes, a nonspecific finding that likely reflects the loss of the anionic charge of the glomerulus and subsequent collapse of the epithelial cell onto the basement membrane. While glomerular deposits are absent, circulating immune complexes of unknown origin have been reported in both children and adults with this disorder. No regular etiological association is known for the disease in children, but some adults with the minimal change lesion are found to have Hodgkin's disease.

The natural course of minimal change nephropathy is that of spontaneous remission and relapse, with eventual disappearance of proteinuria. However, because of the exquisite sensitivity of the proteinuria to corticosteroids, current prognostic categories are based on the response of the nephrotic syndrome to steroids. Steroids are given at an initial dose of about 60 mg/sq m/day of prednisone for 4 weeks, then tapered over 8 to 12 weeks, and discontinued only after the patient has remained free of proteinuria for about 4 weeks.

About two thirds of patients will have complete remission of proteinuria with this regimen. Another 25 per cent of patients will experience remission of the nephrotic syndrome but will continue to have mild proteinuria. However, almost two thirds of the initial responders will ultimately relapse and require subsequent courses of steroids to return to remission.

Of the fewer than 10 per cent who do not respond to the initial course of steroids, some will remit with either prolonged therapy or an increased dose of prednisone. Failure to respond to steroids or persistent steroid dependency has been used as an indication for concomitant therapy with an alkylating agent such as cyclophosphamide. However, the considerable risk of this drug, including the danger of gonadal injury or carcinogenesis in children, makes its use highly controversial in the treatment of a disease with a naturally favorable outcome.

About three fourths of individuals will be free of proteinuria, off treatment, at 10 years. The mortality rate in children is less than 5 per cent and is usually related to vascular complications and occasionally to infections but not to renal insufficiency. Adults have a response to steroids and an eventual outcome similar to that described for children. Nonresponders to steroids will often be found to have a glomerulopathy other than minimal change, often focal sclerosis.

Membranous Glomerulopathy

Membranous GN is the most common cause of nephrotic syndrome in adults, accounting for about 50 per cent of adult cases. Most patients with membranous nephropathy are over 35 years of age, with the peak incidence in the fifth decade; it is not common in children. The disease may be detected as asymptomatic proteinuria, but as many as 80 per cent of patients present with massive proteinuria and the nephrotic syndrome. The majority of cases of membranous GN are idiopathic. However, the membranous lesion is also seen in association with multiple unrelated disorders, including hepatitis B, systemic lupus erythematosus, organic gold exposure, and neoplasia (especially carcinoma).

Proteinuria in excess of 15 to 20 gm/day is not uncommon in membranous GN and is usually nonselective. Microscopic hematuria occurs in a substantial number of patients. Serum complement levels are normal in the idiopathic disease. Renal vein thrombosis is a complication recognized with increasing frequency. A progressive fall in GFR occurs in a majority of patients, and hypertension and azotemia develop late in the disease.

The classic finding on light microscopy is that of uniform basement membrane thickening throughout the glomerulus. Cellular proliferation and infiltration are strikingly absent. Silver stains demonstrate distinctive "spikes" within the basement membrane, causing it to resemble a picket fence. The darkly stained spikes are basement membrane projections between immune deposits. IgG and C_3 are prominent on immunofluorescent microscopy and show a uniform, finely granular pattern outlining the capillary loops (Fig. 34–1E). The extent and progression of the lesion can be classified by electron microscopy. The patterns range from Stage 1 (minimal basement membrane thickening with small subepithelial deposits) to Stage IV (very thick, irregular basement membrane with lucent zones representing former sites of deposits).

While the majority of patients with membranous nephropathy present with the nephrotic syndrome, spontaneous complete remission of proteinuria occurs in about 25 per cent of adults and partial remission in a similar number. However, most of the remaining patients will progress to end-stage renal failure by 10 years. The fall in GFR is usually gradual, so that sudden drops in renal function (see Fig. 31–1) may indicate a secondary problem, such as renal vein thrombosis or drug-induced interstitial nephritis. There continues to be controversy regarding the treatment of membranous nephropathy, but some physicians recommend courses of steroids and/or cytotoxic agents as a means of retarding progression to renal failure.

Focal Glomerular Sclerosis (FGS)

FGS is a cause of the nephrotic syndrome in 10 to 20 per cent of children and young adults. The presentation is usually that of edema with heavy proteinuria.

In children, this disorder may be diagnosed as minimal change nephropathy (MCN) in the absence of a renal biopsy. However, a number of clinical features tend to set focal glomerular sclerosis apart from the more common minimal change lesion. The most striking difference is the steroid resistance of proteinuria in FGS. Only 10 to 15 per cent of patients with FGS remit with steroids, a number similar to the rate of spontaneous remission, compared to a remission rate of more than 90 per cent in MCN. Microhematuria is common in FGS, and gross hematuria occasionally occurs. Hypertension and azotemia are present at the time of diagnosis in a majority of patients with FGS. Serum complement levels are normal. Tubular dysfunction (glycosuria, aminoaciduria, and phosphaturia) is more often seen in this disorder than in other glomerular diseases.

The diagnostic feature of this glomerulopathy on light microscopy is the focal (only some glomeruli involved) and segmental (only parts of each glomerulus affected) finding of hyalin sclerosis in the absence of significant proliferation or necrosis. Typically, the deeper, juxtamedullary glomeruli are first affected and more superficial glomeruli remain normal. Hence, a superficial renal biopsy sample may be mistakenly identified as minimal change nephropathy. There is some predilection for the process to begin near the vascular stalk of the glomerulus. Late in the disease, global sclerosis of individual glomeruli and pronounced tubular atrophy are seen.

Immunofluorescence shows patchy deposits of IgM and C_3 confined to areas of the glomeruli identified as sclerosed on light microscopy. The IgM is believed to be trapped nonspecifically in sclerotic glomeruli but not to be causally related to the development of FGS. On electron microscopy, there are foamy cellular degeneration and hyaline sclerosis in affected areas, and deposits corresponding to the IgM seen by immunofluorescence are evident.

While remissions do occur, the overall course is one of continuous proteinuria with relentless progression to end-stage renal failure. Persistent, nephrotic-range proteinuria has a less favorable prognosis, with at least 50 per cent of these patients having terminal renal failure at 10 years. Steroids do not influence the proteinuria to any significant degree and do not alter the progressive decrease in GFR. Recurrence in transplants does occur.

Nephritic Glomerulopathies

While some glomerular lesions regularly present as the nephrotic syndrome (edema and heavy

TABLE 34–2. GLOMERULOPATHIES ASSOCIATED WITH NEPHRITIC SYNDROMES

Proliferative Glomerulonephritis
  Postinfectious, acute glomerulonephritis
    Streptococcal
    Nonstreptococcal: Staphylococcal, pneumococcal, mumps, varicella, hepatitis B, Ebstein-Barr virus
  Systemic lupus erythematosus
  Anaphylactoid purpura (Schönlein-Henoch purpura)
  Essential cryoglobulinemia
Progressive Crescentic Glomerulonephritis
  Idiopathic rapidly progressive glomerulonephritis
  Anti–glomerular basement membrane disease: Goodpasture's syndrome
Other Glomerulonephritides
  Hemolytic-uremic syndrome
  Hereditary nephritis (Alport's syndrome)
  Vasculitides: Wegener's granulomatosis, periarteritis nodosa

proteinuria), other patterns of renal histopathology present predominantly as nephritic syndromes (hypertension, hematuria, and proteinuria). The common pattern in nephritic glomerular lesions is that of cellular proliferation (mesangial, endothelial, or epithelial cells) and cellular infiltration (polymorphonuclear leukocytes, macrophages). Table 34–2 lists the common histopathological and clinical diseases that present with major manifestations of the nephritic syndrome. Some of these entities are dicussed in subsequent sections.

The clinical presentation of the nephritic syndromes parallels the pattern of glomerular injury. Three general categories of cellular proliferation, each representing one part of the spectrum of clinical nephritis, can be described. *Focal nephritis*, which affects portions of some glomeruli, is most often associated with hematuria and proteinuria but with little or no reduction in GFR. *Diffuse proliferative nephritis* from any etiology, in which nearly all glomeruli show extensive cellular proliferation and/or infiltration, is usually associated with azotemia and hypertension in addition to hematuria and proteinuria. Finally, *glomerulonephritis* with *extensive crescent formation* is almost always associated with progressive deterioration of renal function.

A given case of glomerulonephritis may run its course at any one of the above stages, but crossover from one histological lesion to another is common among most types of glomerulonephritis. The finding of extensive crescent formation on a renal biopsy ($\geq$50 per cent of glomeruli affected) carries an ominous prognosis for reversibility of the renal lesion.

Proliferative Glomerulonephritis

Acute glomerulonephritis (AGN) is the most common nephritic syndrome and can be etiologically divided into post-streptoccocal AGN and nonstreptococcal AGN. In either case, the patient usually presents with oliguria, dependent or facial edema, urine that is grossly bloody or "tea-colored" from hemolyzed RBC's, and a history of a recent or ongoing infectious process. Hypertension is present or develops during the course of the disease in most patients, and the GFR is almost always reduced. Proteinuria is a constant finding but is rarely of sufficient magnitude to produce the nephrotic syndrome. Red blood cell casts are usually present in the urine. Although azotemia is common, the acute renal failure syndrome with uremia occurs in a minority of patients. Complete recovery of renal function after clearing of the infectious process is the rule, although some patients are left with a partial impairment of GFR and fewer still progress to chronic renal failure.

Post-streptococcal AGN is most frequent in children and young adults and follows group A, beta-hemolytic streptococcal infections of either the pharynx or skin (pyoderma). Signs of nephritis usually appear 10 to 20 days after onset of the infection. The antistreptolysin O (ASO) titer is almost always elevated in streptococcal pharyngitis but is elevated in less than one third of patients with streptococcal pyoderma. Antihyaluronidase titers are usually elevated in the latter patients. Total serum complement activity (CH_{50}) and serum C_3 are almost invariably depressed during the acute illness. These return to normal in 3 to 6 weeks as the renal disease disappears. About 2 per cent of patients may have minor urinary sediment abnormalities (protein and/or RBC's) for as long as 7 to 10 years. Progression to chronic renal failure is rare and is usually confined to the older adults who develop AGN.

Nonstreptococcal, postinfectious AGN has been described in association with bacterial endocarditis due to coagulase-positive *Staphylococcus aureus*, with chronically infected ventriculoatrial shunts due to coagulase-negative *S. epidermidis*, and with pneumococcal pneumonia. Acute viral infections such as type B hepatitis, mumps, varicella, infectious mononucleosis, and others have also given rise to AGN. The pattern of the AGN is the same as that for post-streptococcal AGN, and the prognosis for complete renal recovery is favorable in these diseases. A similar syndrome of acute nephritis may be seen in association with other disease processes, most notably with systemic lupus erythematosus (SLE).

Histologically, these cases are characterized on light microscopy by endothelial and mesangial cell proliferation with leukocyte infiltration. Small crescents of proliferating cells adherent to Bowman's capsule may be seen. Immunofluorescent staining is usually strongly positive for IgG and C_3 and shows a granular pattern of deposition around capillary loops. The classic electron microscopic finding in post-streptococcal AGN is that of large "humps" of electron-dense deposits in subepithelial spaces (Fig. 34–1D).

Treatment in all of these cases is directed at eradication, where possible, of the infecting organism and management of the consequences of renal injury until recovery occurs. Corticosteroids and immunosuppressive agents are not useful. Edema and hypertension are best managed by salt restriction and diuretic therapy. The azotemia is usually self-limited, but a few patients will require dialysis. A modest anemia does not require treatment or transfusion.

Anaphylactoid purpura is a chronic recurrent disorder that is most common in young children and is occasionally associated with nephritis. It is characterized by repeated attacks of palpable purpura, chiefly in the lower trunk and legs; variable bouts of abdominal pain; and transient arthralgias. An acute nephritic picture with hematuria, moderate proteinuria, and a modest reduction in GFR occurs in a number of patients. A few patients develop a rapidly progressive course to renal failure, almost always within the first few years of diagnosis of the purpura. Serum C_3 levels are normal, although CH_{50} activity may be mildly depressed.

Light microscopy varies from focal, segmental cellular proliferation to diffuse cellular proliferation with extensive crescent formation; the latter lesion is seen most commonly when renal failure occurs. Immunofluorescent staining for mesangial IgA and C_3 is prominent. Importantly, dermal capillaries of affected or unaffected skin stain strongly for IgA and C_3, so that a skin biopsy may be useful in diagnosing the etiology of nephritis in such patients.

The basic disease is self-limiting, disappearing after a few months to years. Complete renal healing is seen in over half of patients who develop nephritis, but about 10 per cent progress to renal failure. Steroids ameliorate extrarenal symptoms but do not appear to alter the renal component of the disease. Recurrence has been noted in transplants.

Essential cryoglobulinemia, in which IgG/IgM cryoprecipitates having rheumatoid factor activity occur, may cause an acute nephritic syndrome. Acute renal failure with proteinuria and hematuria occurs along with purpura, fever, and Raynaud's phenomenon. Immunofluorescent microscopy typically shows IgG, IgM, and C_3 in granular masses within the mesangium and capillary loops. On electron microscopy, large intracapillary "thrombi" of the cryoprecipitate may be seen. Lowering the circulating level of cryoprecipitate with plasmapheresis often induces a clinical remission of the nephritis.

Progressive Crescentic Glomerulonephritis

Rapidly progressive glomerulonephritis (RPGN) describes a nephritic syndrome that is more common after the third decade of life, has a clinical presentation similar to that of postinfectious AGN, and is characterized by extensive glomerular crescent formation. The major clinical distinction is that RPGN displays a rapid progression (less than six months) to end-stage renal failure. Serum complement levels are normal, a fact that helps in the early distinction of this syndrome from postinfectious or SLE glomerulonephritis.

Two categories of RPGN have been identified, based on the distinctive histopathology and serology of each variety. *Antiglomerular basement membrane* (anti-GBM) glomerulonephritis is diagnosed by the identification of circulating anti-GBM antibodies. Goodpasture's syndrome is a form of anti-GBM nephritis in which pulmonary hemorrhage is a major feature of the clinical disease. *Idiopathic* RPGN has a similar renal course but lacks circulating anti-GBM antibody.

Light microscopy of all forms of RPGN is dominated by the appearance of extensive glomerular crescents in more than 50 per cent of glomeruli. These cellular crescents represent both proliferating urinary epithelial cells and invading tissue macrophages. Crescents are also seen in severe forms of other types of glomerulonephritis, including post-streptococcal and anaphylactoid purpura.

Anti-GBM disease is identified by continuous, linear staining for IgG and C_3 along the basement membranes of glomerular capillaries (Fig. 34–1F). Linear immune staining alone, however, is not pathognomonic and has been seen in diabetic nephropathy and lupus glomerulonephritis. In Goodpasture's syndrome, linear staining of pulmonary capillary basement membranes can also be demonstrated. Idiopathic RPGN has variable immune staining that ranges from patchy, segmental staining for C_3 and IgM to cases in which no immunofluorescence is seen. Electron microscopy does not regularly show deposits in either form of this disorder, but breaks in the glomerular basement membrane are common.

Treatment in anti-GBM nephritis is directed toward lowering the level of circulating anti-GBM antibody. Plasmapheresis to remove circulating antibody, in combination with corticosteroids and immunosuppressive drugs to reduce antibody production, has been successful in halting progression of disease in some patients. Individuals with an initial serum creatinine greater than 5 mg/dl or those having crescents in more than 80 per cent of glomeruli on renal biopsy are not likely to respond to treatment. Anti-GBM disease has been shown to recur in transplanted kidneys. No therapy has been shown to be of consistent benefit in the treatment of idiopathic RPGN.

Other Glomerulonephritides

A number of diseases of diverse etiology display a nephritic syndrome as a major manifestation of their clinical presentation. The glomerular pathology is as varied as the clinical syndromes. Systemic vasculitides that also involve the glomeruli to cause a nephritic syndrome are discussed in the section on vascular disease and the kidney.

The *hemolytic-uremic syndrome* (HUS) chiefly affects children under the age of 10 years and almost always follows a nonspecific gastrointestinal or influenzal syndrome. However, an adult form does occur and is seen primarily in women taking oral contraceptives or those in the postpartum period.

The acute phase of HUS is manifest by sudden onset of severe oligoanuria, hematuria, acute gastrointestinal symptoms, and gastrointestinal bleeding. Hypertension and volume overload are common, as are petechiae and ecchymoses. Oligoanuria and azotemia persist for one to two weeks in children, with spontaneous recovery the rule. Acute dialysis during this period has dramatically increased survival. Recurrence of the syndrome in children is well-documented, and these children may have progressive renal disease. The outcome in adults is much less favorable, with the vast majority of survivors requiring chronic dialysis or transplantation.

The striking feature of this syndrome is the microangiopathic hemolytic anemia, evidenced by fragmented circulating RBC's accompanied by thrombocytopenia. Azotemia is universal and uremia is common. The glomeruli may show fibrin thrombi in capillary loops and segmental fibrinoid necrosis on light microscopy. Bilateral renal cortical necrosis occurs in the most severe cases, mostly in adults. A characteristic lesion is seen on electron microscopy in which capillary endothelial cells are separated from basement membranes by a space filled with finely granular basement membrane–like material.

Thrombotic thrombocytopenic purpura (TTP), which likely shares certain pathogenic origins with HUS, may also present with signs of nephritis and microangiopathic hemolytic anemia. In TTP, the clinical syndrome is dominated by neurological manifestations and the nephritis is evidenced by modest proteinuria, microhematuria, and modest degrees of azotemia. Glomerular pathology is similar to but less extensive than that of HUS.

Hereditary nephritis, or Alport's syndrome, is a chronic GN that seems to follow X-linked inheritance. The clinical manifestations of renal disease are more common and more severe in males. The disease presents in childhood with recurrent bouts of gross hematuria, often with loin or vague abdominal pain. Sensorineural deafness is seen in about half the patients. Proteinuria is usually slight, and the nephrotic syndrome is uncommon. Males are especially prone to develop renal failure by age 20 to 30 years. Treatment does not alter the course of the disease, and it is not known to recur in transplanted kidneys.

Light microscopy findings are nonspecific, but an inflammatory interstitial component with foam cells becomes prominent as the disease progresses. There is no consistent immunofluorescent finding in glomeruli, but electron microscopy shows a distinctive lesion. Widespread glomerular basement membrane alterations are evident, with severe GBM attenuation alternating with thick GBM's split by a central lucent zone.

Mixed Glomerulopathies

Certain glomerular diseases have a mixed clinical presentation (Table 34–3). Either nephrotic or nephritic symptoms may dominate the clinical picture, but signs of both nephrosis and nephritis often occur together. Whatever the initial pres-

TABLE 34–3. GLOMERULOPATHIES WITH NEPHROTIC AND NEPHRITIC FEATURES

Membranoproliferative Glomerulonephritis (Mesangiocapillary GN, Hypocomplementemic GN)
Idiopathic: Type I
           Type II, dense deposit
Secondary: Chronic infections
           Essential cryoglobulinemia
Mesangioproliferative Glomerulonephritis
Idiopathic: IgA/IgG nephropathy (Berger's disease)
           Non-IgA
Secondary: Systemic lupus erythematosus
           Anaphylactoid purpura

entation, these glomerulopathies usually follow a relentless course to end-stage renal failure.

Membranoproliferative Glomerulonephritis (MPGN)

MPGN is a chronic glomerulopathy of unknown etiology that is most common in children and young adults. The majority of patients present with significant manifestations of both nephrosis and nephritis. The presence of glomerular disease is discovered in over one third of patients as a result of finding either hematuria or proteinuria, both of which are present in virtually all patients, on a routine urinalysis. Up to one half of patients present with the nephrotic syndrome and have significant, persistent proteinuria throughout the course of the disease. An acute nephritic picture with hypertension, hematuria, and azotemia is seen in about one third of patients. This presentation, especially in the face of a low serum C_3 value, requires differentiation from post-streptococcal GN by ASO titer measurements and from lupus nephritis by measurement of antinuclear antibody (ANA) titers.

On light microscopy the most prominent features are mesangial cell proliferation and apparent thickening of capillary basement membranes. Electron microscopy serves to separate the disease into two varieties. Type I MPGN is characterized by subendothelial deposits and duplication of capillary basement membranes caused by interposition of mesangium within the basement membrane (Fig. 34–1*B*). Type II, also known as dense deposit disease, displays striking deposits of electron-dense material within the basement membranes of peripheral capillary loops (Fig. 34–1*C*). The early complement components $C1q$ and C_4 are often present in Type I but usually absent in Type II, while C_3 is prominent in both varieties.

Persistent hypocomplementemia in MPGN is often associated with a 7S gamma globulin that is capable of inducing cleavage of C_3 in the absence of calcium or properdin. This C_3 nephritic factor (C_3NeF) is more prevalent in Type II MPGN, but its presence does not appear to influence the prognosis of the disease.

Temporary spontaneous remissions are known to occur, but at least half the patients will have terminal renal failure after 10 years. The rate of progression is somewhat greater in Type II MPGN.

No therapy has proven successful in arresting the progression to renal failure. The presence either of a persistent nephrotic syndrome or of renal insufficiency at the time of diagnosis is associated with rapid deterioration, but neither the occurrence of gross hematuria nor spontaneous remission affects the outcome. Type II, dense-deposit disease almost invariably recurs in transplanted kidneys, while recurrence of Type I is far less common.

Mesangioproliferative Glomerulonephritis

This histopathological pattern may occur in diseases discussed elsewhere but is best exemplified by the idiopathic syndrome of IgA nephropathy. This is a distinctive glomerulopathy found in about half of patients with benign recurrent hematuria, a syndrome predominantly of young adult males. The classic presentation is that of repeated bouts of asymptomatic gross hematuria, which often occur in conjunction with an upper respiratory infection and which are separated by periods when only microscopic hematuria is evident. Proteinuria is usually modest, < 1 gm/day, but up to 10 per cent of patients develop the nephrotic syndrome. Serum complement levels are normal.

The light microscopy is nondiagnostic, but the most typical finding is that of focal, segmental proliferation within glomeruli. The diagnosis is made by the invariable presence of IgA seen by immunofluorescence within the mesangium (Fig. 34–1*G*). IgG and/or IgM are found alongside IgA in about half the cases. Mesangial IgA can also be seen in lupus nephritis and in anaphylactoid purpura. Electron microscopy confirms the presence of deposits within the mesangium.

Originally thought to represent a benign disorder, mesangioproliferative glomerulonephritis is now known to progress to terminal renal failure in 10 to 15 years in 10 to 20 per cent of patients, especially those with heavy proteinuria. The course of the disease is not known to be altered by corticosteroids or immunosuppressive agents. Mesangial deposits of IgA, sometimes associated with hematuria, occur regularly in transplanted kidneys.

TUBULAR AND INTERSTITIAL DISEASE

Clinical Presentation

Dysfunction of the renal tubules can have myriad clinical manifestations, reflecting the many regulatory functions of the different nephron segments. Tubular disorders may present as alterations in osmotic balance (nephrogenic diabetes insipidus), in acid-base regulation (renal tubular acidosis), in extracellular fluid volume homeostasis (salt-losing nephropathy), and in mineral metabolism (primary phosphaturia). In each case, the function of the segment of the nephron most affected determines the clinical manifestations of the syndrome. Some tubular disorders are purely functional and do not directly affect glomerular filtration. Renal failure, expressed as a reduction in the GFR, occurs only as an indirect effect of altered body homeostasis (see Chapter 29) in these disorders.

Other diseases, however, originate in the tubulointerstitial compartment of the kidney and, because of the destructive nature of the lesion, do lead to reductions in GFR. Such disorders include the hereditary cystic diseases of the kidney (polycystic kidney disease) and the chronic interstitial nephritides (lead nephropathy, analgesic nephropathy). The initial presentation of these disorders also reflects the loss of specific tubular functions, and only when far-advanced do they display characteristics of a reduction in GFR. Table 34–4 outlines the diseases discussed in this section.

Pathogenic Mechanisms

The great majority of tubulointerstitial disorders occur as a result of one of three general mechanisms: heredity, toxic injury, or a change in tubule regulation by drugs or hormones. Polycystic kidney disease, familial nephrogenic diabetes insipidus, and Fanconi's syndrome are disorders of hereditary origin. The specific genetic defects are unknown. Analgesic nephropathy, lead nephropathy, and some types of renal tubular acidosis are representative of toxic injuries. Pituitary diabetes insipidus (ADH deficiency), adrenal salt wasting (deficient mineralocorticoid), and diuretic administration are examples of the last category (see Chapter 29).

TUBULOINTERSTITIAL DISEASE

Polycystic Kidney Disease (PKD)

This familial disorder is the most significant of a number of renal cystic disorders (Table 34–5). Inherited as an autosomal dominant trait with high penetrance, PKD is a relatively common cause of end-stage renal failure in the fourth and fifth decades of life. Virtually 100 per cent of persons inheriting the disorder will have cystic

TABLE 34–4. TUBULOINTERSTITIAL DISORDERS

Structural Disorders
  Cystic Diseases
    Polycystic kidney disease
    Medullary cystic disease
    Medullary sponge kidney
    Simple renal cysts
  Chronic Interstitial Diseases
    Analgesic nephropathy
    Heavy metal nephropathy
    Radiation nephropathy
    Others: nephrosclerosis, diabetic nephropathy
  Renal Tumors
    Benign tumors
    Renal cell carcinoma
Functional Disorders
  Proximal Tubular
    Fanconi syndrome
    Aminoacidurias (cystinuria)
    Renal glycosuria
    Vitamin D–resistant rickets (familial hypophosphatemia)
    Proximal (type II) renal tubular acidosis
  Distal Tubular
    Nephrogenic diabetes insipidus
    Bartter's syndrome
    Liddle's syndrome
    Distal (types I and IV) renal tubular acidosis

changes, but not necessarily renal failure, by age 80 years. A separate, infantile form of the disease occurs in association with congenital hepatic fibrosis and causes death from renal failure in the first year of life. In adults, benign multiple renal cysts may present a similar radiographic appearance but are not associated with renal dysfunction or failure.

Clinical manifestations of PKD rarely occur before the ages of 20 to 25 years. This accounts for the frequent passage of the genetic trait to offspring by asymptomatic, yet affected, individuals of child-bearing age. Nonspecific, dull lumbar pain is the most frequent initial symptom and usually occurs when the kidneys are sufficiently enlarged to be palpable on examination of the abdomen. Sharp, localized pain may result from cyst rupture or infection or from passage of a renal cal-

TABLE 34–5. CYSTIC DISEASES OF THE KIDNEY

DISORDER	DIAGNOSTIC FEATURES	CLINICAL MANIFESTATIONS	OUTCOME
Polycystic			
Infantile	Palpable abdominal masses at birth	Hepatic fibrosis	Death in infancy
Adult	Multiple, bilateral renal cysts on IVP or renal sonography in large kidneys	Hematuria, polyuria, hypertension, abdominal pain	Chronic renal failure (40 to 50 years old)
Medullary Cystic	None	Polyuria, enuresis	Chronic renal failure (15 to 20 years old)
Medullary Sponge	Nephrocalcinosis, radial medullary cysts on IVP	Recurrent renal calculi and urinary infections	Benign
Simple	Single or multiple cysts in normal-sized kidneys	Asymptomatic	Benign

culus. Microhematuria without RBC casts is frequently the initial sign of PKD; gross hematuria may also occur.

Hypertension occurs commonly in PKD at early stages of the disease. Polycystic disease may thus be discovered in the course of evaluating hypertension in a young adult. Nocturia due to a urinary concentrating defect is often present at the time of diagnosis, and most patients are unable to conserve salt on a salt-restricted intake. Urinary tract infection and pyelonephritis are common complications. Up to one third of patients with polycystic renal disease have multiple, asymptomatic hepatic cysts, and cerebral aneurysms are more prevalent than in unaffected persons.

The diagnosis of polycystic kidney disease is made on the basis of radiographic evidence of multiple cysts distributed throughout the renal parenchyma. The nephrogram phase of intravenous urography (IVP) shows the lucent cysts surrounded by attenuated strands of functional renal tissue. Renal ultrasonography is another valuable tool in demonstrating the distribution and size of the cystic lesions. Both studies can be employed to screen younger (>16 years of age) family members of patients in order to identify the asymptomatic lesion at a time when genetic counseling may be useful. Failure to concentrate the urine above 800 mOsm/kg H_2O after dehydration is highly predictive of PKD in adolescents at risk for the disorder.

Therapy for polycystic kidney disease is directed toward control of hypertension and prevention and early treatment of urinary tract infections. Nephrectomy is occasionally indicated for persistent gross hematuria or for an infected renal cyst. Decompressing cysts by surgical "unroofing" is associated with a high incidence of complications, including complete renal failure. End-stage renal failure is managed by either dialysis or transplantation. Bilateral nephrectomy may be required prior to transplant in patients with inordinately large kidneys or in those with a history of frequent or persistent urinary tract infection.

Other Cystic Diseases

Cysts of the renal medulla are features of two grossly disparate disorders. *Medullary cystic disease* (nephronophthisis) occurs either as a rare, autosomal recessive disease or as a feature of some cases of retinitis pigmentosa. *Medullary sponge kidney* is a more common, benign disorder that may be discovered incidentally on abdominal radiographs.

Medullary cystic disease regularly results in end-stage renal failure during adolescence or early adulthood. Prolonged enuresis in childhood due to a urinary concentrating defect is one early indication of the renal disease. Anemia is another early manifestation of the disease. Neither radiography nor renal biopsy has a high rate of success in demonstrating the small medullary cysts.

Medullary sponge kidney is a benign disorder that often presents as a result of passage of a renal calculus. Colicky renal pain, hematuria, or urinary tract infection may herald the disorder; each symptom is the result of renal stone formation. Nephrocalcinosis occurs in about half the patients and accounts for discovery of asymptomatic patients on routine abdominal radiographs. The diagnosis is made on IVP by the characteristic radial pattern of contrast-filled medullary cysts. Treatment for urinary tract infection and renal calculus formation is indicated. Renal failure does not occur as part of the basic disease.

Chronic Interstitial Nephritis

Distinct causes of chronic interstitial nephritis include analgesic abuse, heavy metal ingestion, and radiation exposure. Diabetes mellitus, multiple myeloma, and essential hypertension, diseases that affect multiple organs, may also cause significant renal interstitial disease. No specific etiology is identifiable for up to one half of all cases of chronic interstitial nephritis. In each case the disease process may be wholly asymptomatic, with azotemia discovered incidentally on a laboratory screening panel. Hypertension is a regular feature of these disorders and can be the initial, presenting sign of renal disease. Sterile pyuria and microscopic hematuria are presenting signs in some patients. A large number of cases are recognized only when end-stage renal failure occurs and a retrospective diagnosis is made based on a history of toxic exposure.

Analgesic nephropathy follows the ingestion over years of time of combination analgesics, usually a salicylate plus either phenacetin or acetaminophen. Use of the single agents alone is not associated with renal injury. The lesion is first seen in the renal medulla and may reflect a toxic effect of acetaminophen that is intensified by medullary concentration. Salicylates appear to be permissive to the effect, perhaps by blocking production of vasodilator prostaglandins that support medullary blood flow. The disease process may be halted if analgesic intake is stopped early in the course.

Decreased urinary concentrating ability results from the medullary lesion, but frank polyuria is uncommon. Papillary necrosis, visible on renal radiography (IVP) and causing passage of tissue in the urine, is a hallmark of the disease. Treatment consists of withdrawing combination analgesic preparations, rigorously controlling blood pressure, and maintaining surveillance for urinary tract obstruction from sloughed papillary tissue.

Heavy metal nephropathy occurs chiefly with chronic lead ingestion, leaded paints and illicit alcohol being prominent sources. Aside from the coexistence of an anemia disproportionate to the degree of renal insufficiency, prominent peripheral neuropathy, and a high incidence of gouty arthritis, lead nephropathy is clinically similar to analgesic nephropathy. Interstitial nephritis previously attributed to urate deposition in the kidney (urate nephropathy) is now recognized to be lead nephropathy with saturnine gout. Increased

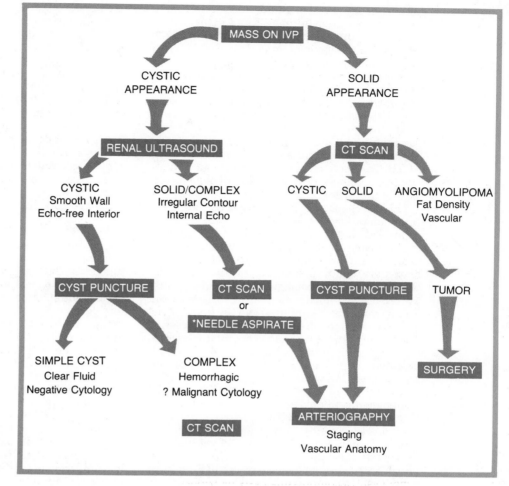

FIGURE 34-2. Scheme for work-up of renal mass.

urinary lead excretion following EDTA administration is a useful diagnostic test, but EDTA infusion may cause toxic renal failure and is not useful in treating this disorder.

Chronic radiation nephritis may follow some years after local retroperitoneal irradiation. It, too, is associated with progressive, often silent, renal insufficiency; accelerated hypertension is a common complication. Proteinuria of modest proportion may be seen. There is no treatment for the nephropathy, but strict management of hypertension is important.

Renal Tumors

Most renal tumors appear to originate from the tubulointerstitial components of the kidney. Renal cell carcinoma, for instance, is thought to be of proximal tubular origin. The evaluation of a patient for any renal mass may proceed according to the scheme given in Figure 34-2. This plan attempts to differentiate benign cystic lesions from solid masses and to identify malignant characteristics in solid renal masses.

Benign tumors of the kidney include cortical adenomas and angiomyolipomas (hamartomas). The former are more common in older males and frequently harbor rests of malignant cells. Therefore, adenomas are usually diagnosed after sur-

gical evaluation of a solid renal mass. Angiomyolipomas are highly vascular fatty tumors that mimic renal cell carcinomas in both presentation and angiographic appearance. A fact of diagnostic significance is the occurrence of over half of these hamartomas in patients with tuberous sclerosis. In patients without tuberous sclerosis, surgical exploration may be necessary for differentiating angiomyolipoma from renal cell carcinoma if CT scan results are equivocal.

Renal cell carcinoma, or hypernephroma, is the most frequent malignant renal neoplasm in adults and accounts for about 2 per cent of cancer deaths in both sexes. The term hypernephroma originated from the gross appearance of most of these tumors, which, because of their high lipid content, resemble adrenal tissue.

The classic clinical presentation of renal cell carcinoma is that of a triad of hematuria, flank pain, and palpable flank mass. Actually, only about 10 per cent of patients present with all these features, but any one of these features is present in well over half of all patients as an initial manifestation of the tumor. A sizable number of patients will present with nonurinary symptoms, including fever of unexplained origin, weight loss, and anemia.

Renal cell carcinoma is notable for the large

number of extrarenal manifestations of the tumor. Fever is seen in about one fifth of cases and an elevated erythrocyte sedimentation rate (ESR) is seen in half the patients. Anemia is seen in about one third of patients, but polycythemia is a striking finding in some cases. Reversible hepatic dysfunction has been described, as has peripheral neuropathy. Ectopic hormone syndromes associated with renal cell carcinoma include hypercalcemia from osteoclast-stimulating factors (either parathyroid hormone or prostaglandins) and a Cushing syndrome from tumor production of an ACTH-like factor. Hypercalcemia in renal cell carcinoma is frequently associated with bone metastasis of the tumor.

The tumors usually have three cell types: clear cells, granular cells, and spindle cells. Tumors composed chiefly of spindle cells and those having extensive nuclear anaplasia carry a poor prognosis. The tumors are highly vascular, supplied by vessels with thin, amuscular walls. Extension of the tumor into normal renal veins and even into the vena cava is not uncommon. Metastatic spread is chiefly via vascular routes, and the lungs, bone, and liver are most frequently sites of metastasis. The tumors often undergo cystic, internal degeneration, thus mimicking benign renal cysts. Calcification within a renal mass is a significant radiographic indicator of malignancy.

As shown in Figure 34–2, needle aspiration of a sonographically cystic lesion is useful in confirming the diagnosis of a simple renal cyst. Sonographically solid masses should not undergo needle puncture owing to a risk of rupture of a degenerating carcinoma. Computerized tomography (CT scan) is the preferred means of examining solid renal masses. Renal cell carcinomas are highly vascular tumors, while avascular masses may be carcinomas (<5 per cent of renal cell tumors) or may represent abscesses. Careful needle aspiration for culture may be performed if renal abscess is judged to be likely. Renal arteriography may be important when the CT results are indeterminate or for delineation of tumor vascular supply.

Treatment of renal cell carcinoma requires surgical excision. Vena caval angiography may be valuable preoperatively to ascertain the presence of venous tumor thrombus. Survival is related to cellular morphology, local extension, and distant metastases and ranges from about 10 per cent to about 50 per cent 10-year survival based on these factors.

DISORDERS OF TUBULAR FUNCTION

The Fanconi Syndrome

This disorder represents a generalized failure of specialized proximal tubular reabsorption. The Fanconi syndrome is identified by a broad range of aminoaciduria, glycosuria, phosphaturia, uricosuria, and bicarbonaturia. The tubulopathy itself does not lead to renal failure, but the condition in which Fanconi's syndrome occurs may cause renal insufficiency.

The Fanconi syndrome is commonly seen as a part of some hereditary disorders, is rarely seen as a single hereditary defect, and may occur as an acquired defect in association with an underlying disease or drug. The most common cause of the syndrome in children is the hereditary disease cystinosis, a disorder characterized by the cellular accumulation of cystine in various organs, including the kidney. Proximal tubular cystine accumulation may play a role in the tubulopathy but is certainly the cause of eventual renal failure. Wilson's disease, characterized by excess body copper accumulation, is also a cause of hereditary Fanconi syndrome. The tubulopathy may be acquired as a feature of such diseases as multiple myeloma, amyloidosis, and Sjögren's syndrome.

Aminoaciduria

Abnormal excretion of amino acids may occur as a single defect in proximal tubular reabsorptive function. The aminoacidurias are grouped according to the class of amino acids affected, i.e., basic, neutral, or acidic, and reflect a specific defect in the cellular transport system for each group. The most significant of these many disorders is cystinuria, which is actually a failure of reabsorption of the dibasic amino acids lysine, ornithine, arginine, and cystine. Cystine is singled out because of its very low solubility over the urinary pH range of 4.5 to 7.0. Renal stone formation is the most prominent feature of the disease, although only half the stones are pure cystine. Renal failure due to repeated bouts of urinary tract obstruction and/or urinary tract infection is a common outcome of untreated cystinuria. No cellular accumulation of cystine occurs, a reflection of the fact that cystinuria represents a defect in cellular transport of cystine, whereas cystinosis represents a defect in cellular processing of the amino acid.

The disease can be recognized on urinalysis by the flat, hexagonal cystine crystalluria. A definitive diagnosis is made by the demonstration of the isolated appearance of the four dibasic amino acids in the urine. Urinary cystine excretion of more than 400 mg/gm creatinine is characteristic. The most effective treatment is forced intake of 5 L or more of water daily to keep urine cystine concentrations below saturation levels.

Renal Glycosuria

The persistent urinary excretion of glucose at normal blood glucose levels and, therefore, normal filtered loads of glucose, is a benign disorder. The specific proximal tubular defect is inherited by either autosomal dominant or autosomal recessive genetics. Renal glycosuria is not associated with a risk of developing diabetes mellitus and requires no treatment.

Vitamin D—resistant Rickets

Also called familial hypophosphatemia, this is an X-linked hereditary disorder characterized by hypophosphatemia (usually <2.5 mg/dl), inappropriate phosphaturia (phosphate/creatinine clearance ratio >0.25), rachitic bone disease, and normal serum calcium and PTH levels. The primary defect is not known, but a decrease in intestinal calcium and phosphate absorption accompanies the renal phosphate "leak." Vigorous treatment with both high doses of vitamin D (20,000 to 50,000 IU/day) and oral phosphate is required to heal the rachitic bone lesions.

Nephrogenic Diabetes Insipidus (NDI)

NDI is a specific defect in the response of the collecting tubule to ADH. ADH release in response to osmotic or volume stimulation and circulating levels of ADH are normal, yet the urine is persistently hypotonic to plasma. Aside from this specific concentrating defect, renal function is normal. NDI may occur either as a rare, X-linked hereditary disorder or as an acquired defect secondary to lithium or demeclocycline therapy.

Hereditary NDI presents in infancy as repeated bouts of fever and altered mental status. These symptoms are the result of hypertonic volume depletion and encephalopathy. In later life, incessant thirst and persistent polyuria dominate the clinical picture. Urinary tract dilation may result from the massive volumes of urine excreted daily, 15 to 20 L in adults. Neurological deficits may be seen as a result of repeated bouts of hypertonic encephalopathy.

The diagnosis is made by family history, a failure to concentrate the urine after 12 to 18 hours of dehydration, and a failure to raise urine osmolality above that of plasma in response to exogenous ADH. Treatment consists of assurance of ready access to and intake of water, plus a thiazide diuretic. Thiazide diuretics plus salt restriction cause a modest reduction in ECF volume, which causes a greater volume of the glomerular filtrate to be absorbed as isotonic fluid in the proximal nephron. Therefore, a lesser volume of hypotonic fluid is generated in the loop of Henle, delivered to the ADH-unresponsive collecting duct, and excreted in the final urine.

Acquired NDI is generally incomplete and is expressed as a dramatic reduction in maximal urinary concentration. The defect almost always disappears with cessation of the demeclocycline or lithium.

Bartter's Syndrome

This rare disorder affects mostly women, who present with stunted growth plus symptoms of polyuria and recurrent muscular weakness. The biochemical profile is that of hypochloremic metabolic alkalosis, profound hypokalemia (1.5 to 2.5 mEq/L), hyper-reninemia, and hyperaldosteronism. Despite high renin values the patients are normotensive and are insensitive to the pressor effect of angiotensin II (AII). Urinary excretion of potassium and chloride remains high despite the hypochloremic, hypokalemic state. Juxtaglomerular apparatus hyperplasia is the distinguishing renal lesion.

The renal manifestations of Bartter's syndrome are associated with excessive renal prostaglandin

E_2 (PGE_2) activity and excretion. PGE_2 has been shown to stimulate renin secretion, to block vasoconstriction produced by AII, and to inhibit salt absorption in the thick ascending limb of Henle. Suppression of PGE_2 production with cyclo-oxygenase inhibitors (aspirin, indomethacin) reduces urinary PGE_2 excretion, restores vascular sensitivity to exogenous AII, and reduces urinary chloride losses. The lack of total correction of hypokalemia by these drugs has led to the notion that Bartter's syndrome is due to a primary defect in the tubular handling of chloride or of potassium, and that the increased PGE_2 production is secondary to hypokalemia.

Liddle's Syndrome

As in Bartter's syndrome, hypokalemia, hyperkaliuria, and hypochloremic metabolic alkalosis characterize this rare disorder. However, in sharp contrast to Bartter's syndrome, aldosterone levels are normal, renal avidity for sodium is increased, and patients are hypertensive in Liddle's syndrome. A primary increase in distal nephron sodium absorption, which can be blocked by the diuretic triamterene but not by the aldosterone antagonist spironolactone, appears to be the cause of the unusual clinical syndrome.

Renal Tubular Acidosis

The term renal tubular acidosis (RTA) describes a group of disorders whose individual features reflect the site and mechanism of failure in tubular hydrogen ion transport (Fig. 34–3). Type I, or classic distal RTA, represents an inability of the collecting duct to maintain a gradient of free hydrogen ion between the blood and the urine. This failure to maintain a hydrogen ion gradient may be due to increased backleak of hydrogen ion from the tubular lumen to blood or to a failure in the hydrogen secretory mechanism. Type I RTA is expressed as an inability to lower urine pH (the free hydrogen ion concentration) in the face of an acid challenge. Type II, or proximal RTA, involves an impairment in the rate of hydrogen ion secretion and therefore bicarbonate reabsorption in the proximal tubule. Proximal RTA is expressed as bicarbonaturia that persists until the serum bicarbonate concentration and the filtered load of bicarbonate fall to levels that match the reduced proximal tubular absorptive capacity. Finally, Type IV RTA designates a defect in mineralocorticoid-dependent hydrogen ion secretion in the distal nephron. Type IV RTA usually accompanies some form of renal interstitial disease (as in lead or diabetic nephropathies) and results either from diminished aldosterone secretion or from a failure of collecting duct response to aldosterone.

Distal RTA may occur sporadically as an isolated disorder or may be secondary to a systemic disease or toxin. Prominent causes of distal RTA include primary and secondary hypergammaglobulinemias, nephrocalcinosis, amyloidosis, sickle cell disease, and amphotericin B administration.

Children often present with lethargy, anorexia, stunted growth, and bone disease. Adults have

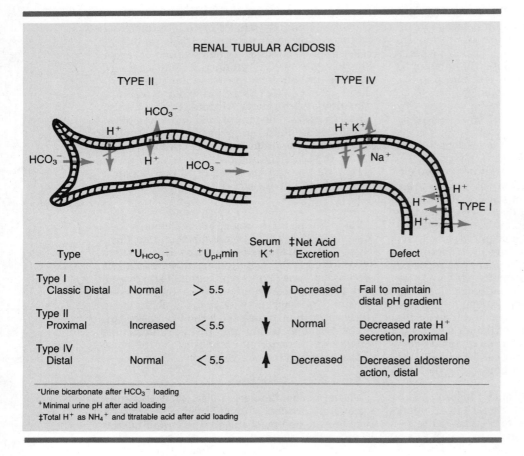

RENAL TUBULAR ACIDOSIS

TYPE II

TYPE IV

TYPE I

FIGURE 34–3. Differentiation of varieties of renal tubular acidosis.

Type	*$U_{HCO_3^-}$	+U_{pH}min	Serum K$^+$	‡Net Acid Excretion	Defect
Type I Classic Distal	Normal	> 5.5	↓	Decreased	Fail to maintain distal pH gradient
Type II Proximal	Increased	< 5.5	↓	Normal	Decreased rate H$^+$ secretion, proximal
Type IV Distal	Normal	< 5.5	↑	Decreased	Decreased aldosterone action, distal

*Urine bicarbonate after HCO_3^- loading

+Minimal urine pH after acid loading

‡Total H$^+$ as NH_4^+ and titratable acid after acid loading

similar symptoms, often with bone pain or pathological fractures, and a high incidence of renal stones. The origin of these symptoms appears to be bone buffering of hydrogen ion over an extended period. This leads to bone calcium loss and hypercalciuria in the presence of an alkaline urine. Disordered calcium metabolism is expressed as rickets in children and osteomalacia, nephrocalcinosis, and nephrolithasis in adults. The distinguishing laboratory features include hyperchloremic metabolic acidosis with hypokalemia and a urinary pH that is consistently above pH 6.0 to 6.5.

An inability to lower urine pH below 5.3 in the face of spontaneous acidosis or an acid load (given as oral NH_4Cl) is diagnostic. Administration of a single dose of the loop diuretic furosemide also aids in the diagnosis of distal RTA. Normal individuals and those with Type I, gradient-limited RTA increase urinary acid secretion concomitant to the increased delivery of Na$^+$ to the distal nephron.

Treatment of distal RTA is accomplished by oral alkali replacement, either as sodium bicarbonate or as Shohl's solution, at the rate of 1 to 3 mEq/kg/day. The 60 to 70 mEq of bicarbonate required to treat Type I RTA correspond to the normal contribution of the distal nephron to H$^+$ excretion. Correction of acidosis by this means leads to cessation of hypercalciuria and renal stone formation and correction of hypokalemia, but

normal growth and bone development in children require administration of several hundred milliequivalents of bicarbonate daily.

Proximal RTA occurs rarely as an isolated lesion and is most often seen as a part of the Fanconi syndrome. Proximal RTA is a self-limiting process in that normal acidification of urine, measured both as a maximum reduction in urine pH and as a normal excretion of ammonia and titratable acid, is seen when the serum bicarbonate level reaches a reduced, steady-state value. This value is usually 14 to 18 mEq/L and represents the maximal resorptive capacity of the proximal tubule in the disorder. At this moderate level of extracellular buffer reduction, daily H$^+$ excretion is complete and long-term buffer deficits do not develop as in distal RTA.

Clinical signs and symptoms are few in proximal RTA and relate to growth retardation. Hyperchloremic metabolic acidosis is evident in all cases. Hypokalemia, the result of increased delivery of sodium bicarbonate to the distal nephron, is prominent. Hypercalciuria, nephrocalcinosis, and nephrolithiasis are absent. The urine pH can reach values of 4.5 to 5.0 as long as the serum bicarbonate level is below the proximal tubular resorptive threshold. The diagnosis is confirmed by the infusion of bicarbonate and observation of an increase in urine pH and bicarbonaturia at subnormal levels of serum bicarbonate.

The treatment of proximal RTA with alkali replacement is virtually impossible because any elevation of the serum bicarbonate above the absorptive capacity of the proximal tubule results in quantitative urinary excretion of the added bicarbonate. Modest salt depletion, thereby increasing general proximal tubular absorption, will aid in raising the serum bicarbonate concentration.

Type IV RTA results from a diminished mineralocorticoid effect in the distal nephron and is expressed as a decrease in the secretory rates of potassium and hydrogen. There are two forms of the disorder. Aldosterone levels may be reduced, either from primary adrenal disease, in which case renin levels are elevated, or from renal interstitial disease, in which case renin levels are grossly reduced. Alternatively, adequate levels of aldosterone may be present but the distal nephron is unresponsive to its effect. This type of the disorder may be caused either by disease of the distal nephron; by the aldosterone-blocking diuretic, spironolactone; or by the potassium-sparing diuretics, triamterene and amiloride.

Since both potassium and hydrogen secretion are blunted, hyperkalemia accompanies the hyperchloremic metabolic acidosis of Type IV RTA. This is in contrast to the hypokalemia seen in Types I and II. A mild degree of renal insufficiency is present in many of these patients. They often demonstrate relative salt wasting, that is, an inability to reduce urinary sodium excretion during salt restriction. Hyperkalemia decreases the renal generation and excretion of the major urinary buffer, ammonium. Therefore, patients with Type IV RTA have a decrease in total acid excretion, although the urine pH may be appropriately acidic. Basal and stimulated renin plus aldosterone levels should be measured in these patients.

Mineralocorticoid replacement, as fludrocortisone, is effective therapy in patients with an absolute reduction in aldosterone. Because increased sodium delivery to the distal nephron augments potassium and hydrogen secretion even in the absence of aldosterone, a high-salt diet plus a loop diuretic (furosemide) will increase both potassium and hydrogen excretion in all these patients. Reduction of the serum potassium alone increases urinary ammonium excretion and net urinary acid excretion and restores the hydrogen balance in some of these patients.

DISORDERS OF RENAL VESSELS

Two major classes of renovascular disorders can be defined based on the size of the vessel involved. Large vessel disease, thromboembolic occlusion of the renal arteries or veins, occurs with greatest frequency in particular clinical circumstances and has dramatic effects on renal function. Stenosis of one or both renal arteries is the most common cause of curable, secondary hypertension. Small vessel diseases include nephrosclerosis, the sclerotic narrowing of small, intrarenal vessels, which is a frequent complication of long-

standing hypertension and is a major factor leading to end-stage renal failure in these patients. In addition, systemic vasculitic diseases frequently involve the smaller intrarenal vessels to produce distinctive renal syndromes.

Renal Artery Occlusion

This is most often an embolic phenomenon. Clot emboli originate in the heart in atrial fibrillation or after myocardial infarction, or atheromatous emboli originate from the aorta after aortic manipulation during angiography or vascular surgery. Both types of embolization are obviously more prevalent in elderly patients.

Renal artery occlusion does not invariably cause renal infarction or symptoms. However, when symptoms occur, they usually reflect tissue ischemia and death. Sudden renal infarction may cause severe localized flank pain, nausea and vomiting, and oliguria, but rarely hematuria. A sudden onset or exacerbation of hypertension may occur. A leukocytosis may be seen along with elevations of lactate dehydrogenase (LDH) in serum and urine. Segmental or unilateral renal infarction may be asymptomatic without an evident effect on renal function.

Renal vascular scintiradiography is a most useful initial test in suspected cases of renal infarction. Total lack of renal blood flow in a dynamic study, or defects in activity on a static image, are highly compatible findings. Renal arteriography may be needed to visualize the extent or location of the occluding embolus/thrombus. Renal artery embolectomy has been successful in restoring blood flow and renal function even if performed two to four days after embolization.

Atheromatous embolization from an aortic plaque usually follows manipulation of an atherosclerotic aorta. The process presents as acute, oliguric renal failure following a surgical or angiographic procedure of the aorta. Although abdominal aortic aneurysms rarely extend into the renal arteries, the manipulation required for surgical repair of the aneurysm may dislodge occluding emboli. Asymptomatic atheromatous embolization to segmental arteries may occur spontaneously, as evidenced by local, healed renal infarcts discovered incidentally at autopsy.

Renal Venous Occlusion

Renal vein occlusion is a thrombotic event. The incidence of renal vein thrombosis (RVT) is high in nephrotic glomerulopathies, especially membranous nephropathy, and in certain neoplastic diseases. Renal vein thrombosis may occur in children who develop severe volume depletion accompanying a gastrointestinal disorder.

Renal vein thrombosis most often occurs in the absence of direct clinical symptoms. However, two distinct patterns of clinical presentation have been recognized. Acute renal failure is often seen in children or in patients with the nephrotic syndrome who have a reduced but stable baseline GFR. The second mode of presentation is that of acute pulmonary embolism and infarction, seen most often in patients with the nephrotic syndrome.

Renal vein thrombosis can often be diagnosed safely with renal ultrasonography, but renal venography may be required for definitive diagnosis in some patients. Prophylactic anticoagulant therapy in patients with nephrotic glomerulopathies, the group at highest risk for RVT, is not of proven use. Acute anticoagulant therapy is indicated in cases of proven or threatened pulmonary embolism; an improvement in renal function may occur.

Renal Artery Stenosis

The consequences of renal artery stenosis are two-fold: the development of secondary hypertension, which is usually renin-dependent, and the progressive loss of renal function through ischemia. Renal artery stenosis (RAS) probably accounts for no more than 2 to 3 per cent of all cases of hypertension in the general population. However, two distinct clinical circumstances point to the high likelihood of RAS as the etiology of the hypertension. First, the onset of significant hypertension in a young female (<35 years old) is highly likely to be due to fibromuscular dysplasia of the renal arteries. Second, the onset of hypertension in a previously normotensive patient older than 55 years of age is often associated with atherosclerotic renal artery stenosis.

Fibromuscular hyperplasia of the renal artery may involve the intima, media, or adventitia of the vessel. The middle and distal thirds of the renal artery are usually involved, the disease is often bilateral, and the lesion tends to progress with time. Renal arteriography demonstrates a typical beaded appearance of the renal arteries. The stenosis can be successfully relieved in about 90 per cent of patients either by surgery or by percutaneous vascular dilation.

Atherosclerotic renal artery stenosis is an extension of atheromatous disease of the aorta. Thus, the renal artery ostium and the proximal third of the renal vessels are most affected. Both renal arteries tend to be involved, but the lesions rarely advance in severity. A number of tests have been devised to predict either improvement of renal function or relief of hypertension following surgical correction of the stenosis. One of the more popular tests, measurement of individual renal vein renin values, depends on the stimulation of renin in the stenosed, ischemic kidney and the suppression of renin in the unaffected kidney. Based on this and similar tests, one can expect improvement in the hypertension in greater than 90 per cent of patients in whom the tests are positive. However, at least one third of patients who have negative test results will have a similarly favorable response to surgery. Therefore, clinical factors such as patient age, operative risk, success of medical therapy, and adequacy of renal function are important in the decision to operate in any particular case of renal artery stenosis. Percutaneous dilatation of atherosclerotic stenosis has a lasting success rate of only 15 to 20 per cent.

Nephrosclerosis

Nephrosclerosis is one of the most common complications of essential hypertension and is a significant cause of end-stage renal failure. Two forms of the process can be described based on the severity and duration of the hypertension, the pathology of the vascular lesion in the kidney, and the eventual effect on renal and patient survival.

Benign nephrosclerosis is a misnomer that is used to describe a slow process of intrarenal vascular sclerosis and ischemic change that complicates the course of long-standing essential hypertension. The kidneys become progressively shrunken and the renal surfaces exhibit a fine, progressing to coarse, granular appearance.

Although all the intrarenal arteries show some signs of sclerotic thickening, the dominant lesion is at the level of the afferent arteriole. Hyaline thickening of the afferent arteriolar wall leads to a homogeneous, eosinophilic appearance of the vessel. The glomeruli have ischemic wrinkling of the basement membranes and become progressively sclerotic, while the tubules undergo atrophy and are replaced by fibrotic tissue in the absence of inflammation.

Minimal proteinuria occurs in some patients, but the urinary sediment is usually normal. A slow decline in GFR is generally the only feature of the disorder. End-stage renal failure due to nephrosclerosis is more common in males and blacks, and nephrosclerosis has been estimated to account for between 5 and 25 per cent of all cases of end-stage renal failure. Treatment is directed at early control of blood pressure elevations, but even late intervention may slow the progression of renal failure.

Malignant nephrosclerosis is the result of a generalized necrotizing arteritis that is seen in conjunction with accelerated hypertension. Proteinuria, often with hematuria, occurs together with acute decreases in GFR. The diastolic blood pressure is usually, but not necessarily, above 120 mm Hg, and neuroretinal signs of encephalopathy, retinal arteriolar hemorrhage, and papilledema are almost always present. The entire syndrome is most common in black males and most often occurs as an acute exacerbation of essential hypertension.

The kidneys are generally contracted in size and have petechial hemorrhages on the surfaces. Two renal vascular lesions characterize malignant nephrosclerosis. The first lesion consists of fibrinoid necrosis, without inflammation, in the renal arterioles and sometimes extending into the glomerular tufts. The second distinguishing lesion is the "onion skin" endothelial proliferation in small arteries. Concentric layers of collagen and proliferating endothelial cells contribute to this appearance. Similar changes are seen in the renal vessels in the hemolytic-uremic syndrome and the accelerated hypertension of scleroderma.

Prior to effective antihypertensive therapy, more than 75 per cent of persons with accelerated hypertension died of renal failure or cardiac failure within one year. With effective control of the blood pressure, the prognosis is reversed, with less than 25 per cent of the patients suffering a renal or cardiac death within one year. Prompt and strict control of blood pressure is essential, and the course of renal failure can be arrested and even reversed. With long-term blood pressure normalization, the vascular lesions heal, demonstrating the contributory role of pressure per se to the pathogenesis of the disorder.

Systemic Vasculitides

Polyarteritis nodosa (PAN) is a multisystem disorder associated with fibrinoid necrosis of medium-sized arteries. The kidneys are commonly involved at the level of lobular and interlobular arteries, particularly at bifurcations of these vessels. A renal arteriogram demonstrating aneurysms of these vessels is virtually diagnostic of the disorder. Chronic hepatitis B antigenemia is seen in a significant number of patients with PAN.

Mild azotemia and microhematuria, but without hypertension, are seen in over 75 per cent of patients with PAN. Glomeruli show only ischemic changes and sclerosis in these patients. A more dramatic nephritic syndrome, associated with a rapid decline in GFR and frequently associated with accelerated hypertension, occurs in about one third of patients. Fibrinoid necrosis, cellular proliferation, and crescent formation are seen in glomeruli of these patients. Corticosteroids and/or cytotoxic agents can arrest or slow the progression of disease in a significant number of patients.

The course of *progressive systemic sclerosis* (PSS), or scleroderma, culminates with accelerated hypertension associated with a rapid decrease in renal function in 10 to 20 per cent of cases. The clinical presentation is similar to that of rapidly progressive glomerulonephritis, with the added neuroretinal features of malignant hypertension. The primary renal lesion is that of extensive intimal proliferation in interlobular arteries and fibrinoid necrosis of small arteries and glomeruli. This lesion may be evident in patients who exhibit no clinical signs of renal disease. Treatment is directed toward rigorous control of hypertension, but renal failure is usually inevitable.

Wegener's granulomatosis is a vasculitis of small arterioles of the respiratory tract and kidneys. The typical clinical presentation includes destructive sinusitis with nodular pulmonary infiltrates and nephritis. The renal lesion is that of a focal, necrotizing glomerulonephritis with extensive cellular proliferation. The diagnosis should be made on the basis of the clinical presentation plus evidence of a granulomatous vasculitis of the respiratory tract. Differentiation from Goodpasture's syndrome can be made on the basis of the sinus involvement and nodular, as opposed to diffuse, pulmonary radiographic changes in Wegener's. Renal biopsies are rarely diagnostic because the diagnostic granulomatous lesion is found in vessels not commonly sampled by renal biopsy. Remarkable responses, including

a high rate of total cures, have been seen with aggressive cytotoxic therapy using cyclophosphamide.

DISEASES OF THE URINARY CONDUITS

There are three disease processes that primarily affect the urinary drainage system: obstruction, infection, and urinary tract stone formation. These processes are closely interactive and often share a cause-effect relationship.

Urinary Tract Obstruction

Obstruction to urine flow may occur at any point from the renal pelvis to the urethral meatus. The causes of obstruction are manifold but may be classified into a few general groups, as given in Table 34–6. The age and sex of the patient obviously influence the likelihood of a given pairing of etiology and site.

The obstruction may occur suddenly, as with a lodged calculus, and be associated with flank and radiating groin pain; or occur slowly, as with compression by cervical carcinoma, and be associated with no symptoms until uremia from renal failure appears. So long as urine formation proceeds, the urinary tract proximal to the obstruction dilates (hydronephrosis). However, long-standing obstruction causes tubular and interstital atrophy and eventual glomerular sclerosis, and urine formation ceases. Urinary tract dilation may no longer be evident at that time.

A change in urinary habits is often the presenting sign of urinary tract obstruction. Complete urinary tract obstruction is the most common cause of true anuria. However, polyuria, especially nocturia, is not uncommon in partial obstruction and may occur as a consequence of defective urinary concentration. Overflow incontinence is a common occurrence in lower tract obstruction.

Unilateral ureteral obstruction usually causes no detectable change in urinary flow nor in total

---

TABLE 34–6. CAUSES OF URINARY TRACT OBSTRUCTION

Congenital Urinary Tract Malformation
  Meatal stenosis
  Ureterocele
  Posterior urethral valves
Intraluminal Obstruction
  Calculi
  Blood clots
  Sloughed papillary tissue
Extrinsic Compression
  Pelvic tumors
  Prostatic hypertrophy
  Retroperitoneal fibrosis
Acquired Anomalies
  Urethral strictures
  Neurogenic bladder
  Intratubular precipitates

renal function, and the asymptomatic loss of one kidney in this manner is not unusual. Azotemia or renal failure occurs only if the drainage of both kidneys is significantly compromised. Urinary tract infection is common in urinary tract obstruction. While red and/or white blood cells are frequently found in the urinalysis of patients with urinary tract obstruction, the combination of a completely normal urinalysis and acute azotemia correlates highly with the presence of urinary tract obstruction.

The diagnosis of urinary tract obstruction rests on a renal imaging study. Renal sonography is the preferred means of diagnosing urinary tract obstruction and depends on identification of hydronephrosis. Since dilation of the urinary tract may not be evident within the first 24 hours of obstruction, IVP can provide valuable diagnostic information. A prolonged nephrogram phase with delayed filling and visualization of collecting structures is seen on IVP. A 24-hour or 48-hour film may show contrast media concentrated either in dilated calyces or in the renal pelvis. Retrograde examination of the ureters is rarely required to make the diagnosis but may be necessary to define the anatomy of the obstruction before surgical intervention.

Long-term partial obstruction is associated with functional defects in urinary acidification and urinary concentration. Total obstruction eventually leads to tubular atrophy and glomerular sclerosis, grossly dilated and distorted calyces, and profound cortical thinning. Recovery of renal function after relief of obstruction is adversely affected by the presence of superimposed urinary tract infection or by a lengthy duration of obstruction. Total urinary tract obstruction is a significant cause of end-stage renal failure.

Management of urinary tract obstruction is directed toward identification of the site and cause of obstruction, and removal of the obstruction, usually through surgical intervention. Elimination of obstruction is at times associated with a postobstructive diuresis. This is partially due to a solute diuresis from salt and urea retained during obstruction and partially due to the renal concentrating defect. In some cases, definitive relief of obstruction is not possible and urinary diversion may be required. This may be as simple as an indwelling urethral catheter or more complex, such as an ileal conduit. In all cases, control of urinary tract infection is of paramount concern. Urinary tract infection in an obstructed kidney constitutes a urological emergency and requires prompt relief of the obstruction. A number of conditions cause renal failure by mechanisms that include intrarenal tubular obstruction. These conditions include multiple myeloma, rhabdomyolysis, and acute uric acid nephropathy.

Acute uric acid nephropathy is a unique form of obstruction in which uric acid crystals precipitate within the collecting ducts and renal pelvis. The phenomenon of hyperuricemia plus hyperkalemia and hyperphosphatemia occurs as part of a tumor lysis syndrome. In this syndrome, massive cell death follows chemotherapy for exquisitely sensitive tumors, often lymphomas. The poorly soluble uric acid "sludge" may be flushed from the kidney and renal pelvis by a forced alkaline diuresis if renal function is not severely compromised. Dialysis is indicated to reduce the uric acid load and/or life-threatening levels of hyperkalemia.

Urinary Tract Infection

Bacterial infection of the lower urinary tract is one of the more common infectious processes (see Chapter 32). However, considering the frequency of lower tract infection, renal parenchymal infection (pyelonephritis) is not common.

Infection of the renal parenchyma, *pyelonephritis*, is caused by bacteria ascending the ureters from the bladder. Parenchymal infections originating from the blood are almost always abscesses and are frequently seen in intravenous drug abusers. The syndrome of acute pyelonephritis almost always includes symptoms of lower tract infection plus bacteriuria. The diagnosis of chronic pyelonephritis has been used to describe the histological finding of renal interstitial inflammation and scarring in persons with histories of recurrent or chronic urinary tract infection. However, there is no clear evidence that long-standing renal parenchymal infection occurs or that significant renal damage follows such infection except in certain susceptible hosts. These include persons with diabetes mellitus, chronic renal insufficiency, and chronic urinary tract obstruction. The more common pathological finding of interstitial inflammation and scarring is usually due to a sterile, toxic renal injury (as in analgesic nephropathy).

Simple urinary tract infection usually presents as dysuria, urinary urgency, and frequency. Fever may be present but is frequently absent. Flank pain or tenderness at the costovertebral angle may be present in uncomplicated infection of the lower urinary tract; these are nonspecific findings. High fever, often with nausea and vomiting, in addition to the above findings more often indicates true pyelonephritis. In either case, the urinalysis consistently reveals pyuria, but microscopic hematuria or minimal proteinuria may also be present. The standard test for diagnosis of urinary tract infection is growth of greater than 10^5 colonies/ml of a recognized pathogen from a clean-catch, midstream urine specimen. Urinary tract infection in the male demands an examination of the urinary tract, preferably by IVP, for structural abnormalities.

For the vast majority of uncomplicated urinary tract infections, especially in females, treatment may be started immediately after a urine specimen for culture is obtained. Any of a number of antibiotics with activity against coliform bacteria is acceptable: ampicillin, a tetracycline, or a sulfa compound. However, urinary tract infections acquired in the hospital, infections associated with obstruction or stones, and cases of acute pyelonephritis often require addition of an antibiotic effective against noncoliform, gram-negative rods; aminoglycoside antibiotics are the most frequent choice.

Prompt treatment of urinary tract infection is critical in several circumstances. Pregnancy is associated with a 10 per cent incidence of urinary tract infection. Untreated, about half of these otherwise simple infections will progress to acute pyelonephritis in the pregnant female. Surveillance for and prompt treatment of bacteriuria is thus an important part of prenatal care. While diabetics have no clear increase in frequency of urinary tract infections, they do have more complications, including pyelonephritis and sepsis, arising from simple infections of the urinary tract. Patients with known urinary tract obstruction, polycystic kidney disease, or renal calculi should be monitored closely and receive prompt, vigorous treatment for urinary tract infection.

Urolithiasis

Renal stone formation and its significant morbidity are common, affecting up to 5 per cent of the general population at least once during a lifetime. Calcium, usually as calcium oxalate or calcium phosphate, is the most common constituent of renal calculi. Calcium is present in some form in almost 90 per cent of all renal stones. Uric acid, cystine, and magnesium are the other major stone constituents. Up to 75 per cent of all stones, composed predominantly of calcium oxalate, occur in the syndrome of idiopathic urolithiasis. About 5 per cent of calcium stone formation is attributable to hyperparathyroidism. Some degree of uric acid lithiasis is contributory to about 20 per cent of all renal calculi.

Urinary stone formation depends on a number of factors. The saturation of urine with a mineral is governed by the amount excreted and the volume of urine in which it is contained. Urine is frequently supersaturated with respect to calcium. Crystallization from solution requires a nidus, or "seed," upon which to grow, and crystal precipitation may be inhibited by certain compounds. Each of these elements is thought to be of importance in formation of renal calculi, but other mechanisms contribute to the process of urolithiasis.

Idiopathic urolithiasis, in which no underlying metabolic or infectious etiology is evident, accounts for the majority of cases of renal stone formation. Hypercalciuria, defined as the excretion of greater than 4 mg calcium/kg/24 hours, is seen in the absence of hypercalcemia in about 80 per cent of these cases. At least two subtypes of hypercalciuria appear to exist: in "renal" hypercalciuria, a deficiency in renal calcium reabsorption appears to drive increased intestinal calcium absorption, whereas in "absorptive" hypercalciuria, there is a primary increase in intestinal calcium absorption necessitating an increase in urinary calcium excretion. In both circumstances, serum calcium and phosphate levels are normal. Stone formation in idiopathic hypercalciuria is believed to depend heavily on the constant supersaturation of urine with calcium.

The cause of stone formation in patients with normal levels of urinary calcium excretion is less certain. However, hyperuricosuria has been observed in a large number of patients with idiopathic urolithiasis and may coexist with hypercalciuria in up to 20 per cent of patients. The finding of uric acid in calculi composed predominantly of calcium salts has led to the notion that uric acid crystals may serve as a nidus for calcium stone growth.

Secondary hypercalciuria, in which the serum calcium concentration may be found to be elevated, occurs in only 5 to 7 per cent of recurrent stone formers. Hyperparathyroidism, distal RTA, sarcoidosis, and hypervitaminosis D account for a large number of these cases.

Chronic urinary tract infection with urea-splitting organisms (i.e., *Proteus* species) is associated with struvite (triple phosphate) stones containing magnesium and calcium. These frequently form as "staghorn" calculi, outlining the renal calyces. A vicious dependency develops in which urinary tract infection cannot be cleared owing to the presence of the foreign body (calculus) and stone formation continues as long as the urine is infected.

Passage of a renal stone is often the initial manifestation of renal stone disease and presents as ureteral colic, sharp unilateral flank pain that radiates to the groin. Hematuria is characteristically present in the urinalysis and crystalluria may be obvious. A plain abdominal radiograph will demonstrate the densely opaque calcium stones and the faintly opaque, sulfur-containing cystine stones. Only pure uric acid stones are radiolucent. An excretory urogram (IVP) may be required to demonstrate small stones or the site along the urinary tract at which a stone has lodged.

The work-up for renal calculus is indicated in Table 34–7. Serial plain abdominal radiographs identify changes in stone size and number, serum calcium determinations identify hypercalcemic disorders associated with stone formation, and urine cultures identify etiological (urea-splitting) and complicating bacterial involvement. Hypercalciuria and hyperuricosuria are identified by appropriate 24-hour urine collections. Any stone

TABLE 34–7. PATIENT EVALUATION IN UROLITHIASIS

INITIAL	SECONDARY
Blood: Serum calcium	Serum PTH
Serum uric acid	Serum 1,25(OH)$_2$
Serum phosphate	vitamin D$_3$
Alkaline phosphatase	
Urine: Urinalysis for crystalluria	24-hour urine calcium
Urinalysis for pyuria	24-hour urine uric acid
	Urine culture
Radiography: Plain film (KUB)	Serial KUB's
IVP	

passed in the urine should be subjected to analysis to determine its mineral composition.

Treatment of urolithiasis may be as simple as the promotion of a *brisk* diuresis to enhance spontaneous passage of a stone. Surgical removal of stones may be required, especially when the urine is chronically infected or when renal compromise secondary to obstruction is evident. The major effort of medical management is directed toward reducing the likelihood of stone growth and recurrent formation.

In all cases, prevention of urolithiasis includes forced hydration with water to produce a dilute urine. This suffices to prevent recurrence in some individuals, especially in hot climates. If hypercalcemia is present, parathyroidectomy for hyperparathyroidism or specific therapy for the elevation in serum calcium is indicated. In cases of idiopathic hypercalciuria, dramatic reductions in urinary calcium excretion and stone formation can be achieved with thiazide diuretics and salt-restricted diet. Thiazide therapy should reduce the 24-hour urinary calcium excretion by almost half. If hyperuricosuria coexists, the addition of allopurinol to reduce the uric acid load is advantageous. In fact, allopurinol may reduce calcium stone formation even in the absence of clear hyperuricosuria. Successful treatment of struvite stones may require specific, long-term antibiotic therapy in combination with surgical lithotomy.

MULTISYSTEM DISEASE WITH RENAL INVOLVEMENT

There are a number of systemic conditions and diseases that are associated with a significant incidence of renal dysfunction. In some cases, the appearance of renal disease carries dire consequences for the outcome of the primary disorder. Each of the diseases or processes discussed in this section usually affects more than one element of the kidney.

Diabetes Mellitus (DM)

The metabolic and physiological consequences of diabetes mellitus regularly involve the kidney and lead to renal dysfunction. Although diabetes almost inevitably affects all elements of the kidney simultaneously, any given patient may present with features typically associated with one of the clinical patterns discussed above. Therefore, renal disease in some patients will present as an interstitial process, typically with hypertension and Type IV RTA. Others will have glomerular proteinuria as the initial clinical manifestation of the diabetic renal lesion. In either group, urinary tract infections and pyelonephritis frequently complicate the course of the diabetes.

Diabetic glomerulosclerosis is one of the more significant of the diabetic renal lesions and is the most frequent cause of end-stage renal failure in these patients. Glomerular disease occurs in about half of persons with juvenile-onset, insulin-dependent (Type I) diabetes mellitus. The onset of clinically apparent glomerular involvement occurs, in most patients, between 15 and 20 years after the initial diagnosis of DM. Renal disease in DM is first seen as asymptomatic, episodic proteinuria, but progression to fixed, moderate to heavy proteinuria occurs rapidly, within one to two years. Glomerulopathy develops uncommonly in Type I diabetics who are free of proteinuria 20 years after diagnosis of DM.

Once proteinuria becomes established, a rapid fall in GFR follows, with the course to end-stage renal failure being complete within five years. Although the incidence of the nephrotic syndrome is low in DM, the prevalence of Type I DM in the population makes diabetic glomerulopathy a significant cause of adult nephrotic syndrome. The appearance of hypertension usually parallels that of proteinuria. Diabetic retinopathy is an invariant finding in patients with diabetic glomerulopathy and has led to the designation of the retinorenal syndrome for persons so affected. The onset of the nephrotic syndrome in an individual having Type I DM for less than 10 years, or in the absence of diabetic retinopathy, should alert one to consider a nondiabetic etiology of the renal disease.

The classic glomerular lesion in DM is Kimmelstiel-Wilson nodular glomerulosclerosis. This appears as hyalin nodules lying in the center of peripheral capillary loops, causing the capillaries to lie in a ring surrounding the nodule. This pattern is actually seen in less than 25 per cent of cases of diabetic glomerulopathy. The more typical finding, seen most often when heavy proteinuria is present, is that of diffuse glomerulosclerosis associated with arteriosclerosis of *both* afferent and efferent arterioles. Basement membrane thickening and interstitial atrophy may be prominent. Immunofluorescent staining may show linear IgG and/or C_3 deposition along capillaries, but this is thought to represent nonspecific trapping. Electron microscopy reveals diffuse increases in mesangial matrix material and generalized thickening of basement membranes by BM-like material.

A metabolic etiology is believed to be responsible for diabetic glomerulopathy. The renal lesion of diabetes may be related to a generalized alteration of basement membranes caused by addition of disaccharide units to the collagen matrix. In glomerular capillaries this may lead to the hyperfiltration seen in early Type I DM, when the GFR may be 20 to 30 per cent above normal. This structurally abnormal basement membrane, together with altered glomerular capillary hemodynamics, may lead to nonimmune glomerular injury and sclerosis. This superimposed physical injury is like that which follows some cases of immune-mediated glomerular injury.

End-stage renal failure is usually seen in diabetic glomerulopathy within two to three years of the first appearance of azotemia. Control of hypertension may slow the rate of deterioration of renal function. While strict control of hyperglycemia does not affect the course of established renal insufficiency, evidence is now accumulating that such control might prevent early metabolic changes in basement membranes in newly diagnosed diabetics.

Renal insufficiency is the major limit to survival in diabetics under 40 years of age. Treatment of end-stage renal disease in diabetics is more difficult than in nondiabetic patients, and the survival of diabetics on hemodialysis is less than that for nondiabetics. Continuous ambulatory peritoneal dialysis (CAPD) offers a better prognosis for many diabetics with renal failure. Death from cardiovascular complications is highly likely for the diabetic on dialysis. The most promising treatment for diabetic renal failure appears to be renal transplantation from a living, related donor. The diabetic lesion does recur in transplanted kidneys but has not been a significant cause of transplant kidney failure.

A significant number of diabetics display a prominent and characteristic interstitial lesion that appears related to ischemic injury. The syndrome of hyporeninemic hypoaldosteronism is a feature of this lesion and is a major cause of Type IV renal tubular acidosis. These patients will typically present with hyperkalemia and hyperchloremic metabolic acidosis with only a modest reduction in GFR. Hypertension is prominent in this syndrome. The clinical features of the interstitial lesion almost inevitably merge into the glomerular syndrome of diabetic glomerulosclerosis as the patient approaches end-stage renal failure.

Two other renal conditions frequently complicate the course of diabetic nephropathy. Papillary necrosis, especially in conjunction with renal infection, is common in diabetics. The sloughing of papillary tissue may cause acute ureteral obstruction with colic, may be associated with hematuria and passage of tissue in the urine, and may be identified by the calyceal irregularity seen on IVP. Although bacteriuria is no more prevalent in diabetics than nondiabetics, the syndrome of acute pyelonephritis, especially in the presence of urinary obstruction with papillary tissue, is a more frequent outcome of untreated bacteriuria in the diabetic.

Multiple Myeloma

This plasma cell dyscrasia, which often presents with bone pain and/or paraproteinuria, is associated with renal dysfunction at some time in about half of all patients (Table 34–8). The etiologies of renal insufficiency in multiple myeloma include a specific renal lesion known as "myeloma kidney," hypercalcemia, and an increased susceptibility to nephrotoxins.

"Myeloma kidney" refers to a unique renal lesion that is associated with Bence-Jones proteinuria, the excretion of kappa and lambda light chains of immunoglobulins. The histopathology is that of tubular occlusion by broad, waxy casts composed of the paraproteins. A prominent tubular reaction with giant cells and atrophy is accompanied by widespread round cell infiltration in the interstitium. Amyloid deposits may be seen

TABLE 34–8. RENAL DISEASE IN MULTIPLE MYELOMA

Functional Disorders
  Paraproteinuria—filtered Bence-Jones protein
  Fanconi syndrome—secondary to amyloidosis
  Vasopressin-resistant polyuria—secondary to amyloidosis or hypercalcemia
Acute Renal Failure
  Prerenal azotemia—secondary to polyuria plus anorexia/vomiting of hypercalcemia
  Vasomotor nephropathy—secondary to severe hypercalcemia
  Nephrotoxic acute tubular necrosis—secondary to increased susceptibility to nephrotoxins, intratubular protein precipitation
Chronic Renal Failure
  Myeloma kidney—Intratubular obstruction and interstitial scarring
  Amyloidosis

in glomeruli and tubules. Renal insufficiency is common with this lesion.

Hypercalcemia is seen in at least one third of myeloma patients and often causes a vasopressin-resistant hyposthenuria with polyuria. Volume depletion from the polyuria may cause reversible renal insufficiency. Levels of serum calcium greater than 12 to 13 mg/dl are commonly observed.

A common phenomenon in multiple myeloma is the increased occurrence of acute renal failure after exposure to agents such as radiocontrast media or aminoglycoside antibiotics. Patients with multiple myeloma should be kept well-hydrated, with intravenous saline if necessary, whenever exposed to a nephrotoxic agent.

Amyloidosis

Amyloidosis is a systemic disease that is classified as either primary (idiopathic) or secondary—that is, accompanying a chronic inflammatory (tuberculosis, leprosy, osteomyelitis), neoplastic (multiple myeloma), or hereditary (familial Mediterranean fever) process. Renal involvement is highly prevalent and follows the same course in either form of amyloidosis. Glomerular, tubular, and vascular deposits of amyloid occur throughout the kidneys.

The majority of patients are over 50 years of age at the time of diagnosis. The most common renal presentation is that of asymptomatic proteinuria, often with paraproteinuria (e.g., Bence-Jones proteinuria). However, about one third of patients have the full nephrotic syndrome. Fanconi's syndrome (see above), an indicator of concomitant tubular dysfunction, is not uncommon. Signs of amyloid deposits in other organs, such as macroglossia, cardiomyopathy, hepatosplenomegaly, malabsorption, or peripheral neuropathy, may aid in diagnosing the etiology of the glomerulopathy. A positive rectal biopsy for amyloidosis correlated highly with renal involvement. Enlarged kidneys may be found on intravenous urography (IVP) or renal ultrasonography.

Routine light microscopy may show only bland eosinophilic deposits in the mesangium or in capillary loops. Special staining by Congo red reveals pink deposits in mesangium, capillary loops, and blood vessel walls; the deposits show green birefringence under polarized light. Immunofluorescent staining is not helpful. On electron microscopy, the diagnosis can be established by identification of characteristic, noncollagen fibrils of 8 to 10 nm deposited randomly or in bundles within the mesangium or capillary basement membranes.

A course leading to terminal renal failure is seen in most patients. Asymptomatic proteinuria may persist for some years, but the occurrence of the nephrotic syndrome usually heralds a rapid progression of renal failure. Steroids have no effect on the disease, nor do alkylating agents seem to alter the course. Colchicine therapy appears promising in patients with familial Mediterranean fever.

Sickle Cell Anemia (SS)

Renal damage occurs in almost all patients homozygous for this hereditary disease, but SS is a most unusual cause of renal failure. The primary injury occurs in the renal medulla, where frequent vascular occlusion from erythrocyte sickling in the hypertonic medullary environment causes obliteration of vasa recta. Hematuria and a reduction in urinary concentrating ability are prominent manifestations of this phenomenon.

Hematuria, usually in the microscopic range, occurs in most SS patients, but dramatic and prolonged bouts of gross hematuria may be seen. Hematuric patients with sickle hemoglobin are most often heterozygotes. This is due simply to the greater number of patients with SS trait. Bleeding originates in the left kidney in most cases. Bed rest, forced hydration, and transfusions are the standard treatment for gross hematuria; nephrectomy is rarely indicated.

A decreased concentrating ability is a very common defect in SS but is not usually of a magnitude sufficient to cause clinically apparent polyuria. Since these patients dilute urine normally, the defect is likely caused by a failure to maintain medullary hypertonicity due to an alteration in medullary blood flow. The pathology of SS is that of vasa recta obliteration with medullary interstitial edema and fibrosis. There is a pronounced tendency for papillary necrosis to occur.

Hepatic Diseases

Renal dysfunction associated with liver disease ranges from glomerulopathies, as seen with hepatitis B, to azotemic syndromes, as seen with cirrhosis of the liver. The latter conditions usually occur in decompensated cirrhosis associated with an elevated serum bilirubin and ascites. The azotemia is most often due to a reduction in the effective circulating volume and in renal blood flow. This situation occurs in the face of a reduction in serum albumin and oncotic pressure with third-spacing of extracellular fluids in ascites.

The *hepatorenal syndrome* is, almost by definition, a terminal event identified by oliguria, a declining GFR, and tremendous renal sodium av-

idity. The urinary sodium concentration is almost always less than 10 mEq/L, and there is a disproportionately high BUN/creatinine ratio in most cases. The decline in renal function usually follows one of three events in a cirrhotic patient with ascites: sepsis, a vigorous attempt to reduce ascites with diuretics, or a large-volume paracentesis. The kidneys are normal as judged from their recovery of function if transplanted into a noncirrhotic host. It is not known if the functional renal defect is induced by a hepatic toxin.

Ascites and edema in cirrhotic patients represent cosmetic rather than medical problems in most cases. When it is necessary to reduce ascites or edema in these patients, sodium restriction and the sparing use of diuretics are indicated in order to reduce the risk of a decline in renal function. Acute expansion of intravascular volume may reverse azotemia in some cirrhotic patients. Dialysis is generally not indicated unless there is a reasonable expectation of improved hepatic function.

Disorders of Pregnancy

Three important relations exist between renal disease and the pregnant state: the effect of existing renal disease on the outcome of the pregnancy; the effect of the normal hemodynamic, endocrinological, and immunological changes of pregnancy on pre-existing renal disease; and the occurrence of distinct renal syndromes in association with pregnancy.

Since uremia causes a disruption in normal hormonal cycles, fertility in women is greatly diminished when the BUN is greater than 40 to 50 mg/dl. However, those patients with mild renal insufficiency (BUN <25 mg/dl) have about a 75 per cent chance of completing a normal, full-term pregnancy. Fetal loss is significant at higher levels of azotemia and when hypertension is a prominent part of the renal disease. The nephrotic syndrome, without azotemia, does not usually affect the outcome of pregnancy, but the birth weight of the infant is decreased in the face of significant maternal hypoalbuminemia.

In most cases, pregnancy does not appear to adversely affect the course of pre-existing renal disease. Of particular note is the case of lupus nephritis (see below), in which the renal activity of the disease is generally decreased during pregnancy. However, some patients with more severe glomerular disease experience an exacerbation of nephritis in the first trimester of pregnancy and a significant number of patients have an increase in nephritic signs with a decrease in GFR after delivery. Increased doses of steroids may prevent this occurrence. Finally, patients with scleroderma will often experience a significant decline in GFR and an increase in blood pressure during pregnancy.

Hypertension in pregnancy requires careful consideration. Blood pressure usually falls in the first weeks of a normal pregnancy and returns to pregestational values only near term. Normal pregnancy is characterized by ECF volume expansion, an increased cardiac output, a decreased systemic vascular resistance, and resistance to the vasopressor effects of angiotensin II. Therefore, any absolute elevation of blood pressure or a pattern of rising blood pressure in early pregnancy is abnormal. At least three categories of pregnancy-related hypertension exist.

Toxemia is a syndrome of hypertension, proteinuria, hyperuricemia, and edema that is seen in the third trimester of pregnancy. It occurs predominantly in young primagravidas or in women over the age of 40. The signs may be deceptive, since mild edema is common in normal pregnancies, and the elevated blood pressure and serum uric acid concentrations must be interpreted in light of the values for a normal pregnancy. A blood pressure of 130/80 may be abnormal at 30 weeks gestation. Likewise, the serum uric acid concentration is often reduced to less than 3 mg/dl in a normal pregnancy, so that a value of 5 to 6 mg/dl is distinctly abnormal.

The renal lesion in toxemia is known as endotheliosis and is totally reversible. The histopathology consists of endothelial cell swelling in an ischemic glomerulus with fibrin deposited between the endothelial cell and the basement membrane. Treatment of toxemia consists of vigorous control of blood pressure and delivery of the fetus as soon as it is judged to be viable. Modest azotemia may be seen, but renal failure is rare. Complete normalization of blood pressure and cessation of proteinuria occur following delivery. There is no increased risk of developing sustained hypertension after the single occurrence of toxemia in a young woman.

Essential hypertension may be present before pregnancy and may have little effect on the outcome of the pregnancy. Hypertensive patients are more prone to develop toxemia. Only when diastolic blood pressures remain above 100 mm Hg is there significant fetal loss.

A final group of patients consists of those in whom hypertension develops in late (third trimester) pregnancy in successive gestations. These patients seem to have an increased likelihood of developing sustained hypertension later in life.

Besides toxemia, two other distinct renal syndromes may be seen in association with pregnancy. *Bilateral renal cortical necrosis* is a rare syndrome that almost always follows a dire obstetric complication; abruptio placentae, retained fetal fragments, or septic abortion. The presentation is usually that of a scant output of bloody urine, followed by sudden, virtually complete anuria. Renal failure is always present, and evidence of disseminated intravascular coagulation is common. The renal histopathology is that of frank necrosis throughout the cortex. The degree of necrosis ranges from patchy areas to confluent cortical necrosis. Oligoanuria is prolonged in all cases, but a few patients recover sufficient renal function to stop dialysis after weeks to months of treatment.

Postpartum renal failure, or the adult hemolytic-uremic syndrome, is a rare disorder that has its onset from two to three days up to eight to nine weeks postpartum. The preceding pregnancy and delivery are usually normal. A microangiopathic hemolytic anemia with prominent fragmentation of red blood cells is evident. The kidneys show marked deposition of fibrin in arterioles and glomeruli and intimal proliferation in blood vessels. The vascular proliferative lesion is the same as that seen in accelerated hypertension, although patients with postpartum renal failure are typically normotensive. About 75 per cent of patients have permanent renal failure and require dialysis or transplantation.

Systemic Lupus Erythematosus (SLE)

This disease chiefly affects young females and is diagnosed by serological evidence of autoantibodies to cell nuclear components (ANA's) and by clinical evidence of inflammatory processes in multiple organs (skin, joints, brain, and kidneys). Five major categories of glomerular histopathology have been described for SLE nephritis (Table 34–9). Virtually all cases of lupus nephritis display a degree of interstitial inflammation uncommon for other glomerulopathies. One subset of patients with SLE renal disease has a dominant interstitial lesion with little or no glomerular involvement.

In general, the clinical presentation and severity of renal disease in SLE correlate to the underlying histological lesion. About two thirds of patients will have some clinical evidence of renal disease (proteinuria, microhematuria, or azotemia) at the time SLE is diagnosed. Virtually all patients will have some evidence of SLE renal disease if studied with renal biopsy.

Renal disease in SLE may present clinically as

TABLE 34–9. RENAL HISTOPATHOLOGY IN SYSTEMIC LUPUS ERYTHEMATOSUS*

CLASS	RENAL SURVIVAL
Type I—Normal Kidneys	~100%
No histological changes	
Type II—Mesangial Glomerulonephritis	~85%
Increased cellularity and immune deposit confined to mesangium	
Type III—Focal Proliferative Glomerulonephritis	~70%
Mesangial changes plus segmental cellular proliferation and necrosis in <50% of glomeruli	
Type IV—Diffuse Proliferative Glomerulonephritis	25–40%
Changes of Type III involving nearly all glomeruli	
Type V—Membranous Glomerulonephritis	~85%
Diffuse, uniform basement membrane thickening due to small subepithelial deposits; normal cellularity	
Type VI—Interstitial Lupus Nephritis	?
Marked interstitial inflammation with minimal or no glomerular changes	

*World Health Organization classification of renal histopathology of SLE. Three additional types may be defined as combinations of these basic categories.

either nephrosis or nephritis. The former presentation is more common, with the nephrotic syndrome occuring in over half of all patients. Even in these patients, however, considerable overlap of clinical manifestations occurs, and hematuria, hypertension, and azotemia are frequent findings. A smaller number of patients present with a full-blown nephritic picture with a clinical course resembling that of RPGN. Renal function may deteriorate rapidly over a period of only a few weeks. Serum complement activity, both CH_{50} and C_3, are reduced with active renal disease. The serum C_4 may be strikingly depressed, indicating activation of the classic complement pathway.

As shown in Table 34–9, the glomerular histopathology in SLE is similar to that seen in non-SLE diseases for any given lesion. For instance, Type IV, diffuse proliferative lupus glomerulonephritis, has similarities to postinfectious AGN. Likewise, Type V, membranous lupus glomerulopathy, is indistinguishable from idiopathic membranous nephropathy. It is believed that the pattern of glomerular injury relates to the presence or absence of circulating immune complexes; the ability of free antigens to fix to, or lodge in, glomerular structures; and the intensity and pattern of the immune response.

The clinical course and prognosis of lupus nephritis correspond to the glomerular lesion. As seen from Table 34–9, the five-year renal survival in untreated patients ranges from more than 80 per cent in patients with Type V, membranous lesion to about 25 per cent in patients with the Type IV, diffuse proliferative lesion. Progression of the renal lesion, for example, from Type III, focal proliferative, to Type IV, diffuse proliferative, has been documented. Regression of lesions to a less ominous pathological picture is also known to occur, especially after vigorous therapy. The indications for renal biopsy either to determine the renal prognosis or to define the need for treatment with steroids or immunosuppressive drugs remain unclear.

Corticosteroid therapy is the mainstay of treatment for lupus nephritis. In the absence of advanced renal failure (serum creatinine >6 mg/dl) and extensive glomerular sclerosis, high-dose steroid therapy (prednisone, 40 to 60 mg/day for 6 to 12 months) has had a dramatic effect on survival. The renal survival in diffuse proliferative SLE glomerulopathy with such treatment is up to 80 per cent in five years versus the 25 per cent survival without steroids. There is some evidence to support treatment of Types II and III lupus nephritis with low doses (<40 mg prednisone/day) of steroids in an attempt to normalize serum CH_{50} activity and to prevent progression to Type IV, diffuse proliferative, nephritis. The addition of a cytotoxic drug, such as azathioprine, may allow use of lower doses of prednisone, avoiding complications of high-dose steroid therapy but adding those of a cytotoxic agent. The membranous lesion has been successfully treated with steroids to reduce proteinuria, but an effective treatment to halt the slow progression to renal failure has not been demonstrated.

REFERENCES

Andriole VT: Current concepts of urinary tract infections. In Weinstein L, and Fields BN (eds): Seminars in Infectious Disease. Vol 3. New York, Thieme-Stratton, Inc, 1980, pp 89–130.

Appel GB, Silva FG, Pirani CL, Meltzer JI, and Estes D: Renal involvement in systemic lupus erythematosus. Medicine 57:371–410.

Arnaout MD, Rennke HG, and Cotran RS: Membranous glomerulonephritis. In Brenner BM, and Stein JH (eds): Contemporary Issues in Nephrology. Vol 9. New York, Churchill Livingstone, 1982, pp 199–235.

Beirne GJ, Wagnild JP, Zimmerman SW, Macken PD, and Burholder PM: Idiopathic crescentic glomerulonephritis. Medicine 56:349–381.

Cameron JS, Turner DR, Heaton J, Williams DG, Ogg CS, Chantler C, Hycock GB, and Hicks J: Idiopathic mesangiocapillary glomerulonephritis. Am J Med 74:175–192, 1983.

Coe FL: Prevention of kidney stones. Am J Med 71:514–516, 1981.

Culpepper RM, and Andreoli TE: Pathophysiology of the glomerulonephropathies. Adv Int Med 28:161–206, 1983.

Dzau VJ, Gibbons GH, and Levin DC: Renovascular hypertension: An update on pathophysiology, diagnosis, and treatment. Am J Nephrol 3:172–184, 1983.

Friedman EA: Diabetic nephropathy: Strategies in prevention and management. Kidney Int 21:780–791, 1982.

Hoyer JR: Idiopathic nephrotic syndrome with minimal glomerular changes. In Brenner BM, and Stein JH (eds): Contemporary Issues in Nephrology. Vol 9. New York, Churchill Livingstone, 1982, pp 145–174.

Kanwar YS: Biophysiology of glomerular filtration and proteinuria. Lab Invest 51:7–21, 1984.

McSherry E: Renal tubular acidosis in childhood. Kidney Int 20:799–809, 1981.

Murray TG: Analgesic use and kidney disease. Arch Intern Med 141:423–424, 1981.

Richie JP, and Skinner DG: Renal neoplasia. In Brenner BM, and Rector FC Jr (eds): The Kidney. 2nd ed. Philadelphia, WB Saunders Co, 1981, pp 2109–2134.

Rodriguez-Iturbe B: Epidemic post-streptococcal glomerulonephritis. Kidney Int 25:129–136, 1984.

Suki WN: Polycystic kidney disease. Kidney Int 22:571–580, 1982.

Tisher CC, and Alexander RW: Focal glomerular sclerosis. In Brenner BM, and Stein JH (eds): Contemporary Issues in Nephrology. Vol 9. New York, Churchill Livingstone, 1982, pp 175–197.

Wright FS, and Howards SS: Obstructive injury. In Brenner BM, and Rector FC Jr (eds): The Kidney. 2nd ed. Philadelphia, WB Saunders Co, 1981, pp 2008–2244.

RENAL PHARMACOLOGY

Renal insufficiency is associated with significant alterations in the metabolism of drugs. In addition, drug-associated renal dysfunction is one of the most common reasons for requesting a nephrological consultation in an acute care hospital. Finally, the principles of extracorporeal removal of metabolic waste products have been applied to the removal of drugs from the body in cases of drug overdose.

RENAL METABOLISM OF DRUGS

A large number of drugs are eliminated from the body by renal excretion. Excretion of drugs by the kidney may involve filtration, secretion, and reabsorption depending upon the agent in question. Filtration of a drug through the glomerulus depends on the chemical characteristics of the drug itself and the degree of binding of the drug to plasma proteins. Drugs that are highly bound to plasma proteins are poorly filtered, while those that are bound less avidly or not at all can gain access to the tubular fluid. Drugs that are organic anions or cations can be secreted from the peritubular capillary blood into the lumen of the tubule by specific transport mechanisms in renal tubular cells. Some drugs that gain access to the tubular fluid by filtration and/or secretion may be reabsorbed back into the systemic circulation by mediated or passive transport mechanisms. For some drugs, bidirectional transport across renal tubules is known to occur, so that the net rate of excretion is dependent on the relative activities of the secretory and absorptive processes. For organic anions and cations whose pK is in the range of the pH normally attainable in the tubular fluid, any change in the pH of the urine may have a

TABLE 35–1. DRUGS WHOSE RENAL EXCRETION IS AFFECTED BY URINE pH

Augmented Excretion in Acidic Urine (Weak Bases)
  Amphetamines
  Chloroquine
  Diazepam
  Meperidine
  Morphine
  Quinidine
  Trimethoprim
Augmented Excretion in Alkaline Urine (Weak Acids)
  Acetazolamide
  Cephaloridine
  Diazoxide
  Furosemide/ethacrynic acid
  Hydrochlorothiazide
  Methotrexate
  Penicillin
  Phenobarbital
  Acetyl salicylic acid
  Sulfonamides

profound and clinically important effect on the rate of excretion of the drug. These principles are known as the effects of "nonionic diffusion" and indicate the differences in the permeabilities of drugs across renal membranes when the drug is in its ionized or un-ionized form (Table 35–1). Alkalinization of the urine significantly increases the excretion of organic anions such as aspirin and phenobarbital. Acidification of the urine increases the renal excretion of organic bases such as amphetamines.

In addition to modulating the rates of excretion of drugs, the kidney accumulates certain drugs. The kidney is also capable of metabolizing specific types of pharmaceutical agents. Owing to an effect on specific transport pathways, drug-drug interactions may occur. For example, probenecid, an inhibitor of organic anion secretion, inhibits the tubular secretion of penicillin. Such an interaction may have clinical utility when it is necessary to achieve high blood concentrations of this antibiotic.

PHARMACOKINETICS OF DRUGS IN RENAL INSUFFICIENCY

Metabolism of Drugs in Patients with Renal Insufficiency

With the development of renal insufficiency, there is a decrease in glomerular filtration as well as a loss of secretory and absorptive transport functions of the kidney. These changes in renal function may have a major effect on the kinetics of drugs that are excreted by the kidney. In addition, renal failure is characterized by the retention of endogenous organic compounds in the blood. Some of these compounds may compete with the pharmacological agents for specific renal transport systems.

Renal insufficiency may affect the metabolism of drugs not only by decreasing the rates of excretion in the urine, but also by a number of nonrenal mechanisms. Renal disease is associated with alterations in the binding of drugs by plasma proteins and, as a consequence, may affect the bioavailability of some drugs. An example of such a change in bioavailability is the pharmacokinetics of Dilantin (phenytoin) in renal failure patients. Presumably owing to occupancy by some products retained in uremia, Dilantin is less avidly bound by plasma proteins and the free concentration of the drug is increased. Renal insufficiency may be associated with a change in the volume of distribution of certain drugs. The absorption of drugs form the gastrointestinal tract may be impaired in patients with renal disease. The secondary consequences of renal failure may also alter the metabolic pathways of drugs in other organs.

Alterations in Drug Doses in Patients with Renal Failure

A considerable number of commonly used drugs require alterations in the amount or timing of administration in patients with renal failure. In patients who are undergoing dialysis, the clinical problem is further compounded. Owing to differences in the permeability of the membranes involved and the duration of the procedures, there are differences in the kinetics of drugs in patients undergoing hemodialysis as compared to those treated by peritoneal dialysis.

Drugs such as those listed on Table 35–2 require no alteration in dose in the patient with renal insufficiency. The metabolism of these drugs is predominantly by nonrenal routes and is not significantly altered by the presence of renal failure or the "uremic" environment. Table 35–3 lists drugs that should not be administered to patients with renal failure. Table 35–4 provides a partial listing of clinically important drugs whose metabolism is significantly altered in the patient with renal

TABLE 35–2. DRUGS REQUIRING LITTLE OR NO ALTERATION IN DOSE IN PATIENTS WITH RENAL FAILURE

ANTIBIOTICS	OTHERS
Cloxacillin	Codeine
Nafcillin	Morphine
Clindamycin	Propoxyphene
Erythromycin	Benzodiazepines
Rifampin	Lidocaine
Isoniazid	Quinidine
Chloramphenicol	Propranolol
Amphotericin B	Hydralazine
	Clonidine
	Prazosin
	Phenytoin
	Theophylline

TABLE 35–3. DRUGS THAT SHOULD BE AVOIDED IN PATIENTS WITH RENAL FAILURE

ANTIBIOTICS	OTHERS
Tetracycline	Aspirin
Nitrofurantoin	Oral hypoglycemics
Nalidixic acid	Lithium carbonate
	Acetazolamide
	Spironolactone
	Triamterene

TABLE 35–4. DRUGS REQUIRING SIGNIFICANT DOSE ADJUSTMENT IN PATIENTS WITH RENAL FAILURE

ANTIBIOTICS	OTHER
Aminoglycosides	Digoxin
Cephalosporins	Procainamide
Carbenicillin/ticarcillin	Cimetidine
Penicillin G	
Sulfonamides	
Vancomycin	

disease. For drugs that are eliminated from the body exclusively by renal excretion, the adjustment in dosing correlates with the degree of renal impairment. For drugs that are only partially excreted by the kidney, other formulas and nomograms are used.

In general, two methods are used to adjust drug regimens in patients with renal disease who are receiving drugs whose metabolism is altered. Either the amount of drug administered is reduced but the dosing interval is held constant or the amount of drug administered per dose is held constant but the dosing interval is lengthened. The choice between these two methods depends upon the characteristics of the drug in question and the clinical effect desired. For the drugs in common usage, drug-dosing nomograms for use in patients with renal failure have been published and these nomograms provide a useful tool in the ordering of drugs. It is important to note, however, that the changes in drug metabolism in the patient with renal failure are complex and that exclusive reliance on a nomogram alone is fraught with considerable danger. Careful clinical and laboratory assessment of the patient is required. If available, blood levels of the drug or drugs should be obtained. The above points can be illustrated by considering the administration of an aminoglycoside antibiotic to a patient with sepsis and renal dysfunction. Use of any of the published drug-dosing nomograms for a specific aminoglycoside antibiotic is associated with a significant number of patients who achieve blood levels of drug below that required to achieve a therapeutic effect. There is also a significant number of patients whose blood concentrations of drug are in the "toxic" range. This may be associated with the development of overt toxicity. In the case of the aminoglycosides, toxicity may be manifest by further deterioration in renal function. While therapeutic blood levels of drugs do not necessarily insure that drug-related toxicities will not occur, when used in conjunction with clinical assessment of the patient, the possibility of drug-related disease may be minimized.

DRUG-ASSOCIATED RENAL INJURY

Renal dysfunction associated with the administration of pharmaceutical agents is a common clinical problem. The classification of drug-related renal dysfunction is somewhat arbitrary, and several drugs are associated with more than one mechanism of injury. The classification shown in Table 35–5 indicates a primary separation into those drugs that are associated with an acute change in kidney function and a clinical picture of prerenal azotemia or the "acute renal failure" syndrome and those that lead to chronic renal disease and a clinical profile of end-stage renal disease. The acute category is further subdivided into drugs that affect kidney function as a secondary consequence and those that directly alter the anatomy or function of the kidney. This

TABLE 35–5. DRUG-INDUCED NEPHROTOXICITY

Acute Renal Dysfunction
Indirect Injury
 Prerenal azotemia
  nonsteroidal anti-inflammatory agents
  vasodilators
 Postrenal azotemia
  methysergide
  practolol
  sulfonamides
Direct Injury: Immunological Mechanism
 Hypersensitivity vasculitis
  penicillins
  sulfonamides
  allopurinol
 Glomerulonephritis
  gold
  penicillamine
  nonsteroidal anti-inflammatory agents
 Tubulointerstitial nephritis
  penicillins—particularly methicillin
  sulfonamides
  cephalosporins
  rifampin
  cimetidine
  phenytoin
  nonsteroidal anti-inflammatory agents
Direct Injury: Nonimmunological Mechanism
 Tubular damage
  Aminoglycosides
  cis-platinum
 Renal tubular acidosis
  amphotericin B
  lithium carbonate
  nonsteroidal anti-inflammatory agents
 Nephrogenic diabetes insipidus
  lithium carbonate
  demeclocycline
  methoxyflurane
Chronic Renal Disease
Chronic Interstitial Nephritis
 phenacetin-aspirin combination
 lithium carbonate
 nitrosoureas

latter category may properly be considered "toxic nephropathy." Although the toxic nephropathy variant of the acute renal failure syndrome is usually taken to imply drug-associated injury to the renal tubules, the term has been extended in recent years to include drugs that cause immunological injury to the kidney (glomerulonephritis and acute interstitial nephritis) and drugs that adversely affect renal function by virtue of their effects on renal blood flow regulation. The terminology and overlapping types of injury may be a source of confusion. Nonetheless, a number of drug-related injuries present a relatively fixed clinical picture. Examples of the more common forms of toxic nephropathies are discussed separately.

ACUTE DRUG-RELATED RENAL DYSFUNCTION

Indirect

Drugs that affect the systemic vascular resistance, the blood pressure, and/or the extracellular fluid volume may cause a decrease in renal blood flow and in the glomerular filtration rate. These hemodynamic changes can result in the development of prerenal azotemia. In individuals whose blood flow autoregulation is impaired and in those in whom the drug inhibits the autoregulatory response of the kidney, the acute renal failure syndrome may evolve. Nonsteroidal anti-inflammatory drugs, as well as vasodilator drugs, may cause this type of renal injury.

Although less common, a postrenal or obstructive pattern of renal injury is associated with a number of drugs. Retroperitioneal fibrosis and obstructive nephropathy have been reported following the administration of methysergide and the beta-blocker practolol. Intratubular precipitation of crystals may result in acute renal dysfunction. Sulfonamide crystalluria was an important cause of renal dysfunction when the sulfa drugs were initially introduced. This drug-related renal dysfunction is now rarely seen, as the newer sulfonamides are more soluble. Acute renal failure may develop from intratubular precipitation of uric acid in patients receiving chemotherapy for cancer. Renal dysfunction due to precipitation of oxalic acid crystals within the renal tubule has been observed in patients ingesting ethylene glycol and occasionally in patients exposed to the anesthetic agent methoxyflurane.

Direct (Toxic Nephropathy)

Immunological Drug-Associated Renal Disease. Drugs such as penicillins, sulfonamides, phenytoin, and allopurinol may be associated with the development of hypersensitivity vasculitis. This is a systemic disorder characterized by the deposition of immune complexes in the small blood vessels of the kidney and the skin. The renal histopathology is that of a proliferative glomerulonephritis. The renal prognosis of this disease is good, and the lesion usually resolves when the offending agent is discontinued.

By contrast to systemic immunological disease with glomerular involvement, primary glomerular injury is associated with drugs such as gold salts and penicillamine. The histological lesion is that of membranous glomerulonephritis. The clinical manifestations of proteinuria and hematuria as well as the histological abnormalities frequently resolve when the drugs are stopped.

The interstitium of the kidney may also be involved in an immunologically mediated renal inflammatory response associated with the ingestion of certain drugs. Agents such as the penicillin derivatives, particularly methicillin, are associated with the development of acute interstitial nephritis. Allopurinol, cimetidine, phenytoin, rifampin, and sulfonamides, as well as a variety of other drugs, have been associated with the development of acute interstitial nephritis. On histological examination of the kidney, there is an interstitial inflammatory response characterized by infiltration of eosinophils. The patient may have fever, rash, and eosinophilia in addition to renal dysfunction. Many patients with this drug-related syndrome, however, manifest only the renal functional impairment. The prognosis is generally good, and renal function improves when there is no longer an exposure to the offending agent. Occasionally, a short course of corticosteroids is indicated to hasten the resolution of the disease.

Nonsteroidal anti-inflammatory drugs have also been associated with the development of acute interstitial nephritis. The inflammatory cell seen on histological examination of the kidney is the lymphocyte. Nonsteroidal anti-inflammatory drug–induced interstitial nephritis may also be accompanied by the development of the nephrotic syndrome. Discontinuance of the drug, with or without the administration of corticosteroids, usually results in resolution of the injury.

Direct Tubular Toxicity. Certain classes of drugs appear to have the capability of causing direct damage to the renal tubular cells. The clinical presentation is that of the acute renal failure syndrome. The aminoglycoside antibiotics and the cancer chemotherapeutic agent, *cis*-platinum, are common causes of the acute renal failure syndrome. The clinical characteristics of this syndrome are discussed in Chapter 32. Although the mechanism of injury differs with different drugs, there is, ultimately, a disturbance in the function of the renal tubular cells.

In addition to the morphological and functional disturbances associated with the development of acute renal insufficiency, a number of drugs are associated with impairments of specific tubular functions. In these conditions, the glomerular filtration rate may or may not be normal. Derangements in proximal tubular function occur with exposure to heavy metals and outdated tetracycline. The manifestations may include renal tubular acidosis, phosphaturia, and glycosuria. Impairment in the ability to concentrate the urine may be seen in patients taking lithium carbonate, demethylchlortetracycline, or amphotericin B. Diabetes insipidus is the clinical expression of this defect. Drugs such as vincristine, cyclophosphamide, and chlorpropamide may be associated with impairment in the ability to excrete a water load and to dilute the urine. Hyperkalemia and distal renal tubular acidosis may be seen in patients receiving amphotericin B, beta-adrenergic blocking agents, and nonsteroidal anti-inflammatory drugs.

Chronic Renal Failure Due to Drugs

A common form of end-stage renal disease is that related to the long-term ingestion of analgesics, particularly drug combinations containing aspirin and phenacetin. The prototypic patient is one with long-standing complaints of chronic pain such as headache or backache. There may be a history of peptic ulcer disease. There is usually a history that indicates ingestion of analgesics in kilogram amounts over a period of years. Obtaining the drug history may be difficult owing to the personalities of such patients and because aspirin and aspirin-containing drugs are not considered

medications by some individuals. The pathogenesis of analgesic abuse nephropathy is uncertain but is likely related to the fact that the aspirin component decreases total and papillary blood flow to the kidney and phenacetin metabolites accumulate in the interstitium and papillae. The incidence of analgesic abuse nephropathy varies widely among different countries and among different regions of the same country. The reasons for these differences are unknown. The clinical presentation is that of renal insufficiency and hypertension. Some patients manifest papillary necrosis. Histological examination of the kidney reveals interstitial fibrosis and atrophy of tubules. It has been suggested that the deterioration in renal function may be slowed or reversed when the drugs are stopped. Since there are no specific characteristics of this disease entity, a strong clinical suspicion and a careful drug history are mandatory.

Important Nephrotoxins

Aminoglycoside Antibiotics. Although there are differences in nephrotoxic potential between specific types of aminoglycoside antibiotics, all agents of this type can cause renal injury. The aminoglycosides are not metabolized. These drugs can be transported across both the luminal and antiluminal borders of the cells of the proximal tubule. They accumulate in these cells and induce a change in lipid metabolism. The histological hallmark of this alteration in lipid metabolism is the presence of lipid cytosegresomes in the cells of the proximal tubules. Nephrotoxicity of the aminoglycosides is related to the cumulative dose of the drug administered. The potential for developing nephrotoxicity from exposure to an aminoglycoside antibiotic is increased in patients who have underlying renal disease, vascular instability, depletion of the extracellular fluid volume, exposure to other potentially nephrotoxic drugs, and hypokalemia. The use of drug-dosing nomograms can be of value, but frequent monitoring of renal function and measurement of the blood concentrations of the drugs is required. If decreases in renal function develop during administration of these drugs, the drug should be discontinued if possible. If the drug is required for the management of the patient, the dose of the agent must be altered. Although the renal dysfunction induced by aminoglycoside antibiotics is usually mild and reversible, when combined with other nephrotoxic insults, it can lead to acute tubular necrosis requiring dialytic support.

Cancer Chemotherapeutic Agents. A number of drugs used in the treatment of patients with cancer can be associated with the development of renal injury and/or specific defects in the function of the kidney. *Cis*-diamminedichloroplatinum (*cis*-platinum) is a potent renal nephrotoxin. The pattern of injury from this agent appears to resemble that seen with other heavy metals such as lead, arsenic, and mercury. Depending upon the magnitude of the injury, the acute renal failure syndrome due to the administration of *cis*-platinum may not be reversible. Vigorous prehydration and administration of mannitol may reduce the risk of developing renal injury.

Nonsteroidal Anti-inflammatory Drugs (NSAID). Renal toxicity due to NSAID has emerged as a very common form of drug-related nephrotoxicity. In some clinical settings it is the most common drug-related cause of renal dysfunction. NSAID are potent inhibitors of prostaglandin synthesis and the toxicity of these drugs derives from this pharmacologic property. Several distinct patterns of nephrotoxicity have been reported (Table 35–6). Administration of NSAID has been associated with fluid retention and a picture of prerenal azotemia. Particularly in patients whose maintenance of renal blood flow is dependent on the action of vasodilating prostaglandins, administration of NSAID may precipitate the development of the acute renal failure syndrome. Because of the relationship between prostaglandins and the renin-angiotensin-aldosterone axis, NSAID may cause a hyperchloremic hyperkalemic metabolic acidosis. In addition, NSAID have been associated with the development of acute renal insufficiency due to acute interstitial nephritis. A peculiarity of this entity is the co-development of the nephrotic syndrome. The histological lesion is that of minimal change glomerulopathy.

HEMODIALYSIS AND HEMOPERFUSION IN THE TREATMENT OF DRUG OVERDOSES

The vast majority of drug overdoses can be managed by routine supportive measures. The excretion of drugs that are eliminated from the body by the kidney can be augmented by increasing the urine flow rate and expanding the extracellular fluid volume. Alteration of the pH of the urine may increase the renal excretion of some organic anions and cations (see Table 35–1). The use of extracorporeal methods to remove drugs is a valuable and potentially life-saving procedure in some patients with drug overdoses.

Principles of Hemodialysis/Hemoperfusion. Hemodialysis is most effective for the removal of small molecular weight species that are water-soluble and not highly protein-bound. Hemodialysis may also be useful in the correction of severe metabolic acidosis induced by an overdose of aspirin or by intoxication with methanol or ethylene glycol (see Table 35–5). Hemoperfusion removes solutes by a process of adsorption onto an activated charcoal column or other resin adsorbents (e.g., Amberlite). Hemoperfusion is most useful for removing lipid-soluble or highly protein-bound species (Table 35–7).

Complications and Indications. Use of these ancillary means of removal of drugs and toxins is not without risk, particularly in the patient who is unstable. Both hemodialysis and hemoperfu-

TABLE 35–6. THE SPECTRUM OF RENAL TOXICITY ASSOCIATED WITH NONSTEROIDAL ANTI-INFLAMMATORY DRUGS (NSAID)

TYPE	PATHOPHYSIOLOGY	FEATURES	ASSOCIATED CONDITIONS
Acute renal failure	↓ Renal blood flow	Prerenal azotemia, sodium retention	Congestive heart failure, cirrhosis, volume depletion, renal insufficiency
Hyperchloremic metabolic acidosis	↓ Renin/aldosterone production	$\uparrow K^+$, $\uparrow Cl^-$, $\downarrow CO_2$	Interstitial renal disease
Acute interstitial nephritis	Lymphocytic infiltration of renal interstitium	Acute renal failure, +/− heavy proteinuria	Unknown

sion require systemic heparinization and insertion of vascular catheters. Vascular instability may be a problem during hemoperfusion, as the extracorporeal volume of blood is about 500 ml. Adherence of platelets to the resin column in hemoperfusion may result in significant thrombocytopenia.

The use of these modalities in the management of drug intoxications should be undertaken only when there are clear indications. The general indications are outlined below. A patient with a drug overdose and with any of the following features should be considered for treatment with hemodialysis or hemoperfusion:

1. A severe intoxication associated with hypotension, hypoventilation, or hypothermia and poorly responsive to usual supportive measures.

2. The presence of prolonged coma, particularly in patients with underlying pulmonary disease.

3. The presence of significant hepatic or renal disease that might interfere with drug metabolism or elimination.

4. The presence of a drug or substance that is either directly toxic to tissues or is metabolized to a direct tissue toxin (e.g., methanol, ethylene glycol).

5. The presence of a potentially fatal blood level of a drug or a toxin.

TABLE 35–7. DRUG AND TOXIN REMOVAL BY HEMODIALYSIS AND HEMOPERFUSION

HEMODIALYSIS	HEMOPERFUSION
Aspirin	Digoxin
Lithium carbonate	Glutethimide
Phenytoin	Ethychlorvinyl
Aminoglycosides	Benzodiazepines
Ethanol	Meprobamate
Methanol	Methaqualone
Ethylene glycol	Phenobarbital
	Theophylline

REFERENCES

Bennett WM, Arnoff GR, et al: Drug prescribing in renal failure: Dosing guidelines for adults. Am J Kidney Dis 3:155, 1983.

Clive DM, and Stoff JS: Renal syndromes associated with nonsteroidal anti-inflammatory drugs. N Engl J Med 310:563, 1984.

Roxe DM: Toxic nephropathy from diagnostic and therapeutic agents. Am J Med 69:759, 1980.

Winchester JF, Gelfand MD, et al: Dialysis and hemoperfusion of poisons and drugs. Trans Am Soc Artif Intern Organs 23:762, 1977.

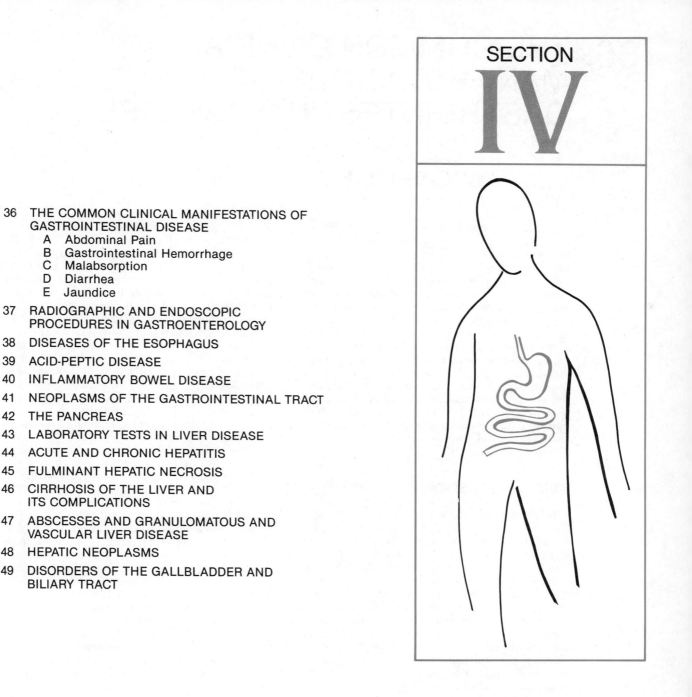

SECTION IV

GASTROINTESTINAL DISEASE

36 THE COMMON CLINICAL MANIFESTATIONS OF GASTROINTESTINAL DISEASE

A. ABDOMINAL PAIN

Pain, a subjective sensation that generally heralds tissue damage, is the most frequent symptom of gastrointestinal disease and the one that usually brings the patient to the physician. Specific patterns of pain are often helpful in suggesting or establishing a correct diagnosis and may be the most sensitive and specific sign of abdominal disease. For example, the diagnosis of acute appendicitis is established on clinical findings alone; a characteristic, localized, right lower quadrant pain and tenderness occur at a time when the most sophisticated imaging studies, such as computed tomography, are normal. This section will review the etiology, characteristics, and patterns of abdominal pain, concluding with a discussion of the approach to the patient with acute abdominal pain and a brief overview of the irritable bowel syndrome.

ORIGIN OF ABDOMINAL PAIN

Afferent nociceptive (pain-sensitive) neurons from the viscera accompany bilateral efferent sympathetic neurons, eventually reaching spinal dorsal root ganglia and spinal sensory neurons. The latter also receive input from peripheral non-pain nerves, thus establishing the basis for referred pain to extra-abdominal sites. Pain signals from the parietal peritoneum and the abdominal wall are carried by lateralized neurons in the somatic sensory nerves. Abdominal organs are insensitive to stimuli such as cutting, tearing, and burning. Generally only three processes produce pain in the alimentary tract: (1) stretching or tension in the wall of a hollow organ or the capsule of a solid organ as a result of forceful muscular contraction, muscle spasms, distention, or traction; (2) inflammation with associated release of substances, such as bradykinin, prostaglandins, histamine, and serotonin, that stimulate or sensitize nerve endings; (3) ischemia, which releases noxious tissue metabolites.

CHARACTERISTICS OF ABDOMINAL PAIN

Abdominal pain usually takes one or a combination of three patterns: (1) Visceral pain is usually dull, poorly localized due to the multisegmental bilateral innervation of abdominal organs, and often midline in location. It originates in an abdominal viscus and may have a crampy or gnawing quality. (2) Parietal (somatic) pain is intense, often well-localized and lateralized. The pain is due to stimulation, usually inflammatory in nature, of the parietal peritoneum. (3) Referred pain is localized superficial or deep pain perceived in areas remote from the diseased viscus and innervated by the same spinal segment. The pain is sometimes associated with hyperesthesia.

Although visceral pain is usually poorly localized, certain useful generalizations can be made. Pain from the esophagus is usually substernal, may be discretely localized, and, if severe, may penetrate to the middle of the back or the left arm. Pain from the stomach, duodenum, and pancreas is epigastric, often with radiation to the back. Liver, gallbladder, and bile duct pain may be epigastric but is usually located in the right upper quadrant. Gallbladder or biliary pain may be referred to the tip of the scapula. Pain from a subphrenic abscess or hepatic abscess may be referred to the shoulder tip. Jejunal and ileal pain is often periumbilical, although terminal ileal pain may be felt in the right lower quadrant. Colonic pain is poorly localized but is usually felt in the lower abdomen or hypogastric area, as is pain from the pelvic organs. Finally, rectal pain may be felt over the sacrum. Unusual but diagnostically important patterns of abdominal pain include angina-like left upper quadrant discomfort from the transverse colon, and left back/hip pain resembling L_4 root disease or ovarian disease but emanating from the transverse or the descending colon. Posterior appendiceal rupture sometimes produces similar pain in the right lumbar-gluteal area.

The quality and progression of pain may also be helpful. The pain of esophageal reflux (heartburn) is usually burning in nature, whereas the characteristic pain of peptic ulcer disease gnaws or burns and often subsides following ingestion of food or antacids. Pain due to bowel obstruction is described as recurrent, severe, and cramping (colic), often interposed with short periods of little or no pain. Furthermore, patients with bowel colic pain are often restless. In contrast, the term biliary colic is a misnomer, as the pain associated with cystic duct obstruction is usually steady rather than intermittent in nature. Pain due to inflammation, particularly of the parietal peritoneum, transmits a steady quality, felt locally, if the peritoneum is irritated focally by an underlying diseased organ such as an inflamed appendix or gallbladder, or diffusely if material such as gastric juice, intestinal contents, blood, or pus has leaked into the peritoneal cavity. Peritoneal irritation is accompanied by tenderness, by guarding (voluntary tensing) and rigidity (involuntary spasm) of the overlying abdominal muscles, and by rebound tenderness. Such patients usually lie still to minimize the discomfort. Pain due to intestinal ischemia is usually severe, poorly localized and steady, often with little abdominal tenderness in the early stages. The pain related to dissection of an abdominal aortic aneurysm occurs suddenly and is severe and often described as "tearing."

Some types of abdominal pain change charac-teristically with time. For example, sudden severe pain that subsequently becomes generalized concomitant with the appearance of signs of peritoneal irritation suggests that a hollow viscus has perforated to cause generalized peritonitis. In contrast, the pain of acute appendicitis or cholecystitis may begin as a poorly localized midline pain that later moves directly over the inflamed organ as localized peritoneal inflammation develops.

The characteristic pain patterns of those abdominal diseases for which pain is an important clinical clue are summarized in Table 36–1.

TABLE 36–1. PAIN PATTERNS OF ABDOMINAL DISEASE

DISEASE	ONSET OF PAIN	PAIN LOCATION	PAIN QUALITY	PAIN REFERRAL	PAIN PROGRESSION	ASSOCIATED FINDINGS
Reflux esophagitis	Chronic One hour after meals	Substernal	Burning	None	Into upper chest	Bitter or sour fluid in the mouth
Duodenal ulcer	Chronic Between meals and at night	Epigastric	Gnawing, burning	Occasionally to the back	—	Relief with food or antacids
Perforated duodenal ulcer	Sudden	Epigastric	Severe	Back	Rapidly progresses over the entire abdomen	Abdominal guarding Free air in peritoneal cavity on x-ray
Acute cholecystitis	Rapid	Epigastric	Colicky or steady	Tip of scapula	Pain intensity steadily increases over hours Pain localizes to right upper quadrant	Fever Localized tenderness Gallstones visible on ultrasound examination ^{99m}Tc-HIDA scan fails to visualize gallbladder
Acute pancreatitis	Rapid	Epigastric	Steady Boring	Back	Peritoneal signs may appear later in severe cases	Nausea and vomiting Epigastric tenderness
Small bowel obstruction	Rapid or gradual	Periumbilical	Cramping	Back	—	Hyperactive bowel sounds Nausea and vomiting Dilated bowel loops with air-fluid levels on x-ray Abdominal distention
Appendicitis	Rapid or gradual	Periumbilical Right lower quadrant	Crampy Steady	—	Pain localizes to right lower quadrant	Localized tenderness on abdominal and rectal examinations
Diverticulitis	Gradual	Left lower quadrant	Steady Aching	Back	—	Palpable inflammatory mass Constipation Fever, leukocytosis
Colon obstruction	Rapid or gradual	Lower quadrants	Crampy	Back	—	Vomiting Constipation Abdominal distention Hyperactive bowel sounds
Intestinal angina	Chronic After meals	Periumbilical	Colicky	—	Pain remits in 1–2 hours	Weight loss
Intestinal infarction	Sudden or rapid	Diffuse	Severe Aching	—	Progresses to peritonitis	Occult blood in feces Decreased or absent bowel sounds Initial examination may be unimpressive Shock
Dissecting aortic aneurysm	Sudden	Periumbilical Lower quadrants	Severe Boring Tearing	Flank Inguinal regions	—	Abdominal bruit Abdominal mass
Irritable bowel syndrome	Chronic Intermittent	Lower quadrants	Crampy Steady	—	—	Alternating diarrhea and constipation

NAUSEA AND VOMITING

Nausea and vomiting are often associated with abdominal pain, and their presence may provide clues to the underlying diagnosis. Vomiting most commonly occurs with obstruction and distention of the stomach or intestine (pyloric stenosis, small bowel obstruction), motility disorders (diabetic gastroparesis), or irritation and inflammation of the peritoneum. In these disorders, vagal afferents are thought to stimulate the medullary chemoreceptor trigger zones, which in turn induce vomiting. Drugs and gastric mucosal irritants may also induce vomiting via this pathway. Other disorders associated with vomiting include increased intracranial pressure, psychogenic vomiting, hypersecretion of gastric acid (Zollinger-Ellison syndrome), and the early morning vomiting of alcoholics, pregnant women, and uremics.

APPROACH TO THE PATIENT WITH ACUTE ABDOMINAL PAIN

The evaluation and care of patients with acute abdominal pain ("acute abdomen") provide one of the great challenges in clinical medicine because of the potentially lethal nature of many of the causes and the frequent need for prompt surgical or medical intervention. Although one can enlarge the differential diagnosis, the most common causes are acute appendicitis, cholecystitis or pancreatitis, bowel obstruction, perforated viscus, intestinal infarction, strangulated viscus, acute diverticulitis, ruptured ectopic pregnancy, and ruptured aortic aneurysm. During the evaluation of these patients, it is essential to remember that pulmonary (pneumonia), pelvic, renal (renal stone), hematologic (sickle cell crisis), hepatic (acute hepatitis), and metabolic (acute porphyria) disorders can cause acute abdominal pain.

The history of patients with acute abdominal pain should focus on the onset, nature, and radiation of pain, and the presence of associated symptoms such as fever, nausea, vomiting, constipation, and diarrhea. Crucial facts also can come from the patient's medical history. For example, prior surgery or peptic ulcer disease might suggest possible bowel obstruction (adhesions) or perforation (ulcer). The physical examination includes observation of the patient for restlessness (more common with intestinal colic) or immobility (more common with diffuse peritonitis), as well as examination for the typical signs of peritonitis, bowel obstruction, shock, and cardiovascular collapse (due to hypovolemia from acute peritonitis, bowel obstruction, or hemorrhage). The chest examination must rule out pulmonary causes of abdominal pain such as pneumonia or hepatic congestion due to congestive heart failure. The abdominal examination particularly addresses the following: (1) the nature of bowel sounds, (2) the presence of localized or diffuse severe tenderness, (3) the presence of masses or incarcerated hernias, and (4) the presence of fluid in the abdomen. Evidence for peritoneal tenderness and abdominal guarding is best sought with gentle palpation and light percussion. Vigorous palpation and maneuvers to elicit rebound are extremely painful and usually unnecessary. Adequate rectal and pelvic examinations are essential and provide important clues to genitourinary, colonic, and appendiceal disease.

Useful laboratory tests include a hematocrit, white blood count and differential, urinalysis, and examination of the stool for blood or pus. Tests for serum amylase, bilirubin, and transaminases and inspection for gross lipid are usually rapidly available and may be helpful. The diagnosis of acute pancreatitis is one of exclusion because an elevated serum amylase can accompany other causes of abdominal pain, including bowel ischemia, biliary tract disease, perforated ulcer, and ruptured ectopic pregnancy.

Helpful radiographic procedures include plain films of the abdomen in a supine and upright position (to evaluate intestinal gas patterns and search for free intra-abdominal air), as well as a chest x-ray. Certain other tests such as barium or Gastrografin studies of the small bowel or colon, CT imaging, ^{99m}Tc-HIDA scans, ultrasound, and endoscopic procedures are useful in selected patients.

Adequate pain relief should be provided to all patients even while awaiting a definitive diagnosis. Ultimate management depends upon the underlying disease process. Because many disorders causing abdominal pain require prompt surgical intervention, surgical consultation should be obtained early. Few pathognomonic signs or symptoms exist for many of the processes under consideration, and an early diagnostic laparotomy may sometimes be necessary.

IRRITABLE BOWEL SYNDROME

The term irritable bowel syndrome (IBS) refers to a common symptom complex, including abdominal pain and altered bowel habits, usually constipation or alternating diarrhea and constipation, for which no organic cause can be demonstrated. IBS is extremely common, constituting up to 50 per cent of referrals to gastroenterologists in the United States. Symptoms usually begin during adolescence or young adulthood, last for many years, and affect women more than men. Although the etiology and pathogenesis of IBS are not well-understood, the syndrome probably is derived from a variety of disorders. For example, patients with lactase deficiency were previously thought to have IBS. Current concepts of the pathogenesis of IBS focus on two major factors: (1) abnormal colonic motility, including high-amplitude segmental contractions, particularly after stimulation by meals, emotion, mechanical distention, or pharmacological agents; and (2) increased inherent sensitivity to physiological levels of discomfort produced by normal amounts of intestinal gas or intraluminal sigmoid pressures.

Abdominal pain, the most frequent symptom of

IBS, varies widely in pattern and degree, ranging from dull, aching discomfort in the lower quadrants to sharp, knifelike hypogastric pain. Pain is often related to meals, possibly reflecting an exaggeration of the normal food-stimulated increase in colonic motility, and may be relieved by passing flatus or stool. The pain rarely occurs at night. Some disturbance of bowel habit is always present in the form of constipation, diarrhea, or a combination of the two. Stools are often described as marble- or pellet-like and may be accompanied by mucus. Bleeding does not occur except perhaps from accompanying hemorrhoids; IBS is never an explanation for occult fecal blood. Certain personality characteristics, such as rigidity, meticulousness, obsessive-compulsiveness, as well as emotional lability, lethargy, and headaches have been associated with IBS.

Evaluation includes a history, physical examination, stool analysis, screening laboratory tests, proctosigmoidoscopy, and barium enema to eliminate the possibility of underlying organic disease.

Most importantly, treatment should include education regarding the benign nature of the condition and the pathophysiological nature of the symptoms, as well as sympathetic reassurance. Drug treatment has little place, and narcotic analgesics must be avoided. Bulk agents such as Metamucil and increased dietary fiber are useful adjuncts in the therapy of constipation. Anticholinergic spasmolytics sometimes may relieve pain. Special diets (aside from increased dietary fiber) offer little or no help, unless it is evident that specific foods repeatedly cause symptoms.

Complications of IBS include potential drug abuse, sigmoid hypertrophy, and the formation of diverticula.

REFERENCES

Connell AM: Motility and its disturbances. Clin Gastroenterol 11:3, 1982.

Schuster MM: Irritable bowel syndrome. In Sleisenger MH, and Fordtran JS (eds): Gastrointestinal Disease. 3rd ed. Philadelphia, WB Saunders Co, 1983, pp 880–895.

Wyngaarden JB, and Smith LH Jr: Cecil Textbook of Medicine. 17th ed. Philadelphia, WB Saunders Co, 1985, pp 645–802.

B.   GASTROINTESTINAL HEMORRHAGE

DEFINITION

Bleeding from the gastrointestinal (GI) tract is an important and common clinical problem. Blood loss may be massive and acute or occult and chronic from a large variety of pathological lesions. A few common lesions, however, account for the bulk of GI bleeding episodes. Although in approximately 80 per cent of patients acute GI bleeding stops spontaneously, bleeding may recur, often during hospitalization, or persist to constitute a life-threatening emergency.

The goals of management in the patient with GI hemorrhage, in order of priority, are to (1) correct hypovolemia, (2) arrest hemorrhage by the least invasive means, and (3) prevent recurrent hemorrhage. The latter two goals are more rationally attained by accurate identification of the site and pathological nature of the bleeding lesion. However, prompt and adequate hemodynamic resuscitation of the patient takes priority over all diagnostic procedures.

PRESENTATION OF GI HEMORRHAGE

Blood loss from the GI tract may be either (1) *acute*, implying sudden or massive bleeding, often with accompanying signs of hypovolemia, or (2) *chronic*, in which case blood loss is usually occult.

Acute bleeding may present in several ways:

Hematemesis. Vomiting of bright red blood or blood altered by contact with gastric acid (which displays a "coffee-grounds" appearance) is called hematemesis. It is an extremely valuable clinical clue that narrows down the field of search for a bleeding site considerably, since it denotes bleeding proximal to the ligament of Treitz.

Melena. Melena, the passage of black, tarry stools, usually implies blood loss greater than 500 ml originating anywhere between the oropharynx and the left hemicolon. Melena may be the only manifestation of upper GI bleeding.

Hematochezia. Passage of bright red or maroon-colored stool is termed hematochezia. This generally results from a lesion in the GI tract distal to the ligament of Treitz, but may also result from rapid, massive GI bleeding proximal to this point.

Chronic gastrointestinal blood loss may present as an incidentally discovered positive test for fecal occult blood or with the manifestations of iron-deficiency anemia: fatigue, dyspnea, syncope, and, not infrequently, angina in older patients with underlying ischemic heart disease. A history of intermittent melena may often be elicited, although confirmation of GI blood loss will usually require a positive guaiac test (e.g., Hemoccult test) for occult blood in the stool. Occasionally, a bleeding lesion in a patient may result in both chronic and acute blood loss, which may present either simultaneously or separated in time.

TABLE 36–2. CAUSES OF GI BLEEDING

UPPER GI	UPPER OR LOWER GI	LOWER GI
Duodenal ulcer	Neoplasm	Hemorrhoids
Gastric ulcer	Carcinoma	Anal fissure
Anastomotic ulcer	Leiomyoma	Diverticulosis
Esophagitis	Sarcoma	Ischemic bowel disease
Gastritis	Hemangioma	ease
Mallory-Weiss tear	Lymphoma	Inflammatory bowel
Esophageal varices	Melanoma	disease
Hematobilia	Polyps	Meckel's diverticulum
	Arterial-enteric fistulas	Solitary colonic ulcer
	las	Intussusception
	Vascular anomalies	
	Angiodysplasia	
	(vascular ectasia)	
	Osler-Weber-Rendu	
	disease	
	Arteriovenous malformations	
	formations	
	Hematologic disease	
	Elastic tissue diseases	
	Pseudoxanthoma	
	elasticum	
	Ehlers-Danlos syndrome	
	drome	
	Vasculitis syndrome	
	Amyloidosis	

ETIOLOGY OF GASTROINTESTINAL BLEEDING

Many lesions in the GI tract may produce bleeding (Table 36–2), although comparatively few account for the vast majority of encountered cases and are discussed here. Bleeding is defined as upper or lower according to its origin above or below the ligament of Treitz.

Upper GI Bleeding

Up to 90 per cent of upper GI bleeding is attributable to peptic ulceration, erosive gastritis, or esophagogastric varices.

Peptic Ulcer. Bleeding may occur from duodenal, gastric, and post-surgical anastomotic ulcers. A typical history of ulcer pain or dyspepsia may be absent, with bleeding being the first manifestation of peptic ulcer disease.

Gastritis. Erosive gastritis may result from ingestion of alcohol or anti-inflammatory drugs, such as aspirin or indomethacin. Gastric erosions also frequently develop as so-called stress gastritis in hospitalized patients with major trauma, severe systemic illness, extensive burns, or head injury. Since the risk of bleeding from erosive gastritis is recognized as being high (about 20 per cent) with a high mortality rate in such severely ill hospitalized patients, preventive measures aimed mainly at raising gastric pH above 4 are usually instituted through the hourly administration of antacids. Although clearly successful in preventing bleeding, these measures do not affect mortality in these critically ill patients.

Esophagogastric Varices. Bleeding occurs most frequently from varices in the esophagus and is characteristically abrupt and massive. Varices arise mainly as a result of portal hypertension secondary to cirrhosis. Alcoholic cirrhosis is by far the commonest cause of variceal bleeding in the United States, although any cause of portal hypertension (e.g., portal venous thrombosis, schistosomiasis) may lead to variceal hemorrhage. Three factors complicate the course of GI bleeding in *patients with cirrhosis.* (1) Although varices are usually suspected as the cause of bleeding, other causes (e.g., gastritis, ulcers) actually account for up to 50 per cent of bleeding lesions in these patients. These other causes of bleeding must invariably be considered in the diagnostic work-up of the cirrhotic patient. (2) Sustained portal hypertension leads to recurrent bleeding in 70 per cent of patients with cirrhosis. Thus portal decompression by means of a surgically created portosystemic shunt is the only absolutely effective means for preventing recurrence of bleeding. This in turn carries a high morbidity and appreciable mortality, especially when performed as an emergency procedure. (3) Cirrhosis often leads to the development of encephalopathy, which may manifest or exacerbate during bleeding, as well as to the development of coagulation defects, which contribute to continued bleeding. Because of these three factors, GI bleeding in patients with cirrhosis often poses difficult therapeutic problems.

Other Lesions. The Mallory-Weiss syndrome, which refers to hemorrhagic laceration of the mucosa of the esophagogastric junction produced by vomiting, is characterized by a history of retching and nonbloody vomiting followed by hematemesis. Several other lesions of the upper GI tract, including esophagitis, carcinoma, and other tumors of the stomach, generally cause chronic blood loss but may also produce massive bleeding. Arterial-enteric fistulae may occur as a result of the use of synthetic bypass grafts for aortic aneurysms and must be suspected in any patient who has had such a bypass and presents with GI bleeding.

Lower GI Bleeding

Lesions of the anorectum and colon are by far the commonest causes of lower GI bleeding.

Non-neoplastic Anorectal Lesions. Small amounts of bright red blood on the stool and toilet tissue usually arise from hemorrhoids, anal fissures, and fistulae. Proctitis from a variety of infectious causes is seen most frequently in male homosexuals and may give rise to hematochezia.

Neoplastic Lesions of the Colon and Rectum. Carcinoma of the colon and colonic polyps usually present with chronic blood loss but may produce brisk bleeding as well.

Ulcerative, Bacterial, and Ischemic Colitis. Bleeding may accompany diarrhea in ulcerative colitis as well as in infectious diarrhea due to *Entamoeba histolytica, Shigella,* and *Campylobacter.* In these cases, diarrhea is usually prominent, with mucus and leukocytes in the stool along with constitutional symptoms (e.g., malaise, fever). Ischemic colitis may cause bloody diarrhea in the elderly.

Colonic Diverticula. The sigmoid colon is the most common site in which large numbers of colonic diverticula occur. Those that bleed, however, are most frequently located in the ascending colon and constitute the commonest cause of massive lower GI bleeding. Diverticulitis, in contrast to diverticulosis, is an uncommon source of blood loss.

Angiodysplastic Lesions. Relatively small, acquired submucosal arteriovenous malformations called angiodysplastic lesions have become increasingly recognized as a common source of bleeding from the cecum and right colon in the elderly. Angiodysplastic lesions may also occur in the upper GI tract and are often difficult to diagnose either endoscopically or radiographically because they are flat, are located in the submucosa, and may be completely obscured by even minor bleeding. These lesions appear to develop with aging and may be responsible for a substantial proportion of bleeding previously ascribed to right-sided diverticula. There seems to be an increased association of these lesions with calcific aortic stenosis.

Small Intestinal Lesions. Small intestinal lesions rarely cause GI hemorrhage. Meckel's diverticulum is present in the distal ileum of 2 per cent of the population and is the commonest discrete lesion of the lower small bowel to bleed acutely.

Bleeding Diatheses

Blood dyscrasias (leukemia, thrombocytopenia), disorders of coagulation (hemophilia, disseminated intravascular coagulation), vascular malformations (Osler-Weber-Rendu disease), vasculitides (Henoch-Schönlein purpura), and connective tissue disorders (pseudoxanthoma elasticum) may all produce GI blood loss originating from upper or lower sites.

THE APPROACH TO THE PATIENT WITH GASTROINTESTINAL HEMORRHAGE

Steps in the approach to the patient who presents with GI bleeding are considered in this section in order of priority, i.e., (1) initial assessment, (2) resuscitation, (3) diagnosis, and (4) treatment. The management of GI bleeding must be individualized according to the nature and extent of bleeding. Thus in cases of massive, continuous bleeding, for example, more urgent diagnostic and therapeutic intervention may be called for, as transfusions may fail to keep pace with the rapid rate of blood loss.

Initial Assessment

If it is established or suspected that a patient has bled acutely from the gastrointestinal tract, pulse and blood pressure are noted and large-bore intravenous lines inserted for the initial infusion of saline or other plasma expanders prior to any further inquiry or examination. Blood is sent for typing and cross-matching, a complete blood count, prothrombin time, and platelet count. The latter two help to rule out a bleeding diathesis, which commonly accompanies bleeding in patients with cirrhosis, and establish a baseline for assessment of coagulation disturbances that may supervene with massive transfusion. Blood sent for electrolytes, BUN, creatinine, and liver function tests at this stage will aid in evaluating renal function, which may become compromised as a result of hypovolemic shock, as well as the presence of liver disease, which would alert the physician to a variceal source of hemorrhage.

Vital signs are the most reliable means for assessing the degree of volume loss. An orthostatic fall in blood pressure of greater than 10 mm Hg usually signifies a 20 per cent or greater loss of blood volume. Hypotension is usually accompanied by tachycardia, but heart rate alone is unreliable. When blood loss approaches 40 per cent of blood volume, signs of shock are usually present with pallor, cool extremities, pronounced tachycardia, and hypotension. A small amount of hematemesis or melena is misleading in that it may represent only a small proportion of the blood lost into the gastrointestinal tract, while even small losses may seriously compromise an elderly patient or a patient with pre-existing anemia or dehydration. The hematocrit is initially unreliable for evaluating acute blood loss, because a fall in hematocrit following acute blood loss requires equilibration of the contracted intravascular space with the extravascular space, which takes several hours. Thus, soon after even substantial bleeding, the hematocrit may be normal. An initially low hematocrit may suggest pre-existing chronic blood loss, and this may be confirmed by the presence of microcytic red cell indices.

Resuscitation

Unless bleeding is mild or chronic, patients are placed in an intensive care unit. Although initial management is usually conducted by internists, surgical consultation at this stage is mandatory, as surgical intervention may be urgently required, and the decision to intervene surgically is greatly facilitated by the patient's being jointly followed by both medical and surgical teams. Resuscitation is directed toward maintaining the intravascular volume and providing adequate tissue oxygenation. Nasal oxygen may be used, particularly in the elderly or in patients with cardiac or pulmonary disease. Vital signs, urine output, and, in some cases, central venous or pulmonary wedge pressure are monitored.

Actively bleeding patients are given whole blood to replace volume losses. However, if the patient is hemodynamically stable as a result of plasma volume restoration from the extravascular space and intravenous administration of crystalloids, packed cells may be given.

Blood is given according to the volume lost, the presence of continued bleeding, pre-existing anemia, and the ability of the patient to withstand blood loss. Thus, severe active bleeding may require whole blood administration under pressure via several intravenous lines. On the other hand, an otherwise healthy young person who is hemodynamically stable and who has stopped bleeding from a duodenal ulcer may tolerate a hematocrit of 25 per cent quite well and may be treated with oral iron. In general, evidence of hypotension, diminished tissue perfusion, or continued bleeding is an indication for transfusion.

Diagnosis

The first step in the diagnosis of the cause of gastrointestinal bleeding is to differentiate between upper and lower bleeding. The patient's *history* may be of considerable value in this differentiation. Hematemesis, for example, suggests bleeding proximal to the ligament of Treitz, and recent ingestion of anti-inflammatory drugs or alcohol suggests gastritis. A typical history of peptic ulcer pain may be helpful, as will a prior or family history of GI bleeding. Recent retching followed by hematemesis points to the possibility of a Mallory-Weiss syndrome. A change in bowel habits may suggest colonic cancer, and acute abdominal pain with bleeding may indicate ischemic colitis. The history may also reveal the presence of an aortic bypass graft.

Physical examination may reveal stigmata of chronic liver disease, suggesting a variceal source of bleeding, whereas enlargement of lymph nodes or an abdominal mass may reflect an intra-abdominal malignancy. Examination of the skin may show the telangiectasia characteristic of Osler-Weber-Rendu disease. Rectal examination will help to rule out a mass.

A simple and expedient diagnostic procedure is the passage of a nasogastric tube. A clear aspirate rules out active bleeding proximal to the pylorus. Active bleeding from a duodenal ulcer may be missed but is ruled out if clear bile is aspirated. If bleeding from an upper GI source is intermittent, the aspirate may be negative. An elevated BUN also suggests upper, as opposed to lower, GI bleeding.

Further *diagnostic procedures* are selected according to the clinical suspicion of upper versus lower GI bleeding and the rate of blood loss. In acute bleeding, barium studies are generally inappropriate, and if very rapid bleeding is present, particularly if the source is colonic, endoscopic examination may fail to visualize the site of bleeding. Under such conditions, angiography is often the procedure of first choice and may be preceded by a radiolabeled red-cell scan to localize further the region of blood loss. If bleeding is moderate, angiography often fails to show extravasation of contrast at the site of bleeding, and endoscopic procedures are preferred.

In most cases of suspected upper GI bleeding, upper GI endoscopy will provide a rapid, safe, definitive means for diagnosis of the site of blood loss. If bleeding has stopped, a double-contrast barium upper GI series is an inexpensive procedure that will detect most malignancies and peptic ulcers, although gastritis is often missed. Endoscopy is a more specific and sensitive diagnostic tool that has occasional therapeutic advantages as well as the advantage of allowing biopsy of lesions suspicious of malignancy. Thus endoscopy is preferred by many physicians for upper GI hemorrhage even in the patient who has stopped bleeding.

Bleeding from the lower GI tract is first evaluated by anoscopy and proctosigmoidoscopy, which will detect lesions in the rectosigmoid region, including hemorrhoids, polyps, carcinoma, and inflammatory bowel disease. More proximal colonic lesions may be detected by colonoscopy after colonic cleansing, but if bleeding is brisk, colonoscopy may prove futile and recourse to angiography may be necessary. If bleeding has stopped, double-contrast barium enema studies may be considered, but they are often inconclusive and make colonoscopy and angiography difficult to perform in the event of early recurrent bleeding. Colonoscopy is thus often performed even after lower GI bleeding has stopped. If evaluation of presumed lower GI bleeding is unrewarding, an upper GI source should always be excluded. Small bowel lesions below the ligament of Treitz are difficult to detect, but may be seen with a small bowel barium series.

For patients with chronic GI blood loss, the approach is usually more leisurely and the initial search for a responsible lesion is undertaken with barium studies followed, as indicated, by endoscopic evaluation and biopsy of lesions suspicious of malignancy. Angiography is occasionally employed, particularly to search for vascular lesions of the bowel.

In spite of the use of sophisticated diagnostic techniques, the site of bleeding is not established in many patients with GI bleeding. Sometimes this reflects a subtle or inaccessible lesion, at other times a multitude of lesions without identification of the one responsible for the bleeding. This does not necessarily compromise the patient, although repeated hospitalization for bleeding from an undiagnosed site is the lot of an unfortunate few and represents a difficult challenge to the physician.

Treatment

Approximately 80 per cent of patients presenting with gastrointestinal hemorrhage will stop bleeding spontaneously. In such cases, management is directed toward prevention of further bleeding by either medical or surgical treatment. Thus, following bleeding from a duodenal ulcer, treatment with antacids, sucralfate, or an H_2-reception blocker is often initiated. Conservative management is usually undertaken in cases of gastritis, Mallory-Weiss tears, angiodysplasia, or diverticulosis in which bleeding ceases spontaneously. On the other hand, malignant lesions and polyps are resected either surgically or endoscopically when possible. If bleeding does not cease or recurs, further management will depend upon the site and nature of the lesion as well as upon the assessed ability of the patient to withstand surgery. For example, most cases of peptic ulcer that fail to cease bleeding will require urgent surgery.

Several nonsurgical techniques for arresting gastrointestinal hemorrhage have been widely used, although their role is far from clear. These include radiological procedures such as intra-arterial infusion of vasopressin, a powerful vasoconstrictor, and selective embolization of bleeding arterial foci. Endoscopic electrocoagulation and laser photocoagulation are also becoming increasingly used, particularly for elderly, poor-risk patients with angiodysplastic lesions.

Variceal hemorrhage requires special consideration. Most patients with variceal bleeding are poor operative candidates and run a high risk of rebleeding. Additional precautions and supportive measures are required in these patients, as bleeding may precipitate hepatic encephalopathy while renal function may deteriorate rapidly (see Chapter 45). Cleansing of blood from the bowel using enemas as well as administration of lactulose helps to lessen the risk of encephalopathy. Volume should be replaced using blood or blood products, with care taken to avoid overtransfusion, which can worsen variceal bleeding. Since these patients often retain sodium and water avidly, infusion of large volumes of saline should

be avoided as far as possible, as this will invariably aggravate ascites. Initial measures to arrest hemorrhage nonoperatively include intravenous infusion of vasopressin (which is as effective as, but safer than, intra-arterial administration) and clotting factor replacement, usually in the form of fresh frozen plasma and platelets. Balloon tamponade is resorted to when bleeding fails to cease, but it is often only a temporary measure. Currently, continued bleeding is usually treated by endoscopic injection of the varices with sclerosant solutions (sclerotherapy), which is successful in arresting bleeding in up to 90 per cent of cases. Emergency decompression of the portal system by means of portosystemic shunt surgery is, at times, the only means for arresting acute variceal hemorrhage. Prevention of recurrent bleeding from varices may be achieved through either repeated endoscopic sclerotherapy or elective portosystemic shunt surgery. Both options carry distinct advantages and disadvantages, which are discussed more fully in Chapter 46.

REFERENCES

Peterson WL: Gastrointestinal bleeding. In Sleisenger MH, and Fordtran JS (eds): Gastrointestinal Disease. Pathophysiology, Diagnosis, and Management. Philadelphia, WB Saunders Co, 1983, pp 177–201.
Wyngaarden JB, and Smith LH Jr: Cecil Textbook of Medicine. 17th ed. Philadelphia, WB Saunders Co, 1985, pp 791–796.

C. MALABSORPTION

The gastrointestinal tract has as its main purpose the digestion and absorption of nutrients, either macronutrients required predominantly for energy or micronutrients, for example, trace elements and vitamins. Only 1 μg of vitamin B_{12} needs to be absorbed daily in a highly specific and complex process in the terminal ileum. Conversely, the gastrointestinal tract may be called upon to digest, solubilize, transport, and resynthesize 80 grams of fat daily. Beyond the net absorption of dietary components, the gut has a large daily internal circulation of water, electrolytes, and bile salts that are secreted in gastric juice, pancreatic juice, bile, and succus entericus and then reabsorbed in the small intestine and colon for reutilization. The gastrointestinal tract must first prepare for subsequent absorption of the crude mixtures of nutrients and non-nutrients ingested as "food." These preparatory processes of digestion consist of (a) the controlled release into the intestine of food that has been fragmented to small particle size by the grinding action of the stomach; (b) the release of appropriate amounts of enzymes, cofactors, buffers (bicarbonate), detergents (bile salts), and water into the lumen under hormonal

control to allow digestion of food to an isotonic mixture of simple components; and (c) further digestion of disaccharides and oligopeptides by brush border–bound enzymes. All of these steps must precede actual absorption.

Absorption of nutrients occurs from an enormous surface area supplied by the intestinal villi and microvilli during an average transit time of approximately $1\frac{1}{2}$ to 2 hours between the stomach and the ileocecal valve. (Colonic absorption consists largely of salvage of fluid and electrolytes only.) The absorption of a given substance may occur diffusely throughout the intestine or be localized to specific sites (e.g., vitamin B_{12} and bile salts in the terminal ileum). In view of the complexities of the above coordinated chemical and physiological processes, it is not surprising that a large number of disorders can result in maldigestion or malabsorption, either with considerable specificity or more globally. The purpose of this section is to present a general classification of the disorders of maldigestion and malabsorption, based on current knowledge of pathophysiology, together with a rational approach to their differential diagnosis.

NORMAL ABSORPTION

Malabsorption can be understood only in the context of normal absorption. Only the absorption of the three major classes of caloric nutrients will be described here. The intestinal absorption of water and electrolytes is described in Section D of this chapter, since this analogous form of "malabsorption" largely results in diarrhea. The important specific mechanisms for the absorption of iron (ferrous and heme forms), calcium (under the control of vitamin D), and vitamin B_{12} are described elsewhere.

Digestion and Absorption of Fat (**Fig. 36–1**). Most dietary fat is in the form of triglycerides of long-chain fatty acids (e.g., saturated—palmitic and stearic; unsaturated—oleic and linoleic). Fat from the stomach enters the duodenum as an oil-liquid emulsion; its presence in the stomach stimulates the flow of bile (via cholecystokinin [CCK]) and pancreatic juice (via secretin and CCK) (see Fig. 36–1). Pancreatic lipase, bound to the lipid surface by colipase in the presence of the detergent action of amphophilic bile salts, releases two free fatty acids from each molecule, leaving a 2-monoglyceride. These products of lipolysis are incorporated into complex mixed micelles with bile salts, which enhance their solubility and allow them to traverse the unstirred water layer that overlies the surface of the epithelial cells. The fatty acids and 2-monoglycerides then diffuse from the micelles into the cell cytosol, where they are largely resynthesized into triglycerides and packaged into chylomicrons and very low density lipoproteins (VLDL) for transport via lymphatics. The bile salts remain in the intestinal lumen for reutilization and are finally reabsorbed from the terminal ileum. The process of fat absorption is normally highly efficient; approximately 95 per cent of ingested neutral fat is absorbed. Fat soluble vitamins are probably "carried along" in this same general process.

Digestion and Absorption of Proteins. The digestion and absorption of proteins are simpler than those for fat, which may explain why malabsorption of fat figures more prominently in most malabsorptive syndromes. Hydrolysis of proteins begins in the stomach with pepsin but continues more completely in the upper small intestine catalyzed by pancreatic trypsin, chymotrypsin, and carboxypeptidase. The products of hydrolysis are free amino acids, dipeptides, and oligopeptides, the latter of which may undergo further hydrolysis by dipeptidases or oligopeptidases in the brush border of microvilli on the surface of the enterocytes. Many amino acids are absorbed as dipeptides, which are subsequently hydrolyzed to the free amino acids in the mucosal cells. There are several specific transport systems for amino acids: (a) the dibasic amino acid system, which is often abnormal in cystinuria; (b) the neutral amino acid system, which is abnormal in Hartnup disease; (c) the imino acid–glycine system; and (d) the dicarboxylic acid system. Amino acids are absorbed by active cotransport with sodium, predominantly in the jejunum.

Digestion and Absorption of Carbohydrates. Ingested carbohydrates consist largely of starch (a complex hexose polysaccharide) and the disaccharides sucrose and lactose. Salivary and pancreatic amylases hydrolyze starch intraluminally to oligosaccharides and disaccharides. In contrast to dipeptides, disaccharides cannot be absorbed. The final stages of digestion are catalyzed by specific enzymes in the microvillous surface—limit dextrinase, sucrase, lactase, and maltase. The released glucose and galactose are absorbed by active transport in association with sodium; fructose absorption is by facilitated diffusion.

CLASSIFICATION OF THE MALABSORPTION SYNDROMES (Table 36–3)

A very large number of disorders can produce or be associated with intestinal malabsorption, varying from specific genetic defects to acquired diffuse mucosal diseases. It will not be possible to discuss all of these entities in this section, which is devoted to a general understanding of malabsorption, but they are described in detail in

FIGURE 36–1. Schematic of intestinal absorption, showing the participation of pancreas, liver, and intestinal mucosal cells in fat absorption. (From Wilson FA, and Dietschy JM: Gastroenterology 61:911, 1971. Copyright 1971, The Williams & Wilkins Company, Baltimore.)

the articles to which reference is made at the end of this section. In general it is useful to think of malabsorption as resulting from abnormalities in one or more of the normal processes of digestion and absorption described earlier.

Inadequate Digestion. Ingested food must be broken down to its proper components for absorption through intraluminal or surface enzymatic processes. The exocrine secretion of the pancreas, described in Chapter 42, is of particular importance in the supply of lipase, colipase, and certain proteases, especially trypsin. One of the cardinal manifestations of chronic pancreatitis, either acquired or secondary to cystic fibrosis, is malabsorption. Even in the presence of normal pancreatic secretion of lipase, however, a gastrinoma (the Zollinger-Ellison syndrome) may stimulate enough gastric acid to lower the duodenal pH sufficiently to impair the activity of lipase and produce fat malabsorption.

The pancreatic component of fat digestion must be supplemented with a sufficient concentration of intraluminal bile salts for normal lipolysis and micelle formation. Inadequacy of bile salts can result from (a) decreased synthesis by the liver, although this is rarely severe enough to result in major malabsorption; (b) prolonged cholestasis (see Chapter 49) especially in biliary cirrhosis; (c) deconjugation of the bile salts within the intestine by bacterial action in the bacterial overgrowth syndrome; or (d) interference in the ileal reabsorption of bile salts for recycling, either due to the use of cholestyramine or more commonly in the presence of ileal disease or an ileal bypass. In these circumstances, the liver is not able to synthesize enough bile salts de novo to maintain critical intraluminal levels so that maldigestion and malabsorption of fat and fat-soluble substances (e.g., vitamins A, D, E, and K) occur.

In addition to these more global disorders of digestion associated with deficiencies of pancreatic enzymes or bile salts, more selective defects in digestion can occur. For example, deficiency of lactase, an intestinal brush border enzyme that normally hydrolyzes lactose to glucose and galactose, impairs the absorption of this disaccharide and may result in milk intolerance with symptoms of flatulence, distention, and diarrhea. Lactase deficiency may be inherited (lactase deficiency is common in certain ethnic groups such as blacks and Orientals) or may occur secondary to other causes of diffuse mucosal injury (e.g., celiac disease).

Inadequate Absorption. The components of food may not be adequately absorbed even after they have been normally digested. This may result from an insufficient available absorptive surface even though that remaining is normal. The simplest example is that of the postsurgical short bowel syndrome, which may follow surgery for mesenteric infarction or bypass surgery for morbid obesity or Crohn's disease.

Conversely, the absorptive surface may be normal in area but be defective in function. This type of defect can be within the mucosal cell and then

TABLE 36–3. CLASSIFICATION OF THE MALABSORPTION SYNDROMES

Inadequate Digestion
  Pancreatic exocrine deficiency
    primary—e.g., chronic pancreatitis, cystic fibrosis, carcinoma of the pancreas
    secondary—gastrinoma with acid inactivation of pancreatic lipase
  Intraluminal bile salt deficiency
    liver disease—especially biliary cirrhosis
    disease or bypass of the terminal ileum—impaired recycling mechanism
    bacterial overgrowth syndrome—increased deconjugation of bile salts
  Specific abnormalities—disaccharidase deficiencies
Inadequate Absorption
  Inadequate absorptive surface—e.g., short bowel syndrome, bypass fistulas, extensive Crohn's disease
  Specific mucosal cell defects
    genetic—abetalipoproteinemia, Hartnup disease, cystinuria, monosaccharide absorptive defects
    acquired—hypovitaminosis D
  Diffuse disease of the small intestine
    immunologic or allergic injury—celiac disease (gluten-sensitive enteropathy), ? eosinophilic enteritis, ? Crohn's disease
    infections and infestations—Whipple's disease, giardiasis, tropical sprue, bacterial overgrowth syndrome
    infiltrative disorders—lymphoma, mastocytosis, amyloidosis
    fibrosis—systemic sclerosis, radiation enteritis
Lymphatic Obstruction
  Lymphangiectasia
  Whipple's disease
  Lymphoma
Multiple Mechanisms
  Postgastrectomy steatorrhea
  Bacterial overgrowth syndrome
  Disease or bypass of the distal ileum
  Scleroderma, lymphoma, Whipple's disease
  Diabetes mellitus
Drug-induced Malabsorption
  Neomycin, cholestyramine, antacids, ethanol, chronic ingestion of laxatives, biguanides
Hyperabsorptive Malabsorption
  Hemochromatosis, hypervitaminosis D
  Enteric hyperoxaluria

is usually highly specific and genetic in origin. Examples are selective absorptive defects for certain amino acids in cystinuria and Hartnup disease and for fat in abetalipoproteinemia, due to defective intracellular synthesis of apolipoproteins. Selective defects can also be acquired, such as the reduced absorption of calcium when there is insufficient synthesis of 1,25-dihydroxycholecalciferol.

More frequently malabsorption, especially that of fat, is found in conditions in which there is a diffuse disease process involving the small intestinal mucosa and/or submucosa. Several causes of such diffuse injury are recognized although the mechanisms involved are often obscure:

IMMUNOLOGIC OR ALLERGIC INJURY. It is thought that gluten-sensitive enteropathy (to be discussed subsequently) falls in this category, as well as possibly some forms of the rare disorder eosinophilic enteritis.

INFECTIONS AND INFESTATIONS. Whipple's disease is a systemic disorder, the presumed bacterial etiology of which has not been clearly defined. In this disorder marked by malabsorption, the intestinal submucosa is packed with macrophages containing PAS-staining granules. Patients may also have fever, arthralgias, lymphadenopathy, pigmentation changes, and neurological manifestations. Whipple's disease is rare, but the diagnosis is important, since it usually responds to prolonged antibiotic therapy. Infestation with *Giardia lamblia* may be sufficient to cause malabsorption, although flatulence, nausea, and diarrhea are more common symptoms. In addition to causing deconjugation of bile salts, bacterial overgrowth may also produce diffuse mucosal injury.

INFILTRATIVE DISORDERS. The mucosa and/or submucosa may be diffusely infiltrated in a number of disorders sufficient to impair its absorptive function. Examples include primary lymphoma of the bowel, particularly important as a cause of malabsorption in certain parts of the world such as the Near East, and such rare disorders as systemic mastocytosis and amyloidosis.

FIBROSIS. The intestinal wall may become thickened and fibrotic in such disorders as systemic sclerosis and radiation injury. The causes of impaired absorption may be complex in these entities, however, and may result in part from abnormal motility and bacterial overgrowth.

LYMPHATIC OBSTRUCTION. After their absorption, long chain fatty acids are largely resynthesized as triglycerides and secreted into the lymphatics as chylomicrons or as very low density lipoproteins (VLDL). Diffuse obstructive lesions of the mesenteric lymphatics can therefore impair fat absorption. This is not infrequently a second cause of malabsorption in diffuse intestinal lymphoma and may also occur in Whipple's disease and in the rare congenital disorder lymphangiectasia. The latter entity more commonly presents as protein-losing enteropathy with secondary hypoalbuminemia.

Multiple Mechanisms. In view of the complexity of the digestive and absorptive processes, it is not surprising that a number of disorders may impair two or more steps. For example after subtotal gastrectomy with a gastroenterostomy (Billroth II procedure) a modest degree of malabsorption is very common. This may result from rapid gastric emptying and rapid intestinal transit, poor mixing of the pancreatic and biliary secretions from the blind duodenal loop with intestinal contents, decreased stimulus for pancreatic and biliary secretion due to decreased release of secretin and cholecystokinin, and bacterial overgrowth due to stasis in the afferent blind loop. As noted, bacterial overgrowth itself not only deconjugates bile salts but may cause diffuse injury to the intestinal epithelium. In diabetes mellitus there may be an associated exocrine deficiency of the pancreas and/or a motility disorder of the small intestine presumed to be due to diabetic neuropathy of the autonomic nervous system. This may be associated with bacterial overgrowth due to stasis.

Drug-induced Malabsorption. A number of

TABLE 36–4. SOME DRUG-INDUCED ABSORPTIVE DEFECTS

DRUG	SUBSTANCE MALABSORBED
Ethanol	Folates, vitamin B_{12}
Antacids	Phosphate
Phenytoin	Folates
Neomycin	Fatty acids, vitamin B_{12}
Cholestyramine	Bile acids, thyroxine
Tetracycline	Iron

drugs have been shown to cause malabsorption of specific dietary elements, some of which are listed in Table 36–4.

Hyperabsorptive Malabsorption. Although we are accustomed to think of malabsorption as too little absorption, it can also represent too much absorption. In hemochromatosis, for example, there is inherited continued excessive absorption of iron. In hypervitaminosis D there is excessive absorption of calcium. Enteric hyperoxaluria is an acquired abnormality characterized by excessive absorption of dietary oxalate, largely in the colon, and results in a tendency to form calcium oxalate kidney stones.

CLINICAL MANIFESTATIONS OF MALABSORPTION

There are a large number of diseases associated with malabsorption, only some of which are listed in Table 36–3. In many of these diseases the major clinical manifestations may not be related directly to malabsorption. In others the defects are highly specific, such as pernicious anemia with selective malabsorption of vitamin B_{12} or osteomalacia or rickets with poor absorption of calcium. In this brief discussion we shall be concerned only with the symptoms and signs associated with the more general forms of malabsorption, especially those forms including malabsorption of fat.

Early Manifestations. The early manifestations of malabsorption may be subtle and easily missed. There is usually a change in bowel habits with somewhat more bulky and sometimes oily stools that are difficult to flush (they are sticky and tend to float because of increased gas content). This may be associated with some weight loss, fatigue, depression, and a sense of bloating. Nocturia may be noted, thought to be caused by nocturnal reabsorption of excessive intestinal fluid. It is important to consider the diagnosis at this early stage in order to define the cause of malabsorption and to institute appropriate treatment.

Late Manifestations. The major late manifestations of the malabsorption syndrome are summarized in Table 36–5. By and large they represent the results of specific deficiencies secondary to malabsorption. Typically these patients are wasted with poor muscle mass but have distended abdomens with hyperactive bowel sounds. They tend to be hypotensive and often have increased pigmentation of the skin. Abdominal pain is un-

TABLE 36–5. CORRELATION OF DATA IN MALDIGESTION AND MALABSORPTION*

CLINICAL FEATURES	LABORATORY FINDINGS	PATHOPHYSIOLOGY
Wasting, edema	↓ Serum albumin	↑ Albumin loss (gut), ↓ protein ingestion, ↓ protein absorption
Weight loss, oily bulky stools	↑ Stool fat excretion, ↓ serum carotene	↓ Ingestion and absorption fat, CHO, protein
Paresthesias, tetany	↓ Serum Ca^{++}, ↑ alkaline phosphatase, ↓ mineralization bones (x-ray), ↓ serum Mg^{++}	↓ Absorption Ca^{++}, vitamin D, Mg^{++}
Ecchymoses, petechiae, hematuria	↑ Prothrombin time	↓ Absorption vitamin K
Anemia	Macrocytosis, ↓ serum vitamin B_{12}, ↓ absorption vitamin B_{12} and/or folic acid, microcytosis, hypochromia, ↓ serum iron, no iron in marrow	↓ Absorption vitamin B_{12} and/or folic acid, ↓ absorption iron
Glossitis	↓ Serum vitamin B_{12}, folic acid	↓ Absorption B vitamins
Abdominal distention, borborygmi, flatulence, watery stools	↓ Xylose absorption, ↓ disaccharidases in intestinal biopsy, fluid levels, small intestine (x-ray)	↓ Hydrolysis disaccharides and ↓ absorption, monosaccharides and amino acids

* From Gray GM: Maldigestion and malabsorption: Clinical manifestations and specific diagnosis. In Sleisenger MH, and Fordtran JS (eds): Gastrointestinal Disease. 3rd ed. Philadelphia, WB Saunders Co, 1983, p 230.

common except in the presence of certain specific disorders, e.g., chronic pancreatitis or primary intestinal lymphoma. At this time the clinical diagnosis is easy to make. The determination of the specific cause of the malabsorption may be more difficult.

CLINICAL TESTS OF DIGESTION AND ABSORPTION

A large number of tests of varying degrees of complexity and specificity are potentially useful in the study of patients suspected of having abnormalities of digestion and/or absorption. Some of the most useful of these tests will be described briefly.

Fecal Fat Analysis. As a screening measure a qualitative test for stool fat using a Sudan III stained smear is useful in the detection of steatorrhea. The standard, however, is to measure quantitatively the amount of fat in a three-day stool specimen after the patient has ingested a diet containing 80 to 100 grams of fat daily. Normal fat excretion in these circumstances is less than 6 grams per 24 hours (usually 2.5 grams). Values higher than this reliably indicate fat malabsorption (steatorrhea) but do not indicate the pathogenesis of the abnormality.

Triolein Breath Test. This test using ^{14}C-triolein reflects the rate of absorption of this radioactive triglyceride rather than the amount not absorbed, but otherwise its use is comparable to that of quantitative fecal fat analysis. Expired $^{14}CO_2$ is measured hourly for six hours, and normally more than 3.5 per cent of the radioactivity administered as the triolein is recovered under these conditions.

Tests of Pancreatic Exocrine Function. These tests are described in Chapter 42 (see Table 42–1). They are rarely required for the clinical diagnosis of chronic pancreatic insufficiency, however.

Xylose Absorption-excretion Test. The absorption of D-xylose, a poorly metabolized 5-carbon sugar, reflects the integrity of carbohydrate absorption by the proximal small intestine. Since no enzymatic digestion or solubilization is required prior to absorption, the rate of absorption is unaffected by pancreatic or hepatic (biliary) disease and is a more selective test of mucosal integrity. Usually 25 grams of D-xylose are given orally to a well-hydrated subject, and the amount of the sugar excreted in the subsequent five-hour urine is measured. Normal values exceed 4.5 grams per 5 hours, but this figure may be reduced by age, decreased renal function, excessive body fluid (ascites, edema), or intestinal bacterial overgrowth. In the latter case the test should return to normal with the use of antibiotics. As a variation the plasma xylose can be measured one hour after xylose is ingested and should exceed 30 mg/dl.

Radiographic Studies. All patients with malabsorption should have radiographic studies of the stomach and small intestine. Often the findings are nonspecific, with thickening of the mucosal folds, modest dilatation of the intestinal lumen, and clumping and segmentation of the barium in a so-called moulage pattern. Occasionally the study may be diagnostic with the demonstration of a stricture, a fistula, or a "blind-loop" (e.g., a small bowel diverticulum). The findings may guide the use of other studies such as biopsy.

Small-intestinal (Jejunal) Biopsy. Peroral biopsy of the small intestinal mucosa is frequently indicated in the investigation of malabsorption. Table 36–6 summarizes the conditions in which the biopsy is likely to be diagnostic and those in which it is often abnormal but in a nonspecific way.

Vitamin B_{12} Absorption (the Schilling Test). Vitamin B_{12} (cobalamin) is selectively absorbed in association with intrinsic factor in the distal ileum. An abnormality in its absorption usually represents one or more of four abnormalities: (a)

TABLE 36—6.   UTILITY OF SMALL BOWEL BIOPSY SPECIMENS IN MALABSORPTION

Often diagnostic

Whipple's disease	Giardiasis
Amyloidosis	Abetalipoproteinemia
Eosinophilic enteritis	Agammaglobulinemia
Lymphangiectasia	Mastocytosis
Primary intestinal lymphoma	

Abnormal but not diagnostic

Celiac sprue	Bacterial overgrowth syndrome
Systemic sclerosis	Tropical sprue
Radiation enteritis	Crohn's disease

disease of the distal ileum (e.g., Crohn's disease), (b) deficiency of intrinsic factor, (c) deficient pancreatic exocrine function (pancreatic trypsin is necessary to release cobalamin from a binding "R-protein" of gastric juice so that it is free to combine with intrinsic factor), and (d) increased utilization of cobalamin during transit (e.g., bacterial overgrowth). In the usual form of the test, radioactive vitamin B_{12} is given orally either alone, with intrinsic factor, or after therapy with a broad-spectrum antibiotic in suspected bacterial overgrowth, and its urinary excretion is measured over 24 hours. A flushing dose of 1.0 mg vitamin B_{12} is given simultaneously to prevent its hepatic storage and to enhance excretion. Normally more than 7 per cent of the orally administered radioactive vitamin B_{12} will be recovered in the urine. The pattern of abnormalities found in the se-

quential Schilling test may suggest (a) all three stages abnormal—intrinsic intestinal disease or pancreatic exocrine insufficiency; (b) stage 1 abnormal, stage 2 normal—intrinsic factor deficiency (pernicious anemia); (c) stages 1 and 2 abnormal, stage 3 normal—bacterial overgrowth.

Other Breath Tests. Several breath tests that assess abnormal rates of intraluminal bacterial metabolism of specific compounds have been developed. In the bile acid breath test, a ^{14}C–glycine conjugate of a bile acid is given orally and the rate of expired $^{14}CO_2$ is measured. Normally most bile salts are recycled intact in an enterohepatic circulation involving ileal reabsorption. Rapid metabolism of the conjugated glycine to CO_2 reflects either bacterial overgrowth within the small intestine or a blind loop from it, while a delayed but increased production of $^{14}CO_2$ indicates ileal dysfunction with increased spillage of the bile salt into the colon. In an analogous fashion, intraluminal bacterial metabolism of sugars releases free hydrogen, which can be measured in expired air. Most frequently this test is used to assess specific disorders of carbohydrate digestion and absorption, such as lactase deficiency, in which expired H_2 is measured after the ingestion of 50 grams of lactose.

Miscellaneous Tests. There are many other important although nonspecific tests that may reflect malabsorption, such as body weight, serum albumin, the prothrombin time (absorption of the fat-soluble vitamin K), and serum levels of cholesterol, carotene, folic acid, calcium, and magnesium. All of these tests measure only the results of malabsorption and are, in general, of little help in its differential diagnosis.

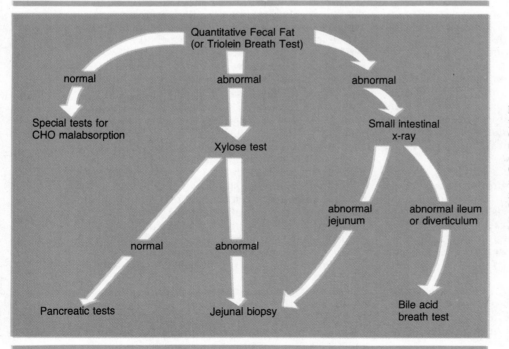

FIGURE 36—2. Approach to the patient with suspected maldigestion or malabsorption. (Modified from Gray GM: Maldigestion and malabsorption: Clinical manifestations and specific diagnosis. In Sleisenger MH, and Fordtran JS (eds): Gastrointestinal Disease. 3rd ed. Philadelphia, WB Saunders Co, 1983, p 239.)

APPROACH TO THE PATIENT WITH SUSPECTED MALDIGESTION AND/OR MALABSORPTION

In view of the large number of tests that are available to study patients suspected of having malabsorption, a logical sequence in their use is indicated in order to arrive at a diagnosis most expeditiously (Fig. 36–2). In general the diagnosis of malabsorption of fat is best established by a quantitative 72-hour fecal fat analysis. If this is normal, the patient may still have a selective abnormality for the absorption of carbohydrates, especially if symptoms are largely those of watery diarrhea, cramps, and excessive flatus. The most frequent causes of abnormal carbohydrate absorption are shown in Table 36–7. Specific tests for carbohydrate malabsorption include oral tolerance tests with the suspected carbohydrate associated with measurement of H_2 in expired air or the level of the sugar in the blood, checking also to see if the symptoms are reproduced. Typically the feces have a low pH (<6) and there is a significant fecal osmotic gap due to the high concentration of fecal short chain fatty acids produced by colonic bacteria from unabsorbed carbohydrates.

If malabsorption for fat is demonstrated (>6 grams/24 hours in the stool), a next logical step would be an upper gastrointestinal radiographic study, including the small bowel, and a xylose absorption-excretion test. A normal xylose test makes a diffuse mucosal abnormality highly unlikely and suggests an abnormality in digestion, such as pancreatic deficiency or deficiency of bile salts. A radiographic study may demonstrate either diffuse or segmental disease, including fistulas, blind loops, or other areas of stasis. A truly abnormal xylose test (see description of the test for its limitations) may be caused by bacterial overgrowth with direct metabolism of the sugar, but more frequently it is caused by some form of diffuse mucosal abnormality. If the latter is suspected, a peroral jejunal biopsy should be performed. The approach to the patient suspected of having bacterial overgrowth is described later in this section.

This sequence of tests is usually sufficient to establish the cause of malabsorption, although other tests, such as the response to a gluten-free diet for celiac disease or the study of pancreatic exocrine function, may also be indicated.

TREATMENT OF MALABSORPTION

The treatment of malabsorption is too diverse to be summarized in general terms and depends in considerable measure on the stage at which the defect occurs as well as its direct causation. Treatment may include cimetidine or ranitidine for a gastrinoma; the daily use of pancreatic enzyme preparations; antibiotics for the bacterial overgrowth syndrome or Whipple's disease; the use of a gluten-free diet for celiac disease; the use of median chain fatty acids, which are more readily absorbed; surgical repair of biliary obstruction, blind loops, or fistulas; or the chemotherapy of lymphoma. It may also require replacement therapy with fat-soluble vitamins and other specific nutrients. Rarely total parenteral nutrition may be indicated (e.g., for the short bowel syndrome).

DISORDERS ASSOCIATED WITH MALABSORPTION

A very large number of disorders may result in intestinal malabsorption of varying degrees of severity. Some but not all of these have been listed in Table 36–3 as examples of the potential causes of the syndrome. This section will discuss only two of these entities, celiac sprue and the bacterial overgrowth syndrome. Other specific disorders are discussed elsewhere in this book or are discussed in detail in the appended references.

Celiac Sprue (Gluten-sensitive Enteropathy, Nontropical Sprue). Celiac sprue is a chronic, seemingly familial disorder associated with a lifelong sensitivity to dietary gluten, a protein found in wheat and wheat products. When this protein (or certain peptides derived from it) is ingested, a diffuse mucosal injury results that is characteristic but nonspecific. The villi are shortened and blunted with decreased absorptive surface area, the crypts are hyperplastic, and the lamina propria is usually heavily infiltrated with lymphocytes.

PATHOGENESIS. The pathogenesis of the injury has not been established, although the best evidence suggests an immunological mechanism. Patients with celiac sprue have a high prevalence of certain histocompatibility types (HLA-B8 and Dw3), suggesting a linkage on chromosome 6 and strengthening the possibility of an immunological origin. On careful examination as many as 10 per

---

TABLE 36–7. DISORDERS OF CARBOHYDRATE ABSORPTION*

Intraluminal digestion of starch
  Neonatal period
  Pancreatic duct occlusion
Membrane digestion
  Lactase deficiency
    Acquired } Probably genetic
    Congenital
    Secondary to mucosal injury
  Sucrase-isomaltase deficiency
  Trehalase deficiency
  Generalized disaccharidase deficiency—mucosal disease
Monosaccharide transport
  Congenital glucose-galactose malabsorption
  Acquired glucose-galactose malabsorption

*From Olsen WA: A pathophysiologic approach to diagnosis of malabsorption. Am J Med 67:1011, 1979.

cent of first-degree relatives of patients with celiac sprue may have the disorder. A second hypothesis postulates that an incomplete hydrolysis of peptides derived from gluten leads to the accumulation of toxic intermediates that directly injure the mucosal cell and that the immunological phenomena are secondary to this direct cell injury. Whatever the cause, it is known that the lesion is locally produced, disappears when gluten is withdrawn, and recurs within a few days when gluten is reintroduced. The pathogenesis of the resulting malabsorption is largely that of a diffuse mucosal abnormality. It has also been suggested that the abnormal mucosa has a reduced ability to secrete secretin and cholecystokinin-pancreozymin and therefore that pancreatic and biliary functions are secondarily impaired.

SYMPTOMS AND SIGNS. The symptoms and signs of celiac sprue are largely those that have been described for malabsorption in general. Symptoms tend to be more severe in childhood, diminishing after adolescence. Once again it must be emphasized that the gastrointestinal symptoms may be very mild and the patient may present with other manifestations such as anemia (iron or folate deficiency), a bleeding diathesis (vitamin K deficiency), or metabolic bone disease (vitamin D or calcium deficiency).

DIAGNOSIS. Patients with sprue usually exhibit fat malabsorption, an abnormal xylose test, and an abnormal pattern of dilated intestinal loops with thickened mucosal folds and flocculation of barium on radiographic examination. The Schilling test is usually normal but may be abnormal if the disorder extends to the ileum. Peroral biopsy shows the characteristic but not pathognomonic lesion. Finally, and most importantly, there is a clinical and histological response to a gluten-free diet.

TREATMENT AND PROGNOSIS. Treatment is by lifelong adherence to a gluten-free diet. Corn flour and rice products can safely be substituted for wheat, barley, and oats. A clinical response usually begins within a few weeks and the patient may continue to improve over a number of months. Reversion to a regular diet usually leads to a rapid return of symptoms. The long-term prognosis is excellent, although patients with celiac sprue appear to have a higher incidence of non-Hodgkin's lymphoma in later life.

Bacterial Overgrowth Syndrome. The small intestine usually harbors very few microorganisms ($<10^4$ colonies per ml). This comparatively sterile sanctuary is thought to result from the combined effects of gastric acidity, the rapid sweeping action of normal intestinal motility, and the secretion into the intestine of immunoglobulins. When bacteria are present in increased numbers in the small intestine, malabsorption is a frequent consequence. Loss of the normal sweeping function of the gut due to motility disorders or to "blind loops" (e.g., spontaneous or surgically created diverticula) is the most common cause of upper intestinal bacterial overgrowth.

PATHOGENESIS. As noted previously the malabsorption associated with bacterial overgrowth may result from three mechanisms: (a) deconjugation of bile salts, leading to impaired micelle formation; (b) a patchy injury to mucosal cells thought to be due to direct injury by bacteria or bacterial products; and (c) direct utilization of nutrients by bacteria, best established for vitamin B_{12}.

CONDITIONS ASSOCIATED WITH BACTERIAL OVERGROWTH. A large number of disorders may be associated with bacterial overgrowth. In addition to such gross structural derangements as blind loops, fistulas, or strictures, this syndrome may be found in the impaired intestinal motility of systemic sclerosis, amyloidosis, diabetes mellitus, and chronic pseudo-obstruction. It may also occur in hypogammaglobulinemia and in pancreatic insufficiency.

DIAGNOSIS. The initial approach to a patient with malabsorption of any cause has been described above and in Figure 36–2. If bacterial overgrowth is suspected based on anatomical abnormalities or on the finding of an abnormal xylose test in the presence of a normal jejunal biopsy, this can be confirmed in one of several ways: (a) by an abnormal bile acid breath test (if there is no ileal disease), (b) by a positive three-stage Schilling test, (c) by direct culture of jejunal fluid (usually $>10^7$ organisms/ml with a mixed culture of anaerobes for significant bacterial overgrowth), or (d) more simply by a 10- to 14-day therapeutic trial using a broad-spectrum antibiotic.

TREATMENT. The treatment depends upon the anatomical and functional cause of the impaired sweeping function of the intestine. Sometimes surgery is indicated. More often patients will require chronic or intermittent antibiotic therapy on an indefinite basis. The most frequently used agents are tetracycline, ampicillin, and trimethoprim-sulfamethoxazole. In some forms of malabsorption, parenteral nutrition may be required. This form of therapy will not be described in this introductory textbook.

REFERENCES

Glickman RM, and Sleisenger MH: Malabsorption. In Wyngaarden JB, and Smith LH Jr (eds): Cecil Textbook of Medicine. 17th ed. Philadelphia, WB Saunders Co, 1985, pp 719–740.

Gray GM: Maldigestion and malabsorption: Clinical manifestations and specific diagnosis. In Sleisenger MH, and Fordtran JS (eds): Gastrointestinal Disease. 3rd ed. Philadelphia, WB Saunders Co, 1983, p 228.

Sleisenger MH, and Brandborg LL: Malabsorption. Philadelphia, WB Saunders Co, 1977.

Sleisenger MH (ed): Malabsorption and nutritional support. Clin Gastroenterol 12:323, 1983.

Toskes PP, and Donaldson RM Jr: The blind loop syndrome. In Sleisenger MH, and Fordtran JS (eds): Gastrointestinal Disease. 3rd ed. Philadelphia, WB Saunders Co, 1983, p 1023.

Trier JS: Celiac sprue. In Sleisenger MH, and Fordtran JS (eds): Gastrointestinal Disease. 3rd ed. Philadelphia, WB Saunders Co, 1983, p 1050.

DEFINITION

Diarrhea is best defined as an increase in stool liquidity and weight (>200 grams per day) that may be associated with increased stool frequency, urgency, perianal discomfort, and/or fecal incontinence. This chapter will discuss normal water and solute handling by the intestine, the pathophysiology of diarrhea, the evaluation of diarrhea, and finally, infectious causes of diarrhea and food poisoning. Other specific clinical entities that lead to diarrhea are discussed in Section C of this chapter and Chapter 40.

NORMAL INTESTINAL PHYSIOLOGY

The intestine normally receives 8 to 10 liters of fluid per day, 1500 to 2000 ml from injested food and liquids and the rest from salivary, gastric, pancreatic, biliary, and small intestinal secretions. The small bowel absorbs all but about one liter of this fluid, and the colon absorbs 90 per cent of the remaining fluid, resulting in a fecal output of 100 to 150 ml per day.

The mechanisms responsible for solute and fluid absorption differ in different regions of the gut. All obey the general principle, however, that solutes (salts and other substances) are absorbed by specific mechanisms, while water follows passively according to osmotic gradients. Many of the cellular mechanisms responsible for small intestinal solute transport, shown in Figure 36–3, appear to be sodium-coupled processes; i.e., they use the energy of the sodium gradient (established by the sodium pump) to drive entry or exit of a wide range of compounds, including protons, chloride, glucose, amino acids, and bile acids across cell membranes. Bicarbonate secretion, driven by sodium/hydrogen exchange, accounts for the relatively alkaline nature of ileal and colonic contents. Thus, jejunal and ileal fluid typically contains Na^+, 140 mM; K^+, 6.0 mM; Cl^-, 100 mM; and HCO_3^-, 30 mM.

Colonic solute transport is limited to electrolytes and occurs through slightly different mechanisms. Sodium absorption, which occurs via a specific sodium channel, generates an electrical potential across the colon wall, which in turn drives both chloride absorption and potassium secretion, leading to the typically high potassium concentration of colonic contents. In addition, organic acids, produced by colonic bacteria from nonabsorbed carbohydrate or fat, react with bicarbonate to produce organic anions and CO_2. Thus, colonic fluid typically contains Na^+, 40 mM; K^+, 90 mM; Cl^-, 15 mM; HCO_3^-, 30 mM; and organic anions, 85 mM.

Both small bowel and colon also secrete electrolytes and water. In the small bowel, secretion

FIGURE 36–3. Active transport mechanisms in the human ileum. (1) Luminal sodium-coupled glucose carrier; (2) double-exchange carriers for neutral NaCl uptake; (3) serosal sodium pump (Na,K-ATPase).

probably originates in crypt cells and may be due to sodium-coupled entry of anions (Cl^-) across the serosal cell membrane, followed by secretion of chloride across the luminal cell membrane. Sodium and water are thought to follow chloride passively according to electrical and osmotic gradients (Fig. 36–4). Colonic chloride secretion may

FIGURE 36–4. Model of cyclic AMP–induced changes in intestinal transport. Active anion secretion (**) is stimulated concomitant with inhibition of neutral NaCl absorption (*). The sodium-coupled glucose carrier and the sodium pump are unaffected. Cations and water move passively via junctions between cells (paracellular pathway).

possibly occur via a similar mechanism in which chloride uptake across the serosal membrane is coupled to both sodium and potassium entry.

Although intestinal water movement is passive, it is not inconsequential. Since water absorption is linked to solute absorption, the presence of poorly absorbed, osmotically active solutes such as Mg^{+2}, SO_4^{-2}, and PO_4^{-2} in the gut lumen will impair water absorption or cause water secretion.

CLASSIFICATION AND PATHOPHYSIOLOGY

Diarrhea may result if one or more of the following occur: (1) decreased normal solute and water absorption; (2) increased electrolyte secretion; (3) presence of poorly absorbed, osmotically active solutes in the gut lumen; (4) abnormal intestinal motility; and (5) inflammation with exudation of mucus, blood, or pus.

Secretory Diarrhea. Secretory diarrhea, usually due to abnormalities in both absorption and secretion of electrolytes, is a common cause of watery diarrhea (Table 36–8). For many of the disorders listed here, the ultimate cause of intestinal secretion is an increase in cellular cyclic AMP (cAMP) levels. As shown in Figure 36–4, cAMP has two effects: it inhibits neutral NaCl absorption and stimulates chloride secretion without altering other solute transport mechanisms. For example, cholera, the archetypal secretory diarrhea, is due solely to the action of a small, heat-labile toxin that binds to intestinal mucosal cells and specifically stimulates the enzyme adenylate cyclase to produce cAMP. Since other sodium-coupled transport mechanisms function normally, hydration can be maintained by oral administration of sodium-glucose solutions.

Other causes of secretory diarrhea exist but remain poorly understood. Ion secretion in some cases may be due to increases in intracellular calcium or other cyclic nucleotides (cGMP). Small bowel disorders that produce villus atrophy ("flat

TABLE 36–8. SOME CAUSES OF SECRETORY DIARRHEA

Agents that activate the adenylate cyclase–cAMP system
Cholera toxin
Escherichia coli heat-labile toxin
Vasoactive intestinal polypeptide (VIP)
Prostaglandins
Salmonella enterotoxin
? Dihydroxy bile acids and fatty acids
Agents that probably do not activate the adenylate cyclase–cAMP system
Escherichia coli heat-stable toxin
Serotonin
Enterotoxins of *Clostridium perfringens*, *Pseudomonas aeruginosa*, *Klebsiella pneumoniae*, and *Shigella dysenteriae*
Calcitonin
Castor oil, phenolphthalein
Villus atrophy (e.g., celiac sprue)

TABLE 36–9. SOME CAUSES OF OSMOTIC DIARRHEA

Disaccharidase deficiencies
Glucose-galactose or fructose malabsorption
Lactulose, mannitol, sorbitol ("chewing gum diarrhea") ingestion
Magnesium ingestion (antacids, laxatives)
Sulfate, phosphate ingestion (laxatives)
Sodium citrate ingestion
Steatorrhea (pancreatic insufficiency)
Generalized malabsorption
Small bowel mucosal disease (celiac disease)
Bacterial overgrowth (bile acid deconjugation, villus atrophy)

gut"), such as celiac disease, are often associated with electrolyte secretion, probably due to unopposed secretion from the remaining crypt cells. Finally, disorders that cause malabsorption (see Section C of this chapter) and osmotic diarrhea (see below) may also be associated with secretory diarrhea. Nonabsorbed bile acids and fatty acids may stimulate ion secretion by colonic mucosal cells.

Secretory diarrhea usually presents as copious watery diarrhea that persists during a two-day fast. Because the diarrheal fluid is composed of electrolytes and water, fecal osmolality can be entirely accounted for by the usual cations and anions (Na^+, K^+, Cl^-, HCO_3^-, and organic anions) and there is little or no fecal solute gap [solute gap = fecal or plasma osmolality − $2(Na^+ + K^+)$]. The factor of 2 is to account for the anions in stool.

Osmotic Diarrhea. Osmotic diarrhea is due to the accumulation of poorly absorbed solutes in the gut lumen. This may occur by (1) ingestion of poorly absorbed solutes such as lactulose, Mg^{+2}, SO_4^{-2}, or PO_4^{-2}; (2) generalized malabsorption; or (3) failure to absorb a specific dietary component such as lactose. Examples of osmotic diarrhea are listed in Table 36–9.

Osmotic diarrhea typically stops when the patient fasts (or stops ingesting the responsible solute). Because osmotic diarrhea is due to the presence of poorly absorbed, unmeasured solutes, fecal fluid exhibits a large solute gap (>50 $mOsm \cdot L^{-1}$). In this case, the measured stool electrolytes [$2(Na^+ + K^+)$] usually do not account for all of fecal fluid osmolality. However, in the case of ingestion of anions such as SO_4^{-2} or PO_4^{-2}, the fecal solute gap will be low (normal) and specific measurement of stool SO_4^{-2} and PO_4^{-2} must be performed. In individuals with carbohydrate malabsorption, stool pH is acidic owing to products of fermentation, and reducing substances are readily measured in the stool.

Abnormal Intestinal Motility. At least three types of motility disorders may result in diarrhea: (1) reduced peristalsis leading to bacterial overgrowth (see Section C of this chapter); (2) increased small bowel motility leading to decreased contact time between small bowel mucosa and intestinal contents and thus delivery of increased volume to the colon; and (3) increased colonic emptying with decreased contact time and increased stool liquidity. Diarrhea due mainly or in part to motility disorders includes that associated with irritable bowel syndrome, postvagotomy and postgastrectomy syndromes, diabetic neuropathy, scleroderma, and thyrotoxicosis.

EVALUATION OF DIARRHEA

The evaluation of diarrhea requires attention to the history and physical examination and careful selection and interpretation of laboratory tests.

History and Physical Examination

The patient's description (or better yet, the physician's observation) of the diarrheal stool is often informative. Large, voluminous stools suggest a small bowel or proximal colon source, whereas small stools associated with frequent urges to defecate suggest disease in the left colon or rectum. Blood suggests mucosal inflammation, whereas frothy stools and flatus suggest carbohydrate malabsorption. Greasy, foul-smelling stools with visible oil or fat indicate severe steatorrhea. A thorough drug history is also important as antibiotics, antacids, antihypertensive agents, thyroxine, digitalis, propranolol, quinidine, colchicine, lactulose, ethanol, and laxatives may be associated with diarrhea. Other pertinent information includes the time course of the present illness (acute or chronic), previous surgery, systemic complaints, recent travel, family history, and sexual orientation (male homosexuals have a high incidence of intestinal infections; see below). For example, acute diarrhea is usually due to infectious agents or toxins (food poisoning) whereas chronic diarrhea is not.

The physical examination may provide clues to the diagnosis of diarrhea, many of which are given in Table 36–10.

Although the cause of diarrhea may be apparent from information obtained through the history and physical examination, selected laboratory tests are often needed to establish or confirm a diagnosis. Table 36–11 lists a number of tests that may be useful in evaluating diarrhea, although for most patients only a few of these will be necessary. In selecting appropriate tests, it is useful to categorize patients into two categories: (1) Those with acute diarrhea, generally due to infection, drugs, food poisoning, and fecal impaction. Traveler's diarrhea is a specific subset of this group which occurs within two weeks of travel to a tropical or developing area and runs a self-limited course of one to ten days. (2) Those with chronic diarrhea, which in turn may be divided into (a) secretory diarrhea, generally due to drugs, hormones, bile acids, or fatty acids; (b) osmotic diarrhea, generally due to drugs, laxatives, or malabsorption; (c) inflammatory diarrhea due to inflammatory bowel disease (ulcerative colitis, Crohn's disease), ischemic colitis, or parasitic infection; (d) motility disorders such as irritable bowel syndrome, scleroderma, and diabetic autonomic neuropathy.

TABLE 36–10.   CLUES TO THE DIFFERENTIAL DIAGNOSIS OF DIARRHEA*

SYMPTOM OR SIGN ASSOCIATED WITH DIARRHEA	DIAGNOSES TO BE CONSIDERED
Arthritis	Ulcerative colitis, Crohn's disease, Whipple's disease, enteritis due to *Yersinia enterocolitica*, gonococcal proctitis
Liver disease	Ulcerative colitis, Crohn's disease, bowel malignancy with metastases to liver
Fever	Ulcerative colitis, Crohn's disease, amebiasis, lymphoma, tuberculosis, Whipple's disease
Marked weight loss	Malabsorption, inflammatory bowel disease, cancer, thyrotoxicosis
Eosinophilia	Eosinophilic gastroenteritis, parasitic disease (particularly *Strongyloides*)
Lymphadenopathy	Lymphoma, Whipple's disease
Neuropathy	Diabetic diarrhea, amyloidosis
Postural hypotension	Diabetic diarrhea, Addison's disease, idiopathic orthostatic hypotension
Flushing	Malignant carcinoid syndrome, pancreatic cholera syndrome
Proteinuria	Amyloidosis
Collagen vascular disease	Mesenteric vasculitis
Peptic ulcers	Zollinger-Ellison syndrome
Chronic lung disease	Cystic fibrosis
Systemic arteriosclerosis	Ischemic injury to gut
Frequent infections	Immunoglobulin deficiency
Hyperpigmentation	Whipple's disease, celiac disease, Addison's disease
Antibiotic ingestion	Pseudomembranous colitis, antibiotic-associated diarrhea
Good response to corticosteroids	Ulcerative colitis, Crohn's disease, Addison's disease, eosinophilic gastroenteritis, celiac disease
Good response to antibiotics	Blind loop syndrome, tropical sprue, Whipple's disease

* From Krejs GJ, and Fordtran JS: Diarrhea. In Sleisenger MH, and Fordtran JS (eds): Gastrointestinal Disease. 3rd ed. Philadelphia, WB Saunders Co, 1983.

Tests that should be performed on all patients include examination of the stool for consistency, fecal leukocytes (Wright's stain), and blood. In patients with acute diarrhea, fecal leukocytes suggest either infection with invasive organisms such as *Shigella*, *Escherichia coli*, *Entamoeba histolytica*, gonococci, or *Campylobacter*, or antibiotic-associated colitis. In patients with chronic diarrhea, pus suggests colitis such as ulcerative colitis, Crohn's disease, or ischemic colitis. Pus is not seen in toxin-induced secretory diarrhea, malabsorption, laxative abuse, or giardiasis. Fecal blood generally indicates inflammation and has the same significance as pus.

The physician selects further tests depending upon the clinical picture. Patients with acute diarrhea, in whom an infectious cause is likely, should have stools examined for ova and parasites and appropriately cultured for bacterial pathogens. Proctosigmoidoscopy is generally of little help in acute diarrhea except to visualize pseudomembranes in antibiotic-associated diarrhea.

TABLE 36–11. TESTS THAT MAY BE USEFUL IN THE WORK-UP OF DIARRHEA*

Stool
  Consistency
  Frequency/24 hr
  Volume/24 hr
  WBC's by Wright's stain
  Blood
  Sudan stain for fat
  Quantitative fat/24 hr
  NaOH for phenolphthalein and
    other laxatives
  Cultures for enteric pathogens
  Ova and parasites
  Clostridium difficile toxin
  Osmolality
  Na, K, Cl
  pH
  Reducing substances
  Mg, SO_4, PO_4
Proctoscopy
  Mucosal appearance
  Biopsy
Blood
  Electrolytes
  Immunoglobulins, albumin
  T_3, T_4
  Ameba serology
  Folate, vitamin B_{12}
  Ca, Mg, PO_4
  Erythrocyte sedimentation rate
  Eosinophil count
Special Assays
  Vasoactive intestinal
    polypeptide (VIP)
  Calcitonin
  Gastrin
  Prostaglandins
  Other

Gastric Analysis
X-ray Studies
  Upper GI, small bowel, barium
    enema
  Abdominal and pelvic
    sonogram, CT scan
  Abdominal angiogram
Small Bowel Studies
  Aspirate (O and P, colony
    count, cultures)
  Biopsy
  Mucosal disaccharidase assay
  D-Xylose absorption test
  Schilling test with intrinsic
    factor
  ^{14}C–bile acid absorption
  Carbohydrate breath tests
Exocrine Pancreatic Function
Upper Endoscopy
Colonoscopy
Urine
  5-Hydroxyindoleacetic acid (5-
    HIAA)
  Metanephrines,
    vanillylmandelic acid (VMA)
  NaOH (for phenolphthalein)
  Heavy metals, drug screen
Room Search for Drugs
Intestinal Perfusion Studies
Therapeutic Trials

* From Krejs GJ, and Fordtran JS: Diarrhea. In Sleisenger MH, and Fordtran JS (eds): Gastrointestinal Disease. 3rd ed. Philadelphia, WB Saunders Co, 1983.

Blood cultures and a white blood cell and differential count may be useful in individuals with signs of systemic infection, while serological tests for amebiasis are helpful as they are usually positive in the presence of tissue invasion.

In evaluating chronic diarrhea, the initial selection of tests is designed to answer the following questions: (1) Is diarrhea secretory or osmotic? Evaluate the effect of fasting and measure the fecal osmotic gap. (2) Is malabsorption present? Evaluate stool fat and D-xylose absorption. (3) Are structural, mucosal, or motility abnormalities present? Evaluate appearance with radiographic or endoscopic procedures and biopsies if appropriate. The answers to these questions will determine selection of the more specific and specialized tests listed in Table 36–11. Certain of these tests deserve brief discussion.

Stool examination and culture should always precede enemas or radiographic studies, as fluid or barium may interfere with demonstration of pathogens. Similarly, proctosigmoidoscopy, which rapidly allows examination and biopsy of the distal colon, should be performed without enemas or other preparation, as these may distort or obscure evidence of disease. Mucosal smears may be obtained at sigmoidoscopy for culture and examined for pus. Rectal biopsies may be performed to detect amyloidosis, Whipple's disease, inflammation, or schistosomiasis.

Quantitative fecal fat determination (see Section C of this chapter) is one of the most sensitive tests for steatorrhea and, if elevated, the differential diagnosis of malabsorption should be pursued. Test results must be interpreted in light of dietary fat intake, which is usually standardized at 100 grams per day for the entire three days of the collection. Other tests for malabsorption are discussed in Section C of this chapter.

Hormone assays (vasoactive intestinal polypeptide, prostaglandins, calcitonin, gastrin, and others) are likely to be helpful only in the rare subgroup of patients with chronic, severe (>1 liter per day) secretory diarrhea in whom laxative abuse and intrinsic gastrointestinal tract disease have been ruled out.

Therapeutic trials may also be indicated in certain cases as diagnostic tests, including pancreatic enzymes (for pancreatic exocrine insufficiency), antibiotics (for bacterial overgrowth), metronidazole (for giardiasis), cholestyramine (for bile acid malabsorption), and various diets (lactose-free).

Therapy

Optimal therapy is to cure the underlying disorder. However, if this is not possible, certain drugs may ameliorate the disease (prednisone in inflammatory bowel disease) or treat the diarrhea (cholestyramine to bind bile acids). Specific antisecretory drugs are not yet available; however, supportive and symptomatic therapy is often required. Fluid and electrolyte replacement is an important aspect of therapy for diarrhea, particularly in infants and elderly individuals. Oral sodium-glucose solutions or intravenous fluids may be required. Opiates (codeine, diphenoxylate, or loperamide) reduce urgency, frequency, and stool volume in a wide range of diarrheal illnesses, probably via decreased gut motility and increased contact time. Opiates should not be used in patients with severe ulcerative colitis and impending toxic megacolon, and they may actually prolong illness in patients with infectious diarrhea (shigellosis). However, they are extremely useful agents in patients with chronic, disabling diarrhea.

Antibiotics are generally not indicated for acute or traveler's diarrhea, as these are self-limited processes and antibiotics usually do not shorten the duration of the illness.

SPECIFIC CLINICAL DISORDERS

Infectious causes of diarrhea, the "gay bowel syndrome," and food poisoning will be discussed briefly. The evaluation and differential diagnosis of malabsorption is covered in Chapter 36C and inflammatory bowel disease in Chapter 40.

Bacterial and Viral Infections. Acute watery

diarrhea in the United States is most commonly due to viruses (rotavirus, Norwalk agent, coronavirus, parvovirus, and adenovirus) or enterotoxin-producing *Escherichia coli. Campylobacter fetus* (ss jejuni), *Shigella, Salmonella,* or *Yersinia enterocolitica,* less commonly seen, may produce either watery (secretory) diarrhea or dysentery with mucosal invasion, bloody diarrhea, chills, fever, tenesmus, and crampy pain. All of these agents, as well as the classic *Vibrio cholera,* also may be responsible for traveler's diarrhea (all of these agents are discussed more fully in Chapter 92). Elaborate diagnostic studies and antibiotic therapy are warranted only for severe, protracted illness or when fever and signs of toxicity indicate bacteremia. Daily prophylaxis for traveler's diar-

rhea with antibiotics (doxycycline, 100 mg) or bismuth subsalicylate (Pepto-Bismol, 60 ml qid) is effective. However, use of antibiotics in this regard should be discouraged in order to (1) avoid emergence of resistant strains, (2) prevent antibiotic-associated side effects, and (3) prevent pseudomembranous enterocolitis.

Antibiotic-associated Diarrhea. Five to 25 per cent of individuals receiving broad-spectrum antibiotics will develop diarrhea, usually within 2 to 20 days. The antibiotics most frequently implicated include ampicillin, clindamycin, lincomycin, and cephalosporins. Diarrhea is usually due to an enterotoxin produced by *Clostridium difficile,* a bacterium that proliferates in the colon when the normal flora is disrupted. Diarrhea may

TABLE 36–12. TYPES OF FOOD POISONING

AGENT	SETTING	INCUBATION PERIOD	CLINICAL MANIFESTATIONS
Staphylococcus aureus: heat-stable toxin	Cooked, inadequately cooled foods	2-7 hr	Salivation, nausea, vomiting, abdominal cramping, diarrhea < 24 hr
Bacillus cereus: heat-resistant spores, heat-stable toxin	Cooked, unrefrigerated food (rice)	2-14 hr	(1) emetic form (like *S. aureus*) (2) diarrheal form: enterotoxin which stimulates cAMP, abdominal cramps, diarrhea < 24 hr
Clostridium perfringens, Type A: heat-resistant spore, ? toxin	Inadequately cooked (< 100°C) meat, beans	8-14 hr	Abdominal cramps, diarrhea < 24 hr
Vibrio parahaemolyticus: water-borne infection of shell fish and crustaceans	Raw seafood	12-24 hr	Nausea, vomiting, abdominal cramps, explosive watery diarrhea; usually < 48 hr
Chinese restaurant syndrome	Monosodium L-glutamate (MSG)	minutes to hours	Burning skin, facial pressure, chest pressure, headaches
Fish poisoning	Cinguatoxin	minutes to hours	Nausea, vomiting, abdominal cramps, diarrhea, paresthesias of face and extremities, cranial nerve palsies, hypotension, bradycardia, respiratory paralysis; recovery may be prolonged
	Scombrotoxin	minutes	Histamine-like reaction; flushing, headache, dizziness, abdominal cramps, nausea, vomiting, diarrhea, urticaria, and pruritus; antihistamines useful; < 4 hr
	Tetrodotoxin	30 min	Paresthesias, muscle weakness, paralysis
Paralytic shellfish poisoning	Dinoflagellate neurotoxin (*Gonyaulax cantanella, Gonyaulax tamarensis*)	30 min	Like tetrodotoxin
Mushroom poisoning	Amanitine Phalloidin	6-24 hr	Abdominal pain, nausea, vomiting, diarrhea; later renal and hepatic failure; 40-90% mortality

be mild but can be quite severe, with development of pseudomembranous colitis, characterized by inflammation, mucosal necrosis, ulceration, and pseudomembrane formation. The diagnosis is readily confirmed by assay of the stool for *C. difficile* toxin and by sigmoidoscopy to visualize the characteristic pseudomembranes. Oral vancomycin is effective in eliminating the toxin-producing organism. Oral metronidazole may also be effective (and is less expensive), and oral cholestyramine has been used to bind the toxin. Relapses, associated with persistence of *C. difficile*, occur in up to 20 per cent of individuals and respond to a second course of therapy.

Parasitic Infection. *Giardia lamblia*, a protozoon that resides on the mucosal surface in the proximal small bowel, usually causes acute, self-limited, watery diarrhea. It is spread via contaminated water and may infect travelers, particularly in the Rocky and Sierra Nevada Mountains. Chronic infection may cause malabsorption. *Entamoeba histolytica*, another water- or food-borne parasite, resides in the colon, where it may invade the mucosal wall, producing inflammation, characteristic undermined ulcers, and bleeding, a picture that may resemble idiopathic ulcerative colitis. Another complication of *E. histolytica* is hepatic abscess (see Chapter 47). Other parasitic diarrheas are rare in the United States; however, *Strongyloides stercoralis* may occur in travelers.

Sexually Transmitted Diarrheal Diseases. Acute diarrhea is encountered as a sexually transmitted disease, often in homosexual males, and may be due to infection with one or more organisms, including *Campylobacter*, *Shigella*, *Chlamydia*, herpes, gonococci, *E. histolytica*, *Salmonella*, *Giardia*, and cryptosporidium. Indeed, 40 per cent of male homosexuals harbor gastrointestinal pathogens. These patients often present with proctitis (herpes, gonococci), colitis, or enteritis. The evaluation of these patients usually requires careful inspection of the perianal area for uclers (herpes, syphilis), anoscopy and sigmoidoscopy to evaluate the extent and severity of rectal and colonic mucosal disease, smears for Gram's stain (gonococci), culture and examination of smears or stool specimens for bacteria or ova and parasites, and VDRL serology. Those in whom anoscopy is normal and fecal leukocytes are absent but who have complaints of diarrhea, bloating, and abdominal cramps should be considered to have small bowel infection or enteritis.

Enteric protozoan infections should be looked for, especially *Giardia lamblia*. Since multiple pathogens are often present, an extensive evaluation should be undertaken and all identified pathogens treated. Homosexual men are also frequently colonized with nonpathogenic parasites (such as *Entamoeba nana*), which do not require therapy.

Food Poisoning. Food poisoning is defined as a set of clinical syndromes resulting from the ingestion of food that is contaminated either with (1) bacteria or their toxins, (2) poisonous chemicals, or (3) poisonous plants or animals. Although some types of food poisoning are recognizable by their unique extraintestinal manifestations, others are only identifiable if they occur in outbreaks where a number of individuals develop a similar illness. The most common types of food poisoning are summarized in Table 36–12.

Bacterial food poisoning may be due to ingestion of preformed toxin, such as the heat-stable toxins of *Clostridium botulinum*, *Staphylococcus aureus*, and *Bacillus cereus*. *C. botulinum* is an anaerobic organism that produces a neurotoxin in improperly canned foods (see Chapter 92). *S. aureus* and *B. cereus* grow in cooked food that is inadequately cooled. Other types of bacterial food poisoning result from infection with live organisms or spores (*Clostridium perfringens* and *Vibrio parahaemolyticus*). The bacterial food poisonings are generally short, self-limited illnesses that often end about the time the patient seeks medical help. Therapy is supportive and symptomatic, the primary goal being to restore extracellular fluid volume, with parenteral fluids if necessary. Antibiotics are usually not indicated. In protracted cases of *V. parahaemolyticus* infection, treatment with tetracycline or ampicillin may shorten the illness.

REFERENCES

Field M, Fordtran JS, and Schultz SG (eds): Secretory Diarrhea. Bethesda, MD, American Physiological Society, 1980.
Fordtran JS: Diarrhea. In Wyngaarden JB, and Smith LH Jr: Cecil Textbook of Medicine. 17th ed. Philadelphia, WB Saunders Co, 1985, pp 712–719.
Horowitz MA: Specific diagnosis of food bourne disease. Gastroenterology 73:375, 1977.
Krejs GJ, and Fordtran JS: Diarrhea. In Sleisenger MH, and Fordtran JS (eds): Gastrointestinal Disease. 3rd ed. Philadelphia, WB Saunders Co, 1983, pp 257–279.

E. JAUNDICE

DEFINITION

The term jaundice or icterus describes the yellow pigmentation of skin, sclerae, and mucous membranes produced by increased serum bilirubin (hyperbilirubinemia). Because jaundice is the most colorful and often the earliest sign of a variety of liver and biliary diseases, it has become a starting point for evaluating many of these disorders. Normal serum bilirubin concentrations range from 0.5 to 1.0 mg/dl. Jaundice usually becomes clinically evident at levels exceeding 2.5

mg/dl and is most readily detected in the sclerae and mucous membranes.

BILIRUBIN METABOLISM

About 4 mg/kg of bilirubin is produced each day, mainly (80 to 85 per cent) derived from the catabolism of the hemoglobin heme group of senescent red blood cells. The heme group is cleaved in the reticuloendothelial system to form biliverdin, which in turn is oxidized to bilirubin, a water-insoluble, linear tetrapyrrole (Fig. 36–5). A smaller proportion of bilirubin (15 to 20 per cent) is derived from the destruction of maturing erythroid cells in the bone marrow (ineffective erythropoiesis) and from the heme groups of predominantly hepatic hemoproteins such as cytochrome P-450 and cytochrome c.

Bilirubin liberated into the plasma is transported to the liver bound tightly but reversibly to albumin. Three phases of hepatic bilirubin metabolism are recognized: (1) uptake, (2) conjugation, and (3) excretion into the bile, the last step

FIGURE 36–6. Pathway of bilirubin (BR) movement across the liver cell. Bilirubin dissociates from albumin in the space of Disse and diffuses across the plasma membrane (uptake). Once inside the cell, bilirubin is bound to cytoplasmic acceptor proteins and is transported to the endoplasmic reticulum (E.R.), where it undergoes conjugation with glucuronic acid. Conjugated bilirubin is then secreted into the bile canaliculus.

being overall rate-limiting (Fig. 36–6). Uptake is reversible and follows dissociation of bilirubin from albumin. Unconjugated bilirubin is insoluble in water and is virtually incapable of being excreted in bile. This apolar molecule, however, dissolves in lipid-rich environments and readily traverses the blood-brain barrier and placenta.

The major physiological process for rendering bilirubin water-soluble, and hence capable of being excreted in the aqueous bile, is its conjugation with the sugar glucuronic acid. Mono- and diglucuronides of bilirubin are formed in the hepatic endoplasmic reticulum catalyzed by the enzyme UDP-glucuronyl transferase. If the biliary excretion of conjugated bilirubin is impaired, the pigment from hepatocytes regurgitates into plasma. Conjugated bilirubin is both water-soluble and less tightly bound to albumin than unconjugated pigment, so that it is readily filtered by the glomerulus and appears in the urine when plasma levels are increased. Unconjugated bilirubin is not excreted in urine. With sustained conjugated hyperbilirubinemia (e.g., obstructive jaundice), a proportion of the conjugated bilirubin becomes covalently bound to albumin and is therefore unavailable for renal or biliary excretion.

Conjugated bilirubin excreted in the bile is not reabsorbed by the intestine but is converted by bacterial action in the gut to colorless tetrapyrroles termed urobilinogens. Up to 20 per cent of urobilinogen is reabsorbed and undergoes an enterohepatic circulation, a proportion being excreted in the urine. Thus, both impaired hepato-

FIGURE 36–5. Formation of bilirubin from heme.

cellular excretion and marked overproduction of bilirubin lead to increased appearance of urobilinogen in the urine.

LABORATORY TESTS FOR BILIRUBIN

The van den Bergh reaction is the most commonly used test for bilirubin in biological fluids. When carried out in an aqueous medium, the test shows a colored reaction only with water-soluble bilirubin derivatives (called the *direct* van den Bergh fraction). The addition of methanol enables a colored reaction to take place with water-insoluble bilirubin (called the indirect van den Bergh fraction). Direct and indirect van den Bergh fractions provide clinically useful estimations of conjugated and unconjugated bilirubin, respectively, but the correlation is only a rough approximation in that levels of conjugated bilirubin are overestimated by the direct reaction. Normal plasma actually contains only unconjugated bilirubin.

Qualitative estimation of bilirubin in urine is carried out with Ictotest tablets or dipsticks, which are positive in cases of conjugated hyperbilirubinemia.

CLINICAL CLASSIFICATION OF JAUNDICE

A logical first step in the study of a jaundiced patient is to determine whether there is an unconjugated or a conjugated hyperbilirubinemia. This question is usually easily resolved by testing the urine for bilirubin. If positive, conjugated hyperbilirubinemia is present and is confirmed by finding greater than 50 per cent conjugated bilirubin on serum testing.

Classification of jaundice according to this distinction is shown in Table 36–13. Mechanisms contributing to predominantly unconjugated hyperbilirubinemia include (1) overproduction, (2) decreased hepatic uptake, and (3) decreased conjugation. Conjugated hyperbilirubinemia implies either (1) a defect in hepatocellular secretion of bilirubin or (2) mechanical obstruction to the major extrahepatic bile ducts. Apart from hemolysis and rare conditions, such as Crigler-Najjar syndrome (decreased or absent conjugation) and Dubin-Johnson syndrome (defective hepatocellular excretion of bilirubin), defects in the pathway of bilirubin production to excretion leading to jaundice are more likely to be multiple than isolated ones. For example, the jaundice occurring in patients with hepatocellular disease (i.e., hepatitis, cirrhosis) may result from a combination of diminished red cell survival and impairment of all three stages of hepatocellular bilirubin transport and metabolism.

Unconjugated Hyperbilirubinemia

Overproduction. Hemolysis from a variety of causes may lead to bilirubin production sufficient to exceed the clearing capacity of the liver with subsequent development of jaundice. This *hemolytic jaundice* is characteristically mild; serum bilirubin levels rarely exceed 5 mg/dl. Up to 15 per cent of the serum bilirubin may be direct-reacting, a phenomenon that mainly reflects an artifact of the van den Bergh reaction. Ineffective erythropoiesis, which may be substantially increased in megaloblastic anemias, may also lead to mild jaundice.

Impaired Hepatic Uptake. Impaired uptake is very rarely encountered as an isolated cause for clinical jaundice, but may play a role in the mild jaundice following administration of radiographic contrast media (competition for bilirubin uptake) and in Gilbert's syndrome (see below).

Impaired Conjugation. A genetically determined decrease or absence of UDP-glucuronyltransferase is encountered in the Crigler-Najjar syndrome, whereas mild, acquired defects in the enzyme may be produced by drugs (e.g., chloramphenicol).

Neonatal Jaundice. All steps of hepatic bilirubin metabolism are incompletely developed in the neonatal period, while increased production is also present. The major defect is in conjugation, however, leading to unconjugated hyperbilirubinemia between the second and fifth days of life. When increased production of bilirubin occurs in the neonatal period, usually as a result of hemolytic disease secondary to blood-group incompatibility, severe unconjugated hyperbilirubinemia may occur, carrying the risk of neurological damage (kernicterus).

Gilbert's Syndrome. This very common disorder affects up to 7 per cent of the population, with a marked male predominance. It commonly manifests during the second or third decade of life as a mild unconjugated hyperbilirubinemia, exacerbated by fasting, and noted clinically or as an incidental laboratory finding. The mechanism appears to involve increased production, diminished uptake, and defective conjugation of bilirubin to varying proportions in different individuals. Nonspecific gastrointestinal symptoms and fatigue are commonly associated, but this condition is entirely benign. The diagnosis is strongly suggested by unconjugated hyperbilirubinemia with normal hepatic enzymes and the absence of overt hemolysis. Liver biopsy is always normal and is rarely, if ever, indicated to confirm the diagnosis.

Conjugated Hyperbilirubinemia

Determining the cause of unconjugated hyperbilirubinemia rarely poses difficulty. Usually, the major difficulty in evaluating jaundice is encountered in differentiating an intrahepatic excretion defect from obstruction in a patient with predominantly conjugated hyperbilirubinemia. This clinical situation is often described as *cholestatic jaundice*, and the approach to its differential diagnosis is discussed in detail below.

Cholestasis implies that, clinically and biochemically, there is impairment of bile formation or flow. Typically, a patient with cholestatic jaundice has predominantly conjugated hyperbilirubinemia and an elevated alkaline phosphatase, usually to at least three to four times normal. When prolonged, cholestasis may lead to hypercholesterolemia, fat and fat-soluble vitamin malabsorption, and retention of bile salts, which may lead to pruritus. Biochemical evidence of liver cell damage (elevated transaminases, prolonged prothrombin time uncorrected by administration of vitamin K) may be minimal or marked, depending upon the cause of the cholestasis. An important corollary is that all the features of cholestasis may be present in some patients *without* jaundice.

Impaired Hepatic Excretion. This pathogenetic category of jaundice, also called intrahepatic cholestasis, is applied to all disorders in the transport of conjugated bilirubin from the hepatocyte up to the radiologically visible bile ducts. Thus it includes a wide range of conditions from drug-induced cholestasis (impaired canalicular transport) to primary biliary cirrhosis (destruction of the small intrahepatic bile ductules). The following are some important causes of intrahepatic cholestasis.

DRUG-INDUCED CHOLESTASIS. Typical cholestatic jaundice may be produced by phenothiazines, oral contraceptives, and methyltestosterone. Eosinophilia may accompany drug-induced jaundice.

SEPSIS. Systemic sepsis, mainly due to gram-negative organisms, may produce a predominantly conjugated hyperbilirubinemia, usually accompanied by mild elevation of serum alkaline phosphatase levels.

POST-OPERATIVE JAUNDICE. This increasingly recognized syndrome has an incidence of 15 per cent following heart surgery and 1 per cent following elective abdominal surgery. Occurring one to ten days postoperatively, the jaundice is multifactorial in origin but predominantly of the conjugated variety with increased alkaline phosphatase and minimally abnormal transaminases.

HEPATOCELLULAR DISEASE. Hepatocellular disease (i.e., hepatitis and cirrhosis) from a variety of causes (see Chapters 44 and 46) may result in a typical cholestatic jaundice. Evidence of hepatocellular damage and dysfunction is usually prominent and includes marked elevation of transaminases, prolonged prothrombin time, hypoalbuminemia, and clinical features of hepatic dysfunction (see Chapter 45). In hepatocellular disease there is interference with all three steps of hepatic bilirubin metabolism. Excretion, the rate-limiting step, is usually the most profoundly disturbed, leading to a predominantly conjugated hyperbilirubinemia. Jaundice may be profound in acute hepatitis (see Chapter 44) without prognostic implications. On the contrary, in chronic liver disease, jaundice is a sign that usually implies severe decompensation of hepatic function with a poor prognosis.

Extrahepatic Biliary Obstruction. Complete or partial obstruction of the extrahepatic bile ducts

TABLE 36–13. CLASSIFICATION OF JAUNDICE

Predominantly Unconjugated Hyperbilirubinemia
  Overproduction
    Hemolysis (spherocytosis, autoimmune, etc.)
    Ineffective erythropoiesis (e.g., megaloblastic anemias)
  Decreased hepatic uptake
    Gilbert's syndrome
    Drugs (e.g., flavaspidic acid, radiographic contrast agents)
    Sepsis
  Decreased conjugation
    Gilbert's syndrome
    Crigler-Najjar syndrome types I and II
    Neonatal jaundice
    Hepatocellular disease
    Sepsis
    Drug inhibition (e.g., chloramphenicol)
Predominantly Conjugated Hyperbilirubinemia
  Impaired hepatic excretion
    Familial disorders (Dubin-Johnson syndrome, Rotor syndrome, benign recurrent cholestasis, cholestasis of pregnancy)
    Hepatocellular disease
    Drug-induced cholestasis
    Primary biliary cirrhosis
    Sepsis
    Postoperative
  Extrahepatic ("mechanical") biliary obstruction
    Gallstones
    Tumors of head of pancreas
    Tumors of bile ducts
    Tumors of ampulla of Vater
    Biliary strictures (post-cholecystectomy, primary sclerosing cholangitis)
    Congenital disorders (biliary atresia, Caroli's syndrome)

may result from a variety of causes, including impaction of gallstones, carcinoma of the head of the pancreas, tumors of the bile ducts, bile duct strictures, and chronic pancreatitis with bile duct compression. In complete obstruction, conjugated hyperbilirubinemia is prominent and usually plateaus at 30 to 40 mg/dl in the absence of renal failure, hepatocellular damage, or infection within the bile ducts, all of which may antedate or develop during the course of mechanical obstruction. Stools may become clay colored as a result of the failure of bile to enter the intestine. In partial obstruction, jaundice may be mild or even absent, becoming prominent when infection of the ducts complicates the obstruction.

APPROACH TO THE DIAGNOSIS OF JAUNDICE

A careful history and physical examination are of paramount importance in obtaining clues to the nature and cause of jaundice. A history of darkened urine invariably implies a conjugated hyperbilirubinemia, while pale stools and pruritus suggest a cholestatic process. An inquiry into drugs, alcohol, exposure to jaundiced persons (drug or viral hepatitis), recurrent abdominal pain and nausea (gallstones), epigastric pain radiating into the back accompanied by weight loss and a distended gallbladder (carcinoma of the head of the pancreas), and pre-existing liver disease will

FIGURE 36–7. Approach to the patient with cholestatic jaundice. The algorithm demonstrates the systematic consideration of the available diagnostic options.

often go far in delineating the probable cause for the jaundice. Routine laboratory tests are helpful in that serum transaminases are usually less than 10- to 15-fold elevated in patients with bile duct obstruction, while alkaline phosphatase levels are usually greater than two to three times normal. Conversely, a greater than 10- to 15-fold elevation of serum transaminases indicates hepatocellular disease. Serological tests for hepatitis may be helpful (see Chapter 43), whereas autoantibodies, if strongly positive, may be of diagnostic value, e.g., the antimitochondrial antibody in primary biliary cirrhosis.

Clinical evaluation and routine laboratory tests serve to identify the cause of jaundice in up to 85 per cent of cases. More sophisticated diagnostic procedures are often needed, however, to determine the cause, especially whether the cholestatic jaundice in a given patient is intrahepatic or due to extrahepatic obstruction.

A diagnostic approach to this question is illustrated in Figure 36–7. If extrahepatic obstruction is suspected, it is necessary to determine first by noninvasive means whether or not the major bile ducts are dilated. Dilatation of the ducts occurs when a mechanical obstruction is present, but is absent in cases of intrahepatic cholestasis. Either ultrasound or CT scanning may be used to determine the caliber of bile ducts, the former generally preferred because of lesser cost and absence of radiation. Additional definitive clues, such as the

presence of stones in the common duct or gallbladder, may be obtained as well. However, both imaging techniques may give rise to false-positive and false-negative results in a small number of patients and cannot be regarded as truly definitive. Thus, in a patient with cholestatic jaundice, the absence of dilated ducts on ultrasound might not dissuade the clinician from proceeding to cholangiography if the suspicion of extrahepatic obstruction based on clinical evaluation is high. If dilated ducts are found on noninvasive imaging, direct cholangiography provides the most reliable approach to nonoperative diagnosis of cholestatic jaundice. This may be accomplished by either percutaneous puncture of the intrahepatic biliary tree with a thin needle (percutaneous transhepatic cholangiography) or by means of endoscopic retrograde cholangiography. The percutaneous route is simpler technically, has a success rate of close to 100 per cent in the presence of dilated ducts, is less expensive, and is thus the procedure of choice when dilated ducts are found on noninvasive imaging. The endoscopic route, although more demanding both technically and in terms of time and cost, is of value in demonstrating duct pathology when the bile ducts are not dilated (in which case the percutaneous route may often fail) or when associated pancreatic disease is present. It may also permit direct biopsy of lesions at the ampulla of Vater and sphincterotomy and stone extraction in appropriate instances.

Liver biopsy may be indicated when an intrahepatic cause for cholestasis is strongly suspected on clinical grounds or when extrahepatic obstruction is ruled out by definitive cholangiography. Liver histology itself is often a poor guide to whether cholestasis is intra- or extrahepatic. The decision to perform a biopsy thus will rest on the certainty with which extrahepatic obstruction has been excluded in a patient with cholestasis and on the clinical course of the disease. Thus, for example, in a patient with cholestatic jaundice in whom recent ingestion of chlorpromazine is documented and in whom the jaundice is beginning to resolve following cessation of the drug, the best course may be to observe without further investigation.

REFERENCES

Blanckaert N, and Schmid R: Physiology and pathophysiology of bilirubin metabolism. In Zakim D, and Boyer TD (eds): Hepatology: A Textbook of Liver Disease. Philadelphia, WB Saunders Co, 1982, pp 246–284.

Scharschmidt BF: Bilirubin metabolism and hyperbilirubinemia. In Wyngaarden JB, and Smith LH Jr (eds): Cecil Textbook of Medicine. 17th ed. Philadelphia, WB Saunders Co, 1985, pp 806–812.

Scharschmidt BF, Goldberg HI, and Schmid R: Approach to the patient with cholestatic jaundice. N Engl J Med 308:1515–1519, 1983.

RADIOGRAPHIC AND ENDOSCOPIC PROCEDURES IN GASTROENTEROLOGY

Over the past few years a wide variety of techniques have been introduced in radiology for the detection of disease in the gastrointestinal tract. There has been a concomitant explosion of new endoscopic techniques designed to address many of the same diagnostic (and therapeutic) problems. Indeed, often the most difficult task for the physician is selecting the most appropriate procedure(s) to use in each clinical setting. This chapter will review briefly the various radiographic and endoscopic procedures currently available and their optimal use.

RADIOGRAPHIC PROCEDURES

Table 37–1 summarizes the radiographic procedures in general use.

Plain Radiographs and Barium Contrast Studies

Plain radiographs of the abdomen in the supine and upright or lateral decubitus positions are simple to obtain and relatively inexpensive; unfortunately, they provide information of value in only a few select circumstances. They are highly sensitive for clinical entities that involve abnormal gas patterns such as bowel obstruction, perforation of a hollow organ (free intraperitoneal air), and infections with gas-forming organisms (emphysematous cholecystitis) and are usually the first test obtained when these entities are considered. Plain films are also useful in detecting intra-abdominal calcifications such as gallbladder or renal stones or pancreatic calcifications in chronic alcoholic pancreatitis.

Contrast studies using barium sulfate (or occasionally the water-soluble iodinated contrast agent Gastrografin) provide more information about the anatomy of the tubular gastrointestinal tract. Single-contrast studies are performed using a bolus of contrast material and generally detect mass lesions but frequently miss small or mucosal lesions. Double-contrast studies, in which barium is administered first followed by a radiolucent substance such as air to produce a thin layer of barium coating the mucosa, are better able to detect all types of lesions, including those confined to the mucosa.

Single- and double-contrast barium swallows detect esophageal strictures and masses, and double-contrast studies may detect lesions of the mucosa such as ulcerations or varices. Endoscopy, which may miss submucosal mass lesions, is much more sensitive for mucosal lesions. Use of fluoroscopy during a barium swallow, particularly when combined with cine or video recordings, allows evaluation of esophageal motility disorders.

The standard single- or double-contrast examination of the upper gastrointestinal tract (upper GI series) is widely used to detect gastric mass lesions, gastric ulcers, and duodenal ulcers. Major changes in gastric motility can be evaluated using fluoroscopy, and markedly reduced motility may provide the first clue to a submucosal gastric cancer, a disease often difficult to detect by endoscopy. Most gastric ulcers (benign and malignant) are visualized radiographically; however, it is not possible to identify correctly all malignant ulcers on the basis of their radiographic appearance, so that biopsy is generally recommended. Double-contrast upper GI examinations may detect mucosal disorders such as erosive gastritis, Mallory-Weiss tears, stress ulcers, and anastomotic ulcers; however, endoscopy is more sensitive for such lesions. Overall, in the initial evaluation of common clinical problems such as dysphagia and epigastric pain, the upper GI series remains a primary diagnostic imaging test.

Satisfactory radiographic examination of the small bowel is more difficult to achieve owing to pooling and dilution of barium during passage through the small bowel and to obscuring of bowel segments by overlapping loops. The standard small bowel series can evaluate the caliber of the small bowel and provide some information regarding bowel mucosa, wall thickness, and fluid transit time, particularly in the proximal bowel. Mass lesions, obstructions, and fistulas are usually detected. An improved view of the entire small bowel can be obtained by performing a small bowel enema (enteroclysis) in which barium, followed by radiolucent methylcellulose solution, is delivered directly into the jejunum via an orogastric tube. A small bowel series is generally utilized when evaluating malabsorption, inflammatory bowel disease, or bowel obstruction. Endoscopic techniques to visualize the small bowel beyond the C-loop of the duodenum are not available.

Single- and double- (pneumocolon) contrast (or "air-contrast") radiographs of the colon have long been the standard for identifying lesions in the colon. With the use of pneumocolon, radiographic detection of even subtle lesions such as polyps and early inflammatory bowel disease is excellent, although generally colonoscopy detects more lesions and allows a more thorough examination of the rectum. Therefore, the choice of double-contrast barium enema or colonoscopy to evaluate patients with occult fecal blood, suspected inflammatory bowel disease, a tumor, diarrhea, or obstruction often depends upon the need

TABLE 37–1. RADIOGRAPHIC AND ENDOSCOPIC PROCEDURES

PROCEDURE	ADVANTAGES	DISADVANTAGES	COST*
Plain film of the abdomen	Identifies gas, calcifications	Few specific features	$119–166
Barium swallow	Shows mass lesions and motility disorders well	Misses many superficial mucosal lesions	$179
Double-contrast barium examination of the upper gastrointestinal tract ("UGI series")	Delineates ulcers and tumors well	Misses some superficial mucosal lesions Misclassifies 9-17% of malignant gastric ulcers	$246
Small bowel series	Simple to perform Evaluates transit time, caliber, proximal mucosa and often shows mass lesions	May miss distal or subtle lesions	$176
Enteroclysis (small bowel enema)	Improved definition of mucosa and bowel wall of entire small bowel	Requires peroral intubation	$204
Double-contrast barium enema ("pneumocolon")	Shows polyps, tumors, fistulas, diverticula and other structural changes (e.g., inflammatory bowel disease) well	Uncomfortable for some patients Impossible in those with lax anal sphincter May miss superficial mucosal lesions and rectal lesions Misses angiodysplastic lesions	$279
Oral cholecystography	Outlines most gallstones May delineate tumors or polyps	Will not visualize gallbladder in jaundiced patients and often fails to visualize the inflamed gallbladder	$117
Percutaneous transhepatic cholangiography	Excellent definition of intrahepatic bile ducts Option for therapeutic intervention	Extrahepatic bile ducts may not be well visualized Nondilated ducts may be missed	$461
Angiography	Demonstration of acutely bleeding lesions Definition of vascularity of mass lesions	Invasive Large contrast load Bleeding lesions visualized only if blood loss exceeds 0.5 ml/min	$1066–2050
Ultrasound	Real-time examination Best for fluid-filled lesions and gallstones	Gas obscures examination Bowel poorly visualized	$120–262
Computed tomography	Excellent anatomical definition Density changes may indicate nature of diffuse parenchymal disease	Expensive Radiation exposure Bowel poorly visualized	$639–954
Liver-spleen scan	Demonstrates mass lesions > 1-2 cm in size Increased bone marrow uptake suggests portal hypertension	Limited anatomical definition	$326
^{99m}Tc-HIDA liver scan	Best test for cystic duct obstruction	Will not visualize if bilirubin > 6 mg/dl Poor anatomical definition	$333
^{99m}Tc-RBC scan	Approximate localization of intermittently bleeding lesion	Poor anatomical definition	$470
Esophagogastroduodenoscopy	Direct visualization of upper gastrointestinal tract. Identifies virtually all mucosal lesions. Permits biopsy, electrocautery	Expensive Invasive May miss motility and compressive lesions	$584
Colonoscopy	Direct visualization of large bowel. Permits biopsy and polypectomy, electrocautery and laser treatment of bleeding	Expensive Invasive Higher rate of complications than barium enema	$948
Endoscopic retrograde cholangiopancreatography	Only method for visualizing pancreatic ducts. Permits biopsy of ampullary lesions and sphincterotomy for common duct stones	Requires considerable skill Expensive	$1109

* Costs are those charged at the University of California, San Francisco, in 1984.

for tissue for histological examination and the availability, cost, and comfort of the procedure.

The studies discussed thus far are usually performed using barium sulfate as the contrast agent. Water-soluble iodinated compounds, which pro- duce images of lesser quality and are more expensive, are generally used only when a perforation is suspected (as barium is toxic when it escapes into body cavities) or when a colonic obstruction is suspected (barium caught above a colonic obstruction will dehydrate and possibly worsen the obstruction, whereas the water-soluble agents will not).

Ultrasound and Computed Tomography

Ultrasound (US) and computed tomography (CT) markedly extend the diagnostic capacity of the radiologist far beyond that which was possible with barium studies alone. Indeed, organs such as the pancreas, which were previously radiologically invisible, are now readily imaged. The information provided by US and CT is complementary to that provided by barium studies: US and CT are most useful in examining the solid abdominal organs (liver, spleen, pancreas, kidney, retroperitoneal lymph nodes) and gallbladder, whereas barium studies excel in depicting the tubular gastrointestinal tract. Table 37-2 outlines the relative merits of US and CT.

Ultrasound, which employs high-frequency sound waves rather than x-rays, allows the examination of solid and fluid-filled structures noninvasively. Air or gas obscures the ultrasound beam; thus, structures under gas-filled loops of bowel cannot be visualized. US requires great skill on the part of the operator; however, real-time images allow examination of dynamic as well as static processes. Images, like those of CT, are displayed in cross-section. US has the ability (1) to detect abdominal masses as small as 2 cm in diameter, particularly in the right and left upper quadrants and pelvis; (2) to differentiate fluid-filled cysts from solid masses; (3) to identify gallstones rapidly and more efficiently than is possible with oral cholecystography or CT; (4) to identify dilated bile ducts; and (5) to detect ascites and some vascular abnormalities such as abdominal aortic aneurysms.

Computed tomography uses multiple x-ray beams and detectors in conjunction with computer analysis to identify and display small differences in tissue density. Anatomical definition is more precise with CT than with US and imaging quality is not affected by bowel gas, but the equipment is very expensive. CT is primarily used for the detection of mass lesions (tumors, cysts, abscesses), although it also detects dilated bile ducts, pancreatic inflammation, and some gallstones. Some diffuse hepatic parenchymal lesions that alter liver density, such as fatty liver or hemochromatosis, can also be identified by CT. Finally CT is better than US in detecting retroperitoneal lesions and parenchymal processes such as ruptures or hematomas of the liver, spleen, and kidney.

Both US and CT also offer the option of performing guided thin needle aspiration of lesions virtually anywhere in the abdomen to obtain cells or fluid for cytological examination and culture.

Radionuclide Imaging

Improvements in radiopharmaceuticals and imaging devices have resulted in new techniques that are of value in selected circumstances. The

TABLE 37–2. COMPARISON OF ULTRASOUND AND COMPUTED TOMOGRAPHY

	ULTRASOUND	COMPUTED TOMOGRAPHY
Organs best visualized	Kidney Gallbladder Liver and bile ducts Pancreas Spleen Blood vessels	Liver and dilated bile ducts Retroperitoneal lymph nodes Gallbladder Spleen Pancreas Kidney Pelvic organs
Lesions best visualized	Fluid-filled masses/cysts Gallstones Dilated bile ducts Aortic aneurysms Pancreatic tumor Ascites	Tumors/cysts/abscesses Mass lesions Fatty liver Hepatic iron overload (hemochromatosis) Trauma or parenchymal hematoma of liver, spleen, and kidney
Advantages	Real-time examination Noninvasive Guided needle aspiration	Less dependent upon a skilled operator Guided needle aspiration
Disadvantages	Skilled operator necessary Gas obscures deeper organs	Radiation exposure Absence of fat makes examination more difficult
Cost	$262	$954

traditional liver-spleen scan, using ^{99m}Tc-sulfur colloid that undergoes phagocytosis by reticuloendothelial cells, has largely been supplanted by US or CT but is still useful in the evaluation of benign hepatic neoplasms (see Chapter 48) and, when combined with a lung scan, subphrenic abscesses. Newer agents, such as ^{99m}Tc-HIDA, which are taken up by hepatic parenchymal cells and excreted in bile, outline the shape of the liver and are useful in the evaluation of acute cholecystitis (see Chapter 49) or of biliary atresia in infants. In general, they are not useful in other biliary tract disorders, as anatomical definition is poor. The affinity of ^{99m}Tc-pertechnetate for gastric mucosa makes this agent useful for the detection of Meckel's diverticula, 85 per cent of which contain ectopic gastric mucosa. Finally, ^{99m}Tc-labeled red blood cells have been used in some centers to detect the site of bleeding in patients with slow and/or intermittent gastrointestinal hemorrhage.

Visceral Angiography

Specially trained radiologists are now able to introduce catheters into virtually any artery or vein and, by injecting contrast agents, to visualize the vasculature of most organs. Because angiography is an invasive procedure with a small but significant morbidity, angiography is generally reserved for the detection of vascular tumors (e.g., hepatoma, angioma, angiosarcoma) and acutely bleeding lesions of the gastrointestinal tract, particularly of the colon or small bowel, that cannot be visualized endoscopically. Angiography also offers the option to treat bleeding by intra-arterial infusion of vasopressin or occlusion of bleeding vessels.

Magnetic Resonance Imaging (MRI)

Cross-sectional images of the body can also be obtained without x-ray by the use of a magnetic field and radiofrequency radiation combined with computer analysis. Current detectors, available in only a few centers, detect protons and thus display organs by their chemical composition rather than x-ray density. MRI may offer better resolution than CT and also offers the opportunity to follow in situ chemical reactions. The equipment is even more expensive than that used for CT, however, and the role of MRI in clinical medicine is not yet established.

Visualization of the Biliary Tree

Oral cholecystography (OCG), the time-honored method for imaging the gallbladder, involves the oral administration of an iodinated compound, which is concentrated in the gallbladder, followed 12 hours later by a radiograph of the gallbladder. The technique identifies most gallstones in patients with a functioning gallbladder. However, in many patients with chronic cholecystitis, and in all patients with a serum bilirubin greater than 2 mg/dl, the gallbladder will not opacify. US is more sensitive (> 98 per cent verus 90 per cent) in detecting gallstones and is replacing the OCG in many centers.

Bile ducts and disorders involving them are well seen only when contrast material is used to fill them. Contrast may be injected into the biliary tree from the upstream side via a thin (23-gauge) needle introduced percutaneously into the hepatic parenchyma (percutaneous transhepatic cholangiogram, PTC) or from below via a small catheter placed endoscopically into the papilla of Vater (endoscopic retrograde cholangiopancreatography, ERCP, see page 289). Table 37–3 compares these two procedures, both of which provide an excellent view of the biliary tree, although PTC is generally preferred for intrahepatic bile duct lesions and ERCP for extrahepatic duct lesions.

ENDOSCOPIC PROCEDURES

Endoscopic examination of the gastrointestinal (GI) tract was first achieved using rigid, multi-lensed instruments that were difficult to use, permitted limited visualization, and were often traumatic to the patient. The development of fiberoptic instruments has revolutionized gastrointestinal endoscopy and hence the management of many gastrointestinal disorders. Currently, a wide range of instruments is available, some tailor-made for specialized applications. The modern fiberoptic endoscope provides a true extension of the eyes and hands of the physician. These instruments combine wide-angle visualization of the GI tract with flexibility and ability to

control the movement of the tip of the scope up to 360 degrees, as well as good patient tolerance.

Most endoscopes include multipurpose channels for passage of air and water, as well as for aspirating fluid out of the GI tract. They also permit the passage of a number of instruments, including cytology brushes, biopsy forceps, injection needles, electrocautery snares, wire baskets, electrocautery, and laser probes.

As discussed earlier, endoscopy has certain distinct advantages over barium contrast radiological examination of the GI tract: (1) It has greater sensitivity for mucosal lesions often missed by barium studies. (2) Endoscopy allows greater diagnostic specificity in certain situations. For example, in a patient with gastrointestinal hemorrhage, a lesion identified by barium contrast radiology will not necessarily be responsible for the bleeding. This uncertainty is eliminated by the direct visualization of actively bleeding lesions permitted by endoscopy. (3) Endoscopy permits biopsy or cytology of lesions at the time of visualization. (4) Endoscopy combines therapeutic capabilities with direct visualization of the gastrointestinal tract, e.g., enabling injection of bleeding esophageal varices at the time of diagnosis. Endoscopy carries the two disadvantages of higher cost (upper gastrointestinal endoscopy costs over $500 as opposed to $246 for an upper GI series—see Table 37–1), and higher patient morbidity and mortality, although the latter is extremely small for nontherapeutic endoscopy (0.001 per cent). Endoscopy is also often inferior to radiology in identifying submucosal or compressive lesions of the gastrointestinal tract as well as disorders of esophageal motility.

Whether endoscopic or radiological examination should be undertaken as a first procedure depends upon the clinical problem (e.g., acute bleeding versus abdominal pain), the range of likely diagnoses, the possible need for therapeutic intervention, and cost factors, as well as the fact that radiological and endoscopic techniques are often complementary to one another in obtaining a diagnosis.

Endoscopic examination is generally performed under sedation with parenteral diazepam and meperidine, with topical anesthetic spray applied to the pharynx for upper endoscopy

Esophagogastroduodenoscopy

Visualization of the GI tract up to the duodenum is also referred to as upper GI endoscopy or panendoscopy. Major indications are diagnosis of suspected upper GI hemorrhage and upper GI malignancy. Endoscopy is the diagnostic procedure of first choice in virtually all instances of upper GI hemorrhage (see Chapter 36B); even when bleeding is brisk, responsible lesions are readily visualized by experienced endoscopists. Endoscopic biopsy and cytology yield a diagnostic accuracy for upper GI cancer of close to 100 per cent, although accuracy is less in submucosal and/or infiltrative lesions. Other indications include investigation of some cases of abdominal

TABLE 37-3.   COMPARISON OF PERCUTANEOUS TRANSHEPATIC CHOLANGIOGRAPHY AND ENDOSCOPIC RETROGRADE CHOLANGIOPANCREATOGRAPHY

	PERCUTANEOUS TRANSHEPATIC CHOLANGIOGRAPHY	ENDOSCOPIC RETROGRADE CHOLANGIOPANCREATOGRAPHY
Lesions best visualized	Intrahepatic ductal lesions Multiple lesions in a single duct system Several punctures may be made to examine ducts in all lobes	Extrahepatic ductal lesions Pancreatic duct Ampulla of Vater
Therapeutic implications	Temporary external drainage of bile Placement of stents through bile duct obstructions Balloon dilation of biliary stricture	Sphincterotomy for removal of common duct stones Placement of stents Biopsy of ampullary lesions

Success rate
  dilated ducts
  nondilated ducts
	
	100%
	60-80%
		
		75-80%
		75-80%

Disadvantages	Experienced operator required May miss additional lesions in left lobe	Experienced operator required May not visualize ducts proximal to a lesion
Complications	Bleeding Biliary infection/sepsis	Pancreatitis Biliary infection/sepsis Bile duct perforation

pain, esophageal symptoms, removal of foreign bodies, and injection of varices.

Endoscopic "Retrograde" Cholangiopancreatography (ERCP)

Cannulation of the ampulla of Vater is carried out using a special side-viewing endoscope. This is technically the most difficult endoscopic examination to perform. Once cannulation is achieved, selective intubation of the pancreatic and common bile ducts is undertaken followed by injection of a radiographic contrast medium. Radiographs are taken of the contrast-outlined ducts. Indications for ERCP include the diagnosis of pancreatic cancer, investigation of obstructive jaundice, placement of biliary stents, and performance of endoscopic sphincterotomy. In obstructive jaundice, ERCP is preferred to percutaneous cholangiography if duct dilatation is absent, if there is associated pancreatic or duodenal pathology, or if a coagulation defect is present. Detailed comparison of ERCP with percutaneous cholangiography is given in Table 37-3.

Endoscopic sphincterotomy entails an electrocautery incision into the duodenal papilla and is used to release retained common duct gallstones in patients who have already undergone cholecystectomy (and who would otherwise require a second operation) and in those patients considered poor surgical risks. The morbidity rate from sphincterotomy is 8 per cent, and the mortality rate is 1 per cent.

Sigmoidoscopy and Colonoscopy

Both rigid and flexible fiberoptic sigmoidoscopes are employed in clinical practice. Rigid sigmoidoscopy is a rapid, inexpensive procedure, but it is less well tolerated by the patient and permits less extensive examination of the rectosigmoid area. Sigmoidoscopy is commonly used to evaluate the cause of bloody diarrhea and to look for neoplastic disease of the rectosigmoid area. When the rectosigmoid area is involved, sigmoidoscopic biopsy will often suffice in making the diagnosis of inflammatory bowel disease without the need for colonoscopy. Colonoscopy enables visualization of the entire colon to the level of the cecum and is optimally employed in conjunction with barium contrast studies of the colon. Indications for colonoscopy include investigation of suspected colonic neoplastic disease, surveillance for the development of malignancy in ulcerative colitis and polyposis syndromes, and diagnosis and evaluation of the extent of inflammatory bowel disease.

Removal of colonic polyps for bleeding or to exclude malignancy is an important therapeutic application of colonoscopy. Colonoscopy has little use in patients with acute lower gastrointestinal bleeding, as considerable blood within the relatively narrow confines of the colon tends to completely obscure vision (see Chapter 36B). Angiography is usually preferable in this situation.

Laparoscopy

Laparoscopy is a procedure occasionally used in gastroenterology. Its major value is in permitting biopsy under direct vision of suspected metastatic tumor nodules on the hepatic or peritoneal surface.

REFERENCES

Berk RN: Diagnostic imaging procedures in gastroenterology. In Wyngaarden JB, and Smith LH Jr (eds): Cecil Textbook of Medicine. 17th ed. Philadelphia, WB Saunders Co, 1985, pp 650–658.

Berk RN, Ferrucci JT, Fordtran JS, et al: The radiological diagnosis of gallbladder disease, an imaging symposium. Radiology 141:49, 1982.

Federle MP, and Goldbert HI: Conventional radiography of the alimentary tract. In Sleisenger MH, and Fordtran JS (eds): Gastrointestinal Disease: Pathophysiology,

Diagnosis and Management. 3rd ed. Philadelphia, WB Saunders Co, 1983, pp 1634–1667.

Mueller PR, Harbin WP, Ferrucci JT, et al: Fine needle transhepatic cholangiography: Reflections after 450 cases. Am J Roentgenol 136:85, 1981.

Pykett IL: NMR imaging in medicine. Sci Am 246:78, 1982.

Sherlock P: Gastrointestinal endoscopy. In Wyngaarden JB, and Smith LH Jr (eds): Cecil Textbook of Medicine.

17th ed. Philadelphia, WB Saunders Co, 1985, pp 658–662.

Sleisenger MH, and Fordtran JS (eds): Gastrointestinal Disease: Pathophysiology, Diagnosis and Management. 3rd ed. Philadelphia, WB Saunders Co, 1983, pp 1599–1634.

Wittenberg J: Computed tomography of the body. N Engl J Med 309:1160, 1983.

38 DISEASES OF THE ESOPHAGUS

Although the esophagus appears to be a simple organ, esophageal disease is common and ranges from trivial complaints of heartburn to major clinical problems of aspiration, obstruction, and hemorrhage. This chapter will briefly outline normal esophageal function and describe a group of unique symptoms characteristic of most esophageal disorders. The major benign categories of esophageal disorders, gastroesophageal reflux disease and motility disorders, will be discussed with a brief review of other common esophageal diseases. Malignant disease of the esophagus will be discussed in Chapter 41.

NORMAL ESOPHAGEAL PHYSIOLOGY

The esophagus serves a single function: conveying solids and liquids from the mouth to the stomach while preventing aspiration and movement of gastric contents in the opposite direction (gastroesophageal reflux). Swallowing is a complex and well-coordinated motor activity that includes (1) movement of a food bolus into the pharynx concomitant with protection of the airway, (2) relaxation of the upper esophageal sphincter, (3) initiation and distal propagation of peristaltic contractions by the esophageal muscle, and (4) re-laxation of the lower esophageal sphincter. After passage of the food bolus, the lower esophageal sphincter re-establishes a tonic contraction, thereby preventing regurgitation of gastric contents.

CLINICAL SYMPTOMS OF ESOPHAGEAL DISEASE

Dysphagia, the sensation that a food bolus arrests ("sticks") during swallowing, indicates esophageal disease, and the patient can often indicate the exact site. Dysphagia may be due to motility disorders or to narrowing of the esophageal lumen by benign or malignant disease (Table 38–1). A motility disorder is more likely if dysphagia occurs with both liquids and solids, or if the patient can force the bolus down by altering posture, performing a Valsalva maneuver, or repeated swallowing.

Heartburn (pyrosis), a common esophageal symptom, is a burning pain that radiates up behind the sternum. It is due to reflux of acidic gastric contents into the esophagus. It is often relieved by antacids, is precipitated by bending over or lying down, and may be accompanied by regurgitation of sour- or bitter-tasting material. Nocturnal reflux and regurgitation may present as recurrent aspiration pneumonia, wheezing, or hoarseness.

Odynophagia, or pain on swallowing, is usually associated with esophageal obstruction or mucosal disease such as reflux esophagitis, radiation-induced damage, or infection by viral or fungal agents.

Severe substernal chest pain that is often indistinguishable from angina pectoris may result from abnormal esophageal motor function, such as diffuse esophageal spasm.

GASTROESOPHAGEAL REFLUX DISEASE

Definition. Gastroesophageal reflux disease (GERD) refers to a spectrum of clinical manifes-

TABLE 38–1. ETIOLOGY OF DYSPHAGIA

TYPE	EXAMPLE
Esophageal motility disorder	Achalasia
	Aperistalsis (scleroderma)
	Diffuse esophageal spasm
Luminal narrowing	Inflammatory disease (reflux, *Candida* infection)
	Extrinsic compression (mediastinal mass, aberrant artery, cardiac enlargement)
	Malignant tumor (squamous cell or adenocarcinoma)
	Benign stricture (reflux, lye ingestion)
	Benign tumor (leiomyoma)
	Esophageal web

tations due to reflux of stomach and duodenal contents into the esophagus. (See Chapter 39 for a general discussion of acid-peptic disease.)

Etiology and Pathogenesis. The esophagus is normally protected from prolonged exposure to acid, pepsin, bile acids, and pancreatic enzymes by three mechanisms: (1) the antireflux barrier provided by tonic contraction of the lower esophageal sphincter, (2) rapid clearance of refluxed material via secondary peristalsis, and (3) alkalinization of acidic material by swallowed saliva. Patients with symptomatic GERD usually exhibit one or more of the following: decreased or absent tone in the lower esophageal sphincter, inappropriate relaxation of the lower esophageal sphincter unassociated with swallowing, and decreased acid clearance due to impaired secondary peristalsis. Other factors such as abnormal saliva and reflux of bile salts and pancreatic enzymes may be implicated in some patients.

Clinical Manifestations. Heartburn, ranging in degree from mild to severe, is the most common symptom of GERD and is often associated with regurgitation of acidic material. Aspiration pneumonia, nocturnal wheezing, and hoarseness may be seen in patients with frequent regurgitation, occasionally in the absence of heartburn. Dysphagia, bleeding from esophageal erosions, and stricture formation also occur. Smoking, alcohol or caffeine intake, and pregnancy, all of which decrease lower esophageal sphincter tone, may precipitate or exacerbate GERD.

Diagnosis. The diagnosis of GERD is best made based on the history and clinical manifestations. Objective tests are useful to quantify the extent and severity of disease and to address three questions: (1) Does reflux exist? (2) Is acid reflux responsible for the patient's symptoms? (3) Has reflux led to esophageal damage? Reflux may be demonstrated during a barium swallow or by a radionuclide scintiscan after placement of ^{99}Tc-sulfur colloid in the stomach. Esophageal manometry is useful to demonstrate abnormal peristalsis and lower esophageal sphincter tone but will not show reflux per se. More sensitive tests for the presence of acid reflux include monitoring esophageal pH with a luminal pH probe for periods of 30 minutes to 24 hours either after instillation of HCl in the stomach (Tuttle test) or under near-physiological conditions. The presence of reflux per se does not necessarily mean that reflux is responsible for the patient's symptoms. If chest pain is not typical of heartburn, the Bernstein test may be performed to determine whether acid, but not saline, dripped into the esophagus via a nasogastric tube reproduces the patient's symptoms. Finally, symptoms due to acid reflux do not always correlate with the extent of damage to the esophageal mucosa. Severe esophageal damage, such as a stricture or deep ulcer, can be assessed by barium swallow. However, endoscopy with suction biopsy is the most sensitive test for reflux-induced mucosal damage, which ranges from increased epithelial turnover and mild polymorphonuclear infiltration to frank ulceration. A few

patients will exhibit Barrett's esophagus, the presence of gastric columnar epithelium in the esophagus, which indicates severe chronic reflux and a greater risk of malignant transformation.

Treatment and Prognosis. Medical management of GERD is successful in all but the most severe cases, and, as outlined in Table 38-2, consists of maneuvers designed to decrease reflux and administration of antacids or H_2-receptor blockers to decrease acid secretion. Chronic therapy may be necessary in patients with severe reflux. Surgical management, which is reserved for those few patients with objective evidence of reflux who fail to respond to an adequate trial of medical management, attempts to restore lower esophageal sphincter function by wrapping the lower esophagus with a cuff of gastric fundal muscle. These procedures are often successful but cannot be performed in patients with aperistalsis (e.g., scleroderma), who may have severe GERD.

Complications. GERD complications include esophageal (peptic) stricture, esophageal ulcer, Barrett's esophagus, pulmonary aspiration, and upper gastrointestinal hemorrhage.

MOTOR DISORDERS OF THE ESOPHAGUS

Definition and Pathogenesis. Motility disorders may arise from disease of smooth muscle (scleroderma) or of the intrinsic nervous system (achalasia, Chagas' disease). In achalasia, degeneration of the ganglion cells in Auerbach's plexus leads to increased tone and impaired relaxation of the lower esophageal sphincter, which is often associated with decreased peristalsis. The etiology of other motility disorders, such as diffuse esophageal spasm, is uncertain.

Clinical Manifestations. The three most common motility disorders are achalasia, scleroderma, and diffuse esophageal spasm, each of which exhibits a unique pattern of symptoms (Table 38-3).

Diagnosis. The clinical history is often characteristic, and a cine esophagogram (Fig. 38-1) combined with esophageal manometric studies

TABLE 38–2. TREATMENT OF GASTROESOPHAGEAL REFLUX DISEASE

Simple Measures
1. Elevation of the head of the bed
2. Avoidance of food or liquids before bedtime
3. Liquid antacid (aluminum hydroxide–magnesium hydroxide), 30 ml one hour and three hours after meals and at bedtime
4. Avoidance of cigarettes, alcohol
5. Weight loss

Measures for Resistant Cases
1. H_2-receptor blockers (cimetidine 300 mg four times a day or ranitidine 150 mg twice a day)
2. Bethanechol (urecholine) 10 or 15 mg four times a day
3. Alginic acid-antacid (Gaviscon) 15 ml four times a day
4. Antireflux surgery (Nissen fundoplication, Hill repair, Belsey repair)

ACHALASIA NORMAL DIFFUSE ESOPHAGEAL SPASM

FIGURE 38–1. Radiological appearance of achalasia (*left*) and diffuse esophageal spasm (*right*). In achalasia the esophageal body is dilated and terminates in a narrowed segment or "bird beak." The appearance of numerous simultaneous contractions is typical of diffuse esophageal spasm. (Courtesy of Drs. FE Templeton and CA Rohrmann. From Pope CE II: In Sleisenger MH, and Fordtran JS (eds): Gastrointestinal Disease. 3rd ed. Philadelphia, WB Saunders Co, 1983.)

(Table 38–3) will confirm the diagnosis in most cases.

Treatment and Prognosis. Achalasia often responds to brisk dilation of the lower esophageal sphincter with a pneumatic bag, a procedure thought to rupture some of the sphincter muscle fibers. Surgical myotomy (Heller procedure) may be beneficial for those few who do not respond to pneumatic dilation. Therapy for scleroderma includes chronic treatment of GERD with H_2 blockers or antacids (see Table 38–2). Patients with diffuse esophageal spasm may respond to nitroglycerin, anticholinergic agents, or calcium-channel blocking drugs, although results are often disappointing. Occasionally, good long-term results have been obtained from a longitudinal myotomy.

OTHER ESOPHAGEAL DISORDERS

Tumors. Carcinoma of the esophagus is discussed in Chapter 41. Benign neoplasms (leiomyoma, lipoma, papilloma, and fibrovascular polyps) are very rare and usually are asymptomatic or present as dysphagia.

Rings and Webs. Congenital rings and webs may occur in the proximal or distal (Schatzki's ring) esophagus. The Plummer-Vinson syndrome consists of an upper esophageal web, dysphagia, and iron-deficiency anemia. Most rings and webs are asymptomatic or may present as intermittent dysphagia for a bolus of meat. They can be disrupted mechanically with peroral dilators.

Esophageal Injury. Caustic ingestion causes severe esophageal injury leading to necrosis and eventual stricture formation. Steroids and broad-spectrum antibiotics are often used to treat caustic injuries, although their efficacy is uncertain. Strictures often respond to peroral dilation.

Trauma. Vomiting may lead to mucosal (Mallory-Weiss) or full-thickness (Boerhaave's syndrome) tears of the lower esophagus. Mallory-Weiss tears usually occur just below the gastroesophageal junction. They often present with hemorrhage and will heal spontaneously. Esophageal rupture often occurs just above the gastroesophageal junction into the mediastinum and requires immediate diagnosis and surgical repair.

Infection. Esophageal infection with *Candida* or *Herpesvirus* can occur, particularly in the immunosuppressed host, often with severe mucosal inflammation and ulceration. Severe odynophagia is a common symptom and dysphagia may occur. Diagnosis is best made by endoscopic visualization and biopsy.

TABLE 38–3. ESOPHAGEAL MOTOR DISORDERS

	ACHALASIA	SCLERODERMA	DIFFUSE ESOPHAGEAL SPASM
Symptoms	Dysphagia Bolus often passes with time or various maneuvers	Gastroesophageal reflux disease Dysphagia	Substernal chest pain (angina-like) Dysphagia with pain
X-ray appearance	Dilated, fluid-filled esophagus Distal "bird beak" stricture	Aperistaltic esophagus Free reflux Peptic stricture	Simultaneous noncoordinated contractions
Manometric findings			
Lower esophageal sphincter	High resting pressure No or incomplete relaxation with swallow	Low resting pressure	Normal pressure
Body	Low amplitude, simultaneous contractions after swallow	Low amplitude peristaltic contractions or no peristalsis	Some peristalsis Diffuse and simultaneous nonperistaltic contractions, often of high amplitude

REFERENCES

Pope CE II: Diseases of the esophagus. In Wyngaarden JB, and Smith LH Jr (eds): Cecil Textbook of Medicine. 17th ed. Philadelphia, WB Saunders Co, 1985, pp 667–677.

Richter JE, and Castell DO: Gastroesophageal reflux. Ann Intern Med 97:93, 1982.
Vantrappen G, Janssens J, Hellemans J, and Coremans G: Achalasia, diffuse esophageal spasm and related motility disorders. Gastroenterology 76:450, 1979.

ACID-PEPTIC DISEASE

39

The normal stomach can secrete H^+ at 1000 times its concentration in extracellular fluid in association with potent proteolytic enzymes. It is not surprising, therefore, that gastric juice is fully capable of injuring the host as well as digesting components of the diet. Acid-peptic disease, which refers nonspecifically to disorders associated with such injury, includes peptic ulcer of the duodenum and stomach (and rarely of the jejunum or of a Meckel's diverticulum), some forms of gastritis, and reflux esophagitis. The latter entity has been discussed in Chapter 38.

NORMAL GASTRIC PHYSIOLOGY

The stomach serves as a reservoir in which ingested food is churned and fragmented into small particles prior to its timed release into the duodenum. Beyond these important mechanical functions, the stomach also initiates the processes of digestion by the secretion of HCl and pepsinogen, which in the presence of HCl is rapidly converted to proteolytic pepsin. Acid-peptic disease occurs when there is an imbalance between the processes of secretion and the normal processes of defense against chemical self-injury.

Normal Secretion. HCl is secreted by the parietal cells and pepsinogen by the chief cells, both found in the gastric mucosa, predominantly in the body and fundus of the stomach. These two agents are secreted in parallel; no condition is known in which there is selective secretion of either HCl or pepsinogen. Three endogenous chemicals stimulate the secretion of acid: gastrin, histamine, and acetylcholine (Fig. 39–1). Acetylcholine is released locally from vagal (cholinergic) nerve terminals in the stomach, stimulated by stretch reflexes within the stomach or by the cephalic phase of gastric secretion. Gastrin is released from "G cells" in the antrum of the stomach and in the duodenum, stimulated largely by the products of protein digestion and by alkalinization. It circu-

FIGURE 39–1. The parietal cell with three receptors, histamine, gastrin, and acetylcholine. All act to stimulate a potassium-hydrogen ATPase (the hydrogen pump at the luminal side of the cell). However, the characteristics of each compound differ enough to suggest that each compound acts at a different receptor. Histamine causes increases in intracellular adenylcyclase and cyclic AMP, which in turn activate or increase the amount of the potassium-hydrogen ATPase. Cholinergic drugs and gastrin cause influx of Ca^{++}, which in turn activates the potassium-hydrogen ATPase. (From Deveney CW: The stomach. In Smith LH Jr, and Thier SO (eds): Pathophysiology: The Biological Principles of Disease. 2nd ed. Philadelphia, W.B Saunders Co, 1985.

Parietal Cell

$*^A_C$ = Adenylcyclase

FIGURE 39–2. Model illustrating mechanisms maintaining mucosal integrity. Superficial epithelial cells secrete mucus and bicarbonate that aid in maintaining a pH gradient between lumen and mucosa and protect the underlying epithelial cells from damage by acid and pepsin. Mucosal blood flow is also believed to be a mechanism important in maintaining mucosal integrity. (From Richardson CT: Peptic ulcer: Pathogenesis. In Wyngaarden JB, and Smith LH Jr (eds): Cecil Textbook of Medicine. 17th ed. Philadelphia, WB Saunders Co, 1985, p 682.)

lates as a hormone before acting on the parietal cell. Histamine is found in mastlike cells in the gastric wall in close proximity to the chief cells. The role and control of local histamine release are unknown, but histamine and its structural analogues are powerful gastric secretagogues when administered systemically, and the use of H_2-receptor antagonists markedly inhibits HCl (and pepsinogen) secretion by the stomach. There is also evidence of a nongastrin gut-derived secretagogue stimulated by the products of protein digestion, but its structure has not been defined. The interaction of these various agents at the final common parietal cell pathway for acid secretion is unclear. In brief, gastric secretion seems to result largely from the cephalic phase (via the vagus), the gastric phase (stretch stimulation of the vagus; protein and alkalinization stimulation of gastrin release), and the intestinal phase (further release of gastrin and of the nongastrin secretagogue). Secretion of pepsinogen seems to be controlled through acetylcholine and possibly the other described mechanisms as well.

Basal secretion of acid averages about 1.0 to 2.0 mEq per hour in men but less in women. The normal range, however, varies widely from 0 to 10.5 mEq per hour for men and from 0 to 5.6 mEq per hour for women. When maximally stimulated with a secretagogue—usually betazole (a histamine analogue) or pentagastrin—the secretory rate may rise as high as 50 mEq per hour for men and 30 mEq per hour for women. The ratio of basal to maximal acid output (MAO) is sometimes determined in the study of patients with suspected abnormal secretory drives.

Normal Defense. The stomach and the duodenum have developed several defense mechanisms to protect the mucosa from the acid-pepsin mix of gastric juice (Fig. 39–2). A thin coating of mucus is continuously formed and spreads out protectively over the mucosal cells. This diminishes the exposure of these cells to luminal gastric juice. The surface apical cells secrete bicarbonate within and under the mucin layer, which serves to neutralize the H^+ that diffuses back from the lumen. The epithelial cells are constantly being shed and renewed so that damaged cells are replaced. Prostaglandins may play a role in stimulating all of these repair mechanisms, including an increase in mucosal blood flow. As a result the average individual can secrete more than 100 mmol of HCl daily throughout life without significant mucosal injury.

PEPTIC ULCER DISEASE OF THE STOMACH AND DUODENUM

For convenience peptic ulcer of the stomach and duodenum will be discussed together, although there are a number of differences that will warrant comment.

Incidence. Peptic ulcers are very common causes of morbidity but rare causes of death. As many as one fourth of men and one sixth of women develop a peptic ulcer sometime during life, as judged by typical scars at autopsy, but far fewer (5 to 10 per cent) develop symptomatic ulcers during life. Furthermore, the incidence seems to be declining in the United States. Duodenal ulcers are more frequent than gastric ulcers; men have a higher incidence of duodenal ulcers but the same incidence of gastric ulcers when compared to women.

Pathogenesis. Peptic ulcers are presumed to represent some breakdown in the balance of acid-pepsin secretion and the relevant mucosal defense mechanisms (Fig. 39–2). The mechanisms involved may be multifactorial for a given individual and certainly are so in different patients with peptic ulcers. Patients with duodenal ulcer tend as a group to have increased basal and maximal acid output rates of HCl secretion, but there is a large overlap with normal controls, and patients with gastric ulcers usually have normal or even reduced rates of acid secretion. Basal levels of serum gastrin are normal with duodenal ulcers, but the level tends to rise excessively following a protein meal. The acid response to graded doses of gastrin or pentagastrin also tends to be enhanced, thought possibly to represent a greater number of gastric parietal cells. Overall the evidence of hyperacidity as the cause of duodenal ulcer is marginal, and for gastric ulcer it is nonexistent.

Genetic factors seem to be important in some patients with peptic ulcer. There is an increased incidence in first-degree relatives of patients with duodenal ulcers and a positive association with high levels of serum pepsinogen I, which appears to be inherited as a dominant trait and may reflect total chief cell mass. There are weaker associations with blood group O and with HLA-B5. Familial gastrinomas will be discussed later.

There is a strong association of peptic ulcer with cigarette smoking, possibly due to diminished bicarbonate secretion by the pancreas for duodenal ulcers and to diminished pyloric sphincter tone with reflux for gastric ulcers. Furthermore, peptic ulcer has been reported to be increased in uremia, chronic obstructive pulmonary disease, alcoholic cirrhosis, hyperparathyroidism (hypercalcemia), mastocytosis (histamine), cluster headaches (Horton's cephalgia), and polycythemia vera. The use of nonsteroidal anti-inflammatory agents definitely increases the incidence of superficial gastric mucosal erosions, but the possible role of these agents, and of glucocorticoids, in the pathogenesis of chronic peptic ulcers is more controversial. Reflux of bile and pancreatic juice from the duodenum through an incompetent pyloric sphincter has been postulated to play a role in some cases of gastric ulcer. The possible role of psychological factors is unclear, but emotional distress may increase gastric secretion.

Clinical Manifestations. The cardinal manifestation of peptic ulcer is epigastric pain that is relieved by the ingestion of food or antacids. The pain, frequently described as burning or gnawing, most typically occurs one to three hours after eating. This is related to gastric emptying, when the continuing secretion of gastric acid is unbuffered and presumably produces pain by direct irritation of nerve endings in the ulcer or, as some think, by inducing spasm. The pain tends to occur in clusters, perhaps over several weeks, with sub-

sequent periods of remission of varying duration. The pain of peptic ulcer may be atypical in location, in character, and in its relationship to meals. It may also be absent despite the presence of an active peptic ulcer demonstrated radiographically or endoscopically.

In addition to pain, patients with peptic ulcer tend to have a variety of symptoms that can be best summarized as "dyspepsia"—bloating, nausea, anorexia, excessive eructations, and epigastric discomfort. Not infrequently patients present with one of the complications of peptic ulcer.

In the absence of complications, the physical examination is rarely of help in the diagnosis of peptic ulcer disease. Most frequently there is a moderate amount of epigastric tenderness. The physical examination may give evidence of one of the diseases associated with ulcer diathesis as noted above.

Complications. Complications are not infrequent in peptic ulcer disease. It has been estimated that as many as one third of patients in whom the diagnosis is made in life will have one or sometimes more than one of these complications during the course of illness. These complications are also the main indications for surgery for peptic ulcer disease, to be discussed subsequently.

Bleeding from peptic ulcer disease, the most common cause of upper gastrointestinal bleeding, occurs in about 10 to 15 per cent of patients. It may be the first manifestation of the disease, and carries an overall mortality rate of about 7 per cent. Death from peptic ulcer bleeding is more likely to occur in older patients (above age 60), in those with other illnesses, with gastric ulcers, or with severe and recurrent bleeding (> 3 units of blood required per day), and when there is an exposed bleeding vessel in the ulcer visualized endoscopically. The approach to the patient with upper gastrointestinal bleeding is described in Chapter 36B. In approximately 85 per cent of patients, bleeding from peptic ulcer disease will stop under medical therapy; about 15 per cent of patients require emergency surgery. This usually consists of ligation of a bleeding vessel for duodenal ulcer together with a truncal vagotomy and a gastric antrectomy or pyloroplasty. Distal gastrectomy is usually indicated for emergency surgery for gastric ulcer in the distal stomach and biopsy, ligation of bleeding vessels, and distal gastrectomy for more proximal ulcers. Patients who have bled once from a peptic ulcer have an increased chance of bleeding again (30 to 50 per cent chance).

Perforation occurs when a peptic ulcer has eroded through the entire wall of the duodenum or stomach. Sometimes this leads to penetration of an adjacent organ such as the pancreas, with resulting pancreatitis and intractable pain. More frequently, especially with anterior duodenal ulcers and lesser curvature gastric ulcers, there is free perforation into the peritoneal cavity. This complication occurs in 5 to 10 per cent of patients with duodenal ulcers and 2 to 5 per cent with gastric ulcers of sufficient severity to be diagnosed during life. Not infrequently there is associated hemorrhage. Rarely perforation is the first symptom of a peptic ulcer; more frequently the patient has a long history of more typical symptoms. The presentation is typically that of an acute abdomen with the sudden onset of severe abdominal pain, peritoneal signs (abdominal muscle rigidity, rebound tenderness), and hypotension with tachycardia. Free air in the abdominal cavity can usually be demonstrated by an upright radiograph. In most patients with free perforation, emergency surgery is indicated to repair the site and to wash out the peritoneal cavity. Depending upon the state of the patient, more definitive surgery (truncal or selective vagotomy and antrectomy, for example) may be carried out at the same operation. In some poor-risk patients the perforation is allowed to seal spontaneously while the patient is maintained on nasogastric suction, fluids, and antibiotics.

Obstruction of the gastric outlet may be caused by the inflammation, spasm, and fibrosis induced by an ulcer. This complication is most frequent in ulcers involving the pyloric channel. The symptoms are usually those of early satiety, nausea, vomiting after eating, epigastric pain, and fullness. On physical examination the patient may present with a succussion splash and signs of dehydration. Laboratory studies may show metabolic alkalosis and hypokalemia. Most patients with this complication, which occurs in about 5 per cent of patients diagnosed as having peptic ulcer, have had long-standing clinical illness. It is very unusual for this complication to be the initial presentation. Obstruction can be readily demonstrated by a positive saline load test (> 400 ml of gastric juice recovered 30 minutes after instilling 750 ml of saline by nasogastric tube into an empty stomach). This test may not be necessary if there is 200 ml of gastric juice in the stomach after an overnight fast. The obstruction can be directly demonstrated by endoscopy or indirectly by an upper GI series. An attempt should be made to treat all patients with gastric outlet obstruction initially by medical means—nasogastric tube drainage, repair of fluid and electrolyte deficits, cimetidine or ranitidine (to reduce HCl loss by the drainage), and parenteral nutrition. At least half of patients so treated, presumably those in whom spasm and edema are of particular importance, will respond to this therapy over several days and can be spared surgical therapy.

Intractable pain as a complication of a peptic ulcer is fortunately rare if the patient is compliant with a treatment regimen. When present it may represent penetration posteriorly or into an adjacent viscus.

Diagnosis. The diagnosis of a peptic ulcer can be established only by the demonstration of the ulcer by direct inspection endoscopically (the most sensitive and specific method) or indirectly by radiographic studies (an upper GI series). An upper GI series is usually the first screening study because it is usually much less expensive than

endoscopy and less difficult for the patient. If no ulcer is found radiographically, however, and the suspicion of peptic ulcer is still high, endoscopic examination may still be indicated, since as many as one fifth of such ulcers may be missed by an upper GI series. If a gastric ulcer is found radiographically, it is imperative to demonstrate that it is benign rather than malignant. A number of findings make a malignant ulcer more or less likely (age of the patient, location and size of the ulcer, the topography of the mucosal folds around the ulcer, the presence or absence of achlorhydria), but this can be established with acceptable clinical accuracy only by inspection and biopsy of the lesion endoscopically. Some physicians supplement this approach by cytological examinations.

When the presence of a typical peptic ulcer has been established radiographically or endoscopically, other studies are rarely indicated, since the pathogenesis of these lesions is still obscure in most cases. In only a few clinical situations is the measurement of serum gastrin or of the basal and peak acid outputs of the stomach indicated (Table 39–1), primarily for the suspicion of a gastrinoma (to be discussed subsequently).

In addition to the occasional need to rule out a gastrinoma, after the presence of a peptic ulcer has been demonstrated, the nonspecific symptoms of peptic ulcer must be differentiated from those of functional dyspepsia, gastric cancer, biliary tract disease, pancreatitis, and a wide variety of other abdominal disorders.

Treatment. Most patients with peptic ulcer can be treated successfully by medical methods. Surgery is usually required only for the complications of the disease noted above: bleeding, perforation, gastric outlet obstruction, and intractable pain. In addition to the specific measures to be described, all patients with peptic ulcer disease should be advised to reduce markedly or discontinue cigarette smoking, to drink alcohol only in moderation, and to limit the use of nonsteroidal anti-inflammatory agents. Although diet was once considered to be of great importance in the treat-

TABLE 39–1. CLINICAL SITUATIONS IN WHICH MEASUREMENT OF SERUM GASTRIN LEVELS IS INDICATED

Family history of peptic ulcer
Ulcer associated with hypercalcemia or other manifestations of multiple endocrine neoplasia Type I
Multifocal peptic ulcer
Peptic ulceration of postbulbar duodenum or jejunum
Peptic ulceration associated with diarrhea*
Chronic unexplained diarrhea*
Enlarged gastric folds on upper GI x-ray
Before surgery for "intractable" ulcer
Recurrent ulcer after ulcer surgery

* Not due to antacid ingestion. (From Schiller LR: Peptic ulcer: Epidemiology, clinical manifestations, and diagnosis. In Wyngaarden JB, and Smith LH Jr (eds): Cecil Textbook of Medicine. 17th ed. Philadelphia, WB Saunders Co, 1985, p 687.)

ment of peptic ulcer, there is no good evidence that changes in diet influence the rate of healing. Patients are best advised simply to avoid foods that in their personal experience lead to dyspeptic symptoms and to limit eating between meals and at bedtime, since eating during that time may further enhance gastric secretion.

Medical management of peptic ulcer is in general directed either toward reducing the concentration of gastric acid or toward reducing mucosal damage from acid-pepsin exposure.

REDUCTION OF GASTRIC ACID. A number of agents can reduce substantially the rate of secretion of acid by acting at various sites in the normal or hyperstimulated parietal cell (Fig. 39–3). Of these agents only the H_2-receptor antagonists are being currently used as primary therapy in the United States. Cimetidine (in a usual dose of 300 mg four times daily) or ranitidine (150 mg twice daily) is highly effective in blocking the secretion of HCl. Cimetidine in its usual doses may cause confusion in some older patients, especially in the presence of renal insufficiency, and sometimes has an antiandrogenic effect characterized by gynecomastia and impotence. It may also inhibit the metabolism of certain other drugs by the liver as an important example of drug interaction. Ranitidine is thought to be less likely to cause mental symptoms in susceptible patients, is not antiandrogenic, and inhibits the metabolism of other drugs less markedly. The substituted benzimidazoles show considerable promise but have not as yet come into general use.

The concentration of gastric acid can be reduced not only by inhibiting its secretion but also by neutralizing it intraluminally with antacids. The antacids more frequently used contain magnesium and/or aluminum hydroxide as their main ingredient. Calcium-containing antacids are no longer in favor because of the effect of ionized calcium in stimulating the secretion of gastrin, and sodium-containing antacids are generally too brief in their effectiveness and often add too much sodium to the diet with the danger of edema, hypertension, or metabolic alkalosis. The aluminum- and magnesium-containing antacids have comparatively few side effects (constipation for Al, diarrhea for Mg, the potential for phosphate depletion due to its enteric trapping), but they are often inconvenient to the patient. In general 15 to 30 ml of the liquid antacid should be taken one and three hours after meals and also at bedtime.

IMPROVEMENT OF MUCOSAL DEFENSE. Mucosal defense is a general concept that covers many aspects of susceptibility that cannot be readily measured, as can the secretion and concentration of HCl. Only one drug is widely used currently in the United States for this purpose, sucralfate. This agent, an aluminum hydroxide salt of sucrose that has been modified by sulfation, is unabsorbed following its usual dose of 1 gram four times daily. Its mechanism of action is unclear, but it is thought to adhere to and protect the surface of the ulcer as an artificial mucin and may also locally stimulate prostaglandin synthesis. Exogenous

FIGURE 39–3. Sites of action of four drugs employed to inhibit acid secretion. (From Peterson WL: Peptic ulcer: Medical therapy. In Wyngaarden JB, and Smith LH Jr (eds): Cecil Textbook of Medicine. 17th ed. Philadelphia, WB Saunders Co, 1985, p 688.)

prostaglandins may also be useful in this mechanism of treatment in the future.

The four main first-line agents—cimetidine, ranitidine, antacids, and sucralfate—have been roughly equally effective in bringing about the healing of peptic ulcer, and all tend to be more effective with duodenal than with gastric ulcer. It has been shown that ranitidine given as a single 300-mg dose at bedtime is as effective as the other less convenient regimens. Treatment for four to six weeks will be associated with healing in approximately 90 per cent of patients. Treatment is then discontinued unless symptoms recur.

If this initial approach to treatment of a duodenal ulcer is not successful, care should be taken to assure that the patient is compliant and that an unhealed ulcer is actually present endoscopically. Other doses or combinations of the above agents can then be tried. True intractability, or the development of a complication, may then indicate the need for surgery.

A gastric ulcer requires special consideration because of the danger of carcinoma and should be carefully followed until healing. If healing does not occur on one of the above regimens by eight weeks, it is usually advisable to carry out endoscopy again with further biopsies and cytological studies. If they prove negative, a trial of another eight weeks on a different regimen may be indicated prior to the consideration of elective surgery.

The indications for long-term maintenance therapy are not certain. In many patients with primary healing and without complications, treatment can be discontinued. In those who are considered at high risk for recurrence or who have had complications of peptic ulcer disease, long-term therapy is probably indicated (Fig. 39–4).

SURGICAL MANAGEMENT. Surgery for peptic ulcer is indicated usually for complications of the disease and when medical management has failed. The surgical procedures most frequently employed are shown in Figure 39–5. In various combinations they are devised to decrease acid secretion by re-

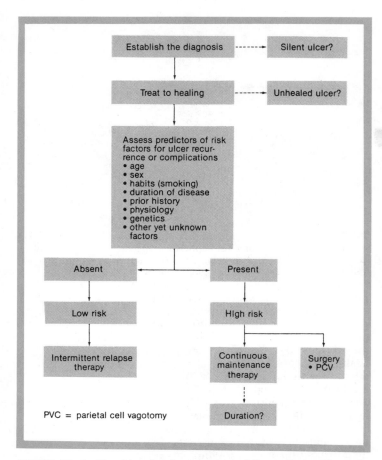

FIGURE 39—4. Algorithm for the treatment of the patient with peptic ulcer disease. (From Van Deventer GM: Approaches to the long-term treatment of duodenal ulcer disease. Am J Med 77(5B):15, 1984.)

ducing the cephalic phase of gastric secretion (vagotomy) or the gastric phase of gastric secretion (antrectomy to remove a major source of gastrin). Various drainage procedures are then employed to maintain gastric emptying in the postvagotomy state. Increasingly proximal ("superselective") vagotomy rather than truncal vagotomy is being employed to reduce acid secretion more selectively without the adverse effects on gastric motility and emptying. In patients with intractable benign gastric ulcers, vagotomy may not be required, since acid production is usually normal or low. Antrectomy or subtotal gastrectomy may be the treatment of choice.

Complications of Treatment. Although surgical treatment of peptic ulcer is usually successful in relieving symptoms and preventing recurrence and carries a low mortality rate, there are not infrequently late complications that are distressing to the patient:

THE DUMPING SYNDROME. With disruption of the normal storage function of the stomach, for which the pylorus is the gatekeeper, ingested food may be prematurely dumped in excessive amounts into the small intestine, leading to nausea, vomiting, abdominal pain, and diarrhea. These symptoms occur soon after eating. More rarely there are late symptoms (one to three hours after eating), which probably result from reactive hypoglycemia from excessive rapidity of carbohydrate absorption followed by an overshoot of insulin release.

WEIGHT LOSS. Many patients lose weight after partial gastric resection procedures. In part this is due to early satiety, but sometimes there is an associated malabsorption syndrome of complex pathogenesis (see Chapter 36C).

POSTVAGOTOMY DIARRHEA. Many patients have diarrhea after truncal vagotomy for reasons that are unclear. In a very few these symptoms may persist and be incapacitating.

AFFERENT LOOP SYNDROME. When the afferent loop formed in a Billroth II procedure (Fig. 39–5) becomes partially occluded, pancreatic and biliary secretions accumulate and cause distention and pain. This is typically followed by opening up of the obstruction to release these secretions back into the gastric remnant where they commonly cause vomiting. This complication may require reconstructive surgery.

ANEMIA. Anemia is common after reconstructive surgery for peptic ulcer and is often complex in pathogenesis—iron deficiency, vitamin B_{12} deficiency, and/or folate deficiency.

THE ZOLLINGER-ELLISON SYNDROME

The Zollinger-Ellison syndrome, usually caused by a functioning islet cell tumor that se-

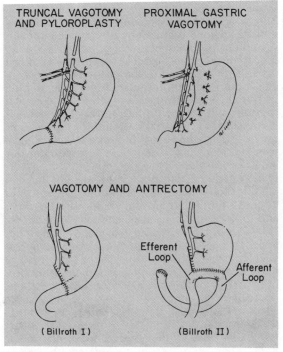

FIGURE 39—5. Model illustrating surgical procedures for peptic ulcer disease. (From Thirlby RC: Peptic ulcer: Surgical therapy. In Wyngaarden JB, and Smith LH Jr (eds): Cecil Textbook of Medicine. 17th ed. Philadelphia. WB Saunders Co, 1985, p 691.)

cretes gastrin, accounts for well under 1 per cent of clinically diagnosed peptic ulcers. The possibility of this rare entity should be considered in several circumstances: (1) ulcers in unusual locations such as the second or third portions of the duodenum or the jejunum, (2) unusually severe peptic ulcer disease that is refractory to treatment or that is recurrent after surgery, (3) ulcer disease accompanied by diarrhea and sometimes malabsorption (see Chapter 36), and (4) a strong family history of ulcer disease, especially if there is evidence of other endocrine tumors.

Pathogenesis. Single or often multiple gastrinomas in the pancreas, or more rarely in other abdominal but extrapancreatic sites, secrete excessive amounts of gastrin. This hormone drives acid secretion by the parietal cells as well as having a trophic effect in increasing their number (as much as three to five times). Although these tumors are slow-growing, most are histologically and biologically malignant with early metastases regionally and to the liver. In approximately one fourth of patients the gastrinoma is associated with other endocrine adenomas, most commonly in the pattern known as the multiple endocrine neoplasia Type II syndrome (MEN II) in which adenomas or hyperplasia may involve the islet cells, the parathyroid glands, the thyroid, and the pituitary.

Clinical Manifestations. The clinical manifestations are usually those of severe peptic ulcer disease as noted above. Rarely diarrhea may precede peptic ulcer formation or be a more prominent part of the symptomatology.

Diagnosis. The diagnosis of the Zollinger-Ellison syndrome is not usually difficult if it is considered. In general it depends on the demonstration of an elevation of serum gastrin in the presence of increased basal secretion of gastric acid. The diagnosis may require use of a stimulation test with pentagastrin to show that basal acid secretion is greater than 40 per cent of that under maximal stimulation.

Treatment. An attempt should be made to find and remove a resectable tumor, although this can be done in only about one quarter of patients. If not successful, patients should be treated with full doses of an H_2-receptor antagonist such as cimetidine or ranitidine.

GASTRITIS

Gastritis does not represent, strictly speaking, an acid-peptic group of diseases, but it will be discussed here for convenience, since it does reflect a breakdown in the interaction of injurious agents and mucosal defense mechanisms. Gastritis can be acute or chronic, specific or nonspecific.

Acute Gastritis. In acute gastritis there is infiltration of the lamina propria by inflammatory cells, often accompanied by superficial erosions that may be diffuse or localized. The mechanism of the mucosal injury is often unclear. Certain drugs, especially aspirin, nonsteroidal anti-inflammatory agents, and ethanol, are thought to disrupt the mucosal barrier to back-diffusion of acid and thereby to initiate chemical injury. "Stress ulcers" represent acute erosive injury to the stomach in many severe surgical or medical conditions with complicating bleeding. Stress ulcers are thought to result from ischemia, but again back-diffusion of acid may be the common final pathway of injury. Gastritis can sometimes be attributed to specific events such as irradiation, ingestion of alkali, or rarely bacterial infection (phlegmonous gastritis). Following surgery, reflux of bile salts and/or pancreatic enzymes may produce acute gastritis.

Most cases of acute gastritis are probably mild and escape diagnosis. The diagnosis is established by endoscopic examination. When present, symptoms are usually those of dyspepsia, epigastric pain, nausea, and vomiting. The most important complication of acute gastritis is that of bleeding from the superficial erosions. This usually responds to conservative management and omission of the precipitating agent if known (aspirin, alcohol). Antacids and/or cimetidine or ranitidine is often used as well but has not been shown to affect healing. The overall prognosis of acute, erosive gastritis is excellent with rapid healing of the lesions within days.

Chronic Gastritis. Chronic gastritis has been classified by the histological severity of the process (superficial, atrophic, or gastric atrophy) and by the anatomical location in the stomach where it is most manifest (Type A—fundus and body of the stomach; Type B—antrum). In most patients no pathogenesis can be firmly established, although chronic use of the same drugs implicated in acute gastritis and chronic exposure to bile salts and pancreatic enzymes are postulated to be of importance in some patients. In Type A atrophic gastritis there are usually circulating antibodies against parietal cells whether or not pernicious anemia is present; in some patients with Type B atrophic gastritis antibodies against gastrin-producing cells have been reported.

There are no definite clinical manifestations of idiopathic chronic gastritis. Patients with Type A gastritis may have pernicious anemia alone or linked with one or more other autoimmune diseases. Chronic gastritis may be associated with a higher incidence of benign gastric ulcer and gastric cancer. No specific treatment is indicated for idiopathic chronic gastritis.

REFERENCES

Feldman M: Peptic ulcer: Complications. In Wyngaarden JB, and Smith LH Jr (eds): Cecil Textbook of Medicine. 17th ed. Philadelphia, WB Saunders Co, 1985, p 693.

Grossman MI (ed): Peptic Ulcer: A Guide for the Practicing Physician. Chicago, Year Book Medical Publishers, Inc, 1981.

Jensen RT, Gardner JD, Raufman J-P, et al: Zollinger-Ellison syndrome: Current concepts and management. Ann Intern Med 98:59, 1983.

Legerton CW Jr (ed): Management of the ulcer patient, therapeutic advances. Am J Med 77(5B):1, 1984.

Peterson WL: Peptic ulcer: Medical therapy. In Wyngaarden JB, and Smith LH Jr (eds): Cecil Textbook of Medicine. 17th ed. Philadelphia, WB Saunders Co, 1985, p 688.

Richardson CT: Gastritis. In Wyngaarden JB, and Smith LH Jr (eds): Cecil Textbook of Medicine. 17th ed. Philadelphia, WB Saunders Co, 1985, p 677.

Richardson CT: Peptic ulcer: Pathogenesis. In Wyngaarden JB, and Smith LH Jr (eds): Cecil Textbook of Medicine. 17th ed. Philadelphia, WB Saunders Co, 1985, p 681.

Richardson CT: Peptic ulcer: Zollinger-Ellison syndrome. In Wyngaarden JB, and Smith LH Jr (eds): Cecil Textbook of Medicine. 17th ed. Philadelphia, WB Saunders Co, 1985, p 696.

Schiller JR: Peptic ulcer: Epidemiology, clinical manifestations, and diagnosis. In Wyngaarden JB, and Smith LH Jr (eds): Cecil Textbook of Medicine. 17th ed. Philadelphia, WB Saunders Co, 1985, p 684.

Soll AH, and Isenberg JI: Peptic ulcer diseases. In Sleisenger MH, and Fordtran JS (eds): Gastrointestinal Disease. 3rd ed. Philadelphia, WB Saunders Co, 1983, p 625.

Thirlby RC: Peptic ulcer: Surgical therapy. In Wyngaarden JB, and Smith LH Jr (eds): Cecil Textbook of Medicine. 17th ed. Philadelphia, WB Saunders Co, 1985, p 691.

Weinstein WM: Gastritis. In Sleisenger MH, and Fordtran JS (eds): Gastrointestinal Disease. 3rd ed. Philadelphia, WB Saunders Co, 1983, p 559.

40 INFLAMMATORY BOWEL DISEASE

Definition

Inflammatory bowel disease (IBD) refers to both idiopathic ulcerative colitis and Crohn's disease, important chronic medical disorders of unknown etiology. For convenience, ulcerative colitis (UC) and Crohn's disease will be discussed together as IBD in order to emphasize their similarities and to point out their differences. In general IBD is more common in whites than in nonwhites, is equal in men and women, and is most common in Ashkenazic Jews. The incidence of UC is somewhat greater than that of Crohn's disease, but the latter seems to be increasing in incidence. Symptoms characteristically begin in early adult life (15 to 30 years) but may begin at any age. A comparison of the pathological and clinical features of UC and Crohn's disease is given in Table 40–1.

Etiology and Pathogenesis

The cause of IBD is not known; therefore speculations abound:

Genetic Factors. The marked difference in incidence in ethnic groups, the occasional occurrence in monozygotic twins, and the tendency of IBD to cluster in families have suggested genetic or host factors, but no consistent genetic markers have been found.

Infectious Origin. Despite many reports, no agent has been consistently isolated.

Immunological Origin. The extraintestinal manifestations (see below), the reported presence of antibodies to colonic epithelial cells and of cytotoxic T cells, and the clinical and histological responses to immunosuppressive agents have suggested an immunological basis for intestinal injury. Many of the immunological abnormalities described are quite likely to be secondary, however.

Psychological Origin. Few believe that emotional factors are etiologic, but they may exacerbate symptoms and impair the ability to cope with the chronicity and debility of IBD.

In brief there may indeed be important inherited factors determining host susceptibility, but environmental factors (infectious?, noninfectious antigens or toxins?) are probably immediately causative. With increasing technological development in Asia, for example, the incidence of IBD is increasing.

Pathology

The pathology is of particular importance in IBD. It is the basis for the clinical manifestations

TABLE 40–1. COMPARISON OF THE PATHOLOGICAL AND CLINICAL FEATURES OF ULCERATIVE COLITIS AND CROHN'S DISEASE

FEATURE	ULCERATIVE COLITIS	CROHN'S DISEASE
Pathology		
Discontinuous involvement	0	+ +
Transmural inflammation	0/ + *	+ + +
Deep fissures and fistulas	0	+ +
Confluent linear ulcers	0	+ +
Crypt abscesses	+ + +	+
Focal granulomas	0	+ +
Clinical		
Rectal bleeding	+ + +	+
Malaise, fever	+	+ + +
Abdominal pain	+	+ + +
Abdominal mass	0	+ +
Fistulas	0	+ + +
Endoscopic		
Diffuse, continuous involvement	+ + +	0/ +
Friable mucosa	+ + +	0/ +
Rectal involvement	+ + +	+
Cobblestoning	0	+ + +
Linear ulcers	0	+ +

* In toxic megacolon.

described below and also for the distinction that is made between UC and Crohn's disease.

Ulcerative Colitis. The acute lesion is a *diffuse* (without skip areas), *superficial* (mucosal and submucosal) inflammation that almost always involves the rectum (>95 per cent) and may extend from the rectum throughout the colon. With pancolitis the terminal ileum may be slightly involved (a "backwash ileitis"), but UC is essentially a colonic disease. Infiltrated with neutrophils, the epithelium is typically diffusely inflamed, granular, and friable and may show small superficial ulcerations or occasionally deep linear ulcers. Multiple microabscesses may develop around the crypts. When severely inflamed, the colon may become markedly distended (diameter >6 cm) with attenuation of its walls, a condition known as "toxic megacolon." This is associated with an immediate danger of perforation. In chronic UC gradual deposition of connective tissue and hyperplasia of the muscularis mucosae secondary to the continuous processes of injury and repair may produce a smooth, foreshortened colon with loss of normal haustral markings (the lead-pipe colon radiographically). Heaped-up, rounded patches of mucosa develop as outcroppings between areas of ulcerative injury; they are called pseudopolyps, since they are not neoplastic. Ultimately with long-standing disease the epithelial cells may show dysplastic changes that are considered to be harbingers of malignancy. Unless carcinoma occurs UC rarely produces an obstructive lesion or results in fistula formation.

Crohn's Disease. In Crohn's disease, also termed regional enteritis, the inflammation is *transmural* (involving all layers of the bowel and the serosal surface), may be *discontinuous* (with skip areas of normal bowel between), and involves the rectum in fewer than 50 per cent of cases. In contrast to UC, it is not exclusively a colonic disease: approximately one third is colonic; one third is ileal; and one third is ileocolonic. Rarely the more proximal small bowel, the stomach, or even the mouth may be involved. With transmural and even mesenteric involvement, inflamed loops of bowel may become adherent to each other or to other organs, producing palpable masses, fistulas, or obstruction. The mucosa may appear grossly normal or exhibit a cobblestone appearance. Deep linear ulcers may be present, most characteristically in the long axis of the bowel. The infiltrate in the thickened, stiffened walls contains not only neutrophils but also lymphocytes and macrophages, with granuloma formation in about 50 per cent of cases. As noted, fistula formation, including perirectal disease, is common, but dysplasia of epithelial cells is not noted.

Clinical Manifestations

The clinical manifestations of IBD can be conveniently considered as those relating directly to the bowel disease and the systemic response to it and those that are extraintestinal and of more obscure origin.

Intestinal Manifestations. The cardinal manifestations of acute UC are diarrhea, rectal bleeding, fever, weight loss, and abdominal pain. The disease can be mild with only a gradual slight increase in the number of stools and can be limited anatomically to the rectum (ulcerative proctitis). Conversely in a minority of patients (10 to 15 per cent) it begins explosively, so that the patient is acutely ill and requires immediate hospitalization to prevent complications of toxic megacolon such as shock, hypokalemia, and colonic perforation. Depending upon the severity of the diarrhea and the extent of ulceration and inflammation, the patient may exhibit electrolyte abnormalities (particularly hypokalemia), anemia, leukocytosis, fever, and all of the symptoms and signs of toxicity—e.g., weakness, anorexia, tachycardia, and hypotension. The abdomen may be distended and diffusely tender, but generally no masses are felt. Most patients with UC have remissions of their symptoms that may last for months or even years, followed by recurrent acute exacerbations.

In *Crohn's disease* the onset of symptoms is often more subtle than in UC, and the type of presentation is influenced by the anatomical site of the major lesion. If the ileum is primarily involved, the symptoms may suggest low-grade intestinal obstruction with postcibal colicky pain, modest diarrhea, and sometimes the presence of a right lower quadrant palpable mass. Rectal bleeding is rare in all forms of Crohn's disease, although occult blood loss is not uncommon. The onset of Crohn's ileitis may simulate acute appendicitis in a young person. With colonic involvement diarrhea may be more prominent as well as perirectal disease, comprising fissures, fistulas, and perirectal abscesses. Colonic Crohn's disease is also associated with a higher incidence of the extraintestinal manifestations described below. Because of the thickened intestinal wall in Crohn's disease, "toxic megacolon" does not occur and free perforation as opposed to fistula formation is uncommon. In brief, consistent with their respective pathological lesions, Crohn's disease is more likely to produce fistulas or obstruction and less likely to produce hemorrhage or perforation than is UC.

Extraintestinal Manifestations. Similar extraintestinal manifestations may occur with UC and with Crohn's disease of the colon (Table 40–2). These will be considered together and discussed briefly. *Nutritional deficiencies*, occurring secondary to anorexia, fever, diarrhea, and blood loss, may result in growth retardation or severe weight loss. IBD may be associated with two forms of *arthritis*: (a) nondeforming acute inflammatory arthritis of unknown cause affecting large joints more frequently, and (b) sacroiliitis and ankylosing spondylitis, which occur in those patients who also have HLA-B27. The former tends to parallel the colonic disease; the latter generally persist, even after colectomy for UC. *Hepatobiliary abnormalities* are diverse in nature and severity. Many patients have fatty liver and mild pericholangitis, often manifested chemically only by an

TABLE 40–2. EXTRAINTESTINAL MANIFESTATIONS OF INFLAMMATORY BOWEL DISEASE*

1. Nutritional abnormalities
   weight loss, hypoalbuminemia, vitamin deficiencies, deficiencies of calcium, zinc, magnesium, phosphate
2. Hematologic abnormalities
   anemia (Fe loss, folate deficiency), leukocytosis, thrombocytosis
3. Skin and mucous membranes
   pyoderma gangrenosum, erythema nodosum, stomatitis with aphthous ulcers
4. Arthritis
   ankylosing spondylitis and sacroiliitis (B27-associated), peripheral large joint involvement
5. Hepatic and biliary abnormalities
   fatty liver, pericholangitis, sclerosing cholangitis, gallstones, carcinoma of the bile ducts
6. Renal abnormalities
   kidney stone diathesis (calcium oxalate, uric acid), obstructive uropathy, fistulas to urinary tract
7. Eye abnormalities
   iritis, conjunctivitis, episcleritis
8. Miscellaneous
   fever, increased thrombophlebitis

* Modified from Rosenberg IH: Crohn's disease. In Wyngaarden JB, and Smith LH Jr (eds): Cecil Textbook of Medicine. 17th ed. Philadelphia, WB Saunders Co, 1985, p 794.

elevated serum alkaline phosphatase. Rarely sclerosing cholangitis involving both intrahepatic and extrahepatic ducts may develop, presenting the full picture of obstructive jaundice and leading to cirrhosis. There is an increased incidence of cholelithiasis, especially with Crohn's disease of the ileum, thought to be secondary to deficient ileal reabsorption of bile salts. Primary carcinoma of the bile ducts is rare but is increased in incidence. *Ocular manifestations* of IBD include episcleritis, iritis, and uveitis. *Erythema nodosum* may occur in about 5 per cent of patients, especially in women, and a peculiar indolent necrotic skin lesion termed *pyoderma gangrenosum* may be found in about 1 to 2 per cent, especially with active UC. *Aphthous ulcers* of the buccal mucosa are not infrequent, particularly in Crohn's disease. *Renal lesions* may include (a) kidney stone diathesis, especially calcium oxalate stones due to absorptive hyperoxaluria in Crohn's disease, (b) obstructive uropathy or fistulas to the urinary tract in Crohn's disease, (c) kaliopenic nephropathy, or, very rarely, (d) amyloidosis. An increased tendency to develop *thrombophlebitis* has also been noted.

These extraintestinal manifestations may rarely precede overt bowel symptoms or may be the most important source of disability. Most of them tend to remit with improvement of colitis or following colectomy except for sclerosing cholangitis, cirrhosis, and sacroiliitis/spondylitis.

Diagnosis

The diagnostic challenge is to determine whether a patient who presents with diarrhea, abdominal pain, rectal bleeding, fever, or any of the other manifestations listed above has IBD or not and, if so, whether the disease represents UC or Crohn's disease. The list of disorders that must be considered varies with the clinical presentations and may be a long one: acute bacillary dysentery, amebiasis, pseudomembranous colitis, ischemic colitis, colonic neoplasms, angiodysplasia, and many others. Laboratory studies are generally not helpful in the diagnosis of IBD except to exclude other possibilities. The diagnosis rests on (1) direct visualization of the colonic mucosa by sigmoidoscopy or colonoscopy, with biopsy of an abnormal area if indicated; (2) a radiological study of the colon, and of the ileum if indicated, preferably using an air-contrast barium enema technique; (3) exclusion of other possibilities by appropriate studies (bacterial cultures, or the search for trophozoites of *Entamoeba histolytica*, for example).

The characteristic endoscopic findings in acute UC are those described under "Pathology" above: a friable, granular, diffuse uniform lesion of the mucosa that may exhibit superficial ulcerations or that bleeds easily when rubbed with a cotton swab. With more chronic disease, deeper ulcers and pseudopolyps may be found. In Crohn's disease the mucosa is often patchily involved and may even appear normal except for a "cobblestone appearance" due to distortions caused by submucosal inflammation and linear ulcerations. When present, ulcers may be shallow and superficial or deep and longitudinal and may be found in areas of mucosa that look otherwise normal. A biopsy confirms submucosal inflammation and may demonstrate granulomas in up to 50 per cent of patients.

Radiographic studies are of particular importance in the diagnosis of IBD and in demonstrating the extent of its involvement. An air-contrast barium enema usually demonstrates the diffuse lesions of UC and may show the presence of small or large pseudopolyps (Fig. 40–1). The study may be normal in early disease, however, and is less sensitive than direct visualization of the mucosa by endoscopy. Late in the disease a smooth "lead-pipe" foreshortened colon with loss of haustral markings may be noted. Radiographic studies of Crohn's colitis most typically show skip areas, rectal sparing, longitudinal ulcers, and segmental narrowing of the bowel. Fistulas may be present. In the small bowel, especially the terminal ileum, there is usually loss of the normal mucosal pattern and reduction in the size of the lumen to produce the characteristic "string sign."

Although the classic differences between UC and Crohn's disease of the colon as described above usually allow this distinction to be made, these two entities are sometimes difficult to distinguish at the time that IBD is diagnosed.

Treatment and Prognosis

The treatment of UC and Crohn's disease is similar in that both disorders require chronic, nonspecific therapeutic programs employing many of the same agents. In addition, the general treatment of the patient's nutrition, psychological problems, anemia, and other systemic disabilities may be similar. Therapy and prognosis differ enough, however, to warrant separate brief discussions.

FIGURE 40–1. Double-contrast barium enema in a patient with ulcerative colitis demonstrating (A) pseudopolyps and (B) multiple, irregular serrations in the transverse colon representing mucosal ulcerations. (From Sleisenger MH, and Fordtran JS (eds): Gastrointestinal Disease. 3rd ed. Philadelphia. WB Saunders Co, 1983, pp 1134–1135.)

Ulcerative Colitis. Mild to moderate acute colitis may respond to supportive measures supplemented by sulfasalazine (4 to 6 grams daily) alone. Sulfasalazine is split by bacterial action in the colon to yield sulfapyridine and 5-aminosalicylate, the latter considered to be the active agent through its local inhibition of prostaglandin and leukotriene synthesis. If this regimen is insufficient, it can be supplemented by corticosteroid therapy, given either as oral prednisone 10 to 20 mg daily or, especially for left-sided colonic involvement, as hydrocortisone (100 mg) administered as a bedtime enema. When the acute exacerbation is over, the use of sulfasalazine alone is usually sufficient to control disease and prevent recurrence.

Acute, severe UC merges into the entity of toxic megacolon, described below. This represents a medical emergency requiring immediate hospitalization, close attention to replacement of blood and electrolytes, systemic corticosteroids in large doses, coverage by broad-spectrum antibiotics, and surgical consultation. Emergency colectomy may be required for failure of toxic megacolon to improve clinically and radiographically in 36 to 48 hours, excessive hemorrhage, or perforation. The medical regimens for the individual patient must be determined within this spectrum for intensity and for duration.

Surgical treatment for UC is usually that of total colectomy with a permanent ileostomy and is ultimately required in approximately 20 to 25 per cent of patients. The operation is "curative" in that UC as a disease is confined to the colon. The indications for elective as opposed to emergency colectomy described above are generally the following: (a) Failure of medical management. This can be either during the first acute episode or after some years of treatment during which therapy is insufficiently effective in suppressing the disease or suppression requires unacceptably large amounts of corticosteroids. (b) Concern about the presence or future development of carcinoma. This may arise because of the detection of dysplastic, presumably premalignant changes in the epithelium or of gross changes on radiographic or endoscopic examination that are suspicious for carcinoma. Of course colectomy may also be indicated for demonstrated carcinoma complicating UC.

Few patients (<5 per cent) die during an acute attack of UC. Most patients (>90 per cent) respond to therapy or have spontaneous remissions, but unfortunately most have recurrence of the disease months or even years later. Most patients with UC have a reasonably normal life span. Death from UC usually results either from an acute complication (perforation, hemorrhage, sepsis, shock) or from the late development of carcinoma of the colon.

Crohn's Disease. The medical treatment of Crohn's disease is similar to that for UC, with sulfasalazine and corticosteroids being the main agents used beyond general supportive and dietary measures. Crohn's disease is seldom acute, in contrast to UC, although it may present acutely as intestinal obstruction, for example. The response to treatment tends to be less striking than that of UC, and remissions are not as complete. Sulfasalazine is not effective in preventing exacerbations of Crohn's disease, as documented in long-term trials. Some success has been noted with ileal disease in putting the bowel to rest by use of parenteral hyperalimentation.

Surgical treatment of Crohn's disease is not curative and is always undertaken with reluctance, since the disease tends to recur proximal to the site of excision and the patients are especially prone to forming postoperative adhesions. Surgery is most frequently required for obstruction, fistula formation, or abscesses (especially perirectal disease).

The prognosis for Crohn's disease is generally less favorable than for UC, since it responds less well to medical management and cannot generally be cured by surgery. As is the case with UC, most patients with Crohn's disease live a normal life span. Death from Crohn's disease is usually from sepsis rather than from hemorrhage or carcinoma of the colon.

Complications

The complications associated with IBD have been largely discussed as part of the clinical manifestations or of the extraintestinal manifestations of these diseases. In addition to the more specific and acute complications such as hemorrhage or perforation, one must be concerned about some of the long-term nonspecific problems such as retardation of growth in children, malnutrition, weakness, lassitude, recurrent pain, and depression. These are complications of many chronic debilitating diseases. Two other complications, alluded to previously and found mostly but not exclusively with UC, will be further described in brief.

Toxic Dilatation of the Colon (Toxic Megacolon). This complication, which represents perhaps the extreme range of acute UC, describes the presence of a markedly distended atonic colon with attenuation of its wall thickness, usually associated with signs of systemic toxicity—hypotension, tachycardia, fever, and leukocytosis. Diarrhea may be diminished rather than enhanced, because of loss of colonic motor function. Hypokalemia and hypoalbuminemia are common. Toxic megacolon may occur spontaneously or be induced by injudicious use of drugs given to diminish diarrhea, by preparation for a barium enema examination, or by hypokalemia. The diagnosis is usually made with a plain film of the abdomen showing a colonic diameter greater than 6 cm, usually seen in the transverse colon. There is an immediate and continuing danger of perforation until the dilatation is reversed. The treatment of this medical emergency has been described above.

Carcinoma of the Colon. A general discussion of carcinoma of the colon is found in Chapter 41. There is a special danger of neoplasia in IBD, particularly in chronic UC. The incidence of carcinoma in UC relates to two variables: (a) the presence of extensive mucosal disease, i.e., pancolitis, and (b) the duration of active colitis. The incidence begins to rise steeply after 10 years of active disease. Carcinoma complicating UC has the following characteristics as compared to that occurring spontaneously: (a) it is distributed more evenly in the colon, (b) it is more likely to occur in multiple sites, (c) it is usually discovered at a more advanced stage and has a worse prognosis,

and (d) it is more difficult to diagnose because its associated symptoms are mimicked by those of the underlying disease. Because of this it is imperative to institute long-term follow-up protocols in patients with chronic pancolitis, using colonoscopy and biopsies of suspicious lesions and of the colonic mucosa in general. The latter may show the development of dysplastic changes, thought to be premalignant, and therefore suggest the advisability of preventive colectomy.

ISCHEMIC COLITIS

In older patients inflammatory bowel disease may be simulated by ischemic injury to the colon. This ischemic injury, which may be acute or chronic, usually occurs as a complication of severe atherosclerosis. More rarely it results from vascular injury secondary to surgery or a dissecting aneurysm, from a low cardiac output state, from vasculitis, or from a hypercoagulable state. The ischemia is more likely to occur in "watershed areas" between the distributions of two major vessels (splenic flexure, rectosigmoid area) and is usually secondary to hypoperfusion rather than to complete obstruction. The rectum is almost always spared because of its collateral blood supplies. The clinical picture may be acute or chronic, with all gradations between.

Acute ischemic colitis is usually manifested by the sudden onset of localized abdominal pain, tenderness, and rectal bleeding, which is sometimes associated with fever, hypotension, tachycardia, and peritoneal signs. Sigmoidoscopy or colonoscopy may show no abnormalities but more frequently shows multiple ulcers or bulging areas of submucosal hemorrhage. Barium enema examination is hazardous during the acute phase, but when carried out later most characteristically shows areas of narrowing and the changes in the bowel outline called "thumbprinting" caused by mucosal hemorrhage and edema. Acute ischemic colitis may be difficult to distinguish from IBD or diverticulitis. Most acute ischemic episodes resolve over the subsequent several weeks with general supportive measures. Angiography is rarely indicated, and surgery is reserved for patients with clear evidence of perforation and/or infarction. The patient who recovers from an acute episode may remain well subsequently or may enter a more chronic phase of the illness.

Subacute or chronic ischemic colitis may lead to longer periods of vague abdominal pain and diarrhea with or without significant bleeding. This may closely simulate IBD in older people clinically as well as endoscopically. Over a period of time fibrosis may follow ischemic injury, leading to areas of narrowing of the colon. If such strictures lead to obstruction, surgery may be required. Rarely are attempts at revascularization indicated.

DIVERTICULITIS

Diverticula, serosa-covered saccules that include mucosa, extend from the lumen through the colonic muscular layer and are very common in later life in Western societies. These small herniations occur usually through areas of the colonic wall weakened by penetration of an arteriole. The incidence of diverticula is thought to be enhanced by any factor that chronically increases intraluminal pressure, particularly by refined diets of low fiber content that yield stools of small bulk. Most diverticula are found in the sigmoid area and are asymptomatic. They become important because of two complications: bleeding and infection. Vessels in or around a diverticulum may bleed briskly in older people, and diverticular bleeding must be differentiated from bleeding from other causes, especially from angiodysplasia or carcinoma. The differential diagnosis of gastrointestinal bleeding is discussed in Chapter 36B.

Diverticulitis refers specifically to infection in or around diverticula, thought to result usually from obstruction by fecoliths or inspissated feces with impairment of the blood supply and drainage. This walled-off, localized infection, caused by intestinal organisms, may produce a microabscess that heals spontaneously, may perforate to cause localized or more rarely generalized peritonitis, or may extend to cause larger abscesses that may be local or that may rarely penetrate other adjacent organs. Acute diverticulitis is said to simulate "left-sided appendicitis" with left lower quadrant pain (often exacerbated during defecation), tenderness, fever, leukocytosis, and sometimes a palpable inflammatory mass. Bleeding during the acute illness, if present at all, is usually microscopic. Rectal examination may reveal a tender mass; sigmoidoscopy characteristically shows extrinsic narrowing of the colonic lumen and inflamed mucosa. Barium enema,

which is hazardous during the acute phase, generally confirms the presence of an inflammatory mass and often shows leakage of barium beyond the lumen of a diverticulum. The acute illness is treated by withholding solid food and by the use of broad-spectrum antibiotics. Surgical treatment may be required acutely for perforation, fistula formation, or a large abscess and electively for recurrent attacks of diverticulitis, especially when these result in fibrosis and obstruction. Many physicians recommend high-fiber diets to reduce colonic intraluminal pressures in an attempt to prevent the progression of diverticulosis and the recurrence of diverticulitis.

REFERENCES

Cello JP: Ulcerative colitis. In Sleisenger MH, and Fordtran JS (eds): Gastrointestinal Disease. 3rd ed. Philadelphia, WB Saunders Co, 1983, p 1122.

Donaldson RM Jr: Crohn's disease. In Sleisenger MH, and Fordtran JS (eds): Gastrointestinal Disease. 3rd ed. Philadelphia, WB Saunders Co, 1983, p 1088.

Greenstein AJ, Janowitz HD, and Sachar DB: The extraintestinal complications of Crohn's disease and ulcerative colitis: A study of 700 patients. Medicine 55:401, 1976.

Grendell JH, and Ockner RK: Vascular diseases of the bowel. In Sleisenger MH, and Fordtran JS (eds): Gastrointestinal Disease. 3rd ed. Philadelphia, WB Saunders Co, 1983, p 1543.

Kirsner JB, and Shorter RG: Recent developments in "nonspecific"inflammatory bowel disease. N Engl J Med 306:775, 837, 1982.

Rosenberg IH, and Levin B: Inflammatory bowel disease. In Wyngaarden JB, and Smith LH Jr (eds): Cecil Textbook of Medicine. 17th ed. Philadelphia, WB Saunders Co, 1985, p 740.

NEOPLASMS OF THE GASTROINTESTINAL TRACT

41

Neoplasms of the gastrointestinal tract are among the most common and important malignant tumors. Only the most important tumors will be discussed in this chapter. Tumors of the pancreas and of the liver are described in the chapters devoted to those organs.

CARCINOMA OF THE ESOPHAGUS

Tumors of the esophagus are usually malignant squamous cell carcinomas; less than 10 per cent are benign (most frequently leiomyomas). Adeno-

carcinomas account for about 5 per cent; all other malignant lesions are exceedingly rare.

Incidence

The incidence of esophageal carcinoma in white men is about 5 per 100,000, about three times that in white women. It is about four times higher in blacks and more than 30 times higher in certain other parts of the world (North China, Caspian Sea area).

Etiology and Pathogenesis

The cause of carcinoma of the esophagus is not known, but there are certain important associations. The incidence varies widely geographically as noted above, but the presumed environmental factors have not been established with certainty. The incidence of esophageal carcinoma is increased in those who smoke or drink alcohol to excess and in those who have or have had squamous cell tumors of the head and neck. Injury due to lye ingestion, irradiation, or long-term stasis (usually achalasia) increases the incidence. Adenocarcinoma is strongly associated with columnar (Barrett's) epithelium, a complication of long-term gastric reflux. A rare inherited disorder with thickened skin in the palms and soles (tylosis) and gluten-sensitive enteropathy are both associated through unknown mechanisms with an increased incidence of esophageal carcinoma.

Clinical Manifestations

Dysphagia is the most frequent and important symptom of esophageal carcinoma (see Chapter 38). This symptom usually begins with difficulty in swallowing solids and then progresses steadily over six to nine months to involve liquids as well. *Anorexia* and *weight loss* commonly occur simultaneously. Regurgitation and aspiration may lead to coughing after swallowing fluids or to recurrent episodes of bronchopneumonia.

Substernal pain usually follows dysphagia and most frequently reflects extension of the tumor into mediastinal structures. These tumors rarely bleed briskly (about 5 per cent) but may result in slow, steady blood loss. With extension of the tumor the recurrent laryngeal nerve may be involved, resulting in hoarseness. Nail clubbing may occur, and very rarely paraneoplastic endocrine abnormalities (hypercalcemia, Cushing's syndrome) have been described.

Complications

A number of the clinical manifestations are in effect complications of the disease, such as pain, aspiration pneumonia, and bleeding. Esophagotracheal or esophagobronchial fistulas may occur, resulting in more frequent episodes of pulmonary infection. Metastases are most frequently to regional nodes, the liver, and the lung.

Diagnosis

Dysphagia occurring in anyone over the age of 40 must be assumed to be secondary to carcinoma of the esophagus until proved otherwise. The diagnosis depends on biopsy of a suspicious lesion or more rarely on cytological examination. An esophagogram, preferably a double-contrast study, is the first step in the evaluation of a patient suspected of having an esophageal carcinoma. If a suspicious area is noted, fiberoptic esophagoscopy is then carried out in order to obtain a number of biopsy specimens from deep within the abnormal area, sometimes supplemented by brush cytology specimens. The distinction between a tumor and a benign stricture can be very difficult to make on radiographic grounds alone, so that esophagoscopy should be carried out in most cases.

CT of the chest is very useful in delineating the extent of the tumor and its mediastinal spread, as part of staging. Ultrasound or isotopic scans of the liver are indicated as well as part of staging if the diagnosis has been established. Early results suggest that gallium-67 is picked up by some tumors and their metastases and may prove useful in staging.

Treatment and Prognosis

Unfortunately esophageal tumors spread and metastasize early; not more than 25 per cent are surgically resectable at the time of diagnosis. The results of surgery, which is usually carried out only for carcinomas of the lower third of the esophagus, are highly unsatisfactory for cure. There is an operative hospital mortality of about 20 to 30 per cent, and only about 5 per cent survive for five years. On the other hand, resection with reanastomosis often gives considerable palliation from dysphagia, pain, and aspiration. Tumors of the upper and middle thirds of the esophagus are most frequently treated for palliation by irradiation using about 600 rads. Symptomatic relief can sometimes be obtained by dilating a malignant stricture or by placing a plastic prosthetic tube across the site of obstruction.

CARCINOMA OF THE STOMACH

Most tumors of the stomach are adenocarcinomas. Only about 5 per cent are primary lymphomas of the stomach, and other malignant lesions (e.g., leiomyosarcoma) are rarer still. Since the clinical characteristics and diagnostic measures are similar for all malignant tumors of the stomach, this chapter will focus on adenocarcinoma. Benign tumors (e.g., leiomyomas and adenomas) are rarely the cause of symptoms, most often being found incidentally.

Incidence

The incidence of gastric carcinoma in the United States (now about 20,000 cases annually) has declined dramatically for unknown reasons during the past 30 to 40 years from being the single most common malignant disease to its current rank of approximately seventh. Similar but lesser declines have occurred in Western European and in other Anglo-Saxon countries, but the incidence remains very high in some parts of the world, especially in Japan, certain parts of South America, and Eastern Europe. When population groups emigrate from areas of high incidence to those of low incidence, they tend to attain over several generations the usual rates found in their new environment. An interesting inverse relationship has been noted between the incidence of carcinoma of the stomach and carcinoma of the colon in population groups.

Etiology and Pathogenesis

Because of the marked geographical differences in the incidence of gastric carcinoma cited above, together with the change in incidence in migrant populations, it is assumed that there are important environmental factors in the etiology of this disease, but none has been clearly demonstrated. Some association patterns can be described however (Table 41–1). Gastric cancer is more common in men than women, blacks than whites, those with a positive family history, those with blood group A, and those of a lower socioeconomic status. Diet is thought to be an important determinant of risk, possibly relating to high nitrate and salt content. Nitrates can be reduced to nitrites by bacterial action (perhaps more readily in achlorhydric stomachs, since more bacteria are present), which in turn can react with a number of amines to form nitroso compounds. The latter have been demonstrated to be gastric carcinogens in animals. Gastric cancer seems to have a positive association with a diet high in salted fish and meat and pickled vegetables and a negative association with ascorbic acid and fresh vegetables. It is increased in patients with atrophic gastritis (with or without pernicious anemia) and with large (>2 cm) gastric polyps, and after partial gastrectomy for peptic ulcer disease. None of these factors can be clearly related to the decreasing incidence of gastric cancer in the United States cited above.

Pathology

Adenocarcinomas of the stomach derive from mucous cells, not from parietal or chief cells. Subtypes have been described related to differentiation and characteristics of growth and spread: the *intestinal type* (resembling colonic carcinoma) has a better prognosis that the *diffuse type*; the *expanding type* (cells maintaining a close relationship) has a better prognosis than the *infiltrative type*. The tumors are most frequently found in the distal third of the stomach and may be exophytic (with or without a stalk), diffusely infiltrative throughout the stomach (sometimes termed linitis plastica), or ulcerated.

Clinical Manifestations (Table 41–1)

Gastric carcinoma usually presents with nonspecific symptoms and signs. *Epigastric pain* is highly variable. In about one quarter of patients it may resemble the pain of peptic ulcer. More frequently it is a dull epigastric discomfort that may be exacerbated rather than relieved by food and may be associated with *nausea* and *early satiety*. Almost all patients have *anorexia* and *weight loss. Vomiting* may be prominent, especially with distal tumors leading to pyloric obstruction. Tumors arising in the cardia may infiltrate into the gastroesophageal junction and cause *dysphagia.* The tumors commonly bleed, producing iron deficiency anemia and more rarely hematemesis with corresponding symptoms of weakness, fatigue, and shortness of breath. More rarely the patient may present when symptoms and signs relating to metastases, direct extension, or paraneoplastic syndromes are prominent. These include, for example, obstructive jaundice, malignant ascites, a gastrocolic fistula. Trousseau's syndrome (thrombophlebitis), dermatomyositis, and acanthosis nigricans.

TABLE 41–1. ADENOCARCINOMA OF THE STOMACH

ASSOCIATED WITH	CLINICAL MANIFESTATIONS
Environment—geographical differences	Anorexia, early satiety, weight loss
Diet—? nitrosamines	Dysphagia, vomiting, weakness
Blood group A	Epigastric distress to severe, boring pain
Atrophic gastritis (pernicious anemia)	Anemia, occult blood in stools
Adenomatous polyps (>2 cm)	Epigastric mass, signs of metastases
Subtotal resection for benign ulcer disease	Rare—Virchow's node, Blumer's shelf, Trousseau's syndrome, acanthosis nigricans

From Sherlock P: Neoplasms of the stomach. In Wyngaarden JB, and Smith LH Jr (eds): Cecil Textbook of Medicine. 17th ed. Philadelphia, WB Saunders Co, 1985, p 698.

Physical examination may reveal an epigastric mass, evidence of one or more of the complications noted above, or other evidence of metastasis, such as a left supraclavicular Virchow's node, a Blumer's shelf (a mass in the perirectal pouch), or Krukenberg tumors (metastases to the ovaries) on pelvic examination.

Diagnosis

The first diagnostic study in a patient with the symptoms noted above is usually a radiographic examination of the stomach, preferably using a double-contrast technique and multiple projections for adequate demonstration of mucosal detail. The radiographic appearance of the tumor may vary considerably, from an ulcerated or nonulcerated exophytic mass to simply a thickened, nondistensible gastric wall. There are certain characteristics that suggest malignancy in an ulcer—an irregular ulcer base, an ulcer within a mass, the type of convergent folds—but the true differentiation can only be made by biopsy.

Endoscopic examination with multiple biopsies of a suspicious area is now the standard means of diagnosing carcinoma of the stomach. This should be supplemented with brush cytology obtained at the time of endoscopy, since cytology will sometimes (about 15 per cent) be positive even when the biopsy specimens do not reveal carcinoma. No other laboratory studies are diagnostic.

Treatment and Prognosis

Surgery offers the only chance for cure of gastric cancer, but it is a rare chance (Fig. 41–1). After the diagnosis is established, staging must be carried out to determine insofar as possible if there is distant spread or local spread (beyond the wall of the stomach but confined to adjacent nodes) or whether the tumor seems to be confined to the stomach. This staging is usually carried out by biopsy of suspected nodes, liver function tests, and scans, ultrasonography, and increasingly CT of the abdomen. Occasionally laparoscopy and biopsy are indicated. If distal spread is found, surgery should be confined to palliative procedures,

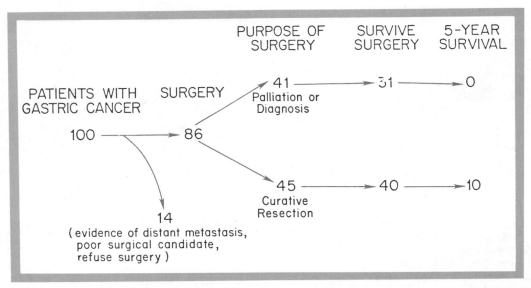

FIGURE 41–1. This scheme, which summarizes the survival results of several large series, suggests what happens to 100 patients with the diagnosis of gastric cancer. (From Davis GR: Neoplasms of the stomach. In Sleisenger MH, and Fordtran JS (eds): Gastrointestinal Disease. 3rd ed. Philadelphia, WB Saunders Co, 1983, p 587.

usually for obstruction. If the tumor is localized, subtotal gastrectomy is usually carried out for tumors of the distal or middle third and total gastrectomy for the proximal third. In either case extensive resection of regional lymphatics is indicated. The results of surgical treatment are summarized in Figure 41–1.

Irradiation of gastric carcinoma is generally unsatisfactory and has been palliative at best. A number of chemotherapeutic programs have been tried with very modest effects, if any, on survival. A current program that combines 5-fluorouracil, mitomycin-C, and doxorubicin shows some promise for both palliation and increase in survival.

No method of preventing gastric carcinoma is known. Careful surveillance of patients at increased risk, especially with pernicious anemia, known atrophic gastritis, and following subtotal gastrectomy, may be indicated.

CARCINOMA OF THE COLON

Adenocarcinoma is the most important malignant disease of the large bowel and will be considered to include rectal cancer as well for purposes of discussion. Other tumors of the large bowel, other than polyps (to be discussed subsequently), are much rarer and will not be considered here.

Incidence

Carcinoma of the large bowel is the third most common cancer in the United States (after carcinoma of the lung and breast) and is second in frequency in both men and women. Approximately 120,000 new cases are diagnosed annually, accounting for about 15 per cent of all malignant tumors in both men and women. The incidence

is much higher in North America, Western Europe, Australia, and New Zealand than in Japan, South America, or Africa. Population groups that emigrate tend to acquire the risk characteristic of their new environment.

Etiology and Pathogenesis

The cause of colonic cancer is not known, but there are certain interesting associations. The geographical differences in incidence noted above, together with shifts in incidence in migrant groups, strongly suggest environmental factors. Particular attention has been directed to diet, since the incidence seems to be greater in those whose diet is low in fiber but high in animal fat and protein, perhaps particularly that derived from beef. It is thought that the type of colonic flora associated with such a diet may produce carcinogens that are in contact with colonic mucosa for longer periods of time due to the prolonged colonic transit times of low-fiber diets. These speculations, and those concerning the possible protective effect of dietary selenium, ascorbic acid, and alpha-tocopherol, await confirmation.

In addition to these possible environmental factors within populations, a number of risk factors are known for the individual (Table 41–2). The risk of colorectal carcinoma begins to increase

TABLE 41–2. RISK FACTORS FOR CARCINOMA OF THE COLON

Increasing age
Inflammatory bowel disease
History of colonic cancer or adenoma
Familial polyposis syndromes (adenomatous polyps)
History of breast or female genital cancer
Peutz-Jeghers syndrome (hamartomas)
Acromegaly

around age 40 and roughly doubles for each succeeding decade. A number of conditions associated with increased mucosal cell turnover may lead to increased risk, e.g., inflammatory bowel disease, especially ulcerative colitis (see Chapter 40), and certain familial polyposis syndromes (to be discussed subsequently). A history of previous cancer or adenoma of the colon, a history of colon cancer in a first-degree relative, and the "family cancer syndrome" (multifocal cancers in other organs, especially the female sex organs, as well as the colon) carry increased risk for carcinoma of the colon as well.

Pathology

Adenocarcinomas of the colon vary considerably in histological appearance (scirrhous, papillary, medullary, or colloid), but the prognosis relates to the degree of invasion of the wall or spread at the time of discovery rather than the pathological description. The distribution of tumors in the colon (Fig. 41–2) is predominantly left-sided, with fully 50 per cent being within reach of a sigmoidoscope, although there seems to be an increasing tendency for tumors to be found more proximally in the colon.

Clinical Manifestations

The early symptoms of carcinoma of the colon are often mild and nonspecific, especially with tumors in the area of the cecum or ascending colon where obstruction is rare and where blood that is lost is well mixed with feces and therefore less apparent. A change in bowel habits, especially with left-sided lesions, may be the first symptoms. This can be diarrhea, constipation, alternation of diarrhea and constipation, a change in the caliber of the stool, or tenesmus. Pain with left-sided tumors usually results from partial obstruction, but pain with right-sided tumors may represent invasion of the colonic wall or adjacent structures. Hematochezia is common, as is constant occult bleeding, leading to iron deficiency anemia with its associated symptoms of weakness, fatigability, and shortness of breath. The generalized symptoms of many malignancies—weight loss, anorexia, and malaise—are usually present late in the illness. Rarely patients may present with peritonitis due to tumor invasion and perforation of the colonic wall or with complications from metastases such as jaundice or ascites.

Diagnosis

Carcinoma of the bowel must be suspected in any patient over age 40 who presents with change of bowel habits or in the caliber of stools, ill-defined abdominal pain, hematochezia, or iron deficiency anemia. Bright red blood on the stools should not be attributed to hemorrhoids or diverticulosis until malignancy has been carefully excluded. If the patient has any of the special risk factors listed in Table 41–2, the threshold for suspicion is further lowered. Even in the absence of such symptoms or findings, careful testing of

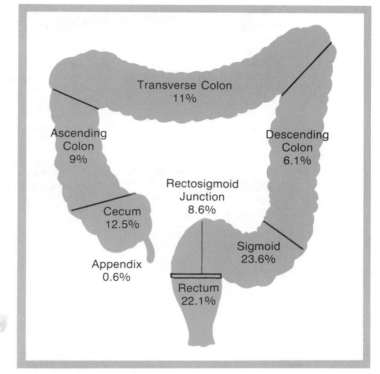

FIGURE 41–2. Distribution of large bowel cancer by anatomical segmen according to the third national cancer survey (segment unspecified). (From Shottenfeld D, and Fraumeni J Jr (eds): Cancer Epidemiology and Prevention. Philadelphia, WB Saunders Co, 1982, pp 703–727.

stools for occult blood (using the Hemoccult test, for example) may pick up early malignant lesions.

Diagnostic studies usually start with a careful digital rectal examination followed by proctoscopy or sigmoidoscopy, since radiographic studies are often not satisfactory for the rectum or lower sigmoid. If no lesion is found, a double-contrast barium enema is performed after careful bowel cleansing. If a suspicious lesion is noted, or indeed even if the study is normal and the suspicion is high, colonoscopy is performed with multiple biopsies and brush cytological preparations from abnormal sites. These combined studies are successful in the detection of the vast majority of carcinomas of the colon. Measurement of carcinoembryonic antigen (CEA) is not useful in diagnosis but may be of value in following a patient after resection of a tumor, as a rise in CEA may then herald recurrence.

The differential diagnosis includes a large number of diseases associated with any of the above symptoms, particularly diverticulitis, ischemic colitis, angiodysplasia, inflammatory bowel disease, and benign polyps.

Treatment and Prognosis

The only effective treatment is surgical removal of the tumor and the adjacent colon and mesentery. Hemicolectomy is usually performed for right-sided and left-sided tumors; anterior resection with anastomosis to the rectal stump for sigmoid or upper rectal tumors; and a combined abdominal-perineal resection with a permanent colostomy for lesions within 5 cm of the anal verge. Surgery may also be indicated for palliation even in the presence of obvious metastatic disease when there is obstruction, perforation, or hemorrhage. Radiation therapy is used most frequently for pelvic recurrences or painful metastases, particularly in bone and sometimes in liver. Chemotherapy, usually with 5-fluorouracil, has been used in the treatment of hepatic metastases, but with only modest success.

The results of the surgical treatment of early carcinoma of the large bowel are excellent, with 80 to 90 per cent 10-year survival for mucosal lesions, 60 to 80 per cent with bowel wall invasion, and as high as 50 to 60 per cent even when regional nodes are involved. Postoperatively each patient must be followed closely for recurrence using colonoscopy, radiographic procedures, and measurements of CEA in a regular schedule over many years.

Screening and Prevention

The process of colonic carcinogenesis probably evolves over years. Neoplastic polyps and early localized carcinomas can be resected readily with excellent long-term results. There is therefore considerable interest in screening certain populations for colonic polyps and carcinomas using annual testing for occult fecal blood and periodic (every three to five years) proctosigmoidoscopy beginning at age 40 to 50. The finding of occult blood in the stool should be followed up rigorously with radiological or endoscopic examination of the entire colon. There is still some debate about the cost effectiveness of this approach in the general population. Quite clearly, however, individuals known to be at high risk for developing carcinoma of the colon (familial polyposis syndrome, prior colonic polyp or cancer, longstanding ulcerative colitis) should be screened even more frequently than the schedule noted above.

POLYPS OF THE GASTROINTESTINAL TRACT

A polyp, a mass of tissue that arises from the surface and extends into the lumen of the gastrointestinal tract, usually represents an overgrowth of epithelial cells. Polyps can be single or

TABLE 41–3. POLYPS OF THE COLON

Neoplastic Polyps
   Benign adenomatous polyps (tubular, mixed, or villous)
      random occurrence
         familial—familial polyposis of the colon, Gardner syndrome (Fig. 41–3), Turcot's syndrome
   Malignant polyps—carcinomatous changes, in situ or invasive
Non-neoplastic Polyps
   Inflammatory "pseudopolyps"
   Peutz-Jeghers syndrome—hamartomas
   Mucosal polyps with normal epithelium
   Juvenile polyps

multiple, sporadic or familial, pedunculated (on a stalk) or sessile (flat based), neoplastic or non-neoplastic, as well as benign or malignant. They can also occur virtually anywhere in the gastrointestinal tract. The polyps of greatest importance, however, are those found in the colon, so these will receive primary attention. A simplified classification of colonic polyps is given in Table 41–3. Only the neoplastic polyps and those benign polyps associated with the familial polyposis syndromes will be discussed here.

Incidence

Colonic adenomatous polyps, usually less than 1 cm in diameter, are very common and are found with increased frequency with age. After the age of 65, for example, two thirds of individuals will have at least one polyp. Patients with one demonstrated polyp have a considerably enhanced chance of having another coincident one or of developing an additional polyp subsequently.

Etiology and Pathogenesis

Nothing is known directly about the cause of colonic polyps other than the role of inheritance in the familial polyposis syndromes to be noted later. There is considerable evidence, albeit most of it indirect, that most if not all carcinomas of the colon derive from previously benign polyps, most commonly after at least 10 to 15 years. If this is so, one would expect that the risk factors that have been defined for colonic carcinoma (Table 41–2) might also prove to pertain to benign polyps as well. Clearly only a very small percentage of benign polyps progress to malignancy, although the definite existence of this potential usually makes it advisable to remove any demonstrated colonic adenomatous polyp.

Clinical Manifestations

As might be expected from lesions that vary so widely in size, shape, number, and location, the associated clinical manifestations are diverse. In fact most polyps cause no symptoms and are found incidentally at autopsy or on radiographic or colonoscopic studies done for other purposes. The most frequent abnormalities are those of *bleeding* (hematochezia, anemia) or more rarely *abdominal pain*, if the polyp is large enough to obstruct the bowel partially. With large polyps patients may note a *change in bowel habits* with diarrhea or constipation. Very rarely large villous adenomas may produce *watery diarrhea* containing enough potassium to produce significant hypokalemia.

Diagnosis

The diagnosis of a colonic polyp is readily made with use of a double-contrast barium enema, or even more effectively by colonoscopy. The nature of the polyp is documented by biopsy, preferably by excisional biopsy.

Treatment

Although only a few polyps in the colon undergo malignant transformation, a polyp that has been discovered should usually be removed. Fortunately this can now be readily accomplished in most patients with smaller polyps (<2 cm in diameter) by colonoscopic polypectomy. Larger polyps may require surgery, especially if the suspicion of malignancy is high. Patients who have required polypectomy should be closely followed (colonoscopy or double-contrast barium enema every two to three years) in order to detect the development of new polyps.

THE FAMILIAL POLYPOSIS SYNDROMES

The familial polyposis syndromes are rare, dominantly transmitted disorders in which multiple polyps are found within the gastrointestinal tract (Table 41–3). Some of the best delineated syndromes will be described briefly here.

Familial Polyposis of the Colon

In this rare genetic disorder (1 in 8000 births) multiple adenomatous polyps develop gradually during childhood such that they characteristically carpet the entire colon. More than 1000 grossly visible polyps may form with many other nascent polyps demonstrable microscopically. Very rarely the ileum may be involved as well. The symptoms are those of bleeding and diarrhea, but the main

clinical consequence is that of the virtual 100 per cent occurrence of carcinoma of the colon by age 40. When the diagnosis of familial polyposis is made, therefore, elective complete colectomy is required (usually after full growth has been attained). Because of its dominant transmission, other members of the family must be carefully surveyed.

Gardner's Syndrome

This rare entity resembles familial polyposis of the colon with certain other associated features, especially osteomas and benign soft-tissue tumors (see Fig. 41–3 for illustration of the complete syndrome). The stomach and small bowel (especially the duodenum) may also be involved. Because of the malignant potential of the colonic polyps, total colectomy is indicated.

Peutz-Jeghers Syndrome

In this familial disorder the polyps are more generally distributed throughout the gastrointestinal tract and are associated with characteristic mucocutaneous pigmentation, especially in the buccal mucosa, the lips, the soles of the feet, and the dorsum of the hands (see Fig. 41–3). The polyps are hamartomas rather than adenomas and therefore have a much lower incidence of neoplastic transformation, although this complication may occur, especially in the small intestine.

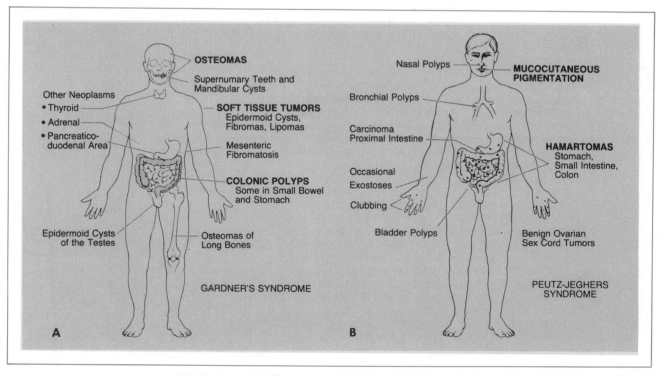

FIGURE 41–3. *A*, Schematic representation of Gardner's syndrome. The triad of colonic polyposis, bone tumors, and soft tissue tumors (heavy print) are the primary features; other features are indicated in lighter print. *B*, Schematic presentation of the Peutz-Jeghers syndrome. Mucocutaneous pigmentation and benign gastrointestinal polyposis (heavy print) are the primary features of this syndrome. Lighter print shows the secondary features. (From Boland CR, and Kim YS: In Sleisenger MH, and Fordtran JS (eds): Gastrointestinal Disease. 3rd ed. Philadelphia, WB Saunders Co, 1983.)

Surgery is usually indicated only for complications from the polyps—bleeding, pain or obstruction.

REFERENCES

Boland CR, and Kim YS: Colonic polyps and the gastrointestinal polyposis syndromes. In Sleisenger MH, and Fordtran JS (eds): Gastrointestinal Disease. 3rd ed. Philadelphia, WB Saunders Co, 1983, p 1196.

Davis GR: Neoplasms of the stomach. In Sleisenger MH, and Fordtran JS (eds): Gastrointestinal Disease. 3rd ed. Philadelphia, WB Saunders Co, 1983, p 578.

Diehl JJ, Hermann RE, Cooperman AM, et al: Gastric carcinoma. A ten-year review. Ann Surg 198:9, 1983.

Pope CE II: Tumors (of the esophagus). In Sleisenger MH, and Fordtran JS (eds): Gastrointestinal Disease. 3rd ed. Philadelphia, WB Saunders Co, 1983, p 479.

Sherlock P: Neoplasms of the stomach. In Wyngaarden JB, and Smith LH Jr (eds): Cecil Textbook of Medicine. 17th ed. Philadelphia, WB Saunders Co, 1985, p 697.

Stearns MW Jr: Neoplasms of the Colon, Rectum, and Anus. New York, John Wiley & Sons, 1980.

Winawer SJ: Neoplasms of the large and small intestine. In Wyngaarden JB, and Smith LH Jr (eds): Cecil Textbook of Medicine. 17th ed. Philadelphia, WB Saunders Co, 1985, p 761.

Winawer SJ, and Sherlock P: Malignant neoplasms of the small and large intestine. In Sleisenger MH, and Fordtran JS (eds): Gastrointestinal Disease. 3rd ed. Philadelphia, WB Saunders Co, 1983, p 1220.

42 THE PANCREAS

NORMAL STRUCTURE AND FUNCTION

The pancreas is a relatively small (70 to 110 grams) but versatile organ containing two specific and seemingly independent components: (a) *the endocrine pancreas* and (b) *the exocrine pancreas.* The endocrine pancreas consists of the islets of Langerhans, packets of endocrine cells peppered randomly throughout the pancreas that secrete insulin, glucagon, and other polypeptide hormones. The endocrine pancreas will be discussed in other chapters and will not be considered further here. The cells of the exocrine pancreas cluster into acini that are further grouped in lobules. Acinar cells are drained by ductules that converge into ducts of increasing size, terminating in the duct of Wirsung, which drains through the sphincter of Oddi and the papilla of Vater into the second portion of the duodenum. The head of the pancreas lies within the curvature of the duodenum, and the body and tail extend for about 12 to 15 cm retroperitoneally toward the hilum of the spleen (Fig. 42–1). The head of the pancreas is in close anatomical relationship with a number of vital structures, including the common bile duct, the inferior vena cava, the aorta and the origin of the superior mesenteric artery, the splenic artery and vein, and the right adrenal gland and kidney. The exocrine pancreas, with its myriads of acini, is depicted schematically in Figure 42–2.

The normal pancreas secretes a large volume (up to 1500 ml per day) of a distinctive fluid.

Electrolyte Composition. Acinar cells secrete fluid that resembles extracellular fluid: ductular cells progressively add a bicarbonate-rich liquid so that the relative amount of bicarbonate increases and may reach as high as 120 mEq/L. Pancreatic bicarbonate may be an important factor in neutralizing gastric acid.

Protein Content. Pancreatic fluid is protein-rich, more than 90 per cent of which represents enzymes or proenzymes secreted by acinar cells: (1) active form—lipase, amylase, and ribonuclease, and (2) inactive form—proteases and phospholipase. The inactive proenzymes are activated in cascade fashion in the gut: enterokinase converts trypsinogen to trypsin; trypsin then activates all of the other proenzymes. Other proteins in pancreatic juice are colipase, which binds to and enhances lipase activity, and trypsin inhibitors.

Control of Secretion. The small basal secretion of the exocrine pancreas is stimulated by a variety of factors, the relative importance of which is un-

FIGURE 42–1. Connections of the ducts of the gallbladder, liver, and pancreas. (Reproduced, with permission, from Bell GH, Emslie-Smith D, and Paterson CR: Textbook of Physiology and Biochemistry. 9th ed. Edinburgh, Churchill Livingstone, 1976.)

FIGURE 42–2. Diagram of pancreatic acinus and duct system ("pancreon"). Sodium bicarbonate is probably also secreted in the acinus. The effects of inhibitors of sodium transport suggest that active transport of sodium occurs proximally. Secretin stimulates a bicarbonate "pump" to add a solution of bicarbonate in the extralobular ducts. (From Swanson CH, and Solomon AK: A micropuncture investigation of the whole tissue mechanism of electrolyte secretion by the in vitro rabbit pancreas. J Gen Physiol 62:426, 1973.)

FIGURE 42–3. Normal pancreas demonstrated by computed tomography. (Courtesy of Dr. Eugene P. DiMagno, Mayo Medical School, Rochester, Minnesota.) (Reprinted from Grendell JH: The pancreas. In Smith LH Jr, and Thier SO (eds): Pathophysiology: The Biological Principles of Disease. 2nd ed. Philadelphia, WB Saunders Co, 1985, p 1225.)

known (Fig. 42–2). Most pancreatic secretion occurs postprandially in response to one or more of three stimuli: (1) *hormones.* Two hormones seem most important and potentiate each other: secretin, which stimulates ductular cells to increase water and bicarbonate; cholecystokinin (CCK), which stimulates acinar cells to secrete enzymes and proenzymes. (2) *Cephalic stimulation.* Vagal, cholinergic pathways stimulate an increase in enzyme-rich fluid. (3) *Intestinal stimulation.* Chyme and acid stimulate pancreatic secretion, probably largely through secretin and CCK release. The role of pancreatic fluid in digestion is further considered in the chapter on Malabsorption (Chapter 36C).

Studies of Pancreatic Structure and Function

The pancreas until recently was frustratingly difficult to study in the presence of suspected disease. It can now be successfully imaged noninvasively by ultrasonography and computed tomography (CT) (Fig. 42–3) and invasively by endoscopic retrograde cholangiopancreatography (ERCP). Biopsy by fine needle with ultrasound or CT guidance and selective angiography are also useful in selected cases, and imaging by nuclear

magnetic resonance (MRI) may prove useful in the future.

Acute injury to the pancreatic acini is reflected by leakage of the enzyme amylase into blood, which can be measured as an increase in serum amylase or more rarely as urinary amylase. Normal serum amylase (25 to 125 U/L) largely originates in salivary glands. Pancreatic secretion is estimated, with considerable error, by aspiration of duodenal contents through a tube following stimulation with secretin, secretin-CCK, or a test meal, as summarized in Table 42–1. Such quantitative studies of secretion are rarely clinically indicated.

ACUTE PANCREATITIS

Definition. Acute pancreatitis is an acute, inflammatory disorder of the pancreas associated

TABLE 42–1. RANGE OF NORMAL RESPONSES TO SECRETORY TESTS OF THE PANCREAS

Secretin test*
    Volume (ml/80 min): 117–392
    HCO_3^- concentration (mEq/liter): 88–137
    HCO_3^- output (mEq/80 min): 16–33
    Amylase output (units/80 min): 439–1921
Secretin + CCK*
    Volume (ml/80 min): 111–503
    HCO_3^- concentration (mEq/liter): 88–144
    HCO_3^- output (mEq/80 min): 10–86
    Amylase output (units/80 min): 441–4038
Lundh Test
    Mean tryptic activity (IU/liter): 61

* Modified from Dreiling DA, Janowitz HD, and Perrier CV: Pancreatic Inflammatory Disease. A Physiologic Approach. New York, Hoeber Medical Division, Harper & Row, Publishers, 1964. (Reprinted from Meyer JH: The pancreas. In Sleisenger MH, and Fordtran JS (eds): Gastrointestinal Disease. 3rd ed. Philadelphia, WB Saunders Co, 1983, p 1426.)

with edema, swelling, and various amounts of autodigestion, necrosis, and hemorrhage. It is usually defined clinically by a symptom complex with an associated elevation of serum amylase. It is useful to consider acute pancreatitis as a single clinical entity, although it may be of diverse etiologies, may vary greatly in severity, and may shade into chronic relapsing pancreatitis and chronic pancreatitis (to be considered subsequently).

Etiology and Pathogenesis. The disorders most commonly associated with acute pancreatitis in the United States are listed in Table 42–2. Of these, alcoholism and biliary tract disease are the most important. The pathogenesis of acute pancreatitis is thought to be autodigestion due to inappropriate intrapancreatic activation of proteases (Fig. 42–4). Just why this occurs usually is unknown, although it is speculated that alcohol produces obstructive inspissated proteinaceous plugs in pancreatic ducts and that gallstones, passing through the sphincter of Oddi, cause obstruction and possibly bile regurgitation into the pancreatic duct. Simply ligating the pancreatic duct does not usually cause acute pancreatitis, however, so that other unexplained factors are probably involved. Knowledge of the association of acute pancreatitis with the conditions listed in Table 42–2 is important for two reasons: (a) it sug-

TABLE 42–2. RISK FACTORS IN ACUTE PANCREATITIS

Alcohol abuse
Gallstones
Abdominal trauma
Infections: mumps, coxsackie, hepatitis, other viruses
Ischemic vascular disease
Hyperlipoproteinemias
Hypercalcemia
Drugs: steroids, diuretics, isoniazid, immunosuppressives
Immunological disorders: polyarteritis, systemic lupus erythematosus
Cancer of the pancreas
Pancreas divisum
Hereditary: several forms
Posterior penetration of a duodenal ulcer
Endoscopic retrograde cholangiopancreatography (ERCP)

Modified from Brooks FP: Diseases of the Exocrine Pancreas. Philadelphia, WB Saunders Co, 1980, p 8.

gests the possibility in a given patient, and (b) preventing recurrent pancreatitis often depends on reversal of these associated abnormalities.

Clinical Manifestations. The most important symptom of acute pancreatitis is abdominal *pain*,

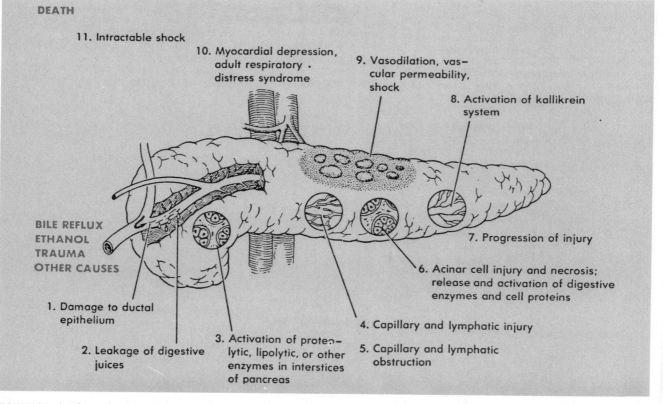

FIGURE 42–4. The pathophysiology of acute pancreatitis is not fully understood, but, as the schematic above implies, a cascade of events seems likely, beginning with the release of toxic substances into the parenchyma and ending with shock and death. Damage to the ductal epithelium or acinar cell injury may result from bile reflux, increased intraductal pressure, alcohol, or trauma. (Reprinted from Grendell JH: The pancreas. In Smith LH Jr, and Thier SO (eds): Pathophysiology: The Biological Principles of Disease. 2nd ed. Philadelphia, WB Saunders Co, 1985, p 1228.)

which is characteristically steady, severe, and epigastric in location with later radiation to the back and partially relieved by leaning forward. The pain is highly variable, however, and may be relatively mild or diffuse. The abdomen is usually tender, without signs of peritoneal irritation, and nausea and vomiting are absent. Severe cases distend the abdomen with ileus and produce high fever, confusion, tachycardia, and, sometimes, impending shock. Rarer features are (1) discoloration in the flanks (Grey-Turner's sign) or around the umbilicus (Cullen's sign) in hemorrhagic pancreatitis, (2) subcutaneous fat necrosis presenting as tender, red subcutaneous nodules, (3) ascites, (4) atelectasis and/or left-sided pleural effusion, (5) adult respiratory distress syndrome, (6) jaundice, and (7) an epigastric mass representing a pseudocyst.

Diagnosis. The diagnosis of acute pancreatitis must be entertained in any patient with the acute onset of severe, noncolicky epigastric pain, especially in the presence of one of the known associated disorders (Table 42–2). The differential diagnosis usually includes biliary colic, a perforated viscus (especially a duodenal ulcer), acute cholecystitis, abdominal vasculitis, acute bowel infarction, renal colic, and a number of other causes of "the acute abdomen."

Most patients with clinically defined acute pancreatitis have an enlarged pancreas as defined by ultrasonography and/or CT, but the diagnosis cannot be made without concomitant evidence of acinar cell injury as reflected in an elevation of serum amylase. Conversely, other causes of an elevated serum amylase must be considered also (Table 42–3). After the onset of symptoms serum amylase rises early (2 to 12 hours) and usually remains elevated for three to five days. Some believe that in the face of an elevated serum amylase, an associated increased renal clearance of amylase (amylase clearance > 4 per cent of that of creatinine) is a useful indication of the presence of pancreatitis, but the test is not diagnostic.

Other laboratory abnormalities may include hyperglycemia, hypocalcemia, and leukocytosis.

Treatment and Prognosis. The treatment of acute pancreatitis is largely supportive: (1) careful monitoring and volume replacement for fluids lost retroperitoneally; (2) relief of pain, preferably using meperidine; (3) nasogastric suction—this traditional approach to "putting the pancreas at rest," however, will not affect outcome in mild to moderate cases; (4) treatment of complications as they arise—calcium for hypocalcemia, insulin for

TABLE 42–3. SOME CONDITIONS OTHER THAN ACUTE PANCREATITIS THAT MAY BE ASSOCIATED WITH HYPERAMYLASEMIA

Macroamylasemia	Mesenteric infarction
Diabetic ketoacidosis	Parotitis, mumps
Renal insufficiency	Opiate administration
Burn injury	Peritonitis
Postoperative state	Cholecystitis
Peptic ulcer	

TABLE 42–4. COMPLICATIONS OF ACUTE PANCREATITIS

Pancreatic—phlegmon, pseudocyst, abscess, ascites, hemorrhage
Contiguous organs—portal venous thrombosis, bowel necrosis, intraperitoneal bleeding, obstruction of common duct
Systemic
  Cardiovascular—hypotension, nonspecific ST-T changes, pericardial effusion
  Pulmonary—pleural effusion, shock lung, atelectasis
  Renal—acute renal failure
  Gastrointestinal—gastritis
  Hematologic—disseminated intravascular coagulation
  Metabolic—hypocalcemia, hyperglycemia, hypertriglyceridemia
  Fat necrosis—subcutaneous, bone
  Central nervous system—confusion or delirium

Reprinted from Levitt MD: Pancreatitis. In Wyngaarden JB, and Smith LH Jr (eds): Cecil Textbook of Medicine. 17th ed. Philadelphia, WB Saunders Co, 1985, p 774.

excessive hyperglycemia, etc. Other measures that have been advocated, including administration of cimetidine, aprotinin, and glucagon, appear to be without benefit.

About 90 per cent of patients recover, usually within one to two weeks. About 10 per cent die despite therapy, most frequently from the adult respiratory distress syndrome or from shock.

Complications. The complications most frequently seen in the course of acute pancreatitis are listed in Table 42–4. A phlegmon is a solid mass of inflamed pancreas, which usually subsides spontaneously. A pseudocyst is a liquified collection of necrotic debris surrounded by a rim of pancreatic tissue and/or other tissue. Small pseudocysts may disappear, but large ones may persist to cause pain or bleeding, erode into adjacent tissues, or become infected, requiring surgical drainage.

CHRONIC PANCREATITIS

Definition. Chronic pancreatitis and chronic relapsing pancreatitis can be considered together, since both represent a slowly progressive destruction of pancreatic acini, varying amounts of inflammation, fibrosis, and dilatation and distortion of the pancreatic ducts. In chronic relapsing pancreatitis there are associated episodes of acute inflammation. The end result is that of varying degrees of pancreatic destruction and exocrine insufficiency.

Etiology and Pathogenesis. By and large the same conditions listed in Table 42–2 as being associated with acute pancreatitis may also lead to chronic pancreatitis. Biliary tract disease, however, is rarely associated with chronic pancreatitis. In the United States the major associated conditions are alcoholism in adults and cystic fibrosis in children; in the developing countries the most common cause seems to be protein-calorie malnutrition. The cause is unknown in many cases. Injury is presumed to be secondary to autodigestion, as in acute pancreatitis (Fig. 42–4), but this has not been established.

Clinical Manifestations. The most important symptoms and signs of chronic pancreatitis are

TABLE 42–5. SYMPTOMS AND SIGNS OF CHRONIC PANCREATITIS

Abdominal pain	Jaundice
Weight loss	Palpable pseudocyst
Diabetes mellitus	Pancreatic ascites
Steatorrhea	Gastrointestinal bleeding

summarized in Table 42–5. In general, severe, intractable abdominal *pain* is the cardinal symptom, although pain may be mild or even absent in a minority of patients or episodic with relapsing pancreatitis. The pain may go through to the back, be partially relieved by sitting up and leaning forward, be exacerbated by eating or drinking alcohol, or exhibit none of these features. Patients usually lose weight because of anorexia and/or an associated malabsorption (steatorrhea and azotorrhea). Encasement of the common bile duct in fibrous tissue may produce obstructive jaundice. The islets of Langerhans often become sufficiently destroyed to produce diabetes mellitus. Gastrointestinal bleeding may rarely result from thrombosis of the splenic vein, leading to gastric varices, or more commonly from gastritis, resulting from the associated excessive use of ethanol or aspirin (in an attempt to relieve pain). Rarely, an abdominal mass representing a pseudocyst may be palpated.

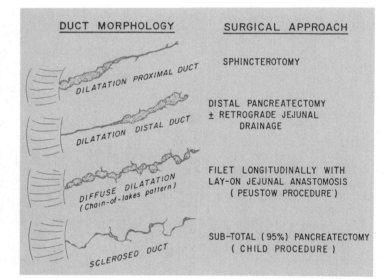

FIGURE 42–5. Pathologic changes in the pancreatic ducts of patients with chronic pancreatitis as demonstrated by endoscopic retrograde cholangiopancreatography (ERCP) in relation to the selection of appropriate operative procedures. (Reproduced with permission from Stone LB, Eaton SB Jr, and Ferrucci JT Jr: Inflammatory disease of the pancreas. In Moseley RD, et al: Current Problems in Radiology. Copyright © 1975 by Year Book Medical Publishers, Inc, Chicago.)

TABLE 42–6. COMPLICATIONS OF CHRONIC PANCREATITIS

Pseudocyst formation	Peptic ulcer
Pancreatic abscess	Drug addiction
Obstruction of the common bile duct	Exocrine insufficiency
Diabetes mellitus	Carcinoma (rare)

Diagnosis. The diagnosis of chronic pancreatitis as a cause of pain is usually easy in the presence of the classic triad of pancreatic calcification, pancreatic exocrine deficiency (malabsorption), and diabetes mellitus, especially if any of the known risk factors are present. However, only a minority of patients present with this complete clinical picture. The differential diagnosis usually includes abdominal malignancy, especially carcinoma of the pancreas or of the stomach or colon. Biliary tract disease, peptic ulcer disease, mesenteric vascular disease, and functional abdominal complaints may occasionally simulate the pain of chronic pancreatitis.

Measurement of serum amylase is of no help in the diagnosis of chronic pancreatitis, since it is usually elevated only during acute exacerbations of chronic, relapsing pancreatitis. Three structural features may be of help: (1) the demonstration of pancreatic calcification by a plain abdominal radiograph or, with greater sensitivity, by CT; (2) the demonstration of dilated, distorted ducts, best shown by ERCP (Fig. 42–5); (3) the demonstration of pseudocysts by ultrasonography and/or CT.

Malabsorption can be demonstrated by fecal analysis for fat, and its pancreatic origin can be deduced by the tests described in Chapter 36C. In chronic pancreatitis pancreatic stimulation tests characteristically show reductions in pancreatic juice volume, bicarbonate content, amylase output, and tryptic activity.

Treatment and Prognosis. The treatment of chronic pancreatitis is directed toward (1) prevention of further injury, (2) relief of pain, and (3) replacement of lost exocrine function. Prevention of further injury usually depends upon attempting to reverse one or more of the factors listed in Table 42–2, especially alcoholism. The replacement of lost exocrine function is described in Chapter 36C on Malabsorption. The treatment of pain is usually the most difficult and important challenge. There are three general approaches:

ANALGESICS. Attempts should be made to begin with nonaddictive analgesics before resorting to narcotics. Many patients unfortunately become addicted because of the severity and duration of the pain.

"PUTTING THE PANCREAS AT REST." The ingestion of large amounts of pancreatic enzymes may reduce pain, presumably by diminishing stimuli to its exocrine secretion. Avoiding large meals and alcohol also may help.

SURGICAL THERAPY. Surgery to relieve a ductal obstruction or drainage of a pseudocyst may be effective in selected cases of intractable pain, although the results are often unsatisfactory. Fortunately, the pain of chronic pancreatitis tends to diminish over time, presumably because of the destruction of most of the residual functioning exocrine cells. Patients seldom die of uncomplicated chronic pancreatitis.

Complications. The complications that may be associated with chronic pancreatitis are listed in Table 42–6. An increased incidence of carcinoma of the pancreas probably occurs only in rare forms of hereditary pancreatitis.

CARCINOMA OF THE PANCREAS

Definition. Carcinoma of the pancreas is an almost universally fatal malignancy, over 90 per cent representing an adenocarcinoma arising from ductal cells. Much rarer are islet cell tumors (not discussed here), epidermoid tumors, or adenocarcinomas arising from acinar cells. Carcinoma of the pancreas seems to be increasing in incidence and is now the fourth most common malignant tumor (after tumors of the lung, colon, and breast), accounting for about 5 per cent of deaths from cancer.

Etiology and Pathogenesis. The cause of carcinoma of the pancreas is not known. Epidemiological studies have suggested the following risk factors: advancing age, smoking, diabetes mellitus, some forms of chronic pancreatitis, and certain dietary habits (increased consumption of animal fat and protein). A reported association with excessive consumption of coffee is unconfirmed.

Clinical Manifestations. The clinical manifestations tend to be nonspecific and are often insidious in onset, so that the malignancy reaches an advanced stage by the time diagnosis is made. The cardinal manifestations are *epigastric pain* and *weight loss.* The pain is usually persistent, dull, and noncolicky and may radiate to the back but can be individually variable. Anorexia, nausea, and vomiting occur frequently, sometimes in association with a strange aversion to meat. Emotional disturbances (anxiety, depression) have been described as occurring more frequently and earlier than in other malignancies. Obstructive jaundice results commonly from carcinoma of the head of the pancreas, sometimes in association with a large, palpable gallbladder. A number of other abnormalities can accompany the illness: migratory thrombophlebitis (Trousseau's sign), acute pancreatitis, diabetes mellitus, paraneoplastic endocrine syndromes (Cushing's syndrome, hypercalcemia), upper gastrointestinal bleeding (direct invasion of stomach or duodenum, involvement of the splenic vein with production of varices), or an abdominal mass. Rarely, with adenocarcinoma of acinar cells, fat necrosis may produce painful nodules subcutaneously or bone pain from intramedullary involvement.

Diagnosis. Carcinoma of the pancreas must be considered in older patients with unexplained abdominal pain, excessive weight loss, the sudden onset of diabetes mellitus without obesity or appropriate family history, acute pancreatitis without a known risk factor (Table 42–2), or obstructive jaundice. Laboratory studies, including the serum tumor markers carcinoembryonic antigen (CEA), α-fetoprotein (AFP), and galactosyltransferase isoenzyme II (GT-II), rarely help because of their nonspecificity.

The diagnosis is made most frequently by a combination of imaging and fine needle biopsy. Figure 42–6 provides an algorithm for using these modalities. The diagnostic sensitivity for carcinoma of the pancreas by these techniques is ultrasonography 70 to 90 per cent, CT approxi-

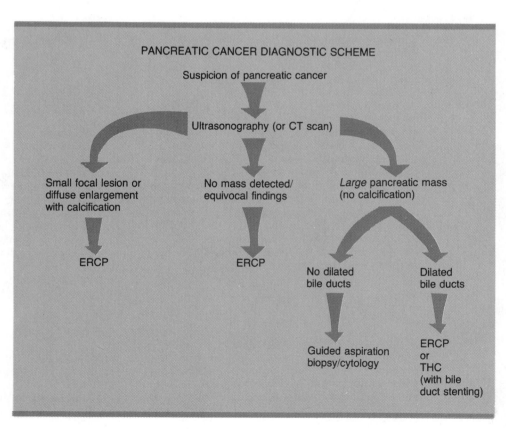

FIGURE 42–6. Pancreatic cancer diagnosis. (Reprinted from Cello JP: Carcinoma of the pancreas. In Wyngaarden JB, and Smith LH Jr (eds): Cecil Textbook of Medicine. 17th ed. Philadelphia, WB Saunders Co, 1985, p 780.)

PANCREATIC CANCER DIAGNOSTIC SCHEME

Suspicion of pancreatic cancer

Ultrasonography (or CT scan)

Small focal lesion or diffuse enlargement with calcification → ERCP

No mass detected/ equivocal findings → ERCP

Large pancreatic mass (no calcification)

No dilated bile ducts → Guided aspiration biopsy/cytology

Dilated bile ducts → ERCP or THC (with bile duct stenting)

mately 80 per cent, and ERCP 75 to 85 per cent. Selective arteriography rarely may be required.

Treatment and Prognosis. The treatment of pancreatic carcinoma is inadequate and disappointing. Only about 10 to 20 per cent of tumors are resectable at the time of diagnosis, and surgical treatment of even this group produces no demonstrated increase in five-year survival. Surgery is often confined to palliative decompression of the biliary system to relieve obstructive jaundice or severe pruritus or cholangitis. This can now be effected in many patients by percutaneous transhepatic stenting of the common bile duct with internal or external drainage. Stents may be placed also during ERCP. Supravoltage radiation or multidrug chemotherapeutic programs may somewhat palliate symptoms but do not prolong survival. Approximately 10 per cent of patients survive diagnosis by one year and only 1 to 2 per cent by five years.

Complications. The complications of pancreatic carcinoma have largely been listed as part of the clinical manifestations. In addition, there may be extensive local invasion of vital structures and metastases, especially to the liver.

REFERENCES

Brooks FP: Diseases of the Exocrine Pancreas. Philadelphia, WB Saunders Co, 1980.
Cello JP: Carcinoma of the pancreas. In Sleisenger MH, and Fordtran JS (eds): Gastrointestinal Disease. 3rd ed. Philadelphia, WB Saunders Co, 1983, p 1514.
Cello JP: Carcinoma of the pancreas. In Wyngaarden JM, and Smith LH Jr (eds): Cecil Textbook of Medicine. 17th ed. Philadelphia, WB Saunders Co, 1985, p 777.
Grendell JH, and Cello JP: Chronic pancreatitis. In Sleisenger MH, and Fordtran JS (eds): Gastrointestinal Disease. 3rd ed. Philadelphia, WB Saunders Co, 1983, p 1485.
Levitt MD: Pancreatitis. In Wyngaarden JB, and Smith LH Jr (eds): In Cecil Textbook of Medicine. 17th ed. Philadelphia, WB Saunders Co, 1985, p 771.
Soergel KH: Acute pancreatitis. In Sleisenger MH, and Fordtran JS (eds): Gastrointestinal Disease. 3rd ed. Philadelphia, WB Saunders Co, 1983, p 1462.
Van Dyke JA, Stanley RJ, and Berland LL: Pancreatic imaging. Ann Intern Med 102:212, 1985.

43 LABORATORY TESTS IN LIVER DISEASE

The liver, the largest organ in the body, has a wide array of metabolic functions. Indeed, it plays a central role in many essential physiological processes, including glucose homeostasis, plasma protein synthesis, lipid and lipoprotein synthesis, bile acid synthesis and secretion, and vitamin storage (B_{12}, A, D, E, and K), as well as biotransformation, detoxification, and excretion of a vast array of endogenous and exogenous compounds. The clinical manifestations of liver disease are, likewise, varied and may be quite subtle. Clues to the existence, severity, and etiology of liver disease may be obtained from a careful history and physical examination or by routine laboratory screening tests. Clinical clues to the presence of liver disease will be briefly mentioned here and are discussed more fully in other chapters. This chapter will focus on the use of laboratory tests in the evaluation of liver disease.

CLINICAL APPROACH TO LIVER DISEASE

Table 43–1 outlines useful clinical clues to the presence of liver disease that may be elicited from the history and physical examination. Other important information to be obtained includes a history of jaundice or liver disease in family members, recent travel, exposure to individuals or animals with liver disease, sexual promiscuity, use of intravenous drugs, and exposure to alcohol, toxins, or drugs.

LABORATORY TESTS OF LIVER FUNCTION AND DISEASE

Unlike tests used to assess function of other organ systems (e.g., arterial blood gas, creatinine clearance), "liver function" tests often do not measure liver function, nor do they accurately reflect etiology or severity of a disease process. Nevertheless, if their limitations are understood, they can be very useful. In general, the tests currently available can be divided into two categories: (1) tests of hepatic function or capacity, and (2) screening tests that suggest the presence and/or type of liver disease. Specific diagnostic tests such as serological tests for hepatitis B infection are covered in other chapters.

TESTS OF HEPATIC FUNCTION

Although the liver performs a great variety of presumably testable functions, it has proved difficult to devise a test that is simple, cheap, reproducible, and noninvasive and that accurately reflects hepatic capacity for all functions. Instead,

TABLE 43–1. CLINICAL MANIFESTATIONS OF LIVER DISEASE

SIGN/SYMPTOM	PATHOGENESIS	LIVER DISEASE
Constitutional		
Fatigue, anorexia, malaise, weight loss	Liver failure	Severe acute or chronic hepatitis
		Cirrhosis
Fever	Hepatic inflammation or infection	Liver abscess
		Alcoholic hepatitis
		Viral hepatitis
Fetor hepaticus	Abnormal methionine metabolism	Acute or chronic liver failure
Cutaneous		
Spider telangiectasias, palmar erythema	Altered estrogen and androgen metabolism	Cirrhosis
Jaundice	Diminished bilirubin excretion	Biliary obstruction
		Severe liver disease
Pruritus	—	Biliary obstruction
Xanthomas and xanthelasma	Increased serum lipids	Biliary obstruction/cholestasis
Endocrine		
Gynecomastia, testicular atrophy, diminished libido	Altered estrogen and androgen metabolism	Cirrhosis
Hypoglycemia	Decreased glycogen stores and gluconeogenesis	Liver failure
Gastrointestinal		
Right upper quadrant abdominal pain	Liver swelling, infection	Acute hepatitis
		Hepatocellular carcinoma
		Liver congestion (heart failure)
		Acute cholecystitis
		Liver abscess
Abdominal swelling	Ascites	Cirrhosis, portal hypertension
Gastrointestinal bleeding	Esophageal varices	Portal hypertension
Hematological		
Decreased red cells, white cells, and/or platelets	Hypersplenism	Cirrhosis, portal hypertension
Ecchymoses	Decreased synthesis of clotting factors	Liver failure
Neurological		
Altered sleep pattern, subtle behavioral changes, somnolence, confusion, ataxia, asterixis, obtundation	Hepatic encephalopathy	Liver failure, portosystemic shunting of blood

currently available tests of liver function are indirect, static measurements of serum levels of compounds that are synthesized, metabolized, and/or excreted by the liver. In interpreting these tests, it is important to remember that the liver has a large reserve capacity, and therefore "function" tests may remain relatively normal until liver dysfunction is severe. Table 43–2 outlines the most available and useful liver function tests. The serum albumin level and prothrombin time both reflect the hepatic capacity for protein synthesis, although changes in these proteins are not specific for liver disease. The prothrombin time responds rapidly to altered hepatic function because the serum half-lives of Factors II and VII are short (hours). In contrast, the serum half-life of albumin is 14 to 20 days, and serum levels fall only with prolonged, severe liver dysfunction.

Serum bile acid levels, particularly when measured two hours after a meal, have proved to be the most sensitive test of liver disease, and this is due to the high efficiency with which the liver normally extracts bile acids from portal blood. Small changes in hepatic blood flow, portosystemic shunting, or liver function all result in a substantial elevation of serum bile acid levels, while terminal ileal dysfunction (e.g., Crohn's disease) leads to fecal loss of bile acids and decreased serum levels. Although exquisitely sensitive, bile acid levels are nonspecific and fail to reflect accurately overall liver function.

The ^{14}C-aminopyrine breath test was originally developed as a true test of liver function. It measures the rate at which the liver metabolizes ^{14}C-labeled aminopyrine to $^{14}CO_2$, which is collected and measured in exhaled breath. This test is performed in some academic centers and may be useful in following the progression of liver disease in an individual patient.

SCREENING TESTS OF HEPATOBILIARY DISEASE

Screening tests of hepatobiliary disease, which are listed in Table 43–2, are conveniently divided into two categories: (1) tests of biliary obstruction, and (2) tests of hepatocellular damage, based on the mechanisms responsible for the abnormal test. However, none of the tests is specific for either category, and it is the pattern and magnitude of abnormalities that often provide diagnostic clues to the type of liver disease present.

The *serum bilirubin level* is the result of bilirubin production, bilirubin conjugation, and excretion of bilirubin into bile. Its bright orange

TABLE 43–2. CLINICAL LIVER TESTS

	PROPERTY EXAMINED	SIGNIFICANCE OF ABNORMAL RESULTS
Tests of Hepatic Function		
Serum albumin	Protein synthetic capacity (over days to weeks)	Decreased synthetic capacity Protein malnutrition Increased protein loss (nephrotic syndrome, protein-losing enteropathy) Increased extracellular fluid volume
Prothrombin time	Protein synthetic capacity (hours to days)	Decreased synthetic capacity (especially Factors II and VII) Vitamin K deficiency
Serum bile acids	Extraction from blood and biliary excretion of bile acids	Diffuse liver disease Cholestasis Terminal ileal disease Portosystemic shunting of blood
^{14}C-aminopyrine breath test	Drug-metabolizing capacity	Decreased metabolic capacity (diffuse liver disease) Severe portosystemic shunting of blood
Screening Tests of Hepatobiliary Disease		
Tests of Biliary Obstruction		
Serum bilirubin	Extraction of bilirubin from blood, conjugation and excretion into bile	Hemolysis Diffuse liver disease Cholestasis Extrahepatic bile duct obstruction Congenital disorders of bilirubin metabolism
Serum alkaline phosphatase (also 5'-nucleotidase and gamma glutamyl transpeptidase)	Increased synthesis and release of membrane enzyme by increased serum bile acids	Bile duct obstruction Cholestasis Infiltrative liver disease (neoplasms, granulomas) Bone destruction/remodeling Pregnancy
Tests of Hepatocellular Damage		
Aspartate aminotransferase (AST; SGOT)	Release of intracellular enzyme	Hepatocellular necrosis Cardiac or skeletal muscle necrosis
Alanine aminotransferase (ALT; SGPT)	Release of intracellular enzyme	Same as AST, but more specific for liver cell damage

color made it the first, and the most striking, of liver tests. However, the differential diagnosis of hyperbilirubinemia is extensive (see Chapter 36E) and includes hematologic disorders, congenital abnormalities of bilirubin metabolism, and a wide array of liver diseases. It is nonspecific and only moderately sensitive as a test of liver function. Striking elevations of serum bilirubin, however, should prompt a search for potentially treatable biliary obstruction. Serum bilirubin levels may not return promptly to normal after relief of biliary obstruction or improvement in liver disease, because some bilirubin binds covalently to albumin and is removed from the circulation only as albumin is catabolized (half-life 14 to 20 days).

Serum *alkaline phosphatase* activity reflects a group of isoenzymes derived from liver, bone, intestine, and placenta. Serum levels are elevated in association with cholestasis, partial or complete bile duct obstruction, and bone regeneration, and also with neoplastic, infiltrative, and granulomatous liver diseases. An isolated elevated alkaline phosphatase level may be the only clue to partial obstruction of the common bile duct, to obstruction of ducts in a single lobe or segment of liver, or to neoplastic or granulomatous disease. Alkaline phosphatase is located on

the plasma membrane of hepatocytes. Bile duct obstruction, accompanied by increased serum and tissue levels of bile acids, results in solubilization into the blood stream of bits of hepatocyte membrane containing alkaline phosphatase. Increased hepatic bile acid levels also stimulate synthesis of alkaline phosphatase, contributing to the elevation of serum levels. 5'-Nucleotidase and gamma glutamyl transpeptidase are other hepatocyte plasma membrane enzymes that are similarly released into the circulation during bile duct obstruction or cholestasis.

Aspartate (AST) and alanine (ALT) aminotransferases are intracellular amino-transferring enzymes present in large quantities in liver cells. Following injury or death of liver cells, they are released into the circulation. In general, the serum transaminases are sensitive (albeit nonspecific) tests of liver damage, and the height of the serum transaminase activity reflects the severity of hepatic necrosis, but there are important exceptions. Both enzymes require pyridoxal 5-phosphate as a cofactor, and the relatively low serum transaminase values seen in patients with severe alcoholic hepatitis (often <300 IU/L) may reflect deficiency of this cofactor. Although transaminase levels are increased in a wide array of liver diseases, high

TABLE 43–3. CHARACTERISTIC PATTERNS OF LIVER FUNCTION TESTS

DISORDER	BILIRUBIN	ALKALINE PHOSPHATASE	PROTHROMBIN TIME	AST	ALT
Gilbert's syndrome	↑	nl	nl	nl	nl
Bile duct obstruction (pancreatic carcinoma)	↑ ↑ ↑	↑ ↑ ↑	↑ - ↑ ↑	↑	↑
Acute viral or toxic hepatitis	↑ - ↑ ↑ ↑	↑ - ↑ ↑	nl - ↑ ↑ ↑	↑ ↑ ↑	↑ ↑ ↑
Cirrhosis	nl - ↑	nl - ↑	nl - ↑ ↑	nl - ↑	nl - ↑

nl = normal

levels (>15 times the upper limit of normal) are rare in bile duct obstruction and almost always indicate acute hepatocellular necrosis (e.g., viral or toxic hepatitis).

The commonly available liver tests usually do not indicate the nature of the underlying liver disease; however, the *pattern* of liver test abnormalities may provide insight in this regard. Table 43–3 outlines the most common patterns of liver test abnormalities.

LIVER BIOPSY

Biopsy and histological examination of liver tissue is of value in the differential diagnosis of diffuse or localized parenchymal diseases (e.g., cirrhosis, hepatitis, hemochromatosis) or hepatomegaly. Liver biopsy is safe (serious complications <0.5 per cent); however, it is contraindicated in uncooperative patients and those with coagulation abnormalities or thrombocytopenia.

REFERENCES

Kaplowitz N, Eberle D, and Yamada T: Biochemical tests for liver disease. In Zakim D, and Boyer T (eds): Hepatology: A Textbook of Liver Disease. Philadelphia, WB Saunders Co, 1982, pp 583–611.

Ockner RK: Laboratory tests in liver disease. In Wyngaarden JB, and Smith LH Jr (eds): Cecil Textbook of Medicine. 17th ed. Philadelphia, WB Saunders Co, 1985, pp 809–811.

ACUTE AND CHRONIC HEPATITIS

44

DEFINITION

The term hepatitis is applied to a broad category of clinicopathological conditions that result from the damage produced by viral, toxic, pharmacological, or immune-mediated attack upon the liver. The common pathological features of hepatitis are hepatocellular necrosis, which may be focal or extensive, and inflammatory cell infiltration of the liver, which may predominate in the portal areas or extend out into the parenchyma. Clinically, the liver is enlarged and tender with or without jaundice, and laboratory evidence of hepatocellular damage is invariably found in the form of elevated transaminase levels. Independent of its cause, the clinical course of hepatitis may range from mild or inapparent to a dramatic illness with evidence of severe hepatocellular dysfunction, marked jaundice, impairment of coagulation, and disturbance of neurological function. Hepatitis is further divided into acute and chronic types on the basis of clinical and pathological criteria.

Acute hepatitis implies a condition lasting less than six months, culminating either in complete resolution of the liver damage with return to normal liver function and structure or in rapid progression of the acute injury toward extensive necrosis and a fatal outcome.

Chronic hepatitis is defined as a sustained inflammatory process in the liver lasting longer than six months.

Differentiation of acute from chronic hepatitis on histological criteria alone may be impossible. Extension of inflammatory cells beyond the limits of the portal tracts surrounding isolated nests of hepatocytes (piecemeal necrosis) and connection of portal and/or central areas of the hepatic lobules by swaths of inflammation, necrosis, and collapse of architecture (bridging necrosis) are seen in liver biopsies taken from patients with severe forms of chronic hepatitis. These features may also be seen, however, in uncomplicated acute hepatitis that will ultimately undergo complete resolution. A purely histological diagnosis of chronic hepatitis usually requires evidence of

TABLE 44—1. CAUSES OF ACUTE HEPATITIS

Viral Hepatitis
  Hepatitis A virus
  Hepatitis B virus
  Hepatitis non-A, non-B viruses
  Delta (δ) agent
  Epstein-Barr virus
  Cytomegalovirus
Alcohol
Toxins
  Amanita phalloides mushroom poisoning
  Carbon tetrachloride
Drugs
  Acetaminophen
  Isoniazid
  Halothane
  Chlorpromazine
  Erythromycin
Other
  Wilson's disease

progression toward cirrhosis such as significant fibrous scarring and disruption of the hepatic lobular architecture.

ACUTE HEPATITIS

Agents causing acute hepatic injury are listed in Table 44–1. The mechanisms whereby these agents produce hepatic damage include direct toxin-induced necrosis (e.g., acetaminophen, *Amanita phalloides* toxin) and host immune-mediated damage, which probably plays an important, but not well understood, role in viral hepatitis. In the case of frank hepatotoxins such as *Amanita* poisoning, massive hepatic necrosis is the dominant process, and the clinical course is more aptly described as fulminant hepatic failure (see Chapter 45) rather than acute hepatitis. Such a course is less common, but well recognized, with all the causative agents listed in Table 44–1.

Acute Viral Hepatitis

Etiology. Viral hepatitis is caused by three main viruses: hepatitis viruses A and B and the so-called non-A, non-B agents, of which there appear to be at least two. Cytomegalovirus and Epstein-Barr virus occasionally cause hepatitis. An incomplete RNA virus, the delta (δ) agent, causes hepatitis either simultaneously with the B virus or in individuals already chronically infected with the B virus. Of these agents, the B virus has been most extensively characterized, whereas least is known regarding the non-A, non-B agents. The three major viruses are compared in Table 44–2. The complete B virus (Dane particle) consists of several antigenically distinct components (Fig. 44–1), including a surface coat (hepatitis B surface antigen, HB_sAg) and a core of circular DNA, DNA polymerase, hepatitis B core antigen (HB_cAg), and hepatitis e antigen (HB_eAg). HB_sAg may exist in serum either as part of the Dane particle or as free particles and rods. Surface antigen as well as HB_cAg and HB_eAg each elicit distinct antibody responses from the host, which are of value in serological diagnosis and characterization of the state of B virus replication in the liver.

Transmission. Hepatitis A virus (HAV) is excreted in the feces during the incubation period (Fig. 44–2) and is transmitted by the fecal-oral route. It is thus implicated in most instances of water-borne and food-transmitted cases and in epidemics of viral hepatitis. The hepatitis B virus is present in virtually all body fluids and excreta of carriers and is transmitted mainly by parenteral routes. Thus, transmission occurs most commonly via blood and blood products, contaminated needles, and intimate personal contact. Persons at high risk of infection with the B virus therefore include sexual partners of acutely as well as chronically infected individuals, with male homosexuals being at particularly high risk; health professionals, particularly surgeons, dentists, and workers in clinical laboratories and dialysis units; intravenous drug abusers; and infants of infected mothers ("vertical transmission"). Patients with increased exposure to blood or blood products and/or with impaired immunity (e.g., dialysis patients, patients with leukemia or Down's syndrome) are also highly susceptible to B virus infection.

TABLE 44—2. CHARACTERISTICS OF COMMON CAUSATIVE AGENTS OF ACUTE VIRAL HEPATITIS

	HEPATITIS A	HEPATITIS B	HEPATITIS NON-A, NON-B (TWO OR MORE AGENTS)
Causative agent	27-nm RNA virus	42-nm DNA virus; core and surface components	Apparent similarities to hepatitis B virus
Transmission	Fecal-oral; water-, food-borne	Parenteral inoculation or equivalent; direct contact	Same as for B; rarely water- or food-borne
Incubation period	2–6 weeks	4 weeks–6 months	2–20 weeks
Period of infectivity	2–3 weeks in late incubation and early clinical phase	During HB_sAg-positivity (occasionally only with anti-HB_c positivity)	Unknown
Massive hepatic necrosis	Rare	Uncommon	Uncommon
Carrier state	No	Yes	Yes
Chronic hepatitis	No	Yes	Yes
Prophylaxis	Hygiene; immune serum globulin	Hygiene; hepatitis B immune globulin; vaccine	Hygiene; ? immune serum globulin; avoid commercial blood

FIGURE 44—1. Different types of hepatitis B virus particles in plasma. The locations of the various antigenic components are indicated.

Non-A, non-B hepatitis, similar to hepatitis B, is largely a parenterally transmitted disease. Since no diagnostic marker exists for this group of viruses as yet, non-A, non-B hepatitis is currently the main cause of post-transfusion hepatitis.

Clinical and Laboratory Manifestations. Acute viral hepatitis typically begins with a prodromal phase lasting several days characterized by constitutional and gastrointestinal symptoms including malaise, fatigue, anorexia, nausea, vomiting, myalgia, and headache. A mild fever may be present. Symptoms suggestive of "flu" may be prominent; arthritis and urticaria, attributed to immune complex deposition, may be present, particularly in hepatitis B. Smokers often describe an aversion to cigarettes. Jaundice soon appears with bilirubinuria and a loss of stool color, often accompanied by an improvement in the patient's sense of well-being. Jaundice may be absent (anicteric hepatitis); in such cases—probably the majority of cases of acute viral hepatitis—medical attention is often not sought. The liver is usually tender and enlarged; splenomegaly is found in about one fifth of patients.

Transaminases (ALT and AST) are released from the acutely damaged hepatocytes and serum transaminase levels rise, often to levels exceeding 20-fold normal. Bilirubinuria and an elevated serum bilirubin are found, with mild elevations in serum alkaline phosphatase levels. The white cell count is normal or slightly depressed.

The icteric phase of acute viral hepatitis may last from days to weeks, followed by gradual resolution of symptoms and laboratory tests.

Complications

POSTHEPATITIS SYNDROMES. In some patients, prolonged fatigue and malaise may persist for months after return of liver function tests to normal. Reassurance is all that is required, and normal activity is encouraged. Isolated elevation of unconjugated serum bilirubin may persist (an expression of Gilbert's syndrome; see Chapter 36E) and requires no treatment.

CHOLESTATIC HEPATITIS. In some patients, a prolonged, although ultimately self-limited, period of cholestatic jaundice may supervene with marked

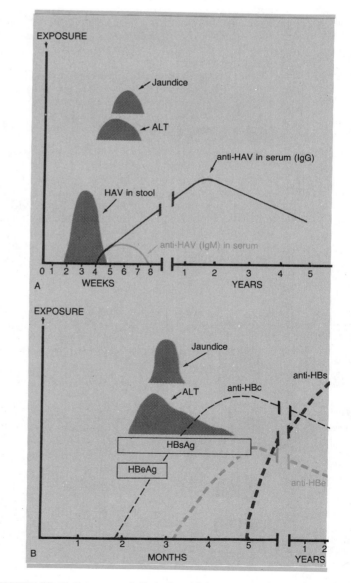

FIGURE 44—2. Sequence of clinical and laboratory findings in (A) a patient with hepatitis A and (B) a patient with hepatitis B.

conjugated hyperbilirubinemia, elevation of alkaline phosphatase, and pruritus. Investigation may be required to differentiate this condition from mechanical obstruction of the biliary tree (see Chapter 49).

FULMINANT HEPATITIS. Massive hepatic necrosis occurs in less than 1 per cent of patients with acute viral hepatitis leading to a devastating and often fatal condition called fulminant hepatitis. This is discussed in detail in Chapter 45.

CHRONIC HEPATITIS. This may develop following acute hepatitis B, non-A, non-B, or delta. Hepatitis A never progresses to chronicity. Persistence of transaminase elevation beyond six months suggests evolution to chronic hepatitis, although a slowly resolving acute hepatitis may occasionally lead to abnormal liver function tests well beyond six months with eventual complete resolution. Chronic hepatitis is considered in detail later in this chapter. Hepatitis B virus infection without evidence of any liver damage may persist, resulting in asymptomatic or healthy hepatitis B carriers. In Asia and Africa, many such carriers appear to have acquired the virus from infected mothers during infancy.

RARE COMPLICATIONS. Rarely, acute viral hepatitis may be followed by aplastic anemia, while vasculitis, cryoglobulinemia, glomerulonephritis, and vasculitis may complicate the course of hepatitis B. Pancreatitis with elevation of serum amylase may also occur.

Serodiagnosis. The ability to detect the presence of viral components in hepatitis B and antibodies to components of hepatitis A, B, and delta agent has enabled considerable progress to be made in the study of the epidemiology of viral hepatitis. These so-called viral markers can be diagnostic of the cause of acute viral hepatitis. An etiological diagnosis is of great importance in planning preventive and public health measures pertinent to the close contacts of infected patients and in evaluating the prognosis. The commonly available serological tests for viral hepatitis and their interpretation are shown in Table 44–3. The time course of appearance of these markers in acute hepatitis A and B is shown in Figure 44–2. Epstein-Barr virus and cytomegalovirus hepatitis may also be diagnosed by the appearance of specific antibodies of the IgM class. No reliable markers have as yet been described for non-A, non-B hepatitis, which is currently diagnosed by exclusion of all other causes of hepatitis. In acute hepatitis B, HB_sAg and HB_eAg are present in serum. Both are usually cleared within a period of three months, but HB_sAg may persist in some uncomplicated cases for six months to one year. Clearance of HB_sAg is followed after a variable "window" period by emergence of anti-HB_s, which confers long-term immunity. Anti-HB_c and anti-HB_e appear in the acute phase of the illness, but neither provides immunity. During the serological window period, anti-HB_c may be the only evidence of hepatitis B infection, and IgM anti-HB_c is suggestive of recent infection. Delta virus infection superimposed on B virus infection may be detected by antibody to delta agent, but this is not yet commercially available.

Management. There is no specific treatment for acute viral hepatitis. Management is largely supportive, including rest in proportion to the severity of symptoms, maintenance of hydration, and adequate dietary intake. Most patients show a preference for a low-fat, high-carbohydrate diet. Vitamin supplementation is of no proven value, although vitamin K administration may be indicated if prolonged cholestasis occurs. Activity is restricted to limit fatigue. Alcohol should be avoided until liver enzymes return to normal. Measures to combat nausea can include small doses of metoclopramide and hydroxyzine. Hos-

TABLE 44–3. SEROLOGICAL MARKERS OF VIRAL HEPATITIS

AGENT	MARKER	DEFINITION	SIGNIFICANCE
Hepatitis A (HAV)	Anti-HA	Antibody to HAV	
	IgM type		Current infection or convalescence
	IgG type		Current or previous infection
			Confers immunity
Hepatitis B (HBV)	HB_sAg	HBV surface antigen	Positive in most cases of acute or chronic infection
	HB_eAG	"e" antigen; a component of the HBV core	Transiently positive in acute B hepatitis
			May persist in chronic infection
			Reflects presence of viral replication and whole Dane particles in serum
			Reflects high infectivity
	Anti-HB_e	Antibody to "e" antigen	Transiently positive in convalescence
			May be persistently present in chronic cases
			Reflects low infectivity
	Anti-HB_c	Antibody to HBV core antigen	Positive in all acute and chronic cases
			Reliable marker of infection, past or current
			Not protective
	Anti-HB_s	Antibody to HBV surface antigen	Positive in late convalescence in most acute cases
			Confers immunity
Hepatitis delta	Anti-δ	Antibody to δ	Acute or chronic infection

pitalization is indicated in patients with severe nausea and vomiting, or with evidence of deteriorating liver function such as hepatic encephalopathy (Chapter 45) or prolongation of the prothrombin time. In general, hepatitis A may be regarded as noninfectious after two to three weeks, whereas hepatitis B is potentially infectious to intimate contacts throughout its course, although the risk is very small once HB$_s$Ag has cleared.

Prevention. Both feces and blood from patients with hepatitis A contain virus during the prodromal and early icteric phases of the disease. Raw shellfish concentrate the virus from sewage pollution and may serve as vectors of the disease. General hygienic measures should include handwashing by contacts and careful handling, disposal, and sterilization of excreta and contaminated clothing and utensils. Close contacts of patients with hepatitis A should receive immune serum globulin (ISG) as soon as possible. Travelers to endemic areas where sanitation facilities are poor may be protected by administration of ISG.

Hepatitis B is rarely transmitted by the fecal-oral route, but it is still prudent to avoid contact with the excreta of infected patients. Far more important is the meticulous disposal of contaminated needles and other blood-contaminated utensils.

ISG is of very limited value in preventing hepatitis B. However, administration of immune serum globulin enriched in anti-HB$_s$ (hyperimmune globulin, hepatitis B immune globulin, HBIG) may afford protection after a needlestick exposure or mucosal exposure (e.g., during pipetting of infectious serum in a clinical laboratory or following eye splash). It also appears to be protective to neonates born to mothers who are acutely or chronically infected. The usefulness of HBIG in household or sexual contacts is less well-established.

An important advance in the field of hepatitis B prevention has been the development of a safe, highly effective vaccine. The current vaccine, manufactured from triple-inactivated HB$_s$Ag obtained from the serum of chronic carriers of the B virus, is given in three doses over six months and confers immunity in close to 100 per cent of recipients for a period of at least five years. The vaccine is currently recommended for high-risk groups and individuals, including health professionals, dialysis patients, hemophiliacs, residents and staff of custodial care institutions, and sexually active homosexual males. It appears also to be of value in combination with HBIG after acute exposure to the virus, e.g., accidental needlestick and particularly in infants born to HB$_s$Ag-positive mothers.

Alcoholic Fatty Liver and Hepatitis

Alcohol is the most common cause of liver disease in the Western world. Three major pathological lesions resulting from alcohol abuse are: (1) fatty liver, (2) alcoholic hepatitis, and (3) cirrho-

sis. The first two lesions are potentially reversible, may sometimes be confused with viral hepatitis, and are described in this chapter. Alcoholic cirrhosis is discussed in Chapter 46.

Mechanism of Injury. Alcohol appears to produce liver damage by several mechanisms that are still incompletely understood. Fatty liver may be related to increased NADPH generated during alcohol metabolism, which promotes fatty acid synthesis and triglyceride formation. Since alcohol also impairs the release of triglyceride in the form of lipoproteins, fat accumulates in hepatocytes. Acetaldehyde produced from oxidation of alcohol may be directly hepatotoxic and is implicated in the production of the more severe hepatic lesions seen in alcoholics. Immune-mediated hepatic damage may also play a role in producing the lesion of alcoholic hepatitis.

Although individuals vary considerably in their ability to withstand the effects of alcohol on the liver, consumption in excess of 40 grams of ethanol per day carries a substantial risk of the development of alcoholic liver disease. Malnutrition may potentiate the toxic effects of alcohol on the liver, and genetic factors may contribute to individual susceptibility.

Clinical and Pathological Features. Alcoholic fatty liver may present as an incidentally discovered tender hepatomegaly. Some patients will consult a physician because of right upper quadrant pain. Jaundice is very rare. Transaminases are invariably elevated to a mild degree (less than five times normal). Liver biopsy shows diffuse or centrilobular fat occupying most of the hepatocyte. This is in contrast to the severe and prognostically ominous lesion of alcoholic hepatitis, which is characterized by the histological triad of (1) alcoholic hyalin, an eosinophilic aggregate usually seen near or around the cell nuclei; (2) infiltration of the liver by polymorphonuclear leukocytes; and (3) a network of intralobular connective tissue surrounding hepatocytes and central veins. Patients with this histological lesion may be asymptomatic or extremely ill with hepatic failure. Anorexia, nausea, vomiting, weight loss, and abdominal pain are common presenting symptoms. Hepatomegaly is present in 80 per cent of patients with alcoholic hepatitis, and splenomegaly is often present. Fever is common, but bacterial infection should always be excluded, since patients with alcoholic liver disease are prone to develop pneumonia as well as infection of the urinary tract and peritoneal cavity. Jaundice is commonly present and may be pronounced with cholestatic features (Chapter 36E). Cutaneous signs of chronic liver disease may be found, including spider angiomata, palmar erythema, and gynecomastia. Parotid enlargement, testicular atrophy, and loss of body hair may be prominent (see Chapter 46). Ascites and encephalopathy may be present and indicate severe disease. The white cell count may be strikingly elevated, whereas transaminases are invariably only modestly raised, an important differentiating feature from other forms of acute hepatitis. The AST/ALT ratio frequently exceeds 2, in contrast to viral hepatitis in which the transaminases are usually increased in parallel. A prolonged prothrombin time, hypoalbuminemia, and hyperglobulinemia may be found.

Diagnosis. A history of excessive, prolonged alcohol intake is often difficult to elicit from patients with alcoholic liver disease, whereas others suspected of imbibing to excess are often found to have liver disease from causes other than alcohol. Liver biopsy is extremely helpful in establishing the diagnosis.

Complications and Prognosis. Alcoholic fatty liver will revert to complete histological normality with cessation of alcohol intake. Alcoholic hepatitis can also revert to normal but more commonly either progresses to cirrhosis, which may already be present at the time of initial presentation, or runs a rapid course to hepatic failure and death. Not infrequently its course is complicated by the development of encephalopathy, ascites, and deteriorating renal function with increasing BUN and creatinine levels (hepatorenal syndrome) or gastrointestinal bleeding from varices.

Treatment. Treatment of acute alcoholic hepatitis is supportive. Attempts should be made to treat the underlying alcoholism, although this is often unrewarding. A high-caloric diet is instituted and may require administration by nasogastric tube in severely anorectic patients. Protein should be included, but may need to be restricted in patients with encephalopathy (see Chapter 46). The use of corticosteroids is of no proven benefit.

TABLE 44–4. CLASSIFICATION OF DRUG-INDUCED LIVER DISEASE

CATEGORY	EXAMPLES
Predictable hepatotoxins with zonal necrosis	Acetaminophen Carbon tetrachloride
Nonspecific hepatitis	Aspirin Oxacillin
Viral hepatitis–like reactions	Halothane Isoniazid Phenytoin
Cholestasis Noninflammatory	Estrogens 17α-substituted steroids
Inflammatory	Chlorpromazine Antithyroid agents
Fatty liver Large droplet	Ethanol Corticosteroids
Small droplet	Phenylbutazone Allopurinol
Chronic hepatitis	Methyldopa Nitrofurantoin
Tumors	Estrogens Vinyl chloride
Vascular lesions	6-Thioguanine Anabolic steroids
Fibrosis	Methotrexate
Granulomas	Allopurinol Sulfonamides

Drug- and Toxin-Induced Hepatitis

A broad spectrum of hepatic pathology may result from a variety of therapeutic drugs and nontherapeutic toxins. The types of hepatic damage and the drugs that typically produce each variety are summarized in Table 44–4. The pathophysiological mechanisms whereby this wide variety of hepatic lesions is produced is complex. At one end of the spectrum is a predictable, dose-dependent, direct toxic effect upon hepatocytes leading to frank hepatocellular necrosis. This is typified by the effects of acetaminophen and carbon tetrachloride, both of which will produce centrilobular hepatocellular necrosis in virtually all individuals in whom a sufficient quantity is ingested. Other reactions are generally not predictable and usually occur for unknown reasons in susceptible individuals (idiosyncratic drug reaction). Immune-mediated hepatic damage appears to be responsible in some, possibly resulting from the drug acting as a hapten on the surface of hepatocytes. In others, subtle, genetically determined differences in pathways of hepatic drug metabolism may result in metabolites with greater toxic potential. Examples include viral hepatitis–like reactions (halothane, isoniazid), cholestatic hepatitis (chlorpromazine), granulomatous hepatitis (allopurinol), chronic hepatitis (methyldopa), and pure cholestasis without inflammatory cell infiltration or hepatocellular necrosis (estrogens, androgens). A few important examples of drug-induced hepatitis are discussed here.

Acetaminophen. Acetaminophen is converted by the hepatic cytochrome P-450 drug-metabolizing system to a potentially toxic metabolite that is subsequently rendered harmless through conjugation with glutathione. When massive doses are taken (in excess of 10 to 15 grams), the formation of excess toxic metabolites depletes the available glutathione and produces necrosis. Acetaminophen overdose, commonly taken in a suicide attempt, leads to nausea and vomiting within a few hours. These symptoms subside and are followed in 24 to 48 hours by clinical and laboratory evidence of hepatocellular necrosis (raised transaminases) and hepatic dysfunction (prolonged prothrombin time, hepatic encephalopathy). Extensive liver necrosis may lead to fulminant hepatic failure and death. Severe liver damage may be predicted on the basis of blood levels of the drug from 4 to 12 hours after ingestion. Early treatment of patients at high risk with N-acetylcysteine (within 16 hours of the ingestion), which is thought to promote hepatic glutathione synthesis, may be life-saving.

Isoniazid (INH). INH as a single-drug prophylaxis against tuberculosis commonly produces subclinical hepatic injury (20 per cent incidence) as evidenced by raised serum transaminase levels. This appears to be transient and self-limiting in most cases. There is, however, a 1 per cent incidence of overt hepatitis with clinical and pathological features of viral hepatitis, which progresses to massive, fatal hepatic necrosis in one tenth of affected patients. The incidence of severe hepatic damage increases with age, such that significant elevation of transaminases in persons over the age of 35 is an indication for discontinuing the drug.

Halothane. The commonly used anesthetic agent halothane rarely causes a viral hepatitis-like reaction in susceptible individuals within a few days of exposure. Complete recovery is the rule, but massive hepatic necrosis may occur, usually following repeated exposure.

Chlorpromazine. Chlorpromazine produces a cholestatic reaction, often weeks to months after the drug is begun. Fever, anorexia, and a rash may accompany jaundice and pruritus. Eosinophilia is common. Erythromycin may produce a similar picture, but right upper quadrant pain, mimicking acute cholecystitis, is usually prominent.

CHRONIC HEPATITIS

An inflammatory process within the liver that fails to resolve after six months is called chronic hepatitis.

Etiology. Many of the causes of acute hepatitis can ultimately lead to chronic hepatitis (Table 44–5). A notable exception is hepatitis A. Hepatitis B is a common cause of chronic hepatitis worldwide, and it is thought that superimposition of delta (δ) agent infection may produce a more severe outcome. Several drugs may produce a chronic hepatitis, the best recognized being methyldopa. In contrast to acute hepatitis, an etiological agent is frequently difficult to identify in cases of chronic hepatitis. The pathogenesis of these idiopathic forms of chronic hepatitis is probably autoimmune in some cases, whereas others are likely to have a viral origin.

Pathology, Clinical and Laboratory Manifestations

CHRONIC PERSISTENT HEPATITIS. Chronic persistent hepatitis is defined as a chronic inflammatory process confined to the portal areas without involvement of the periportal region. This is the commonest form of chronic hepatitis, particularly following hepatitis B. The prognosis is generally excellent, with nonprogression or resolution being the rule. Patients with this lesion may be asymptomatic or complain of fatigue and/or right upper quadrant pain. Laboratory abnormalities are usually confined to mildly raised transaminase levels.

CHRONIC LOBULAR HEPATITIS. Chronic lobular hepatitis, an uncommon form of chronic hepatitis, consists of scattered necrosis throughout the hepatic lobule similar to a late-resolving acute viral hepatitis. Most cases are of viral etiology; progression is uncommon.

CHRONIC ACTIVE HEPATITIS. Chronic active hepatitis, the most serious form of chronic hepatitis, may progress to cirrhosis and liver failure. Histologically, the portal areas are expanded with lymphocytes and plasma cells, with spillover into the adjacent lobule (periportal hepatitis, piecemeal necrosis). Bridging necrosis, collapse, and

TABLE 44–5. CAUSES OF CHRONIC HEPATITIS

Viral Infections
  Hepatitis B
  Hepatitis B with superimposed δ-agent
  Hepatitis non-A, non-B
Drugs and Toxins
  Methyldopa
  Oxyphenisatin
  Isoniazid
Idiopathic
  Idiopathic with prominent autoimmune features (lupoid hepatitis)
  Idiopathic with minimal or no autoimmune features
Metabolic Liver Disease
  Wilson's disease
  α_1-Antitrypsin deficiency

fibrosis, as well as the features of cirrhosis (see Chapter 46), may be present. Twenty per cent of cases are caused by chronic hepatitis B infection; others may follow non-A, non-B hepatitis. Drugs (Table 44–5) may cause an identical picture. Some cases show marked associated features of autoimmunity ("lupoid hepatitis").

The clinical course ranges from asymptomatic disease to a severe illness with constitutional symptoms, cutaneous signs of chronic liver disease, jaundice, and hepatosplenomegaly. The variety of chronic active hepatitis called *lupoid hepatitis* predominates in young females and is often accompanied by prominent extrahepatic manifestations, including amenorrhea, skin rashes, acne, vasculitis, thyroiditis, and Sjögren's syndrome. In chronic active hepatitis, transaminase levels are elevated over a wide range and are characteristically accompanied by polyclonal hypergammaglobulinemia. Laboratory evidence of liver failure may be present (hyperbilirubinemia, prolonged prothrombin time, hypoalbuminemia). Antibodies to smooth muscle and antinuclear antibodies may be found, particularly in lupoid hepatitis. Wilson's disease may present clinically and histologically as a chronic active hepatitis and should be excluded in patients under the age of 35 (Chapter 46).

Liver biopsy is of great value in making the diagnosis of chronic active hepatitis, in differentiating it from milder forms of chronic hepatitis, and in determining the progression of the disease to cirrhosis. Liver biopsy is considered prerequisite to any attempt to treat the disease with immunosuppressive agents.

Treatment. In certain, selected cases of chronic active hepatitis, corticosteroid therapy may lead to dramatic improvement in clinical, laboratory, and histological features of the disease as well as to reduced mortality. Azothioprine is also used, but mainly for its steroid-sparing effect. Patients likely to benefit from corticosteroids are those with severe symptoms, a fivefold or greater elevation in transaminases, and marked necroinflammatory activity on liver biopsy. In patients with HB_sAg-positive chronic active hepatitis, immunosuppression will enhance viral replication and corticosteroids appear to have little benefit on the course of the liver disease. Patients with drug-induced chronic hepatitis or Wilson's disease also will not respond to corticosteroids. Non-A, non-B chronic hepatitis is often mild and may undergo spontaneous improvement; patients with non-A, non-B hepatitis are therefore not usually considered candidates for immunosuppressive therapy.

Patients successfully managed with corticosteroids frequently relapse on discontinuation of the drug and will require its reinstitution.

REFERENCES

Ockner RK: Acute viral hepatitis. In Wyngaarden JB, and Smith LH Jr (eds): Cecil Textbook of Medicine. 17th ed. Philadelphia, WB Saunders Co, 1985, pp 813–820.

Ockner RK: Chronic hepatitis. In Wyngaarden JB, and Smith LH Jr (eds): Cecil Textbook of Medicine. 17th ed. Philadelphia, WB Saunders Co, 1985, pp 824–827.

Ockner RK: Toxic and drug-induced liver disease. In Wyngaarden JB, and Smith LH Jr (eds): Cecil Textbook of Medicine. 17th ed. Philadelphia, WB Saunders Co, 1985, pp 820–824.

Seeff LB: Diagnosis, therapy and prognosis of viral hepatitis. In Zakim D, and Boyer TD (eds): Hepatology: A Textbook of Liver Disease. Philadelphia, WB Saunders Co, 1982, pp 911–971.

Tong MJ: Chronic hepatitis. In Zakim D, and Boyer TD (eds): Hepatology: A Textbook of Liver Disease. Philadelphia, WB Saunders Co, 1982, pp 972–990.

Zakim D, Boyer TD, Montgomery CM, and Kanas N: Alcoholic liver disease. In Zakim D, and Boyer TD (eds): Hepatology: A Textbook of Liver Disease. Philadelphia, WB Saunders Co, 1982, pp 739–789.

45 FULMINANT HEPATIC FAILURE

Fulminant hepatic failure is defined as hepatic failure with Stage III or IV encephalopathy which develops in less than eight weeks in a patient *without pre-existing liver disease.* It results from severe widespread hepatic necrosis, commonly due to acute viral hepatitis with B, A, delta, or non-A, non-B viruses. It may also result from fatty liver of pregnancy, ischemic necrosis or exposure to hepatotoxins such as acetaminophen, isoniazid, halothane, valproic acid, tetracycline, mushroom toxins (e.g., those of *Amanita phalloides*), or carbon tetrachloride. Reye's syndrome, a disease predominantly of children that is characterized by microvesicular fatty infiltration and little hepatocellular necrosis, often resembles fulminant hepatic failure.

Diagnosis

The diagnosis rests on the combination of hepatic encephalopathy, acute liver disease (elevated serum bilirubin, transaminases), and liver failure, the latter usually indicated by hypoprothrombinemia.

Treatment

Treatment of fulminant hepatic failure remains supportive, as the underlying etiology of liver failure is rarely treatable. However, most processes that result in widespread liver cell necrosis and fulminant hepatic failure are transient events, and liver cell regeneration with recovery of liver function often occurs if patients do not succumb to the complications of liver failure in the interim. Meticulous supportive treatment in an intensive care unit setting has been shown to improve survival. Patients with fulminant hepatic failure should be cared for in centers with experience with this disease. Numerous complications, listed in Table 45–1, attend fulminant hepatic failure, and careful identification and treatment of each are essential.

Hepatic encephalopathy is the sine qua non of fulminant hepatic failure, and it is often the first and most dramatic sign of liver failure. The pathogenesis of hepatic encephalopathy, discussed in Chapter 46, remains unclear; however, most clinical observations suggest a role for protein- and gut-derived toxins that are normally taken up and detoxified by the liver. Abnormal neurotransmitters synthesized from excess aromatic amino acids may also play a role in hepatic encephalopathy. Hepatic encephalopathy that accompanies fulminant hepatic failure differs from that associated with chronic liver disease in two important aspects: (1) It is rarely due to a reversible precipitating factor (see Table 46–6) and often responds to therapy only when liver regeneration occurs. (2) It is frequently associated with two other, potentially treatable, causes of coma—hypoglycemia and cerebral edema. Therapy for hepatic encephalopathy follows the principles outlined in Chapter 46. Because these patients are severely ill, all protein intake is stopped, intravenous glucose (1000 to 1500 calories per day) is administered, and lactulose is administered orally, per nasogastric tube, or by enema to cleanse the colon.

Hypoglycemia is a common complication of liver failure. All patients should receive 10 per cent glucose IV infusions with frequent monitoring of blood glucose levels. Other metabolic abnormalities commonly occur, including *hyponatremia, hypokalemia, respiratory alkalosis,* and *metabolic acidosis.* Thus frequent monitoring of blood electrolytes and pH is indicated.

Gastrointestinal hemorrhage may occur from stress ulcers, particularly in the face of impaired synthesis of clotting factors. All patients should receive vitamin K and prophylactic oral antacids or IV cimetidine to maintain gastric pH above 5. Fresh frozen plasma should be used only if clinically significant bleeding occurs.

Renal insufficiency is common in patients with

TABLE 45–1. MANAGEMENT OF FULMINANT HEPATIC FAILURE

COMPLICATION	PATHOGENESIS	MANAGEMENT
Hepatic encephalopathy	Liver failure	Stop protein, cleanse gut, administer lactulose or neomycin
Hypoglycemia	Decreased gluconeogenesis	Monitor blood sugar 10% glucose IV infusion 50% glucose IV if needed
Hemorrhage	Decreased synthesis of clotting factors Stress ulcers	Vitamin K Prophylactic oral antacids or IV cimetidine to maintain alkaline gastric pH
	Disseminated intravascular coagulopathy	Fresh frozen plasma if serious bleeding occurs
Hyponatremia	Impaired free water clearance	Monitor blood electrolytes and fluid balance Water restriction
Hypokalemia	—	Potassium supplementation
Respiratory alkalosis	Hyperventilation	No therapy required usually
Metabolic acidosis	Lactic acidosis	IV bicarbonate if necessary
Cerebral edema	—	Consider intracranial pressure monitoring and treatment with IV mannitol
Azotemia	Hypovolemia Hepatorenal syndrome Acute tubular necrosis	Identify and correct hypovolemia
Infection	Impaired synthesis of complement	Prevent aspiration and catheter-related infection
Hypotension, hypoxia, pulmonary edema	Reduced systemic vascular resistance Pulmonary right-to-left shunts	Employ standard measures as needed

liver failure (see Chapter 32). It is essential that hypovolemia be excluded as a cause of azotemia; central venous pressure measurements may be required in some patients to do so. Survival of patients with either hepatorenal syndrome or acute tubular necrosis does not appear to be improved by dialysis.

Cerebral edema, the pathogenesis of which is unknown, is a particularly common complication of fulminant hepatic failure in children and young adults. It may result in intracranial herniation and generally portends a fatal outcome. Corticosteroid therapy is not useful; however, improved survival has been reported with intracranial pressure monitoring and IV administration of mannitol in selected patients.

Many other forms of therapy for fulminant hepatic failure have been tried, including corticosteroid administration, exchange transfusion, plasmapheresis, hemodialysis, charcoal hemoperfusion, and extracorporeal perfusion through a human cadaver or pig liver. None has been shown to offer any advantage over conventional supportive therapy, however. Liver transplantation is not usually an option because of the dif-

ficulties inherent in procuring a donor liver within a short period of time and also because of the complications of carrying out such major surgery in these desperately ill patients.

Prognosis

Short-term prognosis is very poor, with the average reported survival being about 20 per cent. Long-term prognosis for those who survive is excellent. Follow-up studies have shown normal liver function and histology in virtually all surviving patients, regardless of the cause of the fulminant hepatic failure.

REFERENCES

Jones EA, and Schafer DF: Fulminant hepatic failure. In Zakim D, and Boyer TD (eds): Hepatology: A Textbook of Liver Disease. Philadelphia, WB Saunders Co, 1982, pp 415–445.
Scharschmidt BF: Acute and chronic hepatic failure with encephalopathy. In Wyngaarden JB, and Smith LH Jr (eds): Cecil Textbook of Medicine. 17th ed. Philadelphia, WB Saunders Co, 1985, pp 845–848.

CIRRHOSIS OF THE LIVER AND ITS COMPLICATIONS 46

DEFINITION

Cirrhosis is the irreversible end result of fibrous scarring and hepatocellular regeneration that con-

stitute the major responses of the liver to a variety of long-standing inflammatory, toxic, metabolic, and congestive insults. In cirrhosis, the normal hepatic lobular architecture is replaced by inter-

TABLE 46–1. CAUSES OF CIRRHOSIS

Alcohol
Hepatitis viruses (B and non-A, non-B)
Drugs
    Methyldopa
    Methotrexate
Autoimmune chronic active hepatitis
Biliary cirrhosis
    Primary biliary cirrhosis
    Secondary biliary cirrhosis
        bile duct strictures
        sclerosing cholangitis
        biliary atresia
        tumors of the bile ducts
        cystic fibrosis
Chronic hepatic congestion
    Budd-Chiari syndrome
    Chronic right-heart failure
    Constrictive pericarditis
Genetically determined metabolic diseases
    Wilson's disease
    Hemochromatosis
    α_1-Antitrypsin deficiency
    Galactosemia
Cryptogenic

connecting bands of fibrous tissue surrounding nodules derived from foci of regenerating hepatocytes.

Regenerative nodules may be small (<3 mm, micronodular cirrhosis), a typical feature of alcholic cirrhosis, or large (>3 mm, macronodular cirrhosis). The latter, also termed postnecrotic cirrhosis, is more commonly seen as a sequel to chronic active hepatitis. The pathology of cirrhosis determines its natural history and clinical manifestations. Thus, fibrous scarring and disruption of the hepatic architecture distort the vascular bed, leading to portal hypertension and intrahepatic shunting. Normal hepatocyte function is disturbed by the resulting inadequacy of blood flow and ongoing direct toxic, inflammatory, and/or metabolic damage to the hepatocytes.

ETIOLOGY

Most of the conditions that may lead to cirrhosis (Table 46–1) are rarely encountered. Alcohol is by far the commonest cause of cirrhosis in the Western world, while hepatitis B is a major cause in the Third World. Cryptogenic cirrhosis is a diagnosis of exclusion, but many cases are likely to be an end result of chronic non-A, non-B infection. Causes of hepatic fibrosis alone (e.g., schistosomiasis, which leads to fibrosis of portal venous radicles and portal hypertension) are not classified as causes of cirrhosis, because the hepatic lobular pattern is well preserved and hepatocellular dysfunction (e.g., disordered protein synthesis) is usually lacking.

CLINICAL AND LABORATORY FEATURES

The presence of cirrhosis may remain undetected until autopsy. Individuals with cirrhosis who experience no symptoms and show little clinical evidence of hepatocellular dysfunction are often said to have *well-compensated* cirrhosis. As evidence of complications develops, particularly signs implying disturbed hepatocellular function, the clinical condition is referred to as *decompensated* cirrhosis. Where the disease process leading to cirrhosis primarily affects the hepatocytes, e.g., alcohol (parenchymal liver disease), evidence of failing hepatocellular function may be prominent in the clinical presentation. On the other hand, if the biliary system is primarily affected, as occurs in primary or secondary biliary cirrhosis, the clinical features of cholestasis predominate and hepatocellular function is often well-preserved until late in the course of the disease.

It is convenient to divide the main clinical and laboratory features of cirrhosis into four categories (Table 46–2):
1. *Size and consistency of the liver.*
2. *Features attributable to hepatocellular dysfunction.* These result from both intrinsically "sick" hepatocytes and the shunting of portal blood away from hepatocytes with consequent failure to extract toxins and metabolites.
3. *Features attributable to portal hypertension.*
4. *Extrahepatic features related to specific diseases causing cirrhosis.*

Liver size depends upon the underlying pathological process. In end-stage hepatitis B virus liver disease, the liver is often small, scarred, and shrunken. In alcoholic cirrhosis, fat infiltration may lead to marked enlargement of the liver. Impaired hepatic detoxification of estrogens, as well as disturbed hypothalamic-pituitary function,

TABLE 46–2. CLINICAL AND LABORATORY FEATURES OF CIRRHOSIS

CLINICAL	LABORATORY
Size and Consistency of the Liver	
Hepatomegaly, or small shrunken liver	
Firm to hard consistency	
Hepatocellular Dysfunction	
Jaundice	Hyperbilirubinemia
Spider angiomata	
Palmar erythema	
Gynecomastia	
Loss of body hair	
Testicular atrophy	
Dupuytren's contracture	
Muscle wasting, edema	Hypoalbuminemia, low BUN
Bruising	Prolonged prothrombin time
Signs of hepatic encephalopathy	
Fetor hepaticus	
Portal Hypertension	
Splenomegaly	Thrombocytopenia, leukopenia
Ascites	
Caput medusa	
Variceal bleeding	
Signs of Specific Diseases	

produces several cutaneous signs (often called "stigmata" of cirrhosis, e.g., spider angiomata, palmar erythema). Marked jaundice in the absence of complete bile duct obstruction is often a grave prognostic sign implying advanced hepatocellular dysfunction. Impaired hepatocellular protein synthesis leads to hypoalbuminemia and hypoprothrombinemia.

SPECIFIC CAUSES OF CIRRHOSIS

Alcohol. Alcoholic cirrhosis may coexist with alcoholic hepatitis. Features of hepatocellular dysfunction are thus often marked and may improve with abstinence. Micronodular cirrhosis is the rule but is not specific for alcohol. Evidence of malnutrition and vitamin deficiency is frequently found, particularly in the severely alcoholic patient. Anemia of mixed etiology is common, often with macrocytic indices.

Chronic Active Hepatitis. Chronic active hepatitis from any cause may progress to cirrhosis. The liver is typically small with a macronodular pattern. Evidence of continued inflammatory activity is often present, including moderate elevation of transaminase levels and hypergammaglobulinemia. HB_sAg is usually persistently positive in cirrhosis due to hepatitis B virus.

Primary Biliary Cirrhosis. Almost exclusively a disease affecting women, primary biliary cirrhosis manifests mainly between the ages of 30 and 65 and results from a progressive, probably immune-mediated, destruction of the intralobular bile ductules. Cholestatic features predominate with high serum levels of alkaline phosphatase and cholesterol. Pruritus is a major early symptom, followed later in the course of the disease by xanthomas, pigmentation, and bone pain. Commonly associated conditions include Sjögren's syndrome, scleroderma, and the CREST syndrome (calcinosis, Raynaud's syndrome, esophageal dysfunction, sclerodactyly, telangiectasia). Antimitochondrial antibodies are present in high titer, and serum IgM levels are elevated. Liver biopsy may show characteristic destructive lesions of the bile ductules and is of value in confirming the diagnosis. Jaundice is a prominent feature late in the course of the disease.

Hemochromatosis. Hemochromatosis is a genetically determined disorder of inappropriate iron absorption. Hepatic iron overload eventually leads to fibrosis and cirrhosis. Iron deposition occurs in other tissues as well, leading to skin pigmentation, diabetes, cardiac failure, hypogonadism, and arthropathy. Hepatomegaly is usually found, and the risk of developing hepatocellular carcinoma is high. The diagnosis is supported by findings of high serum iron and ferritin levels with increased transferrin saturation. Liver biopsy shows increased iron in hepatocytes, and direct estimation of liver iron in biopsy specimens is of value in making the diagnosis. Treatment consists of removal of excess body iron stores through phlebotomy at weekly intervals, or more rarely through the use of chelating agents.

Wilson's Disease. Wilson's disease is an autosomal recessive abnormality in hepatic copper excretion. Copper accumulates in the liver, central nervous system, and other tissues. Wilson's disease may eventualy lead to cirrhosis or may present as acute, fulminant hepatic failure or chronic active hepatitis. Deposition of copper in the central nervous system leads to a predominantly extrapyramidal form of motor disorder (basal ganglia damage) with rigidity, tremor, chorea, and dysarthria. Psychiatric disorders are also common. Copper deposited in Descemet's membrane of the cornea manifests as the characteristic Kayser-Fleischer rings, which are best seen on slit-lamp examination. Typical laboratory findings are low serum levels of ceruloplasmin and increased urinary copper excretion. Direct measurement of copper in liver biopsy specimens may be of great value in diagnosing Wilson's disease and monitoring its response to therapy. Copper chelation therapy with D-penicillamine arrests progression of the disease and may prevent its manifestations if instituted early enough.

MAJOR COMPLICATIONS OF CIRRHOSIS

The major sequelae of cirrhosis are:
1. Portal hypertension, with its attendant complications of (a) variceal hemorrhage, and (b) splenomegaly and hypersplenism.
2. Liver failure.
3. Ascites, which may be further complicated by spontaneous bacterial peritonitis.
4. The hepatorenal syndrome.
5. Portosystemic (hepatic) encephalopathy.
6. Hepatocellular carcinoma.

The pathophysiological interrelationships among these complications are shown diagrammatically in Figure 46–1.

Portal Hypertension

The normal liver offers little resistance to portal venous blood flow (about 1 L/min), and portal pressure is normally less than 5 mm Hg above inferior vena caval pressure. The distortion of hepatic architecture in cirrhosis leads to a marked increase in resistance to portal venous flow, which in turn leads to an increase in portal venous pressure.

Although cirrhosis is the most important cause of portal hypertension, any process leading to increased resistance to portal blood flow into or through the liver or to hepatic venous outflow from the liver will result in portal hypertension (Table 46–3). Since the pressure within any vascular system is proportional to both resistance and blood flow, a marked increase in blood flow will also result in portal hypertension, although such situations are rare.

Portal hypertension leads to the formation of venous collaterals between the portal and systemic circulations. Collaterals may form at several

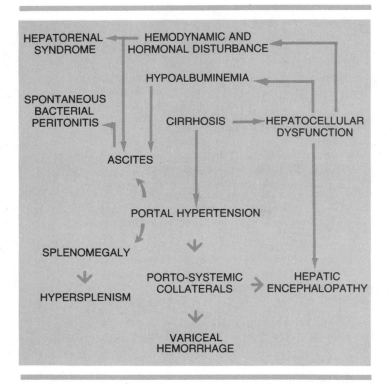

FIGURE 46–1. Interrelationships among the complications of cirrhosis.

sites, the most important clinically being those connecting the portal to the azygos vein which form dilated, tortuous veins (varices) in the submucosa of the gastric fundus and esophagus.

Variceal Hemorrhage. Hemorrhage occurs most frequently from varices in the esophagus and is a common and serious complication of portal hypertension, with a mortality rate of 30 to 60 per cent. What leads to variceal rupture is unknown, but reflux esophagitis and the presence of ascites do not appear to be important. Bleeding may present as hematemesis, hematochezia, melena, or any combination of these (see Chapter 36B). Bleeding may lead to shock, stop spontaneously, or recur.

TABLE 46–3. CAUSES OF PORTAL HYPERTENSION

Increased resistance to flow
  Presinusoidal
    Portal vein occlusion (thrombosis, tumor)
    Schistosomiasis
    Congenital hepatic fibrosis
    Sarcoidosis
  Sinusoidal
    Cirrhosis (all causes)
    Alcoholic hepatitis
  Postsinusoidal
    Veno-occlusive disease
    Budd-Chiari syndrome
    Constrictive pericarditis
Increased portal blood flow
  Splenomegaly not due to liver disease
  Arterioportal fistula

Impaired hepatic synthesis of coagulation factors (hepatocellular dysfunction) and thrombocytopenia (hypersplenism) may further complicate the management of variceal bleeding. The management of variceal bleeding has been discussed in Chapter 36B, and here we will emphasize a few important details.

VASOPRESSIN. When given by intravenous infusion, this posterior pituitary hormone causes constriction of splanchnic arterioles and a reduction in portal flow and pressure. Bleeding may be controlled by this measure but recurs in about 50 per cent of patients. The use of vasopressin does not reduce mortality.

BALLOON TAMPONADE. Compression of the varices by inserting a tube with inflatable gastric and esophageal balloons (Sengstaken-Blakemore tube) is an effective, although often temporary, measure. Complications such as aspiration and esophageal rupture may occur, and rebleeding occurs in up to 60 per cent of patients after the tube is removed.

ENDOSCOPIC INJECTION SCLEROTHERAPY. During endoscopy, varices may be injected with sclerosing solutions. This has become a popular and effective method for arresting acute bleeding. Repeated courses of injection can lead to variceal obliteration, and this approach has been used to prevent recurrent bleeding. However, bleeding frequently recurs prior to complete variceal obliteration, and esophageal strictures are a common complication.

PORTOSYSTEMIC SHUNT SURGERY. Portal decompression may be achieved by a variety of operative procedures aimed at creating a large connection between the high-pressure portal and low-pressure systemic venous system. Nonselective shunts (e.g., portocaval anastomoses) decompress the entire portal system. Selective shunts (e.g., the distal splenorenal shunt) decompress the varices only. Survival is not improved by shunt surgery, and hepatic encephalopathy is a major complication. Shunt surgery is usually performed electively to prevent recurrent bleeding in patients with good preservation of liver function. Emergency shunt surgery carries a 50 per cent mortality and is rarely undertaken.

OTHER THERAPEUTIC MEASURES. Propranolol has been shown to reduce portal pressure, but its use in preventing bleeding is still experimental.

Splenomegaly. Portal hypertension leads to *congestive splenomegaly*, which is often, but not always, clinically apparent. Thrombocytopenia and, less commonly, leukopenia occur due to sequestration of platelets and leukocytes in the enlarged spleen (hypersplenism).

Liver Failure

The derangement of hepatocellular function that occurs in cirrhosis manifests as impaired hepatic protein synthesis (hypoalbuminemia, impaired synthesis of coagulation factors) and failure of normal hepatic detoxification processes. The latter accounts for the development of signs such as spider angiomata and contributes to the development of hepatic encephalopathy, as well as to poorly understood hemodynamic and hormonal disorders that foster the development of ascites and the hepatorenal syndrome.

Ascites

Ascites is the accumulation of excess fluid in the peritoneal cavity. Although cirrhosis is the commonest cause of ascites, it may result from numerous other causes (Table 46–4). Ascites due to cirrhosis is commonly a transudate (protein concentration <3 grams per dl), whereas inflammatory and neoplastic causes usually lead to formation of an exudate (protein >3 grams per dl). Ascites becomes clinically detectable when more than 500 ml has accumulated. Shifting dullness to percussion is the most sensitive clinical sign of ascites, the presence of which can be confirmed by ultrasound examination.

Ascites in cirrhosis is the result of several pathogenetic factors, including portal hypertension, increased hepatic and splanchnic lymph production and transudation, and impaired renal sodium and water excretion secondary to hyperaldosteronism, increased levels of antidiuretic hormone, and other less well-understood factors.

Treatment of ascites consists initially of bed rest with restriction of sodium intake. Restricted fluid intake may be necessary if hyponatremia is present. These measures are commonly inadequate, and administration of spironolactone, an aldosterone antagonist, supplemented with a loop diuretic (e.g., furosemide) is often effective. Diuresis should be promoted cautiously, as aggressive diuretic therapy may result in hypokalemia and a depleted plasma volume, leading to hepatic encephalopathy and impaired renal function. Some patients may be extremely refractory to medical measures and may benefit from a surgically implanted plastic shunt between the peritoneal cavity and the superior vena cava (LeVeen shunt).

Two important complications occur in patients with cirrhotic ascites: spontaneous bacterial peritonitis and the hepatorenal syndrome.

Spontaneous Bacterial Peritonitis. Infection of ascites may occur in patients with cirrhosis, usually with coliform bacteria. Fever, abdominal pain, and tenderness may be present or the infection may be clinically silent. Hepatic encephalopathy may be precipitated. The diagnosis is strongly suspected if the ascitic fluid white cell count is greater than 500/cu mm with greater than 50 per cent polymorphonuclear leukocytes, and is confirmed by Gram's stain and culture. Vigorous antibiotic treatment is indicated, but mortality from this complication is high.

Hepatorenal Syndrome

Serious liver disease from any cause may be complicated by a form of renal failure termed the hepatorenal syndrome. It almost invariably occurs in the presence of severe ascites. Typically, the kidneys are histologically normal, with the capacity of regaining normal function in the event of a recovery of liver function. The renal dysfunction is characterized by oliguria, low urine sodium (<10 mEq/L), and azotemia.

TABLE 46–4. CAUSE OF ASCITES

Exudative Ascites
  Tuberculous peritonitis
  Pancreatitis
  Ruptured viscus (including bile peritonitis)
  Tumors (most commonly metastatic to liver and peritoneal lining)
Transudative Ascites
  Cirrhosis
  Chronic hepatic congestion
    Budd-Chiari syndrome
    Constrictive pericarditis
    Right-heart failure
  Nephrotic syndrome
  Myxedema
  Meigs' syndrome
Chylous Ascites
  Thoracic duct or abdominal lymphatic trauma
  Mediastinal tumors

Differential diagnosis of ascites: ovarian cyst, pancreatic cyst, mesenteric cyst, urinary tract rupture

The hepatorenal syndrome is usually progressive and fatal. It should only be diagnosed after plasma volume depletion (a common cause of reversible, prerenal azotemia in patients with cirrhosis, particularly with diuretic use) and other forms of acute renal injury have been ruled out.

Hepatic Encephalopathy

Hepatic encephalopathy (also called hepatic coma or portosystemic encephalopathy) is a complex neuropsychiatric syndrome that may complicate advanced liver disease and/or extensive portosystemic collateral formation (shunting). Two major forms of hepatic encephalopathy are recognized:

Acute hepatic encephalopathy usually occurs in the setting of fulminant hepatic failure. Cerebral edema plays a more important role in this setting: coma is common and mortality is very high (see Chapter 45).

Chronic hepatic encephalopathy usually occurs with chronic liver disease, commonly manifests as subtle disturbances of neurological function, and is often reversible.

The pathogenesis of hepatic encephalopathy is unknown but is thought to involve the inadequate hepatic removal of predominantly nitrogenous compounds or other toxins ingested or formed in the gastrointestinal tract. Inadequate hepatic removal results from impaired hepatocyte function as well as the extensive shunting of splanchnic blood directly into the systemic circulation via portosystemic collaterals. Nitrogenous and other absorbed compounds are thought to gain access to the central nervous system, leading to disturbances in neuronal function. Ammonia, derived from both amino acid deamination and bacterial hydrolysis of nitrogenous compounds in the gut, has been strongly implicated in the pathogenesis of hepatic encephalopathy. However, blood levels of ammonia correlate poorly with the presence or degree of encephalopathy. Other proposed neurotoxins include gamma-aminobutyric acid, mercaptans, and short chain fatty acids. Mercaptans are also thought to produce the characteristic breath odor (fetor hepaticus) of patients with chronic liver failure. Another hypothesis suggests that an imbalance between plasma branched-chain and aromatic amino acids, a common consequence of severe liver disease, leads to decreased synthesis of normal neurotransmitters and to increased formation of "false neurotransmitters" from aromatic amino acids in the central nervous system.

The clinical features of hepatic encephalopathy include disturbances of higher neurological function (intellectual and personality disorders, dementia, inability to copy simple diagrams [i.e., constructional apraxia], disturbance of consciousness), disturbances of neuromuscular function (asterixis, hyperreflexia, myoclonus), and rarely, a Parkinson-like syndrome and progressive paraplegia. As with other metabolic encephalopathies (which may show many of the signs of hepatic encephalopathy) asymmetrical neurological findings are unusual but can occur, and brain stem reflexes (e.g., pupillary light, oculovestibular, and oculocephalic responses) are preserved until very late. Hepatic encephalopathy is usually divided into stages according to its severity (Table 46–5). Subtle disorders of psychomotor function may exist in many patients with cirrhosis in whom conventional neurological examination is normal. Such subclinical encephalopathy (termed stage 0 encephalopathy) is of importance in that it may impair work performance.

The differential diagnosis of hepatic encephalopathy includes hypoglycemia, subdural hematoma, meningitis, and sedative drug overdosage, all of which are common in patients, particularly alcoholics, with liver disease.

Treatment

Treatment of hepatic encephalopathy is based on four simple principles:

TABLE 46–5. STAGES OF HEPATIC ENCEPHALOPATHY

STAGE	CLINICAL MANIFESTATIONS
I	apathy restlessness reversal of sleep rhythm slowed intellect impaired computational ability impaired handwriting
II	lethargy drowsiness disorientation asterixis
III	stupor (arousable) hyperactive reflexes, extensor plantar responses
IV	coma (response to painful stimuli only)

Stage 0 encephalopathy is used to describe subclinical impairment of intellectual function.

TABLE 46–6. HEPATIC ENCEPHALOPATHY: PRECIPITATING FACTORS

Gastrointestinal bleeding
Increased dietary protein
Constipation
Infection
CNS-depressant drugs (benzodiazepines, opiates)
Deterioration in hepatic function
Hypokalemia ⎫
Azotemia ⎪ most often induced by diuretics
Alkalosis ⎬
Hypovolemia ⎭

IDENTIFICATION AND TREATMENT OF PRECIPITATING FACTORS. Table 46–6 lists several important factors that may precipitate or severely aggravate hepatic encephalopathy in patients with severe liver disease. Gastrointestinal bleeding and increased protein intake may provide increased substrate for the bacterial or metabolic formation of nitrogenous compounds that induce encephalopathy. In patients prone to develop hepatic encephalopathy there is a markedly increased sensitivity to central nervous system–depressant drugs, and their use should be avoided in these patients.

REDUCTION AND ELIMINATION OF SUBSTRATE FOR THE GENERATION OF NITROGENOUS COMPOUNDS. (a) **Dietary protein restriction.** Patients in coma should receive no protein, whereas those with mild encephalopathy may benefit from restriction of protein intake to 40 to 60 grams per day. Vegetable protein diets also appear to be less encephalopathogenic. (b) **Bowel cleansing.** This is important mainly in patients with encephalopathy precipitated by gastrointestinal bleeding or constipation, and is achieved by administration of enemas.

REDUCTION OF COLONIC BACTERIA. Neomycin administered orally reduces the number of bacteria that are responsible for production of ammonia and other nitrogenous compounds.

PREVENTION OF AMMONIA DIFFUSION FROM THE BOWEL. This is achieved by administration of lactulose, a nonabsorbable disaccharide, which, when fermented to organic acids by colonic bacteria, leads to a lower stool pH. This lowered pH traps ammonia in the colon as nondiffusible NH_4^- ions, but other mechanisms such as inhibition of bacterial ammonia production may also be important.

Hepatocellular Carcinoma

Hepatocellular carcinoma and its relationship to cirrhosis are discussed in Chapter 48.

REFERENCES

Boyer TD: Cirrhosis of the liver. In Wyngaarden JB, and Smith LH Jr (eds): Cecil Textbook of Medicine. 17th ed. Philadelphia, WB Saunders Co, 1985, pp 835–840.
Boyer TD: Major sequelae of cirrhosis. In Wyngaarden JB, and Smith LH Jr (eds): Cecil Textbook of Medicine. 17th ed. Philadelphia, WB Saunders Co, 1985, pp 840–845.

Boyer TD: Portal hypertension and its complications. In Zakim D, and Boyer TD (eds): Hepatology: A Textbook of Liver Disease. Philadelphia, WB Saunders Co, 1982, pp 911–971.

Bleeding oesophageal varices. Lancet (Editorial) 1:139–141, 1984.

Hoyumpa AM, and Schenker S: Perspectives in hepatic encephalopathy. J Lab Clin Med 100:477–487, 1982.

Scharschmidt BF: Acute and chronic hepatic failure with encephalopathy. In Wyngaarden JB, and Smith LH Jr (eds): Cecil Textbook of Medicine. 17th ed. Philadelphia, WB Saunders Co, 1985, pp 845–848.

ABSCESSES AND GRANULOMATOUS AND VASCULAR LIVER DISEASE

47

LIVER ABSCESS

Pyogenic Liver Abscess. Pyogenic liver abscess represents a macroscopic collection of pus within the liver parenchyma due to bacterial infection. Liver abscess is an uncommon disorder in the United States, a surprising observation in view of the rich blood supply of the liver and its position upstream from the bacteria-laden intestine. The most common predisposing cause of pyogenic liver abscess is biliary tract disease, especially bile duct obstruction with cholangitis or acute cholecystitis. Less frequent predisposing factors include infection in areas drained by the portal system (e.g., appendicitis and diverticulitis), direct extension from subphrenic or perinephric abscesses, abdominal trauma, and infection in necrotic tumor deposits. Abscesses may be single or multiple, large or small. Enteric flora such as *Escherichia coli* or *Klebsiella* and pyogenic gram-positive cocci such as *Staphylococcus aureus* are the most common causes of pyogenic liver abscesses, although anaerobes either alone or in combination with aerobes may account for up to 50 per cent of all pyogenic abscesses. Hepatic abscesses generally present as a febrile illness lasting days to weeks, often associated with right upper quadrant abdominal pain and tenderness. Pulmonary symptoms, including cough and pleuritic chest pain as well as pulmonary rales and a pleural effusion, are seen in 20 to 40 per cent of cases. Jaundice may be seen in up to 20 per cent of patients, usually due to concomitant biliary disease. Laboratory tests are generally not helpful, although most patients exhibit a leukocytosis and elevated serum alkaline phosphatase activity. Lesions can be localized by radionuclide scan, ultrasound, or computed tomography (see Chapter 37), and the diagnosis is established by percutaneous or surgical aspiration of material for Gram's stain and culture (including anaerobic culture techniques). Blood cultures, which are positive in up to 40 per cent of patients, should also be obtained prior to antibiotic treatment. Broad-spectrum antibiotic therapy directed against an-

aerobes and aerobes should be initiated immediately and, once culture results are available, appropriately tailored according to the sensitivities of the isolated organisms. After a diagnostic aspiration, most abscesses can be treated with antibiotics alone for four to six weeks or in combination with percutaneous drainage. Surgical therapy is generally necessary for those patients with concomitant intra-abdominal sepsis or biliary tract obstruction. Complications of pyogenic abscesses include sepsis, pleuropulmonary involvement via direct extension or embolization, and peritonitis due to abscess rupture. The mortality of treated abscesses is high; however, that of untreated abscesses is 100 per cent.

Amebic Liver Abscess. Amebic liver abscess is rare in the United States, but common in parts of the world where sanitation is poor. Amebic liver abscesses arise in individuals who harbor ameba in the colon, although the colonic infection may be asymptomatic. The clinical and laboratory features of amebic liver abscess are quite similar to those of pyogenic liver abscess, and the two disorders can be definitively distinguished only by examination and culture of aspirated abscess contents (amebic abscesses contain "anchovy paste" material that is free of bacteria) and serological tests. Because ameba are found only at the edge of the abscess, it is *important to examine the last few drops of aspirated material for organisms*. Indirect hemagglutination and gel diffusion precipitin tests for ameba are positive in over 90 per cent of individuals with amebic abscesses, although they may be negative when the patient first presents. Medical therapy is curative and should be instituted promptly in all patients suspected of having an amebic abscess. Metronidazole (750 mg t.i.d. for 10 days) followed by diiodohydroxyquin (650 mg t.i.d. for 20 days) to eliminate intestinal cysts are the drugs of choice, although the combination of dehydroemetine and chloroquin followed by diiodohydroxyquin is also effective. Surgical drainage is usually unnecessary unless the abscess has ruptured into the pleural, pericardial, or peritoneal space.

GRANULOMATOUS LIVER DISEASE

Hepatic granulomas are common, being found in 2 to 10 per cent of all liver biopsies, often in association with an elevated serum alkaline phosphatase level. However, they are rarely a specific finding and have been reported in association with a wide variety of infections, systemic illnesses, hepatobiliary disorders, drugs, and toxins, some of which are listed in Table 47–1. Although granulomas are a nonspecific finding, occasionally specific features are seen, such as acid-fast bacilli in tuberculosis, ova in schistosomiasis, larvae in toxocariasis, and birefringent granules in starch, talc, or silicone granulomas. The differential diagnosis of hepatic granulomas is one of the most extensive in medicine, and the work-up requires meticulous attention to details of the history, physical examination, and laboratory tests. Indeed, in 20 per cent or more of patients, no cause for granulomas is found despite extensive investigation. A subset of these patients, who have a syndrome consisting of fever, hepatomegaly, and hepatic granulomas which responds to administration of corticosteroids, has been described as having granulomatous hepatitis, although some feel that these individuals have a variant of sarcoidosis.

Conversely, liver biopsy (and culture, particularly of acid-fast bacteria) is of considerable value in the diagnosis of sarcoidosis, miliary tuberculosis, and histoplasmosis, as virtually all patients with these disorders will have hepatic granulomas. Similarly, characteristic granulomas are seen in many patients with primary biliary cirrhosis, and granulomas may be the first clue to Hodgkin's disease.

VASCULAR DISEASE OF THE LIVER

Portal vein thrombosis, hepatic vein thrombosis (Budd-Chiari syndrome), and veno-occlusive disease are uncommon disorders of hepatic vasculature that usually present with portal hypertension with or without associated liver dysfunction.

Portal vein thrombosis may develop after abdominal trauma, umbilical vein infection, sepsis, or pancreatitis or in association with cirrhosis or hypercoagulable states; in most cases, however, and particularly in children, the cause is unknown. The disease presents with the manifestations of portal hypertension (see Chapter 46); however, liver histology is usually normal. The diagnosis is established by angiography. Surgical management is difficult owing to the absence of suitable patent vessels for portal-systemic shunting.

The Budd-Chiari syndrome is associated with abdominal trauma, use of oral contraceptives, polycythemia vera, paroxysmal nocturnal hemoglobinuria, other hypercoagulable states, and congenital webs of the vena cava. Illness may be acute or chronic with abdominal pain, hepatomegaly, ascites, and portal hypertension as prominent features. The diagnosis is usually suspected when centrilobular necrosis is seen on liver biopsy and is established angiographically by inability to catheterize the hepatic veins. Although elevation of serum bilirubin and transaminases is often mild, liver function is often poor and mortality rates of 40 to 90 per cent are reported. Anticoagulants have not proven useful; however, recent studies have suggested that the side-to-side portacaval shunts, performed to relieve hepatic congestion, may improve survival.

Veno-occlusive disease or nonthrombotic occlusion of hepatic venules is a small-vessel variant of the Budd-Chiari syndrome. Veno-occlusive disease develops in man and animals exposed to native medicinal teas containing pyrrolozidine alkaloids from *Senecio* and *Crotalia* genera of plants. Cases have also been reported in association with the use of certain chemotherapeutic agents and with bone marrow transplantation. The occluded venules can be seen on liver biopsy, and a distinctive abnormal vascular pattern may be seen when contrast is injected into the hepatic vein. Patients with alcoholic liver disease also frequently exhibit some degree of hepatic venule sclerosis or occlusion. No specific treatment is available. Some patients appear to recover spontaneously, whereas others require therapy for the complications of portal hypertension.

TABLE 47–1. DISEASES ASSOCIATED WITH HEPATIC GRANULOMAS

Infections	Hepatobiliary Disorders
Bacterial, spirochetal	Primary biliary cirrhosis
Tuberculosis and atypical	Granulomatous hepatitis
mycobacteria	Jejunoileal bypass
Tularemia	**Systemic Disorders**
Brucellosis	Sarcoidosis
Leprosy	Wegener's granulomatosis
Syphilis	Inflammatory bowel disease
Whipple's disease	Hodgkin's disease
Listeriosis	Lymphoma
Viral	**Drugs/Toxins**
Infectious mononucleosis	Beryllium
Cytomegalovirus	Parenteral foreign material
Rickettsial	(starch, talc, silicone, etc.)
Q fever	Phenylbutazone
Fungal	Alpha methyldopa
Coccidioidomycosis	Procainamide
Histoplasmosis	Allopurinol
Cryptococcus	Phenytoin
Actinomycosis	Nitrofurantoin
Aspergillosis	Hydralazine
Nocardiosis	
Parasitic	
Schistosomiasis	
Clonorchiasis	
Toxocariasis	
Ascariasis	
Toxoplasmosis	
Amebiasis	

REFERENCES

Adams EB, and MacLeod MI. Invasive amebiasis. Medicine 56:315–334, 1977.

Harrington PL, Gutierrez JJ, Ramirez-Ronda CH, Quinones-Soto R, Bermudex RH, and Chaffey J: Granulomatous hepatitis. Rev Infect Dis 4:638, 1982.

McDonald MI, Corey GR, Galus HA, and Durack DT: Single and multiple pyogenic liver abscesses. Medicine 63:291–302, 1984.

Scharschmidt BF: Parasitic, bacterial, fungal, and granulomatous liver disease. In Wyngaarden JB, and Smith LH Jr (eds): Cecil Textbook of Medicine. 17th ed. Philadelphia, WB Saunders Co, 1985, pp 827–832.

Zakim D, and Boyer T (eds): Hepatology: A Textbook of Liver Disease. Philadelphia, WB Saunders Co, 1982, pp 464–498, 723–738.

HEPATIC NEOPLASMS 48

Hepatic neoplasms can be divided into three groups (1) benign neoplasms, (2) primary malignant neoplasms, and (3) metastatic malignant neoplasms. The latter category, that of metastatic tumors, constitutes the bulk of hepatic neoplasms in this country. This chapter will briefly review all three categories of hepatic neoplasms and will conclude with a brief discussion of the diagnostic approach to these lesions.

BENIGN NEOPLASMS

The group of benign neoplastic lesions includes hepatocellular adenoma, focal nodular hyperplasia, hemangioma, bile duct adenoma, and other rare tumors of mesenchymal origin (e.g., fibromas, lipomas, leiomyomas). Hepatocellular adenomas occur almost exclusively in women, and there is strong circumstantial evidence to implicate estrogens, especially oral contraceptives, in their development and growth. Adenomas consist of a monotonous array of normal hepatocytes without bile ducts, portal tracts, or Kupffer cells. Although they are not regarded as premalignant lesions, they have a predilection for hemorrhage, tumor infarct, and rupture. Patients usually present with signs and symptoms of an abdominal mass or hemorrhage (pain, fever, circulatory collapse). The latter individuals usually require emergency surgery and resection of the adenoma.

Adenomas usually appear as cold spots on ^{99m}Tc-sulfur colloid scans and as vascular lesions on angiography. Management of asymptomatic lesions is controversial, although elective surgical excision is usually performed. A trial period of observation may be warranted if oral contraceptives can be discontinued, and some adenomas have been noted to regress under this regimen.

HEPATOCELLULAR CARCINOMA

Although hepatocellular carcinoma is rare in the United States (accounting for less than 2.5 per cent of all malignancies), in other areas of the world, including sub-Sahara Africa, China, Japan, and Southeast Asia, it is one of the most frequent malignancies and is an important cause of mortality, particularly in middle-aged males. Hepatocellular carcinoma usually arises in a cirrhotic liver and is closely associated with chronic hepatitis B virus infection, particularly in those parts of the world, enumerated above, where infants acquire persistent infection with hepatitis B from chronically infected mothers at birth. The advent and widespread use of vaccination to prevent infection with hepatitis B virus is expected to reduce markedly the incidence of this disease. The risk of hepatocellular carcinoma is low in cirrhosis associated with primary biliary cirrhosis and Wilson's disease and intermediate in cirrhosis due to alcohol. Other risk factors for development of hepatocellular carcinoma, as well as its clinical manifestations, are listed in Table 48–1. Diagnosis of small, potentially treatable lesions, even in high-risk areas, is difficult, as the efficacy of screening for elevated α-fetoprotein levels has been mixed. Most patients present with widespread, often multifocal disease, and the median survival from the time of diagnosis is less than six months. Hepatic resection can be attempted in patients with small, solitary lesions if the remaining liver is not cirrhotic. Chemotherapy, radiation

TABLE 48–1. HEPATOCELLULAR CARCINOMA

Incidence From 1–7 per 100,000 to >100 per 100,000 in high-risk areas **Sex** 4:1 to 8:1 male preponderance **Associations** Chronic hepatitis B infection Hemochromatosis (with cirrhosis) Cirrhosis (alcoholic, cryptogenic) Aflatoxin ingestion Thorotrast α_1-Antitrypsin deficiency Androgen administration **Common Clinical Presentations** Abdominal pain Abdominal mass Weight loss Deterioration of liver function	**Unusual Manifestations** Bloody ascites Tumor emboli (lung) Jaundice Hepatic or portal vein obstruction Metabolic effects: erythrocytosis, hypercalcemia, hypercholesterolemia, hypoglycemia, gynecomastia, feminization, acquired porphyria **Clinical/Laboratory Findings** Hepatic bruit or friction rub Serum α-fetoprotein level >400 ng/ml

therapy, and hepatic transplantation have yielded disappointing results.

Other primary hepatocellular malignancies include cholangiocarcinoma, angiosarcoma (related to exposure to vinyl choride, arsenic, or Thorotrast), hepatoblastoma, and cystadenocarcinoma.

TUMOR METASTASES TO THE LIVER

Metastases constitute the bulk of hepatic malignancies and most commonly derive from tumors of the stomach, pancreas, colon, lung, oropharynx, and bladder and from melanoma. The liver is also a frequent site of involvement by Hodgkin's disease, non-Hodgkin's lymphoma, and malignant histiocytosis.

DIAGNOSTIC APPROACH TO HEPATIC NEOPLASMS

Most hepatic neoplasms present with right upper quadrant abdominal pain or an abdominal mass. Hemorrhage, systemic manifestations, and biliary obstruction (from strategically located tumors) may also occur. Visualization of discrete focal lesions and histological examination of tissue are generally required for diagnosis. Thus evaluation employs one or more imaging proce-dures followed by percutaneous, laparoscopic, or surgical biopsy of one or more lesions. Radionuclide scanning is a reasonable first step in the work-up, although imaging by computed tomography or ultrasound may be more sensitive in detecting small lesions and offers the advantage of performing guided percutaneous biopsy or aspiration cytology. Localization of lesions is generally followed by biopsy; however, additional factors must be considered. Percutaneous biopsies of vascular lesions such as hemangiomas, angiosarcomas, and perhaps hepatocellular adenomas are potentially dangerous, whereas cells obtained by aspiration cytology frequently fail to differentiate hepatocellular adenoma, hepatocellular carcinoma, and normal hepatocytes. Thus, the choice of procedures will depend on the diagnostic and therapeutic options under consideration.

REFERENCES

Kew MC: Tumors of the liver. In Zakim D, and Boyer T (eds): Hepatology: A Textbook of Liver Disease. Philadelphia, WB Saunders Co, 1982, pp 1048–1083.

Kew MC, and Geddes EW: Hepatocellular carcinoma in rural South African blacks. Medicine 61:98, 1982.

Margolis S, and Homcy C: Systemic manifestations of hepatoma. Medicine 51:381, 1972.

Scharschmidt BF: Hepatic tumors. In Wyngaarden JB, and Smith LH Jr (eds): Cecil Textbook of Medicine. 17th ed. Philadelphia, WB Saunders Co, 1985, pp 848–851.

49 DISORDERS OF THE GALLBLADDER AND BILIARY TRACT

The liver produces 500 to 1500 ml of bile per day. The major physiological role of the biliary tract and gallbladder is to concentrate this material and to conduct it silently and efficiently, in well-timed aliquots, to the intestine. In the intestine, biliary bile acids participate in normal fat digestion while cholesterol and a wide variety of other endogenous and exogenous compounds carried in bile are excreted in the feces. Normally unobtrusive, the gallbladder and biliary tree are the source of considerable pain and disability when they become infected or obstructed. This chapter will briefly outline the normal physiology of the biliary system and then focus on the pathophysiology and clinical consequences of gallstones, the most important biliary tract disorder, closing with a brief discussion of neoplasms and other causes of bile duct obstruction. The reader is referred to Chapter 36E for a detailed discussion of the diagnostic approach to jaundice and biliary obstruction, and to Chapter 37 for a review of the various imaging techniques used to study the biliary tract.

NORMAL BILIARY PHYSIOLOGY

Bile, a complex fluid secreted by hepatocytes, passes via the intrahepatic bile ducts into the common bile duct. Tonic contraction of the sphincter of Oddi during fasting diverts about half of hepatic bile into the gallbladder where it is stored and concentrated. Cholecystokinin, released after food ingestion, causes contraction of the gallbladder and relaxation of the sphincter of Oddi, allowing delivery of a nicely timed bolus of bile, rich in bile acids, into the intestine. Bile acids, detergent molecules possessing both fat-soluble and water-soluble moieties, convey phospholipids and cholesterol from the liver to the intestine, where the latter undergoes fecal excretion. In the intestinal lumen, bile acids solubilize dietary fat and promote its digestion and absorption. Bile acids are, for the most part, efficiently reabsorbed by the small intestinal mucosa, particularly in the terminal ileum, and are recycled to the liver for re-excretion, a process termed the enterohepatic circulation.

PATHOPHYSIOLOGY OF GALLSTONE FORMATION (CHOLELITHIASIS)

Gallstones, the most common cause of biliary tract disease in the United States, occur in 20 to 35 per cent of people by the age of 75 and are of two types: 75 per cent consist primarily of cholesterol, whereas 25 per cent, termed pigment stones, are composed of calcium bilirubinate and other calcium salts. Cholesterol, which is insoluble in water, normally is carried in bile solubilized by bile acids and phospholipids. However, in many individuals, not all of whom will develop gallstones, bile contains more cholesterol than can be maintained in stable solution (Fig. 49–1); i.e., it is supersaturated with cholesterol. In the supersaturated bile of many, but not all, such individuals, microscopic cholesterol crystals form.

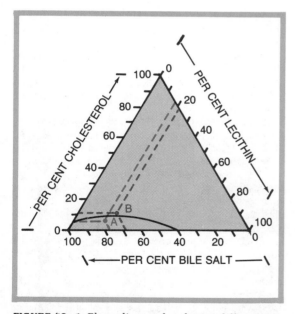

FIGURE 49–1. Phase diagram for plotting different mixtures of bile salt, lecithin, and cholesterol. The curved line represents the boundary of the micellar zone for aqueous solutions containing 4 to 10 per cent solids. Any mixture, such as A, falling within this area contains all its cholesterol in solution. Any mixture, such as B, falling outside this area has excess cholesterol as a precipitate or supersaturated solution. The points A and B actually depict the average composition of gallbladder bile obtained from normal persons and patients with cholesterol gallstones, respectively.

Gradual deposition of additional layers of cholesterol leads to the appearance of macroscopic cholesterol gallstones. The gallbladder is key to gallstone formation; it constitutes an area of bile stasis where slow crystal growth can occur and it also may provide mucus, bacteria, or other material to act as a nidus to initiate cholesterol crystal formation. Many of the recognized predisposing factors for cholelithiasis can be understood in terms of the pathophysiological scheme just outlined: (1) biliary cholesterol saturation is increased by estrogens, multiparity, oral contraceptives, obesity, and terminal ileal disease (which decreases the bile acid pool); (2) bile stasis is increased by bile duct strictures, parenteral hyperalimentation, fasting, and choledochal cysts.

The pathophysiology of pigment stones is less well understood; however increased production of bilirubin (hemolytic states), cirrhosis, and bacterial deconjugation of bilirubin to a less soluble form are all associated with pigment stone formation.

CLINICAL MANIFESTATIONS OF GALLSTONES

Many individuals with gallstones are asymptomatic. Duct obstruction is the underlying cause of all manifestations of gallstone disease. Obstructin of the cystic duct distends the gallbladder and produces biliary pain, while superimposed infection or inflammation leads to acute cholecystitis. Obstruction of the common duct may produce pain, jaundice, infection (cholangitis), and/or pancreatitis, whereas reflux of biliary contents (and bacteria) back into the liver can produce sepsis or hepatic damage and biliary cirrhosis. The natural history of cholesterol gallstone disease is outlined in Figure 49–2.

Asymptomatic Gallstones. Approximately 30 to 50 per cent of patients with gallstones in the United States are asymptomatic, and over a 20-year period it appears that only about 18 per cent of these individuals will develop biliary pain and only 3 per cent will require a cholecystectomy. Asymptomatic patients should be followed expectantly, with prophylactic cholecystectomy considered in three high-risk groups: (1) diabetics, who have a greater mortality (10 to 15 per cent) from acute cholecystitis; (2) persons with a calcified gallbladder, which is often associated with carcinoma of the gallbladder; and (3) persons with sickle-cell anemia in whom hepatic crises may be difficult to differentiate from acute cholecystitis. Attempts to dissolve cholesterol gallstones by orally administered chenodeoxycholic acid or ursodeoxycholic acid have been successful in some patients; however, a policy of expectant management followed by cholecystectomy is probably more cost-effective.

Chronic Cholecystitis and Biliary Colic. The term chronic cholecystitis is used to denote non-acute symptoms due to the presence of gallstones. A better term is biliary "colic," as there is only a loose correlation between the presence of symp-

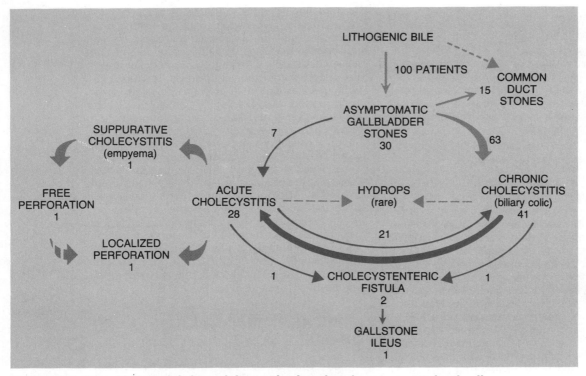

FIGURE 49—2. Natural history of cholecystolithiasis. The clinical syndromes associated with gall-stones are shown here, and the numbers represent the approximate percentage of patients with gallstone disease who present in that way.

toms and pathologic findings such as inflammation in the gallbladder wall. Gallbladders from symptomatic patients may be grossly normal with mild histological inflammation or may exhibit shrinking, scarring, and thickening, often as a result of previous attacks of acute cholecystitis. Symptoms arise from contraction of the gallbladder during transient obstruction of the cystic duct by gallstones. Biliary colic usually produces a steady, cramplike pain in the epigastrium or right upper quadrant which comes on quickly, reaches a plateau of intensity over a few minutes, and begins to subside gradually over 30 minutes to several hours. Referred pain may be felt at the tip of the scapula or right shoulder. Nausea and vomiting may accompany biliary colic, whereas fever, leukocytosis, and a palpable mass (signs of acute cholecystitis) do not. Attacks occur at variable intervals (days to years) and may be associated with ingestion of large or fatty meals. Other symptoms such as dyspepsia, fatty food intolerance, flatulence, heartburn, and belching may occur in patients with chronic cholecystitis; however, they are nonspecific and frequently occur in individuals with normal gallbladders. Gallstones are the sine qua non of chronic cholecystitis and can be demonstrated by either oral cholecystography (which demonstrates stones in two thirds of patients; the gallbladder is not visualized in one third of patients, a finding taken to indicate gallbladder disease) or ultrasound (which demonstrates gallstones in more than 95 per cent of patients). Cholecystectomy, which carries a

mortality of less than 0.5 per cent, is the treatment of choice, and is accompanied by examination of the common duct for concomitant choledocholithiasis. Surgery relieves symptoms in virtually all patients and will prevent development of future complications such as acute cholecystitis, choledocholithiasis and cholangitis, and gallbladder carcinoma.

Acute Cholecystitis. Acute cholecystitis refers to acute right subcostal pain and tenderness due to obstruction of the cystic duct and subsequent distention, inflammation, and secondary infection of the gallbladder. Acalculous cholecystitis, accounting for 5 per cent of cases, is associated with prolonged fasting, e.g., trauma, surgery, or parenteral hyperalimentation, and gallbladder bile that is viscous or "sludgelike." Acute cholecystitis usually begins with epigastric or right upper quadrant pain that gradually increases in severity and usually localizes to the area of the gallbladder. Unlike biliary colic, the pain of acute cholecystitis does not subside spontaneously. Anorexia, nausea, vomiting, fever, and right subcostal tenderness are commonly present, as is Murphy's sign (increased subhepatic tenderness and inspiratory arrest during a deep breath). In approximately one third of patients, a tender, enlarged gallbladder may be felt. Mild jaundice occurs in about 20 per cent of patients due to concomitant common duct stones or bile duct edema. Complications of acute cholecystitis include emphysematous cholecystitis (bacterial gas present in gallbladder lumen and tissues), empyema of the gallbladder, gangrene, and perforation. Approximately 10 per cent of patients will present with or develop one of these complications and require emergency surgery. The onset of severe fever, shaking chills, increased leukocytosis, increased abdominal pain or tenderness, or persistent severe symptoms all indicate progression of disease and suggest development of one of these complications.

Radionuclide scanning following intravenous administration of ^{99m}Tc-HIDA is the most accurate test with which to confirm the clinical impression of acute cholecystitis (cystic duct obstruction). If the gallbladder opacifies, acute cholecystitis is unlikely, whereas if the bile duct opacifies but the gallbladder does not, the clinical diagnosis is strongly supported. An ultrasound examination that shows the presence of gallstones (or sludge in acalculous cholecystitis) and localized tenderness over the gallbladder also provides strong supportive evidence for acute cholecystitis. Oral cholecystograms are of no value in this clinical setting, as they are unreliable in the acutely ill patient.

Most patients with acute cholecystitis will improve over one to seven days with conventional expectant management, which includes nasogastric suction, intravenous fluids and judicious pain medication, and patients may resume oral feedings after a few days. Antibiotics are useful in conjunction with surgery to treat suppurative complications; however, their efficacy in uncomplicated acute cholecystitis is unclear. Because of the high risk of recurrent acute cholecystitis, it is recommended that most patients undergo elective cholecystectomy within four to eight weeks of an acute episode.

An alternative course of management, outlined in Figure 49–3, is to perform early (acute) cholecystectomy. This approach is becoming common practice, as it is less costly and involves no increase in morbidity or mortality. In general, emergency surgery is performed on those patients with advanced disease and complications, usually associated with infection and sepsis. Cholecystostomy, rather than cholecystectomy, may be a useful temporizing measure in emergent circumstances in patients with a high operative risk. Patients who are good operative risks and in whom the diagnosis is certain are scheduled for prompt cholecystectomy within 24 to 48 hours. Expectant management is reserved for those with uncomplicated disease who are not good operative candidates or those in whom the diagnosis is not clear.

The mortality of acute cholecystitis of 5 to 10 per cent is almost entirely confined to patients over 60 years of age with serious associated diseases and to those with suppurative complications. Complications of acute cholecystitis include infectious complications already listed and gallstone ileus (intestinal obstruction due to a gallstone that has eroded through the gallbladder and duodenal walls into the intestinal lumen).

Choledocholithiasis and Acute Cholangitis. In the United States, most gallstones in the com-

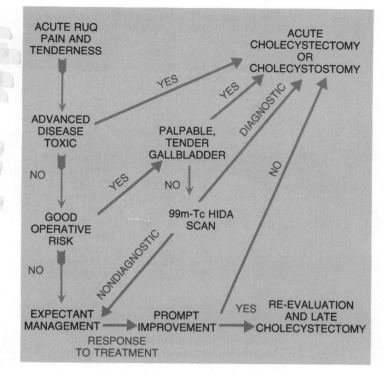

FIGURE 49–3. Scheme for managing patients with right upper quadrant pain and tenderness who are thought to have acute cholecystitis. This scheme is based on a policy of early operation for appropriate patients.

mon duct come from the gallbladder; this occurs in up to 15 per cent of persons with cholelithiasis. Less commonly, stones may form de novo in the biliary tree, usually behind a partial obstruction. Ductal stones may be asymptomatic (30 to 40 per cent) or may produce biliary colic, jaundice, cholangitis, pancreatitis, or a combination of these. Secondary hepatic effects include biliary cirrhosis and hepatic abscesses.

Intermittent cholangitis, consisting of biliary colic, jaundice, and fever plus chills (Charcot's triad) is the most common manifestation of choledocholithiasis, although it may also occur in patients with previous biliary surgery. Biliary infection may be mild or it may be severe, with suppurative cholangitis, sepsis, and shock. Diagnosis is based on a compatible clinical picture and radiological or endoscopic evidence of ductal stones. Treatment includes hospitalization, treatment of infection, and removal of stones. The latter may be accomplished surgically in patients with an intact gallbladder by cholecystectomy and choledochotomy. In individuals with a previous cholecystectomy or those who are poor surgical candidates, endoscopic sphincterotomy, which opens the sphincter of Oddi and allows passage of gallstones up to 1 cm in size, is an alternative approach.

The severest form of cholangitis, suppurative cholangitis, rapidly results in life-threatening sepsis. Initially, the patients may have only mild signs of biliary obstruction, yet they require rapid evaluation and treatment, including intravenous fluids and antibiotics and emergency surgery to drain the biliary tree. The high mortality of 50 per cent for this disease reflects the age of the patients generally affected, the speed with which sepsis develops, and the frequent failure to identify the biliary tree as the source of sepsis.

Other Disorders of the Biliary Tree. A number of other processes, all of which may present with biliary obstruction, jaundice, or infection, may involve the biliary tree. The approach to evaluating these entities is outlined in Chapter 37.

Benign biliary strictures usually result from surgical injury and may cause symptoms days to years later. Early diagnosis is important, as strictures that partially obstruct and are clinically asymptomatic may cause secondary biliary cirrhosis. Biliary stricture should be suspected in anyone with a history of right upper quadrant surgery and a persistently elevated serum alkaline phosphatase level. A similar type of benign stricture is seen in alcoholics in whom the intrapancreatic portion of the common bile duct is compressed by pancreatic fibrosis. Surgical repair or bypass of these lesions is successful in 75 per cent of patients. Balloon catheter dilation may be useful in selected individuals.

Sclerosing cholangitis is an idiopathic condition of nonmalignant, nonbacterial chronic inflammatory narrowing of the intra- and extrahepatic bile ducts. It most commonly occurs in males in the third and fourth decades of life, often in association with ulcerative colitis. Patients usually present with pruritus or jaundice, and percutaneous transhepatic cholangiography or endoscopic retrograde cholangiopancreatography shows characteristic changes ("beading") of the extrahepatic bile ducts. Therapy is supportive.

Structural abnormalities such as choledochal cysts, Caroli's disease (saccular intrahepatic bile duct dilation), and duodenal diverticuli may also cause bile duct obstruction, often with secondary choledocholithiasis. Hemobilia and intermittent bile duct obstruction by blood clots are caused by hepatic injury, neoplasms, or hepatic artery aneurysms.

Biliary neoplasms are rare, but include carcinoma of the gallbladder, scirrhous or papillary adenocarcinoma of the bile ducts, and carcinoma of the ampulla of Vater. The latter two neoplasms usually present as unremitting painless jaundice, although necrosis and sloughing of tumor may cause intermittent obstruction and the appearance of occult fecal blood. The term "Klatskin tumor" specifically refers to an adenocarcinoma located at the bifurcation of the common bile duct. Carcinoma of the gallbladder often presents as advanced disseminated disease, although symptoms also may resemble acute or chronic cholecystitis or bile duct obstruction. Resection of most of these tumors is difficult or impossible and prognosis is poor. For patients with unresectable tumor the goal is palliation, and for those with severe symptoms due to obstruction, percutaneous or endoscopic stenting of the biliary tree may be helpful. Stents should not be used in patients with benign disease because complications due to biliary infection and plugging of the stent invariably occur; rather, definitive surgical repair or bypass is preferred.

Motility disorders of the biliary tree have not been well recognized in the past. With the use of newer endoscopic techniques for measuring biliary pressures and motility, it has become apparent that a small group of patients with biliary pain may have symptoms due to hypertension, dysmotility, and/or stenosis of the sphincter of Oddi. However, at this time there is only limited evidence to suggest that surgical or endoscopic treatment (sphincterotomy) is of value.

REFERENCES

Malet PF, and Soloway RD: Diseases of the gallbladder and bile ducts. In Wyngaarden JB, and Smith LH Jr (eds): Cecil Textbook of Medicine. 17th ed. Philadelphia, WB Saunders Co, 1985, pp 845–865.

Sleisenger MH, and Fordtran JS (eds): Gastrointestinal Disease: Pathophysiology, Diagnosis and Management. 3rd ed. Philadelphia, WB Saunders Co, 1983, pp 1346–1414.

Wiesner RH, and LaRusso NF: Clinicopathological features of the syndrome of primary sclerosing cholangitis. Gastroenterology 79:200, 1980.

Zakim D, and Boyer T (eds): Hepatology: A Textbook of Liver Disease. Philadelphia, WB Saunders Co, 1982, pp 297–350, 1261–1273.

HEMATOLOGY

SECTION

V

Bone marrow in the adult occupies the vertebrae, sternum, ribs, pelvic bones, and, to a lesser extent, the long bones and skull, and comprises about 1 kg of tissue. In the child, hematopoiesis is more prominent in the long bones and skull, whereas in adulthood fatty tissue replaces the hematopoietic marrow in these peripheral areas. In addition, liver and spleen, primary sites of hematopoiesis in the fetus, may regain hematopoietic acitivity in certain adult diseases, including severe anemias, skeletal marrow failure, myelofibrosis, and hematologic malignancies such as leukemia.

Normal bone marrow consists of about 50 per cent hematopoietic cells and 50 per cent fat, with the hematopoietic cells being arranged in cords around sinusoids; blood vessels are abundant (Figs. 50–1 and 50–2). The space occupied by fat increases during adulthood, although hematopoietic tissue can replace it under appropriate conditions at any age. The hematopoietic cells include a small pluripotential stem cell compartment, consisting of small cells resembling lymphocytes, a large compartment of proliferating cells of committed lineage (the ratio of myeloid:erythroid precursors is normally 3 to 5:1) and a large compartment of postmitotic maturing cells of both myeloid and erythroid lineage. Smaller numbers of megakaryocytes, which differentiate into platelets, plasma cells (which produce immunoglobulins), reticulum cells, and lymphocytes are also present. It requires about one week for a stem cell to differentiate into mature daughter cells of either erythroid or myeloid type; the marrow additionally contains about one week's worth of mature leukocytes and erythro-

FIGURE 50–1. Photomicrographs of bone marrow biopsies. *Upper left*, Normal bone marrow: 50 per cent cellular, 50 per cent fat. Heterogeneous cell population can be seen at low power (×100) including megakaryocytes. *Upper right*, Aplasia. Marked hypocellularity is present. *Lower left*, Myelofibrosis and myelosclerosis. Cellular marrow is replaced with fibrous tissue and spicules of bone are thickened. *Lower right*, Acute myelogenous leukemia. Marrow is completely replaced by a homogenous population of cells and fat is obliterated.

FIGURE 50—2. Photomicrographs of peripheral blood smears. *Upper left*, Spherocytes, round dense cells lacking a central pallor. *Upper right*, Sickle cells. *Lower left*, Target cells. *Lower right*, Schistocytes, or red cell fragments.

cytes. The circulating half-life of polymorphonuclear leukocytes is about 6 hours, of platelets 8 to 10 days, and of erythrocytes 120 days; thus, the granulocyte pool is released much faster than the erythrocyte pool, which is renewed at a rate of 0.8 per cent per day. Because the ratio in the peripheral blood of granulocytes:erythrocytes:platelets is about 1:5000:100, approximately equal numbers of these three cell types are released from the bone marrow each day.

Erythropoiesis is under the control of the hormone, erythropoietin, released from the kidney under the stimulus of tissue hypoxia. A glycoprotein of molecular weight 46,000, erythropoietin may also be produced in the liver. It stimulates primitive pluripotential or stem cells into erythropoietic differentiation, acting mainly on the CFU-E (colony forming unit-erythroid) to promote differentiation into proerythroblasts. The earliest recognizable red cell precursor, the *erythroblast*, eventually gives rise to eight or more mature erythrocytes. The erythroblast is a large cell with abundant endoplasmic reticulum, which decreases in size as it matures, incorporates trans-

ferrin-bound iron via specific membrane receptors, and begins to form hemoglobin. In more mature stages the developing erythroblasts, the basophilic, then polychromatophilic, then orthochromic *normoblasts*, lose the capacity to divide. Their nuclei become pyknotic and are finally extruded prior to release of the erythrocytes from the bone marrow. Newly released erythrocytes, or *reticulocytes*, have active mitochondrial function and retain the capacity to form hemoglobin; about 25 per cent of hemoglobin is synthesized after these cells leave the bone marrow, but the mature erythrocyte in the circulation lacks the capacity for protein synthesis and is anucleate. Its energy is supplied by glycolysis.

The earliest recognizable granulocyte precursor is the *myeloblast*, although developmentally committed stem cells, CFU-C, can be identified in tissue culture. Colony stimulating factors (CSF) produced by monocytes and lymphocytes in response to stimuli such as bacterial endotoxin stimulate mitosis in granulocyte precursors. Prostaglandin E_2 inhibits granulocyte production. *Promyelocytes*, the next stage of myeloblast differentiation, are the largest marrow cells except for megakaryocytes. They contain primary lysosomal granules and give rise to neutrophilic, eosinophilic, or basophilic *myelocytes*, which display the specific granules that identify each myeloid subtype. Myelocytes form the most abundant type of myeloid cell in the marrow and represent the last proliferating cell pool; their descendants, *metamyelocytes, bands,* and *neutrophils* (or eosinophils or basophils) are incapable of cell division but show increasing functional activity concomitant with maturation of membrane functions: chemotaxis, phagocytosis, bactericidal action. After extrusion from the bone marrow, granulocytes occupy two geographic pools in free equilibrium: a marginated pool of cells adhering to blood vessel walls and a circulating pool of roughly equal size. Once in the peripheral blood, granulocytes, like erythrocytes, do not normally re-enter the bone marrow. They follow a "one-way traffic" pattern, spending a relatively short time in the peripheral blood (average, 6 hours) and exiting into the tissues.

The *megakaryocyte*, the only giant, multinucleated cell in the hematopoietic lineage, also derives from the primitive stem cell, and undergoes endomitosis, reaching DNA contents of 32 to 64 n. Specific surface markers characteristic of mature platelets appear at very early stages in megakaryocyte differentiation and persist through maturation. Megakaryocytes tend to stay near marrow sinusoids, where they mature, developing internal membranes that mark off platelet fields. Each megakaryocyte eventually breaks up, releasing some 5000 *platelets* at the edge of a marrow sinusoid into the blood. Some megakaryocytes circulate and may release their platelets in the lung. Although platelets are anucleate fragments of megakaryocytes, they possess a highly organized structure and glycogen energy stores (and some mitochondria) and circulate for 7 to 10 days.

Marrow lymphocytes are mainly of B cell origin, arising also in spleen and lymph nodes. Primitive T cell precursors arise in the marrow, travel to the thymus, where they undergo further differentiation, and thence to spleen, lymph nodes, or marrow as fully functional mature T cells. Lymphocytes are generally much longer-lived than other marrow cells and may survive for years.

Bone marrow functions include hematopoiesis, the differentiation of antibody-producing plasma cells, and the monitoring of hematopoietic cell quality. Normal bone marrow has an 8- to 10-fold capacity to increase blood cell production in response to humoral signals, which include erythropoietin, colony-stimulating factors, and prostaglandins. Normal bone marrow function depends upon intact marrow architecture, the availability of key nutrients including iron, folic acid, and vitamin B_{12}, and regulatory hormones.

Two types of injury can induce marrow failure: damage that affects the capacity for stem cells to undergo differentiation (e.g., in aplastic anemia) and damage that alters the marrow microenvironment (e.g., invasion of marrow by infection or tumor).

REFERENCES

Golde DW, and Takaku F (eds): Hematopoietic Stem Cells. New York, Marcel Dekker, Inc, 1984.

Williams WJ, Beutler E, Erslev AJ, and Lichtman MA (eds): Hematology. 3rd ed. New York, McGraw-Hill Book Co, 1983.

51 ANEMIA

Definition

Anemia represents a decrease in red cell mass or hemoglobin content of blood below physiological need as set by tissue oxygen demand. The conventional limits for normal range of hemoglobin represent the values obtained for 95 per cent of a normal, healthy population, assuming a normal distribution of individuals (Table 51–1). In physiological terms, different ranges exist for men and women, for infants and growing children, and for different metabolic states. Anemia is an expression of many pathological conditions and is not itself a disease state but a clinical sign of such disorders. Therefore, analysis of any anemia should follow a tripartite logical pathway: (1) seek mechanisms by which the anemia occurs, e.g., bleeding, lack of red cell production, or excessive red cell destruction; (2) identify associated dis-eases that cause anemia; (3) evaluate morphologically the peripheral blood smear.

Determinants of the normal range for hemoglobin, hematocrit, and red cell count include age, sex, and ambient altitude. Newborn infants have high values, which soon decline with rapid growth in infancy. Prepubertal boys and girls have similar values. At puberty, male sex hormones produce a rise in erythropoiesis so that adult males have hemoglobin levels approximately 2 to 4 gm/dl higher and hematocrits 5 to 7 per cent higher than adult females. The healthy elderly normally suffer no decline in hemoglobin or hematocrit values; however, because of increased incidence of chronic diseases, elderly populations may show slight decreases in these values. Populations living at altitudes over 4000 feet above sea level show increased hematocrits, which appear to represent physiological adaptation to the desaturation resulting from diminished atmospheric oxygen tension.

Clinical Assessment of Anemia

Signs and symptoms of anemia vary with the rapidity of onset and with underlying disease of the cardiovascular system (Table 51–2). Thus, rapid blood loss, especially if plasma volume decreases rapidly, or brisk hemolysis may result in cardiovascular compensatory reactions, including tachycardia, postural hypotension, vasoconstriction in skin and extremities, dyspnea on exertion, and faintness. Slowly developing anemias, such as those resulting from nutritional deficiency, permit gradual expansion of the plasma volume so that increased cardiac output gradually compensates. The subject may remain asymptomatic, noting only slight exertional dyspnea or, in the case of pre-existing coronary artery disease, increased angina. Pallor of skin and mucous membranes, jaundice, cheilosis (fissuring of the angles of the mouth), a beefy red, smooth tongue, and koilonychia (spoon-shaped nails) are signs that accompany more advanced anemias of different types. The level of anemia at which signs of cardiovascular decompensation occur varies considerably with underlying disease, age, level of activity, and the individual's stoicism. For example, in the sedentary elderly person, a change in mentation can be an important clue to anemia, whereas decreased activity can mask exercise intolerance.

Evaluation of the anemic patient is best served by a systematic evaluation of the clinical and laboratory findings together (Fig. 51–1). First, is the patient truly anemic? Increased plasma volume, fluid overload, or congestive heart failure may produce a dilutional anemia that disappears when fluid balance is restored. Second, is the anemia acquired or inherited? Family history is important, especially in hemolytic anemias, and a positive family history of jaundice, splenomegaly, or gallstones may suggest such a condition. Hemoglobinopathies are frequent in Mediterranean, African, and Far Eastern populations, making ethnic background pertinent. For the immediate problem, a lifelong history versus recent onset is a key differential point. Third, is there evidence for blood loss? The most common reason for anemia is iron loss and iron deficiency. While in growing children and pregnant women iron deficiency may result from dietary lack, the overwhelming cause of iron deficiency in adults is loss of blood from the gastrointestinal or genitourinary tract. Fourth, is there evidence for nutritional deficiency or malabsorption? In the urban Westerner, folic acid deficiency is a common form of malnutrition, seen especially in the elderly living alone and in alcoholics. Fifth, is there evidence for hemolysis? Inherited hemolytic anemias are common in certain populations, whereas acquired hemolytic anemia is rare, occurring mainly in settings of autoimmune disease and drug ingestion. Sixth, is there evidence for toxic exposure or drug ingestion that could cause bone marrow depression and anemia? Finally, does the patient have

TABLE 51–1. NORMAL VALUES FOR HEMOGRAM IN ADULTS

	MALE	FEMALE
Hemoglobin (gm/dl)	13.5–17.5	11.5–15.5
Hematocrit (%)	40–52	36–48
Red cell count ($\times\ 10^{12}$/L)	4.5–6.5	3.9–5.6
Mean cell hemoglobin (MCH) (pg)	27–34	
Mean cell volume (MCV) (fl)	80–95	
Mean cell hemoglobin concentration (MCHC) (gm/dl)	30–35	
White blood cell count ($\times\ 10^9$/L)	4–11	
Platelet count ($\times\ 10^{12}$/L)	150–450	
Reticulocyte count (%)	0.5–1.5	

a chronic inflammatory disease, renal insufficiency, or cancer, each of which is associated with secondary mild anemias, the "anemia of chronic disease"?

Laboratory Evaluation of Anemia

Laboratory evaluation of anemia starts with the hemogram, that is, the complete blood count (hemoglobin, hematocrit, white blood cell count, differential, platelet count, and red cell indices) plus the peripheral blood smear. In addition, initial evaluation should include a reticulocyte count, examination of the stool for occult blood, and urinalysis. Automated cell counters directly determine the number and size (volume) of blood cells and measure hemoglobin chemically; the hematocrit is then derived from these values. This complete examination can be carried out on capillary blood from a fingerstick. Automated differential counters are available that report the white cell differential in absolute numbers based on scanning of large populations of leukocytes either on fixed smears or in cell suspensions. Nevertheless, the visual differential performed on stained smears remains an important method and permits evaluation of the morphology of individual leukocytes and of erythrocytes and platelets. Direct examination of the morphology of a stained pe-

TABLE 51–2. CLINICAL CLUES IN EVALUATION OF ANEMIA

History
1. Family history: anemia, splenomegaly, jaundice, splenectomy
2. Rejection as blood donor
3. Exercise intolerance, syncope, easy fatigue
4. Pallor, jaundice
5. Blood loss or bleeding tendency
6. Malnutrition, malabsorption, alcoholism
7. Chronic disease
8. Transfusion or iron therapy
9. Multiple pregnancy, menorrhagia

Physical Examination
1. Skin and mucous membranes: pallor, jaundice, purpura, smooth or beefy tongue, cheilosis, koilonychia, telangiectasia
2. Adenopathy
3. Hepatomegaly or splenomegaly
4. Tachycardia, cardiomegaly, murmurs
5. Bone tenderness
6. Neuropathy
7. Stool exam (for blood)

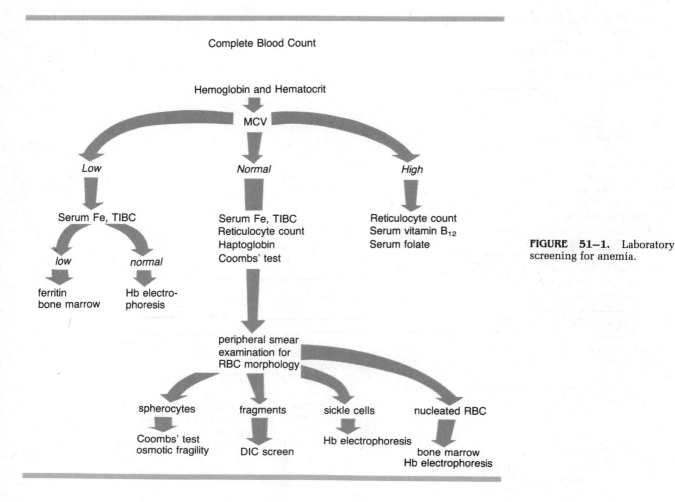

Complete Blood Count

Hemoglobin and Hematocrit

MCV

Low

Serum Fe, TIBC

low

ferritin
bone marrow

normal

Hb electro-
phoresis

Normal

Serum Fe, TIBC
Reticulocyte count
Haptoglobin
Coombs' test

peripheral smear
examination for
RBC morphology

spherocytes

Coombs' test
osmotic fragility

fragments

DIC screen

sickle cells

Hb electrophoresis

nucleated RBC

bone marrow
Hb electrophoresis

High

Reticulocyte count
Serum vitamin B$_{12}$
Serum folate

FIGURE 51–1. Laboratory screening for anemia.

ripheral blood smear is particularly important in evaluating abnormal cells, as in leukemia. An advantage of automated cell counting is the ability to use the standard deviation of the variable being measured, e.g., red cell volume, to provide information on population heterogeneity, an important factor in certain disease states.

The *red cell indices* give information about the average red cell volume (MCV, mean corpuscular volume) and red cell hemoglobin content (MCH, mean corpuscular hemoglobin) or concentration (MCHC, mean corpuscular hemoglobin concentration). The MCV is the most useful, since it permits separation of microcytic anemia (MCV <80 cu μm) from normocytic (MCV 80 to 100) and macrocytic anemias (MCV >100 cu μm). These morphologic categories correlate well with several common types of anemia. *Microcytosis* most commonly occurs in iron deficiency, thalassemia trait, and chronic renal insufficiency, whereas normocytosis accompanies acute blood loss. *Macrocytosis* is characteristic of nutritional anemias, including folic acid deficiency and vitamin B$_{12}$ deficiency. Mild macrocytosis (MCV 100 to 110) may also be associated with hemolytic anemias with a raised reticulocyte count and with the refractory anemias found in myelodysplastic syndromes. The MCH is generally low in thalassemia

trait, thalassemia, and iron deficiency; the MCHC may be high in spherocytic hemolytic anemias.

Inspection of the peripheral blood smear gives information about individual blood cells not readily obtained from the average values reported by the automated blood counters. The appearance and heterogeneity of red cells can be of diagnostic importance. For example, the microcytes of iron deficiency are relatively homogeneous, whereas in thalassemia major much more diversity in red cell size and shape occurs. In general, the further red cells diverge from the ideal shape (biconcave disc) and size (8 μm diameter), the shorter their lifespan in the circulation. The appearance of sickle cells, cells with inclusion bodies, e.g., Howell-Jolly bodies (nuclear remnants) or basophilic stippling (RNA remnants), parasitized cells (e.g., malaria), microspherocytes, and schistocytes (e.g., microangiopathic anemias, disseminated intravascular coagulation) is rapidly appreciated by inspection of the peripheral blood smear. Similarly, the appearance of individual leukocytes discloses blasts, hypersegmented polymorphonuclear cells, atypical lymphocytes, toxic granulation, and other morphologic abnormalities of disease generally inaccessible to machine recording. Platelet clumping versus true thrombocytopenia and the appearance of very large or small platelets also adds clinically relevant information to the numerical counts.

Evaluation of the leukocyte and platelet counts is an integral part of investigating anemia, since low counts may signify marrow failure or replacement, and high counts may be associated with leukemia or infection. Suspicion of pancytopenia or of marrow invasion with a pathological process should lead to a bone marrow examination.

The *reticulocyte count* measures the per cent of newly released erythrocytes in the circulating blood; these are larger than mature red blood cells and contain traces of endoplasmic reticulum, signifying the continuing capacity for hemoglobin synthesis. After one to two days in the circulation, these methylene blue–stained traces of RNA disappear. Since the normal red cell lifespan is 120 days, the normal reticulocyte count is approximately 1 per cent. Anemia increases the apparent reticulocyte count by decreasing the denominator by which the reticulocyte percentage is calculated (reticulocytes/1000 RBC); hence reticulocyte counts should be corrected to a "normal" hematocrit of 45 (corrected reticulocyte count = retic count × patient's hematocrit/45). Further corrections may be needed during severe anemias when reticulocytes circulate for longer than 24 hours. An elevated reticulocyte count (corrected) signifies increased erythropoietic activity, which may represent a normal response to bleeding, replacement of an appropriate hematinic such as iron, folate or vitamin B_{12}, or a response to hemolysis. A very low reticulocyte count or absence of reticulocytes occurs after transfusion or in aplastic states.

Blood loss from the gastrointestinal tract is such a common cause of anemia that any initial evaluation of anemia should include testing one to three stool specimens for occult blood. Because bleeding is often intermittent, it is best to obtain several stool specimens on different days. While blood loss into the urine is less common, it is nevertheless desirable to examine the urine for the presence of red cells or blood as well.

ANEMIAS REPRESENTING BONE MARROW FAILURE

Primary disorders of bone marrow function are rare causes of anemia except as a result of drug or toxin action. These disorders include aplastic anemia, pure red cell aplasia, marrow replacement with fibrotic tissue or tumor (myelophthisis and myelodysplastic syndromes), and certain anemias secondary to cancer.

Aplastic anemia is characterized by a peripheral pancytopenia and markedly decreased hematopoietic activity in the bone marrow without a change in normal marrow architecture or replacement with other cell types. The disorder is considered to be severe when the corrected reticulocyte count is less than 1 per cent, platelets are less than 20,000 per cu mm, neutrophil count is less than 500 per cu mm, and marrow cellularity

is less than 25 per cent of marrow space. Aplastic anemias, or the tendency toward their development, may be inherited (e.g., Fanconi's anemia) or may develop after a viral infection or as a reaction to a drug. Some drugs, such as cytostatic agents used in cancer chemotherapy, regularly cause marrow hypoplasia as part of their cytotoxic action; such aplasia is dose-dependent and usually reversible. The effect of cycle-specific agents such as cytosine arabinoside and methotrexate on more rapidly dividing mature stem cells tends to spare the earlier, pluripotent stem cells, so that marrow recovery occurs after the drug is stopped. Other drugs induce idiosyncratic marrow hypoplasia or aplasia that is unrelated to drug dose and tends to be less reversible. Chloramphenicol, which also induces a dose-related suppression of erythropoiesis, and phenylbutazone are examples of drugs that produce idiosyncratic marrow aplasia in 1:24,000 to 1:40,000 of exposed individuals. An inherited stem cell sensitivity or defect is postulated in such cases because of the findings in family and twin studies. A variety of environmental toxins, including solvents such as benzene and insecticides, also can cause a long-lasting marrow aplasia. Radiation exposure of bone marrow also can produce aplastic anemia. Viral infections, particularly hepatitis, Epstein-Barr virus infection, and parvovirus, can result in severe aplasia. An increased incidence of acute leukemia is observed in patients who have had aplastic anemia, and preleukemia may present as marrow hypoplasia.

Pure red cell aplasia, producing a severe anemia with absent reticulocytes, but normal leukocyte and platelet counts, is characterized by selective absence of erythroid precursors in the bone marrow. It is associated with immunological deficiency states, including thymoma.

Two mechanisms have been postulated for aplastic anemia: immunological suppression of hematopoiesis and damage to marrow stem cells. Suppressor T cells as well as immunoglobulins that inhibit erythropoietin or block differentiation of hematopoietic stem cells in vitro have been demonstrated in some cases. Immunosuppressive therapy has led to remission in certain of these cases, especially in pure red cell aplasia. In other cases, no inhibitory immunological mechanisms can be demonstrated, and patients respond to bone marrow transplantation, which presumably repopulates the marrow by new stem cells. Early transplantation of normal, HLA-matched bone marrow, before the patient becomes alloimmunized to blood cells given as supportive therapy, is the treatment of choice in young patients, especially if the patient has an HLA-compatible donor. For patients in whom transplantation is not possible, prednisone (in low dosage for its hemostatic effect), androgens, and etiocholanolone have been used, in addition to supportive transfusion therapy. Recent studies indicate that treatment with a course of antithymocyte globulin is effective in 40 to 50 per cent of cases. Availability of commercially prepared antithymocyte globulin now makes this treatment a feasible early step in the

TABLE 51–3. EVALUATION OF HYPOCHROMIC ANEMIA

A. Iron lack or inability to utilize iron in heme production
  1. Iron deficiency
    a. Blood loss
    b. Dietary lack during high demand (childhood, pregnancy)
    c. Poor absorption of food iron (postgastrectomy, small bowel disease, pica)
  2. Poor iron mobilization from body stores
    a. Chronic inflammatory disease
    b. Malignancy
  3. Sideroblastic anemia; failure of iron incorporation into protoporphyrin
  4. Lead poisoning (similar to #3)
B. Defective globin synthesis
  1. Alpha thalassemia
  2. Beta thalassemia

approach to aplastic anemia, especially in the patient who does not have a bone marrow donor.

Marrow invasion by infection (e.g., tuberculosis), tumor, or fibrosis can produce hypoplastic anemias characterized by a normocytic red cell, low reticulocyte count, and the presence of nucleated red blood cells on the peripheral smear: *myelophthisic anemia.* Cancer also can produce a hypoplastic, normocytic anemia without direct marrow invasion. Such anemias involve a subnormal response to erythropoietin and represent one type of the anemia of chronic disease.

HYPOCHROMIC ANEMIAS

Inadequate or defective hemoglobin synthesis results in poorly hemoglobinized erythrocytes in the peripheral blood, a decreased hemoglobin level, and frequently a small erythrocyte volume (microcytosis). Any lesion in the pathway of heme or of globin synthesis can produce a hypochromic anemia. By far, the most common cause of hypochromic anemia throughout the world is iron deficiency resulting from blood loss (at any age) or inadequate dietary iron (mainly in children and pregnant women). Other important causes of hypochromic anemia include poor iron utilization, as in the anemia of chronic disease, defective heme or porphyrin synthesis, as in the porphyrias or lead poisoning, or impaired globin synthesis, as in the thalassemic syndromes (see below). In the thalassemias, abnormal globin synthesis re-

sults in a secondary impairment of heme production and leads to a hemolytic state; this problem will be discussed in the section on hemolytic anemias.

The characteristic findings in iron deficiency anemia reflect exhaustion of body iron stores: absent marrow iron, low plasma iron and ferritin concentrations, a low transferrin saturation (<15 per cent) and high iron binding capacity, and hypochromic, microcytic erythrocytes on the peripheral smear. The reticulocyte count is reduced (Table 51–3).

Normal Iron Metabolism

Iron is the most abundant metal in the human body, yet is a trace metal totalling only 3 to 4 gm. Two thirds of total body iron exists as hemoglobin iron in circulating erythrocytes, about one quarter remains in iron stores, and small amounts are found in myoglobin, enzymes, and the plasma. Body iron is tightly regulated and conserved; the daily absorption from the diet averages 1 to 2 mg, and iron balance is maintained by efficient re-utilization of hemoglobin iron from red cells removed from circulation by the reticuloendothelial system or enzyme iron except for a small amount lost from the body in sweat, shed skin, and intestinal mucosal cells. Elemental iron is extremely toxic and insoluble, and iron within the body is almost entirely bound to protein carriers. The distribution of iron in body compartments is shown in Table 51–4.

Food iron is absorbed in the ferrous form, after being released from foodstuffs by gastric acid. Heme iron is absorbed directly as hemin (Fe^{+++} heme). The duodenum is the optimal locus of absorption, with less occurring further down the small intestine. An active process transports ferrous iron across the intestinal mucosal cell, governed by the iron content of the cells, with local storage as ferritin if the content is high. The average Western diet contains 10 to 30 mg of iron per day, of which only 5 to 10 per cent is absorbed. In iron deficiency states absorption increases to 20 to 30 per cent. Many common foodstuffs and other materials that contain iron-binding substances interfere with iron absorption. These include phytates in cereals and vegetables, casein in milk, clay, and the drug tetracycline. Clay-eating or starch-eating (pica) by children or young

TABLE 51–4. IRON DISTRIBUTION AND TURNOVER

	AMOUNT OF IRON IN AVERAGE ADULT			
	MALE (gm)	FEMALE (gm)	PER CENT OF TOTAL	DAILY TURNOVER
Hemoglobin	2.4	1.7	65	20 mg
Ferritin and hemosiderin	1.0	0.3	31	
Myoglobin	0.15	0.12	3.5	
Heme enzymes	0.02	0.015	0.5	
Transferrin-iron	0.004	0.003	0.1	
Total daily requirement	0.001	0.002*		

* Menstruating and pregnant women require two to three times the daily Fe requirement of adult men because of increased blood loss and the iron requirement of the fetus. One ml of blood contains approximately 0.5 mg iron.

women, many of whom are already iron-deficient, can produce severe iron deficiency.

Absorbed iron is transported from the intestine to storage in the bone marrow complexed to the plasma protein transferrin, each molecule of which binds two iron molecules. Transferrin-bound iron (Fe^{+++}, reoxidized by ceruloplasmin) is delivered to reticuloendothelial macrophages for storage as ferritin and to developing erythroblasts, where it is released intracellularly for incorporation into protoporphyrin. Since 25 mg of iron are needed daily for new red cell production, and only 1 to 2 mg are absorbed from the diet, most of the iron being utilized for erythropoiesis is recycled, derived from effete red cells destroyed by the reticuloendothelial system. The transferrin concentration in plasma (measured as the iron-binding capacity) varies widely diurnally, is decreased in inflammatory diseases or infection, and is increased in iron deficiency.

Iron is delivered to developing erythrocytes by the binding of transferrin to a specific cellular receptor. This step is followed by micropinocytotic internalization of the iron-transferrin complex within acidic vacuoles where the iron is released, and from which the apotransferrin-receptor complex is recycled to the cell surface and the apotransferrin liberated. The iron then enters the mitochondria and is enzymatically incorporated into protoporphyrin to form heme; the heme is bound by globin in the cytoplasm to produce hemoglobin. The level of free heme regulates the uptake of iron by normoblasts and reticulocytes.

Iron is stored as ferritin or hemosiderin. Ferritin consists of a spherical protein shell of apoferritin units surrounding a central core of ferric phosphate; up to 4000 iron molecules may be present per molecule of ferritin. Aggregates of ferritin can be detected in bone marrow smears as ferricyanide-positive granules, having a bright blue-green color. Ferritin circulates at concentrations that generally reflect body iron stores, with a normal range of 12 to 325 ng/ml (mean 125 ng/ml for men, 55 ng/ml for women). In iron deficiency the serum ferritin is less than 10 ng/ml and in iron overload the level may be several thousand ng/ml. Infection tends to reduce the serum ferritin level; liver disease or hepatitis raises the level. Hemosiderin is an insoluble, partially dehydrated derivative of ferritin; iron contained in hemosiderin is less accessible for erythropoiesis than is iron in ferritin, which is readily available. Fixed tissue macrophages also serve as a store of ferritin and hemosiderin, derived from phagocytized aged red blood cells. Such iron is rapidly made available after hemorrhage but is poorly available for hemoglobin production during infection, inflammation, and malignancy.

Iron Deficiency

Iron deficiency anemia is a sign of underlying disease, not a disease in itself. The major cause for iron deficiency in adults is blood loss, whereas in growing children and pregnant women dietary iron lack is more common. Malabsorption also can lead to iron deficiency, for example following partial gastrectomy or in adult celiac disease. Rarer associations include esophageal webs (Plummer-Vinson syndrome) and clay or starch pica.

The usual Western diet provides sufficient iron to cover normal losses of adult men, but for menstruating women (who require twice as much iron daily as adult men) dietary iron intake may not be adequate. Women with repeated pregnancies are also at risk of iron lack, since each fetus requires about 400 mg of iron. Gastric acid facilitates iron absorption, since acid is needed to reduce ferric iron in food to the absorbable ferrous form; gastrectomy not only removes the source of acid but by increasing transit time in the intestine may impair duodenal absorption (this is why delayed release forms of iron are less efficacious).

Gastrointestinal bleeding is the most common cause of iron deficiency in men, and the second after gynecologic bleeding in women. In less developed countries, hookworm infestation is the leading cause of iron deficiency. Both benign and malignant gastrointestinal lesions may produce iron deficiency, and investigation for possible colon cancer is imperative in adults over the age of 40. Peptic ulcer disease, bleeding due to aspirin ingestion, diverticulitis, and chronic hemorrhoidal bleeding are other frequent causes of gastrointestinal blood loss. Hematuria may also produce iron deficiency. Frequent blood donations may deplete iron stores even in males and lead to latent iron deficiency.

Clinical Manifestations. Clinical manifestations may be subtle, if the iron deficiency is gradual in onset. The most common symptoms include fatigue, exercise intolerance, irritability, and dizziness, i.e., symptoms common to any type of anemia. In severe iron deficiency there may be koilonychia, pallor, and cheilosis. Splenomegaly has been reported in about 10 per cent but not in American adults.

Laboratory Findings. Laboratory findings range from a normocytic anemia in mild cases to microcytic, hypochromic anemia in severe cases. The blood smear shows an increased central pale area in red blood cells, and increased anisocytosis and poikilocytosis. If bleeding is chronic or active, the platelet count may be increased. The serum iron is depressed early in iron deficiency and the transferrin level or total iron-binding capacity is increased to more than 350 μg/dl, with a transferrin saturation of less than 15 per cent. The plasma ferritin concentration is low, below 10 ng/ml. Free erythrocyte protoporphyrin is elevated. The reticulocyte count is usually normal. The bone marrow characteristically reveals erythroid hyperplasia, with small, poorly hemoglobinized normoblasts. Iron stores are absent.

The sequence of changes in laboratory variables follows a definite pattern as iron deficiency develops. First, iron stores are depleted and serum ferritin falls. The iron-binding capacity increases, plasma iron concentration falls, and transferrin desaturation follows. The hemoglobin decreases. Red cell morphology initially remains normochromic and normocytic while the total red cell

TABLE 51–5. STAGES IN DEVELOPMENT OF IRON DEFICIENCY ANEMIA

HEMOGLOBIN (gm/dl)	PERIPHERAL SMEAR*	SERUM Fe (μg/dl)	BONE MARROW	SERUM FERRITIN (ng/ml)
13+ (normal)	nc/nc	50–150	Fe 2+	40–340 (male) 14–150 (female)
10–12	nc/nc	↓	Fe absent, erythroid hyperplasia	<12
8–10	hypo/nc	↓ ↓	Fe absent, erythroid hyperplasia	<12
<8	hypo/micro	↓ ↓	Fe absent, erythroid hyperplasia	<12

* nc/nc = normochromic, normocytic; hypo/nc = hypochromic, normocytic; hypo/micro = hypochromic, microcytic.

count falls. Eventually, microcytic, hypochromic red cells appear (Table 51–5).

Diagnostic Evaluation. As iron deficiency represents a manifestation of underlying disease, the cause must be sought. The iron deficiency is easily documented by laboratory tests indicating reduced serum iron, increased transferrin level (or alternatively, a low serum ferritin), and absence of iron stores in the bone marrow. Urinalysis and stool examinations are part of the initial evaluation. In the older patient especially, investigation for a source for gastrointestinal blood loss requires serial examinations of stool for blood, plus, if indicated, appropriate x-rays and endoscopy. Women should have a careful gynecologic history recorded and a pelvic examination.

Therapy. The goals include treating the cause for the iron loss, correcting the anemia, and replenishing body iron stores. Simple iron salts, ferrous sulfate or ferrous gluconate, are effective treatments. Slow-release preparations or enteric-coated tablets are not recommended because they may bypass upper duodenal absorption, thereby reducing absorption. All iron salts are irritating to the gastrointestinal tract in a dose-dependent manner and may cause diarrhea, constipation, or epigastric distress. Accordingly, iron salts are best given in divided doses, gradually increasing to a full dose of 200 mg of elemental iron (about three tablets of ferrous sulfate, 325 mg) daily. This dose provides an optimal response. Iron is best absorbed when the stomach is empty, but gastric irritation may be more common. Absorption after meals is sufficient, and the decrease in GI symptoms is offset by better patient compliance. Ascorbic acid taken with the iron enhances absorption by 20 to 30 per cent but adds to expense. Because of the limited extent of iron absorption even in the iron-deficient patient, it is important to continue therapy for 6 to 12 months, by which time anemia will be corrected and iron stores replenished. Patients should be instructed to continue taking their iron tablets for the full period of time.

Subjective improvement in fatigue or lassitude may occur within a few days, well before a detectable hematologic response, which takes about two weeks. A mild reticulocytosis can be ob-

served, followed by a slow rise in hemoglobin of about 1 gm per two weeks. "Unresponsiveness" to iron therapy is most commonly a sign of poor compliance or continued blood loss. Intercurrent disease, malabsorption, or an ineffective preparation (e.g., sustained-release products) may also impair reponse.

Parenteral iron therapy should be reserved for patients who cannot tolerate oral iron, have malabsorption, fail to comply, or have a rapid and chronic blood loss. An example of the latter condition is hereditary hemorrhagic telangiectasia (Osler-Weber-Rendu), which in some cases demonstrates a frequency or rate of bleeding exceeding the capacity for oral iron absorption. Iron-dextran complex (Imferon) contains 50 mg iron/ml and is the preparation of choice. It can be administered intramuscularly or intravenously. Because of occasional hypersensitivity to the dextran moiety, a test dose of 0.5 ml should be given first and the patient observed for anaphylactic reactions. The replacement total dose is calculated from the patient's hemoglobin level:

$$\text{mg Imferon needed} = [15 - \text{Hgb(gm/dl)}] \times \text{body weight (kg)} \times 3].$$

The amount is administered in divided doses, 2.5 ml injected into each buttock daily in a Z-track manner, to provide about 250 mg iron daily, or is given intravenously as a single infusion at a rate of up to 1 ml/min.

MEGALOBLASTIC ANEMIAS

Definition. Megaloblastic anemias are anemias in which DNA synthesis is impaired, leading to delayed division of all rapidly proliferating cells—skin, gastrointestinal tract, mucosae, hematopoietic cells—and cellular gigantism. Since all hematopoietic cell lines proliferate rapidly, megaloblastic anemias usually manifest not only macrocytic anemia but also pancytopenia. Ineffective hematopoiesis results from intramedullary loss of a large proportion of developing cells, related to the asynchrony of DNA synthesis, hence producing a hemolytic state.

Causes. The major causes of megaloblastic anemias are folic acid or vitamin B_{12} deficiency, which may be related to nutritional deficiency, disease of the stomach or small bowel, pregnancy, alcoholism, or cancer chemotherapy. Rarer inherited defects in DNA synthesis also occur.

Pathophysiology. Pathophysiology of the megaloblastic anemias relates to the interlocking roles of folic acid and vitamin B_{12} in DNA synthesis. Folic acid (in the reduced 5,10-methylene tetrahydrofolate form) is the carrier for one-carbon fragments that are donated to desoxyuridine to form desoxythymidine, the characteristic pyrimidine in DNA. This methylation of desoxyuridine is essential for thymidine synthesis, and subsequent regeneration of 5,10-methylene tetrahydrofolate is necessary for continued delivery of methyl groups to desoxyuridine. Vitamin B_{12} is the cofactor of the reaction that regenerates tetrahydrofolate from 5-methyl tetrahydrofolate, a major form of folate in the body that is unable to donate its methyl group to desoxyuridine. The 5-methyl group is transferred to homocysteine to form methionine in a methyltransferase-catalyzed reaction in which vitamin B_{12} acts as intermediate methyl acceptor. In addition, vitamin B_{12} is the coenzyme in the conversion of methylmalonyl CoA to succinyl CoA, a reaction necessary for myelin metabolism in the nervous system. Thus, deficiency of vitamin B_{12} leads to neurologic changes as well as megaloblastic anemia, whereas folate deficiency leads only to megaloblastic anemia. In folate deficiency, the inadequate generation of thymidylate leads to increased incorporation of uridylate into developing hematopoietic cell DNA. The incorporated uridylate is then enzymatically excised, leading to fragmentation of the DNA, blocking of DNA synthesis at a normal rate, and impaired cell proliferation. RNA and protein synthesis, however, can proceed normally.

The ineffective hematopoiesis that results from the impaired DNA synthesis in vitamin B_{12} or folate deficiency leads to megaloblastosis, the production of giant leukocytic forms and large platelets, and is characterized by early intramedullary death of these abnormal cells and shortened lifespan of circulating blood cells. A hemolytic state involving both intramedullary and extramedullary hemolysis results, accompanied by leukopenia and thrombocytopenia.

Clinical and Laboratory Manifestations. Signs and symptoms of megaloblastic anemia are identical for folic acid and vitamin B_{12} deficiency, whereas effects of these vitamin deficiencies on tissues other than hematopoietic tissue may vary. Thus, a profound and slowly developing macrocytic anemia is observed, with large, oval, well-hemoglobinized red cells, considerable anisocytosis, and frequent nuclear remnants. The reticulocyte count is very low. There is leukopenia with hypersegmentation of polymorphonuclear leukocyte nuclei and thrombocytopenia. The platelets are large. The bilirubin is elevated. The bone marrow is markedly hypercellular with megaloblasts showing "nuclear-cytoplasmic dissociation," that is, normal maturation of the cyto-

plasm in the face of nuclear immaturity, a finely dispersed chromatin pattern, and large nuclear size. Nuclear condensation is delayed in erythroid cells. The myeloid series also shows megaloblastosis, with giant band forms and hypersegmented polymorphonuclear leukocytes. The number of mitotic figures is increased. Megakaryocytes are large and decreased in number and show decreased budding. The iron stores in the marrow are typically increased (because of the intramedullary hemolysis). Epithelial cells of mucosal surfaces such as the mouth, intestinal tract, stomach, and vagina also show gigantism. The gastric and intestinal mucosae tend to atrophy, leading to further malabsorption of folate.

In vitamin B_{12} deficiency neurologic changes may occur, although their presence correlates poorly with the development of the hematologic abnormalities: some patients develop severe neurologic manifestations with only mild anemia, and vice versa. Morphologically, the neurologic abnormality initially produces demyelination, first of the large fibers in peripheral nerves, later of the dorsal and lateral columns of the spinal cord, and sometimes in the cerebrum. Irreversible nerve cell damage is a late complication. Earliest symptoms typically include distal paresthesias in the extremities, with a glove-stocking peripheral neuropathy, and impairment of position and vibration sense in combination with increased deep tendon reflexes. Later a typical spastic ataxia, motor weakness, and paraparesis may occur. Mental changes may also occur with "megaloblastic madness," i.e., dementia in severe cases. Autoimmune phenomena are common with vitiligo, early graying of hair, autoantibody formation, and emergence of other autoimmune diseases.

Vitamin Requirements, Absorption, Metabolism, and Action

FOLIC ACID. Folic Acid (pteroylglutamic acid) is derived from leafy plants, liver, or yeast and exists as a family of compounds consisting of a pteroyl ring, para-aminobenzoic acid, and one or more glutamates in a gamma glutamyl linkage (Table 51–6). Food folate comprises polyglutamates, whereas medicinal folate is pteroylmonoglutamic acid. The daily requirement for folate is 50 to 200 μg; the body stores of folate (in the liver) of 5 to 20 mg suffice only for weeks to three or four months. Folate requirements are increased during growth, pregnancy, and hemolytic anemias.

Food polyglutamates must be cleaved to the monoglutamate form in the intestinal tract by folate conjugases in the intestinal mucosa before efficient uptake by an active transport mechanism. Absorption takes place mainly in the upper portion of the small intestine. Certain drugs, such as Dilantin and oral contraceptives, or intrinsic small bowel disease can impair absorption by interfering with conjugase action. Folate is heat labile and is destroyed by prolonged heating or cooking. Absorbed folate is mainly converted to 5-methyl THF, the main transport and storage form. The rate of folate absorption is dependent

TABLE 51–6. COMPARISON OF FOLIC ACID AND VITAMIN B₁₂

	FOLIC ACID	VITAMIN B$_{12}$
Source	Leafy vegetables, yeast, liver	Animal products
Dietary intake	500–1000 μg	7–30 μg
Effect of cooking	Destroyed	Unchanged
Minimal daily need	100–200 μg	1–2 μg
Body stores	10–12 mg (four months)	2–3 mg (2–4 years)
Absorption	Active transport, upper small bowel	Carrier-mediated (intrinsic factor) terminal ileum
Physiological forms	Reduced polyglutamates	Methylcobalamin, adenosylcobalamin
Serum level	3–15 ng/ml	200–900 pg/ml
Function	Transfer 1-carbon fragments in thymidine synthesis	Regenerate reduced folate from 5-CH$_3$ THF; succinyl CoA formation in CNS

upon tissue stores and on the integrity of the intestinal mucosa. Accordingly, diseases of the small intestine such as sprue and celiac disease can impair folate absorption.

Because of the relatively low body stores of folic acid, dietary deficiency is a common cause of folate-related megaloblastic anemia. Thus, a diet devoid of fresh vegetables or limited mainly to alcohol frequently leads to folate deficiency. In the elderly, "tea and toast" diets frequently result in folate deficiency. In alcoholism, several factors combine to produce folate deficiency: poor diet, a toxic effect of alcohol on the intestinal mucosa, and interference by alcohol with folate utilization in the bone marrow. Increased demands for folate occur during pregnancy, lactation, and rapid growth in childhood. Folate requirements also rise in any chronic hemolytic anemia such as sickle cell anemia, immune hemolytic anemia, or thalassemia, in patients on hemodialysis, and in psoriasis or exfoliative dermatitis. Pregnancy increases the folate requirement 5- to 10-fold. Malabsorption syndromes are commonly accompanied by folic acid deficiency, as food polyglutamates are poorly absorbed by abnormal intestinal mucosa (monoglutamate folic acid is normally absorbed) especially if villous atrophy is present. As a result, celiac disease and nontropical and tropical sprue may result in folate deficiency. Bacterial overgrowth, as in the blind loop syndrome, more commonly causes vitamin B$_{12}$ deficiency. Folate deficiency may lead to low serum B$_{12}$, whereas in B$_{12}$ deficiency serum folate may be high because of underutilization, although red cell folate may be low.

Folic acid is reduced by the enzyme dihydrofolate reductase to forms capable of carrying one carbon fragment. Once fully reduced by dihydrofolate reductase, folate as tetrahydrofolate again can transport the appropriate 5,10-methylene group needed in thymidylate synthesis. Inhibitors of dihydrofolate reductase therefore inhibit DNA synthesis: the first antimetabolite successfully used in leukemia chemotherapy, aminopterin, is an inhibitor of dihydrofolate reductase. Antimalarial drugs such as pyrimethamine also

are dihydrofolate reductase inhibitors. Therefore, megaloblastic changes are observed in patients receiving pyrimethamine for malaria, trimethoprim (present in the drug Bactrim) for bacterial infections, or methotrexate. The toxicity induced by such drugs may be counteracted by administration of folinic acid, which bypasses the need for dihydrofolate reductase by supplying the fully reduced folate.

VITAMIN B$_{12}$. Vitamin B$_{12}$ is synthesized in nature only by microorganisms and is obtained by eating animal foods (Table 51–6). This vitamin consists of a group of cobalamins, which contain a porphyrin-like corrin ring similar in structure to heme but with a central cobalt molecule linked to a nucleoside instead of iron. The normal diet contains a large excess of B$_{12}$ (5 to 30 μg) over the daily requirement of 1 μg; only the strictest vegetarian diet is B$_{12}$-deficient. The chief body storage site for vitamin B$_{12}$ is the liver, where 3 to 5 mg are normally present, representing stores sufficient for several years. The much greater body storage of B$_{12}$ compared to folic acid means that in malnutrition or after GI surgery, vitamin B$_{12}$ deficiency develops much more slowly than does folate deficiency. In the stomach, food vitamin B$_{12}$ is released by pepsin from protein complexes at acid pH and binds with intrinsic factor, a glycoprotein produced by the parietal cells. Other binding proteins, R-factors, present in saliva and gastric juice, also bind vitamin B$_{12}$. These complexes stabilize the vitamin during intestinal transit. In the small intestine, pancreatic proteases and an alkaline pH further convert B$_{12}$ bound to R proteins to intrinsic factor–B$_{12}$ complexes. In the distal small ileum, specific mucosal receptors permit attachment of intrinsic factor–B$_{12}$ complexes necessary for absorption of the vitamin (without the intrinsic factor) across the gut wall. R protein–B$_{12}$ complexes are not absorbed. Plasma B$_{12}$ is complexed to several types of transcobalamins or transport proteins. Only TC II transports B$_{12}$ to hematopoietic and other proliferating cells; TC I (from leukocytes) and TC III bind the vitamin avidly and may be important in preventing its loss. The normal plasma level of vitamin B$_{12}$ ranges between 175 and 725 pg/ml. Most of this represents B_{12} bound to TC I. In myeloproliferative diseases, in which granulocyte production is high, serum levels of TC III and B_{12} are greatly increased.

An enterohepatic circulation of vitamin B_{12}, ensuring recycling of the vitamin, contributes to the low daily requirement. After partial gastrectomy, which may result in loss of intrinsic factor production, this recycling mechanism is interrupted and the requirement increases to 5 to 10 μg/day. The result is that clinical B_{12} deficiency arises earlier after gastric surgery than after dietary depletion. B_{12} deficiency is inevitable after total gastrectomy; after partial gastrectomy, owing to the large amount of intrinsic factor normally produced in the gastric antrum, the development of B_{12} deficiency is variable in time of onset and in rate of occurrence, depending upon the extent of surgery.

Different forms of vitamin B_{12} mediate different chemical reactions. Methylcobalamin, which acquires methyl groups from folate, is the form that acts as a coenzyme for the methyltransferase that converts homocysteine to methionine and is key for the regeneration of biologically active folate. Adenosylcobalamin is the form that is involved in the isomerization of methylmalonyl CoA to succinyl CoA. Medicinal vitamin B_{12} is cyanocobalamin; the binding of cyanate to the B_{12} molecule may represent a natural detoxification mechanism.

Diagnosis. Diagnosis of megaloblastic anemia is usually made from the blood smear and MCV and is confirmed by the finding of a megaloblastic bone marrow and low plasma level of folic acid, vitamin B_{12}, or both (Fig. 51–2). Plasma folic acid falls to low levels (less than 3 ng/ml) quickly, within days to weeks of dietary deprivation, whereas red cell folate better reflects total body stores. Vitamin B_{12} levels fall only when body stores are depleted. Both vitamins were formerly measured by bioassays employing vitamin-requiring microorganisms, which thus assessed biological activity of vitamin; recent development of sensitive radioimmunoassays involving a vitamin B binder have sometimes led to falsely high values for plasma B_{12} because certain assays also measure biologically inactive analogues of B_{12} that bind to R proteins. Assays using intrinsic factor only as the binding protein give true values for plasma B_{12}; the action of the analogues is unknown.

Once a folic acid or vitamin B_{12} deficiency state is verified, the underlying cause must be sought. For folic acid, an accurate dietary history plus an evaluation for possible malabsorption usually uncovers a cause. Vitamin B_{12} deficiency is most commonly seen as a result of pernicious anemia, prior partial gastrectomy, or small bowel disease. Pernicious anemia involves an atrophic gastritis that leads to deficient intrinsic factor secretion, hence vitamin B_{12} malabsorption. The disease is accompanied by numerous autoimmune phenomena (unknown whether primary or secondary), including frequent occurrence of anti–parietal cell and anti–intrinsic factor antibodies. The latter impair the absorption of B_{12}-intrinsic factor complexes in the ileum. Finding anti–intrinsic factor antibodies in the serum is considered diagnostic for pernicious anemia, whereas the presence of anti–parietal cell antibodies is a more common, nonspecific phenomenon found in association with gastric disease in older persons. Impaired absorption of oral vitamin B_{12} occurs in several types of B_{12} deficiency and serves as the basis of the Schilling test, which can be used to distinguish between pernicious anemia, small intestinal bacterial overgrowth, and other malabsorption syndromes. In this test a trace amount (1μg) of radiolabelled B_{12} is administered by mouth, and a large dose of unlabelled B_{12} (1000 μg) is

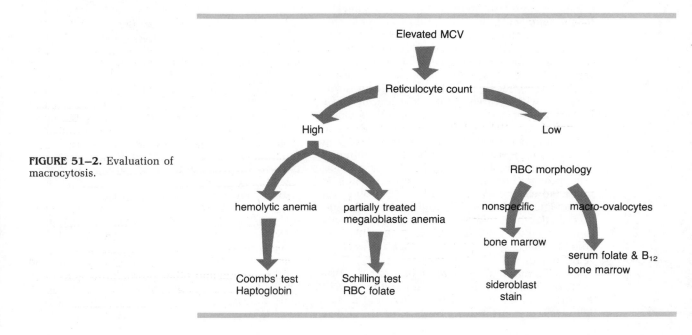

FIGURE 51–2. Evaluation of macrocytosis.

injected intravenously to saturate body stores. The patient's urine is then collected for 48 hours and the amount of excreted labelled B_{12}, representing what was absorbed from the oral dose, is measured. Normally more than 7 per cent of the oral dose is excreted in 48 hours. If the excretion is less than 5 per cent, vitamin B_{12} malabsorption is present. If pernicious anemia is suspected, the test is repeated giving intrinsic factor by mouth together with the radiolabelled B_{12}. If urinary excretion of the radiolabelled B_{12} rises into the normal range, pernicious anemia is confirmed. Villous atrophy caused by the B_{12} deficiency occurs in untreated patients and may prevent normal absorption of B_{12} in the presence of intrinsic factor if the test is carried out before therapy or early after therapy has been started. Repeating part 2 of the Schilling test after one month of replacement therapy, when the gut mucosa has regenerated, gives more accurate results. If small intestinal bacterial overgrowth is suspected as the cause of the B_{12} deficiency, administration of a course of antibiotics before repeating the test will normalize B_{12} absorption and excretion. A special advantage of the Schilling test is that it can be carried out after treatment has begun, because it measures absorption of vitamin independent of therapy.

A therapeutic trial can also be undertaken to determine whether a megaloblastic anemia is due to vitamin B_{12} deficiency. Administration of 1 to 5 μg of vitamin B_{12} intramuscularly daily will lead to a reticulocytosis within three to four days, peaking within ten days. Continuation of the therapy will correct the anemia within a month. Administration of 200 μg of folic acid daily to a patient on a folate-deficient diet will lead to a reticulocytosis in folic acid deficiency but not in vitamin B_{12} deficiency; larger doses of folate will induce a reticulocyte response in the vitamin B_{12}-deficient patient, but will not fully correct the megaloblastic anemia and may lead to worsening or induction of the neurologic abnormalities.

The response to specific therapy of megaloblastic anemia is prompt and follows a predictable pattern. Symptoms improve within 48 hours and the bone marrow red cell morphology reverts to normal in 24 to 48 hours. Serum potassium may fall within 48 hours, representing a return of potassium to intracellular sites. Reticulocytosis is observed within three to four days and may rise to over 25 per cent; leukopenia and thrombocytopenia regress within ten days. Hypersegmented polys and giant bands (in the marrow) disappear within about a week. The elevated bilirubin and LDH, indicating the ineffective erythropoiesis, disappear within one to three weeks. Anemia is corrected within one to two months (if iron stores are adequate). Neurologic improvement in corrected vitamin B_{12} deficiency occurs more slowly and may take 6 to 12 months; long-standing neurologic defects, especially long tract dysfunction, may be irreversible.

Less Common Causes of Megaloblastic Anemia. About 5 per cent of megaloblastic anemias are due to inherited disorders of pyrimidine metabolism such as orotic aciduria, absence of ileal receptors for the intrinsic factor–B_{12} complex (Immerslund's syndrome) or to dyspoietic anemias that may represent preleukemia or may be familial. Megaloblastic anemia may also be induced by antimetabolite therapy that interferes with DNA synthesis, as in cancer chemotherapy.

HEMOLYTIC ANEMIAS

Definition. Hemolytic anemias result from an increased rate of red cell destruction. Because the bone marrow can increase red cell production eight-fold, the rate of red cell destruction may increase considerably without causing anemia (compensated hemolytic state). Normally, red cells survive 120 days in the circulation, gradually losing enzyme activities and becoming denser and less deformable. In hemolytic anemias, the red cell survival ranges from only slightly shortened to a few hours. Hemolytic anemias result from abnormalities of the red cell membrane, enzymes, or hemoglobin, from antibody interactions with the red cell membrane, from toxins or microbial products, or from heat or mechanical trauma. In a hemolytic anemia the red cell morphology may be normal or abnormal, reticulocytes are usually increased, nucleated red cells may be present in the peripheral blood, the bilirubin and LDH increased, urine urobilinogen raised, and red cell survival short. In chronic hemolytic anemias splenomegaly or hepatomegaly may be present, gallstones are common, jaundice and pallor may be present, and the bone marrow shows erythroid hyperplasia.

Hemolysis may be intravascular or extravascular, i.e., takes place in the reticuloendothelial system (Table 51–7). Intravascular hemolysis is relatively rare and occurs with acute transfusion reactions, prosthetic heart valve dysfunction, paroxysmal cold or paroxysmal nocturnal hemoglobinuria (PNH), cold agglutinin disease, heat stroke, and clostridial infections. Hemoglobin is released from injured red cells into the plasma, where it is rapidly bound to haptoglobin, hemopexin, or albumin. Haptoglobin-hemoglobin or hemopexin-hemoglobin complexes are promptly cleared from the circulation by the liver, lowering the plasma levels of these proteins. Methemalbumin (the complex of heme with albumin) circulates for some days. If the binding capacity of these proteins is exceeded, hemoglobinuria occurs. Acute hemoglobinuria is not toxic to the kidney, but the accumulation of red cell stroma in renal vessels can lead to acute renal failure. Chronic hemoglobinuria leads to iron deficiency due to the sloughing of renal tubular cells loaded with hemosiderin derived from reabsorbed heme iron. In acute intravascular hemolysis, serum haptoglobin is very low and lactate dehydrogenase (LDH), an enzyme abundant in red cells, is elevated.

Extravascular hemolysis occurs commonly and represents early removal of red cells sequestered by the fixed phagocytes of the spleen and liver. Only a small amount of the hemoglobin removed reaches the plasma, and the heme iron is recycled for further red cell production, so that serum iron levels tend to be high during active hemolysis. Haptoglobin levels also tend to be reduced, but hemoglobinemia is not present. The level of serum lactic dehydrogenase (LDH), representing LDH released from destroyed red cells, is elevated. The level of unconjugated (indirect) bilirubin reflects the net effect of the briskness of hemolysis and the ability of the liver to process bilirubin.

Differential Diagnosis. Differential diagnosis of hemolytic anemias requires evaluation of whether the process is congenital or acquired, is due to abnormality of the red cell or to an abnormality in the plasma or circulatory system (including red cell antibodies, mechanical trauma, infection, etc.), or reflects other underlying disease, and whether it is acute or chronic. An important differentiating point is whether antibodies against red cell antigens are present on the red cell surface (direct Coombs' test) or in the plasma (indirect Coombs' test). Hence, an accurate family history and knowledge of the patient's prior history of jaundice, anemia, splenomegaly, or gallstones are of great importance. Physical findings depend upon the rate and chronicity of hemolysis, and range from scleral icterus and pallor in mild cases to splenomegaly and bony changes in severe chronic hemolysis.

Hemolysis due to intracorpuscular abnormalities may be caused by intrinsic defects in the red cell membrane, hemoglobin (or hemoglobin production), or enzymes. The most common membrane defect is hereditary spherocytosis, which has an incidence of 1:5000 in northern Europeans and less in other population groups. The peripheral blood smear shows a uniform population of spherocytes lacking central pallor. The mean cellular hemoglobin concentration (MCHC) is increased. The osmotic fragility of the red cells is increased, and red cell survival is short. Splenomegaly is usually present, bilirubin gallstones commonly develop, and intermittent jaundice is frequent, particularly in conjunction with stress states such as infection or pregnancy. Aplastic crises may occur during infection, as with parvovirus, due to bone marrow suppression in the face of a short red cell survival. The pathogenesis of the hemolysis is sequestration of the poorly deformable spherocytes, which require extra expenditure of ATP to maintain membrane flexibility. The underlying molecular defect is not fully understood, although abnormalities of the red cell cytoskeletal protein, spectrin, appear to be responsible. In addition, permeability to sodium ion is excessive, requiring increased ATP-dependent cation pump activity to prevent water accumulation by the red cells. Treatment of hereditary spherocytosis includes folic acid administration and splenectomy, which improves red cell survival without altering the red cell defects. Other membrane abnormalities resulting in hemolytic anemia include hereditary elliptocytosis and hereditary stomatocytosis.

The most common red cell enzyme defect world-wide is *glucose 6-phosphate dehydro-*

TABLE 51–7. MECHANISMS OF HEMOLYSIS

Type of Red Cell Defect
1. Intrinsic (usually inherited)
   a. Membrane (e.g., hereditary spherocytosis)
   b. Enzyme (e.g., glucose 6-phosphate dehydrogenase deficiency)
   c. Hemoglobinopathy (e.g., sickle cell disease, Hb C disease)
   d. Globin synthesis (e.g., thalassemia)
   In all of the above, the red cell defect leads to membrane or cellular rigidity, splenic sequestration, short RBC lifespan.
2. Extrinsic (usually acquired)
   a. Antibody-induced (e.g., Coombs' positive hemolytic anemia)
      1. warm antibody
      2. cold antibody
   b. Drug-induced (e.g., penicillin)
   c. Toxin-mediated (e.g., burns, sepsis)
   d. Red cell fragmentation, mechanical hemolysis (e.g., after heart valve surgery)
   In all of the above, induced changes in red cell membrane leads to splenic removal, and in some, intravascular hemolysis with hemoglobinemia and hemoglobinuria may occur.

Laboratory Features of Hemolysis
1. Increased red cell breakdown
   a. Increased serum bilirubin (unconjugated)
   b. Increased urine urobilinogen
   c. Decreased serum haptoglobin
2. Increased red cell production
   a. Reticulocytosis and polychromasia
   b. Erythroid hyperplasia in bone marrow
   c. Increased requirement for folic acid (low serum folate)
3. Red cell damage
   a. Morphology: fragments, microspherocytes, spherocytes
   b. Increased osmotic fragility
   c. Short red cell survival
   d. Intraerythrocytic inclusions

genase (G6PD) deficiency, which affects over 100 million individuals. Other abnormalities in the Embden-Meyerhof enzyme pathway also lead to hemolytic states, but these are extremely rare (pyruvate kinase and hexokinase deficiencies, the next most common, have been reported in a few hundred cases). Normal red cells depend upon aerobic glycolysis to metabolize 90 per cent of glucose in producing ATP and 2,3-diphosphoglycerate. ATP is necessary to preserve membrane flexibility and to support membrane cation pumps, whereas 2,3-DPG influences the binding of oxygen to hemoglobin so as to facilitate oxygen unloading in tissues. Ten per cent of glucose is metabolized via the hexose monophosphate shunt, which generates NADPH, the major reducing compound produced by the red cell. NADPH is required for regeneration of reduced glutathione, which prevents hemoglobin denaturation, preserves the integrity of red cell membrane sulfhydryl groups, and detoxifies hydrogen peroxide and oxygen radicals in and on the red cell. Since G6PD is the initial enzyme in the hexose monophosphate shunt pathway, functionally abnormal enzyme or a low level of G6PD leads to increased red cell oxidative damage, particularly during periods of oxidant stress. G6PD deficiency is a sex-linked trait that is clinically expressed in male heterozygotes. Over 100 inherited variants of G6PD are recognized; young red cells have higher levels of the enzyme in general than do older cells.

The common A$^-$ variety seen in the black population is less severe than the Mediterranean type, as red cell enzyme levels are about 15 per cent of normal in blacks but less than 5 per cent in the latter group. G6PD deficiency leads to hemolysis in the setting of hepatitis, severe infections, fava bean ingestion, or ingestion of oxidant drugs. Black males with G6PD deficiency and falciparum malaria develop severe intravascular hemolysis (blackwater fever) when treated with antimalarial drugs such as primaquine. G6PD deficiency in persons of Greek or Mediterranean lineage is associated with favism, or hemolysis after ingestion of the fava bean. Acquired G6PD deficiency has been observed in bacterial overgrowth of the bowel and in uremia.

ACQUIRED HEMOLYTIC DISORDERS

Red cell lifespan can become shortened in the course of infectious, malignant, cardiovascular, or immunologic diseases. In most of these, hemolysis results from an extracorporeal abnormality such as altered hemodynamics, antibody against red cell antigens, or exposure to toxins. Rarely, the red cells themselves may undergo membrane changes that lead to hemolysis (e.g., in paroxysmal nocturnal hemoglobinuria). For convenience, acquired hemolytic anemias are divided into two categories: Coombs' positive (antibody-mediated) and Coombs' negative hemolytic anemia.

Antibody-mediated hemolytic anemias represent a wide variety of conditions in which antibodies directed against red cell antigens (or neoantigens) coat the red cells and are directly or indirectly responsible for hemolysis. Antibodies that arise after transfusion or sensitization to foreign red cells, as during pregnancy, are called *alloantibodies*. Antibodies that arise without sensitization, representing abnormalities in the subject's own immune regulation, are called *autoantibodies*. The presence of antibody on the red cell surface can alter the behavior of the red cells, making them less deformable and more susceptible to phagocytosis by macrophages in the spleen or liver. Macrophages ingest antibody- or complement-coated portions of the red cell membrane, via Fc or complement receptors. Red cells that have lost part of their plasma membrane reseal but assume a more spherical shape (spherocytosis) associated with decreased pliability in the circulation and a shortened lifespan.

Autoimmune hemolytic anemias (AIHA) are characterized by antibodies directed against the patient's own red cell antigens (Table 51–8). In contrast to alloantibodies resulting from transfusion of imperfectly matched red cells, autoantibodies can arise spontaneously, in response to drugs acting as haptens, or in 40 per cent of cases as manifestations of systemic disease. Diseases of disordered immunity such as collagen vascular diseases, chronic inflammatory bowel disease, chronic lymphocytic leukemia, or lymphomas manifest an increased incidence of autoimmune hemolytic anemia. Autoantibodies increase in frequency with age, but only a small proportion of red cell autoantibodies actually cause hemolytic anemia. Whether or not hemolysis occurs depends on the density of red cell coating by antibody, the capacity of the antibody to fix complement on the red cell membrane, the thermal amplitude of the antibody, and the tendency for antibody-coated red cells to be phagocytized by splenic macrophages. AIHA fall into two groups, the warm antibody and the cold antibody autoimmune hemolytic anemias.

Warm antibody hemolytic anemias are mediated by IgG antibodies that attach to red cells at body temperature and that may fix complement (Table 51–8). Clinically important antibodies tend to be of the IgG$_1$ and IgG$_3$ subclasses. The

TABLE 51–8. AUTOIMMUNE HEMOLYTIC ANEMIAS

	Ab COATING ON RBC	OPTIMUM TEMPERATURE FOR DETECTING Ab
Warm Type		
Idiopathic	IgG or IgG + C	37°C
Secondary	Rarely, IgA or IgM	
Systemic lupus erythematosus		
Other "autoimmune disease"		
Lymphoma		
Chronic lymphocytic leukemia		
Drug induced		
Cold Type	IgM (in cold only) anti-I or anti-i	4°C
Idiopathic	C3b or C3d	4° or 37°C
Secondary		
Infections		
Mycoplasma pneumoniae		
Infectious mononucleosis		
Lymphoma (diffuse histiocytic lymphoma)		
Paroxysmal cold hemoglobinuria	IgG (anti-P)	4°C—antibody binding 37°C—complement-mediated lysis

AIHA may be associated with collagen vascular disease, lymphoma, chronic lymphocytic leukemia, ovarian teratoma, or ulcerative colitis. Almost half of cases with AIHA are idiopathic, although the hemolytic anemia may be the harbinger of a later-appearing systemic disease; such cases may have a very variable course. The clinical picture relates to the rate of hemolysis; thus, the spectrum varies from a mild asymptomatic jaundice with splenomegaly, when the rate of hemolysis is mild and bone marrow production of red cells can compensate for shortened red cell lifespan, to severe anemia with cardiovascular symptoms, when the rate of hemolysis is rapid. A positive Coombs' (antiglobulin) test using an antiglobulin antiserum detects the coating of the red cell membrane by the autoantibody (Fig. 51–3); if the amount of autoantibody is high, free antibody in the plasma (positive indirect Coombs') is also detected. Complement coating on the red cell, usually the biologically inactive cleavage products of the third component of complement, C3b or C3d, may be detected by specific anticomplement antisera or by broad-spectrum Coombs' antisera that incorporate anticomplement as well as antiglobulin antibodies for screening. AIHA may be accompanied by immune thrombocytopenia (Evan's syndrome). As in other hemolytic anemias, the reticulocyte count is elevated, the serum haptoglobin is low, and spherocytes of varied sizes are present on the peripheral blood smear. The bilirubin may be elevated; usually it is mostly conjugated, but if the total bilirubin exceeds 4 mg/dl, the unconjugated fraction may be increased.

Therapy is directed toward decreasing the rate of hemolysis. The first approach is oral corticosteroids, using 1 to 2 mg/kg/day of prednisolone (or equivalent) and tapering after the hematocrit returns to normal. Steroid therapy diminishes the

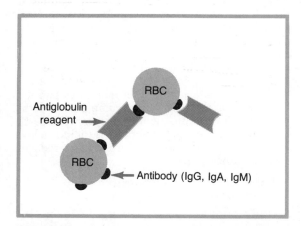

FIGURE 51–3. Coombs' or antiglobulin test. In the Coombs' test, an antibody directed against human immunoglubulin is used to detect the presence of antibody on the surface of the red cells by agglutination. Complement coating on the red cells (C_3) can similarly be detected by an anticomplement Coombs' reagent. Broad-spectrum Coombs' reagents can be prepared which detect either immunoglobulin or complement or both; these are used for screening.

binding of antibody to fixed macrophages and thereby limits the rate of red cell destruction. Steroids have a slower and less marked effect on inhibition of autoantibody production. Splenectomy is helpful in steroid-dependent or unresponsive cases if splenic sequestration of antibody-coated red cells can be demonstrated. Splenectomy also removes an important source of antibody production. Immunosuppressive drugs such as azathioprine or cyclophosphamide are reserved for refractory cases. Transfusion is avoided if possible, as the transfused red cells are usually destroyed as quickly as the patient's own cells. Folic acid supplementation is often necessary because the rapid rate of red cell turnover depletes body stores of this vitamin.

Cold antibody autoimmune hemolytic anemia has a complex etiology. While many naturally occurring antibodies react with red cells in the cold, certain IgM autoantibodies with wide thermal amplitude may mediate autoimmune hemolysis (Table 51–8). The term thermal amplitude describes the temperature range over which these antibodies attach to red cells. Cold agglutinins causing hemolytic anemia are those with a wide thermal amplitude; that is, the capacity to bind to red cells occurs over a broad range from 4°C to a few degrees below body temperature, i.e., at temperatures that may occur in the nose, ears, or extremities during cold exposure. Polyclonal cold-reacting, IgM autoantibodies may arise transiently during infectious mononucleosis, cytomegalovirus infection, mycoplasma pneumonia, or protozoal infections and can cause significant hemolysis. Such polyclonal cold-reacting antibodies tend to be present transiently for days or weeks and resolve spontaneously following convalescence from the infection. In addition, "idiopathic cold agglutinin syndrome," characterized by monoclonal IgM antibodies, may precede the development of lymphoma or Waldenström's macroglobulinemia or may continue for years in the absence of malignant transformation. Unlike the polyclonal IgM cold antibodies, which appear briefly after infections, the monoclonal cold antibodies can persist for years. They show specificity for the I-i antigen system, glycoprotein precursors of ABO antigens. There are two ways in which hemolytic anemia results from the binding of complement to the red cells: these IgM antibodies bind directly to red cells in the cold, fixing complement to the red cell surface; at warmer temperatures the antibodies dissociate from the red cells, leaving only activated complement bound to the red cell membrane. Depending upon the amount of complement bound and the rate of complement inactivation, rewarming blood activates the complement cascade, leading to intravascular hemolysis. This type of hemolysis is rather uncommon; it is more likely that the C3b fixed on the red cell surface leads to removal of the coated red cells by macrophages in the spleen; in addition, bound C3 is converted to inactive C3d on the red cell membrane, which interferes with further binding or activation of C3 and limits the rate of hemolysis.

Paroxysmal cold hemoglobinuria is a rare form of cold-reactive hemolysis in which a polyclonal IgG directed against the red cell P antigen system binds to red cells in the cold and fixes complement, so that when rewarming occurs, the complement cascade is activated and brisk intravascular hemolysis follows. This condition is found uncommonly in syphilis or after viral infections. The hemolysis is self-limited so that protection from cold is the most important therapy.

Drug-induced immune hemolytic anemia is a relatively common disorder that can result from three different mechanisms of hemolysis (Fig. 51–4). (1) *Hapten type.* Haptenic drugs bind to red cell membranes, forming neoantigens to which antibodies develop; a Coombs' positive hemolytic process follows with mainly extravascular destruction of red cells. The drug must be present for hemolysis to occur. Penicillins and cephalosporins are the chief offenders. (2) *Innocent bystander type.* Drugs that bind to plasma proteins elicit antibodies that form circulating immune complexes and activate complement. Red cells as "innocent bystanders" become coated with complement and may undergo intravascular or extravascular hemolysis depending on the rates of activation and inactivation of complement. Red cells show only complement coating. This represents the hemolytic mechanism for most drugs that produce immune hemolysis, including sulfonamides, phenothiazines, quinine, and isoniazid. (3) *Alpha methyldopa type.* Upon chronic use of alpha methyldopa, 15 per cent of patients develop a positive direct Coombs' test, with IgG present on the red cells; only 1 in 10 has hemolysis. The autoantibodies show Rh specificity, suggesting that the drug may somehow modify this red cell antigen system. The positive Coombs' test may persist for months after cessation of the drug. Levodopa and mefenamic acid (an anti-inflammatory drug) may also produce this type of autoimmune phenomenon.

Hypersplenism represents excessive sequestration of blood cells, particularly red cells, by an enlarged or abnormally functioning spleen. While senescent red cells are normally removed by trapping in the tortuous, poorly oxygenated sinusoids of the spleen, an enlarged spleen can randomly remove nonsenescent red cells. Pancytopenia, rather than anemia, may result from hypersplenism, but it appears that platelets and leukocytes are merely sequestered in enlarged spleens rather than being excessively destroyed. Hypersplenism is characterized by the picture of "empty blood and full marrow," which distinguishes this condition from the pancytopenias of marrow failure. It may occur in chronic hemolytic anemias of any cause, chronic infections, chronic leukemias and myeloproliferative diseases, lipid storage diseases, lymphomas, and rheumatoid arthritis (Felty's syndrome).

Paroxysmal nocturnal hemoglobinuria (PNH) is an acquired hemolytic disorder associated with increased susceptibility of a red cell subpopulation to complement-mediated damage. It is extremely rare, is considered a stem cell defect, and is associated with eventual bone marrow aplasia and leukemia. Not only red cells but also granulocytes and platelets are sensitive to the lytic effects of complement and bind increased amounts of C3b compared to normal cells. PNH red cells fail to facilitate inactivation of complement by the plasma C3b inactivator, which may account for their susceptibility to lysis. Clinical manifestations include intravascular hemolysis, back pain, a tendency to venous thrombosis, and iron deficiency secondary to recurrent hemoglobinuria from intravascular hemolysis. Bone marrow may be hypocellular; the Coombs' test is negative. Hemolysis can be demonstrated by placing the patient's red cells in acidified serum (which permits activation of the alternative complement pathway) or in hypotonic medium (sugar-water test). Other markers associated with PNH include a low leukocyte alkaline phosphatase and a low red cell acetylcholinesterase.

Chemical, Toxic, and Parasitic Causes of Hemolytic Anemia

Either inorganic or complex organic toxins, including snake venoms and heavy metals, can cause hemolytic anemia. Arsenic and copper cause hemolysis by binding red cell membrane sulfhydryl groups; copper-induced hemolysis is seen in Wilson's disease and in hemodialyzed patients. Chloramine, generated in urban water supplies purified with chlorine, and alum may cause hemolysis in hemodialysis patients dialyzed against tap water. The lipophilic antifungal drug

Hapten Type
(e.g., penicillin)

Immune
Complex Type
(e.g., quinidine)

Alpha Methyl
Dopa Type

RBC   RBC   RBC

A   B   C

drug = ●   plasma protein = ▨

complement = Ⓒ   antibody = ⋎

FIGURE 51–4. Mechanisms of drug-induced hemolysis. *A,* The drug binds to the red cell membrane as a hapten. Antibodies to the drug-membrane complex can lyse the red cells, but only in the presence of bound drug. *B,* The drug binds to a plasma protein or antibody, and the complex attaches to the red cell membrane. Antibodies produce binding of complement, and lysis follows. *C,* There appears to be a change in the red cell membrane after long-term treatment with the drug, often with Rh specificity. Antibodies develop which bind to the altered membrane, producing a positive Coombs' test and, rarely, hemolysis.

amphotericin can cause hemolysis, and snake venoms are directly lytic to red cells because of their content of lysolecithinases. Patients with advanced cirrhotic liver disease often develop spur cell anemia, a hemolytic disorder in which red cell membranes absorb excessive cholesterol present in abnormal circulating low density lipoproteins that contain an excess of cholesterol compared to phospholipid. Acanthocytes with irregular "spurs" are typically found in the peripheral blood.

Malaria commonly causes hemolytic anemia. Parasitized red cells become metabolically depleted, change membrane permeability and deformability characteristics, and may develop neoantigens that produce a positive antiglobulin test. The parasitized red cells also are prone to adhere to the vascular endothelium, which may contribute to local thrombosis. Babesiosis and bartonellosis also cause hemolytic anemia via red cell parasitism.

Hemolysis Resulting from Red Cell Trauma

Red cells exposed to excessive mechanical stress intravascularly or during extracorporeal circulation can undergo *fragmentation hemolysis*. Abnormal shear forces arise during passage of red cells through prosthetic heart valves, damaged natural valves, or vascular shunts. Chronic intravascular hemolysis due to abnormally functioning heart valves or valve prosthesis is relatively uncommon today, when ball valves are less frequently used. Its occurrence usually signals the existence of valve malfunction. Because of higher shear stresses associated with systemic pressures, malfunctioning aortic valves most often cause this type of intravascular hemolysis, but similar syndromes have occurred with mitral valve pathology. In both acute and chronic intravascular hemolysis, the blood smear shows red cell fragments (schistocytes), microspherocytes, and increased polychromasia (indicating reticulocytosis). The plasma haptoglobin is depressed, and the bilirubin and LDH may be elevated. If the process is chronic, hemosiderinuria and consequent iron deficiency may occur, because the hemolysis is intravascular and iron is lost in the urine. Iron therapy is needed to counteract the urinary losses and to correct the anemia. A similar process may occur acutely during extracorporeal circulation as in cardiopulmonary bypass. Red cell fragmentation also occurs after severe burns covering large areas of body surface, or in heat exhaustion. Intravascular hemolysis, without fragmentation of red cells, develops occasionally after prolonged marching or marathon running (march hemoglobinuria).

Microangiopathic hemolytic anemias result when normal red cells are fragmented while traversing intravascular fibrin strands in microvessels partially occluded by thrombi. Acute causes of microangiopathic hemolytic anemia include disseminated intravascular coagulation (DIC), thrombotic thrombocytopenic purpura, hemolytic-uremic syndrome, malignant hypertension, rejection of renal grafts, and mitomycin C toxicity. Certain vascular malformations such as giant hemangiomas (Kasabach-Merritt syndrome), in which sluggish blood flow through abnormally formed vessels triggers localized DIC, produce microangiopathic hemolytic anemia. In each of these settings, localized shearing of red cells within microthrombi results in intravascular hemolysis, usually accompanied by thrombocytopenia because of the concomitant intravascular clotting. In contrast, the schistocytic (fragmentation) hemolytic anemias related to large vessel pathology generally are not accompanied by thrombocytopenia.

Trousseau's syndrome represents chronic DIC in the setting of visceral cancer, with typical schistocytes and thrombocytopenia on the peripheral smear. Coagulation factor levels may be normal or decreased, depending upon the rate of consumption of clotting factors.

HEMOGLOBINOPATHIES

Hemoglobin, the major protein in the red cell, binds oxygen reversibly and is responsible for the capacity of red cells to transport oxygen to the tissues. Hemoglobin is present as a 5 mM solution in red cells. Each hemoglobin molecule consists of two identical alpha globin chains and two nonalpha chains, which in the adult comprise mainly beta globin, with a small amount of delta globin; in the fetus the main nonalpha polypeptide is gamma globin (Fig. 51–5). Two genes on chromosome 16 code for the alpha chains, whereas the genes for the nonalpha globins are clustered on chromosome 11.

Each polypeptide subunit of hemoglobin holds a single heme group in a hydrophobic pocket. The iron of the heme is bound to the porphyrin ring and is also bound to a histidine residue to the globin chain; its hydrophobic environment protects the Fe^{++} from being oxidized even in the presence of oxygen. Oxygen is bound to each heme group via the central iron atom. The structure of the tetrameric hemoglobin molecule changes with the binding of oxygen so that the interactions of the globin chains alter the sequential release of oxygen from the four heme groups, thereby producing the sigmoidal shape of the oxygen dissociation curve. These interactions facilitate the uptake of oxygen in the lungs and its unloading at the tissues, with the steepest part of the curve lying within the ambient oxygen tensions of these two locations. The synthesis of hemoglobin begins in the erythroblast and continues throughout erythrocyte maturation, with about 25 per cent being synthesized after the red cells leave the bone marrow, in circulating reticulocytes. Normal synthesis of alpha and beta chains is balanced, with little excess of either type produced within red cells. Excess globin chains are unstable and tend to precipitate at the red cell membrane (forming Heinz bodies), shortening red cell lifespan.

During transport of red cells from arterial ox-

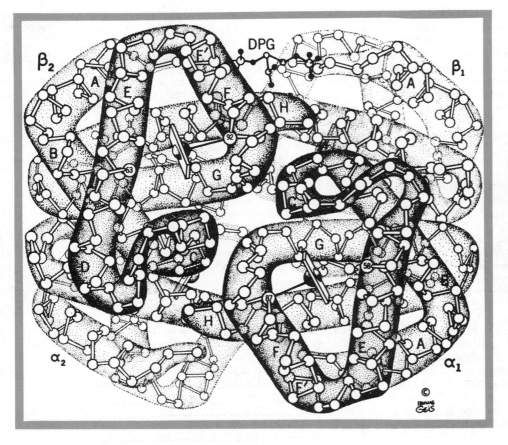

FIGURE 51–5. Hemoglobin structure. The folding of both alpha (α_1, α_2) chains and beta (β_1, β_2) chains is illustrated. A to H indicate helical regions within each globin chain. DPG indicates diphosphoglycerate-binding site. Numbered amino acid residues designate histidines to which the iron is bound. (Copyright 1981 by Irving Geis, 4700 Broadway, New York, New York 10040.)

ygen tension (P_{O_2} 100 mm Hg) to tissue oxygen tension (P_{O_2} 40 mm Hg), the saturation of hemoglobin oxygen decreases from 100 to 75 per cent, although the capacity for O_2 delivery is much greater. Oxygen unloading is facilitated by the binding to hemoglobin of the molecule 2,3-diphosphoglyceric acid (2,3-DPG), an intermediate product of glycolysis; acidic pH and the binding of CO_2 also assist in the release of oxygen from hemoglobin, as do configurational changes in the hemoglobin molecule itself during oxygen release. Changes in the structure of the globin polypeptide chains, or in the heme itself, can affect the oxygen affinity of hemoglobin.

TABLE 51–9. CLINICAL SYNDROMES RELATED TO ABNORMAL HEMOGLOBINS

TYPE OF DEFECT	CLINICAL FEATURES
A. Decreased hemoglobin solubility	
1. Crystalline hemoglobin Hb S, C, D, E	Hemolytic anemia with microvascular occlusion
2. Unstable hemoglobin	Hemolytic anemia
B. Abnormal oxygen transport	
1. Increased O_2 affinity	Polycythemia
2. Decreased O_2 affinity	Normochromic "anemia"
C. Heme oxidation (Hb M)	Cyanosis Methemoglobinemia

Mutations in the DNA sequences controlling globin synthesis either can produce structurally abnormal hemoglobins (hemoglobinopathies) or can decrease the rate of hemoglobin synthesis (thalassemias) (Table 51–9). The term *hemoglobinopathy* connotes structurally abnormal hemoglobins with altered function, whereas *thalassemia* refers to mutations resulting in decreased synthesis of one globin type. Since the alpha globin chain contains 241 amino acids and the beta chain 246, and single amino acid substitutions resulting from single mutations produce abnormally functioning molecules, a very large number of mutant forms are possible. Only mutations of certain types, however, lead to functional alterations in hemoglobin resulting in abnormal oxygen carriage or anemia. Examples of these functionally important mutations include surface substitutions that alter hemoglobin solubility (e.g., Hb S), substitutions in internal nonpolar residues resulting in hemoglobin instability (e.g., Hb Koln), substitution for the histidine that binds iron, permitting oxidation of heme iron (e.g., Hb M), or substitution at the alpha-beta contact points, which alters heme-heme interactions and changes oxygen affinity (Hb Kansas or Chesapeake). Mutations causing thalassemic syndromes include deletions, removal of stop codons, and frameshift mutations leading to nonsense sequences; these all tend to alter globin synthesis and to decrease the rate of normal globin production, a process that secondarily regulates heme synthesis and leads to hemolytic anemias. In addition, mutations affecting the normal sequence of expression of the beta cluster genes may result in hereditary persistence of Hb F synthesis after birth.

Anemias Resulting From Abnormalities in Hemoglobin Structure or Function

Sickle Cell Anemia. By far the most important disease resulting from a mutation to an abnormally functioning hemoglobin is sickle cell disease, in which a single base change in the DNA results in a substitution of valine for glutamic acid at the sixth position in the beta globin chain. The ensuing insolubility of Hb S under deoxygenated conditions results in polymerization of Hb S molecules within the red cells, leading to distortion of shape, membrane changes, cellular dehydration, and decreased deformability. Microvascular occlusion results from the altered behavior of sickle red cells and produces progressive microinfarction of vital organs, painful bony crises, splenic autoinfarction, and renal damage. Patients have a shortened lifespan. The Hb S gene is present in 10 per cent of American blacks and up to 25 per cent of the population in Western Africa. In the heterozygote (Hb S trait, Hb SA), protection against falciparum malaria is associated with the hemoglobinopathy. The heterozygote state usually has 60 per cent Hb A and 40 per cent Hb S; both types of globins are present in the same cell, but not in the same molecule. The homozygous state (Hb SS, sickle cell disease) has over 90 per cent Hb S, with small amounts of Hb F or Hb A_2. The concurrent presence of thalassemia trait or persistence of Hb F tends to ameliorate the clinical course of SS disease, in the first case by decreasing the rate of synthesis of the β^S chain in relation to other globins, and in the second case by introducing a nonaggregating hemoglobin that interferes with Hb S polymerization (Table 51–10).

Clinical manifestations of SS disease begin in infancy, when Hb F levels begin to fall. Major symptoms and signs include painful crises, swelling of the extremities and spleen (in infants and children), bony and pulmonary infarctions, and cerebrovascular accidents. Any organ may be affected. Intrahepatic sickling can produce marked hepatic swelling, dysfunction, and hyperbilirubinemia; intrarenal sickling can cause renal papillary necrosis and hematuria, with loss of renal concentrating ability (usually by age five); intracutaneous sickling produces necrotic skin ulceration, usually of the ankles and feet; retinal sickling can produce neovascularization and retinal detachment; bony sickling can produce aseptic necrosis and predispose to osteomyelitis. Growth is disturbed, with typical elongated limbs and asthenic habitus. Chronic hemolysis results in a markedly increased incidence of cholelithiasis with multiple bilirubin stones and cholecystitis, a tendency to folic acid deficiency, impaired immunity partially due to loss of spleen tissue and partly related to poor IgM production, and an increased tendency to infections. Cardiomyopathy is common, as is delayed puberty.

Typical laboratory findings in sickle cell anemia include Hb ranging from 6 to 8 gm/dl, hematocrit 18 to 24 per cent, and a normal MCV. WBC and platelets are normal to increased. The reticulocyte count is chronically elevated, often to more than 20 per cent, and nucleated red blood cells are frequently present. Sickle-shaped, hollyleaf–shaped, or otherwise distorted red cells appear in variable numbers on the peripheral smear and in large numbers in deoxygenated wet preparations. Hemoglobin electrophoresis shows 90 to 95 per cent Hb S. The serum bilirubin is elevated, with mainly direct-reacting bilirubin; the haptoglobin level is low; and the serum LDH level is elevated. Screening for Hb S is most simply performed with a "sickle cell prep" by mixing the patient's blood with sodium metabisulfite, which deoxygenates the red cells and induces sickling observable with a microscope; commerical tests that demonstrate the insolubility of Hb S (Sickledex) are easier to perform for mass screening, as they do not require a microscope. Hemoglobin electrophoresis after positive screening tests is needed to delineate the specific hemoglobinopathy (Table 51–10).

Other sickle cell syndromes representing concomitant SS-thalassemia trait or a mixed hemo-

TABLE 51–10. COMPARISON OF SICKLE CELL SYNDROMES

GENOTYPE	CLINICAL CONDITION	Hb A	Hb S	Hb A_2	Hb F	Hb C	OTHER FINDINGS
SA	Sickle cell trait	55–60	40–45	2–3	—	—	Asymptomatic
SS	Sickle cell anemia	0	85–95	2–3	5–15	—	Clinically severe anemia Hb F heterogeneous in distribution
S-β⁰thal	Sickle cell–beta thalassemia	0	70–80	3–5	10–20	—	Moderately severe anemia Splenomegaly in 50% Smear: hypo, micro
S-β⁺thal	Sickle cell-beta thalassemia	10–20	60–75	3–5	10–20	—	Hb F distributed heterogeneously
SC	Hb SC disease	0	45–50	—	—	45–50	Moderately severe anemia Splenomegaly; target cells
S-HPFH	Sickle—hereditary persistence of Hb F	0	70–80	1–2	20–30	—	Asymptomatic; Hb F is uniformly distributed

globinopathy (SC, SD) usually have milder clinical courses than does sickle cell anemia (SS). They produce a less severe anemia and may present with splenomegaly rather than an absent spleen. Patients with Hb SC disease, however, can have severe morbidity in pregnancy and a higher rate of ocular complications than patients with SS disease; Hb C, also a β^6 substitution, also results in intracellular hemoglobin polymerization, but anemia and vaso-occlusive manifestations are milder in homozygous Hb C disease than in SS disease. In sickle–beta thalassemia trait, the red cells show microcytosis and hypochromia, the percentage of Hb S is less than 80 per cent, with increased Hb F in a heterogeneous distribution, and some Hb A may be present. If hereditary persistence of Hb F is present, the Hb F distribution among the red cells is homogeneous rather than variable, as it is in beta thalassemia trait.

Management of sickle cell anemia is largely symptomatic and supportive. Painful crises are treated with oxygen administration, intravenous and oral fluids, correction of acidosis, analgesics, and attention to precipitating causes such as dehydration, fever, and infection. Sickle cell crisis itself does not cause fever, but infection or tissue infarction does. Because of the increased risk of infection, pneumococcal vaccine should be administered to all sickle cell patients. Transfusion is not useful in treatment of acute sickle cell crises, but chronic transfusions programs (exchange transfusions are preferred to avoid iron overload) have been tried in patients at high risk of recurrent cerebral infarction. Transfusion prior to surgery appears to help prevent initiation of intraoperative and postoperative crises and perhaps to improve healing. Special attention to good oxygenation during surgery and avoidance of hypothermia are imperative to avoid intraoperative sickling and tissue infarction. Transfusions are also given during the later stages of pregnancy in women with SS disease to counteract placental dysfunction and placental infarction caused by sickling.

Recently, therapies designed to enhance production of Hb F in patients with SS disease have entered clinical trial; these include administration of the drugs 5-azacytidine and hydroxyurea, which may derepress the gene for Hb F or initiate differentiation of more primitive stem cells in which this gene is active. Since the presence of Hb F in SS red cells tends to decrease the intracellular polymerization and precipitation of Hb S, leading to less sickling and improved red cell survival, induction of Hb F production is highly desirable. However, because these drugs are cytotoxic (and 5-azacytidine is potentially carcinogenic), such therapy may depress bone marrow function and have adverse long-term effects. The use of these drugs is considered experimental at present.

Genetic counselling of heterozygotes for Hb S has not been very successful in decreasing reproductive activity of persons at risk of having children with SS disease. Prenatal diagnosis is now possible using restriction enzyme techniques applied to amniocentesis samples, taking advantage of several restriction fragment polymorphisms.

Unstable Hemoglobins. Unstable hemoglobins represent a varied group of disorders, usually autosomal dominant mutants, in which either heme association with globin is defective or the forces holding the globin tetramer together are altered. The result is intracellular precipitation of the denatured hemoglobin as Heinz bodies that bind to the red cell membrane. Such cells are either "pitted" of these inclusions by splenic or hepatic macrophages, resulting in shortened red cell lifespan, or are totally removed in the reticuloendothelial system. Exposure of red cells containing unstable hemoglobin to oxidant stress exacerbates the hemolysis and may cause acute jaundice.

Hemoglobins of Altered Oxygen Affinity. The parital pressure of oxygen at which hemoglobin is half-saturated with oxygen (P_{50}) provides a useful guide to measurement of functional oxygen affinity. The normal P_{50} is about 25 mm Hg. Although more than 80 mutations producing altered oxygen affinity have been found, only a few are of clinical consequence. When hemoglobin is fully oxygenated, it normally assumes the R, or relaxed state, which manifests a high affinity for oxygen; when it is deoxygenated, it is in the T, or tense state, having a low oxygen affinity. Mutations that affect hydrogen bonding or hydrophobic interactions at the $\alpha_1\beta_2$ interface change the R-T balance and alter oxygen affinity. Hemoglobins of high oxygen affinity are clinically associated with erythrocytosis, sometimes with thrombotic tendencies; hemoglobins of low oxygen affinity are associated with apparent anemias, which actually represent a functional marrow response to the increased tissue oxygen delivery. The latter may be accompanied by an asymptomatic cyanosis.

Methemoglobinemia. Methemoglobinemia represents the oxidation of heme iron, which prevents its capacity to transport oxygen, and may result from enzyme deficiency (e.g., NADH-methemoglobin reductase), abnormal hemoglobins with substitutions in the heme pocket (M hemoglobinopathies), or exposure to oxidant drugs. The clinical manifestation is cyanosis without hypoxemia. The blood is brownish and does not turn red upon shaking with air. The reducing agents methylene blue and ascorbic acid can improve the cyanosis in patients with methemoglobinemia due to enzyme deficiency or oxidant drug exposure, but not in patients with M hemoglobinopathies. The drugs that induce methemoglobinemia in normal individuals include nitrites (especially toxic to infants), primaquine, dapsone, aniline dyes, and sulfanilamide.

Thalassemias

As mentioned above, hemolytic anemia in the thalassemias results from mutations that affect globin synthesis (Table 51–11). The hemoglobin that is produced is less than normal in amount but is structurally normal. A decreased synthetic rate of one type of globin chains results in ineffective erythropoiesis, with markedly enhanced

TABLE 51–11. COMPARISON OF THE THALASSEMIA SYNDROMES

GENETIC ABNORMALITY	PER CENT Hb A	PER CENT Hb A$_2$	PER CENT Hb F	OTHER	CLINICAL SYNDROME
Normal β β	90–98	2–3	2–3		None
Beta Thalassemias					
Thalassemia major					
β thal⁰ β thal⁰	0	2–5	95	—	Severe anemia, abnormal growth, iron overload, needs transfusion
β thal⁺ β thal⁺	very low	2–5	20–80	—	
Thalassemia intermedia (varied genetic globin abnormalities)		overlaps with Thalassemia major			Severe hypo/micro anemia with HB 7–9 gm/dl, hepatosplenomegaly, bone changes, iron overload, less need for transfusion
Thalassemia minor					
β β thal⁰ or β β thal⁺	90–95	5–7	2–10		Hypo/micro blood smear, mild to no anemia
Alpha Thalassemias					
Homozygous α-thalassemia − − / − −	—	—	—	Hb H (β₄) Hb Barts (γ₄)	Hydrops fetalis, stillborn
Hemoglobin H disease − − / − α	60–70	2–5	2–5	Hb H 30–40	Hypo/micro anemia, Hb 7–10 gm/dl, Heinz bodies
α-thalassemia trait − α / − α α α / − −	90–98	2–3	2–3		Hypo/micro smear, no anemia
Silent carrier − α / α α	90–98	2–3	2–3		Normal
Hemoglobin Lepore (∂β fusion)					
Heterozygote	70–80	1–2	5–20	Hb Lepore 5–15	Mild hypo/micro anemia
Homozygote	0	0	70–90	10–30	Severe Thalassemia major

intramedullary loss of developing red cells. Several mechanisms are involved: a primary decrease in globin synthesis; the accumulation and precipitation of the other type of globin chain, which is produced in relative excess; and secondarily depressed heme synthesis. The red cells are hypochromic and markedly microcytic and have a shortened circulating lifespan. Because of the complexity of hemoglobin synthesis, thalassemic states can vary clinically from "silent" carrier (heterozygotes for alpha thalassemia) to severely anemic thalassemia major (homozygotes for beta thalassemia) to death in utero from hydrops fetalis (homozygotes for alpha thalassemia). The incidence of beta thalassemia is greatest in persons of Mediterranean and African origin and that of alpha thalassemia in persons of Far Eastern origin; the trait is present in 3 to 5 per cent of such populations. In the United States as many as 20 per cent of blacks and persons of Mediterranean origin carry thalassemia trait.

Beta thalassemia syndromes include thalassemia trait (heterozygous β thalassemia), thalassemia intermedia, and thalassemia major (Cooley's anemia). The genetic alterations that produce these syndromes are many. Mutations of the β-globin gene that depress synthesis of β-globin include the following: deletions, nonsense mutation, or frame shifts that prevent any mRNA production (β°), and mutations affecting promoter or splice sites, which permit reduced levels of mRNA and hence some hemoglobin synthesis (β⁺). The clinical features of thalassemia trait are a mild anemia that is markedly microcytic in relation to the hemoglobin level and is sometimes accompanied by splenomegaly. The MCV is frequently in the 60's, with a hemoglobin level of 10 to 12 gm/dl and marked anisocytosis on the peripheral smear. Serum iron and transferrin levels are normal. Hemoglobin electrophoresis (Fig. 51–6) reveals elevation of Hb A$_2$ to 3 to 5 per cent, and Hb F to 2 to 3 per cent. Morbidity is not associated with thalassemia trait, and iron therapy should not be given.

In contrast to this asymptomatic picture, the homozygous *thalassemia major* is a lethal, severe hemolytic anemia characterized by growth abnormalities, dysfunction of almost all organ systems, and iron overload. Because both β genes are abnormal, very little to no β chain synthesis occurs, and the excess of insoluble α-globin chains in the red cells leads to intracellular precipitation that affects both erythropoiesis and red cell lifespan. The resulting ineffective erythropoiesis causes extreme expansion of marrow space into long bones, skull, and facial bones, as well as the development of extramedullary hematopoiesis in liver, spleen, and around the spinal vertebrae. Growth abnormalities and cortical bone fragility ensue, with an increased rate of fractures. Growth retardation and delay of puberty are universal. The peripheral smear shows severe microcytosis

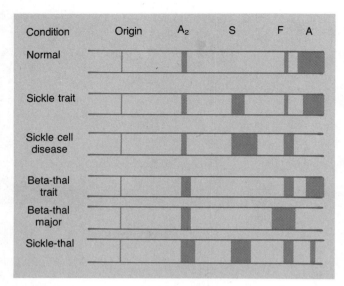

FIGURE 51—6. Common patterns of hemoglobin electrophoresis. Note that in sickle cell anemia, 95 per cent of Hb is S; in sickle trait, 40 per cent is S and 60 per cent is A, but in sickle-thal, 60 to 70 per cent of Hb is A. In beta-thal trait, either Hb A_2 or F (or both) is elevated, whereas in beta-thal major, Hb A is absent and Hb F makes up most of the hemoglobin.

and anisocytosis, many nucleated red blood cells, and hypochromia. The hemoglobin level in the untransfused patient is 3 to 6 gm/dl. Hemoglobin A is very low to absent, and the major hemoglobin is Hb F, with a variably increased amount of Hb A_2. Early death by age two to three years was common before transfusion therapy was instituted. With regular transfusion, the hemoglobin level can be maintained at 8 to 10 gm/dl and many of the growth and bony abnormalities decreased.

An absolute increase in iron absorption, plus severe iron overload from transfusion therapy, has led to a different set of complications, that of tissue fibrosis from iron deposition. This abnormality results in cardiomyopathy, diabetes mellitus, and adrenal, parathyroid, and thyroid hypofunction. Affected children also show increased susceptibility to infection and functional hyposplenism; splenectomy is usually performed in late childhood to lessen the transfusion requirements and adds to the risk of sepsis. Iron chelation therapy with subcutaneous desferrioxamine, now begun in early childhood, appears to decrease the devastating consequences of iron overload if chronically maintained; use of carefully phenotyped frozen blood can decrease alloimmunization and prevent transfusion refractoriness. With the most modern of these supportive therapies, the lifespan of patients with thalassemia major has been extended from early childhood to the 20's. Newer approaches, still highly experimental, include bone marrow transfusion and agents that increase Hb F production, such as 5-azacytidine and hydroxyurea (see above). Prenatal diagnosis by restriction enzyme polymorphism techniques is currently more useful in α than in β-thalassemia, but direct measurement of depressed β-globin synthesis in fetal blood can be made.

Thalassemia intermedia is genetically variable and frequently appears to represent double heterozygosity for two different thalassemic mutations. Affected persons can maintain an untransfused Hb level of 8 to 10 gm/dl. They have more normal growth and sexual maturation, suffer fewer clinical complications than patients with thalassemia major, and frequently live into mid-adulthood. Iron overload, however, may occur, as can the tendency to infections, bony fragility, and organ dysfunction, but with a slower time course.

Alpha thalassemia syndromes depend upon the combination of mutations in the four α-gene loci. In order of increasing severity they are α-thal$_2$ trait, α-thal$_1$ trait, hemoglobin H disease, and hydrops fetalis. The first condition is asymptomatic without anemia, except that the MCV and MCH are decreased, while the second condition results in a mild microcytic anemia. Hb H disease presents a mild, variable degree of hemolytic anemia characterized by red cell inclusions, which result from precipitation of the unstable β_4 hemoglobin. Hydrops fetalis, the absence of all α-globin production, consistently leads to death in utero or to stillbirth. The amount of Hb Bart's (γ_4) present in the blood of an infant with alpha thalassemia corresponds directly to the number of thalassemic α-gene loci. The occurrence of α-thalassemia trait together with another hemoglobinopathy such as Hb SS tends to ameliorate the latter disease, probably by decreasing the intracellular concentration of the abnormal hemoglobin. There is a high incidence of α-thalassemia trait in American blacks, and this factor ameliorates the clinical severity of sickle cell disease in this population. Silent carrier states for both α- and β-thalassemia genes are common and can be detected only by family studies.

REFERENCES

Bunn HF, and Forget BG: Hemoglobin: Molecular, Genetic and Clinical Aspects. Philadelphia, WB Saunders Co, 1984.

Finch CE (ed): Clinical aspects of iron deficiency and excess. Semin Hematol, Vol 19, No 1, 1982.

Lindenbaum J (ed): Nutrition in Hematology. New York, Churchill Livingstone, 1983.

Nienhuis AW, Anagnou NP, and Ley TJ: Advances in thalassemia research. Blood 63:738, 1984.

van Rood J, and Zwann F (eds): Bone marrow transplantation. Semin Hematol, Vol 21, Nos 1–3, 1984.

Williams WJ, Beutler E, Erslev AJ, and Lichtman MA (eds): Hematology. 3rd ed. New York, McGraw-Hill Book Co, 1983.

THERAPY WITH BLOOD PRODUCTS

Human blood is an invaluable resource in the supportive therapy of patients with hemorrhage, severe anemias, and coagulation deficits, and yet a dangerous substance if improperly used. Modern blood banking has been made possible by the science of immunohematology and by the development of special methods for the maintenance and preservation of blood ex vivo. Each unit of 450 ml of blood is mixed with 63 ml of an anticoagulant solution containing citrate to prevent clotting, as well as glucose, phosphate, and adenine to prolong red cell viability. The shelf life is 35 days. Transfusion of whole blood is rarely necessary: it is physiologically and economically more reasonable to separate each unit of fresh blood into components that can be used to treat as many as five different recipients (Table 52–1). These components include red blood cells, platelets, and granulocytes; plasma and its protein constituents including albumin, Factor VIII: antihemophilic factor (AHF), other coagulation factors, and gamma globulin.

Red blood cells can be transfused as packed red cells (most of plasma removed); leukocyte-poor (buffy coat–poor) red cells, from which about 80 per cent of the leukocytes have been removed; or frozen red cells (from which about 90 per cent of leukocytes have been removed). Each unit of red cells transfused should raise the hematocrit by 3 to 5 per cent. Platelets are separated from red cells by differential centrifugation and are administered as concentrates of 4 to 10 units suspended in a small volume of plasma. Platelet transfusion is indicated as therapy for severely thrombocytopenic patients who are bleeding, or as prophylaxis for patients with aplastic anemia or with leukemia during myelosuppressive chemotherapy. A rise in platelet count can be expected for one to three days following transfusion, unless the patient has fever, which shortens the survival of transfused platelets, or immune thrombocytopenia, which destroys transfused platelets as fast as autologous ones. Patients who require repeated platelet transfusion may become allosensitized and refractory to random donor platelets and require HLA-matched platelets. Granulocytes can be separated from whole blood by leukapheresis and administered to neutropenic patients or given as buffy coat preparations; both preparations contain considerable lymphocyte and platelet admixture. Because the effect of granulocyte transfusions is transitory (the half-life is about 6 hours), such therapy is usually reserved for treating life-threatening neutropenia. Fresh frozen plasma supplies several of the labile coagulation factors. Fibrinogen and Factor VIII:AHF can be concentrated in cryoprecipitate prepared from individual units of plasma. At the present time the only approved form of fibrinogen for replacement therapy is cryoprecipitate.

BLOOD COMPATIBILITY TESTING

Over 300 different antigenic determinants have been identified on human red blood cells, the most important being the ABO system (Table 52–2). Almost all human red cells belong to one of the four major blood groups—A, B, AB, or O. Subjects of one type, for example A, carry in their plasma natural IgM antibodies to the B antigen. Serum from type AB individuals contains no such natural antibodies, whereas serum from type O carries both anti-A and anti-B. These antibodies are easily demonstrable in saline solution. The

TABLE 52–1.   BLOOD COMPONENT THERAPY

COMPONENT	VOLUME	SHELF LIFE	EFFECT
Whole blood	500 ml	35 days	Raises Hct 3–5%
			Plasma expansion
Packed red cells	200 ml	35 days	Raises Hct 3–5%
Frozen red cells	200 ml	24 hours after thawing	Raises Hct 3–5%
			Decreases sensitization to HLA and leukocyte ag
Fresh frozen plasma	200 ml		Replaces coagulation factors (1 U/ml); plasma expansion
Plasma protein fraction			Plasma expansion (hepatitis-free)
Cryoprecipitate	20 ml		70 U Factor VIII/bag
			Fibrinogen 300–400 mg/bag
Platelet concentrates	60 ml	1–3 days	4–6 units raises platelet count about 50×10^9/L
Granulocyte concentrates	pooled	nil	Little effect on WBC
Lyophilized Factor VIII concentrates			Raises Factor VIII
Lyophilized prothrombin complex concentrates			Raises Factor IX levels
			Emergency correction of oral anticoagulant effect
"FEIBA"			Bypasses inhibitors to clotting factors

TABLE 52–2. ABO BLOOD GROUP SYSTEM

PHENOTYPE	GENOTYPES	ANTIGENS	NATURAL ANTIBODIES	FREQUENCY*
O	OO	O	anti-A, anti-B	45%
A	AA or AO	A	anti-B	40%
B	BB or BO	B	anti-A	9%
AB	AB	AB	none	3%

* For Caucasian population

ABO types are inherited as autosomal codominant traits. ABO compatibility is essential for blood transfusion. Acquired antibodies against ABO antigens, produced by alloimmunization following transfusion, pregnancy, or exposure to heterologous antigens, usually microbial, are IgG in type.

A second important blood antigen group is Rh, which consists of at least three linked loci—Cc, D, and Ee. IgG antibodies can develop to the Rh antigens after sensitization by prior transfusion or pregnancy. These antibodies are more difficult to detect than the natural ABO isoagglutinins and usually require testing in the presence of protein-containing medium rather than saline. The most clinically important locus in the Rh system is D; the absence of D is called Rh negative. Transfusion of Rh + (D +) blood to a sensitized Rh − person can provoke acute hemolysis. An Rh + fetus carried by a sensitized Rh − mother can develop erythroblastosis fetalis. In the past, maternal sensitization in such cases occurred at the time of delivery of the first child. This problem has been prevented in about 80 per cent of potential cases by treating Rh − mothers immediately after delivery, amniocentesis, or abortion with Rh immune globulin (RhoGAM) to prevent Rh immunization of the mother. In Rh − mothers who incur transplacental hemorrhage during pregnancy (diagnosed by the appearance of Rh alloantibody in maternal blood), Rh immune globulin should be administered during the pregnancy. Intrauterine transfusion of the fetus can also be carried out in those Rh − mothers who become sensitized.

Antibodies to Kell, Duffy, and Kidd antigens occur after sensitization by allogeneic red cells and may cause hemolytic transfusion reactions. Antibodies to many other antigens, such as the MN system, Lewis, P, or Ii, occur commonly but generally are inactive at body temperature and do not usually cause clinical problems (Table 52–3).

Compatibility testing for red cell transfusion consists of several sequential steps. First, the potential recipient's own red cells are typed. Then an antibody screen is performed, i.e., testing the potential recipient's serum against a panel of red cells selected to include the most frequent antigens that cause clinical reactions. Third, cross-matching is carried out, that is, testing the recipient's serum with samples of the red cells from units intended for transfusion. Under emergency circumstances, packed type O red cells can be given to a recipient of any ABO type. Rh + cells can, in an emergency, be transfused to an Rh − recipient if the latter's serum contains no anti-D; the likelihood of sensitizing the recipient is 70 per cent. In the presence of sudden hemorrhage, plasma expanders such as albumin can be used until cross-matched blood becomes available.

HAZARDS OF BLOOD TRANSFUSION

The hazards of administering blood products include transfusion reactions, circulatory overload, transmission of disease, iron overload, coagulation disturbances, and graft-versus-host disease (Table 52–4).

Transfusion reactions include acute hemolytic reactions, anaphylaxis, and febrile reactions. Most commonly, acute hemolytic reactions result from errors made by the persons who label blood samples intended for typing and cross-matching or from administering to one patient a unit of blood intended for another. Most such errors are made on the hospital floor or clinic. Less commonly, such reactions may result from errors made in the blood bank procedures. Hemolytic reactions may also occur when blood has been properly typed and cross-matched by standard techniques but unusual alloimmunization has escaped detection.

Since acute hemolytic reactions may lead to anaphylaxis and renal failure or death, rapid and orderly response to such catastrophes is essential. The blood transfusion must first be discontinued, a tube of blood drawn from the patient for inspection and for evaluation at the blood bank, and intravenous fluids immediately started. Urine output and vital signs must be monitored, and diuretics or mannitol administered in an effort to maintain a brisk urine flow. A hematocrit tube

TABLE 52–3. MAIN BLOOD GROUP SYSTEMS

NAME	FREQUENCY OF ANTIBODIES	CAUSE OF HEMOLYTIC REACTIONS
ABO	Very common	Yes
Rhesus	Common	Yes
Kell	Occasional	Yes
Duffy	Occasional	Yes
Kidd	Occasional	Yes
Lutheran	Rare	Yes
Lewis	Rare	No
P	Rare	Rare
MNS	Rare	No
Ii	Rare	Yes

TABLE 52–4. EVALUATION OF TRANSFUSION REACTIONS

TYPE OF REACTION	CLINICAL SIGNS	MANAGEMENT OF PROBLEM
Major hemolytic (incompatibility)	Shock, back pain, flushing, fever, intravascular hemolysis	1. Stop transfusion. Return blood to blood bank with fresh sample of patient's blood. 2. Hydrate IV; support BP, maintain high urine flow. 3. Check for hemoglobinemia and hemoglobinuria.
Febrile	Fever, urticaria (usually due to sensitization to WBC antibodies)	Pretreat with hydrocortisone, Benadryl or both Use buffy coat—poor RBC
Allergic	Fever, urticaria, anaphylactoid reaction (often due to sensitivity to donor plasma proteins)	Benadryl, hydrocortisone Use washed RBC or frozen RBC

should be immediately centrifuged and the plasma inspected for the presence of hemoglobin; pink plasma confirms an intravascular hemolytic transfusion reaction. Hemoglobinuria also should be sought but may be delayed in time of appearance. If oliguria or anuria occurs, dialysis is warranted. In all cases, fluid and electrolyte balance requires careful monitoring, especially to guard against hyperkalemia.

Hemolytic transfusion reactions may be immediate or delayed. ABO incompatibility can activate the complement cascade and therefore produce acute reactions with intravascular hemolysis. Rh or Kell antibodies do not activate complement at a rapid rate and tend not to produce acute hemolysis. Instead, they cause shortened red cell lifespan and produce extravascular hemolysis. Acute hemolytic transfusion reactions usually present with the sudden onset of back pain, hypotension, sweating, fever, and chills. Patients receiving incompatible blood while under anesthesia fail to exhibit such reactions, and postoperative oliguria, hemoglobinuria, or renal failure may be the first sign that a prior hemolytic transfusion reaction has occurred. Delayed hemolysis is common in the repeatedly transfused patient owing to anamnestic increases in antibody after prior sensitization, and takes place 5 to 10 days after the transfusion. Such delayed transfusion reactions produce a rapid fall in hematocrit accompanied by jaundice or a rise in bilirubin. A previously negative alloantibody screen often becomes positive at this time.

Febrile reactions or urticaria are much more common than hemolytic transfusion reactions. They usually represent alloimmunization to leukocyte antigens, which may be acquired during pregnancy (20 per cent of women) or prior multiple transfusion (70 to 90 per cent of multitransfused recipients). They range in severity from simple fever, to urticaria plus fever and chills, to vomiting and hypotension. These symptoms can usually be prevented by administering leukocyte-poor blood or by pretreatment of the patient with chlorpheniramine and hydrocortisone. Both drug pretreatment and the administration of leukocyte-poor blood may be needed. If these measures do not suffice, then frozen-thawed, washed red cells should be substituted. Anaphylactoid reactions (3 to 5 per cent of transfusion recipients develop ur-

ticaria) may also be caused by recipient antibody to IgA, especially in transfusion recipients who are IgA-deficient. IgA-deficient patients should receive washed red cells and should avoid plasma-containing preparations.

Transmission of disease by transfused blood components rarely involves bacterial infection, because modern blood banking practices utilize closed blood collecting systems that guard effectively against bacterial contamination. Hepatitis transmission, however, remains a serious hazard of blood transfusion, despite the reduction in transmission of hepatitis B. Thanks to the development of sensitive methods of detecting HB Ag positivity, hepatitis B now represents only 10 per cent of all post-transfusion hepatitis. Non-A, non-B hepatitis and delta agent account for the balance of cases. About 7 per cent of patients receiving blood products will develop hepatitis, the highest risk being in recipients of commercial coagulation factor concentrates. Patients receiving red cells, platelets, or plasma also incur considerable risk. Transfusion can also transmit cytomegalovirus infection, particularly to patients undergoing organ grafts who have activated lymphocytes in which this virus multiplies. Malaria and babesiosis can also be transmitted by transfusion, but syphilis is now rare.

Acquired immune deficiency syndrome (AIDS) develops in a small percentage of persons receiving transfusion of red cells, platelets, or commercial coagulation factor concentrates. By the end of 1984, about 100 persons with no risk factors other than transfusion had developed AIDS out of some 7000 total reported cases of AIDS. The risk overall is low, calculated at 1 in 10^6 transfusions. Hemophiliacs who receive coagulation factor concentrates are at highest risk. Several cases of AIDS have been reported in infants following neonatal exchange transfusion. Elimination of high-risk individuals from blood donor pools will reduce this risk further, as will screening for anti-HTLV III antibodies in prospective blood donors.

Circulatory overload, especially with whole blood transfusion, may occur in patients with cardiopulmonary dysfunction or congestive heart failure and can be avoided by using packed red cells or other concentrated components. In patients with congestive heart failure who need red cells, exchange transfusion consisting of removal of a unit of the patient's own blood before administering one to two units of packed red cells may avoid circulatory overload.

Problems Associated with Massive Transfusions

A bleeding tendency may occur in patients receiving multiple units of blood over a short time period. This is due in part to dilutional thrombocytopenia, since blood stored longer than 24 hours contains few viable platelets. Conditions requiring massive transfusion support are often accompanied by disseminated intravascular coagulation, adding the problems of consumption of

platelets and coagulation factors. In such cases, it may be necessary to replace platelets, coagulation factors (using fresh frozen plasma), or fibrinogen (as cryoprecipitate) in addition to red cells. In addition, administration of large amounts of citrated blood may temporarily depress the serum calcium level and require calcium supplementation.

Graft-versus-host disease, representing engraftment of donor lymphocytes in the recipient, can be observed after transfusion of blood products to immunocompromised recipients, such as patients with congenital T cell defects or those being prepared for bone marrow transplantation. Irradiation of the blood products prior to transfusion prevents this complication.

53 LEUKOCYTE DISORDERS

The main function of leukocytes is to maintain host defenses against disease, especially infection. Mononuclear phagocytes (monocytes and tissue macrophages) and granulocytes accomplish this by ingestion and killing of microorganisms and by digestion of tissue debris. Lymphocytes participate in the activation and effector functions of the immune system, and macrophage/monocytes play essential roles in the responses of lymphocytes.

Quantitative disorders of granulocytes are more common than functional disorders; the latter are frequently incompatible with normal lifespan and are mainly confined to children, although some acquired disorders of granulocyte function occur in the setting of hematologic diseases or drug therapy. Acquired leukopenia, especially neutropenia and its extreme form, agranulocytosis, is the most common quantitative disorder of clinical significance.

NEUTROPHIL STRUCTURE AND FUNCTION

Polymorphonuclear leukocytes make up the largest percentage of circulating leukocytes (50 to 70 per cent). They are nondividing, terminally differentiated cells that are motile, phagocytize a variety of microorganisms and inert particles, and release enzymes from cytoplasmic granules both into phagocytic vacuoles, and, under many circumstances, into the extracellular milieu. The three phases of microbial attack by neutrophils include chemotaxis, the directed movement along a concentration gradient of attractant substance toward a target organism; phagocytosis, the engulfment of the microbe in a membrane-lined phagocytic vacuole; and microbial killing, a

chemical attack on the ingested microorganisms via the release of granule contents into the phagocytic vacuoles (bactericidal proteins, myeloperoxidase, cathepsins) plus the formation of oxygen free radicals such as superoxide and hydroxyl ion. In the presence of halides, such as Cl^-, toxic substances are generated that kill the ingested microbes.

Chemotaxis involves the margination of circulating neutrophils along the endothelial lining of vessels, usually in postcapillary venules, their penetration through the vascular wall via intercellular junctions, and their directed migration toward the extravascular source of the infection. The migration of the neutrophils takes place along a chemical gradient of an attracting substance, which may be n-methylated bacterial peptides, complement fragments (C5a), or leukotriene B_4. Leukocyte proteases are responsible for the production of complement-derived chemotaxins, whereas lipoxygenases mediate production of arachidonic acid–derived leukotrienes and hydroxyacids. These latter substances also have chemotactic and leukocyte-activating functions. Chemotactic substances binding to tissue sites may also serve to localize neutrophil accumulation.

Recognition of microorganisms or other particulate substances is required for subsequent ingestion by phagocytes. Opsonins, or proteins that coat microorganisms and promote their avid uptake by neutrophils, include the complement fragment C3b, the large plasma protein fibronectin, and immunoglobulins. These substances adhere to the surface of microorganisms and promote binding to the C3b and Fc receptors on the neutrophil plasma membrane. *Phagocytosis*, the localized invagination of the leukocyte surface membrane to form a vacuole or vesicle, follows, with internalization and then fusion of the phagocytic vacuoles with intracellular enzyme-containing granules.

Microbicidal activity of neutrophils combines two interacting functions: degranulation and activation of the respiratory burst. Neutrophils possess a double set of cytoplasmic granules. The primary or azurophilic granules contain lysozyme, acid hydrolases, neutral proteases including cathepsin G and elastase, myeloperoxidase, and basic proteins. Specific granules contain lysozyme, transcobalamin III, apolactoferrin, collagenase, and the C5-cleaving protease. Azurophilic granules fuse mainly with the phagocytic vesicles, pouring their contents into the acidic interior of the vesicles. Specific granules fuse both with phagocytic vesicles and with the plasma membrane, so that their contents are also released outside the neutrophil. These enzymes aid in the digestion of the bacterial cell wall, dissolve connective tissue, degrade cellular debris, or bind specific substances useful to bacterial metabolism such as iron.

The same stimuli that activate phagocytosis and granule release also initiate the respiratory burst by activating a plasma membrane–bound oxidase that catalyzes one-electron reduction of oxygen to superoxide (O_2^-) in the presence of the electron acceptor NADPH. Interaction of O_2^- with H_2O yields hydroxyl radical OH·, which is directly bactericidal. In addition, H_2O_2 and Cl^- in the presence of myeloperoxidase form the microbicidal hypochlorite ion OCl^-. These reactions are essential for the killing of catalase-positive microorganisms.

Granulocytes have a short lifespan in the circulation (half-life about 6 hours) and undergo one-way traffic from the bone marrow through the blood into the tissues, where they may live for a few days. In the blood, about 50 per cent of granulocytes normally are marginated along vascular endothelium, remaining in dynamic equilibrium with the circulating neutrophil pool. Epinephrine, stress, or certain steroids shift more granulocytes to the circulating pool.

MONOCYTE STRUCTURE AND FUNCTION

Monocytes represent a second type of circulating and fixed (tissue macrophage) phagocyte of even greater functional versatility than neutrophils. They comprise a much smaller fraction of the leukocytes, about 10 per cent, and are longer-lived. Monocytes contain granules that are not clearly divided into subtypes. The circulating monocytes display slower chemotaxis than do neutrophils and appear later at sites of inflammation. Their major phagocytic role relates to the killing of intracellular microorganisms, both bacterial and parasitic. When monocytes are exposed to lipopolysaccharide or gamma interferon, they become "activated" and display increased motility, metabolic activity, size, and microbicidal potency. The three basic functions of mononuclear phagocytes are secretion, ingestion, and interaction with lymphocytes. Monocytes synthesize more than 50 different protein mediators and enzymes, release interleukins that affect lymphocyte function and cause fever, present antigen to T cells for immune responses, and have very active arachidonic acid metabolism resulting in production of prostaglandins (PGE_2, which regulates bone marrow and immunologic cell proliferation), leukotrienes, and thromboxane. In addition to complement and immunoglobulins, fibronectin also serves as an opsonin for mononuclear phagocytes. The process of pinocytosis permits macrophages to ingest and process large volumes of fluid, including plasma. Activated monocytes are also tumoricidal.

A series of reciprocal interactions between monocytes and lymphocytes is necessary for normal immune function. Monocytes and macrophages activate T cells by presenting antigen; special subpopulations of monocytes subserve this function, especially dendritic and Langerhans (skin) cells. Dendritic cells are a recently identified minor population of monocytic cells with long surface processes that appear to be the antigen-presenting cells of the blood, whereas Langerhans cells have a similar function in the skin. Lymphokines secreted by activated T cells cause accumulation and activation of monocytes. One such lymphokine, interleukin 2, is the T cell growth factor that permits expansion of T cell populations in immune responses. In addition, macrophages stimulate proliferation and differentiation of B lymphocytes via secretion of interleukin 1. Prostaglandin E_2 secreted by monocytes and macrophages, in contrast, down-regulates lymphocytic responses.

NEUTROPENIA

The normal white blood cell count varies between 5,000 and 10,000/µl, with 50 to 70 per cent neutrophils. The normal lower limit for neutrophil concentration is approximately 2×10^9/L for Caucasians and 1.5×10^9/L for blacks, the difference resulting from different sizes of marginated pools. Normal bone marrow contains a postmitotic compartment of mature neutrophils sufficient for 7 to 10 days, although under stress, neutrophil transit time in the marrow from early differentiation to the appearance of mature forms in the blood can be as short as five days (Fig. 53–1).

Neutropenia can result from depressed production of leukocytes, increased peripheral destruction, increased pooling in the spleen, or an increased rate of loss into tissues (Tables 53–1 and 53-2). The most common cause of neutropenia is marrow depression caused by drugs or radiation. Idiosyncratic drug reactions, that is, reactions rarely caused by a given drug, may result in sudden marrow suppression (e.g., chlorpromazine) or neutrophil destruction (e.g., amidopyrine); removal of the drug usually results in recovery. The latter situation often involves an antineutrophil antibody or an innocent bystander mechanism, in

FIGURE 53–1. Neutrophil granulocyte maturation and kinetics.

TABLE 53–1. ACQUIRED ABNORMALITIES OF NEUTROPHIL FUNCTION

1. **Adhesiveness**
   Increased: Bacteremia, hemodialysis (early)
   Decreased: Corticosteroids, epinephrine (demargination), aspirin, alcohol

2. **Chemotaxis**
   Increased: Bacterial infection
   Decreased: Diabetes mellitus, uremia, cirrhosis
   Severe burns
   Hodgkin's disease, leprosy, sarcoid
   Neonates
   Myeloproliferative syndromes

3. **Phagocytosis**
   Decreased: Diabetes mellitus, acute infections
   Myeloproliferative syndromes
   Leukemia

TABLE 53–2. CAUSES OF NEUTROPENIA

Benign familial
Drug-induced
  Anti-inflammatory drugs
  Antibacterial drugs (chloramphenicol, cotrimoxazole)
  Anticonvulsants
  Antithyroid drugs
  Phenothiazines
Cyclical
Disease-related
  Viral infection
  Bacterial sepsis
  Anaphylaxis
  Autoimmune
  Felty's syndrome
  Systemic lupus erythematosus
  Bone marrow failure
  Hypersplenism
  Vitamin B$_{12}$ and folic acid deficiency
  Leukemia

which drug-antibody complexes attach to the neutrophil surface (cephalosporins).

In *agranulocytosis*, the bone marrow appears normocellular except for the absence of granulocyte precursors; profound neutropenia is present in the blood, and sore throat and fever are common symptoms. Drugs commonly causing this syndrome include antithyroid drugs, phenylbutazone, chlorpromazine, and sulfonamides.

Neutropenia also is frequent in collagen vascular diseases such as systemic lupus erythematosus, and accompanies hypersplenism, as in Felty's syndrome. It is also seen in vitamin B$_{12}$ or folic acid deficiency, acute leukemia, and viral infections including infectious mononucleosis and viral hepatitis, and it is common in alcoholism. Many types of congenital neutropenias and benign familial neutropenias have been described. A rare form is *cyclic neutropenia*, which is familial or sporadic and is characterized by periodic falls in the neutrophil count to near zero; granulocyte precursors are absent from the marrow at such times. Marrow production spontaneously resumes to restore granulocyte counts to normal levels; then the entire cycle repeats. A defective stem cell is postulated and other blood cells may also cycle, but less dramatically. Fever and sepsis may occur during the granulocyte nadirs. A temporary neutropenia or "pseudoneutropenia" can be found early in hemodialysis, when complement activation on the dialyzer membrane induces neutrophil aggregation and temporary sequestration in the lungs.

Evaluation of neutropenia involves a search for underlying disease, examination of the bone marrow, testing for antibodies directed against leukocytes, and elimination of drugs. An absolute neutrophil count of less than 1000/μl is considered life-threatening. Meticulous oral and anal hygiene, stool softener therapy, and immediate evaluation of fever or any sign of infection are required throughout the duration of neutropenia. Rapid initiation of broad-spectrum antibiotics for fever or infection is needed, with attention to the danger of superinfection. Transfusion of neutrophil concentrates has not proved to be of benefit in recent controlled trials, probably because of a combination of dysfunction of neutrophils that occurs during preparation of the cells for transfusion and the rapid half-life of neutrophils following their infusion.

NEUTROPHIL LEUKOCYTOSIS

Neutrophil leukocytosis, or a persistent increase in circulating neutrophil levels above 7.5 $\times 10^9$ per cu mm, is frequently observed in bacterial infection, inflammatory diseases, and hemorrhage and in association with malignancy or myeloproliferative disease (Table 53–3). There are also familial leukocytoses, which are benign. Transient leukocytosis can be induced by stress or severe exercise. A leukemoid reaction can usually be distinguished from the high white cell count of myeloproliferative disease or leukemia by the maturity of the leukocytes, an orderly "left

TABLE 53–3.   CAUSES OF NEUTROPHIL LEUKOCYTOSIS

Bacterial infections (pyogenic)
Inflammation; tissue necrosis
Acute hemolysis or hemorrhage
Corticosteroid therapy
Lithium therapy
Myeloproliferative disease
Metastatic cancer
Familial

shift" or appearance of band forms and a few metamyelocytes, and an elevated leukocyte alkaline phosphatase.

REFERENCES

Babior BW: The respiratory burst of phagocytes. J Clin Invest 73:599, 1984.
Gallin JI, and Fauci AS (eds): Advances in Host Defense Mechanisms. Vol 1. Phagocytic Cells. New York, Raven Press, 1982.
Williams WJ, Beutler E, Erslev AJ, and Lichtman MA (eds): Hematology. 3rd ed. New York, McGraw-Hill Book Co, 1983.

HEMATOLOGIC MALIGNANCIES 54

The hematologic malignancies include diseases that arise in bone marrow and lymph nodes. The primary bone marrow disorders are the leukemias, the "immunoproliferative diseases" such as multiple myeloma, and the myeloproliferative syndromes such as polycythemia vera and myelofibrosis with myeloid metaplasia. Evidence suggests that all of these diseases arise from single cell mutations that develop into malignant clones having a growth advantage over normal cells in the marrow. The evidence has arisen from different avenues. In chronic lymphocytic leukemia, for example, the malignant lymphocytes all express an identical surface immunoglobulin, and in multiple myeloma the malignant plasma cells express the identical cytoplasmic and secreted immunoglobulin. In chronic myelogenous leukemia, all the cells of the myeloid series as well as the erythroid precursors, the megakaryocytes, and the B lymphocytes bear the same marker chromosome, the Philadelphia chromosome. Further evidence for the clonal nature of the hematologic malignancies has come from the study of females who are heterozygous for the X-linked enzyme, glucose-6-phosphate dehydrogenase (G6PD). Because only one X chromosome is active in any single cell (inactivation of a maternal or paternal X chromosome occurring at random), half of all the somatic cells of a female heterozygote carry the gene for one G6PD type (e.g., G6PD^A) and the other half

carry the gene for the other type (e.g., G6PD^B). Figure 54–1 demonstrates a study of G6PD expression in the cells of such a woman who developed polycythemia vera. Whereas the skin fibroblasts express either one or the other G6PD isoenzyme, the malignant cells express only one isoenzyme. This finding indicates that the malignant cells arise from a single cell that has expanded into a malignant clone.

THE MYELOPROLIFERATIVE DISORDERS

Four diseases are commonly grouped together as the myeloproliferative disorders: polycythemia vera, myelofibrosis with myeloid metaplasia, essential thrombocythemia, and chronic myelogenous leukemia. All represent clinical conditions that result from uncontrolled expansion of all bone marrow elements (Fig. 54–2). The increased production of erythroid, myeloid, and megakaryocytic lines results from a malignant transformation of a pluripotent stem cell. The increased marrow fibrosis often present in these diseases represents a reaction of normal fibroblasts to growth stimuli provided by the neoplastic cells. Present evidence suggests that the fibroblast growth factor is produced by the bone marrow megakaryocytes that are increased in the myelopro-

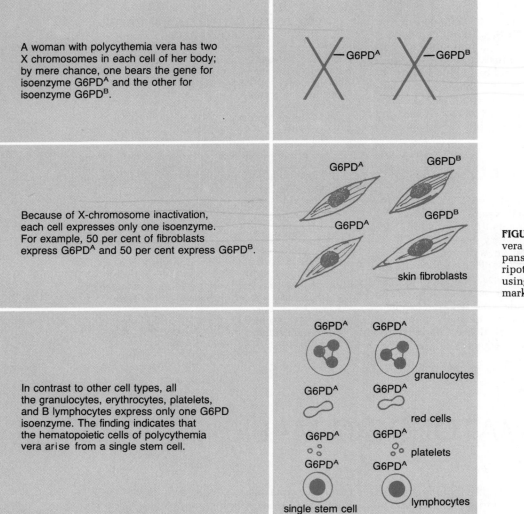

A woman with polycythemia vera has two X chromosomes in each cell of her body; by mere chance, one bears the gene for isoenzyme G6PD^A and the other for isoenzyme G6PD^B.

Because of X-chromosome inactivation, each cell expresses only one isoenzyme. For example, 50 per cent of fibroblasts express G6PD^A and 50 per cent express G6PD^B.

In contrast to other cell types, all the granulocytes, erythrocytes, platelets, and B lymphocytes express only one G6PD isoenzyme. The finding indicates that the hematopoietic cells of polycythemia vera arise from a single stem cell.

FIGURE 54—1. Polycythemia vera represents a clonal expansion of an abnormal pluripotent stem cell: Analysis using G6PD expression as a marker of clonality.

liferative disorders. Chronic myelogenous leukemia will be discussed separately.

The myeloproliferative disorder polycythemia vera is a neoplastic disease of a bone marrow stem cell which affects primarily the erythroid line. Hyperplasia of all bone marrow elements is characteristic, but the increase in erythroid precursors with an elevated red cell mass is the most prominent feature. The increased red blood cell production is autonomous; that is, there is no secondary stimulus such as hypoxia or elevated erythropoietin levels driving red cell production. The typical clinical presentation is that of a patient with an elevated hematocrit. The physician must approach all patients with elevated hematocrits in a systematic way (Table 54–1) to decide first whether the high hematocrit actually represents an increased red cell mass and, if so, whether the increased red cell mass is secondary

FIGURE 54—2. The myeloproliferative disorders represent expansion of all the bone marrow elements with uncontrolled proliferation of hematopoietic cells. The fibrosis is reactive.

to a stimulus external to the bone marrow or whether it represents true polycythemia, polycythemia vera.

A hematocrit above 54 per cent for men or 50 per cent for women should lead the physician to question whether the patient has polycythemia. The hematocrit or per cent packed red cell volume reflects the ratio of red cells to plasma. Thus, the hematocrit may be elevated either if there is truly an excess of red cells or if there is decreased plasma volume, as in dehydration. The best available direct measurement of red cell mass is the ⁵¹Cr-labelled red cell mass. This test will distinguish between absolute polycythemia, in which the red cell mass is truly expanded, and "relative" polycythemia, in which the red cell mass is normal but the plasma volume is contracted (Fig. 54–3).

Relative polycythemia (also called spurious, stress, or Gaisbock's polycythemia) is a chronic condition that typically affects obese, hypertensive, tense men who present with hematocrit values between 55 and 60 per cent. The red cell mass is normal; the plasma volume is contracted for unknown reasons. The pathophysiology of relative polycythemia is not well understood. Because the red cell mass is normal, aggressive phlebotomy is not indicated.

As noted, an elevated red cell mass (men > 36 ml/kg; women > 32 ml/kg) defines *absolute polycythemia*. Absolute polycythemia may be primary, as in the autonomous increase in red cell production that occurs in polycythemia vera, or it may be secondary to a physiological mechanism driving red cell production to a higher than normal level. The most common cause for secondary polycythemia is decreased tissue oxygen delivery, usually due to decreased arterial oxygen saturation, as, for example, in chronic obstructive pulmonary disease. In this setting, the tissue hypoxia causes an increase in renal erythropoietin production. The erythropoietin in turn stimulates the bone marrow erythroid precursors and increases the number of red cells produced in order to in-

TABLE 54–1. EVALUATION OF THE PATIENT WITH AN ELEVATED HEMATOCRIT

1. History
   Family history? Social history (e.g. smoking)?
2. Physical examination
   Splenomegaly? Cardiac or pulmonary disease?
3. Chromium 51 red blood cell mass

NORMAL   ABSOLUTE   RELATIVE
POLYCYTHEMIA POLYCYTHEMIA

Plasma

RBC
mass

Hematocrit-50%   Hematocrit-60%   Hematocrit-60%
(high red cell mass) (low plasma volume)

FIGURE 54–3. The relative volume of plasma to red cell mass in normal and polycythemic patients. In a normal man, the red cell mass represents approximately 50 per cent of the total blood volume and the hematocrit is 50 per cent. In a patient with absolute polycythemia, the plasma volume is normal and the red cell mass is elevated, resulting in a hematocrit of 60 per cent. In relative polycythemia, the plasma volume is contracted and the red cell mass is normal; this results in an elevated hematocrit.

crease tissue oxygen delivery. The increase in red cell mass may be beneficial to the hypoxic tissue; however, the associated increase in total blood viscosity and the marked increase in total blood volume may be clinically detrimental. For example, patients with cyanotic congenital heart disease with a hematocrit of 75 per cent require repeated phlebotomy to decrease the total blood volume and whole blood viscosity. The consequences of the marked hyperviscosity that accompanies a hematocrit greater than 60 per cent include decreased cerebral blood flow, decreased cardiac output, and a tendency to thrombosis.

The approach to the patient with absolute polycythemia should follow a logical pathway to determine whether the patient has secondary or primary polycythemia, polycythemia vera. The history and physical examination may provide the answer. A wheezing, cyanotic, barrel-chested man with severe chronic obstructive pulmonary disease can be distinguished quickly from the plethoric patient with splenomegaly who most likely has typical polycythemia vera. Simple laboratory data will complete the analysis in the majority of patients. White blood count and platelet count are elevated in most patients with polycythemia vera; they are normal in most patients with secondary polycythemia. A low arterial oxygen saturation will indicate that the polycythemia is a compensatory mechanism for hypoxemia. Thus, the history, physical examination, and screening laboratory data should distinguish between primary and secondary polycythemia. Sometimes, however, the cause of the secondary polycythemia may not be obvious and requires further testing for rare causes; these include abnormal hemoglobins with increased oxygen affinity, erythropoietin-secreting renal cysts, cerebellar hemangioblastoma, and hepatocellular carcinoma (Table 54–1).

In *polycythemia vera*, normal control of bone marrow cell production is lost. Although the erythroid line is primarily affected, resulting in an elevated red cell mass, increased granulocyte and platelet production are frequently found as well. Polycythemia vera shares some clinical features with the other myeloproliferative disorders: myelofibrosis with myeloid metaplasia, essential thrombocythemia, and chronic myelogenous leukemia. In all these diseases, there is abnormal (although variable) expansion of all the bone marrow elements: the myeloid precursors, the megakaryocytes, the erythroid precursors, and the fibroblasts of the bone marrow.

The cause of polycythemia vera is not known. The disorder occurs sporadically in both sexes, with a mean age of presentation of about 60 years. Some affected patients are asymptomatic, while others can suffer symptoms due to hypervolemia, hyperviscosity, or platelet dysfunction.

The combination of intravascular hyperviscosity due to a high red cell mass and a high platelet count with functionally abnormal platelets puts patients with polycythemia vera at high risk for stroke, myocardial infarction, and venous thromboembolism.

The metabolic consequences of increased cell turnover also can cause symptoms such as gout or itching (Table 54–2).

The diagnosis of polycythemia vera may be readily apparent or may require extensive laboratory testing to exclude secondary polycythemia (see Table 54–1). Clinical criteria diagnostically useful for the disease are outlined in Table 54–3. If a full evaluation does not convince the physician that a patient has polycythemia vera, two other laboratory tests may be helpful when avail-

TABLE 54–2. CLINICAL MANIFESTATIONS OF POLYCYTHEMIA VERA

Hyperviscosity and/or **hypervolemia** may lead to:
1. Decreased cerebral blood flow with:
   a. Tinnitus
   b. Lightheadedness
   c. Stroke (rarely)
2. Congestive heart failure
3. Thrombosis

Platelet dysfunction may lead to:
1. Thrombosis due to:
   a. Thrombocytosis
   b. Intrinsically abnormal platelets
      (e.g., prolonged bleeding time, absent aggregation to epinephrine, abnormal prostaglandin metabolism, increased Fc receptor expression)
2. Hemorrhage:
   a. Upper gastrointestinal bleeding may occur.
   b. Aspirin aggravates bleeding tendency.
3. Microvascular thrombosis may produce painful toes and fingers.

Increased cell turnover can lead to:
1. Gout (due to hyperuricemia)
2. Itching (due to increased histamine production from basophils)

able: a serum erythropoietin level (which should be zero in polycythemia vera) and an assay of bone marrow erythroid colony growth (which should demonstrate growth of erythroid colonies independent of added erythropoietin in polycythemia vera).

Polycythemia vera, appropriately treated, is compatible with many years of active life. The treatment involves two steps: lowering the hematocrit by phlebotomy and, if necessary, decreasing bone marrow red cell and platelet production by chemotherapy or radioactive phosphorus. Initially, phlebotomy serves to lower the hematocrit, which optimally should be brought to 45 per cent or less. With repeated phlebotomies, bone marrow iron stores (which may be low at the time of diagnosis in polycythemia vera) are further depleted, and red cell production is retarded. In response to repeated phlebotomy, however, platelet production may be increased by as yet incompletely understood mechanisms. If the platelets increase to more than $10^6/\mu l$, the risk of thrombosis or hemorrhage increases. Accordingly, treatment with chemotherapy or radioactive phosphorus may be indicated in this setting. Use of antiplatelet drugs such as aspirin has not proved beneficial in preventing thrombosis in patients with polycythemia vera and may promote hemorrhage.

With appropriate therapy, the median survival for patients with polycythemia vera is at least 10 years. Thrombosis is a major cause of death. Acute leukemia occurs in a small percentage. This tendency to malignant transformation is increased if the patient receives an alkylating agent or radioactive phosphorus for treatment. The current choice of chemotherapy in polycythemia vera is the antimetabolite hydroxyurea, which so far has not been associated with an increased incidence of acute leukemia. Late in the course of polycythemia vera, the "spent" phase may occur. This is marked by increasing bone marrow fibrosis with decreased red cell production and, commonly, the development of anemia and marked splenomegaly. At this stage of the disease, the patient's clinical picture resembles that of myelofibrosis with myeloid metaplasia.

Myelofibrosis with myeloid metaplasia (MMM) (agnogenic myeloid metaplasia) is a myeloproliferative disorder in which, as in the other myeloproliferative disorders, there is expansion of all bone marrow elements due to malignant transformation of a pluripotent stem cell. Bone marrow fibrosis is a reaction to this event and may progress to cause almost complete obliteration of normal marrow space. Extramedullary hematopoiesis in the liver and spleen is a cardinal feature of the disease. The extramedullary hematopoiesis due either to reactivation of a fetal site of hematopoiesis or to new migration of bone marrow stem cells may produce marked hepatosplenomegaly.

The clinical presentation of MMM may be subtle, consisting of no more than nucleated red blood cells detected in a peripheral blood smear. Such cells are a hallmark of extramedullary hematopoiesis. Anemia with teardrop forms and nucleated red cells on peripheral smear, leukocytosis with a shift to the left, and splenomegaly provide additional suggestive features. The diagnosis is strengthened by bone marrow aspiration (usually a "dry tap") and confirmed by biopsy showing fibrosis. The differential diagnosis of MMM includes a leukemoid reaction or chronic myelogenous leukemia as outlined in Table 54–4.

The course of MMM is one of slowly progressive splenomegaly, hepatomegaly, and anemia with thrombocytopenia. The spleen may become so massive that the patient can barely eat or sit comfortably. Portal hypertension due to increased splenic blood flow may become a major clinical

TABLE 54–3. CRITERIA FOR THE DIAGNOSIS OF POLYCYTHEMIA VERA

A1—Elevated red cell mass
  Male: >36 ml/kg
  Female: >32 ml/kg
A2—Normal arterial O_2 saturation (>92%)
A3—Splenomegaly

B1—Thrombocytosis: Platelet count >400,000/μl
B2—Leukocytosis: White cell count >12,000/μl
B3—Elevated leukocyte alkaline phosphatase (LAP): >100
B4—Elevated serum B_{12}: >900 pg/ml

Diagnosis requires:
  A1 + A2 + A3
  or
  A1 + A2 and any two from B category

(Polycythemia Vera Study Group, 1975)

TABLE 54–4. DIFFERENTIAL DIAGNOSIS OF AN ELEVATED WHITE BLOOD COUNT

	MYELOFIBROSIS WITH MYELOID METAPLASIA	CHRONIC MYELOGENOUS LEUKEMIA	LEUKEMOID REACTION
WBC	Usually <100,000/μl with early myeloid forms	May be >100,000/μl with early myeloid forms	Rarely >100,000/μl; promyelocytes or blasts are rare.
RBC morphology	Nucleated RBC and teardrop cells	Occasional nucleated RBC	Usually normal
Leukocyte alkaline phosphatase (LAP score)	Normal or high	Low (<20)	High
Bone marrow	Usually "dry tap" with fibrosis	Panhypercellular	Myeloid hyperplasia
Philadelphia chromosome	Absent	Present (about 90% of cases)	Absent

TABLE 54–5.   DIFFERENTIAL DIAGNOSIS OF AN ELEVATED PLATELET COUNT

	ESSENTIAL THROMBOCYTHEMIA	BENIGN REACTIVE THROMBOCYTOSIS
Platelet number	$>1 \times 10^6/\mu l$; may have bizarre morphology	Usually $>4 \times 10^5$–$1 \times 10^6/\mu l$; may have large platelets
Platelet function	Prolonged bleeding time may be present; absent aggregation response to epinephrine	Normal
Spleen	Usually palpable	Normal
Course	Platelets remain elevated without treatment	Platelets return to normal after inciting event is past (e.g., splenectomy, GI bleeding, infection)
Complications	Hemorrhagic events more common than thrombosis	Rare

problem late in the course of the disease. Unfortunately no treatment alters the natural history of MMM. Supportive care includes treatment with folic acid and iron supplementation when indicated, but most patients eventually require transfusion to counteract anemia. Androgens may decrease the transfusion requirement, at least temporarily. Splenectomy is used cautiously for those selected patients in whom the enlarged organ produces unbearable pressure symptoms, pain, or poor nutrition. The procedure carries a substantial morbidity and mortality. Furthermore, following splenectomy, the liver may enlarge rapidly. Patients may live five or even ten years after the diagnosis of MMM is made, but most suffer serious morbidity during this time.

Essential thrombocythemia is a myeloproliferative disorder characterized by platelet counts consistently elevated over 1 million/μl. The differential diagnosis between essential thrombocythemia and benign reactive thrombocytosis is outlined in Table 54–5. The major presenting symptom of this disease is hemorrhage, although thrombotic events also may occur. Many patients, particularly young ones, remain totally asymptomatic. The optimum therapy is not known. Because the natural history may include a long lifespan, aggressive therapy with alkylating agents usually is not indicated.

THE LEUKEMIAS

Leukemia is a condition in which the bone marrow is replaced by a malignant clone of lymphocytic or granulocytic cells (Fig. 54–4). The course of the disease may be chronic or explosive; if left untreated, all leukemias are fatal.

Chronic Leukemias

Chronic myelogenous leukemia (CML) is often classified as a myeloproliferative disease as well as a leukemia, since it shares the major feature of the myeloproliferative diseases: uncontrolled expansion of all marrow elements. All marrow cell lines in CML express a marker chromosome, the Philadelphia chromosome, pointing to a mutation in a pluripotent stem cell as the initiating event. The Philadelphia chromosome represents a reciprocal translocation of part of the long arm of chro-

mosome 22 to chromosome 9. The biological mechanism behind this rearrangement is not clear, but recent work suggests an association of the Philadelphia chromosome with activation of cellular oncogenes. Cellular oncogenes are human DNA sequences that are homologous to DNA of viruses that cause cancer in other species. Further work is needed to define the meaning of this association.

Although CML is usually a disease of adults, it sometimes affects children as well. The average age at onset is between 40 and 50 years. The disorder is not familial, and most patients have no history of excess exposure to carcinogenic chemicals or increased radioactivity. Nonetheless, the incidence of CML did increase markedly seven years after the atomic bomb explosion in Japan in 1945.

The typical patient with CML presents with few symptoms, and the disease may be discovered on routine blood count. Leukocytosis with early myeloid precursors in the peripheral blood and splenomegaly are almost always present at the time of diagnosis. Thrombocytosis is also common. Table 54–4 outlines the differential diagnosis between CML, MMM, and a leukemoid reaction. Initially, affected patients are managed easily with periodic oral chemotherapy (alkylating agents or hydroxyurea) to normalize the blood count and reduce splenomegaly. This chronic phase of CML lasts three to five years. Subsequently, the course of the disease accelerates. The white count and spleen size become more difficult to control. Anemia and, eventually, thrombocytopenia develop, and fever and increasing weakness may appear. Eventually, white cell maturation ceases, so that the peripheral blood contains increasing numbers of promyelocytes and myeloblasts. This is termed the "blast phase," and it heralds death within three to six months.

The events that transform CML from the chronic to the blast phase are not understood. Hyperdiploidy or other chromosome abnormalities in addition to the Philadelphia chromosome often develop. In approximately 20 per cent of blast crises, the blast cells bear markers of lymphoid cell origin such as the enzyme terminal deoxynucleotidyl transferase (Tdt). This finding is important in therapeutic management, since drugs that are effective in lymphoid malignancies (e.g., vincris-

FIGURE 54—4. Photomicrographs of leukemic bone marrows. *Upper left,* Acute lymphoblastic leukemia. Large primitive cells with prominent nucleoli. *Upper right,* Chronic lymphocytic leukemia. Marrow is almost entirely replaced with small, well-differentiated lymphocytes. *Lower left,* Chronic myelocytic leukemia (chronic phase). Myeloid hyperplasia with "left shift" to predominance of early myeloid forms, but preservation of mature neutrophils as well. *Lower right,* Acute promyelocytic leukemia. Large promyelocytes with prominent cytoplasmic granules replace normal marrow elements.

tine and prednisone) may be useful in a lymphoid type (Tdt-positive) of blast crisis. Overall, however, the treatment of blast crisis is unsatisfactory, and any remissions are short.

New strategies are needed if patients with CML are to be cured. Bone marrow transplantation represents a potentially promising approach. Patients under 40 with an identical twin or HLA-identical sibling should be considered for bone marrow transplantation during the chronic phase, with the goal of producing long-term disease-free survival.

Chronic lymphocytic leukemia (CLL) was described by Dr. William Dameshek as an "accumulative disease of immunologically incompetent lymphocytes," a concise definition that describes the majority of patients. CLL is a disease of older persons, and fewer than 10 per cent of cases are patients under 50 years old. Men develop CLL twice as often as women and, as in all forms of leukemia, the disorder is more common in whites than blacks.

The diagnosis of CLL is based on an absolute and sustained lymphocytosis in the peripheral blood of no less than 15,000 cells/μl. The bone marrow is hypercellular, and more than 40 per cent of the cells are lymphocytes. The lymphocytes in the peripheral blood and marrow are of the small, well-differentiated type. Slowly enlarging lymph nodes and gradual enlargement of the liver and spleen due to the accumulation of neoplastic lymphocytes may occur early or late in the course of the disease. The immunological incompetence of the expanding lymphocyte population expresses itself in hypogammaglobulinemia with predisposition to infections and in the emergence of such autoimmune phenomena as the production of antibodies against host red blood cells, causing Coombs' positive hemolytic anemia. Table 54—6 outlines the immune disorders in CLL.

Lymphocytes in chronic lymphocytic leukemia usually consist of a clonal proliferation of B lymphocytes (Fig. 54—5). The malignant cells all display immunoglobulin molecules on their plasma membranes bearing the same idiotype and the same single light chain type. The most common surface immunoglobulins represented are IgM and IgD. The finding of two heavy chain classes does not preclude the concept of monoclonality, as the IgD and IgM have the same idiotype specificity and presumably reflect an early, frozen

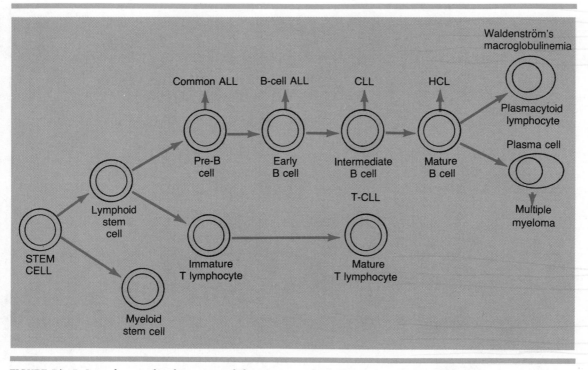

FIGURE 54–5. Lymphocyte development and the stages at which maturation arrest will result in various immunological subtypes of lymphoid leukemia or in an "immunoproliferative" malignancy. B cell = bursa or bone-marrow derived lymphocyte; T cell = thymus-derived lymphocyte; ALL = acute lymphoblastic leukemia; CLL = chronic lymphocytic leukemia; HCL = hairy cell leukemia. (Adapted from Markowitz MJ, Mouradian J, and Moore A: Acute and chronic lymphocytic leukemia. In Molander DW (ed): Disease of the Lymphatic System. New York, Springer-Verlag, 1984.)

stage of differentiation of normal B lymphocytes. CLL lymphocytes also express the Ia antigen, the receptor for C3, and the receptor for the Fc portion of immunoglobulin.

About 1 per cent of patients with CLL demonstrate predominantly T lymphocytes in their peripheral blood. These lymphocytes form rosettes with sheep red blood cells and do not bear surface immunoglobulin. The T cell form of CLL appears to carry a poorer prognosis than the B cell type. Skin involvement is seen frequently in these patients, and standard forms of therapy for CLL are less effective.

TABLE 54–6.   IMMUNE DISORDERS IN CLL

Autoantibody Production
Autoimmune hemolytic anemia
    Coombs' test positive in 20 to 30% of patients with CLL
    Hemolysis rare
    Usually responds to corticosteroids
Autoimmune thrombocytopenic purpura
    Thrombocytopenia may also be due to bone marrow replacement by CLL or to splenic sequestration.
    Usually responds to corticosteroids
Disorder of Immunoglobulin Synthesis
Monoclonal gammopathy
    Monoclonal spike present in 10% of patients with CLL—IgG or IgM.
    Usually not of clinical importance
Hypogammaglobulinemia
    Present in majority of cases, particularly stages III and IV
    Results in increased susceptibility to bacterial infection

The etiology of CLL is unknown. Despite occasional familial clusterings of CLL, no firm genetic basis for the disease has been found, nor does exposure to radiation or other potentially mutagenic agents such as alkylating agents appear to predispose. Consistent chromosomal abnormalities have not been found and, to date, no convincing data support a viral etiology.

A major contribution to understanding the natural history of CLL is the clinical staging system devised by Rai et al., which identifies prognosis according to the state of illness at the time of first diagnosis (Table 54–7). The stages of the disease reflect the concept of the "accumulative" nature of CLL. Stage 0 is lymphocytosis alone. Stages I and II reflect the development of increasing tumor mass (nodes, liver, or spleen), while the anemia and thrombocytopenia of stages III and IV indicate bone marrow replacement interfering with normal hematopoiesis, and splenomegaly causing decreased red blood cell and platelet survival. Most patients are in stage 0, I, or II at the time of diagnosis.

Figure 54–6 plots the median duration of survival from the time of diagnosis of 125 patients studied by Rai et al. As can be seen, although the median survival was 71 months, the duration depended considerably on the clinical stage. Although palliative treatment exists, there is no cure for CLL. Treatment is generally withheld in the asymptomatic stage. When symptoms such as enlarging lymph nodes, splenomegaly, progressive anemia, and/or thrombocytopenia occur, alkylating agents (e.g., chlorambucil) and prednisone prove beneficial. Radiotherapy to the spleen or to areas of bulky adenopathy may be useful.

Hairy cell leukemia (HCL) (also called leukemic reticuloendotheliosis) is a neoplastic disorder characterized by "hairy cells" in the peripheral smear and bone marrow. Hairy cells look like lymphocytes with fine cytoplasmic projections. Unlike B cells, they are capable of phagocytosis. The cells stain positive for tartrate-resistant acid phosphatase (TRAP).

HCL is more common in men than women and usually presents as a slowly developing pancytopenia with splenomegaly. Splenectomy may be useful if the spleen enlarges painfully or severe cytopenia develops. Chemotherapy has not helped most patients with hairy cell leukemia. The median survival for patients with hairy cell leukemia is three to five years; some patients live many years after diagnosis with little treatment.

Acute Leukemias

In acute leukemias immature hematopoietic cells proliferate without differentiation into normal mature blood cells. The proliferating cells, whether myeloblasts or lymphoblasts, do not allow the normal production of erythrocytes, granulocytes, and platelets to take place. This leads to the major clinical complications of the disease: anemia, susceptibility to infection, and bleeding.

In most cases of acute leukemia, one finds no recognizable predisposing condition or event. In a few circumstances, however, an association with a possible leukemogenic agent(s) has been identified. Known agents associated with the development of acute leukemia include radiation, viruses, genetic predisposition, and chemicals (Table 54–8). How these agents interact with normal marrow stem cells so as to produce a malignant clone that lacks the ability to differentiate is not known.

Acute leukemias are divided into two broad categories: *acute lymphoblastic leukemia* (ALL) and *acute myeloblastic leukemia* (AML). ALL is primarily a disease of children, AML primarily of adults. Approximately 20 per cent of adult leukemias, however, are of the lymphoblastic type. Because the natural history and the treatment of these two types of leukemia differ, it is important to distinguish between them. The major distinction lies in bone marrow morphology; histochemical stains and surface and cytoplasmic markers are also useful (Table 54–9). Chromosome analysis of the acute leukemias has not identified a consistent abnormality; however, various abnormal karyotypes are described.

Because of heterogeneity within the two broad categories of acute leukemia, a French, American, and British (FAB) group recently has developed a subdividing classification that has proved useful in studying the course and therapy of the acute leukemias (Table 54–10). Among the myeloblastic leukemias the morphologic subtypes possess rel-

TABLE 54–7. CRITERIA FOR CLINICAL STAGING OF CLL (RAI)

Stage 0:	Lymphocytosis alone
	>15,000/μl in peripheral blood
	>40% marrow lymphocytosis
Stage I:	Lymphocytosis and enlarged nodes
Stage II:	Lymphocytosis and splenomegaly, hepatomegaly, or both
Stage III:	Lymphocytosis and anemia: hemoglobin <11 g/dl
Stage IV:	Lymphocytosis and thrombocytopenia: platelets <100,000/μl

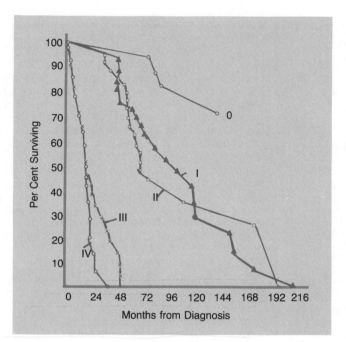

FIGURE 54–6. Chronic lymphocytic leukemia: Median survival from time of diagnosis of 125 patients staged by the Rai criteria. (Adapted from Rai KR, Sawitsky A, Cronkite EP, et al: Clinical staging of chronic lymphocytic leukemia. Blood 46:219, 1975.)

TABLE 54–8. EXAMPLES OF AGENTS ASSOCIATED WITH THE DEVELOPMENT OF ACUTE LEUKEMIA

AGENT	EXAMPLE
Ionizing radiation	Incidence of leukemia increased in persons exposed to atomic bombings in Japan, 1945.
Viruses	A T cell leukemia that clusters in Southern Japan is associated with a human type C retrovirus (HTLV).
Genetic predisposition	An identical twin of a young child with acute leukemia has a 20% chance of developing the disease.
Chemicals	Alkylating agents: Chlorambucil, a treatment for polycythemia vera, leads to increased development of acute leukemia.

TABLE 54–9.   LABORATORY AIDS TO DISTINGUISH BETWEEN AML AND ALL

	AML	ALL
1. Morphology of leukemic blasts	Granules in cytoplasm; Auer rods* may be present	Agranular, basophilic cytoplasm
	Multiple nucleoli	Regular, folded nucleus with one prominent nucleolus
	FAB (see Table 54–10) subclassification, M₁–M₆	FAB subclassification, L₁–L₃
2. Histochemistry	Myeloperoxidase positive	Myeloperoxidase negative; PAS positive
3. Cytoplasmic markers	—	Terminal deoxynucleotidyl transferase (TDT) positive
4. Surface markers (% of cases)	—	B cell markers (5%)
		T cell markers (15–20%)
		CALLA† (50–65% cases)

* Auer rods are a linear coalescence of cytoplasmic granules that stain pink with Wright's stain.
† CALLA = Common acute lymphoblastic leukemia antigen.

atively distinctive clinical correlation. For example, acute promyelocytic leukemia (M_3) is associated with disseminated intravascular coagulation (DIC); the prominent cytoplasmic granules in the promyelocytes release enzymes that stimulate the coagulation cascade and promote intravascular coagulation. Acute monocytic leukemia (M_5) is associated with skin and gum infiltration with leukemic cells. Among lymphoblastic leukemias, the L_1 subtype is found predominantly in children and the L_2 subtype is found primarily in adults. The L_3 subtype is uncommon and carries a poor prognosis.

The diagnosis of acute leukemia is rarely difficult. The patient is usually acutely ill and presents with symptoms that indicate abnormal bone marrow function: infection due to granulocytopenia, bleeding due to thrombocytopenia, and/or anemia due to lack of erythroid maturation. Bone pain due to the expanded leukemic marrow may be present. In ALL, lymphadenopathy and splenomegaly are common. The total white blood count usually is elevated, sometimes above $100,000/\mu l$, but can be normal or even low ($<3000/\mu l$). The blood smear is almost always abnormal, showing predominantly blast cells with only a few normal mature leukocytes present. The hemoglobin and platelet count are almost always depressed. The blood uric acid is usually elevated due to the increased white cell turnover; clinical gout is rare but renal damage due to the hyperur-

icemia may occur. A bone marrow aspirate and biopsy make the diagnosis. The marrow is almost always hypercellular or "packed" with sheets of monotonous undifferentiated cells that replace the normal marrow elements.

The diagnosis of acute leukemia represents a medical emergency. The initial hours or days after diagnosis should be spent stabilizing the patient and preparing him for treatment. If the white blood count is greater than $100,000/\mu l$, the patient is at high risk for cerebral hemorrhage caused by leukostasis, that is, obstruction of and damage to blood vessels plugged with rigid blasts. In this setting, immediate steps should be taken to reduce the white count by initiating chemotherapy, if possible, or performing leukapheresis. Allopurinol, a xanthine oxidase inhibitor, is given concurrently to decrease the uric acid formation that results when treatment begins to destroy leukocytes. Antibiotics may be needed to treat infections, which can be life-threatening when patients have few or no mature granulocytes. Transfusion with red cells to maintain adequate blood hemoglobin levels and/or platelets to prevent hemorrhage is usually required. Acute leukemia is one of the most dreaded diagnoses that a patient can receive. The initial management must include enough time spent with the patient and his family to reassure them and to explain the treatment and support programs.

The specific treatment of acute leukemia consists primarily of chemotherapy; radiotherapy sometimes may be used as an adjunct. The total leukemic cell burden is estimated to be from 10^{11} to 10^{12} cells at clinical presentation. Chemotherapeutic drugs follow first-order kinetics. This means that the drugs kill a constant percentage of cells (e.g., 99 per cent) with each administration. A clinically complete remission with disappearance of all detectable leukemia in the blood and bone marrow may mean a reduction in tumor burden from 10^{12} to 10^9 cells. A similar amount of treatment is needed to reduce the number of cells from 10^9 to 10^7. Thus, the eradication of the last leukemia cell by chemotherapy becomes almost an impossible task.

Chemotherapeutic drugs are administered with the goal of stopping cells from proliferating. The

TABLE 54–10.   FRENCH-AMERICAN-BRITISH (FAB) CLASSIFICATION OF ACUTE LEUKEMIA

Acute Myelocytic Leukemia
M_1—Acute myelocytic leukemia without differentiation
M_2—Acute myelocytic leukemia with differentiation (predominantly myeloblasts and promyelocytes)
M_3—Acute promyelocytic leukemia
M_4—Acute myelomonocytic leukemia
M_5—Acute monocytic leukemia
M_6—Erythroleukemia
Acute Lymphocytic Leukemia
L_1—Predominantly "small" cells (twice the size of normal lymphocyte), homogeneous population
L_2—Larger than L_1, more heterogeneous population
L_3—"Burkitt-like" large cells, vacuolated abundant cytoplasm

TABLE 54–11. A TYPICAL PROGRAM FOR TREATMENT OF ACUTE LYMPHOBLASTIC LEUKEMIA

PHASE	PURPOSE	TREATMENT
Induction of complete remission	To eradicate all detectable leukemia cells	Vincristine, prednisone, daunorubicin, L-asparaginase
Central nervous system prophylaxis	To treat a potential "sanctuary" of leukemia	Intrathecal methotrexate (? cranial radiotherapy)
Intensification or consolidation during remission	To decrease further the leukemic burden	Chemotherapy similar to induction
Maintenance of remission	Continual suppression of the leukemic clone	Methotrexate, 6-mercaptopurine, vincristine and prednisone

drugs are targeted against different phases of the cell cycle, with specific programs designed to follow the kinetics of the cell cycle. An example of a treatment program for acute lymphoblastic leukemia is outlined in Table 54–11. Similar programs are used in the treatment of AML, in which case the major drugs are cytosine arabinoside and daunorubicin.

Cure of acute leukemia with rigorous chemotherapy programs and meticulous supportive care is sometimes possible, although the encouraging results achieved in children with ALL (i.e., over 60 per cent alive in complete remission and probably cured at five years) have not been reproduced in adults. About 30 per cent of adults with ALL may obtain a long-term remission. The percentage is considerably smaller in AML, with only 10 to 20 per cent surviving five years in remission, although 60 to 70 per cent of patients achieve a first remission averaging one year in duration.

Bone marrow transplantation from a related HLA-matched donor is being investigated as a treatment for patients with acute leukemia. Patients under age 30 who achieve an initial complete remission with chemotherapy can be considered possible candidates for this experimental procedure if they have a suitable donor. The complications of bone marrow transplantation are substantial, however, and include acute and/or chronic graft-versus-host disease, interstitial pneumonias, and the infections and hemorrhagic complications expected during an initial period of bone marrow aplasia. Late recurrence of the leukemia is still a major concern and is believed to represent inadequate eradication of the leukemic clone by the initial cytotoxic treatment. Since in one case, however, post-transplant recurrence in a male patient involved a female's donor cells, it appears possible that the recipient passed a transmittable agent to the new cell line.

Other innovative approaches to the cure of acute leukemias include the use of monoclonal antibodies directed to leukemia-associated cell surface antigen. The technology of this approach is progressing rapidly and may be incorporated into future treatment programs.

MYELODYSPLASTIC SYNDROMES

In contrast to the explosive nature of acute leukemia, the myelodysplastic syndromes are characterized by the slow development of an anemia refractory to standard therapy. Affected patients are usually elderly; however, in recent years an increasing number of younger patients have developed myelodysplastic syndromes following prior treatment with radiotherapy, combination chemotherapy, or both, for another neoplasm such as Hodgkin's disease or ovarian carcinoma. Typically, the patient presents with the insidious onset of increasing fatigability and decreasing exercise tolerance; often the patient ascribes the symptoms to "growing old." Physical examination may reveal pallor, and laboratory examination shows an anemia that may be profound. The anemia is typically macrocytic, with an MCV of 100 to 110 μ; the peripheral smear may show a dimorphic erythrocyte population, and the patients may also have leukopenia with or without thrombocytopenia. The bone marrow is hypercellular, with increased iron stores and morphologically abnormal erythroid precursors (dyserythropoiesis) as well as an increased percentage of early myeloid cells. This syndrome has been called "refractory anemia" or "preleukemia" in the past. Because the initial presentation and the course are variable, the condition is now referred to as the myelodysplastic syndrome and further defined according to a classification proposed by the FAB co-operative group mentioned above. Table 54–12 outlines the major clinical features and relative incidence of the five types of myelodysplastic syndromes. For refractory anemia (with or without ringed sideroblasts), the median survival time is approximately three to four years. The other three categories (refractory anemia with excess blasts, chronic myelomonocytic leukemia, and refractory anemia in transformation) carry a survival of one to two years or less. The risk of developing acute leukemia increases with the number of blasts in the bone marrow at presentation; thus, about 20 to 30 per cent of patients with refractory anemia (type 1 or 2) develop acute leukemia, but over 60 per cent of patients with refractory anemia with excess blasts in transformation will develop acute leukemia.

Treatment of the myelodysplastic syndrome is primarily directed toward improving the anemia. Blood transfusions are a mainstay of treatment. A few patients with refractory anemia with ringed sideroblasts respond to large doses of vitamin B_6. Chemotherapy has been used when increased numbers of blasts appear in the bone marrow. The role for chemotherapy, either in conventional doses or in low doses, is still being studied.

TABLE 54-12. CLASSIFICATION OF THE MYELODYSPLASTIC SYNDROMES

DIAGNOSIS (RELATIVE INCIDENCE)	PATIENT CHARACTERISTICS	PERIPHERAL BLOOD	BONE MARROW
Refractory anemia (56%)	Elderly patient; anemia	May have abnormal red cell morphology	<5% blasts
Refractory anemia with ringed sideroblasts (21%)	Elderly; anemia	May have dimorphic picture (microcytic/hypochromic and macrocytic)	Hypercellular; iron stain shows iron in a ring around red cell nuclei.
Refractory anemia with excess blasts (10%)	May have pancytopenia	<5% blasts	5–20% blasts
Chronic myelomonocytic leukemia (11%)	Similar to above	Absolute monocytosis <5% blasts	5–20% blasts
Refractory anemia in transformation (1%)	Any age; symptoms of brief duration	>5% blasts	20–30% blasts

THE LYMPHOMAS

The lymphomas are a group of malignant neoplasms that arise in lymph nodes or extranodal lymphoid tissue. They are a heterogeneous group of malignancies from both a pathological and a clinical viewpoint. The two major subgroups are Hodgkins' disease and the non-Hodgkin's lymphoma. In both these subgroups, the most common clinical presentation is that of a patient who notices an enlarged lymph node. Before the physician considers a biopsy of the enlarged node, he must obtain a thorough history and perform a physical examination and selected laboratory tests to evaluate possible causes of the swollen lymph node. Cervical lymphadenopathy most commonly is associated with infections such as streptococcal pharyngitis, infectious mononucleosis, and toxoplasmosis. Axillary lymphadenopathy, particularly if it is unilateral, should direct the physician to perform a careful breast examination for possible cancer. Inguinal adenopathy may reflect skin infections of the legs or infection of the genitalia or anus such as syphilis. Scrofula,

TABLE 54-13. COMMON CAUSES OF LYMPHADENOPATHY

Infection
  Bacterial: Localized infection with regional adenopathy (e.g., streptococcal pharyngitis, foot ulcer with inguinal adenopathy)
  Viral: Infectious mononucleosis, cytomegalovirus, cat scratch fever
  Parasite: Toxoplasmosis
  Spirochete: Syphilis
  Mycobacterial: Tuberculosis, *Mycobacterium avium* (in immunosuppressed patients)
  Fungal: Actinomycosis, Cryptococcosis (in immunosuppressed patients)
Drug Reaction
  Serum sickness
  Phenytoin (may cause "pseudolymphoma")
Malignancy
  Solid tumors—metastatic patterns:
    Cervical adenopathy: head and neck cancer
    Supraclavicular adenopathy: gastrointestinal tumors
    Axillary adenopathy: breast cancer
    Inguinal adenopathy: carcinoma of the anus
  Lymphoma
Miscellaneous
  Sarcoidosis
  Generalized lymphadenopathy in homosexual men (possible pre-AIDS)

or tuberculous lymphadenitis, may present as asymptomatic isolated lymphadenopathy. Table 54–13 outlines various common causes of lymphadenopathy. If the cause of the enlarged lymph node(s) is not obvious after consideration of the above, the physician should consider lymph node biopsy for diagnosis.

Hodgkin's disease is primarily a disease of young adults but also appears in children and the elderly. The patient usually presents with asymptomatic lymphadenopathy; for example, on a routine pre-employment chest x-ray the radiologist finds mediastinal lymphadenopathy. Some patients with Hodgkins' disease have symptoms of fever, night sweats, or loss of weight; the factor or factors responsible for the production of these symptoms are not known.

Hodgkin's disease is classified by pathological subtype, by clinical stage, and by the presence or absence of symptoms. The four pathological subtypes are nodular sclerosis, lymphocyte predominance, mixed cellularity, and lymphocyte depletion (Table 54–14). In all four subtypes the finding of Reed-Sternberg cells assures the pathologist that the diagnosis of Hodgkin's disease is correct. The typical Reed-Sternberg cell is a large cell with two prominent nuclei. Each nucleus contains a prominent nucleolus surrounded by a "halo." This pattern gives the cell the appearance of "owl's eyes." Pathologists have puzzled over the cell of origin of the Reed-Sternberg cell since it was first described around 1900. At present, the true macrophage or histiocyte rather than a lymphocyte is considered the progenitor of the Reed-Sternberg cell.

Nodular sclerosis is the most common pathological subtype of Hodgkin's disease. Broad bands of fibrosis disrupt the lymph node architecture. "Lacunar" cells and scattered Reed-Sternberg cells are characteristic. This subtype of Hodgkin's disease typically presents as an asymptomatic mediastinal mass in a young woman. Hodgkin's disease of the mixed cellularity subtype demonstrates a pathological picture of a heterogeneous cellular background with lymphocytes, eosinophils, and plasma cells; the Reed-Sternberg cell is present. Young and middle-aged men rather than women are more likely to have this subtype. Lymphocyte-predominant Hodgkin's disease is an un-

TABLE 54–14. HODGKIN'S DISEASE: PATHOLOGIC TYPES

SUBGROUP	RELATIVE FREQUENCY
Lymphocyte predominance	5–15%
Nodular sclerosis	40–75%
Mixed cellularity	20–40%
Lymphocyte depletion	5–15%

common subtype. An asymptomatic young man presenting with an enlarged high cervical node would be a typical patient. The prognosis for this subtype is generally excellent. Lymphocyte-depleted Hodgkin's disease is also uncommon. An older patient with fever, night sweats, or weight loss would be most likely to have this subtype, and the prognosis is generally poor.

Cure of the patient with Hodgkin's disease is the goal of treatment. Treatment is planned once the extent of disease or the stage is known. The definition of stages I, II, III, and IV is outlined in Table 54–15. Figure 54–7 shows examples of the various stages. The presence or absence of systemic symptoms is also part of the staging criteria. The staging process is rigorous, and a basic outline of tests that should be done to establish the stage is shown in Table 54–16. Hodgkin's disease tends to follow a logical anatomical progression of node involvement. For example, a patient with cervical adenopathy may have supraclavicular or mediastinal adenopathy but in the absence of supraclavicular or mediastinal adenopathy is

TABLE 54–15. ANN ARBOR STAGING CLASSIFICATION FOR HODGKIN'S DISEASE

Stage I: Involvement of a single lymph node region (I) or a single extralymphatic site (IE)

Stage II: Involvement of two or more lymph node regions on the same side of the diaphragm (II) or a solitary extralymphatic site and one or more lymph node areas on the same side of the diaphragm (IIE)

Stage III: Involvement of lymph node regions on both sides of the diaphragm (III), accompanied by spleen involvement (IIIs), or solitary involvement of an extralymphatic organ or site (IIIE) or both (IIISE)

Stage IV: Diffuse involvement of extralymphatic sites with or without lymph node enlargement

In addition to above, presence or absence of symptoms (specifically, fever, night sweats, loss of 10% body weight) is designated by B (presence) or A (absence).

TABLE 54–16. STAGING EVALUATION FOR A PATIENT WITH LYMPHOMA

1. Complete history and physical examination
2. CBC, differential, platelet count, urinalysis
3. Screening blood chemistries
4. Chest x-ray, CAT scan of chest, abdomen and pelvis
5. Bone marrow aspirate and biopsy
6. Consider lymphangiogram, gallium scan

NON-HODGKIN'S LYMPHOMA	HODGKIN'S DISEASE
Stage III or IV—Treat with chemotherapy	Stage IIIB or IV—Treat with chemotherapy
Stage I—Treat with radiotherapy	Stage IA—Treat with radiotherapy
Stage II—Treat with radiotherapy and/or chemotherapy	Stage IIA, IIB, IIIA—Consider exploratory laparotomy

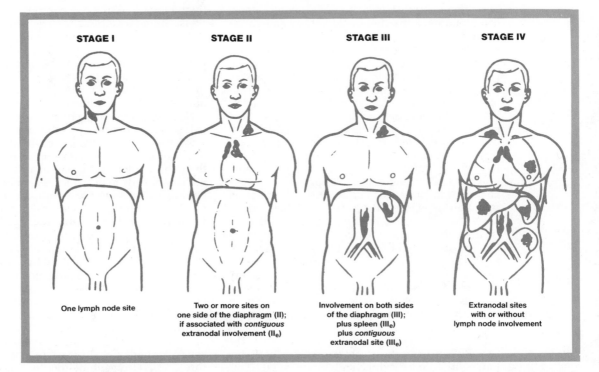

STAGE I — One lymph node site

STAGE II — Two or more sites on one side of the diaphragm (II); if associated with *contiguous* extranodal involvement (IIe)

STAGE III — Involvement on both sides of the diaphragm (III); plus spleen (IIIe) plus *contiguous* extranodal site (IIIe)

STAGE IV — Extranodal sites with or without lymph node involvement

FIGURE 54–7. Malignant lymphoma: Examples of stages I through IV. (Reprinted from Tindle BH: Teaching monograph: Malignant lymphomas. Am J Pathol 116:115, 1984, with permission.)

unlikely to have pelvic adenopathy or liver involvement. This principle is important when considering how far to pursue a staging evaluation. For example, the patient with a high cervical node and no other adenopathy by CTT scan is very unlikely to have abdominal disease. An exploratory laparotomy with liver biopsy, multiple node biopsies, and splenectomy may be necessary to establish an accurate stage for a patient. A laparotomy should be considered in two situations: first, if the findings at laparotomy will alter the treatment plan; and, secondly, if abdominal or pelvic radiotherapy is being considered for a young woman of child-bearing age, the laparotomy would include transposing the ovaries out of the radiotherapy field. If a patient has clinical stage IIIB or stage IV Hodgkin's disease, the treatment is chemotherapy; laparotomy is not necessary because the findings will not change this recommendation. If a patient has a mediastinal mass and cervical node involvement but a lymphangiogram suggests pelvic node involvement, a laparotomy may be necessary to establish whether the patient has stage IIA or stage IIIA disease. Both these stages can be treated with radiotherapy, but the parts would differ according to the findings at laparotomy.

The treatment of Hodgkin's disease is radiotherapy, chemotherapy and, in certain cases, both therapies (Table 54–16). Radiotherapy is the recommended treatment for patients with stages I and IIA. Some patients with stage II or IIIA will have such massive adenopathy that chemotherapy may be used initially to shrink the bulk of the disease before curative radiotherapy. Patients with stage IIB are a controversial group; because of a high relapse rate after radiotherapy alone, combined modality (i.e., radiotherapy and chemotherapy) may be recommended. Patients with stage IIIB or IV are considered to have widespread disease that cannot be cured by radiotherapy; curative chemotherapy is used in these patients.

Radiotherapy is delivered in tumoricidal doses to areas of known disease and to adjacent areas. For example, a patient with stage I Hodgkin's disease in a cervical node receives a "mantle" port designed to treat cervical, supraclavicular, axillary, mediastinal, and hilar lymph nodes. A patient with inguinal node involvement receives an "inverted Y" to encompass the para-aortic, iliac, and inguinal nodes. The immediate side effects of radiation depend on the field irradiated and include sore throat, dysphagia, nausea, and diarrhea. Delayed effects include radiation pneumonitis and hypothyroidism if the thyroid has been included in the field. Ovarian function will be suppressed unless the ovaries are surgically moved out of the radiation field prior to treatment.

A major advance in Hodgkin's disease has been the development of combination chemotherapy that can cure the majority of patients with stages IIIB and IV. The original program was the "MOPP" program (nitrogen-mustard, vincristine [oncovin], procarbazine, and prednisone). This program is still one of the best programs for advanced-stage Hodgkin's disease. The immediate side effects include nausea, vomiting, and bone marrow suppression. The delayed side effects include sterility and the potential for the late development of leukemia. The risk of leukemia increases if the patient is over 40 and also receives radiotherapy.

The long-term prognosis for patients with Hodgkin's disease is related to stage at diagnosis. Patients with stages IA and IIA disease have a five-year survival of over 90 per cent. Most patients with stage IIIA have a five-year survival of over 80 per cent. B symptoms decrease the survival figures at each stage. Stage IIIB and stage IV patients can expect a five-year survival of over 50 per cent. The five-year survival rates can translate to cure rates in most instances.

The non-Hodgkin's lymphomas are a heterogeneous group of neoplasms that arise from a monoclonal proliferation of a malignant cell of lymphoid origin. As in Hodgkin's disease, the cause of lymphoma is not known. Viruses, radiation, immunosuppression, and certain genetic conditions have all been implicated. Burkitt's lymphoma, a rare monoclonal B cell neoplasm, has provided some clues about the pathogenesis of lymphoma. In Africa, there is a "lymphoma belt" in which the development of Burkitt's lymphoma mirrors the endemic area for malaria. This distribution, along with the finding of Epstein-Barr virus in the majority of cases of African Burkitt's lymphoma, suggests a viral pathogenesis. There is an intriguing set of chromosomal translocations in Burkitt's lymphoma that involve chromosomes 8 and 14 and less commonly 2 and 22. These are the chromosomes that carry the genes for the immunoglobulin heavy chains and light chains. With the chromosome translocations, immunoglobulin rearrangements are detected. The translocations also occur at the chromosome site where a cellular oncogene (c-myc) is found. The relationship of the translocation at the site of a cellular oncogene and monoclonal proliferation of this malignant neoplasm is intriguing but is not yet understood.

Non-Hodgkin's lymphomas are classified by pathological subtype and clinical stage. The pathological subtype depends on the overall pattern of nodal architecture and on the morphology of the predominant cell in the neoplastic node. The malignant cells may replace the node in a diffuse pattern obliterating the germinal centers or follicles completely. This pattern defines a "diffuse" lymphoma. Alternatively, the malignant cells may form a pattern of nodules or follicles that defines the lymphoma as a nodular or follicular lymphoma. The predominant cell type further classifies the lymphoma. The major lymphoma cell types are the small, well-differentiated lymphocyte; the slightly larger, poorly differentiated lymphocyte with a cleaved nucleus; and the large lymphoid cell with characteristics of a histiocyte or lymphoblast. Two major lymphoma classification systems use these criteria, nodal architecture, and cell type to define the subtypes of lymphoma. Table 54–17 shows the International Formulation classification of lymphoma next to the classification of Dr. Rappaport. Both these systems have received wide acceptance because of their clarity and clinical applicability. These classifications are morphologic and do not depend on immunological subtyping of the malignant cells. If lymph node biopsies are further subjected to studies of cell origin using surface immunoglobulin markers for B cells, erythrocyte rosettes for T cells, or more sophisticated monoclonal antibodies for B and T cells, most of the lymphomas are of B cell origin. Some lymphomas are of T cell origin; in rare lymphomas, the cell of origin cannot be determined.

Clinical staging of non-Hodgkin's lymphoma is defined by the same criteria as those for Hodgkin's disease (see Table 54–15). Two aspects of the staging process are different from Hodgkin's disease. First, the non-Hodgkin's lymphomas are more likely than Hodgkin's lymphomas to present in an extranodal site (Fig. 54–8). Secondly, the progression of the non-Hodgkin's lymphomas does not follow the orderly anatomical progression described above for Hodgkin's disease. Non-Hodgkin's lymphoma is much more likely to be disseminated at the time of diagnosis. True stage I or stage II non-Hodgkin's lymphomas are rare. The treatment and prognosis of the patient with non-Hodgkin's lymphoma depend on the clinical stage and the pathological classification. Patients with stage I or stage II disease may be treated with radiotherapy alone. The overall cure rate for these patients is less than 50 per cent. This suggests that there may be a role for adjuvant chemotherapy in the treatment of some of these patients. Patients

with stage III or IV disease are treated primarily with chemotherapy. Curability in this group depends on the pathological subtype. Paradoxically, the patients with "high-grade" or "high-intermediate" grade lymphomas in whom the natural history would lead to survival of less than one or two years are now curable with aggressive com-

TABLE 54–17. CLASSIFICATION OF THE NON-HODGKIN'S LYMPHOMAS

INTERNATIONAL WORKING FORMULATION	RAPPAPORT CLASSIFICATION
I. Low-grade lymphoma	
a. Small lymphocytic cell	Diffuse lymphocytic, well-differentiated
b. Follicular, mixed cleaved cell	Nodular lymphocytic, poorly differentiated
c. Follicular, mixed small cleaved and large cell	Nodular mixed lymphocytic-histiocytic
II. Intermediate-grade lymphoma	
d. Follicular, large cell	Nodular histiocytic
e. Diffuse, small cleaved cell	Diffuse lymphocytic, poorly differentiated
f. Diffuse, mixed small cleaved cell	Diffuse mixed lymphocytic-histiocytic
g. Diffuse large cell	Diffuse histiocytic
III. High-grade lymphoma	
h. Large cell immunoblastic	Diffuse histiocytic
i. Lymphoblastic cell	Diffuse undifferentiated
j. Small noncleaved cell (Burkitt and non-Burkitt)	

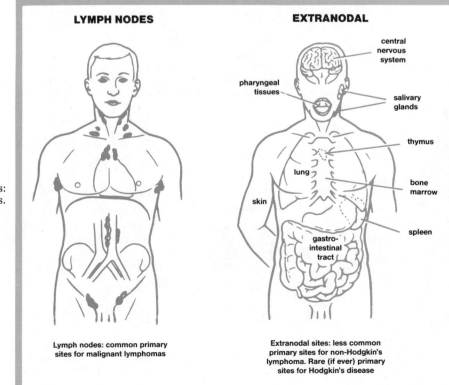

FIGURE 54–8. Malignant lymphomas: Examples of nodal and extranodal sites.

LYMPH NODES

EXTRANODAL

central nervous system

pharyngeal tissues

salivary glands

thymus

lung

bone marrow

skin

spleen

gastro-intestinal tract

Lymph nodes: common primary sites for malignant lymphomas

Extranodal sites: less common primary sites for non-Hodgkin's lymphoma. Rare (if ever) primary sites for Hodgkin's disease bination chemotherapy programs incorporating drugs such as cyclophosphamide, adriamycin, vincristine, prednisone, and bleomycin. Patients with low-grade lymphomas are rarely curable by chemotherapy. The natural history of these lymphomas tends to be an indolent one, with median survivals of five years and sometimes longer. Treatment offers palliation but may not alter survival. Thus, observation alone, less aggressive chemotherapy, and palliative radiotherapy may be used in the management of the patient with an indolent lymphoma.

THE IMMUNOPROLIFERATIVE DISORDERS

The immunoproliferative disorders include a group of neoplasms that arise from a clone of immunoglobulin-secreting cells and produce a monoclonal immunoglobulin (or part of an immunoglobulin). If the monoclonal immunoglobulin (Ig) is of the IgM class, the disease is Waldenström's macroglobulinemia and the malignant cells are plasmacytoid lymphocytes. If the monoclonal immunoglobulin is of the IgG, IgA, IgD, or rarely the IgE class, the disease is multiple myeloma and the malignant cells are plasma cells. Normal plasma cells represent the most specialized cells in the B cell lineage. Figure 54–4 illustrates one scheme of maturation proceeding from a pluripotent stem cell to an early B cell to a well-differentiated plasma cell. The figure also indicates the malignant diseases that can arise from neoplastic proliferation at each stage of B cell maturation.

Plasma cells normally secrete immunoglobulins and are responsible for maintaining humoral immunity. The basic structure of all immunoglobulins is the same and includes two heavy ("H") polypeptide chains and two light ("L") polypeptide chains, bound together by disulfide bonds (Fig. 54–9). Both H chains and L chains have "constant" regions of amino acid sequence and "variable" regions that allow for antibody specificity. The five subclasses of immunoglob-

ulin, immunoglobulin gamma (IgG), mu (IgM), alpha (IgA), delta (IgD), and epsilon (IgE) are determined by the constant region of their H chains. Light chains are of two types: kappa and lambda. Each antibody molecule has two identical H chains and two identical L chains; hybrid molecules are not synthesized. Table 54–18 outlines special properties of the five immunoglobulin classes. Protein electrophoresis provides the first step in detecting a monoclonal immunoglobulin in serum (Fig. 54–10). Analysis of the protein "spike" by agar gel immunoelectrophoresis using specific antibodies (e.g., anti-human IgG, anti-kappa chains, etc.) further defines the exact type of monoclonal immunoglobulin.

Monoclonal immunoglobulin elevations can be found in conditions other than multiple myeloma or Waldenström's macroglobulinemia. Approximately 10 per cent of patients with chronic lymphocytic leukemia have monoclonal IgG or IgM spikes in their serum. In addition, a monoclonal spike on serum electrophoresis may be found in patients with no detectable associated disease. The "spike" is usually not large (i.e., is less than 2 gm/dl) and is accompanied by no other clinical or laboratory evidence of multiple myeloma or Waldenström's macroglobulinemia. This finding, called "benign monoclonal gammopathy," is found in elderly patients (i.e., over 60); approximately 10 per cent of these patients later develop a true immunoproliferative disorder.

Multiple myeloma is a malignant disease of plasma cells that is characterized by the presence of monoclonal immunoglobulin or light chains in the serum and urine and bone destruction. The typical patient is over 50 and presents with back pain, mild anemia, and an elevated sedimentation rate. Initial bone x-rays may demonstrate only osteoporosis, although widespread lytic lesions are typical. Less frequently the patient will have hypercalcemia and renal disease ("light chain nephropathy") at the time of diagnosis. Serum immunoelectrophoresis generally demonstrates a monoclonal elevation of one immunoglobulin (e.g., IgG^k), with reciprocal depression of the other

FIGURE 54–9. Structure of an immunoglobulin molecule: L chain = light chain, mw 22,000; H chain = heavy chain, mw 50,000–70,000; $/\!/$ = sites of cleavage by the enzyme, papain, which results in three fragments: Fc (crystallizable) fragment and two identical Fab (antigen-binding) fragments.

TABLE 54–18. SOME PROPERTIES OF NORMAL IMMUNOGLOBULINS

	IgG	IgA	IgM	IgD	IgE
Molecular weight	150,000	180,000	900,000 (a pentamer)	150,000	200,000
Plasma concentration (mg/ml)	7–15	2.0	1.0	0.03	trace
Biologic half-life (days)	20	6	5	3	–
Complement fixation	+	0	+	–	–
Crosses placenta	+	0	0	0	0
Special properties	4 subclasses (1–4)	Present in external secetions	Synthesized by lymphocytes	—	Important in hypersensitivity

immunoglobulins (e.g., IgA and IgM). Free kappa or lambda light chains (Bence-Jones protein) are usually detected by a 24-hour urine immunoelectrophoresis. About 20 per cent of patients with multiple myeloma will not have a monoclonal serum spike but will have free light chains detectable in urine and serum ("light chain disease"); about 1 per cent of patients with multiple myeloma will have neither monoclonal nor free light chains detectable. These patients with "nonsecretory" myeloma can be shown to have a malignant clonal proliferation of plasma cells by immunofluorescent staining of the bone marrow. The plasma cells will be shown to stain with either the anti-kappa or anti-lambda antiserum, but not with both reagents.

Bone marrow aspiration is essential for the diagnosis of myeloma. Plasma cells usually make up less than 5 per cent of bone marrow cells; greater than 20 per cent plasma cells are required to make a bone marrow diagnosis of multiple myeloma. Some of the plasma cells may have bizarre morphology with binucleated and multinucleated plasma cells. The clinical manifestations of mul-

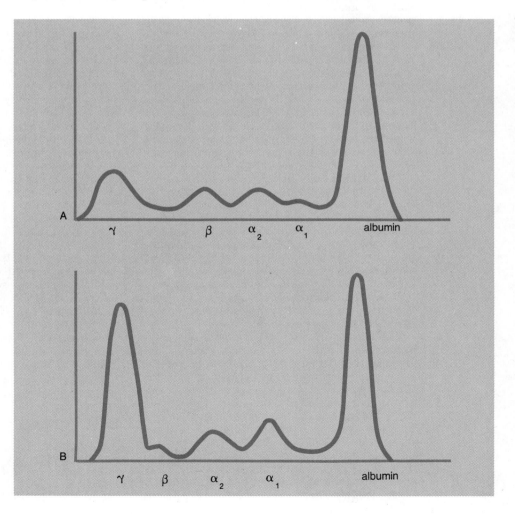

FIGURE 54–10. A, A normal serum protein electrophoresis showing a polyclonal distribution of protein in the gamma (γ) region. B, A serum protein electrophoresis showing a monoclonal spike in the gamma region.

TABLE 54–19. COMMON CLINICAL MANIFESTATIONS OF MULTIPLE MYELOMA

Bone involvement
Malignant plasma cells may secrete osteoclast activating factor leading to:
   a. osteoporosis, pathologic fracture, and bone pain
   b. hypercalcemia
Anemia
Decreased red cell production due to tumor inhibition of erythropoiesis and marrow invasion by plasma cells
Renal disease
  Calcium nephropathy
  Light chain nephropathy
  Uric acid nephropathy
  Amyloidosis (may develop in about 15% of patients)
Elevated sedimentation rate
  The paraprotein causes red cell rouleaux.
Infection
  Normal immunoglobulin production is suppressed.
  Pneumococcal disease is particularly prevalent.

tiple myeloma center on the systemic effects of the monoclonal protein (the paraprotein) and the concomitant humoral immunodeficiency state, as well as the effects of the bone and bone marrow invasion by malignant cells. Table 54–19 outlines the common clinical syndromes associated with multiple myeloma. Despite high levels of paraprotein, syndromes of hyperviscosity are rare in myeloma.

The prognosis of multiple myeloma is a reflection of the tumor cell burden. A poor prognosis is associated with a high tumor cell burden, as reflected by anemia, decreased renal function, hypercalcemia, extensive bony involvement, and large monoclonal protein peaks. A patient without any of these poor prognostic criteria may have a median survival of five years; a patient in the poor prognosis category is likely to have a median survival of less than two years.

The treatment of a patient with multiple myeloma requires meticulous attention to supportive care as well as expertise in the administration of chemotherapy. Cautious exercise and ambulation are important to retard bone resorption. Bone lesions may require local radiotherapy to prevent a pathologic fracture. Adequate hydration and avoidance of intravenous dye injection (e.g., for intravenous pyelography) helps to prevent renal failure. Administration of pneumococcal vaccine and early detection and treatment of infections are important in these susceptible patients.

The current chemotherapy of multiple myeloma centers on the use of alkylating agents (single or multiple) and corticosteroids. Improvement in symptoms ensues in the majority of patients. Clinical remission is associated with a decrease of less than one log of tumor cells (e.g., 10^{12} to 10^{11}). Eradication of all tumor cells aand cure of multiple myeloma is not attainable with available therapy.

Waldenström's macroglobulinemia is a clonal disease of IgM-secreting plasmacytoid lymphocytes. It is a chronic disorder that usually affects older people. The patient commonly presents with anemia and symptoms due to the physical properties of the elevated monoclonal IgM. IgM is a large molecule and remains primarily in the intravascular space. If the IgM level is elevated, plasma viscosity may be high. Nosebleeds, retinal hemorrhages, mental confusion, and congestive heart failure are clinical presentations of the hyperviscosity syndrome. Some IgM molecules precipitate in the cold. The patient with this type of IgM may manifest the clinical picture of cryoglobulinemia. Blue (cyanotic) fingers, toes, nose, and earlobes on exposure to cold are a typical presentation. Foot and leg ulcers may develop, and vascular occlusion with gangrene may ensue. Leukocytoclastic vasculitis is seen on biopsy of these skin lesions. Some IgM molecules may have activity directed against red cells, particularly the "I" antigen (see Hemolytic Anemias). This type of IgM, a cold agglutinin, agglutinates red cells at temperatures below 37°C (e.g., in the extremities). These patients present with Raynaud's phenomenon and a hemolytic anemia. Keeping patients with cryoglobulinemia or the cold agglutinin syndrome warm is a primary part of their treatment. Peripheral neuropathy is a rare presentation of Waldenström's macroglobulinemia. A few patients have been described in whom the IgM monoclonal protein had antimyelin activity. Splenomegaly and lymphadenopathy may develop during the course of Waldenström's macroglobulinemia but are rarely a major cause of disability. Bone pain and hypercalcemia rarely occur.

The treatment of Waldenström's macroglobulinemia is directed to relief of symptoms. If the symptoms are primarily due to the elevated IgM (e.g., hyperviscosity syndrome), plasmapheresis is a useful tool and may be combined with chemotherapy. If the IgM is a cold agglutinin or a cryoglobulin, the plasmapheresis must be done in a warm environment. Chemotherapy (e.g., alkylating agents) may be useful to decrease the lymphadenopathy and splenomegaly but does not alter the natural history of the disease. The median survival is about three years, although some patients may live ten or more years with indolent disease.

Rarely, a patient may present with *heavy chain disease,* a disorder that has some characteristics of myeloma or Waldenström's macroglobulinemia but behaves clinically more like lymphoma. Analysis of the serum reveals only the heavy chain of IgG, IgA, or IgM. Gamma chain disease is associated with lymphadenopathy and edema of the soft palate. Alpha chain disease ("Mediterranean lymphoma") is characterized by intestinal infiltration by lymphoma; mu chain disease is associated with chronic lymphocytic leukemia.

REFERENCES

Adamson JW, Fialkow PJ, Murphy S, Pichal JF, and Steinmann L: Polycythemia vera: Stem cell and probable clonal origin of the disease. N Engl J Med 295:913, 1976.

Bennett JM, Catovsky D, Daniel MT, et al: Proposals for

the classification of the acute leukemias. Br J Haematol 33:451, 1976.

Berk PD, Goldberg JD, Silverstein MN, Balcerzak SP, Berlin NI, Brubaker LH, et al: Increased incidence of acute leukemia in polycythemia vera associated with chlorambucil therapy. N Engl J Med 304:441, 1981.

Berlin NI: Diagnosis and classification of the polycythemias. Semin Hematol 12:339, 1975.

DeVita VJ Jr, Simon RH, Hubbard SM, et al: Curability of advanced Hodgkin's disease with chemotherapy: Long-term follow-up of MOPP-treated patients at The National Cancer Institute. Ann Intern Med 92:587, 1980.

Durie BGM, Salmon SE, and Moon TE: Pretreatment tumor mass, cell kinetics and prognosis in multiple myeloma. Blood 55:364, 1980.

Foon KA, Schroff RW, and Jale RP: Surface markers on leukemia and lymphoma cells. Recent advances. Blood 60:1, 1982.

Koeffler HP, and Golde DW: Chronic myelogenous leukemia—New concepts. N Engl J Med 304:1201, 1269, 1981.

Kyle RA, and Bayrd ED: The Monoclonal Gammopa-thies. Springfield, IL, Charles C Thomas, Publisher, 1976.

Markowitz MJ, Mouradian J, and Moore A: Acute and chronic lymphocytic leukemia. In Molander DW (ed): Disease of the Lymphatic System. New York, Springer-Verlag, 1984.

Non-Hodgkin's lymphoma pathologic classification project. National Cancer Institute sponsored study of classifications of non-Hodgkin's lymphomas: Summary and description of a working formulation for clinical usage. Cancer 49:2112, 1982.

Rai KR, Sawitsky A, Cronkite EP, et al: Clinical staging of chronic lymphocytic leukemia. Blood 46:219, 1975.

Thomas ED: Marrow transplantation for malignant diseases. J Clin Oncol 1:517, 1983.

Tindle BH: Teaching monograph: Malignant lymphomas. Am J Pathol 116:115, 1984.

Ward HP, and Block MH: The natural history of oncogenic myeloid metaplasia (AMM) and a critical evaluation of its relationship with the myeloproliferative syndrome. Medicine 50:357, 1971.

Ziegler JL: Burkitt's lymphoma. N Engl J Med 305:735, 1981.

HEMOSTASIS 55

The arrest of bleeding after blood vessel injury involves a complex interaction among three responding systems: the blood vessel wall, the platelets, and the plasma coagulation proteins. This interaction results in normal *hemostasis*, but if pathologically exaggerated produces *thrombosis*. While hemostasis is initiated within a few seconds after blood vessel injury, it is not completed for minutes to about an hour.

Primary hemostasis involves constriction of the injured vessel, exposure of subendothelial collagen, and the adhesion and aggregation of blood platelets on the damaged surface to form a *primary hemostatic plug* that is completed within 3 to 7 minutes. This process also involves participation of von Willebrand factor (Factor VIII: von Willebrand Factor, Factor VIII: VWF), which mediates platelet adhesion and the release from platelets of vasoactive materials that augment aggregation. Clinical assessment of primary hemostasis is made with the bleeding time, which is a sensitive index of the adequacy of platelet function.

Secondary hemostasis represents the formation of a *fibrin clot* at the site of the initiating primary hemostatic plug. The surface of activated platelets catalyzes the formation of thrombin by its efficient assembly of coagulation factors involved in the prothrombinase complex in the presence of membrane phospholipid and calcium released upon platelet activation. Such localized thrombin activation in turn has several crucial effects. (1) Thrombin catalyzes fibrinogen conversion to fibrin, the fibrous protein that consolidates the platelet plug and entraps erythrocytes to provide bulk for the permanent clot. (2) Thrombin stimulates further platelet activation, prothrombin conversion, platelet release, and thromboxane production. (3) Thrombin activates coagulation Factor XIII, fibrin stabilizing factor, which covalently cross-links and stabilizes the fibrin clot. Measurement of secondary hemostasis is made with the whole blood clotting time, which averages 8 to 10 minutes.

The *third stage of coagulation* is clot retraction, a process in which the loose meshwork of platelet aggregates, fibrin strands, and trapped red cells is formed into a firm clot. This process involves the contraction within individual platelets of the smooth muscle protein, thrombosthenin, which compresses the clot. This stage may be evaluated in vitro and takes about one hour.

EVALUATION OF A BLEEDING TENDENCY

A clinically important bleeding tendency may result from defects in the blood vessels, the platelets, or the coagulation proteins. The defects may be qualitative or quantitative, and single or multiple. Inherited hemorrhagic disorders tend to result from single defects, whereas acquired disorders result from single or multiple deficiencies. Evaluation of a patient for a bleeding tendency is needed in three settings: (1) screening prior to surgery, (2) when prior episodes of spontaneous or traumatic bleeding are reported, and (3) during active bleeding unresponsive to simple measures (Table 55–1).

TABLE 55–1. DIFFERENTIAL DIAGNOSIS OF BLEEDING DISORDERS

	COAGULATION DEFECT	PLATELET DEFECT	VASCULAR DEFECT
Family history	Usually positive	Rarely positive	Usually negative
Sex predominance	Males	Often females	Mainly females
Type of bleeding	"Deep" joint, muscle and visceral; spontaneous and post-trauma	Mucosal skin, mucous membranes	Purpuric or GI
Time sequence	Delayed after trauma followed by prolonged oozing	Immediate, brief	Ecchymoses after trauma
Response to local pressure	Ineffective	Effective	Effective

The personal and family history is essential in evaluation of a bleeding tendency. A positive family history of bleeding in males suggests one of the hemophilias, which make up 95 per cent of congenital coagulation deficiencies. Spontaneous bleeding or bruising or easy bruising and bleeding after minor trauma are important, especially if bruises are large or raised (hematomas). Excessive bleeding after prior surgery or dental extraction, events that stress the hemostatic process, may indicate a bleeding tendency in persons without spontaneous bleeding history. A history of menorrhagia or peripartum hemorrhage in a woman can also signify an underlying bleeding diathesis.

If bleeding has occurred, its timing, location, and clinical setting provide key clues to the type of defect. In platelet disorders, bleeding tends to be immediate and transient and involves mucous membranes or skin (e.g., epistaxes or bruising). In contrast, delayed bleeding after trauma or surgery, or bleeding into joints or muscles, is typical of coagulation disorders. The presence of systemic diseases such as liver disease, hematologic malignancy, or uremia may impair hemostasis. Drug ingestion is the single most common cause for acquired hemostatic defects; a careful drug history should include direct questioning about ingestion of aspirin, nonsteroidal anti-inflammatory compounds, antibiotics, and anticoagulants as well as

alcohol. All of these substances can cause bleeding or exacerbate an underlying bleeding disorder, as can profound nutritional impairment. Some specific bleeding disorders to be considered from the patient's history are listed in Table 55–2.

Pertinent aspects of the physical examination in evaluating possible bleeding disorders include examination of the skin, mucous membranes, and retina for petechiae, ecchymoses, or hematomas and examination of the abdomen for hepatosplenomegaly. Petechiae are pinpoint hemorrhages from microvessels in the skin and are associated with platelet disorders or thrombocytopenia. Because pressure can exacerbate petechial bleeding, these lesions are commonly found on the legs or in other areas of increased hydrostatic pressure (e.g., on the buttocks in a bedridden patient). Purpura (confluent petechiae) are also common in thrombocytopenia. Ecchymoses, especially if spontaneous or raised (hematomas), and hemarthroses suggest defects in plasma coagulation factors as in hemophilia. Hepatomegaly suggests liver disease, and splenomegaly is associated with thrombocytopenia or with hematologic malignancy.

LABORATORY EVALUATION OF HEMOSTASIS

Basic screening for hemostatic integrity can be accomplished with a prothrombin time, partial thromboplastin time, platelet count, and bleeding time (Table 55–3). If all results from these tests are normal, a serious bleeding diathesis is unlikely. Any abnormalities indicate that further investigation for particular defects should be made. Levels of individual coagulation factors, the presence of circulating anticoagulants, the nature of thrombocytopenia, abnormal platelet function, and signs of intravascular consumption of procoagulants can all be assessed.

PLATELET DISORDERS

Normal platelet function and a platelet count greater than 100,000/cu mm in the peripheral blood are needed for normal primary hemostasis (Fig. 55–1). The platelet count represents the net balance between platelet production rate and the rate of loss or peripheral destruction of platelets. Since the bone marrow has the capacity to increase platelet production 8- to 10-fold, and plate-

TABLE 55–2. CLINICAL CLUES TO BLEEDING DISORDERS

CLINICAL SIGN	DISORDER
Lifelong history of easy bruising or bleeding	Congenital coagulopathy (factor deficiency) Von Willebrand's disease
Family history of bleeding in males only	Hemophilia A or B
Family history of bleeding in both sexes	Factor XI deficiency Von Willebrand's disease
Excessive bleeding at surgery	Mild coagulation factor deficiency Von Willebrand's disease Thrombocytopenia
Acquired bruising tendency	Aspirin or other drug ingestion Thrombocytopenia
Delayed bleeding after trauma or surgery	Factor XIII deficiency
Bleeding after dental extraction	If negative, a bleeding disorder is unlikely.
Bruising or bleeding starting during another illness	Drug ingestion Thrombocytopenia Acquired anticoagulant

TABLE 55–3. SCREENING TESTS FOR BLEEDING DISORDERS

TEST	MECHANISM TESTED	NORMAL	WHERE ABNORMAL
Prothrombin time (PT)	Extrinsic and common pathways	< 12 sec	Defect in vitamin K–dependent factors, liver disease, DIC, oral anticoagulants
Activated partial thromboplastin time (APTT)	Intrinsic and common pathways	25–40 sec	Hemophilia, von Willebrand's disease, heparin therapy, DIC; deficient XII, IX, IX circulating anticoagulant
Thrombin time (TT)	Fibrinogen-fibrin conversion	10–15 sec	Third-stage anticoagulant; fibrin split products, DIC; severe hypofibrinogenemia
Bleeding time (BT)	Primary hemostasis, platelet function	3–7 min	Platelet dysfunction, von Willebrand's disease, thrombocytopenia

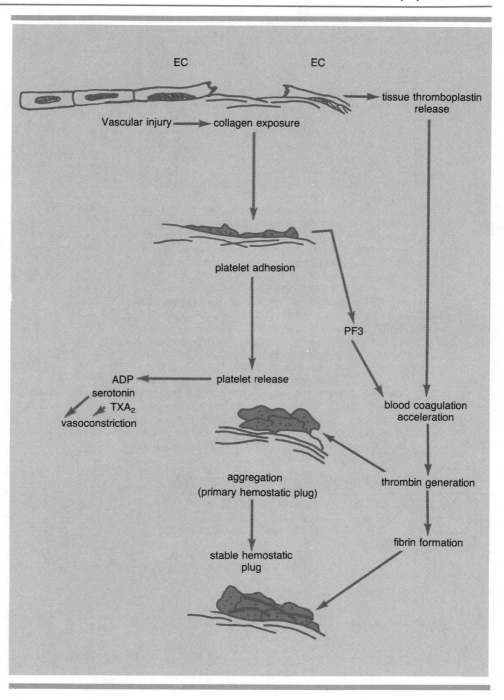

FIGURE 55–1. Hemostasis and platelet interactions with coagulation. Upon vascular injury, collagen fibrils underlying the endothelial cells (EC) are exposed when the endothelium is damaged. Adhesion of single platelets that flatten out and expose PF3 (procoagulant phospholipid) follows, then platelet release and primary aggregation to form a platelet plug. Release of ADP, serotonin and TXA₂ induces vasoconstriction, while the PF3 accelerates blood coagulation, the formation of thrombin, and the generation of fibrin. Fibrin strands stabilize the hemostatic plug. Thrombin also promotes platelet aggregation and vasoconstriction.

lets survive 8 to 10 days in the circulation, the platelet count can be maintained under most circumstances, even if losses or destruction are increased. Young platelets are more metabolically active and more hemostatically effective than older ones. Platelet adhesion, procoagulant activity, and aggregation and release of vasoactive substances must also be normal for hemostatic effectiveness. Impairment of one or several of these functions leads to a bleeding tendency characterized by mucosal and skin bleeding, purpura, and prolonged oozing of blood after trauma or surgery.

Thrombocytopenia

Platelet counts below 100,000/μl portend an increased bleeding risk, which correlates roughly with the depression of the platelet count. Counts above 50,000/μl are rarely associated with spontaneous bleeding, whereas counts below 20,000/μl are frequently associated with spontaneous bleeding, especially if the patient is febrile or anemic. Bleeding is observed more often in a thrombocytopenic patient with a rapidly falling platelet count than in a patient with a low, stable count. The mechanisms for severe thrombocytopenia include (1) decreased or ineffective platelet production, (2) increased peripheral destruction, (3) splenic sequestration, and (4) intravascular dilution (Table 55–4).

Decreased platelet production occurs with systemic infection, nutritional defects (folate or vitamin B$_{12}$), radiation, chemotherapy, or marrow replacement by fibrosis or tumor. Transient decreases in platelet production are common in viral infections and are the rule after radiation therapy to bone or after most types of cancer chemotherapy. Bone marrow megakaryocytes may appear decreased or immature. Numerous drugs can inhibit megakaryocytopoiesis, including alcohol, anticonvulsants, and thiazides. Marrow hypoplasia as in aplastic anemia or Fanconi's syndrome also results in thrombocytopenia.

Increased platelet destruction is a common cause of thrombocytopenia and may be induced by commonly used drugs, including digitalis, quinidine, thiazides, imipramine, phenothiazines, sulfonamides, antibiotics (penicillins and cephalosporins), and gold salts. These agents usually produce thrombocytopenia by an immune mechanism in which a drug–antibody or drug–plasma protein complex adsorbs passively to the platelet surface ("innocent bystander") via the platelet Fc receptor, coating the platelets and resulting in their rapid removal from the circulation by the spleen. Other drugs may directly adsorb to the platelet surface, resulting in neoantigens that provoke antiplatelet antibody formation. Stopping all drugs, if possible, and substituting drugs of different chemical structure if discontinuation is not possible is the first step in the evaluation and treatment of drug-induced immune thrombocytopenia. Unfortunately, direct tests of drug involvement are difficult to perform and often are insensitive, so that clinical assessment after drug discontinuation or switching is the main instrument for detecting drug-related thrombocytopenias.

Idiopathic (or autoimmune) thrombocytopenic purpura (ITP) represents immune thrombocytopenic purpura occurring without toxic or drug exposure. A polyclonal antiplatelet antibody has been demonstrated by transfer experiments. Platelet-associated IgG (and complement) may be elevated, large platelets circulate in the blood, and megakaryocytes are increased in the bone marrow. The spleen is not enlarged. The platelet survival is short. Acute ITP is mainly a disease of childhood, having a sudden onset following acute viral infection and resolving spontaneously in 80 per cent of affected children within a few weeks. In adults, chronic ITP is more common, has an insidious onset, and affects women more often than men. Fewer than 10 per cent of cases resolve spontaneously. In some cases an autoimmune hemolytic anemia is also present (Evan's syndrome). Adult ITP occurs alone or in association with diseases of disturbed immunity such as systemic lupus erythematosus, lymphoproliferative disorders, or AIDS. ITP can herald such diseases, appearing even years in advance of the full blown disease. Pregnant women with ITP can deliver thrombocytopenic infants, as the antiplatelet antibody is usually an IgG$_1$ or IgG$_3$ and thus crosses the placenta. The infant's platelet count does not correlate with the mother's count, so that a mother with ITP by history and a normal platelet count can deliver a thrombocytopenic infant.

Diagnosis of ITP is by exclusion. It is made in a patient with thrombocytopenia, increased megakaryocytes in the bone marrow, and increased platelet-associated IgG in the absence of drug exposure or toxic exposure. Aside from thrombocytopenia marked by large platelets, the blood count is otherwise normal. Platelet function may be entirely normal or may show diminished aggregation responses. Platelet survival is shortened, sometimes to hours compared to the normal survival of 8 to 10 days. Direct measurement of platelet survival can be made with ^{51}Cr or ^{112}In-labelled autologous platelets. This test, however, is not routinely performed because of expense and technical difficulty.

Treatment of both drug-induced thrombocytopenia and ITP is similar. Any suspected drug is

TABLE 55–4. CAUSES OF THROMBOCYTOPENIA

Failure of platelet production	
Selective megakaryocyte depression	Drugs, viral infections
General bone marrow failure	Aplastic anemia, hematologic malignancy
	Myelophthisis
	Megaloblastic anemia
	Radiation
Increased platelet destruction	Drug-induced
	ITP
	Heparin
	DIC, TTP
Abnormal distribution	Hypersplenism
Dilutional	Massive transfusion of bank blood
	Extracorporeal circulation

stopped, and essential drugs are switched to substitutes of different chemical composition. All aspirin-like drugs are avoided. If the thrombocytopenia is severe, with purpura on the mucous membranes or retina, corticosteroids (1 to 2 mg/kg/day prednisolone) are given. Platelet transfusion should be avoided except for treatment of intracerebral bleeding because of the extremely short survival of transfused platelets. Plasmapheresis is generally not effective because of the IgG nature of the antiplatelet antibodies, which are inefficiently removed by this technique. In acute ITP of childhood or drug-induced thrombocytopenia, steroids can be tapered within a few weeks as platelet counts rise. In chronic ITP steroids should be administered for two to three months before tapering the dose or moving to alternative therapy, in order to achieve the maximum number of remissions and responses. In 70 per cent of patients the platelet count will rise toward normal within that period. Once a normal platelet count has been reached, the steroid dosage should be slowly tapered to avoid precipitating a relapse. The probable actions of steroids include inhibition of splenic reticuloendothelial phagocytic activity, decreased immune complex binding to platelets, decreased capillary fragility, and decreased immunoglobulin synthesis. When steroids are tapered following an initial increase in platelet count to the normal range, thrombocytopenia recurs in as many as 80 per cent of initially responding adult patients. Reinstitution of steroids may restore the platelet count, but many patients may require splenectomy for permanent remission. After splenectomy, 60 to 80 per cent of patients with ITP will maintain an adequate platelet count, while the remainder will require further therapy with steroids (at a lower dose) or with immunosuppressive drugs such as vincristine, cyclophosphamide, or azathioprine. For short-term therapy intravenous high-dose gamma globulin can transiently raise the platelet count in patients with refractory ITP (e.g., in preparation for emergency surgery), but adults do not respond well to repeated high-dose IgG therapy. Children with chronic ITP who are refractory to other therapy have been successfully managed with repeated infusion of high-dose intravenous IgG. Anabolic steroids such as danazol have also been reported to raise platelet counts in refractory ITP.

Other Causes of Immune Thrombocytopenia.

Post-transfusion purpura is a rare syndrome that follows the administration of PL^AI-positive blood to patients who lack this common platelet antigen and who have developed anti-PL^AI antibodies after previous transfusion or pregnancy. An explosive thrombocytopenia develops five to eight days after transfusion (anamnestic response) which may require plasmapheresis and exchange transfusion with PL^AI-negative blood. The thrombocytopenia may persist a few weeks but is self-limited. Other platelet antigen systems are occasionally involved. Neonatal purpura may be seen in infants of PL^AI-negative mothers or mothers with ITP. In systemic anaphylactic reactions thrombocytopenia may result from sequestration

of platelets coated with circulating antigen-antibody complexes. Thrombocytopenia may also result from platelet coating with "i"-cold antibodies that arise following viral infections such as rubella or infectious mononucleosis.

Platelet consumption syndromes include disseminated intravascular coagulation (DIC), thrombotic thrombocytopenia purpura, and the hemolytic uremic syndrome or can result from platelet damage during extracorporeal circulation. Intravascular activation of the coagulation mechanism is associated with sepsis, shock, exposure to toxins, or malignancies and may present with hemorrhage or thrombosis (see below). Thrombin-induced platelet aggregation or vascular damage that initiates platelet activation can cause thrombocytopenia. Vascular malformations such as cavernous hemangiomas (Kasabach-Merritt syndrome) sometimes produce localized DIC and platelet trapping, resulting in chronic thrombocytopenia.

Thrombotic thrombocytopenic purpura (Moschkowitz's syndrome) is an acute, relapsing disease affecting the microcirculation. There is a pentad of signs and symptoms including thrombocytopenia, microangiopathic hemolytic anemia, neurologic abnormalities, renal dysfunction, and fever. Two-thirds of affected persons are young women. There is often a history of preceding viral infection. The characteristic lesions are hyaline thrombi, consisting of platelet aggregates and fibrin, plugging small arterioles and capillaries. Endothelial proliferation may be seen, but vasculitis is not present. The blood smear shows schistocytes, increased reticulocytes, and normoblasts, reflecting the microangiopathic and hemolytic nature of the characteristic anemia; thrombocytopenia is usually severe, the serum bilirubin is elevated, and the Coombs' test is negative. Early in the disease DIC is absent, but it appears as renal failure ensues. Abnormal forms of von Willebrand factor have been observed (released by injured endothelium), and some patients possess a plasma factor that promotes platelet activation. TTP is frequently fatal. Treatment by splenectomy, steroids, or platelet-inhibitory drugs such as aspirin and dipyridamole has had variable results. Exchange transfusion, plasmapheresis, and plasma infusion have more recently been used with greater success and represent the current approach of choice.

Hemolytic-uremic syndrome, usually seen in children, involves a Coombs-negative microangiopathic hemolytic anemia, thrombocytopenia, diarrhea, and acute renal failure. Unlike TTP, this disorder does not affect the brain to produce neurologic signs. DIC may be present. The major pathologic lesion consists of hyaline thrombi in the renal microcirculation, probably representing a form of immune complex disease. Renal dialysis is the mainstay of therapy. The role of plasmapheresis has not been defined.

The use of therapeutic extracorporeal circulation frequently produces thrombocytopenia as the result of platelet activation, with subsequent adherence of platelets to the surface of the membrane oxygenator, dialyzer membrane, or other extracorporeal device. Platelet dysfunction induced by such contact may contribute to postoperative hemorrhage, over and above the contribution of thrombocytopenia.

Thrombocytopenia Produced by Platelet Sequestration. Normally the spleen contains about one third of the circulating pool of platelets. Increased splenic sequestration occurs with splenomegaly; very large spleens may sequester up to 90 per cent of the circulating platelets, resulting in a moderate thrombocytopenia of 50,000 to 100,000/cu mm. Platelet lifespan, however, is not shortened in hypersplenism, and severe hemorrhage is unusual.

Dilutional thrombocytopenia can follow massive transfusion of whole blood or plasma and lasts for several days. Platelet transfusions may be needed if the patient's residual platelets are dysfunctional or if bone marrow function is depressed and there is threatened or actual hemorrhage; the condition is transient in patients with normal marrow function.

Thrombocytosis

Elevation of the platelet count above 500,000/µl may be physiologic, secondary to bleeding, trauma, or infection, or can result from a primary bone marrow disease (thrombocythemia or other myeloproliferative disease). Transitory thrombocytosis follows stress or exercise and represents mobilization of platelets from the spleen or lung under the influence of epinephrine (Table 55–5).

Secondary, or reactive, *thrombocytosis* results from increased platelet production in response to hemorrhage, hemolysis, infection (such as tuberculosis), inflammatory disease, or malignancy. The platelets are normal in function and the platelet count may reach 10^6/µl. A similar secondary thrombocytosis follows splenectomy and lasts for several weeks. In general, secondary thrombocytosis does not lead to hemorrhagic or thrombotic complications. Therapy to lower the platelet count or inhibit platelet function is not necessary. Treatment of the underlying disease usually results in a return of the platelet count to normal levels.

Primary thrombocytosis, or thrombocythemia, represents increased platelet production independent of normal regulatory control, except that the platelet count can increase further after hemorrhage. Platelet counts may exceed 1 to 2 $\times$ 10^6/µl. The platelets are large and bizarre in appearance, may appear in clumps on the blood smear, and are dysfunctional. The number of epinephrine receptors is decreased, and platelet aggregation responses to epinephrine are abnormal.

TABLE 55–5. CAUSES OF THROMBOCYTOSIS

Acute stress (release of splenic pool)
Secondary to inflammatory disease or infection: tuberculosis, rheumatoid arthritis, chronic inflammatory bowel disease, malignancy
Postsplenectomy
Myeloproliferative disease (primary thrombocytosis)

Other metabolic abnormalities are also present. Both the platelet mass and megakaryocyte mass are markedly increased, and megakaryocyte morphology may be abnormal. Clusters of megakaryocytes are frequently present in the marrow and may be found in the spleen and lung as well. The clinical course of primary thrombocytosis manifests both hemorrhage and thrombosis, both complications occurring in the same patient and without relation to the actual platelet count. Thrombocythemia usually occurs in myeloproliferative diseases such as chronic myelocytic leukemia, myelofibrosis, and polycythemia but may occur alone (essential thrombocythemia). Because of the high rate of hemostatic complications in these conditions, control of the platelet count with hydroxyurea or busulfan is generally employed. Antiplatelet therapy with low dose aspirin is often used, as the risk of gastric bleeding with higher doses of aspirin is increased. Mucous membrane bleeding and hemorrhage or thrombosis with surgery are common clinical complications. Even when the platelet count is controlled by chemotherapy, platelet dysfunction persists. Plateletpheresis for very rapid control of platelet counts can be used in emergency settings, but it only transiently reduces platelet number. In *erythromelalgia*, aspirin dramatically relieves the painful erythema of the extremities related to intravascular platelet aggregation. This condition is a premyeloproliferative disorder with thrombocytosis.

In thrombocythemias, the increased platelet mass results in several abnormalities in serum values because of release of platelet constituents during blood clotting: serum potassium, lactic dehydrogenase, acid phosphatase, and zinc levels are elevated, while plasma levels are normal.

QUALITATIVE PLATELET DISORDERS

Inherited defects in platelet function are rare and produce mucosal bleeding when severe. Acquired defects in platelet function are common and are chiefly associated with drug ingestion—particularly of aspirin—or with underlying hematologic disease. They become clinically important if accompanied by another hemostatic defect, such as thrombocytopenia, or during therapy with anticoagulants. Acquired platelet function defects may also cause excessive bleeding at surgery. Evaluation of platelet disorders requires specialized testing (Table 55–6).

Congenital platelet disorders include *thrombasthenia* (Glanzmann's syndrome), characterized by a prolonged bleeding time, absent platelet aggregation despite normal platelet adhesion to collagen, and episodes of mucosal bleeding. The disorder is transmitted by an autosomal recessive gene. Thrombasthenic platelets lack two surface glycoproteins (IIb and IIIa) necessary for fibrinogen binding to the platelet membrane and for platelet aggregation. Bleeding may be life-threatening. The only therapy is transfusion of normal platelets. *Platelet-release defects* resulting in impaired platelet aggregation comprise several syn-

TABLE 55–6. LABORATORY EVALUATION OF PLATELET DISORDERS: CBC, PLATELET COUNT, AND PERIPHERAL SMEAR EXAMINATION

Low Platelet Count

1. Bone marrow examination	Increased megas:	ITP, immune purpura
	Decreased megas:	Drug, aplasia, infection
2. Screen for DIC		Sepsis, malignancy
3. Platelet associated IgG		
4. Serum folate and B_{12}		

Normal Platelet Count

1. Bleeding time	if prolonged:	Thrombasthenia, uremia, drug ingestion (aspirin)
2. Platelet aggregation	if depressed:	Aspirin, other drugs, uremia, DIC
3. Platelet agglutination with ristocetin	if depressed:	von Willebrand's disease
4. Factor VIII: AHF and Factor VIII: VWF	if depressed:	von Willebrand's disease
5. Platelet procoagulant activity	if decreased:	Thrombocytopathy, uremia

High Platelet Count

1. Bone marrow examination		Myeloproliferative disease, malignancy
2. Platelet aggregation	if absent to epi:	Myeloproliferative disease
3. Peripheral smear	if normal sized platelets:	Secondary thrombocytosis
	if giant platelets:	Primary thrombocytosis is likely

dromes. First, a mild bleeding tendency results from an "aspirin-like" defect in which all platelet structures are normal, but normal activation does not take place when platelets are exposed to the usual agonists. The causes of this syndrome include defective phospholipase activation or a deficiency in enzymes of the prostaglandin pathway, such as cyclooxygenase or thromboxane synthase. Several types of *storage-pool deficiency* present with impaired platelet-release reactions, associated with poor platelet aggregation, a long bleeding time, and mucosal bleeding. The storage pool deficiencies are varied: they comprise defects in platelet granule storage of ADP or serotonin or abnormalities in platelet granule structure. In the *Hermansky-Pudlak syndrome*, platelet granule abnormalities are associated with albinism. An acquired storage pool defect occurs after exposure of blood to extracorporeal circulation and, rarely, in myeloproliferative disease. Since ADP release is necessary for normal platelet function, defective storage or release results in a hemorrhagic tendency. Bleeding episodes in affected patients are usually limited to trauma, surgery, or childbirth. Aspirin and nonsteroidal aspirin-like drugs should be avoided. As in thrombasthenia, platelet transfusion provides the only therapy.

Platelet adhesion is abnormal in two inherited bleeding disorders: von Willebrand's disease and the Bernard-Soulier syndrome. *Von Willebrand's disease* is a common bleeding disorder that affects both sexes and is transmitted as an autosomal recessive trait. In this condition, platelets are normal in structure and number but fail to adhere to the vascular subendothelium because of the lack of a plasma factor essential for platelet interaction with collagen in the vessel wall. The von Willebrand's factor (VWF), which is synthesized in vascular endothelial cells and in megakaryocytes, normally circulates in a macromolecular complex with coagulation Factor VIII. In addition to decreased, absent, or abnormal VWF, patients with von Willebrand's disease also have decreased coagulation Factor VIII. In von Willebrand's disease, laboratory findings include a prolonged bleeding time, poor platelet adhesion, and normal platelet aggregation, but absent agglutination of platelets by the antibiotic ristocetin, which requires VWF. The clinical manifestations include mucosal bleeding, menorrhagia, and bruising. Both laboratory and clinical abnormalities are corrected by administration of VWF. Further discussion of von Willebrand's disease follows the discussion of hemophilia A.

In *Bernard-Soulier syndrome*, a very rare autosomal recessive disease, giant platelets are observed on the blood smear, the bleeding time is prolonged, and mucosal hemorrhage is common. A platelet membrane glycoprotein (Ib) that mediates VWF binding is absent. Plasma VWF is normal, but VWF cannot correct defective platelet adhesion in the absence of the platelet receptor. Treatment is limited to platelet transfusion.

The gray-platelet syndrome consists of a lack of platelet alpha granules containing VWF, fibronectin and thrombospondin, the proteins necessary for normal platelet adhesion and aggregation. Their deficiency leads to a mild bleeding tendency, correctable by platelet transfusion.

Thrombocytopathy or impaired expression of platelet procoagulant activity, i.e., the acceleration of thrombin formation by the surface of activated platelets, produces a mild bleeding tendency mainly following trauma or surgery.

ACQUIRED DISORDERS OF PLATELET FUNCTION

Aspirin and other nonsteroidal anti-inflammatory drugs inhibit platelet cyclooxygenase, the key enzyme in transformation of platelet arachidonic acid to products that induce platelet aggregation, the cyclic endoperoxides and thromboxane A_2. These substances mediate the normal platelet release reaction initiated by platelet agonists such as ADP, epinephrine, or collagen. After contact with aspirin or similar drugs, platelets exhibit impaired aggregation and release, the bleeding time is moderately prolonged, and the number of microaggregates of platelets detectable in the blood is diminished. The duration of these platelet effects of the nonsteroidal anti-inflammatory drugs varies widely. Only aspirin, by virtue of covalent acetylation of cyclooxygenase at its active site, has a prolonged effect on platelet function (since platelets do not synthesize enzymes as they circulate, one dose of aspirin inhibits platelet function for up to a week); other nonsteroidal anti-inflammatory drugs have antiplatelet effects lasting less than 24 hours. Thrombin-induced platelet activation is unaffected by aspirin or similar drugs, accounting for the limited hemorrhagic tendency produced by these agents. However, when a second defect of hemostasis exists, such as hemophilia, thrombocytopenia, or anticoagulant therapy, ingestion of aspirin may lead to serious bleeding.

Acquired defects in platelet function can accompany several types of systemic diseases. *Uremia* produces a hemorrhagic tendency with epistaxes, ecchymosis, and gastrointestinal bleeding related to platelet dysfunction and often to thrombocytopenia. Platelet aggregation and platelet procoagulant activity are both abnormal and the bleeding time is prolonged. Accumulation of toxic metabolites in the plasma may be partly responsible for these dysfunctions, as may be an inadequate synthesis of thromboxane. Hemodialysis tends to improve platelet function. Infusion of cryoprecipitate or administration of estrogens has been reported to correct the hemostatic abnormalities. *Paraproteinemias* such as *multiple myeloma* can induce bleeding by coating the platelet surface with monoclonal immunoglobulin, which prevents platelet-platelet interaction, and by interfering with fibrin polymerization. In *leukemias* and *myeloproliferative syndromes*, defects in platelet function are common. In DIC, the presence of fibrin split products in the circulating blood also can impair platelet function (Table 55–6).

Laboratory findings distinguish *vascular purpuras* from purpuras directly involving the components of the hemostatic mechanism. The typical findings in vascular purpura include an abnormal tourniquet test (positive Rumpel-Leede test), indicating increased capillary fragility, and prolonged bleeding time in the presence of a normal platelet count, normal platelet function, and normal coagulation screen. Congenital vascular purpura is found in inherited diseases of connective tissue. Acquired vascular purpura can occur in paraproteinemias, scurvy, Cushing's disease or corticosteroid treatment, in association with other drugs, or in old age. In children, *Henoch-Schönlein purpura* is an allergic-type vasculitis manifested by abdominal pain, hematuria and glomerulonephritis, hemorrhagic urticaria and arthralgias.

Bleeding in *hereditary hemorrhagic telangiectasia* (Osler-Weber-Rendu disease) results from fragile, easily bleeding mucosal telangiectases. This disorder is inherited as an autosomal dominant trait in which the vascular abnormalities continue to form throughout life, becoming more prominent after puberty. All mucosal surfaces may be involved, with bleeding commonly originating from the nose and from the respiratory, gastrointestinal, and genitourinary tracts. Pulmonary arteriovenous fistulae are common (15 per cent). Telangiectases may or may not be present on the skin. The mainstays of treatment are cauterization of accessible lesions, vigorous iron replacement therapy to correct continual blood loss, and efforts at maintaining local hemostasis.

REFERENCES

Bachmann F: Diagnostic approach to mild bleeding disorders. Semin Hematol 17:292, 1980.

Colman RW, Hirsh J, Marder V, and Salzman EW (eds): Hemostasis and Thrombosis: Basic Principles and Clinical Practice. Philadelphia, JB Lippincott Co, 1982.

McKee PA: Hereditary disorders of hemostasis. In Stanbury JB, Wyngaarden JB, Frederickson DS, Goldstein JS, and Brown MS (eds): The Metabolic Basis of Inherited Disease. 5th ed. New York, McGraw-Hill Book Co, 1983, pp 1531–1560.

Rickles FR, and Edwards RI: Activation of blood coagulation in cancer. Trousseau's syndrome revisited. Blood 62:14, 1983.

Rosenberg RD, and Rosenberg, JS: Natural anticoagulant mechanisms. J Clin Invest 74:1, 1984.

56 COAGULATION DISORDERS

THE BLOOD CLOTTING MECHANISM

Blood clotting involves the generation of a powerful serine protease, thrombin, which cleaves the soluble plasma protein fibrinogen so that an insoluble meshwork of fibrin strands develops, enmeshing red cells and platelets to form a stable clot (Table 56–1). This process is triggered by injury to the blood vessels and involves the rapid, highly controlled interaction of more than 20 different proteins to amplify initial activation of a few molecules to an appropriately sized, fully developed clot (see Fig. 55–1). Both the injured vessel wall and platelet aggregates provide specialized surfaces that localize and catalyze the coagulation reactions.

Blood coagulation proteins circulate as inactive zymogens in amounts far greater than required for blood clotting. Two activation pathways are rec-

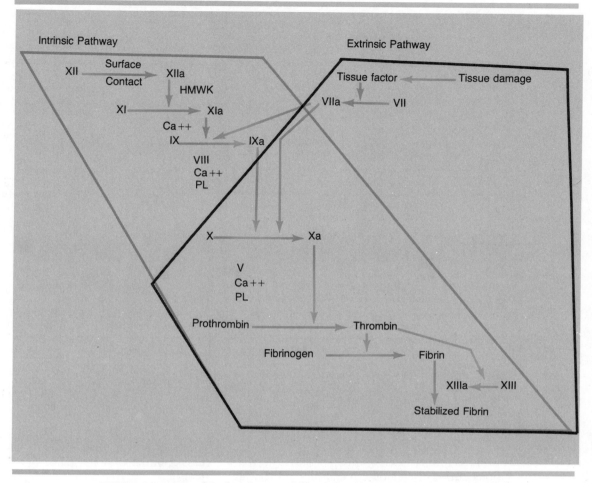

FIGURE 56–1. Simplified pathways of blood coagulation. The area inside the blue line is the intrinsic pathway, measured by APTT. The area inside the black line is the extrinsic pathway, measured by PT. The area encompassed by both lines is the common pathway.

ognized: an intrinsic pathway and an extrinsic pathway; the latter requires participation of a lipoprotein activity released from injured tissues: tissue factor (Fig. 56–1). These pathways converge in the activation of Factor X at the platelet surface. Most of the blood coagulation proteins are serine proteases that show a high degree of homology; others are cofactors without enzyme activity (Factors V and VIII).

The intrinsic pathway of coagulation begins by activation of Factor XII upon the altered vascular surface (endothelium, subendothelium) or another negatively charged surface such as glass. Cofactors or promoters of Factor XII activation include prekallikrein, high molecular weight kininogen (HMWK), and Factor XI. A surface-localized complex is formed which optimally activates Factor XII. Factor XIIa then converts complex-bound Factor XI to its active form XIa and prekallikrein to its active form, kallikrein, which then cleaves HMWK to form bradykinin. In turn, Factor XIa activates Factor IX but may also activate Factor VII (in the extrinsic coagulation pathway) as well as cleaving plasminogen to form plasmin, thus initiating fibrinolysis as well as coagulation.

Factor XIa requires calcium ions (Ca^{++}) to activate Factor IX, which binds to Factor VIII (antihemophilic factor). In the presence of Ca^{++} and phospholipid, IXa activates Factor X to Xa. This activation usually takes place at the plasma membrane of stimulated platelets but also may occur on the vascular endothelium.

In the extrinsic pathway, the release of tissue factor from injured tissues directly activates Factors VII, which then activates Factor X to Xa in the presence of Ca^{++}. In addition, the complex tissue factor–Factor VIII–Ca^{++} can activate Factor XI.

Assembly of the plasma prothrombinase complex on the surface of activated platelets in the presence of Factor V, another cofactor specifically bound to the platelet membrane, enhances the efficiency of prothrombin (Factor II) activation to thrombin on the platelet surface. Thrombin acts upon fibrinogen, a large, asymmetric, soluble protein (MW 340,000) consisting of three pairs of polypeptide chains: Aα, Bβ, and G. Thrombin then

TABLE 56–1. BLOOD COAGULATION FACTORS

GROUP	MODE OF ACTION	PLASMA CONCENTRATION (μg/ml)	HALF-LIFE (hours)	COMMENTS
Contact Factors				
XII (Hageman)	Serine protease	<5	50	Deficiency does not produce bleeding tendency
XI	Serine protease	<5	60	
Prekallikrein	Serine protease	30		Do not require Ca^{++} to act
High molecular weight kininogen	—	80		Do not require Vitamin K Stable, well preserved in plasma
Prothrombin Group				
II (prothrombin)	Serine protease	150	72	All vitamin K–dependent
VII	Serine protease	<1	3–5	Require Ca^{++} for activity
IX (Christmas factor)	Serine protease	3	24	Not consumed in serum (except prothrombin)
X	Serine protease	<5	40	Stable
Protein C	Serine protease			
Protein S	?			
Fibrinogen Group				
I (fibrinogen)	Soluble protein	2500	72–96	All interact with thrombin
V	Cofactor	10	15–30	Activity is lost on clotting
VIII	Cofactor	trace	3–6	Increase in inflammation, pregnancy, birth control pill
XIII	Transglutaminase	10	>100	V, VIII unstable in stored plasma

cleaves small peptides from the Aα chain of fibrinogen to form Fibrin I, which polymerizes end to end; further thrombin cleavage of small peptides from the Bβ chain leads to formation of Fibrin II, which polymerizes side to side and is then cross-linked via the plasma glutaminase (Factor XIII) to form an insoluble fibrin clot.

Thrombin has several different and critical actions during coagulation in addition to the cleavage of fibrinogen to fibrin. It activates platelets, exposing their procoagulant activity (e.g., binding sites for the prothrombinase complex) and inducing the release of platelet-aggregating substances such as thromboxane, Ca^{++}, ADP, von Willebrand factor, fibronectin, and thrombospondin. Thrombin cleaves Factors VIII and Va, augmenting clotting, and Factor XIII, promoting fibrin stabilization. Thrombin acts on the endothelium by binding to the surface protein thrombomodulin to activate protein C, a potent inactivator of Factors Va and VIIIa which also stimulates fibrinolysis. Thrombin also causes endothelial cell contraction. Conversely, endothelium can bind and in-

activate thrombin, and in some cases can generate the vasodilatory substance prostacyclin in response to thrombin. Thus, thrombin activation contributes to the limitation as well as the initiation of clotting.

The final stage of the coagulation process is fibrinolysis, or clot resolution (Fig. 56–2). This process is initiated by the action of thrombin during clotting, including activation of protein C and the initiation of release of plasminogen activators from the blood vessel wall. Protein C, together with protein S, a promoter of its action, inhibits the coagulant activity of Factors Va and VIIIa. The circulating zymogen, plasminogen, is cleaved to the active protease, plasmin, by plasminogen activators. Plasmin then digests fibrin. The activity of tissue plasminogen activators is enhanced by their binding to fibrin, so that plasmin generation is localized to the clot. In addition the plasma protease inhibitors α$_1$-antitrypsin, α$_2$-plasmin inhibitor, and α$_2$-macroglobulin rapidly inactivate any circulating serine protease including thrombin and plasmin. Antithrombin III binds all the serine protease procoagulant proteins (Factor Xa as well as thrombin); its activity is enhanced by heparin or heparin-like substances. Complexes of antithrombin III and protease are rapidly cleared by the liver and the reticuloendothelial system.

The liver is the site of synthesis for most of the coagulation proteins. Factors II, VII, IX, and X and proteins C and S require vitamin K for their synthesis. In the absence of vitamin K, abnormal molecules lacking the γ-carboxyglutamate binding sites for Ca^{++} binding are produced. These abnormal molecules do not function in clotting. Fibrinogen, Factor V, and the protease inhibitors are also produced in the liver, and their levels may be depressed in liver disease. Vitamin K is not

FIGURE 56–2. Fibrinolysis.

required for their synthesis or function. Factor VIII is probably synthesized in the liver, but the precise location of its production is not known. Von Willebrand factor and tissue plasminogen activator are produced in the vascular endothelium. While von Willebrand factor and Factor VIII circulate together as a macromolecular complex, they are produced in different sites, are regulated by different genes, and are completely different in structure and function.

SCREENING FOR DISORDERS OF BLOOD COAGULATION

A history of bleeding upon trauma or surgery, severe epistaxes, muscle or joint bleeding, or large ecchymoses arouse suspicion of a coagulation disorder. A family history of only affected males points to one of the hemophilias, whereas the other congenital coagulation disorders are transmitted as autosomal recessive traits. The most important screening tests are the prothrombin time and activated partial thromboplastin time (see Table 55–3); the bleeding time is generally normal in plasma coagulation disorders except for von Willebrand's disease, in which the deficient factor affects platelet function, and therefore primary hemostasis is also impaired. The prothrombin time measures activity of Factors II, VII, IX, and X; the activated partial thromboplastin time measures Factors XII, XI, IX, VIII, and X. Both tests measure Factors V and II and fibrinogen. A history of delayed bleeding or rebleeding suggests Factor XIII deficiency, which requires specific testing of the stability of the fibrin clot (e.g., in 8M urea) for detection. The pattern of abnormalities and the ability of normal plasma or serum to correct them permits more specific identification of factor deficiencies or circulatory anticoagulants. Specific factor assays are available for confirmation and quantification of the various deficiencies.

INHERITED DISORDERS OF BLOOD COAGULATION

Hemophilia A

Classic hemophilia is the most common severe, inherited coagulation disorder. The gene for Factor VIII has recently been cloned and sequenced. It is an unusually large gene occupying 0.1 per cent of the length of the X chromosome. In 70 per cent of cases of hemophilia A a positive family history of affected males is obtained; the gene appears to have a high rate of spontaneous mutation, accounting for the remaining 30 per cent of cases. Because of the random inactivation of one X chromosome in females, the carrier mother of a hemophiliac has a 50 per cent (on the average) level of Factor VIII. Identification of the carrier state can frequently be made. Prenatal diagnosis can now be carried out in pregnancies at risk, and development of restriction polymorphism techniques for identifying hemophilic fetuses is now possible since the Factor VIII gene has been cloned. Lab-

oratory results in hemophilia A show a normal PT, markedly prolonged APTT corrected by mixing with normal plasma, and a normal bleeding time. Specific assay for Factor VIII shows a deficient level of functional activity. Hemophilia A can represent both a quantitative deficiency and a dysfunctional molecule, so that both functional and immunologic assays need to be combined. About half of affected patients have severe hemophilia with Factor VIII activity less than 1 per cent of normal; they have spontaneous and trauma-induced hemorrhage from infancy. Levels above 5 per cent are associated with a mild clinical course except with trauma or surgery, when supportive therapy is necessary. As the hemophilic child becomes physically active, bleeding into muscles and joints is common, and painful deformities follow. Bleeding is frequently spontaneous or may be related to stress or other illness. Any organ can be affected, and pressure on vital structures from deep hemorrhages can be life-threatening.

Replacement therapy with concentrates of Factor VIII to raise the plasma Factor VIII to hemostatic levels has become a mainstay of treatment. In home therapy programs, the hemophilic patient or his parent administers Factor VIII concentrate according to a preset schedule based on bleeding severity. This approach prevents delay in treatment following onset of bleeding and can reduce morbidity, cost of therapy, and emotional stress. Reconstructive joint surgery and dental care can also be undertaken with such replacement coverage. A high incidence of hepatitis, however, accompanies extensive use of commercial Factor VIII concentrates. Moreover, transmission of more than 80 cases of AIDS to hemophilic patients receiving replacement therapy with Factor VIII concentrates (presumably carrying HLTV-3 virus) has been documented. This requires caution in giving Factor VIII replacement therapy until recombinant Factor VIII becomes available.

Factor VIII has a short half-life (8 to 12 hours); infusion schedules are calculated according to the patient's plasma volume (40 ml/kg), the severity of the bleeding episode, and the per cent of normal Factor VIII level desired to control each type of bleeding. About 20 per cent of patients develop inhibitors to transfused Factor VIII and have accelerated destruction and decreased efficacy of the replacement therapy. Such inhibitory activity must be taken into account when calculating Factor VIII replacement needs.

For milder hemophiliacs or during episodes of less severe hemorrhage, cryoprecipitate may suffice. Epsilon-aminocaproic acid, a potent inhibitor of fibrinolysis, diminishes bleeding after dental procedures. In addition to replacement of Factor VIII, local therapy such as joint immobilization and ice packs is helpful. For relief of pain, hemophiliacs should avoid aspirin and nonsteroidal anti-inflammatory drugs, which impair platelet function and worsen bleeding. Acetaminophen, codeine, or choline-magnesium salicylate should be used, as these analgesics do not affect platelets and thus preserve primary hemostasis.

The long-term complications of hemophilia include (1) hemorrhage; (2) progressive arthropathy; (3) development of inhibitor to Factor VIII; (4) hepatitis; (5) hypertension; and (6) AIDS. While in recent years the lifespan of hemophiliacs has markedly increased and morbidity lessened, hemorrhage still remains the major cause of death.

Von Willebrand's Disease (VWD)

This is one of the most common inherited bleeding disorders. It affects both sexes and is transmitted as an autosomal codominant or recessive trait. A double defect is observed in this disorder: abnormal platelet adhesion in combination with low Factor VIII procoagulant activity. Normal platelet adhesion to vascular subendothelium requires the presence of the plasma glycoprotein, von Willebrand factor (VWF). VWF circulates in the form of high molecular weight multimers (MW $>2 \times 10^6$) complexed with antihemophilic factor (Factor VIII:AHF). In VWD the level of VWF is decreased, absent, or present in a functionally abnormal form. The level of antihemophilic factor may be mildly to severely depressed in VWD. This finding is reflected in the prolonged APTT in addition to the prolonged bleeding time (Table 56–2).

The clinical manifestations of VWD vary widely in the same patient at different times, in different affected members of the same family, and in different families. Mucosal bleeding, ecchymoses, epistaxis, gastrointestinal bleeding, and menorrhagia are common symptoms; severely affected persons may also have hemarthroses and behave like hemophiliacs, with the added complication of defective primary hemostasis. There are several subtypes of von Willebrand's disease. In 75 per cent of patients the bleeding time and APTT are prolonged, with an absolute decrease in the levels of both VWF and Factor VIII:AHF as measured by functional and immunological tests (Type I). Platelet agglutination to ristocetin is impaired but is restored by VWF or normal plasma. Other platelet aggregation responses are normal. All sizes of VWF multimers in plasma are decreased. Infusion of normal plasma (or hemophilic plasma) to Type I VWD patients results in a prolonged rise in VWF levels that is greater and longer lasting than expected from the amount of VWF infused or its half-life. Several variant types of VWD occur in which VWF is only slightly depressed by immunoassay despite a long bleeding time (Type IIA) or in which increased agglutination of platelets by ristocetin is observed and the large multimeric forms of VWF are absent (Type IIB).

Treatment of von Willebrand's disease relies upon cryoprecipitate infusion for severe bleeding episodes and desmopressin for milder disease. The prolonged bleeding time and hemorrhagic diathesis are corrected by transfusion of normal plasma or cryoprecipitate (which is rich in VWF). In mild VWD, infusion of desmopressin (DDAVP, des-amino, des-argininne vasopressin) can raise VWF levels and correct the bleeding tendency. Desmopressin can be used before dental or other surgery in many cases. Most commercial Factor VIII concentrates contain low levels of VWF and are not effective therapy in VWD. In women with severe VWD, menorrhagia can be managed by hormonal suppression. The bleeding tendency may improve during pregnancy when the levels of VWF and antihemophilic factor rise. Aspirin and similar drugs should be completely avoided by patients with VWD.

INHERITED DISORDERS OF OTHER COAGULATION FACTORS

Contact factor deficiencies are rare disorders that produce prolongation of the APTT or clotting time without any clinical bleeding tendency, except for Factor XI deficiency. *Factor XII (Hageman factor) deficiency* is suspected when the clotting time or APTT is prolonged in an asymptomatic patient. This diagnosis is confirmed by mixing experiments, in which the patient's plasma is mixed with plasma from patients with known specific factor deficiencies to determine the type of defect (e.g., in Factor XII deficiency there is no correction of APTT upon mixing with known Factor XII deficient plasma, but the APTT becomes normal after mixing 1:1 with known Factor XI deficient plasma). *Prekallikrein deficiency (Fletcher trait)* and *high molecular*

TABLE 56–2. COMPARISON OF HEMOPHILIA A, HEMOPHILIA B, AND VON WILLEBRAND'S DISEASE

	HEMOPHILIA A	HEMOPHILIA B	VON WILLEBRAND'S DISEASE
Inheritance	X-linked	X-linked	Autosomal dominant or recessive
Factor deficiency	VIII (coagulant) (= VIII:AHF)	IX	von Willebrand's factor and VIII:AHF
Bleeding sites	muscle, joints, surgical	muscle, joints, surgical	mucous membranes, skin, surgical
Prothrombin time (PT)	normal	normal	normal
Partial thromboplastin time (APTT)	prolonged	prolonged	prolonged or normal
Bleeding time	normal	normal	prolonged
Factor VIII coagulant activity	low	normal	low
Factor VIII antigen (VIII:VWF)	normal	normal	low
Factor IX	normal	low	normal
Platelet aggregation	normal	normal	normal
Ristocetin-induced platelet agglutination	normal	normal	impaired

weight kininogen deficiency (Fitzgerald trait) are also asymptomatic, rare conditions. A bleeding tendency, however, does exist in persons with Factor XI (or PTA) deficiency when they undergo trauma, dental extraction, or surgery. This autosomal recessive trait is most common in persons of Jewish or Japanese origin. The APTT is prolonged, the PT normal. The bleeding tendency does not correlate well with the calculated deficiency of Factor XI, and some patients with low values have no bleeding problems. The half-life of Factor XI is about three days, so that treatment of bleeding or prophylaxis for surgery consists of daily infusion of fresh frozen plasma.

Deficiencies of the vitamin K–dependent coagulation factors cause severe bleeding tendencies. The only common example is Factor IX deficiency (hemophilia B, or Christmas disease), an X-linked recessive trait that is clinically similar to hemophilia A, producing muscle, joint, gastrointestinal, and central nervous system bleeding. A quantitative severe deficiency of Factor IX is the usual finding, but some families possess a functionally abnormal Factor IX molecule present in the blood in normal levels when measured by antigenic assay. Diagnosis of hemophilia B is suspected when a normal PT but prolonged APTT is observed and the APTT is corrected by normal serum but not by barium-adsorbed plasma (BaSO$_4$ adsorbs the vitamin K–dependent factors from plasma). The diagnosis is confirmed by specific factor assay. Fresh frozen plasma or prothrombin complex concentrates containing Factor IX correct the deficiency and are used to treat bleeding. The plasma half-life of 20 hours permits twice-daily infusion. Factor IX concentrates carry a high risk of transmitting hepatitis and are contaminated with activated coagulation factors. The latter can cause thromboembolism, so that use of prothrombin complex concentrates should be reserved for severe hemorrhage. Specific antibodies to transfused Factor IX develop in 10 to 15 per cent of patients and may complicate management, similarly to acquired Factor VIII inhibitors in hemophilia A.

Factor VII deficiency is a rare autosomal recessive defect, leading to a lifelong history of bleeding in homozygotes: mucous membrane and gastrointestinal bleeding, epistaxes, hemarthroses, and menorrhagia are observed. Individual patients show varied manifestations of bleeding over time. The PT is prolonged with a normal APTT. Since Factor VII is stable, the prolonged PT is corrected by stored plasma but not by BaSO$_4$-adsorbed plasma. Treatment is with plasma or prothrombin complex concentrates; the half-life of Factor VII is short (two to six hours), requiring frequent administration.

Factor X deficiency is another rare autosomal recessive trait that produces bleeding. Two types exist, a quantitative decrease in the factor or a dysfunctional molecule. Epistaxis, gastrointestinal bleeding, and occasionally joint or muscle hemorrhage result. Postpartum bleeding and menorrhagia may be severe in affected women. Both the PT and the APTT are prolonged; a specific factor assay establishes the diagnosis. Treatment is with fresh frozen plasma.

Afibrinogenemia or congenital dysfibrinogenemia represents a variety of disorders in which the plasma fibrinogen level is very low or abnormal fibrinogens are produced. The latter may lead to either hemorrhage or thrombosis. Both the PT and the APTT are abnormal in these disorders. Over 80 different types of dysfibrinogenemia have been described, varying widely in clinical effects. Current replacement therapy consists of cryoprecipitate, which is rich in fibrinogen, since formerly available fibrinogen concentrates carried a very high risk of transmitting hepatitis. The half-life of fibrinogen is four days, so that infusion to reach a normal plasma level of 150 mg/dl can be readily achieved.

Factor XIII deficiency is a rare, autosomal recessive trait in which only the homozygote shows a bleeding tendency, manifested by delayed bleeding after trauma and impaired wound healing. Affected persons usually have less than 1 per cent of the normal Factor XIII level; heterozygotes are asymptomatic. Absence of the fibrin-stabilizing factor also impairs crosslinking of fibronectin, the cell surface protein, and fibrin, which may contribute to poor wound healing. Since the initial formation of fibrin is unimpaired, PT, APTT, and thrombin time are normal. Dissolution of the patient's fibrin clot in 8M urea indicates a Factor XIII level of less than 1 per cent. Treatment is with fresh frozen plasma or cryoprecipitate to reach a Factor XIII level of 10 per cent. The prolonged half-life of the factor (21 days) makes infrequent replacement infusions (every three weeks) effective.

ACQUIRED DISORDERS OF BLOOD COAGULATION

Acquired coagulation abnormalities can result from several causes, including deficient production or increased consumption of clotting factors, production of functionally abnormal molecules, selective inhibition of factors by acquired anticoagulants, and selective inhibition or adsorption of factors, resulting in functional deficiency. The first three mechanisms are common complications of systemic disease, the last two are rare. For example, the adsorption of Factor X by vascular amyloid, producing a severe bleeding diathesis, has been reported in only a few cases.

Acquired Vitamin K Deficiency

Vitamin K–dependent clotting factors are a group of structurally closely related proteins synthesized in the liver, including prothrombin, Factors VII, IX, and X, and proteins C and S. Vitamin K is required for the post-translational gamma carboxylation of glutamyl residues at the amino terminal regions of these clotting factor zymogens, resulting in formation of calcium-binding sites important for normal hemostatic function. Calcium is required for the binding and activation of these factors from zymogen to active serine proteases on the surface of platelets. Vitamin K deficiency prevents the carboxylation of the glutamyl residues and results in functionally abnormal clotting factors. Because of its short half-life, Factor VII activity is the earliest to decrease in vitamin K deficiency or anticoagulation with vitamin K antagonists, followed by decreases in Factors IX and X and prothrombin.

As vitamin K is not stored in the body but is obtained from green vegetables in the diet and is a fat-soluble vitamin, a deficiency of vitamin K occurs in malabsorption or bile-salt deficiency, when dietary intake is poor, and when the gastrointestinal tract is sterilized by antibiotic therapy. Common clinical states producing vitamin K deficiency include (1) in newborn infants, especially premature infants, liver immaturity and lack of synthesis of vitamin K by intestinal bacteria until the gut is colonized; (2) malabsorption, including biliary tract disease; (3) prolonged parenteral feeding in combination with antibiotic therapy, especially bowel sterilization; and (4) ingestion of oral anticoagulants. Vitamin K absorption depends upon fat absorption, and any condition impairing that process (e.g., celiac disease, oral neomycin, cholestyramine, biliary obstruction, regional enteritis) can result in vitamin K deficiency. Mucosal or gastrointestinal bleeding may develop. Oral administration of vitamin K_1 (2 to 10 mg/day) can correct the vitamin deficiency, and 10 to 25 mg IM can correct an overt bleeding tendency.

Coumarin anticoagulants competitively inhibit the effects of vitamin K on gamma carboxylation of the vitamin K–dependent coagulation proteins and thus produce anticoagulation, which is monitored by the PT. The therapeutic goal is to maintain a PT 1.5 to 2 times greater than a normal control, achieved by administering 2.5 to 10 mg of Coumadin (warfarin) once daily. Since many drugs affect the action of coumarins, either directly enhancing or depressing their effect or altering their metabolic disposition, it is essential to monitor coumarin effects carefully during treatment with multiple drugs. Coumarin drugs possess a narrow toxic/therapeutic ratio. Administration of vitamin K can reverse the effects of coumadin anticoagulation within hours, and administration of fresh frozen plasma (or prothrombin concentrates) reverses anticoagulant effects even more rapidly. In emergency circumstances, such as with brain hemorrhage, severe gastrointestinal bleeding, or need for immediate surgery, anticoagulation can be reversed within minutes by Factor IX concentrates or prothrombin complex.

Liver Disease

In addition to the vitamin K–dependent coagulation factors, the liver synthesizes Factor V, fibrinogen, plasminogen, and Factors XII and XI. Patients with advanced liver disease commonly suffer bleeding tendencies. If these mainly involve deficiencies of vitamin K–dependent clotting factors, they are corrected by administering parenteral vitamin K. Bleeding in severe liver disease also results from dysfibrinogenemias, localized DIC, lack of Factor V, increased fibrinolysis, and thrombocytopenia. Treatment of these deficiencies employs fresh frozen plasma.

Renal Disease

Uremia is associated with mucous membrane, gastrointestinal, and skin bleeding. The cause of the bleeding tendency is complex. Thrombocytopenia may be present as part of depressed bone marrow function or may arise secondary to immunosuppressive drugs. Platelet dysfunction is typical and represents thrombocytopathy (impaired platelet procoagulant activity) with depressed platelet adhesion and aggregation, producing a prolonged bleeding time. In the nephrotic syndrome, urinary loss of plasma proteins may result in Factor IX deficiency. In patients undergoing hemodialysis, inaccurate reversal of heparinization at completion of dialysis may also contribute to uremic bleeding.

Disseminated Intravascular Coagulation

DIC represents the consumption of coagulation factors resulting from intravascular activation of the coagulation process with secondary activation of fibrinolysis. Depending upon the rates of these two processes, the compensatory synthesis of procoagulants, and the nature of the underlying disease, DIC may cause either thrombosis or hemorrhage. DIC is always secondary to another disease process and often resolves when the primary disease is controlled. Intravascular coagulation is initiated by release of procoagulant substances into the blood (amniotic fluid embolism, snakebite, abruptio placenta, malignancy, crush injury), by contact of blood with an abnormal surface (infections, burns, extracorporeal circulation, grafts), or by generation of procoagulants in the blood (promyelocytic leukemia, hemolytic transfusion reactions). The formation of microthrombi within the circulation secondarily activates fibrinolysis, as does the presence of injured endothelium. Circulating plasmin may further deplete Factors V and VIII and cleave fibrinogen. The degradation products of both fibrinogen and fibrin (formed by thrombin or plasmin action) act as circulating anticoagulants, delay fibrin polymerization, and impair platelet function.

TABLE 56–3. CLINICAL SETTINGS FOR DISSEMINATED INTRAVASCULAR COAGULATION

ACUTE	CHRONIC
1. Sepsis	1. Visceral malignancy
2. Obstetric emergencies Abruptio placentae Amniotic fluid embolism	2. Large arteriovenous malformations
3. Burns	3. Toxemia
4. Heat stroke	4. Retained dead fetus
5. Shock	5. Malignant hypertension
6. Snakebite	6. Severe liver cirrhosis
7. Promyelocytic leukemia	
8. Hemolytic transfusion reactions	

TABLE 56–4. SCREENING LABORATORY TESTS FOR DIC

1. Prolonged prothrombin time
2. Prolonged partial thromboplastin time
3. Low fibrinogen
4. Thrombocytopenia
5. Presence of fibrin degradation products
6. Depressed Factors V and VIII

Common clinical settings for DIC (Table 56–3) include sepsis, obstetric emergencies, burns, and liver disease. Chronic DIC is characteristic of Trousseau's syndrome, widespread visceral malignancy presenting as migrating superficial thrombophlebitis.

The diagnosis of DIC depends upon a pattern of laboratory test results (Table 56–4). No single test is diagnostic. In acute DIC the typical laboratory results include thrombocytopenia, a prolonged PT and PTT, decreased fibrinogen level, decreased Factors V and VIII, and increased fibrin split products. The thrombin time is also elevated because of the anticoagulant action of the fibrin split products. A microangiopathic hemolytic anemia may be present, resulting from shear damage to red cells passing intravascular fibrin strands. In chronic DIC, compensatory increases in synthesis of coagulation factors may produce normal levels of fibrinogen, Factors V and VIII, and platelets, and the PT and PTT may be normal or even short. However, fibrin split products are usually elevated. Microangiopathic hemolytic anemia is more likely to be present in chronic DIC. Localized DIC may occur in the liver in severe cirrhotic liver disease and in the kidney during malignant hypertension.

Therapy of DIC should be aimed at the underlying disease, for example, by treating sepsis in the infected patient or by emptying the uterus in the case of abruptio placenta. If the symptoms of bleeding or thrombosis are mild, no specific therapy is needed. If DIC produces significant bleeding, replacement of depleted clotting factors using fresh frozen plasma, cryoprecipitate, and platelets may be necessary. If thrombosis is the clinical problem, heparinization may be required (provided that the patient does not have central nervous system bleeding, is not hypertensive, and has not undergone surgery within the past few days). Replacement of fibrinogen and of antithrombin III (as plasma) may also be required. Heparin is generally reserved for cases that fail to respond to other measures. Special situations in which heparin is used include meningococcemia, acute promyelocytic leukemia, and Trousseau's syndrome. Oral anticoagulation cannot be substituted for heparin in the treatment of DIC.

Acquired Circulating Anticoagulants

Antibodies to procoagulants occur in hemophiliacs receiving replacement therapy (see above) as well as in states of disturbed immunity such as systemic lupus erythematosus, lymphoproliferative diseases, the postpartum period, and old age. Acquired inhibitors to Factor VIII:AHF can produce severe hemorrhagic disease. Several cases of inhibitors of von Willebrand's factor causing an acquired von Willebrand's disease have been reported in patients with lymphoma. Very rarely, a heparin-like anticoagulant molecule can circulate, producing a bleeding tendency. In contrast, the "lupus anticoagulant," which is the most common cause of a prolonged APTT in asymptomatic individuals, is rarely associated with a bleeding tendency unless combined with another hemostatic defect, such as thrombocytopenia. Only about half of "lupus anticoagulants" occur in patients with systemic lupus erythematosus. These antibodies are directed against membrane phospholipids or against the phosphodiester bond structure, which is a common chemical moiety in many diverse compounds including DNA, membrane phospholipids, and organic sugars. This circulating anticoagulant is associated with a tendency to thrombosis rather than hemorrhage.

ONCOLOGY

57 | GENERAL CONSIDERATIONS

Cancer comprises a diverse group of more than 100 epidemiologically and pathologically different malignant neoplasms and is second only to cardiovascular diseases as the leading cause of death in the United States.

A neoplasm is a new growth of cells that originates from normal tissue but is relatively unresponsive to normal body and cellular controls. Malignant neoplasms (cancer) differ from their benign counterparts principally in their ability to metastasize (travel) from their original site to new locations in the body.

Not a new phenomenon, cancer was described in early Greek and Roman writings and has been detected in Egyptian mummies 5000 years old. Current statistics suggest that about 30 per cent of Americans now living eventually will develop cancer. Fifty years ago, fewer than one in five would have survived five years after treatment; modern technology has improved five-year survival to three in eight.

ETIOLOGY

Many types of agents are thought to contribute to the malignant transformation of normal cells in a susceptible host.

Carcinogens

A carcinogen is an agent capable of causing direct malignant transformation of a normal human or animal cell. Chemicals (such as benzene), viruses (such as RNA tumor viruses), and physical agents (such as ionizing radiation) all can serve as carcinogens. In order for such agents to cause heritable neoplastic cell transformation, they must alter the structure and function of the cell's DNA.

Co-carcinogens

Following exposure of a cell to a carcinogen, other agents may serve as co-carcinogens, or promotors. While unable to induce cancer alone, they can act in concert with a carcinogen to promote tumor activity and growth. These agents may interact with cell membranes, enter the cell, and activate a critical effector reaction, such as a protein kinase in the case of the potent phorbol esters.

Host Susceptibility

Another key determinant in the development of cancer is host susceptibility, resulting in part from the host's genetic or acquired hormonal milieu, immunological resistance, ability to metabolize carcinogenic precursors, and ability to repair damage to the DNA molecule.

Examples of hereditary syndromes predisposing to the development of cancer are listed in Table 57–1.

Susceptibilities to other types of cancers are inherited directly as autosomal dominant traits. These include forms of retinoblastoma and the multiple endocrine neoplasias.

CANCER EPIDEMIOLOGY AND PREVENTION

Epidemiology, the study of populations, has contributed substantially to our rudimentary understanding of cancer's etiology. The initial leads to epidemiologic investigation often come from astute clinicians who note an excessive number of patients with the same malignancy and trace the "cluster" to a particular cultural, occupational, or environmental exposure. In the eighteenth century, for example, Percivall Pott observed that chimney sweeps exposed to soot were prone to scrotal cancer.

Population-based tumor registries provide international and regional data on tumor sites, stratified by such patient characteristics as age, sex, and ethnic and geographic background. From compilations of these data emerge patterns of occurrence that suggest that 80 to 90 per cent of all cancers are related to environmental influences, particularly those resulting from personal practices such as sun exposure, the use of tobacco products, and diet—implying that the majority of cancers can be prevented.

The most common malignancies in the United States are skin cancers (including squamous and basal cell carcinomas and malignant melanoma). Exposure to ultraviolet radiation from the sun is the dominant risk factor. Major preventive measures include using protective clothing and sunscreen preparations and avoiding sun exposure between 10 A.M. and 3 P.M., when ultraviolet rays are strongest.

Thirty per cent of cancers in the United States (and about 350,000 premature deaths and $27 billion in medical care costs each year) could be prevented if Americans simply stopped smoking.

Some clues to the dietary causes of cancer are based on international variations in cancer inci-

TABLE 57–1. SOME HEREDITARY SYNDROMES PREDISPOSING TO MALIGNANCY

SYNDROME	NEOPLASMS	PROPOSED MECHANISMS
Ataxia-telangiectasia	Lymphoma, leukemia	Chromosomal fragility, ineffective DNA repair
X-linked lymphoproliferative syndrome	Immunoblastic sarcoma, B cell lymphoma, plasmacytoma	Abnormal response to EBV infection
Xeroderma pigmentosa	Skin cancers	Defective repair of DNA damaged by UV light

dence. For example, colon cancer in Japan is far less common than in the United States. Japanese immigrants to the United States develop colon cancer at rates higher than their relatives remaining in Japan, and the rates in their American-born children approximate those of white Americans. These facts suggest that the lower incidence of colon cancer in Japan results from environmental rather than genetic influences.

Clues from such population-based statistics lead to working hypotheses on the causes of cancer. Some scientists suggest, for example, that the American diet is the primary cause of high colon cancer rates. Compared to the Japanese diet, the lower fiber and higher fat content cause slower transit through the gut, allowing more time and providing both more substrates for the formation of carcinogens and more prolonged contact of those carcinogens with the gut mucosa. Many such nutritional hypotheses are under study, but the mechanisms are complex and will take years to elucidate fully. From current working hypotheses come the following possibilities:

1. Lowering dietary fat may decrease the risk of colon, breast, endometrial, and renal cancers.
2. Adequate amounts of vitamin A, carotene, and selenium may protect against lung cancer.
3. Adequate amounts of vitamin C–rich fruits and vegetables may inhibit the formation of carcinogenic nitrosamines in the stomach.
4. Adequate amounts of indole-rich cruciferous vegetables (e.g., cabbage, Brussels sprouts, cauliflower) may decrease the risk of colon cancer.

Such working hypotheses are further investigated using "case-control" studies (in which past experiences and exposures of persons with cancer are compared to persons who are cancer-free) and by monitoring cancer incidence in laboratory animals exposed to agents and conditions suspected of being carcinogenic.

True cause and effect relationships between environmental factors and the cancers they produce in man can, however, be proven only by "cohort" studies, in which large groups of persons with and without already-defined exposures and characteristics are followed for cancer incidence over very long periods of time.

Examples of environmental agents showing a relation to cancer induction and promotion are listed in Table 57–2.

SCREENING FOR EARLY DETECTION

Even if the means of preventing all cancers were currently available, large portions of the population would already have been exposed to precipitating factors and would continue to develop disease well into the twenty-first century. Since earlier detection may increase the likelihood of cure, improved prognosis could depend upon screening for evidence of asymptomatic, early cancer.

TABLE 57–2. SOME ENVIRONMENTAL CAUSES OF CANCER*

AGENT	SITE
Alcoholic beverages	Mouth, pharynx, esophagus, larynx, liver
Alkylating agents	Leukemia
Androgen-anabolic steroids	Liver
Aromatic amines	Bladder
Arsenic (inorganic)	Lung, skin, liver (angiosarcoma)
Asbestos	Lung, pleura, peritoneum, gastrointestinal
Benzene	Leukemia
Estrogens	
Synthetic (DES)	Vagina, cervix (adenocarcinoma)
Conjugated (Premarin)	Endometrium
Steroid contraceptives	Liver (benign)
Immunosuppressives	Histiocytic lymphoma, squamous carcinoma of skin, soft tissue sarcomas
Ionizing radiation	Nearly all sites
Mustard gas	Lung, larynx, nasal sinuses
Nickel dust	Lung, nasal sinuses
Phenacetin	Renal pelvis
Polycyclic hydrocarbons	Lung, squamous carcinoma of skin
Tobacco products	Mouth, lung, larynx, pharynx, esophagus, bladder, pancreas, kidney
Ultraviolet radiation	Skin (including melanoma)
Vinyl chloride	Liver (angiosarcoma)
Wood dusts	Nasal sinuses

* Adapted from Fraumeni JF Jr: Epidemiology of cancer. In Wyngaarden JB, and Smith LH Jr (eds): Cecil Textbook of Medicine. 17th ed. Philadelphia, WB Saunders Co, 1985, p 1070.

Screening asymptomatic populations must take into account cost-benefit ratios. Costs include not only the dollar cost to society, but also the risk to the individual of the screening procedure itself. Costs can be reduced by using epidemiologically derived data to restrict the screening to (1) those individuals at highest risk of developing cancer and (2) those cancers whose early detection and treatment lead to significantly increased survival.

Using available epidemiologic data and cost-benefit estimates, the American Cancer Society recommends screening as detailed in Table 57–3. Only one of the recommendations results from an adequately controlled, randomized, prospective clinical trial: the annual use of mammography and physical examination to detect breast cancer in women aged 40 to 65. The remaining recommendations are based on evaluation of less complete data.

Note that routine chest x-rays and sputum cytology are not included in these recommendations. Studies have not demonstrated that earlier detection of lung cancer by these means improves survival.

At the time of the routine physical examination, it is reasonable to evaluate simple, readily available, and relatively inexpensive blood and urine tests. A complete blood count might uncover a hypochromic, microcytic anemia suggestive of occult gastrointestinal blood loss. Serum chemistries might reveal tumor-related hypercalcemia. Microscopic hematuria might lead to the diagnosis of surgically curable cancer of the urinary tract.

TABLE 57–3. AMERICAN CANCER SOCIETY RECOMMENDATIONS FOR SCREENING OF ASYMPTOMATIC INDIVIDUALS

TEST	SEX	AGE	FREQUENCY
Sigmoidoscopy	M & F	over 50	every 3–5 years after 2 negative exams 1 year apart
Stool guaiac test	M & F	over 50	every year
Digital rectal exam	M & F	over 40	every year
PAP test	F	20–65; under 20 if sexually active	at least every 3 years after 2 negative exams 1 year apart
Pelvic exam	F	20–40	every 3 years
		over 40	every year
Endometrial tissue sample	F	at menopause if high risk[1]	at menopause as indicated
Breast self-exam	F	over 20	every month
Breast physical exam	F	20–40	every 3 years
		over 40	every year
Mammography	F	35–40	one baseline study
		over 50	every year
		under 50[2]	as indicated
Health counseling	M & F	over 20	every 3 years
Cancer check-up[3]	M & F	over 40	every year

[1] History of infertility, obesity, failure of ovulation, abnormal uterine bleeding, or estrogen therapy
[2] Special high-risk groups
[3] To include examination for cancers of the thyroid, testicles, prostate, ovaries, lymph nodes, oral region, and skin

Tumor Markers

Physical examination and routine radiological diagnostic tests are rarely able to detect tumor masses of less than 1 cu cm, which are composed of approximately one billion tumor cells. Researchers have thus sought more sensitive measures of tumor-specific products—"tumor markers"—in body fluids.

The ideal tumor marker would be absent in normal persons, unequivocably positive and localizing in an otherwise undetectable, specific type of malignancy, and quantitatively reflective of total tumor burden. Such a marker might then be used in screening asymptomatic populations for an occult neoplasm. Unfortunately, no such marker is yet available.

Certain tumor products can be used as markers in a more limited manner, especially in following response to treatment of a known cancer and in providing early evidence of recurrence during or after treatment. The readily available serum markers listed in Table 57–4 can be used in these limited ways but are too insensitive and nonspecific to be used in the screening of asymptomatic populations.

BIOLOGIC EFFECTS OF TUMORS

Whether localized or widely metastatic, cancer eventually produces symptoms. Pain and disa-

TABLE 57–4. TUMOR MARKERS USEFUL IN FOLLOWING KNOWN MALIGNANCIES*

TUMOR MARKER	POSITIVE IN SOME	FALSE POSITIVES IN
Carcinoembryonic antigen (CEA)	GI, lung, breast cancers	Smokers, cirrhotics Inflammatory bowel disease Rectal polyps Pancreatitis
Alpha-fetoprotein (αFP)	Hepatocellular, gastric, pancreatic, colon, and lung cancers Teratocarcinomas Embryonal cell carcinomas of testis, ovary, and extragonadal sites	Pregnancy Ataxia-telangiectasia Alcoholic and viral hepatitis Cirrhosis
Human chorionic gonadotropin (beta subunit of hCG)	Trophoblastic tumors Germ cell neoplasms Adenocarcinomas of ovary Pancreatic, gastric, and hepatocellular cancers	Pregnancy (the alpha subunit cross-reacts with luteinizing hormone)
Acid phosphatase	Some prostatic cancers (especially if bony metastases are present)	Hemolysis Cytolysis of many organs, including liver, spleen, and kidney

* These markers are too nonspecific to be useful in screening asymptomatic populations.

bility can be caused directly by obstruction of respiratory, gastrointestinal, or urinary tracts, by replacing vital organs, or by invading vascular, lymphatic, or neural structures.

Even small, localized tumors can produce widespread systemic effects indirectly through biochemical, hormonal, and immunological mediators, causing a multitude of so-called paraneoplastic syndromes.

Anorexia and Cachexia

Anorexia, malnutrition, and wasting are frequently the most distressing systemic effects of cancer. Malnourishment impairs wound healing, interferes with immunocompetence, and diminishes tolerance to treatment.

Cancer-related cachexia probably has many causes, the details of which are yet to be elucidated. Certainly an important factor is anorexia, which includes aberrations in taste and smell, early satiety, and (in some GI, GU, and head and neck tumors) obstructive symptoms. In addition, rapid tumor growth and infection can produce hypercatabolic states.

Medical factors also contribute to malnutrition. Diagnostic tests frequently require fasting. Surgical extirpation of head and neck or GI tumors can interfere with enteral nutrition perioperatively and may permanently impair chewing, swallowing, or absorption of nutrients. Chemotherapy and radiation can cause nausea and vomiting, diarrhea and subsequent malabsorption, mucositis, stomatitis, esophagitis, and increased aberrations of taste and smell.

Tumor remission frequently reverses the signs and symptoms of malnutrition. Without such remission, however, there is no evidence that aggressive treatment with oral and parenteral nutrition enhances the patient's response to therapy or prolongs meaningful survival.

Hematologic Manifestations

Prominent systemic signs and symptoms can result from the hematologic complications of malignancy listed in Table 57–5. Some can be life-threatening; others can be reversed only by successfully treating the underlying malignancy.

Endocrine Manifestations

Tumor production of bioactive hormones can have widespread systemic effects far out of proportion to the size of the tumor itself. Table 57–6 gives examples of such "ectopic hormones" (those produced by cells outside of the organ usually responsible for that hormone's production, and not responsive to the body's normal homeostatic controls).

Neurologic Manifestations

Malignancies can cause neurologic sequelae directly (by compressing or invading the spinal cord, epidural space, brain tissue, or nerve plexuses) and indirectly (by means of infection and metabolic abnormalities).

Table 123–2 lists some of the remote effects of cancer on the nervous system; these may be the presenting signs of occult malignancy. The mechanisms by which these remote effects are manifested are not yet well-delineated.

TABLE 57–5. SOME HEMATOLOGIC MANIFESTATIONS OF MALIGNANCY

MANIFESTATION	SOME ASSOCIATED TUMORS	CONTRIBUTING FACTORS
Anemia	About 50% of all advanced malignancies	Chronic disease; extrinsic blood loss; bone marrow invasion by tumor or suppression by therapy; autoimmune hemolytic anemia; disseminated intravascular coagulation (DIC); microangiopathic hemolytic anemia; erosion of the tumor into a blood vessel; splenic sequestration
Leukopenia, thrombocytopenia	Any malignancy	Bone marrow infiltration by tumor or suppression by tumor or therapy; DIC; splenic sequestration
Erythrocytosis	Hepatoma, hypernephroma, cerebellar hemangioblastoma	Inappropriate production of erythropoietin
Leukemoid reaction	Carcinomas of lung, pancreas, stomach; hepatoma; lymphomas	Tumor necrosis; tumor elaboration of granulopoietin; marrow invasion by metastases
Eosinophilia	Lymphomas, especially Hodgkin's disease; melanoma; brain tumors	Tumor elaboration of eosinophilopoietin
Thrombocytosis	Hypernephroma; disseminated GI neoplasms	
Bleeding diatheses	Myeloma; Waldenström's macroglobulinemia	Paraprotein coating of coagulation proteins or platelets
	Myeloproliferative diseases	Platelet dysfunction
Disseminated intravascular coagulation (DIC)	Any malignancy	Sepsis
		Hemolytic transfusion reactions
	Mucin-producing adenocarcinomas	Activation of coagulation Factor X
Hypercoagulability	Carcinoma of pancreas, lung; myeloproliferative diseases	

TABLE 57–6. SOME ECTOPIC HORMONES PRODUCED BY MALIGNANCY

HORMONE	MANIFESTATIONS	SOME ASSOCIATED TUMORS
ACTH	Cushing's syndrome (psychosis, hyperglycemia, hypokalemia, generalized weakness)	Lung (especially oat cell); thymus; pancreas; medullary thyroid carcinoma; neural crest tumors (such as pheochromocytoma)
Parathyroid hormone	Hypercalcemia	Carcinomas of lung, kidney, ovary, head, and neck
Growth hormone	Acromegaly	Bronchial carcinoid; pancreatic islet cell tumor
Vasopressin	Syndrome of inappropriate antidiuretic hormone (SIADH)	Carcinoma of lung (especially oat cell)

TABLE 57–7. SKIN LESIONS THAT CAN PRECEDE OTHER EVIDENCE OF MALIGNANCY

LESION	DESCRIPTION	MALIGNANCY
Dermatomyositis (over age 40)	"Heliotrope" eyelid coloration; scaly violet knuckle rash	Carcinomas of breast, lung, GI and GU tracts; lymphomas
Acquired pachydermoperiostosis	Thickened skin of forehead, scalp, hands, feet	Carcinomas of bronchus, stomach, esophagus; thymoma
Acanthosis nigricans	Confluent hyperpigmented, hyperkeratotic areas in skin folds	GI, lung, breast, uterine, ovary, cystic, and hepatic duct carcinomas

Cutaneous Manifestations

Many types of skin changes are associated with malignancies: direct invasion of the skin (such as the infiltrating acute granulocytic leukemic cells in "chloromas"), lesions associated with syndromes predisposing to cancer (as in ataxia-telangiectasia—associated reticuloendothelial malignancies), and lesions that may herald the onset of an occult malignancy such as those listed in Table 57–7.

Renal Complications

Malignancies can infiltrate the kidneys directly or can cause malfunction indirectly by deposi-

tions resulting from hypercalcemia, hyperuricemia, paraproteinemia, or amyloid; they also can obstruct the lower urinary tract.

The nephrotic syndrome can be caused by membranous glomerulopathy resulting from deposition of tumor or oncofetal antigen-antibody complexes, or by the minimal change glomerulopathy associated with Hodgkin's disease.

REFERENCE

DeVita VT, Hellman S, and Rosenberg SA: Cancer: Principles and Practice of Oncology. Philadelphia, JB Lippincott Co, 1982.

58 ONCOLOGIC EMERGENCIES

The natural history of malignancies leads to several types of medical emergencies. Many gastrointestinal and genitourinary tumors present with acute obstruction or hemorrhage. Bone marrow or immunologic involvement by tumor or suppression by therapy can lead to life-threatening infection. Tumor erosion into a blood vessel, or tumor- or treatment-induced thrombocytopenia can precipitate life-threatening hemorrhage. Other types of oncologic emergencies include those summarized in Table 58–1, a few of which are discussed in more detail below.

HYPERCALCEMIA

Hypercalcemia is probably the most common cancer-associated acute medical problem, occur-

ring in 10 to 20 per cent of patients with malignancies. It occurs most frequently in the presence of metastatic bone involvement but can also result from ectopic secretion of parathyroid hormone, increase in osteoclast activity (resulting from increases in osteoclast activating factor—OAF), tumor production of prostaglandins, or multiple benign causes seen in the general population—especially primary hyperparathyroidism, which must be included in the differential diagnosis.

Changes in mental status (ranging from apathy to coma), generalized muscle weakness, nausea and vomiting, abdominal pain, polyuria (resulting from a reversible renal tubular defect in urine concentrating ability), and polydipsia are among the common presenting symptoms. Signs of hypercalcemia include changes in mental status, dehydration, renal insufficiency, hyporeflexia, pan-

TABLE 58–1. SOME ONCOLOGIC EMERGENCIES

	MOST COMMON MANIFESTATIONS	MOST COMMON ETIOLOGIES
Hemodynamic		
Superior vena cava syndrome	Superficial thoracic vein collaterals	Bronchogenic carcinoma
	Neck vein distention	Lymphoma
	Facial edema	
	Tachypnea	
Pericardial tamponade	CHF-like symptoms	Lung carcinoma
	Kussmaul's sign	Breast carcinoma
	Pulsus paradoxus	Lymphoma
	Distant heart sounds	
Hyperviscosity syndrome	Confusion, coma	Waldenström's macroglobulinemia
	Stroke	Myeloma
	Hypervolemia	
	Retinopathy	
Thrombosis	Trousseau's syndrome (migratory thrombophlebitis)	Mucinous adenocarcinomas
		Myeloproliferative disorders
	Local obstructive symptoms and signs	Prostatic carcinoma
	Disseminated intravascular coagulation (DIC)	Acute promyelocytic leukemia
Neurologic		
Increased intracranial pressure	Mental status changes	Brain metastases
	Seizures	Primary brain tumors
	Signs of herniation	Carcinomatous or lymphomatous meningitis
Spinal cord compression	Pain (usually radicular)	Carcinoma of lung, breast, prostate
	Weakness	Lymphoma
	Autonomic dysfunction	Myeloma
	Sensory abnormalities	
Metabolic		
Hypercalcemia	Anorexia, nausea, and vomiting	Carcinoma of breast, lung, kidney, head, and neck
	Abdominal pain	Myeloma
	Apathy, coma	
	Muscle weakness	
	Polyuria, azotemia	
	Cardiac conduction abnormalities	
Hyperuricemia	Acute renal failure	Lympho- and myeloproliferative disorders
	Gouty arthritis	Myeloma
		Widely metastatic carcinoma
Hypoglycemia	Confusion, loss of consciousness	Insulinoma
		Mesenchymal tumors
		Hepatoma
Hyponatremia	Confusion, coma	SIADH (see Table 57–6)
	Seizures	GI loss with hypotonic replacement
	Anorexia	

creatitis, peptic ulcer, hypertension, cardiac arrhythmias, prolonged PR interval, shortened QT interval, and widening of the T wave on EKG.

Definitive treatment of hypercalcemia is aimed at tumor control; in the interim, general measures should be used to lower the ionized calcium temporarily. Intravascular volume must be repleted first.

Either furosemide or ethacrynic acid can be used in conjunction with intravenous normal saline to decrease renal tubular reabsorption of calcium and sodium; fluid and electrolyte (especially potassium and magnesium) balance must be monitored and carefully maintained. Vigorous treatment can decrease serum calcium by 2 to 4 mg/dl in the first 24 hours.

Pharmacologic doses of glucocorticoids are most useful in the hypercalcemia associated with the hematologic malignancies and breast cancer, probably because corticosteroids are effective an-

tineoplastic agents in these diseases. Less important actions of these steroids are to decrease intestinal absorption and increase renal excretion of calcium, to block activation of osteoclasts by OAF, and to reduce prostaglandin synthesis. Decreases in serum calcium begin only after several days.

When other methods of decreasing serum calcium are inadequately effective, mithramycin can be used. This cytotoxic drug directly inhibits bone resorption. Administered intravenously, its effects are usually detectable within 24 to 48 hours and can last for a week or more. The adverse effects of mithramycin (including bone marrow suppression, postural hypotension, and hepatocellular and renal damage) limit its usefulness as a first-line agent.

The fastest acting (and potentially most dangerous) form of therapy is the intravenous use of inorganic phosphate, which acutely precipitates serum ionized calcium in bone, heart, kidney, lens, and other soft tissues. Life-threatening complications of acute hypocalcemia, hypotension, and renal failure are probably dose- and rate-related.

In the face of significant renal insufficiency, peritoneal dialysis or hemodialysis is indicated; serum phosphate must be monitored closely, with repletion if necessary.

Diphosphonates, inhibitors of prostaglandin synthesis (such as indomethacin and aspirin), and calcitonin are occasionally useful in mild hypercalcemia.

Oral phosphates can be used for chronic maintenance of normocalcemia.

SPINAL CORD COMPRESSION

Extradural spinal cord compression (SCC) is the most frequent neurologic complication of systemic cancer, found on autopsy in as many as 5 per cent of patients with malignancy. Most lesions causing SCC are metastatic and involve the extramedullary space. The primary tumor is usually one that arises in or commonly metastasizes to bone, such as lymphoma, myeloma, and carcinomas of lung, breast, and prostate.

Back pain, with or without a radicular component, is the presenting symptom in nearly all patients with SCC; the pain is frequently worse when supine. Later signs and symptoms include weakness, sensory loss, and autonomic dysfunction.

Unless diagnosed and treated early, SCC leads to irreversible neurologic deficits; thus a high index of suspicion must be employed in any older patient presenting with back pain of recent onset, especially if there is a history of malignancy. Once SCC enters into the differential diagnosis of neurologic symptoms, diagnostic and therapeutic measures must be undertaken immediately. Interim medical management includes the use of high-dose steroid therapy in an attempt to decrease pressure on the cord.

Although plain films are likely to demonstrate extensive vertebral involvement or destruction by tumor, myelography is required to diagnose SCC, to demonstrate the number of lesions, and to define the upper and lower margins of the blockage to free flow of spinal fluid. At the time of myelography, spinal fluid should be obtained for cell count and chemical and cytological analysis. In the rare case that myelography is contraindicated, CT scanning with contrast enhancement can be helpful.

Available treatment approaches include radiation therapy and surgery with or without postoperative radiation. Surgery, which may involve more morbidity and mortality, is usually reserved for (1) cases in which there has not been a previous diagnosis of malignancy and there is no more accessible site for biopsy, (2) lesions known to be radioresistant, and (3) tumors involving areas already treated with maximum tolerated doses of radiation. Chemotherapy can be used as an adjuvant, depending on the histology of the lesion; it is not usually recommended as the primary mode of treatment.

In general, neurologic prognosis (sphincter control and independence of ambulation) depends on the degree of impairment when treatment is initiated and on the radiation sensitivity of the primary tumor (even if surgical therapy alone is employed).

INCREASED INTRACRANIAL PRESSURE

Both mass lesions and diffuse infiltrative processes such as lymphomatous or carcinomatous meningitis are among the abnormalities that can present with signs and symptoms of increased intracranial pressure (ICP).

Prompt recognition of the cause of ICP and rapid institution of medical therapy (prior to definitive diagnosis and treatment of the precipitating cancer) are essential to preservation of cerebral function. Early signs of ICP include somnolence, lethargy, confusion and, sometimes, papilledema. Associated focal neurologic lesions can cause hyperreflexia, abnormal reflexes, or seizures. The diagnosis and management of patients with increased intracranial pressure associated with intracranial neoplasms is discussed in Chapter 123. The CT scan has become the safest and most reliable tool for providing information essential to decisions on definitive diagnostic measures and subsequent therapy.

Care must be taken not to make unfounded presumptions without tissue diagnosis unless the patient has a previously diagnosed, widely disseminated malignancy and the CT scan is diagnostic of metastatic tumor. For example, there is an increased incidence of benign meningioma in women with breast cancer, emphasizing that an intracranial mass in a patient with a history of localized breast cancer cannot be assumed to be malignant. Similarly, brain abscesses must be distinguished from CNS involvement by malignancies that depress the immune system.

While definitive diagnostic and therapeutic measures are being planned and executed, medical therapy including pharmacologic doses of intravenous steroids, diuretics, and fluid restriction can temporarily decrease ICP. If the lesion is supratentorial, anticonvulsant therapy should be instituted to prevent seizure activity.

SUPERIOR VENA CAVA SYNDROME

The superior vena cava (SVC) syndrome creates a subacute or acute medical emergency whose diagnosis and treatment usually require the multidisciplinary efforts of the medical oncologist, surgeon, and radiation therapist. The SVC is the major venous channel for blood return from the head, neck and upper extremities, and thorax. A thin-walled vessel enclosed in a relatively unyielding compartment, its low intravascular pressures make it particularly vulnerable to extrinsic compression by the expansion of an adjacent mass.

Patients with SVC syndrome frequently show distended thoracic venous collaterals and neck veins, facial edema, and tachypnea. Less often, they have facial plethora, cyanosis, upper extremity edema, Horner's syndrome, and vocal cord paralysis. Chest x-ray almost invariably shows a mass—usually in the right superior mediastinum. Malignancy causes most cases of the SVC syndrome; fewer than 5 per cent result from benign causes such as thyroid goiter, pericardial constriction, idiopathic sclerosing mediastinitis, and thrombosis of the SVC. Since the 10 to 20 per cent of patients with malignant presentation of SVC syndrome survive longer than two years, definitive diagnosis and treatment are essential.

Unless the clinical presentation is immediately life-threatening, tissue diagnosis should be obtained prior to treatment. The diagnostic procedure of choice will depend upon the accessibility of the lesion and the surgeon's estimate of bleeding risk from the known increase in venous pressures. Table 58–2 shows the yield of procedures employed by Perez and coworkers in diagnosing 84 cases of the SVC syndrome.

The preferred treatment usually consists of radiation, with subjective relief occurring in most cases within one week. Chemotherapy alone may be equally efficacious in lymphoma and small cell lung carcinoma. Failure of patients to respond to either modality can usually be attributed to thrombotic obstruction of the SVC. Efforts at primary surgical treatment with bypass of the obstruction usually fail and carry a high mortality. Supportive medical therapy with steroids, diuretics, anticoagulation, and (in the case of SVC thrombosis) fibrinolytic therapy may be helpful in ameliorating symptoms.

TABLE 58–2.   SVC SYNDROME—YIELD OF DIAGNOSTIC METHODS*

METHOD	NO. PATIENTS	POSITIVE DIAGNOSES (%)
Thoracotomy and biopsy	19	100
Mediastinoscopy and biopsy	11	81
Bronchoscopy and biopsy	45	62
Lymph node biopsy		
Scalene	22	50
Palpable supraclavicular	19	84
Cytology		
Sputum	24	63
Bronchial washings	12	50
Pleural effusion	4	100

* From Perez CA, Presant CA, and Van Amburg AL III: Management of superior vena cava syndrome. Semin Oncol 5:123–134, 1978.

REFERENCE

Yarbrow JW (ed): Oncologic emergencies. Semin Oncol 5(2):123–224 1978.

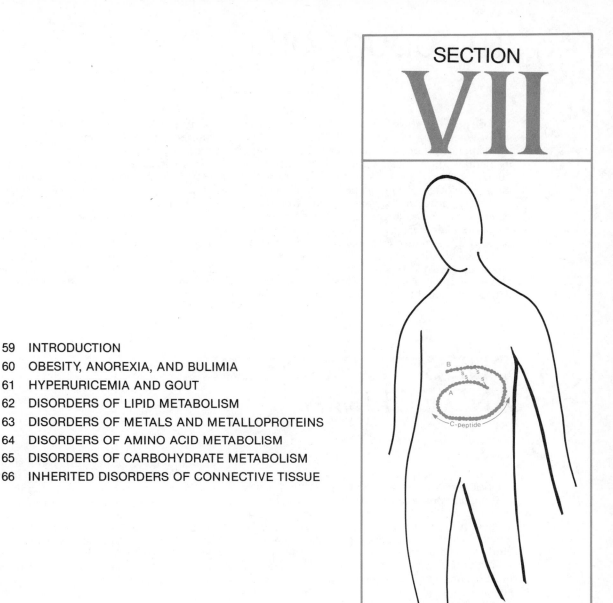

SECTION

VII

METABOLIC DISEASES

59 INTRODUCTION

A disorder is classified as a disease of metabolism when the fundamental pathogenic mechanism includes one of numerous chemical transformations that occur within living organisms. Such chemical reactions are divided into two large categories. *Anabolic* reactions are usually energy-requiring and generally result in the synthesis of molecules larger than those of the initial reactants. *Catabolic* reactions are energy-yielding processes that cause degradation of larger molecules into smaller products. Many diseases of metabolism involve specific enzyme defects that alter anabolic or catabolic processes. Defects that can be attributed to an underlying genetic abnormality are termed *inborn errors of metabolism.* Other metabolic diseases are acquired rather than hereditary.

The diseases discussed in this chapter are chiefly those whose manifestations are multisystemic or in which biochemical and genetic factors dominate the clinical presentation. A complete discussion of all known inborn errors of metabolism falls beyond the scope of this text. Many inborn errors are life-limiting, leading to death in infancy or early childhood. This section focuses upon the more common hereditary or acquired metabolic diseases encountered in adults.

60 OBESITY, ANOREXIA, AND BULIMIA

OBESITY

Obesity can be defined as excess body fat. The pathologic consequences of the overweight syndrome correlate directly with the proportion of adipose tissue in the body and not with body weight per se. Exact measurements of body fat elude quantification, but estimates can be obtained with a variety of indirect techniques. The most accurate methods include measurements of subcutaneous skin folds with standard calipers and the use of various indices incorporating measurements of height and weight. Several studies have shown that the risk of death increases with increased body weight, but this risk becomes statistically significant only above 130 per cent of ideal weight. Using this figure as the criterion, an estimated 15 per cent of the general population in the United States suffer from obesity.

Pathogenesis. Although several rare inherited syndromes, endocrine diseases, and neurologic conditions can cause massive weight gain, over 99 per cent of overweight patients have idiopathic obesity. Fat accumulation results from excessive food intake and/or decreased caloric expenditure. Food intake is regulated by several hypothalamic and extrahypothalamic sites in the central nervous system. Some obese individuals appear to have a stable set point for body weight to which they always return after a temporary weight loss. This observation has led to speculation that some obese patients have a hypothalamic abnormality in which hunger centers function normally, but with an elevated threshold for satiety. Both genetic and environmental factors influence human eating habits. Monozygotic twins show a higher concordance for obesity than dizygotic twins, and children show a higher correlation in body weight with natural parents than with adoptive parents. The social environment strongly influences these genetic tendencies, however. For example, the body weights of identical twins vary to a greater degree when the children are raised in separate families than when raised in the same home. Also, obesity is much more prevalent in American women of low socioeconomic status than in higher socioeconomic groups.

Patients with idiopathic obesity generally fall into one of two broad clinical categories. Those with *lifelong obesity* give a characteristic history of obesity in early childhood, an acceleration of weight gain during puberty, and (in women) a history of successive weight gains with each pregnancy. Such individuals tend to be grossly overweight as adults (more than 150 per cent of ideal body weight) and exhibit both truncal and peripheral obesity. *Adult-onset obesity* is much more common. These individuals are often thin or of average weight until the second to fourth decade, when truncal obesity ensues. All obese patients exhibit enlarged fat cells; those with severe lifelong obesity may have an increased number of fat cells as well. Since insulin receptors are located on adipose cell membranes, patients with increased numbers of fat cells may possess an enhanced proclivity for fat storage and resistance to its loss. By contrast, adult-onset obesity usually reflects only an imbalance between caloric intake and energy expenditure.

Clinical Consequences of Obesity. Massive

obesity greatly increases the risk of several medical diseases. Men aged 25 to 35 who weigh 150 to 300 per cent of their ideal body weight exhibit a mortality rate 12 times that of similarly aged nonobese men. Among 16 reported persons weighing greater than 700 pounds, the average age at death was 34 years. Cardiovascular diseases account for over 50 per cent of these early deaths. Congestive heart failure is common and may be related to the measured increase in blood flow to adipose tissue or to the greatly increased incidence of hypertension and diabetes mellitus among the overweight.

In addition to cardiovascular disorders, several other debilitating conditions affect the obese. Restrictive and obstructive ventilatory abnormalities occur, leading to hypoxemia, carbon dioxide retention, sleep apnea (pickwickian syndrome), and cor pulmonale. Gallbladder disease is three times more common in obese than nonobese persons, and the prevalence of diabetes mellitus is four to seven times higher than normal among the overweight. Venous stasis, thrombophlebitis, renal vein thrombosis, and pulmonary emboli occur more frequently. Osteoarthritis commonly affects the weight-bearing joints in obese persons who exceed 130 per cent of their ideal weight. General anesthesia carries a much higher risk, and operative risks are much greater. Obesity is associated with high plasma concentrations of triglyceride and total cholesterol, as well as elevated LDL and reduced HDL levels, both of which increase the risk of coronary artery disease.

Treatment. The goal of therapy for the obese patient is to achieve a state of negative caloric balance. This may be extremely difficult. Success rates in achieving an initial weight loss of 20 pounds with conventional diets range between 12 and 29 per cent; the success rate for achieving a 40-pound weight loss varies from 3 to 8 per cent. Among obese patients who initially lose weight, "relapses" are common.

Weight reduction diets should be designed to maintain normal body composition as well as to attain normal weight. Despite the popularity of calorically unbalanced "fad" diets, there is little evidence to support the superiority of any single low-calorie diet over others. The rate of weight loss on low-calorie diets high in protein is identical to the rate on diets high in fat or carbohydrate. A minimal quantity of protein and carbohydrate in weight reduction appears necessary, however. Carbohydrate-depleted ("ketogenic") diets enhance weight loss only by promoting transient water excretion; the associated ketosis and acidosis may cause bone demineralization. Total starvation rapidly induces weight loss, but serious complications including anemia, hyperuricemia, gout, ketosis, potassium depletion, cardiac arrhythmias, and sudden death preclude its routine use. High-protein ("protein-sparing") formulae or liquid protein hydrolysates employed to supplement fasting have been associated with increased mortality, probably resulting from hypokalemia-induced cardiac arrhythmias.

More practical recommendations for the long-term management of obesity include a diet that is balanced in carbohydrate, protein, and fat content, provides adequate vitamins and minerals, and promotes a weight loss of no more than one to two pounds per week. Because one pound of fat contains 3500 calories, this rate of weight loss requires a negative caloric balance of 500 to 1000 calories per day. One can calculate a person's caloric expenditure by estimating 10 calories per pound of current weight for basal metabolic needs and adding 20, 35, or 50 per cent for sedentary, average, or above average activity, respectively. For most obese adults, a reasonable initial weight reduction diet would thus consist of 15 to 20 calories per kilogram of ideal body weight, containing 20 per cent protein, 45 per cent carbohydrate, and 35 per cent fat calories.

Exercise programs provide important adjuncts to an effective diet program but should be undertaken gradually, giving attention to the patient's age, physical capabilities, and cardiovascular health. Physical exercise increases calorie expenditure and promotes a sense of well-being without necessarily stimulating appetite. Because the caloric equivalent of most activities is easily nullified by small amounts of food, exercise alone is rarely effective in weight reduction unless the patient concomitantly reduces calorie intake.

Many drugs have been employed in the attempted management of obesity. The use of pharmacological doses of thyroid hormone, digitalis, and diuretics in patients without hypothyroidism, congestive heart failure, or other edematous disorders must be condemned as dangerous and inappropriate. Amphetamine and its congeners rarely lead to more than a 10 per cent weight reduction, generally lose their anorectic properties with time, and carry the risk of addiction. Numerous other medications including mazindol, fenfluramine, and phenylpropanolamine have been promoted for their ability to induce weight loss in obese individuals, but none has been adequately tested in controlled clinical trials.

Behavior modification as a modality for the treatment of obesity can be effective in selected patients, working best in those who are minimally overweight. The long-term efficacy has not been established. Acupuncture and hypnosis have met with minimal success and results with individual or group therapy have been disappointing.

Surgical procedures designed to interfere with ingestion and digestion of food have been effective in producing marked and persistent weight loss, improvement in hypertension, diabetes, congestive heart failure, and hyperlipidemia, as well as a marked improvement in self-image, anxiety, and depression. Surgical intervention is warranted, however, only in patients who exceed 200 per cent of ideal body weight. In patients who are 30 to 100 per cent overweight, the medical risks of obesity are generally outweighed by the risks of surgery. Jejunoileal bypass was the procedure used most frequently in the 1960's and 1970's. Because of the high morbidity associated with this procedure (diarrhea, electrolyte disturbances, gallstones, renal stones, and progressive hepatic fibrosis), surgical treatment of obesity has shifted more recently to procedures that impede gastric filling, all having in common the creation of a physical restriction to the passage of food through the stomach. Gastric "bypass" surgery is technically more difficult than intestinal bypass and is not universally successful.

ANOREXIA NERVOSA

Anorexia nervosa, a complex psychiatric disorder primarily affecting young pubertal women, is characterized by semistarvation and weight loss, a distorted body image, amenorrhea, and hyperactivity. Among women evaluated in amenorrhea clinics, the prevalence of anorexia nervosa ranges between 5 and 14 per cent. There is general agreement that the incidence of anorexia nervosa has increased dramatically over the last decade. A former preponderance of the disease among upper socioeconomic classes has concomitantly shifted to a more even class distribution.

Pathogenesis. The essential feature of anorexia nervosa is the "relentless pursuit of thinness." The patient with anorexia nervosa does not have true loss of appetite in the early stages of the disease, restriction of food intake being voluntary initially. In addition to avoidance of food, attempts to lose weight may include self-induced vomiting, abuse of purgatives, and excessive exercise. Although anorexia nervosa is generally classified as a psychiatric disorder, the psychopathology can be overshadowed ultimately by the effects of starvation and by secondary disturbances of the hypothalamic-pituitary-gonadal axis that lead to amenorrhea in females and decreased libido in the rare males with the syndrome. Mild diabetes insipidus, increased insulin sensitivity, low metabolic rate, and decreased pituitary gonadatropin secretion may also occur. Serum T_3 levels are low and serum reverse T_3 levels increased owing to altered peripheral metabolism of T_4, the levels of which are normal.

Clinical Features. Anorexia nervosa has as its central psychological theme a morbid fear of being unable to control eating and of becoming too fat. Associated features include an obsessional preoccupation with food and a grossly distorted body image that causes emaciated patients to perceive themselves as obese. The illness usually begins in a girl aged 14 to 17 years, but can occur as early as age 10 or up to the age of menopause. There may be a preceding history of food fads or signs of maladjustment such as difficulty in making friendships or fears of meeting strangers. Progressive weight loss is frequently accompanied by irritability, withdrawal, and depression.

Physical findings include signs of severe malnutrition. Disappearance of subcutaneous fat leads to gaunt facial features, atrophic breasts, and wasting of the buttocks. Hypothermia, hypotension, and bradycardia may be noted. The skin is typically dry, and excessive growth of lanugo hair may be detected on the neck and extremities. Mental status examination may reveal signs of depression, agitation, or obsessive-compulsive behavior.

Mortality in anorexia nervosa ranges from 0 to 24 per cent in various series. There is a risk of death from suicide and from complications of malnutrition—especially potassium depletion and hypothermia. The prognosis is poorest in patients with a later age of onset and those in whom the illness has lasted more than five years.

Treatment. Effective treatment of anorexia nervosa requires a combination of techniques with input from specialists of several disciplines. The effects of starvation must be reversed prior to initiating psychotherapy. An open and honest relationship with the patient is essential. Psychotherapy should address specific predisposing factors in individual patients, and the patient's family should be involved in establishing treatment goals and plans.

Hospitalization may be necessary for patients who weigh less than 75 per cent of ideal body weight, but compulsory admission is best avoided because the patient's continued cooperation is essential throughout the course of the illness. Refeeding in a hospital setting is often the only means of restoring body weight in order to facilitate psychotherapy. Oral feeding should be gradually increased from low levels to avoid acute gastric dilatation. No special diets are needed. Parenteral nutrition may be required in emergency situations but carries the risk of infection as well as the metabolic consequences of rapid carbohydrate refeeding, including water retention and acute hypophosphatemia. Behavior modification techniques have been used with variable success to encourage food intake. Nursing personnel must diligently monitor the patient for deceptive behavior such as surreptitious disposal of food or vomiting.

The cornerstone of treatment for anorexia nervosa is long-term individual psychotherapy. Group therapy and family therapy are useful adjuncts. Phenothiazines have been employed in anorexia nervosa to lower anxiety, reduce excessive exercise by sedation, and stimulate the appetite. Results with cyproheptadine, a centrally acting serotonin antagonist, have also been promising. The endocrine and metabolic abnormalities that occur in patients with anorexia nervosa generally resolve following restoration of ideal body weight, but amenorrhea sometimes persists. Relapses requiring hospital readmission occur in about half the patients.

BULIMIA NERVOSA

Bulimia nervosa is a variant of anorexia nervosa with similar psychological themes. The primary symptom consists of recurrent gorging with food, followed by self-induced vomiting. Abuse of laxatives is often combined with self-induced vomiting or may occur on its own. Up to 15 per cent of college students regularly use these methods for weight control. In contrast to patients with anorexia nervosa, those with bulimia exhibit weight fluctuations due to alternating binges and fasts and rarely exhibit signs of malnutrition. Some display other impulsive behavior such as drug or alcohol abuse, shoplifting, and repeated attempts at self-harm. Volume depletion, hypokalemia, and metabolic alkalosis are the chief clinical manifestations of recurrent vomiting. Bulimic patients may present with complications of hypokalemia including muscular weakness, electrocardiographic abnormalities, and renal dysfunction.

Treatment consists of long-term psychotherapy. Bulimic patients are at greater risk of suicide than anorectic patients, and they may die suddenly from hypokalemia-induced arrhythmias. Prognosis for full recovery varies with the severity of the underlying disorder.

REFERENCES

Bierman EL: Obesity. In Wyngaarden JB, and Smith LH Jr (eds): Cecil Textbook of Medicine. 17th ed. Philadelphia, WB Saunders Co, 1985, p 1191.
Bruch H: Eating Disorders: Obesity, Anorexia Nervosa and the Person Within. New York, Basic Books, 1972.
Lew EA, and Garfinkel L: Variations in mortality by weight among 750,000 men and women. J Chron Dis 32:563, 1979.
Russell GFM: Bulimia nervosa: An ominous variant of anorexia nervosa. Psychol Med 9:429, 1979.

HYPERURICEMIA AND GOUT 61

The term *gout* refers to a group of disorders characterized by a derangement in purine metabolism manifested by hyperuricemia, crystalline deposits of monosodium urate monohydrate in tissues (tophi), and recurrent episodes of acute arthritis. Hyperuricemia and gout may be classified as primary or secondary (Table 61–1). *Primary gout* results from inborn errors in the metabolism of purines or inherited defects in the renal tubular secretion of urate. *Secondary gout* occurs in disorders characterized by increased catabolism of nucleic acids or by acquired defects in the renal excretion of urate.

Pathogenesis

The biochemical hallmark of gout is an elevated serum urate, a metabolic end-product formed by the oxidation of both exogenous and endogenous purine bases. The concentration of uric acid in body fluids reflects the balance between rates of production and elimination. Approximately one third of uric acid produced on a daily basis (100 to 300 mg in the adult) is excreted in the gastrointestinal tract, where it is destroyed by bacteria. The remaining two thirds (300 to 600 mg) is excreted in the urine. Hyperuricemia may result from increased production of uric acid, decreased renal excretion, or some combination of these factors.

The risk of developing gout increases with the degree of hyperuricemia; however, the pathogenesis of gout is related more closely to the *solubility* of urate in various body fluids than to its absolute concentration. The solubility of urate is influenced by temperature and pH. At 37°C and pH 7.40, the solubility of urate is 6.4 to 6.8 mg/dl. But solubility is considerably less at the lower temperatures of peripheral joints. A urate concentration of 7.0 mg/dl usually constitutes the physicochemical upper limit of normal beyond which supersaturation occurs and crystal formation increases. Virtually all patients with gout have serum urate levels above 7.0 mg/dl. Occasional patients exhibit lower levels during an acute attack, but hyperuricemia can almost always be demonstrated during quiescent periods.

Overproduction of uric acid, detected clinically by the urinary excretion of more than 600 mg of uric acid per day, accounts for less than 10 per cent of all cases of gout. Increased production of uric acid occurs as the result of an inherited enzyme defect, as the secondary consequence of a disorder in which nucleic acid turnover is in-

TABLE 61–1. CLASSIFICATION OF HYPERURICEMIA AND GOUT

Primary (presumably genetic)
I. Metabolic (overproduction)
  A. Idiopathic (10% of primary gout)
  B. Associated with specific enzyme defects (<1% of primary gout)
    1. PP-ribose-P synthetase overactivity
    2. Partial deficiency of hypoxanthine-guanine phosphoribosyl transferase
    3. "Complete" deficiency of hypoxanthine-guanine phosphoribosyl transferase
II. Renal (idiopathic underexcretion—90% of primary gout)
Secondary (acquired)
I. Metabolic
  A. Increased nucleic acid turnover (e.g., chronic hemolysis, lymphoproliferative or myeloproliferative disorders)
  B. Glucose-6-phosphatase deficiency (i.e., Type I glycogen storage disease)
II. Renal
  A. Acute or chronic renal failure
  B. Volume depletion
  C. Altered tubular handling by drugs or endogenous metabolic products

creased, or as an idiopathic phenomenon probably representing as yet undetected enzyme defects. A review of purine metabolism will clarify the enzyme defects associated with primary gout (Fig. 61—1).

The purine nucleotides, adenylic acid (AMP), inosinic acid (IMP), and guanylic acid (GMP), are products of purine biosynthesis ultimately utilized for the synthesis of nucleic acids, cyclic AMP, ATP, cyclic GMP, and various cofactors. Degradation of purine nucleotides occurs via intermediate purine nucleotide formation of uric acid. The intracellular concentration of 5-phosphoribosyl-1-pyrophosphate (PRPP) controls the rate of uric acid synthesis.

Increased activity of the enzyme PRPP synthetase (Fig. 61—1) results in increased concentrations of PRPP, accelerated purine biosynthesis, and increased production of uric acid. Hypoxanthine-guanine phosphoribosyl transferase (HPRT) catalyzes the salvage conversion of hypoxanthine to IMP and guanine to GMP (Fig. 61—1). Deficiency or reduced activity of HPRT leads to decreased consumption and increased accumulation of PRPP, thus accelerating the *de novo* synthesis of purines and uric acid. Approximately 10 per cent of patients with gout and overproduction of uric acid exhibit partial deficiency of HPRT. Complete or virtually complete deficiency of HPRT results in the Lesch-Nyhan syndrome, a rare infantile disorder characterized by hyperuricemia, gout, choreoathetosis, mental retardation, and self-mutilation. PRPP synthetase overactivity and HPRT deficiency are familial enzyme defects inherited as X-linked traits. Together these inborn errors of metabolism account for less than 15 per cent of all cases of gout associated with uric acid overproduction. In the majority of overproducers of uric acid with gout, the biochemical abnormalities remain undefined.

Uric acid is overproduced whenever there is increased turnover of nucleic acids due to rapid division or lysis of cells. Myeloproliferative and lymphoproliferative diseases, hemolytic anemias, and various hemoglobinopathies are the most common disorders in which this occurs. Hyperuricemia is a prominent feature of the "tumor lysis syndrome" that may follow treatment of patients with lymphoma, myeloproliferative disorders, or carcinomatosis.

Underexcretion of uric acid accounts for more than 90 per cent of all cases of gout. Impaired excretion may result from (1) reduced glomerular filtration of uric acid, (2) enhanced renal tubular reabsorption, (3) reduced tubular secretion, or (4) a combination of defects in filtration and tubular

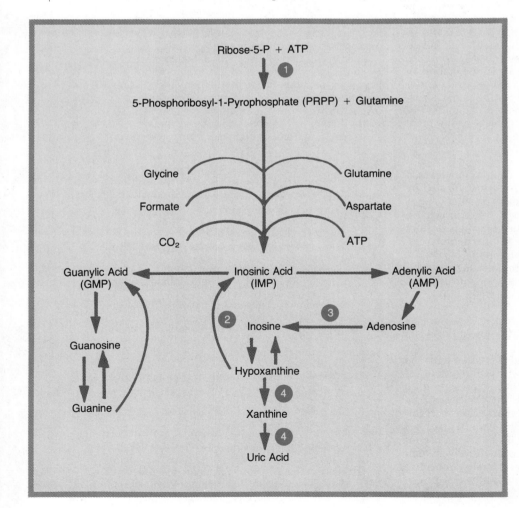

FIGURE 61—1. Purine biosynthetic pathway. (1) 5-Phosphoribosyl-1-pyrophosphate (PRPP) synthetase. (2) Hypoxanthine-guanine phosphoribosyl transferase (HPRT). (3) Adenosine deaminase. (4) Xanthine oxidase.

TABLE 61–2. SOME DRUGS THAT AFFECT SERUM URIC ACID CONCENTRATION

Drugs that Increase Serum Uric Acid
  Thiazides
  "Loop" diuretics (furosemide, ethacrynic acid)
  Small doses of salicylate (< 2 gm per day)
  Acetazolamide
  Pyrazinamide
  Ethambutol
Drugs that Decrease Serum Uric Acid
  Increased renal excretion
    Probenecid
    Sulfinpyrazone
    Phenylbutazone, oxyphenylbutazone
    Large doses of salicylate (4-6 gm per day)
  Decreased production
    Allopurinol

handling. In most instances of primary renal gout the defect remains undefined.

A number of factors can secondarily reduce renal urate excretion and cause gout. In patients with acute or chronic renal failure, reductions in glomerular filtration rate lead to a decrease in the filtered load of uric acid. Although renal disease is a frequent cause of hyperuricemia, clinical gout seldom ensues, perhaps because uremia blunts the inflammatory response to urate crystals. Because renal tubular reabsorption of urate is linked to sodium reabsorption, hyperuricemia frequently accompanies disorders characterized by renal sodium avidity. Extracellular volume depletion of any etiology (e.g., hemorrhage, gastrointestinal losses, adrenal insufficiency, diabetes insipidus) leads to decreased filtration and enhanced renal tubular reabsorption of uric acid. In clinical practice, diuretic therapy is probably the most common cause of secondary hyperuricemia and gout mediated by volume depletion. A number of other drugs can cause hyperuricemia by directly altering renal tubular handling of uric acid (Table 61–2). Some of these (e.g., thiazides, "loop" diuretics) are organic acids that may occupy uric acid secretory sites along the proximal nephron, thus impairing tubular secretion of urate. Competitive inhibition of uric acid secretion by *endogenous* organic acids accounts for hyperuricemia in patients with lactic acidosis and ketoacidosis.

Clinical Features

Gout is chiefly a disorder of adult males; only about 5 per cent of cases occur in women. The natural history encompasses four distinct clinical syndromes: (1) asymptomatic hyperuricemia, (2) acute gouty arthritis, (3) chronic tophaceous gout, and (4) nephrolithiasis. In most patients, these syndromes arise in roughly chronological order; however, nephrolithiasis may precede the development of arthritis in approximately 20 per cent of cases. Clinical gout is uncommon before the third decade of life; its peak age of onset in men is about 45 years, usually after 20 to 30 years of sustained hyperuricemia. *Asymptomatic hyperuricemia* refers to elevation of serum urate prior

to the development of arthritic symptoms, tophi, or nephrolithiasis.

Acute Gouty Arthritis. The primary manifestation of gout is a painful arthritis, usually involving the lower extremities. Ninety per cent of initial attacks are monoarticular, and at least half involve the first metatarsophalangeal joint (podagra). Other initial sites of involvement, in order of frequency, include the ankles, heels, knees, wrists, fingers, and elbows. Acute gouty arthritis may be precipitated by events such as trauma, surgery, alcohol ingestion, or systemic infection. While the course of an untreated attack varies, initial episodes are usually self-limited. Over 50 per cent of patients, however, will experience recurrent arthritis within one year of the first attack. Later attacks tend to be more prolonged and severe and more commonly involve multiple joints.

A presumptive diagnosis of gout can be made if the patient is hyperuricemic and has the classic clinical features described above. Unfortunately, a substantial minority of patients with acute gout exhibit *normal* uric acid levels. A dramatic response to colchicine is highly suggestive but not pathognomonic of acute gout. When the diagnosis is in doubt, acute gouty arthritis can be confirmed by demonstration of negatively birefringent, needle-shaped urate crystals within the white blood cells of synovial fluid examined under a polarizing lens. Synovial fluid analysis otherwise exhibits nonspecific signs of acute inflammation. The leukocyte count ranges from 1000 to over 70,000/cu mm, with a predominance of polymorphonuclear cells. Concentrations of glucose and uric acid in synovial fluid are usually similar to those in serum.

Chronic Tophaceous Gout. In untreated patients, tophaceous deposits of monosodium urate ultimately appear in cartilage, tendons, bursae, soft tissues, and synovial membranes at a rate that parallels the degree and duration of hyperuricemia. Common sites include the external ear and pressure points such as the Achilles tendons and olecranon bursae. Gouty tophi may spontaneously ulcerate and extrude a pasty material consisting of pure urate. Although tophi themselves are painless, their presence in and around joints ultimately can limit joint mobility.

Nephrolithiasis. Three distinct renal syndromes are associated with hyperuricemia. (1) *Acute urate nephropathy* results from the precipitation of urate within renal tubules and occurs almost exclusively in patients with myeloproliferative or lymphoproliferative disorders with severe hyperuricemia (serum uric acid >25 mg/dl), especially following chemotherapy. Intratubular obstruction with uric acid may cause profound reductions of glomerular filtration rate and severe azotemia. (2) *Chronic gouty nephropathy* is characterized by the deposition of monosodium urate crystals in the renal interstitium. More than 90 per cent of patients with chronic tophaceous gout exhibit interstitial urate deposits; however, a cause-and-effect relationship between chronic gout and renal insufficiency has been open to question. Most authorities agree that chronic hyperuricemia per se rarely, if ever, leads to clinically significant renal disease. The finding that renal disease is a common cause of death in patients with gouty arthritis may be explained by the higher than expected occurrence of hyperuricemia in patients with hypertension, diabetes mellitus, abnormalities in lipid metabolism, and/or atherogenesis. Hyperuricemia is also a well-recognized manifestation of lead toxicity. In some patients, the coexistence of hyperuricemia and renal dysfunction may reflect underlying lead nephropathy. (3) *Uric acid urolithiasis* occurs in approximately 20 per cent of patients with a history of gouty arthritis. Increased urinary excretion of uric acid is the main factor favoring the formation of uric acid stones. Both gouty and nongouty uric acid stone formers also exhibit inappropriate urine acidity that favors the precipitation of uric acid. Gouty subjects also have an increased incidence of calcium oxalate stones, perhaps because uric acid crystals serve as a nidus for calcium stone formation.

Treatment

Management of Asymptomatic Hyperuricemia. Controversy surrounds the management of asymptomatic hyperuricemia. Because only 10 to 20 per cent of patients with asymptomatic hyperuricemia develop arthritis, treatment should be withheld unless the patient (1) has a strong family history of gout or uric acid nephrolithiasis, (2) is excreting greater than 1100 mg/day of uric acid, or (3) has a serum uric acid level greater than 11 mg/dl.

Treatment of Acute Gouty Arthritis. Acute gout is treated with one of three types of anti-inflammatory agents: colchicine, nonsteroidal anti-inflammatory drugs, or corticosteroids. Colchicine is the only therapeutic agent with specific diagnostic value in acute gout. An initial oral dose of 0.6 to 1.2 mg should be administered as soon as the diagnosis is suspected. The initial dose should be followed by 0.6 mg every hour until (1) symptoms of arthritis abate, (2) nausea, vomiting, or diarrhea develops, or (3) a maximum dose of 6 mg has been administered. When this regimen is initiated within 12 hours of the onset of symptoms, colchicine is effective in over 90 per cent of cases; however, gastrointestinal side effects preclude administration of optimal doses in a number of patients. Intravenous colchicine is advantageous when a rapid response is desired or when gastrointestinal side effects prohibit oral administration of the drug. Occasionally, intravenous colchicine is effective when the oral preparation is not. The initial intravenous dose of colchicine is 2 mg (injected over two to five minutes), followed by 0.5 mg every six hours until a daily satisfactory response is achieved. The total daily dose of intravenous colchicine should not exceed 4 mg.

Nonsteroidal anti-inflammatory drugs including indomethacin, phenylbutazone, naproxen, fenoprofen, and ibuprofen are also effective in the treatment of acute gouty arthritis. In general, these agents should initially be administered at near maximal doses, with gradual tapering as symptoms subside. For example, indomethacin may be given as an oral dose of 75 mg, followed by 50 mg every 8 hours for three doses, and then 25 mg every 8 hours for three doses.

Corticosteroids should be reserved for patients in whom full doses of colchicine or nonsteroidal agents are either contraindicated or ineffective. Intra-articular injections of steroids (e.g., 5 to 10 mg of triamcinolone) are effective in treating acute gout limited to a single joint. Alternatively, 40 to 80 mg of prednisone administered daily for three to four days may be effective, but rebound attacks of gout are common. Uricosuric agents and allopurinol are of no value in the treatment of acute gouty arthritis. Once an attack subsides, administration of small daily doses of colchicine (0.6 to 1.2 mg per day) is effective in preventing further attacks.

Prevention or Reversal of Urate Deposition and Nephrolithiasis. Antihyperuricemic drugs should be administered to patients with recurrent gouty arthritis, nephrolithiasis, or tophi. The goal is to maintain the serum urate level below 7.0 mg/dl. Reductions to these levels can be achieved by drugs that increase the renal excretion of uric acid or decrease uric acid production. While a number of drugs exhibit uricosuric properties (Table 61–1), only probenecid and sulfinpyrazone are widely employed specifically as antihyperuricemic agents. Uricosuric therapy is accompanied by a transient increase in uric acid excretion, which returns to pretreatment levels a few days later as the total body urate pool is depleted. To avoid overt nephrolithiasis during this transient hyperuricosuric phase, the uricosuric agents should be started at low doses and gradually increased. For example, probenecid is started in doses of 250 mg twice daily and increased over a period of several weeks to the dose necessary to achieve effective reversal of hyperuricemia. Sulfinpyrazone is begun at 50 mg twice daily and increased to maintenance levels of 300 to 400 mg per day in divided doses. In addition, maintaining an ample urine flow with adequate hydration reduces the likelihood of stone formation. Probenecid and sulfinpyrazone are ineffective in patients with impaired renal function (glomerular filtration rate <30 ml/min).

Hyperuricemia may also be controlled by allopurinol, a drug that decreases uric acid production by inhibiting xanthine oxidase, the enzyme that catalyzes the conversion of hypoxanthine to xanthine and xanthine to uric acid (Fig. 61–1). In most patients, 300 mg per day is effective, but the half-life of allopurinol is increased in patients with renal insufficiency so that a smaller dose (100 to 200 mg) may be sufficient. Although uncommon, adverse effects with allopurinol are more severe than with uricosuric drugs and include fever, dermatitis, elevation of hepatic enzymes, diarrhea, and occasional vasculitis. *Initiation of antihyperuricemic therapy with any agent may precipitate acute gouty arthritis, since acute gout may occur whenever there is a rapid change in the serum urate concentration.* It is prudent to begin prophylactic therapy with colchicine just prior to the initiation of antihyperuricemic drugs.

Acute urate nephropathy can be prevented by administration of allopurinol to patients with neoplastic disorders prior to administration of chemotherapy. For prophylaxis during treatment of lymphoproliferative or myeloproliferative disorders, treatment with 600 to 900 mg daily is advisable during the first few days of therapy; thereafter the dose is tapered to 300 mg per day, so long as the serum urate remains less than 7.0 mg/dl. A generous intake of fluids should be maintained to assure a high rate of urine flow. Urinary alkalinization also helps to prevent intrarenal precipitation of uric acid. The pKa of uric acid is 5.75. In urine at pH 5.0, only 15 per cent of uric acid exists in soluble, ionized form. The solubility increases more than 10-fold at pH 7.0 and more than 100-fold at pH 8.0. Administration of sodium bicarbonate and/or the carbonic anhydrase inhibitor, acetazolamide, should be considered in patients at high risk for developing acute urate nephropathy.

OTHER DISORDERS OF PURINE METABOLISM

Xanthinuria is a rare genetic disorder, probably inherited as an autosomal recessive trait, that results from deficiency of the enzyme xanthine ox-

idase. Affected patients exhibit hypouricemia, increased urinary excretion of hypoxanthine and xanthine, and sometimes xanthine kidney stones. They are otherwise asymptomatic.

Immune dysfunction may be associated with certain enzyme deficiencies in the purine pathway. Patients with deficiency of adenosine deaminase, which normally catalyzes the deamination of adenosine to inosine (Fig. 61–1), have severe combined immune deficiency (i.e., severe dysfunction of cell-mediated immunity with milder abnormalities of humoral immunity). Deficiency of purine nucleoside phosphorylase, which catalyzes the conversion of inosine to hypoxanthine and guanosine to guanine, has also been associated with an inherited immune deficiency syndrome.

REFERENCES

Berger L, and Yu TF: Renal function in gout. IV. An analysis of 624 gouty subjects including long-term follow-up studies. Am J Med 59:605, 1975.
Rieselbach RE, and Steele TH: Influence of the kidney upon urate homeostasis in health and disease. Am J Med 56:665, 1974.
Wyngaarden JB, and Kelly WN: Gout. In Stanbury JB, Wyngaarden JB, Fredrickson DS, Goldstein JL, and Brown MS (eds): The Metabolic Basis of Inherited Disease. 5th ed. New York, McGraw-Hill Book Company, 1982.

DISORDERS OF LIPID METABOLISM 62

NORMAL REGULATION OF PLASMA LIPIDS

Dietary fat is hydrolyzed in the gut to form partial glycerides and fatty acids. The latter compounds are absorbed and resynthesized to triglycerides by mucosal cells of the small intestine. Triglycerides are then secreted into the intestinal lymphatics as chylomicrons and enter the blood via the thoracic duct. Chylomicrons are usually present in plasma only during the active absorption of fat. Triglycerides are removed from chylomicrons in extrahepatic capillary beds that contain the enzyme lipoprotein lipase. Free fatty acids and cholesterol are cleaved from triglycerides by this enzyme and diffuse across capillary beds to be stored or oxidized. Chylomicron remnants are rapidly taken up by the liver and repro-

cessed. Mechanisms involved in plasma lipid transport are schematically illustrated in Figure 62–1.

Fatty acids and cholesterol are the major lipids requiring transport in plasma. Both are insoluble in water and must be transported in hydrophilic complexes, collectively referred to as lipoproteins. Fatty acids circulate either bound to albumin or as esters, of which the main transport form is triglyceride. Cholesterol molecules are generally transported as esters of fatty acids. Each spherical lipoprotein particle includes a nonpolar core containing triglyceride and cholesterol esters in varying proportions. A surface coat of polar phospholipids surrounds this core, making the lipoprotein particle more water-soluble. Finally, surface proteins (apoproteins) coat the lipoprotein particle, allowing it to bind to specific en-

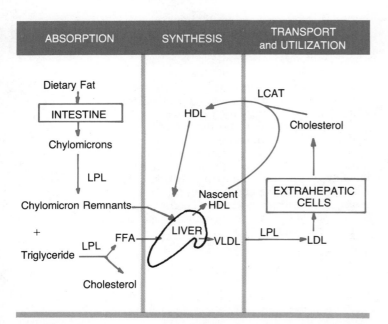

FIGURE 62–1. Normal regulation of plasma lipids. See text for details. LPL = Lipoprotein lipase; FFA = free fatty acids; LCAT = lecithin-cholesterol acyltransferase; VLDL = very low density lipoproteins; HDL = high density lipoproteins; LDL = low density lipoproteins.

which LDL delivers cholesterol to extrahepatic cells, while cholesterol is returned to LDL from extrahepatic cells via HDL.

INHERITED HYPERLIPOPROTEINEMIAS

Familial hypercholesterolemia is a relatively common autosomal dominant disorder characterized by an increased plasma concentration of LDL. In its heterozygous form, this disorder affects approximately one in 500 Americans. Heterozygotes exhibit a two- to three-fold elevation in their total plasma cholesterol concentration, while homozygotes have a six- to eight-fold elevation in plasma LDL–cholesterol levels. Hypercholesterolemia with little or no increase in plasma triglycerides can be detected shortly after birth and is present throughout life. Clinical features include the development of large xanthomas in the Achilles or plantar tendons as well as small xanthomas on the extensor tendons of the hands. Xanthelasma (raised yellow plaques near the inner canthus of the eyelids) and corneal arcus are common findings. Patients with familial hypercholesterolemia have an increased incidence of premature atherosclerotic coronary artery disease and peripheral vascular disease compared to the general population. Homozygotes can develop malignant coronary vascular disease, with death from myocardial infarction often occurring in the third decade of life.

Diagnosis rests on the detection of a greater than normal serum cholesterol concentration and normal plasma triglyceride levels in a patient with characteristic xanthomas. Although a diet restricted in saturated fats and cholesterol will induce some reduction in plasma cholesterol levels, such treatment alone will not reduce lipoprotein levels to normal. Administration of nonabsorbable substances such as cholestyramine that bind bile acids is more effective. The addition of large doses of nicotinic acid may reduce lipoprotein levels to normal. Following such treatment, xanthomatous lesions may regress slowly, but tendinous lesions seldom resolve completely. It has not been established that reducing the lipoprotein level will prevent or delay the onset of ischemic vascular disease.

zymes or transport proteins on cell membranes. Lipoproteins are classified according to their size, density, electrophoretic mobility, and molecular composition (Table 62–1).

Circulating free fatty acids are reconstituted with glycerol in the liver to form endogenous triglycerides that are secreted continuously as *very low density lipoproteins (VLDL)*. VLDL remain in the blood for a considerably longer period of time than chylomicrons. VLDL remnants are converted by a poorly understood mechanism to *low density lipoprotein (LDL)*.

Dietary cholesterol is transported to the liver in the form of chylomicrons. *High density lipoproteins (HDL)* play an important role in the subsequent transport of cholesterol to distant metabolic sites. Within HDL, cholesterol is coupled with fatty acid in an esterification process catalyzed by the plasma enzyme lecithin-cholesterol acyltransferase (LCAT). A large fraction of the cholesterol products of the LCAT reaction are eventually transferred to LDL. A cycle is thus established in

TABLE 62–1. CLASSIFICATION OF LIPOPROTEINS

ULTRACENTRIFUGAL DESIGNATION	ELECTROPHORETIC MOBILITY	MAJOR CORE LIPIDS	NUMERIC DESIGNATION OF HYPERLIPIDEMIA
Chylomicrons	Remain at orgin	Dietary triglycerides	I (alone) V (with VLDL)
VLDL	Pre-beta	Hepatic triglycerides	IV (alone) V (with chylomicrons) IIb (with LDL)
Remnants	Slow pre-beta	Cholesterol esters, triglycerides	III
LDL	Beta	Cholesterol esters	IIa (alone) IIb (with VLDL)
HDL	Alpha	Cholesterol esters	

Familial dysbetalipoproteinemia is an autosomal recessive disorder characterized by accumulation of an abnormal lipoprotein composed of remnant particles derived from the partial catabolism of VLDL and chlyomicrons. The condition has also been called broad beta disease or Type III hyperlipoproteinemia. The molecular defect resides in deficiency of two apoprotein components of VLDL—apoproteins E-3 and E-4. Clinical features include planar xanthomas in the creases of the palms and digits and confluent "tuberous" xanthomas over the knees and elbows and on the buttocks. Affected individuals seldom develop hyperlipidemia or other clinical features until the third decade of life. Premature coronary and peripheral atherosclerotic vascular diseases are common.

Laboratory evaluation of patients with familial dysbetalipoproteinemia reveals elevated plasma concentrations of cholesterol and triglycerides. Lipoprotein electrophoresis shows a broadening of the beta band; definitive diagnosis requires demonstration of apoprotein E-3 and E-4 deficiency. Treatment consists of reduction in dietary intake of simple sugars and cholesterol and weight reduction in obese patients. Clofibrate (500 mg two to four times daily) may be effective in reducing both triglyceride and cholesterol levels.

Primary Hypertriglyceridemias

Lipoprotein lipase deficiency results in the accumulation of triglycerides in the form of chylomicrons. The disorder, inherited as an autosomal recessive trait, is characterized by hepatosplenomegaly, recurrent bouts of pancreatitis, and "eruptive" xanthomas, i.e., small yellow skin papules surrounded by an erythematous halo. Patients exhibit markedly lactescent plasma, and plasma triglyceride levels can exceed several thousand mg per dl. The diagnosis is confirmed by demonstrating reduced lipolytic activity in serum following the administration of heparin. Treatment requires restriction of dietary fat to less than 30 grams per day.

Deficiency of apolipoprotein C-2 is a rare autosomal recessive disorder that also results in increased plasma chylomicron and triglyceride concentrations. In contrast to lipoprotein lipase deficiency, however, deficiency of apoprotein C-2 results in an elevation of plasma VLDL. The disorder also presents with recurrent bouts of pancreatitis, but eruptive xanthomas are much less common. Treatment consists of dietary fat restriction.

Familial endogenous and mixed hypertriglyceridemias are a heterogeneous group of disorders characterized by an increased plasma concentration of VLDL with or without a concomitant increase in plasma chylomicrons. Obesity and glucose intolerance are often present. Affected patients exhibit markedly elevated plasma triglyceride levels and frequently develop premature ischemic vascular disease. Eruptive xanthomas may occur if triglyceride levels are extremely high. The diagnosis is suspected if plasma triglyceride levels are elevated in the presence of normal plasma cholesterol levels. Electrophoresis of the plasma reveals an increase in the pre-beta fraction of lipoproteins. The plasma is typically cloudy and may exhibit a creamy supernatant if high levels of chylomicrons are present. Effective therapy begins with caloric restriction and weight reduction in obese patients. Dietary restriction of simple sugars, saturated fats, and alcohol assists in reducing plasma triglyceride levels. Clofibrate may be effective in patients who do not respond to dietary intervention alone.

Familial multiple lipoprotein-type hyperlipidemia is a relatively common disease, characterized by elevation of both plasma triglycerides and cholesterol. Most affected patients have a strong family history of premature coronary artery disease. Perhaps 10 per cent of patients with a myocardial infarction below age 60 have this disorder. Depending upon a variety of factors, VLDL, LDL, or both lipoprotein fractions may be elevated in the plasma, but the abnormal lipoprotein pattern is generally consistent within a single family. There is no specific diagnostic test, but a strong family history of premature coronary artery disease and lipoprotein abnormalities strongly suggests the diagnosis. Treatment should be individualized and directed at the predominant lipid abnormality. Triglyceride elevations decline with weight reduction, restriction of dietary saturated fats, and clofibrate. Some patients with isolated hypercholesterolemia respond to cholestyramine or nicotinic acid.

ACQUIRED HYPERLIPOPROTEINEMIA

A secondary increase in plasma lipoproteins accompanies numerous clinical disorders. Severe hypercholesterolemia commonly occurs with hypothyroidism and the nephrotic syndrome. Less marked increases in plasma cholesterol concentration may be observed in patients with Cushing's syndrome, anorexia nervosa, hepatoma, Werner's syndrome, and acute intermittent porphyria. The elevations in plasma cholesterol, if sustained, can predispose to premature atherosclerotic vascular disease. Therapy should be directed to correcting the underlying disorder, but persistent and severe hypercholesterolemia may warrant treatment with cholestyramine or nicotinic acid.

Severe forms of secondary hypertriglyceridemia can accompany diabetes mellitus, Von Gierke's disease, chronic alcohol consumption, chronic renal failure, acute hepatitis, and the administration of oral contraceptives. Less severe forms of hypertriglyceridemia have been observed in lipodystrophies, nephrotic syndrome, monoclonal gammopathies, acromegaly, Cushing's syndrome, and with corticosteroid administration. In diabetic patients with prolonged insulin deficiency and ketosis, chronic elevations of both VLDL and chylomicrons may lead to eruptive xanthomas and lipemia retinalis. Treatment of secondary hypertriglyceridemia is directed at correction of the underlying disorder. As with the primary hypertriglyceridemias, weight reduction in obese patients, restriction of dietary saturated fats, and avoidance of simple sugars, including alcohol, may be effective in reducing plasma triglyceride concentrations.

HYPOLIPOPROTEINEMIAS

These rare conditions merit discussion because the selected defects in lipoprotein synthesis shed light on the important normal functions of plasma lipoproteins. *Abetalipoproteinemia* is a rare autosomal recessive disorder that results from defective synthesis of apolipoprotein B, a substance required for the assembly of chylomicrons, VLDL, and LDL. Transport of plasma lipids is severely impaired and patients develop malabsorption, progressive ataxia, nystagmus, distal sensory loss, weakness, and visual impairment early in life. Treatment is limited to restriction of dietary fat, but the prognosis remains poor.

Tangier disease is a rare autosomal recessive disorder characterized by an absence of plasma HDL, resulting in impaired cholesterol transport. Pathologic features include diffuse deposition of cholesterol esters in reticuloendothelial cells and Schwann cells. Clinical manifestations include hepatosplenomegaly, lymphadenopathy, grossly enlarged tonsils, peripheral neuropathy, and premature vascular disease. No specific treatment is available.

Lecithin-cholesterol acyltransferase (LCAT) deficiency is a rare disorder characterized by an inability to form cholesterol esters in serum, resulting in accumulation of free cholesterol in tissues, particularly the bone marrow and kidney. Clinical manifestations include proteinuria, anemia, and renal failure.

LIPID STORAGE DISEASES

The lipid storage diseases result from inherited enzyme defects or deficiencies and are characterized by the abnormal accumulation of specific lipids within various organs (Table 62–2).

Tay-Sachs disease is the most common of the lipid storage diseases and results from deficiency of hexosaminidase A, leading to tissue accumulation of ganglioside. This autosomal recessive disorder occurs 100 times more frequently in Ashkenazi Jews than in other ethnic groups. The diagnosis can be confirmed by rectal biopsy using special histochemical stains to detect excess ganglioside. Homozygous infants exhibit growth retardation, weakness, seizures, blindness, and cherry-red retinal spots and generally die by two years of age.

Gaucher's disease is caused by a deficiency of β-glucocerebrosidase and is characterized by an abnormal accumulation of glucosylceramide in tissues. All forms of this disorder have an autosomal recessive inheritance and are found with increased frequency in Ashkenazi Jews of eastern European origin. The infantile form of Gaucher's

TABLE 62–2. THE LIPID STORAGE DISEASES

TYPE	ENZYME DEFICIENCY	STORED MATERIAL	INHERITANCE	CLINICAL MANIFESTATIONS	DIAGNOSIS
Gaucher	β-glucocerebrosidase	Glucosylceramide	AR*	*Infantile:* rapidly progressive neurologic abnormalities and early death *Juvenile and adult:* hepatosplenomegaly, hypersplenism, bleeding diathesis, bone pain, pathologic fractures	↓ enzyme activity in WBC's. Gaucher's cells in bone marrow or splenic tissue
Fabry	α-galactosidase A	Trihexosylceramide	Sex-linked	Painful neuropathy, telangiectasias, cataracts, progressive renal failure	↓ enzyme activity in renal or small bowel biopsy
Neimann-Pick	Sphingomyelinase	Sphingomyelin	AR*	*Infantile:* hepatosplenomegaly, failure to thrive, mental retardation, retinal degeneration. Less severe forms described	Distinctive foam cells, bone marrow, liver, spleen, and lymph nodes
Tay-Sachs	Hexosaminodase A	Ganglioside	AR*	Growth retardation, weakness, seizures, blindness, death by age 2	Histochemical stains on renal biopsy

AR = autosomal recessive.
*Increased incidence among Ashkenazi Jews.

disease is characterized by rapidly progressive neurologic abnormalities and early death. Juvenile and adult variants of this disorder are less severe, characterized primarily by hepatosplenomegaly and hematologic abnormalities resulting from bone marrow infiltration and hypersplenism. Other clinical manifestations include a bleeding diathesis, bone pain, and pathologic fractures. Decreased activity of β-glucocerebrosidase can be demonstrated in white blood cells and confirms the diagnosis. Diagnosis is also supported by the demonstration of Gaucher's cells in a bone marrow aspirate or in splenic tissue obtained by needle biopsy. These cells are characteristically round, oval, or spindle-shaped and have one or more small, eccentrically placed nuclei and numerous wavy fibrillae in the cytoplasm. The natural history of adult Gaucher's disease is variable, but life span is normal in most patients. Splenectomy may be required in patients with severe hypersplenism.

Fabry's disease results from a deficiency of the enzyme α-galactosidase A and is characterized by accumulation of the glycolipid trihexosylceramide in various tissues, including the liver, kidney, spleen, cornea, blood vessels, and ganglia of the central and peripheral nervous system. The disorder is sex-linked and fully manifest only in males who present in childhood with characteristic telangiectasias, corneal opacities, episodic burning and stabbing pains in the extremities, hypertension, and progressive renal failure. Heterozygous females may exhibit an attenuated form of the disease and often have detectable corneal opacities. Diagnosis is confirmed by the absence of α-galactosidase activity in tissue obtained by renal or small bowel biopsy. Affected males usually develop end-stage renal failure by the fourth decade and require maintenance dialysis. Renal transplantation may be accompanied by biochemical and clinical remission, presumably because the transplanted kidney provides normal α-galactosidase A for substrate metabolism.

Neimann-Pick disease is a group of disorders characterized by a deficiency in sphingomyelinase, resulting in an accumulation of sphingomyelin in various tissues. The infantile forms are characterized by failure to thrive, hepatosplenomegaly, mental retardation, and retinal degeneration with cherry-red spots in the macular area of the optic fundi. Bone marrow biopsy reveals infiltration by large macrophages filled with lipid inclusions (foam cells). The liver, spleen, and lymph nodes are also infiltrated with foam cells. There is no specific treatment for any of the sphingomyelin storage diseases.

REFERENCES

Brunzell JD: The Hyperlipoproteinemias. In Wyngaarden JB, and Smith LH Jr (eds): Cecil Textbook of Medicine. 17th ed. Philadelphia, WB Saunders Co, 1985, p 1109.

Havel RJ: Symposium on lipid disorders. Med Clin North Am 66:317, 1982.

DISORDERS OF METALS AND METALLOPROTEINS | 63

WILSON'S DISEASE (HEPATOLENTICULAR DEGENERATION)

Wilson's disease is a rare autosomal recessive disorder characterized by a defect in hepatic excretion of copper. Toxic levels accumulate in the liver, basal ganglia of the brain, and other tissues. The majority of patients exhibit reduced concentrations of ceruloplasmin in the serum.

Pathogenesis. The primary genetic defect accounting for impaired biliary copper excretion in Wilson's disease is unknown. It has been speculated that hepatocytes of patients with this disorder contain an abnormal protein with an increased affinity for copper. Hepatic lysosomes lack the ability to excrete into bile copper that has been cleaved from circulating ceruloplasmin. This may cause a secondary deficiency of ceruloplasmin, since excess copper inhibits the formation of ceruloplasmin from apoceruloplasmin. The capacity of hepatocytes to store copper is eventually overwhelmed, resulting in release of the metal into blood and accumulation at extrahepatic sites.

Clinical Features. The age of onset and initial signs and symptoms of Wilson's disease are quite variable, clinical manifestations of copper excess being rare before the age of six. Approximately one third of patients present with symptoms of liver disease that may mimic acute viral hepatitis or cirrhosis with portal hypertension. More frequently, patients first present with extrahepatic manifestations of copper excess. Neurologic disturbances, including tremor, dysarthria, muscular rigidity, seizures, personality changes, and dementia, are common initial manifestations.

Other clinical features of Wilson's disease include Kayser-Fleischer corneal rings caused by copper deposition at the margins of the cornea. The rings, which may require slit-lamp detection, are uniformly present in patients with neurologic symptoms but may be absent in patients with isolated hepatic involvement. Like other heavy metals, copper may be nephrotoxic; renal deposition of copper is usually manifest by tubular dysfunction, including glycosuria, phosphaturia, aminoaciduria, renal tubular acidosis, or the complete Fanconi syndrome. Acute or chronic hemolytic anemia in Wilson's disease has been attributed to the release of copper from overloaded tissues, but the exact mechanisms have not been elucidated.

The diagnosis of Wilson's disease is supported in suspected cases by (1) detection of Kayser-Fleischer rings by slit-lamp examination, (2) a serum concentration of ceruloplasmin less than 20 mg/dl, (3) a concentration of copper in a liver biopsy sample greater than 250 µg per gram of dry weight, or (4) urinary excretion of more than 100 µg of copper per day. While none of these criteria is sufficiently sensitive or specific to make an unequivocal diagnosis of Wilson's disease, they serve to corroborate the diagnosis in patients with appropriate clinical signs and symptoms. Although the level of direct-reacting (non–ceruloplasmin-bound) copper in the serum of patients with Wilson's disease is typically elevated, total levels are not consistently altered, so that measurement of serum copper levels serves little purpose in the diagnosis of this disorder.

Treatment. D-Penicillamine is the drug of choice. Daily doses of 1 to 2 gm increase urinary copper excretion more than five-fold over pretreatment levels and can prevent virtually every manifestation of Wilson's disease, provided that treatment is begun as soon as the diagnosis is secure.

HEMOCHROMATOSIS

An increase in the quantity of storage iron in the body is called *hemosiderosis*. The term *hemochromatosis* refers to an increase in total body iron stores with iron deposition in parenchymal tissues that ultimately leads to functional impairment of the most severely affected organs. *Acquired hemochromatosis* results from exogenous iron overload due to excessive dietary iron ingestion or repeated blood transfusions. This section focuses on *familial hemochromatosis*, a genetically determined iron storage disorder resulting from an inappropriate increase in intestinal iron absorption. The clinical and pathologic features of acquired and familial hemochromatosis can be identical.

Pathogenesis. Normally the total body iron content of 3 to 4 gm is maintained by a balance between intestinal absorption and fecal excretion of iron. The amounts of iron absorbed and excreted daily are small, being approximately 1.0 mg in men and 1.5 mg in menstruating women. In familial hemochromatosis, intestinal iron absorption is inappropriately large, usually amounting to more than 3 mg per day. The progressive accumulation of iron produces an early elevation of plasma iron and an increased saturation of circulating transferrin. In advanced disease, total body iron content may exceed 20 gm.

The tendency to absorb iron excessively is inherited as an autosomal recessive trait. Homozygotes have large iron stores and manifest the disease; heterozygotes exhibit minor derangements in iron metabolism but may develop the disease when an added factor such as alcohol consumption or increased oral iron intake enhances the accumulation of iron in excess of their usual stores. Hemochromatosis is observed five to ten times more commonly in men than in women, presumably because menstrual blood losses protect against iron overload.

Excess iron is deposited predominantly in parenchymal cells of the liver, heart, pancreas, and other endocrine organs. In early stages of the disease, deposits of iron in these organs consist of ferritin and hemosiderin stored within lysosomes. Tissue injury results from disruption of lysosomes and lipid peroxidation of subcellular organelles by iron. Varying degrees of fibrosis occur in affected organs. Cirrhosis of the liver is almost invariably present in symptomatic cases. Iron deposition in the liver is initially limited to lysosomes in the pericanalicular cytoplasm of hepatocytes. As the disease progresses, iron is also deposited in bile duct epithelium and in Kupffer cells. In the advanced stage, an irregular multilobular cirrhosis develops, with a paucity of inflammatory cells and prominent bile duct proliferation.

Clinical Features. Signs and symptoms of hemochromatosis usually develop between the ages of 40 and 60. Constitutional symptoms include lassitude and weakness, but the most prominent symptoms relate to iron deposition in specific organs. The liver is usually the first organ to be affected. Although firm hepatomegaly is present in more than 95 per cent of cases at the time of diagnosis, liver function tests may remain normal during early stages of the disease. The spleen is enlarged in approximately half of cases, but other clinical manifestations of portal hypertension occur less commonly than in other forms of cirrhosis. Hepatocellular carcinoma develops in about 35 per cent of cases and is currently the most common cause of death in treated patients.

About 90 per cent of patients exhibit excessive skin pigmentation, developing a characteristic metallic gray appearance from increased deposition of melanin and hemosiderin in the basal layer of the epidermis. Pigmentation is usually greatest on the face, neck, genitalia, and extensor surfaces of the extremities.

Insulin-dependent diabetes mellitus develops in approximately 80 per cent of cases from iron deposition in pancreatic islet cells. Vascular complications of diabetes such as retinopathy, peripheral neuropathy, and nephropathy may develop in long-term survivors.

Cardiac manifestations include congestive

heart failure, a variety of ventricular and supraventricular arrhythmias, and conduction disturbances including heart block. Cardiac involvement is the presenting manifestation in about 15 per cent of cases. Congestive failure in hemochromatosis may be resistant to digitalis therapy. Cardiomyopathy accounts for about one third of deaths.

Loss of libido, sexual impotence, and testicular atrophy are present in more than 50 per cent of cases. Although hypogonadism may result in part from chronic liver disease, the symptoms more often are due to deficient production of trophic sex hormones by the anterior pituitary gland. Adrenal insufficiency and hypothyroidism rarely have been described.

About 25 per cent of patients develop acute attacks of synovitis due to synovial deposition of calcium pyrophosphate (i.e., chondrocalcinosis). In late stages, a progressive polyarthritis involving the hands, wrists, knees, and hips may develop. Radiographic findings include cystic changes in subchondral bone, loss of articular cartilage, and diffuse demineralization. The pathophysiological link between the rheumatologic manifestations of hemochromatosis and the underlying disturbance in iron metabolism is unknown.

Hemochromatosis should be suggested by the above clinical features and confirmed by laboratory tests. Measurements of the plasma iron concentration and the plasma iron-binding capacity provide the best screening tests. Plasma iron is usually greater than 200 µg/dl; total iron-binding capacity is normal or slightly decreased, but the transferrin saturation is greatly elevated, usually between 80 and 100 per cent. Other available measures of excessive parenchymal iron stores include (1) serum ferritin concentration, (2) urinary iron excretion following administration of the chelating agent desferrioxamine, and (3) liver biopsy with measurement of hepatic iron content (Table 63–1).

Treatment and Prognosis. Treatment consists of removing excess body iron and supportive treatment of complications such as diabetes mellitus and heart failure. Body iron is best removed by phlebotomy. Since 500 ml of blood contains 200 to 250 mg of iron, two to three years of weekly phlebotomies may be required to remove 20 gm of iron and to restore normal plasma iron concentrations. Once normal plasma iron levels return, less frequent phlebotomies are continued to maintain a plasma concentration less than 150 µg/dl.

Phlebotomy is more effective and less expensive than administration of chelating agents such as desferrioxamine, but the latter may be useful when anemia precludes frequent venesections. Daily intramuscular injection of 0.5 to 1.0 gm of desferrioxamine removes 10 to 20 mg of iron per day—one tenth or less of the amount mobilized by weekly phlebotomy. Desferrioxamine can also be administered subcutaneously using a small constant infusion pump.

Without treatment, hemochromatosis offers an

TABLE 63–1. IRON INDICES IN NORMAL SUBJECTS AND IN PATIENTS WITH SYMPTOMATIC HEMOCHROMATOSIS

INDEX	NORMAL SUBJECTS	PATIENTS WITH HEMOCHROMATOSIS
Plasma iron (µg/dl)	50–150	180–300
Total iron binding capacity (µg/dl)	250–375	200–300
Per cent transferrin saturation	20–40	80–100
Serum ferritin (ng/ml)	10–200	900–6000
Urinary iron after 0.5 gm desferrioxamine	0–2	9–23
Liver iron (µg/100 mg dry weight)	30–140	600–1800

average life expectancy of four and one-half years following diagnosis. Life expectancy is extended to more than eight years by removal of excessive iron stores. Therapy improves carbohydrate tolerance in almost half of cases, but established cirrhosis is irreversible. Blood relatives of patients with hemochromatosis should be examined by measurements of plasma iron, iron-binding capacity, and serum ferritin levels so as to initiate early therapy in asymptomatic carriers.

PORPHYRIA

The porphyrias are a group of heterogeneous disorders resulting from inherited or acquired disturbances in heme biosynthesis. Porphyrins are pigments that serve as intermediates in this synthetic pathway. Heme, the ferrous iron complex of protoporphyrin IX, serves as a prosthetic group for a number of hemoproteins, including hemoglobin and mitochondrial cytochromes. Each of the porphyrias results from a deficiency of a specific enzyme in the heme biosynthetic pathway and is characterized by a unique pattern of overproduction and accumulation of porphyrin intermediates (Table 63–2). The porphyrias are usually categorized into two main groups, erythropoietic and hepatic, according to the major site at which the metabolic error is expressed.

Pathogenesis. Porphyrins are "side-products" of intermediates in the heme biosynthetic pathway, schematically outlined in Figure 63–1. The precursors glycine and succinyl coenzyme A are converted to δ-aminolevulinic acid (ALA) in a reaction catalyzed by ALA-synthetase. This reaction is the rate-limiting step in heme biosynthesis, subject to feedback regulation by heme, the end-product of the pathway. Two moles of ALA combine to form porphobilinogen. Only protoporphyrin is utilized in heme synthesis. The other porphyrins (i.e., uroporphyrin, coproporphyrin) have no physiological function and must be excreted; their fluorescent properties account for the diagnostic appearance of the urine in some patients.

Clinical Features. Congenital erythropoietic porphyria is a rare disorder resulting from a defect in the activity of uroporphyrinogen III cosynthetase resulting in massive overproduction of uroporphyrinogen III and secondary accumulation of

TABLE 63–2. CLASSIFICATION AND CHARACTERISTICS OF THE PORPHYRIAS: HEME PRECURSORS PRESENT IN ABNORMAL AMOUNTS

TYPE	URINE	PLASMA	ENZYME DEFECT
Erythropoietic			
Congenital erythropoietic porphyria	URO ≫ COPRO	URO	UROgen III cosynthetase
Erythrohepatic			
Protoporphyria	—	PROTO	Ferrochelatase
Hepatic			
Acute intermittent porphyria	ALA < PBG ≫ URO	ALA, PBG	PBG deaminase
Hereditary coproporphyria	ALA < PBG < URO < COPRO	COPRO	COPROgen oxidase
Variegate porphyria	ALA < PBG < URO < COPRO	COPRO, PROTO	PROTOgen oxidase
Porphyria cutanea tarda	URO ≫ COPRO	URO	UROgen decarboxylase

ALA = δ-aminolevulinic acid; PBG = porphobilinogen; URO = uroporphyrin; COPRO = coproporphyrin; PROTO = protoporphyrin.

uroporphyrin and coproporphyrin. Fewer than 100 cases have been described. Patients exhibit hemolytic anemia and severe photosensitivity, with mutilating bullous lesions on light-exposed skin. Treatment relies on avoidance of sunlight.

Protoporphyria results from partial deficiency of ferrochelatase, the final enzyme in heme biosynthesis that catalyzes the conversion of protoporphyrin to heme. The disease is characterized by excess protoporphyrin IX in erythrocytes, plasma, and feces. Cutaneous photosensitivity is the major clinical manifestation. About 10 per cent of patients develop protoporphyrin-contain-

ing gallstones, and some develop mild liver disease. Treatment includes avoidance of sunlight and administration of β-carotene, which blocks light- and porphyrin-induced cutaneous injury.

Three variants of hepatic porphyria can be considered together, since their clinical manifestations and treatment are similar. *Acute intermittent porphyria* results from partial deficiency of porphobilinogen deaminase, leading to accumulation and excess urinary excretion of porphobilinogen and ALA. *Hereditary coproporphyria* is characterized by excess excretion of ALA, porphobilinogen, uroporphoyrin, and coropor-

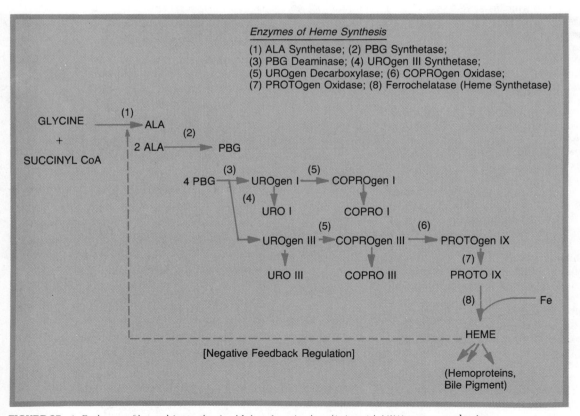

FIGURE 63–1. Pathway of heme biosynthesis. ALA = δ-aminolevulinic acid; URO = uroporphyrin; COPRO = coproporphyrin; PROTO = protoporphyrin; PBG = porphobilinogen. (Reprinted from Bissell DM: Porphyria. In Wyngaarden JB, Smith LH Jr (eds): Cecil Textbook of Medicine. 17th ed. Philadelphia, WB Saunders Co, 1985, p 1154.)

phyrin due to partial deficiency of coproporphyrinogen oxidase. Partial deficiency of protoporphyrinogen oxidase underlies *variegate porphyria* and leads to excess excretion of the entire series of heme precursors. Acute attacks of abdominal pain, seizures, or a severe motor polyneuropathy can occur with each of these disorders. Intense abdominal pain during the first 24 to 48 hours of an attack may suggest acute cholecystitis, appendicitis, or other surgical diagnoses and may provoke unnecessary surgery. Psychiatric disturbances include personality changes and acute delirious reactions, with signs and symptoms resembling delirium tremens. Attacks may be precipitated by a variety of drugs (Table 63–3), especially those such as barbiturates that increase the demand for heme synthesis by induction of cytochrome P-450. Attacks are rare prior to puberty and are more common in women than in men, suggesting that endogenous hormones may play a role. Infection and fasting may also precipitate attacks. Because urinary porphobilinogen is increased in each of these porphyrias, the diagnosis is suspected by qualitative detection of porphobilinogen with the Watson-Schwartz test. Quantitation of urinary and fecal porphyrins identifies the specific variant of porphyria. Treatment includes elimination of possible precipitating drugs, administration of carbohydrate to reverse fasting, analgesia, and supportive management of seizures, delirium, and other neurologic complications. Hematin, a commercial preparation of ferriprotoporphyrin IX, has been administered to patients with prolonged attacks that do not respond to conservative therapy, but its efficacy remains unproven.

Porphyria cutanea tarda is another variant of hepatic porphyria. The condition results from partial deficiency of uroporphyrinogen decarboxylase, leading to increased urinary uroporphyrin

TABLE 63–3. DRUGS THAT MAY PRECIPITATE ACUTE ATTACKS IN HEPATIC PORPHYRIA

Barbiturates	Estrogens
Ethanol	Ergot preparations
Chlordiazepoxide	Methyldopa
Imipramide	Chloroquine
Meprobamate	Griseofulvin
Glutethimide	
Chlorpropamide	

excretion and modest increments of urinary coproporphyrin. Mechanical fragility and photosensitivity of the skin are the primary clinical manifestations. Most affected patients give a history of ethanol abuse and/or chronic liver disease. The liver abnormalities are nonspecific but include increase in stainable iron and fluorescence resulting from the high content of uroporphyrin. Treatment includes avoidance of alcohol and phlebotomy to remove hepatic iron when clinically overt liver disease is present. Beta-carotene offers little or no protection against light-induced injury in this disorder.

REFERENCES

Bissell DM: Heme metabolism and the porphyrias. In Wright R, Alberti KGMM, Karran S, Millward-Sadler GH (eds): Liver and Biliary Disease. London, WB Saunders Co, 1984.

Milder MS, Cook JD, Stray S, and Finch CA: Idiopathic hemochromatosis, an interim report. Medicine 59:34, 1980.

Stein JA, and Tschudy DP: Acute intermittent porphyria. A clinical and biochemical study of 46 patients. Medicine 49:1, 1970.

Sternlieb I: Diagnosis of Wilson's disease. Gastroenterology 74:787, 1978.

Strickland T, and Len ML: Wilson's disease: Clinical and laboratory manifestations in 40 patients. Medicine 54:113, 1975.

DISORDERS OF AMINO ACID METABOLISM

64

Defects in the membrane transport or catabolism of amino acids account for more than 70 inherited or acquired "aminoacidopathies." Each of these disorders is rare, but collectively they occur in approximately 1 in 1000 live births. This section describes selected disorders that illustrate the problems posed by aminoacidopathies.

HYPERAMINOACIDURIA (MEMBRANE TRANSPORT DEFECTS)

Although most of the body's 20 amino acids are contained within various polypeptides and proteins, a small but critical pool of *free* amino acids circulates in extracellular fluid. Most amino acids are freely filtered by renal glomeruli, but more than 95 per cent of the filtered load is actively and specifically reabsorbed in the proximal renal tubule via receptors that recognize and transport individual amino acids or groups of structurally related ones. Aminoaciduria results from either an acquired or hereditary disturbance of cellular metabolism or when the transport of amino acids is impaired by (1) saturation of the receptor sites, (2) competition for the receptor sites by other substrates, or (3) a defect in the function or structural integrity of the receptor. Defects in membrane transport may affect a single amino acid, a group

TABLE 64–1. CLASSIFICATION OF MAJOR HYPERAMINOACIDURIAS

	TRAIT	SUBSTANCE(S) AFFECTED
Substrate-specific	Histidinuria	Histidine
	Hypercystinuria	Cystine
Group-specific	Cystinuria	Lysine, ornithine, arginine, cystine
	Hartnup disease	Neutral amino acids
	Iminoglycinuria	Proline, hydrocyproline, glycine
	Dicarboxylic aminoaciduria	Glutamic acid, aspartic acid
	Hyperdibasic aminoaciduria	Lysine, ornithine, arginine
Generalized	Idiopathic Fanconi's syndrome	Generalized effect on all amino acids, solutes, and water
	Acquired Fanconi's syndrome	Generalized effect on all amino acids, solutes, and water

of structurally related amino acids, or all amino acids (Table 64–1).

Cystinuria, the most common inborn error of amino acid transport, results from an inherited defect in the membrane receptor for the dibasic amino acids lysine, arginine, ornithine, and cystine. The disorder is inherited as an autosomal recessive trait. Cystine is the least soluble of all amino acids, and its excessive excretion in urine predisposes to the formation of calculi. Normally, the maximum solubility of cystine in urine is about 300 mg/L. Affected homozygotes regularly excrete 600 to 1800 mg of cystine per day.

Signs and symptoms of cystinuria are those of urolithiasis: renal colic, hematuria, obstructive uropathy, and secondary infection, usually beginning during the second or third decade of life. Recurrent episodes of urolithiasis and infection can lead to progressive renal insufficiency.

The diagnosis of cystinuria requires either demonstration of the characteristic aminoaciduria by chromatography or electrophoresis or the detection of cystine in a urinary tract calculus. As many as 50 per cent of stones excreted by cystinuric patients, however, have a mixed composition. Uri-

TABLE 64–2. SOME DISORDERS ASSOCIATED WITH ACQUIRED FANCONI'S SYNDROME

1. Systemic or Hereditary Diseases
Multiple myeloma	Wilson's disease
Amyloidosis	Hereditary fructose intolerance
Sjögren's syndrome	Galactosemia
Cystinosis	
2. Heavy Metal Poisonings
Mercury	Uranium
Lead	Strontium
Cadmium	
3. Drugs
6-Mercaptopurine	"Outdated" tetracycline
Streptozocin	

nary cystine crystals have a characteristic hexagonal shape; their discovery in the urine of a patient with signs and symptoms of urolithiasis is often the first clue to the diagnosis of cystinuria.

Treatment of cystinuria consists of efforts to reduce the urinary concentration of cystine. Vigorous hydration, with fluid ingestion of 4 to 8 L per day, is the most important aspect of medical management. Because the solubility of cystine increases sharply as urine pH rises above 7.5, urinary alkalinization may be effective in preventing stone formation; however, vigorous administration of sodium bicarbonate and/or acetazolamide is required to maintain a persistently alkaline urine. Administration of D-penicillamine in doses of 1 to 3 gm per day effectively lowers the urinary concentration of free cystine, prevents new stone formation, and promotes the dissolution of existing calculi. The drug undergoes sulfhydryl-disulfide exchange with cystine to form a mixed penicillamine-cysteine disulfide that is 50 times more soluble than cystine. D-Penicillamine, however, has a number of serious side effects (e.g., exfoliative dermatitis, heavy proteinuria, bone marrow depression), and should be reserved for patients who fail to respond to more conservative measures.

Generalized aminoaciduria reflects a generalized defect in the renal tubular reabsorption of all filtered amino acids and is characteristic of patients with Fanconi's syndrome. The renal loss of amino acids in Fanconi's syndrome is usually outweighed by other disturbances of proximal tubular function, including glycosuria, phosphaturia, bicarbonaturia, and uric aciduria. Presenting manifestations of this disorder may include hypophosphatemic rickets in children, osteomalacia in adults, proximal renal tubular acidosis, or hypouricemia. Fanconi's syndrome may be acquired or associated with an inherited enzymatic disorder (e.g., hereditary fructose intolerance). In addition, a primary hereditary disorder (idiopathic Fanconi's syndrome) has been identified. The common causes of acquired Fanconi's syndrome are listed in Table 64–2.

AMINO ACID STORAGE DISEASES

Cystinosis is a rare idiopathic disorder characterized by the accumulation of cystine crystals in various tissues, including the cornea, bone marrow, lymph nodes, and kidneys. Three clinical forms exist: (1) *infantile cystinosis*, characterized by the Fanconi syndrome and progressive renal failure, occurs during the first decade of life; (2) in *juvenile cystinosis*, renal failure does not occur until the second decade; (3) *adult cystinosis* is a relatively benign disorder in which cystine accumulation is usually limited to the cornea, resulting in photophobia or mild irritation of the eyes.

Adult cystinosis requires no treatment. Treatment of nephropathic cystinosis consists of supportive management of progressive renal failure;

D-penicillamine is ineffective. Renal transplantation has been performed successfully in patients with cystinosis and end-stage renal failure, but reaccumulation of cystine can occur in the transplanted allograft after many years.

Alcaptonuria, a rare disorder of tyrosine catabolism resulting from hereditary deficiency of homogentisic acid oxidase, is associated with the excretion of large amounts of homogentisic acid in the urine and the accumulation of oxidized homogentisic acid in connective tissues. *Ochronosis*, a bluish-grey pigmentation, occurs when homogentisic acid and its oxidized polymers bind to collagen. The earliest clinical manifestations of alcaptonuria include slight pigmentation of the sclerae and external ears during the second and third decades. The urine tends to darken on standing, a finding that frequently goes unnoticed. Most patients develop degenerative joint disease by the fourth or fifth decade, ankylosis of the lumbar spine being a common late finding. The diagnosis is suggested by the triad of degenerative arthritis, ochronotic pigmentation, and the detection of urine that blackens on standing and is confirmed by measurement of urinary homogentisic acid. There is no known specific treatment.

OTHER DISORDERS OF AMINO ACID METABOLISM MEDIATED BY ENZYMATIC DEFECTS

Phenylketonuria is an autosomal recessive disorder resulting from impaired conversion of the essential amino acid phenylalanine to tyrosine due to deficient activity of the enzyme phenylalanine dehydroxylase. This disorder is manifested by accumulation of phenylalanine and its minor metabolites and by severe mental retardation. Infants with phenylketonuria are usually normal at birth, but signs of mental and psychomotor retardation, hyperactivity, tremors, or seizures usually develop within the first year of life. Early recognition of this disorder is imperative, since its devastating consequences can be prevented completely if dietary restriction of phenylalanine is instituted within the first 30 days of life. Most newborns in the United States are

screened for this disorder by determinations of blood phenylalanine concentrations using a bacterial inhibition assay. Quantitative chromatographic assays are employed for definitive diagnosis in infants with abnormal screening results. Treatment of phenylketonuria consists of a diet in which the bulk of protein is replaced by an amino acid mixture low in phenylalanine. Although scrupulous adherence to such a dietary regimen is of critical importance during the early months of life, it is probably wise to continue dietary therapy at least through the first decade, and perhaps indefinitely. Phenylalanine ingestion must be monitored carefully in the pregnant woman with phenylketonuria to prevent central nervous system damage in the fetus.

The term *homocystinuria* refers to a group of biochemically and clinically distinct disorders characterized by accumulation of the sulfur-containing amino acid, homocystine, in blood and urine. Homocystine is the disulfide oxidation product formed by two molecules of homocysteine. Accumulation of homocystine results in impaired collagen formation, a phenomenon that accounts for many of the clinical manifestations of this disorder. The most common variant of homocystinuria results from deficiency of cystathionine β-synthase, resulting in a failure of homocysteine to react with serine to form cystathionine. Deficiency of this enzyme is inherited as an autosomal recessive trait. Patients with homocystinuria and cystathionine β-synthase deficiency exhibit dislocated optic lenses, lax ligaments, and sparse fine hair. They may resemble patients with Marfan's syndrome. Mental retardation occurs in approximately 50 per cent of cases. Thromboembolic disease is the major cause of morbidity and mortality and may be initiated by damage to vascular endothelium.

REFERENCES

Scriver CR, and Rosenberg LE: Amino Acid Metabolism and Its Disorders. Philadelphia, WB Saunders Co, 1973.

Wellner D, and Meister A: A survey of inborn errors of amino acid metabolism and transport in man. Annu Rev Biochem 50:911, 1981.

DISORDERS OF CARBOHYDRATE METABOLISM 65

GALACTOSEMIA

Two inherited enzyme deficiencies impair the metabolic conversion of galactose to glucose and cause accumulation of galactose in the body, or galactosemia. *Classic galactosemia* results from

deficient activity of the enzyme galactose-1-phosphate uradyl transferase; a less common form of galactosemia results from *galactokinase deficiency*. Accumulation of galactose in the ocular lens produces excessive hydration, precipitation of lens protein, and formation of cataracts. Classic galactosemia also features liver disease, mental retardation, and failure to thrive, untreated infants surviving only a few days to weeks. Further details regarding clinical features of these neonatal disorders can be found in pediatric textbooks.

THE GLYCOGEN STORAGE DISEASES

Glycogen is present in virtually all animal cells and constitutes the principal storage form of carbohydrate. In contrast to starch, the storage form of carbohydrate in plants, glycogen has a highly branched structure that enhances its solubility. A variety of inherited enzymatic defects adversely affect the synthesis and degradation of glycogen. In general, such defects produce either an elevated tissue concentration of glycogen or an abnormality in the structure of the carbohydrate. As specific enzyme defects were recognized, the glycogen storage diseases were numbered or assigned eponyms. The diseases are grouped as either hepatic or muscular disorders, according to the major site affected by the metabolic error. The enzyme deficiencies, clinical manifestations, and laboratory findings of the glycogen storage diseases are shown in Table 65–1. Hepatic variants are largely disorders of children and frequently cause death early in life. Clinical features of the muscle glycogen storage diseases are discussed elsewhere in this text.

DISORDERS OF FRUCTOSE METABOLISM

Fructose is an important source of dietary carbohydrate. The monosaccharide is widely distributed in vegetables and fruits and is found in honey and numerous other nutrients as a component of the disaccharide sucrose. The average daily intake of fructose is 50 to 100 grams. The liver, kidney, and small intestine are the main sites of fructose metabolism. Fructose is clearly toxic when given intravenously in high doses and may produce hyperuricemia, hyperlactatemia, and ultrastructural abnormalities in liver and intestinal cells.

Fructokinase catalyzes the first reaction in the major pathway of fructose utilization in man and is normally present only in liver, kidney, and intestinal mucosa. Deficiency of this enzyme is inherited as an autosomal recessive trait and results in a rare condition known as *fructosuria*. The diagnosis of fructosuria is established by a fructose loading test, which produces an excessive rise in the concentration of fructose in blood and urine. The condition is generally benign; its major clinical significance lies in its potential confusion with diabetes mellitus, since urinary fructose produces a positive reaction with Clinitest tablets. Fructose does not, however, react with the urine dipstick test for glucose.

Hereditary fructose intolerance results from a structural mutation of the liver enzyme fructose-1-phosphate aldolase (aldolase B). This autosomal recessive disorder is characterized by severe hy-

TABLE 65–1. THE GLYCOGEN STORAGE DISEASES

NUMERIC TYPE	EPONYM	ENZYME DEFICIENCY	CLINICAL MANIFESTATIONS	LABORATORY FINDINGS	DIAGNOSIS
Hepatic Forms					
I	Von Gierke's	Glucose-6-phosphatase	Massive hepatomegaly, short stature, failure to thrive, severe hypoglycemia, retinal lesions	↑ lactate, pyruvate, triglycerides, cholesterol, uric acid	↓ enzyme activity or ↑ glycogen on liver biopsy
III	Cori's	Debrancher	Similar to Type I, but less severe; myopathy in adults	Normal lactate and uric acid, cholesterol, triglycerides	Enzyme assay on liver, muscle, WBC's or RBC's
IV	Anderson's	Brancher	Cirrhosis, hepatosplenomegaly, ascites, early death from liver failure	Very rare	Very rare
VI	Hers'	Liver phosphorylase	Mild hepatomegaly, mild hypoglycemia	Minimal	Enzyme assay on liver, ↑ liver glycogen
VIII	None	Phosphorylase β-kinase	Marked hepatomegaly, sex-linked disorder	Minimal	Enzyme assay on liver or WBC's
Muscle Forms					
II	Pompe's	α-1,4-glucosidase (acid maltase)	Massive cardiomegaly, hypotonia, early death from cardiorespiratory failure. Milder form in adults	↑ CPK	Enzyme assay on WBC's
V	McArdle's	Muscle phosphorylase	Exercise-induced muscle pain and cramps, rhabdomyolysis	↑ CPK with episodes; no blood lactate with exercise	↑ glycogen and ↓ enzyme activity on muscle biopsy

poglycemia and vomiting following the ingestion of fructose. Infants with this condition initially exhibit vomiting and failure to thrive; continued ingestion of fructose ultimately leads to hepatosplenomegaly, jaundice, ascites, and proximal renal tubular dysfunction manifested by the Fanconi syndrome, i.e., bicarbonaturia, generalized aminoaciduria, phosphaturia, and renal potassium wasting. Untreated children die from complications of hepatic failure. A high degree of clinical awareness is required for prompt diagnosis of this disorder, but suspicion is increased by the detection of a reducing substance (fructose) in the urine of an infant with other manifestations of the Fanconi syndrome. Treatment consists of prompt elimination of fructose from the diet. Infants with the disorder may respond slowly to withdrawal of dietary fructose, but once recovery is made the prognosis is excellent.

PRIMARY HYPEROXALURIA

Primary hyperoxaluria is a rare genetic disorder resulting from excessive synthesis and urinary excretion of oxalic acid. Two variants of this disorder can be distinguished by characteristic excretion of oxalate metabolites in the urine. *Type I primary hyperoxaluria* results from a defect in the enzyme α-ketoglutarate:glyoxalate carboligase and is manifest by increased urinary concentrations of oxalate and glycolate. In *Type II hyperoxaluria*, there is a defect in the enzyme D-glyceric dehydrogenase, resulting in increased urinary excretion of oxalate and L-glycerate. Each of these disorders is characterized by recurrent calcium oxalate nephrolithiasis and/or nephrocalcinosis during childhood, resulting in renal failure and death in patients not supported by dialysis. Once renal failure supervenes, the diagnosis may be difficult to establish because urinary excretion of oxalate metabolites declines as the glomerular filtration rate falls. Calcium oxalate deposition also occurs in other tissues, including the liver, spleen, testes, and bone marrow. Deposition of calcium oxalate in the walls of blood vessels may result in severe peripheral vascular insufficiency. Milder forms of primary hyperoxaluria have been described in adults with calcium oxalate kidney stones. The vast majority of patients with calcium oxalate nephrolithiasis have normal oxalate metabolism.

There is no specific treatment for primary hyperoxaluria. Phosphate or magnesium supplementation and forced diuresis have been variably successful in decreasing urinary stone formation. High doses of pyridoxine (200 to 400 mg/day) may reduce oxalate excretion in Type I hyperoxaluria. Patients with end-stage renal disease can be maintained on chronic dialysis. Successful renal transplantation has been hampered by rapid deposition of calcium oxalate in the transplanted kidney; however, intensive daily hemodialysis in the early post-transplant period may reduce plasma oxalate levels to sufficiently low levels to minimize renal oxalate deposition.

REFERENCES

Howell RR, and Williams JC: The glycogen storage diseases. In Stanbury JB, Wyngaarden JB, Fredrickson DS, Goldstein JL, and Brown MS (eds): The Metabolic Basis of Inherited Disease. 5th ed. New York, McGraw-Hill Book Co, 1982.
Segal S: Disorders of galactose metabolism. In Stanbury JB, Wyngaarden JB, Fredrickson DS, Goldstein JL, and Brown MS (eds): The Metabolic Basis of Inherited Disease. 5th ed. New York, McGraw-Hill Book Co, 1982.
Williams HE, and Smith LH Jr: Primary hyperoxaluria. In Stanbury JB, Wyngaarden JB, Fredrickson DS, Goldstein JL, and Brown MS (eds): The Metabolic Basis of Inherited Disease. 5th ed. New York, McGraw-Hill Book Co, 1982.

INHERITED DISORDERS OF CONNECTIVE TISSUE 66

The genetically transmitted disorders discussed in this section are characterized by histologically or ultramicroscopically demonstrable structural changes in the integumentary system. They are neither inflammatory nor immunological in origin and must be distinguished from acquired immunological diseases such as systemic lupus erythematosus, scleroderma, rheumatoid arthritis, and polymyositis, which have been improperly termed connective tissue diseases.

THE MUCOPOLYSACCHARIDOSES

The mucopolysaccharidoses are a group of disorders resulting from deficiencies of specific lysosomal enzymes involved in the degradation of the glycosaminoglycans, including chondroitin sulfate, dermatan sulfate, heparan sulfate, and keratan sulfate. Clinical manifestations derive from the accumulation of partially degraded glycosaminoglycans in connective tissues, heart, bony skeleton, and central nervous system. Features common to most of the mucopolysaccharidoses include onset in childhood, coarse facial features, corneal clouding, hepatosplenomegaly, joint stiffness, and a tendency to develop inguinal and umbilical hernias. Changes in the body skeleton, collectively referred to as dysostosis multiplex, include short stature, impaired growth of long bones, short stubby hands, and a variety of cranial abnormalities. Enzyme deficiencies and

TABLE 66–1.   THE MUCOPOLYSACCHARIDOSES

ABBREVI-ATION	EPONYM	ENZYME DEFICIENCY	MAJOR STORAGE PRODUCT	INHERI-TANCE	CLINICAL FEATURES
MPS-IH	Hurler's	α-L-Iduronidase	DS + HS	AR	Onset 6–12 months, dysostosis multiplex, progressive mental retardation, cardiac disease, death by age 10
MPS-IS	Scheie's	α-L-Iduronidase	DS + HS	AR	Onset 5–15 years, dysostosis multiplex, normal intelligence, long survival
MPS-II	Hunter's	L-Sulfoiduronate sulfatase	HS + DS	X-linked	May be mild or severe. If severe, similar to MPS-IH, death by age 15. If mild, survival to 30's–60's, depending on cardiac involvement
MPS-III	Sanfilippo's	4 types	HS	AR	Onset 2–6 years, dysostosis multiplex, rapidly progressive mental retardation, death at end of puberty
MPS-IV	Morquio's	N-acetylgalactosamine-6-sulfatase	KS + CS	AR	Severe, distinctive skeletal dysplasia, odontoid hypoplasia, aortic insufficiency, normal intelligence, death in 20's
MPS-VI	Maroteaux-Lamy	N-acetylgalactosamine-4-sulfatase (arylsulfatase B)	DS + ?CS	AR	Onset 2–4 years, dysostosis multiplex, aortic valve disease, normal intelligence, death in 20's (severe) or long survival (mild)
MPS-VII	None	β-glucuronidase	HS, DS, CS	AR	Onset 1–2 years, dysostosis multiplex, granulocyte inclusions, vascular involvement very rare

DS = dermatan sulfate; HS = heparan sulfate; KS = keratan sulfate; CS = chondroitin sulfate; AR = autosomal recessive.

clinical manifestations of the more common mucopolysaccharidoses are summarized in Table 66–1.

MARFAN'S SYNDROME

Marfan's syndrome is inherited as an autosomal dominant trait with ocular, skeletal, and cardiovascular manifestations. Approximately 15 per cent of cases represent new mutations. The exact nature of the molecular defect is unknown. The clinical expression of Marfan's syndrome varies greatly among affected family members, some patients having findings limited to one or two organ systems. The typical patient is tall and thin with long extremities: the arm span measures greater than the height, and the floor-to-pubis measurement exceeds the distance from pubis to crown. The fingers are long, thin, and hyperextensible (arachnodactyly). Kyphoscoliosis, asymmetry of the thoracic cage, and sternal deformities are common. The palate is high and arched, the facies is long and narrow, and the anterior teeth are crowded. Ligamentous weakness may lead to loose- or double-jointedness, and skeletal muscles often are poorly developed and hypotonic. Inguinal and femoral hernias are common, as are recurrent joint dislocations. Weakness and redundancy of the supporting tissues of the ocular lens lead to subluxation, most frequently in an upward and outward direction. Myopia and flattened corneas are common.

About 80 to 90 per cent of patients with Marfan's syndrome develop aortic disease, the most common cause of death. Medial degeneration leads to dilatation or dissection of the proximal aorta and aortic valvular insufficiency. Mitral valve prolapse is also common; either valvular lesion can be complicated by bacterial endocarditis. Surgical repair of aortic lesions has been variably successful. Propranolol has been recommended to decrease myocardial contractility and diminish the stress on the aorta, but results have not been encouraging. Isometric exercises and pregnancy increase the risk of cardiovascular catastrophe in patients with aortic disease.

EHLERS-DANLOS SYNDROME

The Ehlers-Danlos syndrome, a group of inherited connective tissue diseases, causes hyperextensible skin and joints, easy bruisability, friability of tissues, and poor wound healing. Eight variants of Ehlers-Danlos syndrome have been distinguished on the basis of clinical manifestations and purported alterations in collagen biosynthesis. Ehlers-Danlos syndrome Type I is the prototype with the most severe clinical manifestations. The skin is unusually soft, velvety, and hyperextensible, having a rubber-like quality allowing it to be stretched away from the underlying structures, promptly returning to its original position upon release. With aging, the skin may sag and become redundant, particularly over the elbows. Extreme fragility affects the skin so that minor trauma may produce gaping wounds. Minor injuries may also produce large hematomas that may organize into tumor-like calcified masses. Hyperextensibility of the joints allows affected patients to perform unusual contortions. Chronic or recurrent joint dislocations are common, particularly affecting the hips, knees, shoulders, and temporomandibular joints. Many patients suffer inguinal, hiatal, and umbilical hernias as well as gastrointestinal or genitourinary diverticulae. Ophthalmologic changes include blue sclerae, myopia, microcorneas, dislocated lenses, retinal detachment, and the appearance of widely spaced eyes. Cardiovascular manifestations include mitral valve prolapse, myocardial conduction abnormalities, and a variety of congenital cardiac anomalies. Catastrophic cardiovascular complications, including rupture of large arteries, occur most commonly in Ehlers-Danlos syndrome Type IV. Weakness of blood vessel walls or abnormal interaction of platelets with collagen often leads to a hemorrhagic diathesis.

The diagnosis of Ehlers-Danlos syndrome is usually suggested by the combination of hyperextensible skin and hypermobile joints. Additional clinical features and a family history of similar manifestations help in establishing the genetic type. Loose joints may also occur in Marfan's syndrome, several of the chondrodystrophies, and osteogenesis imperfecta. No specific treatment is available. Protection of the skin and joints from trauma is important, and surgery should be undertaken with extreme caution. Pregnancy carries a great risk.

REFERENCES

Hollister D, Byers PH, and Holbrook KA: Genetic disorders of collagen metabolism. Adv Hum Genet 12:1, 1982.

McKusick VA: Heritable Disorders of Connective Tissue. 4th ed. St. Louis, C.V. Mosby Co, 1972.

SECTION VIII

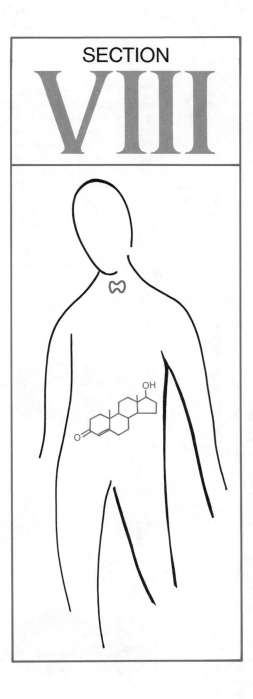

ENDOCRINE DISEASES

67 HYPOTHALAMIC-PITUITARY AXIS

The pituitary gland is a complex endocrine organ located in a bony fossa, the sella turcica, at the base of the brain. It consists of two distinct portions: the anterior pituitary (adenohypophysis) or glandular portion, derived from Rathke's pouch, and the posterior pituitary (neurohypophysis), which is an anatomical extension of the hypothalamus, derived from the diencephalon. Hormonal secretion by both portions of the pituitary gland is under the control of the central nervous system: the posterior lobe by a direct neurosecretory pathway from the anterior hypothalamus; the anterior lobe by a neuroendocrine system in which peptide and monoamine products of cells of the ventral hypothalamus are transported to the anterior pituitary via the hypothalamic-hypophyseal portal system. Owing to its unique location and intimate relationship with the central nervous system, the pituitary gland or, more appropriately, the hypothalamic-pituitary axis, is often referred to as the master gland of the endocrine system.

In this chapter we will review briefly the physiological regulation of anterior and posterior pituitary function as well as the major pathophysiological disorders affecting the hypothalamic-pituitary axis. In view of the intimate relationship between this axis and the function of specific endocrine target organs (i.e., thyroid, adrenal, and gonads), the reader should consult Chapters 68, 69, 70, and 71 for additional treatment of these topics.

HYPOTHALAMIC HORMONES

The hypothalamic secretory products that stimulate the secretion of the anterior pituitary hormones are peptides that vary in length from 3 to 44 amino acids. As an exception dopamine, a monoamine, is thought to provide tonic inhibition of prolactin secretion. Releasing hormones for thyrotropin (thyrotropin-releasing hormone or TRH), gonadotropin (GnRH), corticotropin (CRF), and growth hormone (GRF), and an inhibitory hormone for growth hormone secretion (somatostatin or SRIF) have been sequenced and synthesized. In addition to their roles in regulation of anterior pituitary function, several of these peptides and amines are found elsewhere in the brain and even outside of the central nervous system, particularly in the gut, where they may have neurotransmitter and other regulatory functions.

Hypothalamic hormones are secreted under neural regulation involving a variety of neurotransmitters (e.g., biogenic amines such as catecholamines and serotonin) (Fig. 67–1). Their secretion is also regulated by a blood-borne (closed-loop) feedback system involving the secretory products of pituitary and endocrine target cell origin. The hypothalamic hormones enter the hypophyseal portal system in complex mixtures, but the selectivity of their effects is assured by the presence of highly specific receptors on the various subtypes of trophic cells in the anterior pituitary gland.

ANTERIOR PITUITARY HORMONES

The anterior pituitary gland contains several cell types, each of which is capable of synthesizing, storing, and releasing a specific hormonal product. Six major and distinct secretory products have been recognized, which can be further subdivided into three classes of hormones: somato-

FIGURE 67–1. Neural regulation and feedback control of the hypothalamic-pituitary axis. Solid lines indicate positive and broken lines indicate negative regulation.

mammotropins, corticotropin and related peptides, and glycoproteins.

The somatomammotropins include growth hormone and prolactin as well as a placental secretory product known as chorionic somatomammotropin. These products, which share many structural similarities, have primarily lactogenic and growth-promoting effects. The somatomammotropins differ from the other hormonal products of the anterior pituitary in that they do not have a single classic endocrine target organ through which their effects are mediated. Many actions of growth hormone are mediated by a peptide, somatomedin C or insulin-like growth factor I (IGF-I), that is synthesized in the liver. Prolactin acts directly on the breast to promote synthesis of constituents of breast milk, but it is not responsible for breast development or milk release. The release of breast milk is regulated by oxytocin, a peptide that is released from the posterior pituitary.

Corticotropin (ACTH) is a 39 amino acid peptide that is part of a larger precursor molecule, proopiomelanocortin, which is the actual secretory product of the corticotrope. The larger molecule contains a number of biologically active peptides, including β-lipotropin, β-endorphin, melanocyte-stimulating hormone (MSH), and a large N-terminal fragment containing peptides that may have natriuretic properties. The exact mechanism controlling the differential release of these various fragments is not well understood. The principal effect of ACTH is to stimulate secretion of glucocorticoid (and to a lesser extent mineralocorticoid hormones) by the adrenal cortex. ACTH also has extraadrenal effects such as stimulation of lipolysis in adipose tissue.

The pituitary glycoprotein hormones—thyroid stimulating hormone (TSH), follicle-stimulating hormone (FSH), and luteinizing hormone (LH)—contain an α and a β subunit. The α units are identical, whereas the β units differ and confer thereby the specificity of the biological effects of each of these substances. A gonadotropin of chorionic origin, similar in structure to the glycoproteins of pituitary origin, also possesses an identical α subunit. The glycoprotein hormones exert their biological effects via the secretory products of their target organs: TSH modulates secretion of thyroxine and triiodothyronine by the thyroid gland; FSH and LH in women regulate ovulation and secretion of the steroid products of the ovary, whereas in men these gonadotropins regulate development of the seminiferous tubules and production of testosterone by the Leydig cells.

TESTS OF ANTERIOR PITUITARY FUNCTION

Radioimmunoassays for all of the major secretory products of the anterior pituitary gland are currently available in most clinical laboratories. When measurements of these hormones are used in conjunction with the appropriate physiological maneuvers and pharmacological probes, a precise characterization of states of anterior pituitary hypo- and hyperfunction is generally possible.

ACTH

Because levels of plasma ACTH may be undetectable in normal individuals when obtained under basal conditions, demonstration of ACTH deficiency requires the use of a stimulatory maneuver such as induction of hypoglycemia with insulin (0.1 U/kg intravenously) or of hypocortisolism with the 11β-hydroxylase inhibitor, metyrapone (750 mg orally every six hours for four doses). If ACTH assays are not available, ACTH reserve can be evaluated indirectly by measuring the response of plasma cortisol to the former and of 11-deoxycortisol to the latter stimulus; this approach presupposes that adrenal function is intact. The use of CRF to determine ACTH secretory reserve is currently being evaluated and may soon be available for general use. When used in conjunction with indirect stimuli such as insulin hypoglycemia, CRF testing may identify patients with hypothalamic lesions causing ACTH deficiency.

In states of suspected ACTH excess, suppression tests using exogenous glucocorticoid hormones such as dexamethasone are generally employed (see Chapter 69). Administration of CRF may also prove to be of value in this setting, particularly in distinguishing pituitary from ectopic sources of ACTH.

TSH

In patients with hypothyroidism and normal or undetectable levels of TSH, distinction between hypothalamic and pituitary abnormalities can be made using TRH. In this procedure, TSH levels are obtained before and 15 to 30 minutes after administration of TRH, 500 μg intravenously. Normally, TSH levels will increase to values of 15 to 30 μU/ml in response to this stimulus. Patients with pituitary hypothyroidism have a flat response, whereas TSH levels increase in those with hypothalamic hypothyroidism, although the response may be delayed. A flat TSH response to TRH may also be found in hyperthyroidism, acromegaly, renal insufficiency, and depression and during steroid therapy.

Gonadotropins

Administration of GnRH, 100 μg intravenously, can distinguish between pituitary and hypothalamic etiologies of gonadotropin deficiency. Normally, the response of LH is greater than that of FSH, averaging three to five times the control value. Repeated injections may be required to elicit normal responses in some patients with hypothalamic disorders. In children the pattern of response also differs depending on the age of the patient, and, in particular, the stage of pubertal development. The estrogen antagonist, clomiphene, can stimulate LH and FSH secretion in patients with hypothalamic hypogonadism and may be used as a therapeutic as well as diagnostic agent in this setting.

Prolactin secretory reserve can be evaluated by administration of inhibitors of dopaminergic transmission, such as chlorpromazine, or by dopamine antagonists such as metoclopramide. For evaluation of hyperprolactinemia, tests of suppressibility with L-dopa or water loading are employed. However, the failure of these latter procedures to distinguish readily between prolactin-secreting adenomas and other causes of hyperprolactinemia has reduced their popularity and usefulness.

Growth Hormone

Growth hormone secretory reserve can be evaluated in response to insulin-induced hypoglycemia, as described above, during a 30-minute infusion of arginine (0.5 gram/kg), or in response to L-dopa (0.5 gram orally). Autonomy of growth hormone secretion can be evaluated by oral glucose loading, a maneuver that normally suppresses growth hormone secretion.

ANTERIOR PITUITARY HYPOFUNCTION: HYPOPITUITARISM (Table 67–1)

Etiology

Hypopituitarism, an endocrine deficiency state characterized by diminished or absent secretion of the hormones of the anterior pituitary gland, results either from a primary disorder of the secretory cells of the anterior pituitary gland or as a secondary consequence of reduced stimulation by the releasing hormones of the hypothalamus. When the deficiency of anterior pituitary hormones is generalized, the condition is referred to as panhypopituitarism.

Hypopituitarism can be caused by destruction of the pituitary by tumors or granulomas or by hemorrhagic necrosis of a hypertrophied pituitary

TABLE 67–1. CAUSES OF HYPOPITUITARISM

Neoplasms
1. Pituitary tumors
2. Hypothalamic tumors, e.g., craniopharyngioma
3. Metastatic tumors, lymphoma, etc.

Infections or Granulomas
1. Tuberculosis
2. Sarcoidosis
3. Meningitis
4. Syphilis

Vascular
1. Postpartum necrosis (Sheehan's syndrome)
2. Hemorrhagic infarction of a pituitary tumor
3. Aneurysm of the carotid artery

Infiltrative
1. Histiocytosis X
2. Hemochromatosis

Physical Injury
1. Head trauma
2. Surgery
3. Radiation therapy

Isolated or Combined Hypothalamic-Releasing Hormone Deficiencies

gland in pregnancy as a complication of postpartum hemorrhage and shock (Sheehan's syndrome). Secondary hypopituitarism can result from lesions of the hypothalamus per se, from destruction of the pituitary stalk, or from a deficiency of one or more of the specific hypothalamic-releasing hormones that regulate secretion of the anterior pituitary gland. Isolated growth hormone deficiency in children is a typical example of a secondary form of anterior pituitary deficiency presumed to be due to a selective deficiency of growth hormone–releasing factor.

Clinical Features

The clinical manifestations of hypopituitarism depend upon the rapidity with which the hormonal deficiencies occur, the specific hormones that are deficient, the sex of the patient, and the age at the time of onset of the disease. Often pituitary insufficiency occurs insidiously, and the complaints are vague and nonspecific. Much less commonly, the onset of hypopituitarism occurs with dramatic suddenness in association with acute infarction of a pituitary tumor, a condition referred to as pituitary apoplexy.

In prepubertal children, the deficiencies of growth hormone and gonadotropins result in short stature and delayed puberty. In adults, growth hormone deficiency is of little clinical consequence, so that the predominant clinical features depend upon which of the other anterior pituitary hormones are deficient. Deficiency of ACTH results in findings similar to those of primary adrenocortical insufficiency (Addison's disease), including weakness, malaise, nausea, vomiting, and eventual collapse (see Chapter 69). In contrast to Addison's disease, hyperpigmentation is absent and severe sodium depletion is rare, since aldosterone secretion is maintained at normal or nearly normal levels. Hyponatremia can occur, however, as a consequence of impaired water excretion secondary to cortisol deficiency. Deficiency of TSH results in many of the typical findings of thyroid hormone deficiency, but the severity is generally less than that seen in primary hypothyroidism, and true myxedema is rare indeed. Gonadotropin deficiency results in amenorrhea and atrophy of the breasts in women, testicular atrophy in men, and diminished libido and the absence of pubic and axillary hair in both sexes. Additional findings include a waxy character and color of the skin and a fine wrinkling in the periorbital area that suggests premature aging. Hypothermia, hypotension, and hypoglycemia may also occur.

Diagnosis

Once suspected, the diagnosis of hypopituitarism can usually be established without difficulty, although care must be taken to distinguish the multiple deficiencies of target organ hormone production due to pituitary insufficiency from those due to primary polyglandular deficiency states resulting from autoimmune processes (e.g., Schmidt's syndrome). Demonstration of deficiency of the major target organ products (cortisol, thyroxine, testosterone, estrogen) together with an absence of compensatory increases in levels of the trophic hormones of pituitary origin (ACTH, TSH, FSH, LH) establishes that the abnormality resides in the hypothalamic-pituitary axis.

In patients with hypopituitarism, the finding of increased levels of prolactin, which is normally under tonic inhibition by the hypothalamus, suggests that the lesion is in the hypothalamus or pituitary stalk. Distinction between primary pituitary abnormalities and secondary deficiencies due to impaired hypothalamic function can also be made using the specific hypothalamic-releasing hormones as outlined above.

Treatment

Treatment of patients with panhypopituitarism consists of replacement of the specific hormone deficiencies with glucocorticoid, thyroxine, and the appropriate gonodal steroid. Growth hormone replacement is indicated in children who have not reached adult stature. Growth hormone and prolactin deficiencies in adults require no specific therapy. Restoration of fertility in women with hypopituitarism is theoretically possible with a combination of human menopausal gonadotropin and chorionic gonadotropin and by GnRH therapy in cases in which the lesion is in the hypothalamus or pituitary stalk.

Special precautions are required when initiating hormonal replacement therapy in patients with panhypopituitarism. Administration of thyroxine in patients who have concomitant ACTH deficiency can result in an increase in the metabolic clearance rate of glucocorticoid hormones and the sudden precipitation of an Addisonian crisis. Accordingly, such patients should always receive glucocorticoid therapy at the same time or preceding the onset of thyroid hormone replacement. Initiation of therapy with glucocorticoid hormones and thyroxine can unmask co-existing diabetes insipidus by improving free water clearance in patients with combined anterior and posterior pituitary insufficiency. Such patients may require concomitant treatment with antidiuretic hormone, as discussed in a subsequent section.

SYNDROMES OF ANTERIOR PITUITARY HYPERFUNCTION: THE PITUITARY ADENOMA

Adenomas of the pituitary gland may be nonfunctioning or they may secrete any of the trophic hormones normally produced by the gland. Hypersecretion of prolactin, growth hormone, and ACTH occurs commonly, resulting in the syndromes of amenorrhea-galactorrhea, acromegaly, and Cushing's syndrome, respectively. Hypersecretion of TSH or of gonadotropins from a pituitary adenoma is extremely rare. Whether or not hyperfunction of the anterior pituitary represents a primary disorder therein or is secondary to in-

creased stimulation by hypothalamic releasing factors has still not been resolved. Even the demonstration of a microadenoma and reversal of the clinical abnormalities with removal of the neoplasm does not exclude the latter possibility, since long-term follow-up is necessary to assure that the disease will not recur and pituitary microsurgery is a relatively recent intervention. In the following sections we will discuss the management of pituitary tumors in general as well as the pathogenesis, clinical features, and management of the specific syndromes produced by excess secretion of prolactin and growth hormone. For a discussion of Cushing's syndrome the reader is referred to Chapter 69.

PITUITARY NEOPLASMS: GENERAL CONSIDERATIONS

Pituitary neoplasms are usually benign and slow growing and may remain undetected for many years. Neurologic symptoms, principally headache and visual disturbances, may be the first manifestations, or the patient may present with findings consistent with pituitary insufficiency or with excessive secretion of any of the anterior pituitary hormones. Not infrequently, the presence of a pituitary neoplasm may be discovered in an asymptomatic patient in whom a skull radiograph is obtained for unrelated reasons.

Because of the close proximity of the optic nerves and optic chiasm, visual field defects are often the principal neurologic findings when a pituitary tumor extends beyond the confines of the sella turcica. Typically, this is manifested as bitemporal hemianopsia, often beginning in the upper quadrants of the visual field. Extraocular nerve palsies can also occur when the tumor enlarges laterally into the cavernous sinus. Headache, due in some cases to increased intracranial pressure secondary to obstruction of outflow of cerebrospinal fluid from the third ventricle, may also be a prominent complaint with large tumors. Headache is also common with smaller tumors.

Decisions regarding the management of pituitary tumors should be made in collaboration with a neurosurgeon. The optimal approach usually depends upon the size, location, and whether or not the tumor is endocrinologically active. Large tumors that impinge on extrasellar structures usually require surgical management whether or not they are secretory in nature. Smaller tumors that are actively secreting anterior pituitary hormones, such as prolactinomas, can often be managed medically with bromocriptine (see below).

The finding of an enlarged sella turcica does not of itself indicate the presence of a pituitary tumor. Many patients with an enlarged sella, particularly obese women, have the so-called empty sella syndrome, in which the pituitary gland is displaced by cerebrospinal fluid that enters the sella via a defect in the diaphragm above the sella. These patients rarely have endocrinologic abnormalities. Distinction from pituitary tumor is usually possible with high-resolution CT scans.

HYPERPROLACTINEMIA: GALACTORRHEA-AMENORRHEA SYNDROME

Etiology (Table 67–2)

Prolactin is under chronic inhibitory control by a hypothalamic factor (presumably dopamine). Any pharmacologic agent or lesion of the hypothalamus or pituitary stalk that interferes with dopamine secretion or its action can result in hyperprolactinemia. In view of the wide clinical use of pharmacologic agents that interfere with dopaminergic transmission, such as the phenothiazines, it is not surprising that the majority of patients with hyperprolactinemia do not harbor a pituitary adenoma. Once the use of such an agent can be excluded, however, and mechanical or neurogenic factors eliminated, the frequency with which a pituitary microadenoma is found is quite high. The most common pituitary tumor, chromophobe adenoma, once thought to be nonfunctioning and endocrinologically silent, is frequently a prolactin-secreting adenoma (prolactinoma).

Clinical Manifestations

The clinical manifestations of hyperprolactinemia depend upon the hormone level, the sex of the patient, and individual sensitivity to the lactogenic and mammotropic effects of the hormone. In women, hyperprolactinemia results in the so-called galactorrhea-amenorrhea syndrome. Persistent lactation, unprovoked by breast stimulation, and amenorrhea are the classic features. The syndrome may appear following pregnancy or may be unrelated to pregnancy. In men, galactorrhea can occur, but impotence and loss of libido are more frequent complaints.

Diagnosis

The diagnosis of hyperprolactinemia should be considered in patients with any of the previously described clinical manifestations, i.e., galactorrhea, secondary amenorrhea, and impotence. Serum prolactin determinations are available in most clinical laboratories and are required to establish a diagnosis of hyperprolactinemia. If levels are markedly elevated (>150 ng/dl, normal <20), the presence of a prolactin-secreting adenoma is highly likely. With lower levels a greater degree of overlap with non-neoplastic causes of hyperprolactinemia occurs. Normal levels of serum prolactin can occur in patients with galactorrhea, particularly if the blood sample is drawn at a time between hormone secretory bursts. For this reason, some investigators recommend drawing multiple samples in patients suspected of this disease. Occasionally galactorrhea can occur with persistently normal serum prolactin levels, presumably as a consequence of increased sensitivity to the hormone.

Treatment

For tumors located in the sella, or with minimal suprasellar extension, the treatment of choice is microsurgery via the transsphenoidal approach. This procedure preserves the surrounding normal pituitary tissue and rarely results in hypopituitarism. Pituitary irradiation, using either conventional sources or heavy particle beams, is also frequently successful, but the incidence of hypopituitarism is greater than in patients treated with transsphenoidal hypophysectomy. This may be a very important consideration in women in the child-bearing years or in children who have not yet achieved adult height. Bromocriptine, a dopamine agonist, can be used as a medical alternative to surgical management of patients with hyperprolactinemia. Doses of 10 to 15 mg daily will usually result in cessation of lactation, resumption of menses and fertility, and restoration of libido and potency. Bromocriptine may also result in regression of the tumor per se, although surgical therapy is probably indicated in patients with tumors large enough to produce neurologic symptoms. At the present time bromocriptine should probably be reserved for patients with small tumors and those in whom surgery is contraindicated, or as adjunctive treatment of tumors that cannot be completely resected.

GIGANTISM AND ACROMEGALY

Clinical Manifestations (Table 67–3)

The manifestations of excess growth hormone production are critically dependent on the age of the patient at the time that the abnormality first occurs. If growth hormone is present in excess before the epiphyses close, the increase in linear skeletal growth results in gigantism. After closure of the epiphyses, growth hormone excess results in acromegaly, a disorder characterized by physical changes in the bones and soft tissues as well as metabolic abnormalities reflecting the physiologic actions of this polypeptide.

The typical physical changes of acromegaly result from enlargement of the skeleton and soft tis-

TABLE 67–2. CAUSES OF HYPERPROLACTINEMIA

Physiological
1. Pregnancy and lactation
2. Breast stimulation
3. Estrogen therapy
4. Stress
5. Newborn

Hypothalamic-Pituitary Lesions
1. Prolactinoma
2. Stalk section
3. Hypothalamic disorders—craniopharyngioma, granulomas

Metabolic Disorders
1. Hypothyroidism
2. Renal failure

Chest Wall Injury

Drugs
1. Phenothiazines, haloperidol
2. Alpha methyldopa
3. Reserpine
4. Metoclopramide
5. Opiates

TABLE 67–3. CLINICAL MANIFESTATIONS OF ACROMEGALY IN 100 PATIENTS

Manifestations of GH Excess

Acral enlargement	100*
Soft tissue overgrowth	100
Hyperhidrosis	88
Lethargy or fatigue	87
Weight gain	73
Paresthesias	70
Joint pain	69
Photophobia	46
Papillomas	45
Hypertrichosis	33
Goiter	32
Acanthosis nigricans	29
Hypertension	24
Cardiomegaly	16
Renal calculi	11

Disturbance of Other Endocrine Functions

Hyperinsulinemia	70
Glucose intolerance	50
Irregular or absent menses	60
Decreased libido or impotence	46
Hypothyroidism	13
Galactorrhea	13
Gynecomastia	8
Hypoadrenalism	4

Local Manifestations

Enlarged sella	90
Headache	65
Visual deficit	20

* Percentage of patients in whom these features were present. From Findling JW, and Tyrrell JB: Anterior pituitary & somatomedins: I. Anterior pituitary. In Greenspan FS, and Forsham PH (eds): Basic and Clinical Endocrinology. Los Altos, CA, Lange Medical Publishers, 1983, p 77.

FIGURE 67–2. Typical physical appearance of a 52-year-old woman with end-stage acromegaly. Note the coarsening and enlargement of the facial features, prognathism, and enlargement of the hands. (From Mendeloff AI, and Smith DE (eds): Acromegaly, diabetes, hypermetabolism, proteinuria and heart failure. Clinical pathological conference. Am J Med 20:133, 1956.)

sues and thickening of the skin (Fig. 67–2). Enlargement of the acral parts (fingers and toes), coarsening and enlargement of the facial features, prognathism, frontal bossing, enlargement of the tongue, and deepening of the voice are characteristic findings. Since these changes may occur insidiously, comparisons of pictures of the patient taken serially over the years is often very helpful in recognizing their appearance. An increase in shoe size, hat size, or ring size may be noted by the patient. Additional complaints include headache, weakness, increased perspiration, paresthesias, and bilateral carpal tunnel syndrome. Enlargement of the viscera, hypertension, and congestive heart failure can also occur.

In addition to the physical changes that result from excess growth hormone secretion, a variety of metabolic abnormalities may also occur. Impaired glucose tolerance is present in more than half the cases, but frank diabetes mellitus is not evident unless pancreatic insulin secretion is incapable of responding to the counter-regulatory effect of growth hormone. An increase in glomerular filtration rate and in renal tubular reabsorption of phosphate may also be observed, the latter causing the typical finding of hyperphosphatemia.

Diagnosis

In fully developed acromegaly the physical findings are so characteristic as to provide an unmistakable diagnosis. Confirmation of this diagnosis as well as determination of whether or not the disease is in an active phase requires measurement of growth hormone. Levels of growth hormone obtained under basal conditions generally exceed the upper limit of normal (5 ng/ml) and typically cannot be suppressed by a physiological maneuver such as administration of glucose. A paradoxical increase in growth hormone levels in response to administration of glucose occurs in some patients with acromegaly, whereas administration of L-dopa, which normally stimulates growth hormone, usually reduces the levels. Both TRH and GnRH, which normally have no effect on growth hormone, may cause a paradoxical rise in growth hormone levels in patients with acromegaly. Measurement of plasma concentrations of somatomedin C may also be useful, inasmuch as plasma levels of this mediator of growth hormone action fluctuate less than those of growth hormone and are thought to reflect more accurately the state of disease activity.

Treatment

Treatment of acromegaly depends partially on the size of the tumor, particularly whether or not the mass extends beyond the sella and whether or not the optic nerves are involved. Surgical results are often not as gratifying as with other pituitary neoplasms, presumably because the secretory cells are more widely dispersed and therefore are not entirely removed with the microsurgical technique. External radiation using either standard cobalt or proton beams generally results in a slow decrease in elevated growth hormone levels and eventually arrests the progress of the disease, but at the cost of a high incidence of hypopituitarism. Bromocriptine has been far less effective in the treatment of acromegaly than in the treatment of the amenorrhea-galactorrhea syndrome.

DISORDERS OF THE POSTERIOR PITUITARY

The posterior lobe of the pituitary gland (neurohypophysis) is an anatomical extension of the hypothalamus, containing the axons and axon terminals of neurons whose nuclei originate in the supraoptic and paraventricular areas of the hypothalamus. Two peptide hormones, arginine vasopressin and oxytocin, and their carrier proteins, the neurophysins, are synthesized in the cell bodies of these neurons. These peptides and their carrier proteins travel down the axons to the nerve terminals from which they are released in response to a variety of physiological stimuli.

Oxytocin causes release of breast milk and may promote uterine contractions during labor. There is no known function for this peptide hormone in men. Arginine vasopressin (also known as antidiuretic hormone [ADH]) is the principal hormonal factor regulating water metabolism. Deficiency of ADH or impaired action in its major target organ, the kidney, results in a polyuric state known as diabetes insipidus. Excessive and physiologically inappropriate secretion of ADH results in hyponatremia (the syndrome of inappropriate ADH secretion), as discussed elsewhere in this volume (Chapter 29). Arginine vasopressin, as the name implies, also has pressor activity, the physiological relevance of which is unknown.

PHYSIOLOGICAL REGULATION OF ADH SECRETION

Variations in secretion of ADH by the posterior pituitary occur primarily in response to changes in body osmolality. Normally, osmolality averages approximately 285 mOsm/kg body water. An increase in body osmolality as small as 1 per cent (3 mOsm/kg), such as occurs after 10 to 12 hours of water deprivation, will normally increase ADH secretion (Fig. 67–3). Conversely, reduction in osmolality following administration of an oral water load causes dilution of body fluids and a prompt suppression of ADH secretion. Concomitant stimulation and suppression of the hypothalamic thirst center in response to hypertonicity and hypotonicity, respectively, provides a parallel physiological mechanism for regulating body osmolality.

In addition to osmotic regulation, several nonosmotic factors (Table 67–4) can influence ADH secretion. Most notable among these is the state of the so-called effective extracellular fluid (ECF) volume, perceived by high-pressure baroreceptors in the aorta and by low-pressure volume receptors in the left atrium. Hypotension and/or decreased effective ECF volume result in stimulation of ADH

FIGURE 67–3. The relationship of plasma arginine vasopressin (AVP) to plasma osmolality in normal subjects and patients with various polyuric states. (From Robertson GL, Mahr EA, Athar S, and Sinha T: Development and clinical application of a new method for the radioimmunoassay of arginine vasopressin in human plasma. J Clin Invest 52:2340, 1973.)

secretion via adrenergically mediated signals to the hypothalamus. Although minute-by-minute regulation of ADH secretion is probably through its osmotic control mechanism, nonosmotic factors will predominate in situations in which there is diversion of the two stimuli (e.g., hypovolemia in a hypotonic individual).

The principal site of action of ADH is the distal nephron, where the hormone induces an increase in osmotic water permeability of the collecting tubule and collecting duct. Permeability to urea is also increased in response to ADH. The hor-

TABLE 67–4. NONOSMOTIC STIMULI OF VASOPRESSIN RELEASE

Neural
1. Stress—pain, fright
2. Coitus
3. Suckling

Diminished Effective Extracellular Fluid Volume
1. Hemorrhage
2. Decreased cardiac output
3. Hypoalbuminemia
4. Prolonged quiet standing

Drugs
1. Morphine
2. Barbiturates
3. Acetylcholine
4. Nicotine
5. Clofibrate
6. Vincristine
7. Carbamazepine

Hypoxemia

mone acts through a classic cyclic AMP–dependent mechanism that is initiated by binding to a receptor on the basolateral surface of the target cell. This process is modulated by a number of factors, including calcium, prostaglandins, adrenal corticosteroids, and a variety of adrenergic agents.

DIABETES INSIPIDUS

Etiology

In diabetes insipidus the urinary concentrating mechanism is impaired either as a consequence of a failure to secrete adequate amounts of vasopressin (central diabetes insipidus) or as a consequence of failure of the distal tubule and collecting duct to respond normally to the hormone (nephrogenic diabetes insipidus). Central diabetes insipidus is usually caused by head trauma, surgical hypophysectomy, granulomatous diseases, histiocytosis X, primary or metastatic neoplasms, or following anoxic brain damage or meningoencephalitis. In at least one third of patients no pathological cause is evident. Diabetes insipidus following surgery or head trauma may occur transiently, may be followed by a transient period of hyponatremia due to inappropriate release of ADH from the damaged pituitary tissue, and then may resolve completely or progress to a permanent ADH-deficient state. Rarely central diabetes insipidus is familial, presumably due to hypoplasia of the secretory cells in the hypothalamus. Nephrogenic diabetes insipidus can occur as an inherited disorder, predominantly affecting males, or can be an acquired condition due to a variety of renal diseases, electrolyte disorders (hypokalemia, hypercalcemia), or drug therapies (e.g., lithium).

Diagnosis

In both central and nephrogenic diabetes insipidus the principal findings are polyuria and polydypsia with urinary volumes generally in excess of 3 L per day, and occasionally, depending upon the concomitant water intake, exceeding 5 to 10 L per day. The diagnosis is generally suspected in patients who excrete large quantities of a dilute urine in which the specific gravity is less than 1.010 or osmolality is less than 300 mOsm/kg. The major diagnostic challenge is to distinguish diabetes insipidus of either type from compulsive water drinking (psychogenic polydipsia), in which maximal urinary concentrating ability may be impaired as a consequence of "washout" of the normally hypertonic medulla by continuous excretion of a dilute urine. Demonstration of frank hypertonicity (serum osmolality >295 mOsm/kg) will exclude primary polydypsia, but usually a protocol employing water deprivation (overnight dehydration) followed by administration of aqueous pitressin is required to distinguish between these three polyuric states. In this procedure, water is withheld until the osmolality of hourly voided urines reaches a plateau. In patients with primary polydypsia, urine osmolality is generally much greater than plasma osmolality

and increases minimally in response to the subsequent administration of aqueous vasopressin, 5 units subcutaneously. In patients with severe central diabetes insipidus, urine osmolality is usually much less than plasma osmolality and increases by at least 50 per cent in response to vasopressin; those with nephrogenic diabetes are distinguished by the failure of a low urine osmolality to respond normally to vasopressin. Occasionally, patients with partial defects in ADH secretion will require further investigation using hypertonic saline infusion or more elaborate water deprivation tests.

Treatment

Treatment of central diabetes insipidus depends to a large extent on the severity of the hormone deficiency. In patients in whom the deficiency is only partial, chlorpropamide will potentiate the effect of ADH on the renal tubule. However, hypoglycemia may result, particularly if the dose of chlorpropamide exceeds 250 mg per day. Patients with more complete hormone deficiency require ADH replacement therapy. Long-acting Pitressin Tannate in Oil (warmed and shaken thoroughly), in doses of 5 units intramuscularly every 48 to 72 hours, has been the standard treatment. More recently a synthetic analogue, 1-desamino-8-D-arginine vasopressin (DDAVP), has become the treatment of choice. Devoid of significant pressor activity, DDAVP can be conveniently administered by nasal insufflation in doses of 5 to 10 µg every 12 to 24 hours. No specific treatment is available for patients with nephrogenic diabetes insipidus, but reduction of solute load by salt restriction and administration of thiazide diuretics will reduce the polyuria.

REFERENCES

Andreoli TE: The posterior pituitary. In Wyngaarden JB, and Smith LH Jr (eds): Cecil Textbook of Medicine. 17th ed. Philadelphia, WB Saunders Co, 1985, pp 1266–1273.

Cook DM: Pituitary tumors. Diagnosis and therapy. CA 33:215, 1983.

Daniels DL, Williams AL, Thornton RS, Meyer GA, Cusick JF, and Haughton VM: Differential diagnosis of intrasellular tumors by computed tomography. Radiology 141:697, 1981.

Frohman LA: The anterior pituitary. In Wyngaarden JB, and Smith LH Jr (eds): Cecil Textbook of Medicine. 17th ed. Philadelphia, WB Saunders Co, 1985, pp 1251–1266.

Lufkin EG, Kao PC, O'Fallon WM, and Mangan MS: Combined testing of anterior pituitary gland with insulin, thyrotropin-releasing hormone, and luteinizing hormone-releasing hormone. Am J Med 75:471–475, 1983.

Miller M, Dalakos T, Moses AM, Fellerman H, and Streeten DHP: Recognition of partial defects in antidiuretic hormone secretion. Ann Intern Med 73:721–729, 1970.

Wilson CB, and Dempsey LC: Transphenoidal microsurgical removal of 250 pituitary adenomas. J Neurosurg 48:13, 1978.

Wollesen F, Andersen T, and Karle A: Size reduction of extrasellar pituitary tumors during bromocriptine treatment: Quantitation of effect on different types of tumors. Ann Intern Med 96:281–286, 1982.

THE THYROID

Dysfunction of the thyroid gland causes some of the most common endocrine disorders seen by the physician. Thyrotoxicosis (hyperthyroidism) is a consequence of excess thyroid hormone; a deficiency of thyroid hormone causes hypothyroidism (myxedema). Thyroid dysfunction is frequently manifested clinically by a swelling (enlargement) of the gland, a condition referred to as goiter formation.

The thyroid gland arises embryologically from the fourth pharyngeal pouch. The lateral components combine to develop the easily palpable, butterfly-shaped mature thyroid gland (20 grams). The lateral lobes (2×3 cm), partially hidden by the sternocleidomastoid muscles, are connected by the isthmus, which sits just below the cricoid cartilage. A pyramidal lobe is present in about 30 per cent; it extends upward from the isthmus lateral to the trachea. The gland consists of spherical follicles (acini) lined by epithelial tissue and filled with colloid. This substance consists of thyroglobulin, the storage form of T_4 (thyroxine), T_3 (3,5,3'-triiodothyronine), and the precursors MIT (monoiodotyrosine) and DIT (diiodotyrosine). Other functioning cells of neural crest origin located in the parafollicular area of the thyroid (C cells) secrete calcitonin (see page 508).

THYROID PHYSIOLOGY

Iodide, a substrate for thyroid hormone synthesis, also plays an autoregulatory role in the metabolism of the thyroid gland. The normal gland contains approximately 10,000 μg of iodine, which is predominantly organically bound. The minimal daily requirement of iodide is only about 200 μg (renal loss replacement). Iodide deficiency is a rare occurrence in the iodide-replete western world but remains the commonest cause of goiter (endemic goiter) in the world. Many patients with endemic goiter are mentally deficient owing to hypothyroidism dating from birth (cretinism) or suffer from retarded musculoskeletal development owing to thyroid hormone deficiency during childhood.

The thyroid gland concentrates iodide through a unique trapping mechanism to maintain a cell-to-plasma iodide ratio of about 50 to 1. Trapped iodide is rapidly oxidized by peroxidase to iodine and subsequently undergoes organification by iodinating tyrosine residues on thyroglobulin to form MIT and DIT. Coupling of these compounds results in the formation of T_3 and T_4. The secretory process is initiated by pinocytosis of thyroglobulin from the follicular lumen followed by the release of T_4 and T_3 from their storage form by proteolysis induced by lysosomal enzymes. The active hormones T_4 and T_3 are then secreted into the circulation. The thyroid gland is the only source for T_4, whereas it contributes only about 20 per cent of the T_3 produced daily.

A number of chemicals interfere with thyroid gland metabolism. These effects have been exploited for therapeutic purposes in the case of propylthiouracil (PTU) and methimazole. Both drugs effectively block thyroid hormone synthesis and are utilized clinically in the treatment of hyperthyroidism. Agents that are preferentially trapped by the thyroid (iodide, pertechnetate) are used diagnostically for gland imaging. Pharmacologic amounts of iodide will also inhibit thyroid gland synthesis and release of hormones. This inhibitory effect is generally of short duration in normal people, but if sustained it can lead to hypothyroidism and compensatory goiter formation. Lithium has a similar effect to that of iodide. Its current extensive use in manic-depressive illness has lead to a significant problem with hypothyroidism in this patient group.

Thyroid hormones circulate in two forms, protein-bound and free. Thyronine-binding globulin (TBG), the principal carrier, binds about 70 per cent of the thyroid hormones under normal conditions. Other carrier proteins, thyroxine-binding pre-albumin (TBPA) and albumin, play a lesser role. A small but very important quantity of T_4 (0.03 per cent) and T_3 (0.3 per cent) is free and remains in rapid equilibrium with the protein-bound fraction. The metabolic state of the patient correlates with the free component rather than the total (bound) thyroid hormone level. Alterations in serum TBG concentration are common and account for the majority of changes in serum total T_4 not attributable to hyper- or hypothyroidism (Table 68–1). These changes in serum total T_4 levels are not accompanied by changes in the free T_4 concentration. Thus a measurement of free T_4 or an index of free T_4 is obligatory under these conditions in order to interpret accurately the significance of a change in the total hormone value. During acute illness, however, factors that affect the affinity of TBG for T_4 may reduce the total and occasionally the free T_4 concentration.

TABLE 68–1. ALTERATIONS IN THYRONINE-BINDING GLOBULIN (TBG) CONCENTRATION

TBG Increased (Total $T_4 \uparrow$, $FT_4 \rightarrow$)
  Newborn
  Pregnancy (estrogen effect)
  Acute hepatitis
  Acute intermittent porphyria
  Genetic TBG excess
  Oral contraceptives (estrogens)
  Heroin and/or methadone abuse
  Clofibrate or 5-fluorouracil use
TBG Decreased (Total $T_4 \downarrow$, $FT_4 \rightarrow$)
  Cirrhosis
  Nephrotic syndrome
  Severe nonthyroidal illness
  Genetic TBG deficiency
  Anabolic steroids (androgens)
  Glucocorticoids

T_4 = serum thyroxine level; FT_4 = serum level of free (unbound) thyroxine; TBG = thyronine-binding globulin.

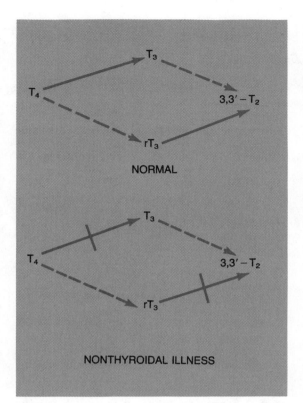

FIGURE 68–1. Sequential deiodination of thyroxine (T_4) to 3,3′-diiodothyronine (3,3′-T_2) via 3,5,3′-triiodothyronine (T_3) and 3,3′,5′-triiodothyronine (reverse-T_3, rT_3), in the normal subject and in a patient with nonthyroidal illness. The solid arrows reflect outer-ring deiodination. The dashed arrows reflect inner-ring deiodination. The changes in serum T_3 and rT_3 associated with nonthyroidal illness are consequent to the indicated lesions in deiodination.

The thyroid gland is the only endogenous source of T_4. Although the thyroid also secretes T_3, 80 per cent of the daily T_3 produced is derived from extrathyroidal T_4 deiodination. Since T_3 is biologically the most active thyroid hormone, this process is regarded as an activation step. In addition, T_4 can be deiodinated to 3,5′,3′-triiodothyronine (reverse-T_3, rT_3). This pathway inactivates T_4, as rT_3 is calorigenically inactive. These balanced pathways for T_4 deiodination are frequently disturbed during acute illness (Fig. 68–1). This results in an impairment in T_3 neogenesis (low T_3 syndrome) and increased levels of serum rT_3. Despite these alterations such patients are currently considered euthyroid, and T_3 replacement is not indicated.

The integrated control of thyroid hormone metabolism is regulated by the hypothalamic-pituitary-thyroid axis (Fig. 68–2). Thyrotropin-releasing hormone (TRH) secreted by the hypothalamus controls the synthesis and secretion of pituitary thyroid-stimulating hormone (TSH). The set point for the pituitary TSH response to TRH is regulated by the feedback inhibitory effect of the thyroid hormones. TSH stimulates all aspects of thyroid gland synthesis and secretion of thyroid hormone.

The metabolic effects of thyroid hormone are mediated through a variety of mechanisms. Assessment of the basal metabolic rate (BMR) was traditionally the method for the determination of thyroid status. Thyroid hormones regulate protein synthesis by binding to specific nuclear receptors. They enhance mitochondrial oxidation and regulate the activity of membrane-bound enzymes. Normal brain maturation during fetal and infant development is dependent on adequate quantities of thyroid hormone. Irreversible mental retardation develops in the absence of thyroid hormone (cretinism). During childhood, deficiency of thyroid hormone results in delay of somatic growth and development. In the geriatric population reversible dementia consequent to hypothyroidism is not an uncommon problem.

THYROID FUNCTION TESTS

Serum Thyroid Hormone Concentration. No one test can specifically determine thyroid status. Thus a variety of tests have been developed. These must be interpreted in an integrated fashion, keeping the patient's clinical presentation clearly in mind. Measurement of serum total T_4 (5 to 11 μg/dl) and free T_4 concentration (1.5 to 3.5 ng/dl) is the best current initial screening mechanism for thyroid dysfunction. Since the serum total T_4 can be altered by changes in carrier-protein concen-

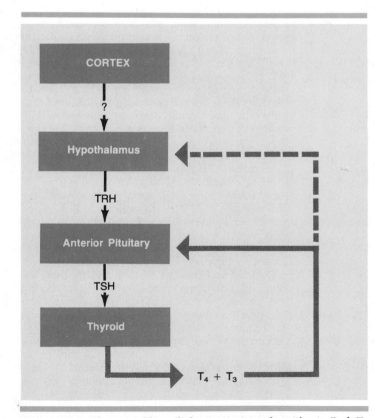

FIGURE 68–2. The normal hypothalamic-pituitary-thyroid axis. Both T_4 and T_3 feed back negatively on the pituitary and inhibit the secretion of thyroid-stimulating hormone (TSH). A similar process may regulate the hypothalamic secretion of thyrotropin-releasing hormone (TRH).

tration as well as by changes in thyroid function, this value must be evaluated in conjunction with a measurement of serum free T_4 or an indirect index of free T_4. Direct measurement of serum free T_4 is preferable. Many centers, however, continue to use indirect methods and derive a "free T_4 index" (0.5 to 1.5) from a combination of serum total T_4 and resin T_3 uptake test (RT_3U). The latter procedure allows an estimation of changes in serum TBG. The patient's serum, a trace amount of radioiodine-labeled T_3, and an anion-exchange resin are co-incubated. The resin-bound T_3 is measured and expressed as a percentage of the total amount of tracer T_3 added (25 to 35 per cent). Values correlate inversely with the concentration of unsaturated TBG. Generally, a parallel increase or decrease in both total T_4 and RT_3U indicates hyperthyroidism or hypothyroidism, whereas opposite changes suggest alterations in TBG binding. The derivation of the free T_4 index from the total T_4 and T_3 uptake generally gives a normal value in the setting of alterations in TBG. The free T_4 index or absolute free T_4 concentration is high or low in the hyperthyroid or hypothyroid subject, respectively. Occasionally free T_4 values may be misleadingly low in patients with severe nonthyroidal illness, "euthyroid sick syndrome." Serial analysis of thyroid function tests will generally resolve this dilemma. Measurement of total and free T_3 values is clinically useful only when T_3-thyrotoxicosis is suspected. In this setting T_4 values are normal and the hyperthyroidism will be missed in the absence of a T_3 measurement. Measurement of serum rT_3 has limited value as a routine clinical test. A measurement of serum TSH is the single best test to detect primary thyroid failure, since the value is invariably elevated in primary hypothyroidism owing to loss of the inhibitory feedback effect of thyroid hormone. Currently the majority of radioimmunoassays for TSH cannot differentiate between a normal TSH and the suppressed value found in hyperthyroidism.

The TSH response to TRH is a very useful test. The normal TSH response ranges between a serum level of 15 and 30 μU/ml at 20 minutes after 500 μg of intravenous TRH. An incremental TSH rise of 5 mU above baseline in response to TRH is consistent with a normal axis. In hyperthyroidism the TSH response is flat. The mildly hypothyroid patient with a borderline high serum TSH value will have an exaggerated response to TRH.

Thyroid Radioiodide Uptake (RAIU) Test. The accumulation of tracer iodide (^{123}I, ^{131}I) in the thyroid can be quantitated at standard intervals (6 to 24 hours) to assess thyroid activity. Owing to the enrichment of western diets with iodide, this procedure is of no value in the differentiation between a normal and a hypoactive gland. In addition the uptake value may be normal in many hyperthyroid patients (approximately 30 per cent), especially with multinodular goiter and with T_3 thyrotoxicosis. Consequently a normal RAIU test does not exclude hyperthyroidism. In patients with thyrotoxicosis associated with thyroiditis, low (<3 per cent) uptake values are usually found in contrast to normal or high values in Graves' disease. A low uptake value is also a feature of thyrotoxicosis consequent to excess thyroid hormone medication.

Immunologic Tests. Autoimmune thyroid disease (Hashimoto's thyroiditis and Graves' disease) is associated with positive tests for antibodies to specific thyroid antigens (antimicrosomal and antithyroglobulin), which are useful in the detection of these autoimmune disorders. The recent availability of a biological assay for thyroid-stimulating immunoglobulin (TSI), a specific marker for Graves' disease, has helped in both the diagnosis and management of this common disorder. A reduction in TSI level during therapy with antithyroid drugs is a good indicator that a remission has been induced and that therapy can be modified or withdrawn.

SCINTISCAN. The RAIU test provides useful information on the anatomy of the thyroid. A scan at 6 hours demonstrates a homogeneous distribution of ^{123}I in the normal gland, whereas ^{123}I activity will be heterogeneous in Hashimoto's thyroiditis and multinodular goiter. Furthermore, this procedure will differentiate a functioning (benign) from a nonfunctioning (possible carcinoma) thyroid nodule. Functioning nodules demonstrate normal (warm) to increased (hot) ^{123}I activity, whereas nonfunctioning nodules fail to concentrate ^{123}I (cold).

SONOGRAPHY. Ultrasound imaging will decisively differentiate whether a nonfunctioning nodule on ^{123}I scan (cold nodule) is cystic or solid. In addition, this noninvasive procedure is very helpful in the serial sizing of the thyroid nodule and provides an objective basis for the evaluation of T_4 suppressive therapy.

NEEDLE BIOPSY. Fine needle aspiration biopsy with cytological analysis of the tissue has now become a routine procedure in the evaluation of a thyroid nodule. The specificity and sensitivity of this procedure are now so reliable that most centers will use needle biopsy as the first step in the evaluation of a thyroid nodule, even before scintiscanning.

THYROTOXICOSIS (HYPERTHYROIDISM)

Thyrotoxicosis, a common clinical condition consequent to excess thyroid hormone, can be caused by a number of different disorders; these

TABLE 68–2. CAUSES OF THYROTOXICOSIS

Grave's disease
Toxic nodular goiter
Thyroiditis
Iodide-induced hyperthyroidism
Factitious thyrotoxicosis
Thyrotoxicosis due to excess TSH
Toxic thyroid carcinoma
Toxic struma ovarii

should be differentiated in the individual patient for proper management (Table 68–2). Graves' disease is the most common cause in young individuals, whereas toxic nodular goiter is more prevalent in the elderly. Transient thyrotoxicosis is frequently associated with thyroiditis. Also exposure to iodide (contrast studies) and iodine-containing drugs (e.g., amiodarone) has become a relatively common cause of thyrotoxicosis. The other conditions listed are relatively rare.

Graves' Disease

This complex autoimmune disorder consists of toxic goiter, ophthalmopathy, and not infrequently dermopathy, which may occur together or separately. The abnormal immunoglobulin(s) responsible for the hyperthyroidism can now be measured by bioassay. Thyroid-stimulating immunoglobulins (TSI) are antibodies to the normal thyroid gland TSH receptor site. They have powerful agonist action and consequently induce hyperthyroidism. The initiating factors in the development of TSI and the role of TSI in the development of the ophthalmopathy or dermopathy have not been elucidated.

Clinical Features. The clinical presentation of the thyrotoxic patient is extremely variable (Table 68–3). The actual features relate to the age at onset, the duration of the condition, and the degree of hormone excess. The patient most frequently presents with a history of nervousness, heat intolerance, sweating, palpitations, tremor, and weight loss. In addition a change in collar size (goiter formation) and eye discomfort (Graves' ophthalmopathy) may be noted.

More prolonged disease is associated with features of chronic catabolism. Skeletal muscle wasting, especially of the limb girdles, induces a proximal myopathy. Patients may experience difficulty in climbing stairs or getting up from the sitting position. Although dyspnea in the absence of cardiac failure is common, more severe disease can be manifested by a severe cardiomyopathy and congestive failure, especially in the elderly.

The mental changes are characterized by anxiety, irritability, poor concentration, restlessness, and emotional lability. In addition, insomnia and forgetfulness may be disturbing features.

Physical Findings (Table 68–3). The majority of young patients with hyperthyroidism have an enlarged thyroid (goiter). Diffuse symmetrical enlargement of the thyroid is characteristic of Graves' disease, whereas asymmetric changes occur in toxic nodular goiter. A bruit over the thyroid indicates extreme vascularity and is generally found only in Graves' disease. In addition, the finding of a palpable pyramidal lobe in a hyperthyroid patient is suggestive of Graves' disease.

The eye changes may be due to excess thyroid hormone or to the ophthalmopathy of Graves' disease. Enhanced sympathetic tone due to excess thyroid hormone causes the characteristic widening of the palpebral fissure (stare) and failure of the upper lid to closely follow globe movement

TABLE 68–3. CLINICAL FEATURES OF THYROTOXICOSIS

SYMPTOMS	SIGNS
Nervousness	Thyroid enlargement
Heat intolerance (sweating)	Eyestare and lid lag
Palpitations	*Proptosis and ophthalmoplegia
Tremulousness	Warm smooth skin
Weight loss (good appetite)	*Pretibial myxedema
Muscle weakness	Fine tremor
Emotional lability	Brisk reflexes
Hyperdefecation	Onycholysis
	Tachycardia or atrial fibrillation

* Graves' disease only

(lag). Proptosis (exophthalmos), forward protrusion of the globe due to retro-orbital deposition of fat, mucopolysaccharides, and lymphocytes, is the cardinal feature of Graves' ophthalmopathy. In addition, extraocular muscle weakness may limit eye movement and result in diplopia.

Smooth, shiny, silky, warm skin is frequently noted in hyperthyroidism. Thinning and loss of hair may be particularly worrisome for women. Hyperpigmentation over extensor surfaces and clubbing (thyroid acropachy) are rare features. Onycholysis, separation of the distal portion of the nail from the nailbed (Plummer's nails), fine tremor of the outstretched hands, and brisk reflexes are commonly noted. Pretibial myxedema may occasionally be seen in Graves' disease.

A spectrum of cardiovascular abnormalities may be detected on physical examination. Sinus tachycardia with a wide pulse pressure may progress to atrial fibrillation and congestive heart failure. Systolic flow murmurs and a forceful apical pulse are common features.

Diagnosis. A typical case of Graves' disease is easily diagnosed. In many instances, however, the typical eye features are minimal, goiter may be moderate (especially in the elderly), and systemic features may be few. Thus the condition may go unrecognized for years. In the majority of cases serum total and free T_4 levels will be high. If normal, a serum total T_3 must be performed as T_3 toxicosis occurs in 5 to 10 per cent of cases. If all other tests are equivocal, the TSH response to TRH should be flat if the patient is indeed hyperthyroid.

The recognition of hyperthyroidism in the elderly is frequently delayed owing to the insidious nature of the disease. These patients have been classically described as "apathetic" owing to the paucity of features of sympathetic overactivity. The dominant features may be reflected in other systems such as the cardiovascular system. Patients present with atrial fibrillation and congestive failure. In the absence of ophthalmopathy and goiter the hyperthyroid state is generally missed. All elderly patients presenting with new-onset cardiovascular disorders should be screened for hyperthyroidism. Beware, however, that patients with nonthyroidal systemic disorders may have a transient rise in serum total and free T_4 values as a byproduct of their disease and require close monitoring with serial thyroid function tests in order to elucidate their thyroid status.

Anxiety neurosis may be difficult to differentiate clinically from hyperthyroidism. These patients may present with tremor, tachycardia, irritability, and fatigue. Typical anxiety neurosis is generally associated with depression, weight loss accompanied by anorexia, cold moist hands, and a normal resting (sleeping) pulse. If the clinical suspicion for hyperthyroidism remains, a baseline screening test with total and free T_4 should clarify the diagnosis. Some patients with psychiatric disorders (10 per cent) have a transient elevation in serum total and free T_4 levels, such that serial analyses may be needed or further detailed testing may be indicated to exclude hyperthyroidism.

Graves' ophthalmopathy may occur in a euthyroid or even a hypothyroid patient. Other diseases of the orbit or retro-orbital space must be considered as a cause of exophthalmos. Orbital pseudotumor may display similar extraocular muscle swelling on CT scan or sonogram. When the ophthalmopathy is bilateral and the TRH test and TSI analysis are positive, the diagnosis of Graves' disease can generally be made. Other features of the disease eventually become evident in most cases.

Hyperthyroidism in the absence of goiter suggests factitious thyrotoxicosis or thyroiditis (or very rarely struma ovarii). In both conditions the RAIU test is suppressed. Serum thyroglobulin is high in thyroiditis but reduced in subjects taking exogenous thyroid hormone.

Therapy. Graves' disease is a self-limiting disease; 30 per cent of cases will go into spontaneous remission within one to two years. Antithyroid drugs can be used for the temporary control of symptoms, or the gland can be ablated with ^{131}I or surgery. The choice of therapy is usually dictated by the patient's age, the size of gland, and the severity of the disease.

DRUGS. The thionamides propylthiouracil (PTU) and methimazole (Tapazole) will control the features of hyperthyroidism in almost all cases. These drugs inhibit the synthesis of thyroid hormone and will restore a euthyroid state in four to eight weeks. The initial dose recommended is 150 to 300 mg every 8 hours for PTU or 20 to 30 mg every 12 hours for methimazole. Once achieved, euthyroidism can generally be maintained by smaller doses of PTU (50 to 100 mg twice daily) or methimazole (5 to 10 mg once daily). Antithyroid drugs are preferred for children, young adults, and the pregnant patient. They are also used in the adult and elderly patient to induce euthyroidism prior to definitive therapy with ^{131}I or surgery. Antithyroid drugs will induce a permanent remission in about 30 per cent of patients with Graves' disease, usually within three to six months of therapy. A reduction in TSI during therapy generally indicates that a remission has occurred and consequently is a good guide for the discontinuation of therapy.

Transient dermatitis, the most common side effect of antithyroid drugs, is not dose-related and generally disappears despite continued therapy. Urticaria and pruritus may also occur. Dose-related leukopenia, myalgia, arthralgia, and elevated serum alkaline phosphatase occur commonly in patients during therapy with PTU. Generally these abnormalities can be controlled by dose adjustment. The most serious side effect (agranulocytosis) is not dose-related. A routine blood count is of no value as a predictor, since this complication occurs acutely. Thus patients should be advised to watch for fever and sore throats and to report such developments immediately to their physician. Fortunately the majority of patients recover from agranulocytosis once the drug is stopped.

Sympathetic overactivity can be controlled with beta-adrenergic blockade. Such therapy with propranolol (40 mg every 6 hours) is indicated for severe agitation, tremor, sweating, and tachycardia. Beta-blockers should not be used in the patient with severe thyrotoxic heart disease.

Radioactive iodine therapy with ^{131}I is the preferred form of therapy for the majority of patients with Graves' disease. An appropriate dose (7 to 12 mCi ^{131}I) will induce euthyroidism in most patients. This form of therapy is inexpensive and easy to administer. Since the gonadal exposure is extremely low (less than a diagnostic radiograph), genetic effects are unlikely. Thus ^{131}I can be used in all adult patients. ^{131}I is contraindicated during pregnancy; thus a pregnancy test should be performed prior to therapy, or the dose should be given during the first half of the menstrual cycle. Long-term hypothyroidism (70 per cent at 10 years) is the major disadvantage of ^{131}I therapy. In addition, dose-related hypothyroidism occurs acutely after therapy (in six months) in a number of subjects. These complications are currently unavoidable, since lower doses may fail to induce euthyroidism.

SURGERY. Surgical ablation is still preferred for children who cannot be controlled with antithyroid drugs and possibly for young adults with extremely large glands. The procedure, subtotal thyroidectomy, should be performed only by an experienced surgeon. In the proper hands it is very effective therapy associated with minimal morbidity. Recurrent laryngeal nerve damage with vocal cord paralysis, permanent hypoparathyroidism, and hypothyroidism may be significant postoperative problems. Long-term hypothyroidism (40 per cent at 10 years) occurs despite the best of surgery, and immediate postoperative hypothyroidism may occur in 5 to 10 per cent of patients. Furthermore, recurrent hyperthyroidism also occurs in about 5 to 10 per cent of cases and should always be treated with ^{131}I therapy, since reoperation is more frequently accompanied by major complications.

Hyperthyroidism During Pregnancy. Graves' disease is responsible for the majority of cases of thyrotoxicosis associated with pregnancy. It should always be treated with antithyroid drugs. Surgery is rarely indicated and ^{131}I therapy should never be used. The dose of antithyroid drug used should be the minimum needed to restore euthyroidism. These drugs freely cross the placenta; thus hypothyroidism and goiter can be induced in the fetus with inappropriate high dosage. In general propylthiouracil is the drug of choice in the pregnant patient needing thionamide therapy, since aplasia cutis has been described in fetuses following methimazole therapy. The maternal thyroid status should be monitored with free T_4 determinations, since the total T_4 concentration is normally elevated during pregnancy because of the estrogen-induced high serum TBG level. The physician caring for the newborn infant of a Graves' mother should carefully monitor for neonatal Graves' disease. Passive transfer of TSI occurs and may produce transient neonatal hyperthyroidism. The cord blood TSI level may predict the infant at risk.

Toxic Nodular Goiter

This common cause of hyperthyroidism in the elderly generally occurs in patients with a long history of nodular goiter, but only a few patients with nodular goiter develop hyperthyroidism. It is not clear why these few nodular goiters progress to the toxic state and become autonomous in function. These patients generally present with symptoms and signs referable to the cerebrovascular, cardiovascular, musculoskeletal, or gastrointestinal system. Their hyperthyroidism is frequently masked by the nonthyroidal manifestations so that the true diagnosis is often delayed. Elderly patients with nodular goiter should be screened for thyroid dysfunction whenever they present with features of a new illness. The majority of these hyperthyroid patients will have an unequivocal increase in serum total and free T_4 values. Since 10 to 15 per cent may have normal T_4 values but a high serum T_3 concentration (T_3 toxicosis), the latter measurement should always be included when hyperthyroidism is clinically suspected in the elderly patient.

The majority of these patients can be treated with ^{131}I, but the effective dose generally ranges from 15 to 30 mCi. Hypothyroidism follows less frequently than in Graves' disease. It is preferable to induce a euthyroid state with antithyroid drugs prior to definitive therapy in order to avoid aggravation of the thyrotoxicosis. Surgery may be indicated in individuals with very large goiters (>100 grams) and in those patients who have pressure complications from goiter.

Thyroiditis

Transient thyrotoxicosis may be a feature of subacute granulomatous and lymphocytic thyroiditis. Subacute granulomatous thyroiditis is viral in origin, whereas lymphocytic thyroiditis probably results from autoimmune injury. The thyrotoxicosis associated with subacute granulomatous thyroiditis is generally mild, and symptomatic therapy is rarely needed. However, patients with subacute lymphocytic thyroiditis may need therapy for more prolonged and severe thyrotoxicosis. The latter condition is estimated to cause 15 to 20 per cent of thyrotoxicosis in adults and is also a common cause of postpartum thyroiditis. Both forms of thyroiditis are characterized by low RAIU tests. It is important to differentiate thyroiditis from Graves' disease, since therapy with ^{131}I or surgery is not indicated and antithyroid drugs (PTU or methimazole) are not effective. These patients are treated symptomatically with beta-blockers (propranolol) until remission occurs.

Hyperthyroxinemia of Acute Illness

Both serum total and free T_4 values are frequently elevated transiently during acute systemic (nonthyroidal) illness, especially in the elderly. This does not represent true hyperthyroidism. Serum T_3 concentrations are usually normal or low, and the TSH response to TRH is usually normal or slightly blunted. Hyperthyroidism can generally be excluded by demonstrating that the T_4 values return to normal during the recovery from the acute disorder. A similar phenomenon can be associated with acute psychiatric illness. It is important not to confuse these features of nonthyroidal illness with the diagnosis of true hyperthyroidism.

Familial Dysalbuminemic Hyperthyroxinemia (FDH)

This autosomal dominant condition may be a relatively common and misleading cause for an elevated total T_4 and free T_4 index. These subjects possess an abnormal albumin that has a high affinity for T_4, resulting in a high serum total T_4. Furthermore, the free T_4 index when derived from the T_3 resin uptake method is also high because the abnormal albumin does not have a high affinity for T_3. Thus an incorrect diagnosis of hyperthyroidism may be made. The serum free T_4 concentration and the total T_3 level are normal in these subjects. Thus in the absence of clinical features of thyrotoxicosis a high free T_4 index should suggest FDH as a differential possibility.

Thyrotoxic Crisis

This medical emergency is due to stress-induced exaggeration of the features of thyrotoxicosis. Additional clinical features include mental disorientation, fever, disproportionate tachycardia, and jaundice. Patients may rapidly deteriorate with shock and coma. The mortality of thyrotoxic crisis (thyroid storm) remains high. The diagnosis is made clinically, as time generally does not permit the laboratory confirmation of hyperthyroidism. Treatment should be initiated based on clinical suspicion.

Supportive measures are as important as specific therapy. Hyperpyrexia is controlled with a cooling blanket (aspirin is contraindicated), and the hypotension is reversed by volume expansion and vasopressor agents. During the extreme catabolic phase, adequate attention to nutritional support is mandatory. Other therapy includes glucocorticoids (hydrocortisone 100 mg t.i.d.),

TABLE 68-4. CAUSES OF HYPOTHYROIDISM

Primary

Autoimmune	Hashimoto's thyroiditis
	Idiopathic myxedema
Iatrogenic	^{131}I therapy for hyperthyroidism
	Subtotal thyroidectomy
Drug-induced	Iodide deficiency or excess
	Lithium, amiodarone
	Antithyroid drugs
Congenital	Synthetic enzyme defect
	Thyroid dysgenesis or agenesis

Secondary

Hypothalamic dysfunction	Therapeutic irradiation
	Granulomatous disease
	Neoplasms
Pituitary dysfunction	Therapeutic irradiation
	Pituitary surgery
	Idiopathic hypopituitarism
	Neoplasms
	Postpartum pituitary necrosis

to cover the severe stress and purported relative adrenal insufficiency. Specific therapy includes propylthiouracil (200 mg q4h), propranolol (40 mg q6h), and iodide (500 to 1000 mg q.i.d.). Iodide is given as a specific blocker of thyroid hormone secretion but not until hormone synthesis has been inhibited by PTU. Iodide initiated before PTU may aggravate the underlying hyperthyroid state. Cardiac decompensation should be treated with conventional doses of digoxin and diuretics. If cardiac failure is the dominant component of the crisis, beta-blockade may be contraindicated. This combined therapeutic approach should provide an effective amelioration of the thyrotoxic crisis within a few days.

HYPOTHYROIDISM

Deficiency of thyroid hormone may occur as a primary thyroid defect or more rarely may be due to pituitary or hypothalamic disease (secondary hypothyroidism). Primary thyroid failure is a common disorder (prevalence 0.8 per cent) whose clinical features range from mild hypothyroidism to severe myxedema. The latter condition develops in the setting of prolonged severe hypothyroidism and is due to the deposition of mucopolysaccharides in the skin and other tissues.

TABLE 68-5. CLINICAL FEATURES OF HYPOTHYROIDISM

SYMPTOMS	SIGNS
Weakness	Dry, coarse, cold skin
Lethargy, fatigue	Perorbital and peripheral edema
Memory impairment	Coarse, thin hair
Cold intolerance	Pallor of skin
Weight gain (anorexia)	Thick tongue
Constipation	Slow speech
Loss of hair	Decreased reflexes
Hoarseness	Hypertension
Deafness	Bradycardia
Dyspnea	Pleural, pericardial effusions
Myalgia, arthralgia	Ascites
Paresthesias	Vitiligo
Precordial pain	
Menstrual irregularity	

Two acquired and possibly related autoimmune disorders, atrophic (idiopathic) and Hashimoto's thyroiditis, are responsible for the majority (45 per cent) of cases of hypothyroidism (Table 68-4). Iatrogenic hypothyroidism consequent to definitive therapy (^{131}I or surgery) for hyperthyroidism constitutes a second major group (35 per cent). More recently drugs (iodide, lithium, and amiodarone) have become increasingly common causes of hypothyroidism in the hospital setting. The congenital causes are rare and generally present in childhood. Secondary causes induce hypothyroidism infrequently (approximately 1 per cent).

Clinical Features (Table 68-5)

The spectrum of clinical presentation depends on the degree, severity, and age at onset of the hypothyroidism. Cretinism, irreversible mental and motor retardation, presents within six months after delivery in the hypothyroid infant. Mass screening at birth should help to eliminate this correctable metabolic deficiency, since prompt replacement therapy with thyroid hormone can prevent or minimize this serious condition. Congenital hypothyroidism occurs in 1 in 5000 newborns. The development of hypothyroidism in childhood is associated with growth retardation and delayed puberty. Bone age is delayed relative to chronological age. In the adult the insidious nature of hypothyroidism may result in its being undetected for years. Symptoms are nonspecific, and in the absence of goiter the primary thyroid defect is frequently overlooked. Fatigue, lethargy, tiredness, cold intolerance, myalgias, and arthralgias are generally the earliest symptoms. The skin is dry and scaly, and hair loss is frequent. Facial puffiness and periorbital edema are characteristic features. The voice becomes hoarse and rough. In older subjects mental changes, confusion, paranoia, depression, and dementia are often attributed to aging per se. Nerve entrapment syndromes are common, such as deafness and hand paresthesia (median nerve distribution) due to the carpal tunnel syndrome.

In severe hypothyroidism (myxedema) the above features are exaggerated and characteristic clinical features develop. Extensive scaling of the skin leads to exfoliation, and diffuse subcutaneous infiltration with mucopolysaccharides gives the skin a thickened or doughy feeling. The edematous change is characteristically nonpitting except when hypoproteinemia develops. Deposition of carotene gives the skin a yellow-orange appearance. Sinus bradycardia may progress to variable degrees of heart block. This in conjunction with myocardial dilatation may lead to decompensation and congestive heart failure. More commonly the heart appears enlarged owing to pericardial effusion. Pleural effusions and ascites may also be prominent.

Deep tendon reflexes show the characteristic delayed relaxation phase (hung-up reflexes). Slow mentation progressing to confusion, disorientation, and coma is not uncommon. Rarely marked cerebellar ataxia occurs.

Myxedema Coma. This severe form of myxedema is frequently fatal. Decompensation is frequently precipitated by stress such as infection, alcohol (drugs), or cold exposure. Severe respiratory failure (CO_2 narcosis), hypothermia, and sluggish cerebral perfusion all contribute to the development of coma. The diagnosis is based on the clinical presentation. Therapy must be instituted before the clinical suspicions are substantiated by laboratory tests, since delay may lead to a fatal outcome in this medical emergency.

Laboratory Findings

Primary thyroid failure can be definitely diagnosed with the demonstration of low serum total T_4 and free T_4 values combined with a high serum TSH level. Measurement of serum T_3 is of no value in the diagnosis of hypothyroidism. Occasionally when the serum TSH value is borderline, the exaggerated TSH response to TRH will substantiate the diagnosis of primary hypothyroidism. Secondary hypothyroidism is associated with a low serum TSH level. The finding of other features of pituitary or hypothalamic disease generally confirms the diagnosis.

In addition to the definitive diagnostic tests noted above, hypothyroidism is associated with other abnormal laboratory tests. Muscle enzymes, especially creatine phosphokinase (CPK), are frequently elevated. In fact CPK isoenzyme analysis may show a modest increase in MB bands (cardiac). This in conjunction with myalgias and arthralgias, especially of the anterior chest wall, should not be mistaken for myocardial infarction. Hyponatremia, consequent to a relative excess of antidiuretic hormone (ADH) and impaired free water clearance, may be difficult to differentiate from the syndrome of inappropriate ADH secretion (SIADH).

Anemia in hypothyroidism is generally normochromic normocytic but may be macrocytic (vitamin B_{12} deficiency due to pernicious anemia) or microcytic because of poor nutrition or blood loss in women (menorrhagia).

The electrocardiogram classically demonstrates bradycardia and low voltage. In addition, variable degrees of heart block may be found, and nonspecific ST/T changes can occur. Blood gas analyses will demonstrate moderate to severe hypoxia and hypercapnia consequent to hypoventilation.

Differential Diagnosis

A clinical awareness of the wide spectrum of presentation and a high index of suspicion for hypothyroidism will generally detect most cases. A number of clinical states may mimic hypothyroidism, e.g., nephrotic syndrome and cirrhosis, including an associated reduction in serum TBG and consequent low serum total T_4 value. However, the serum free T_4 is generally normal. The diagnosis of hypothyroidism during acute illness is complicated by the finding of a low serum total T_4 and free T_4 index in many (10 to 20 per cent) of these patients. Serum T_3 is also low and serum TSH is generally within the normal range. The serum TSH response to TRH is either normal or blunted. These patients do not have primary thyroid failure but appear to have a stress-related form of secondary hypothyroidism. They are currently considered euthyroid ("euthyroid sick syndrome"), and T_4 replacement therapy is not warranted. In the majority of these patients the serum free T_4 concentration is normal and serum rT_3 is elevated. Furthermore, in clinically relevant hypothyroidism the serum TSH will be unequivocally elevated (>20 μU/ml) despite their acute illness.

Treatment

Hypothyroidism should be treated with a synthetic preparation of L-thyroxine. In young healthy individuals with hypothyroidism of recent onset and without cardiac disease, thyroxine replacement may be initiated at full dosage. Elderly subjects with heart disease or a history of pre-existing heart troubles should be slowly corrected to euthyroidism by incremental dose adjustments over several months in order to reduce the risk of cardiac complications. The average full replacement dose of L-thyroxine in the healthy adult ranges between 100 and 150 μg daily. In the elderly patient, thyroxine therapy should begin at 25 to 50 μg daily, with an incremental dose of 25 μg every two to four weeks. The therapeutic response should be monitored clinically and with serial serum T_4 and TSH analyses.

In a patient with myxedema coma, a large dose of thyroxine (300 to 500 μg) is given parenterally as a bolus and followed by 100 μg daily over the succeeding five days. Even elderly subjects with cardiac disorders tolerate these doses under this condition. The underlying stressful, precipitating event (e.g., infection) must obviously be corrected. Furthermore, standard supportive therapy for the comatose patient must be promptly introduced. This is especially important with respect to respiratory support. Many of these patients need mechanical ventilatory assistance, which may persist for some period after improvement in mental status. In addition, because of the associated relative adrenal insufficiency, these patients are treated with glucocorticoids. With proper therapy patients with myxedema coma should improve clinically within 24 to 36 hours. If this does not occur, the clinical diagnosis may not have been correct or the underlying aggravating medical illness may have persisted or advanced. The expected mortality from myxedema coma with adequate therapy remains around 25 per cent.

GOITER

This most common thyroid abnormality means basically an enlargement of the thyroid gland. Patients suffering from goiter are predominantly euthyroid (simple goiter) but may be hyperthyroid (toxic goiter) or hypothyroid. In areas where iodine deficiency is still prevalent, goiter formation is said to be endemic. The development of euthyroid simple colloid goiter, termed sporadic goiter, in an iodide-replete location is predominantly due to congenital defects in thyroid hormone synthesis. Dietary goitrogens such as the thiocarbamides found in cabbage, turnips, and soybeans may also induce sporadic goiter. Thyroid enlargement may be symmetrical and diffuse (simple goiter, Graves', Hashimoto's) or may be asymmetrical and nodular (nodular goiter, Hashimoto's).

Goiter formation is generally a TSH-mediated compensatory enlargement of the thyroid gland that ensures sufficient synthesis and secretion of thyroid hormone and prevents hypothyroidism. In addition, goiter formation may be consequent to an autoimmune process, as in Hashimoto's thyroiditis and Graves' disease.

Pain is unusual with a goiter except in the course of subacute thyroiditis, or consequent to cystic or hemorrhagic degeneration. Most frequently patients with nontoxic goiter present because of the neck swelling or features of obstruction. A large goiter can cause dysphagia, respiratory distress, or hoarseness. The latter symptom generally indicates recurrent laryngeal nerve invasion and most likely thyroid cancer rather than a benign simple goiter. The neck swelling can be readily confirmed as due to enlargement of the thyroid gland by either radioiodine scan or sonogram. In addition, the functional activity of the goiter can be determined from the radioiodine scan.

Most simple nontoxic goiters can be treated with continuous T_4 suppression of TSH, which should prevent further enlargement and eventually induce regression. It is important to determine that the gland is suppressible, since hyperthyroidism may develop from exogenous hormone therapy if the gland is autonomous. Autonomous function is frequent in patients with nontoxic multinodular goiter and patients with euthyroid Graves' disease. Thus a careful monitoring of the serum T_4 response to T_4 suppression is mandatory. If serum T_4 increases inappropriately during standard suppression therapy (150 to 200 μg L-thyroxine daily), the gland is probably autonomous and the dose should be reduced accordingly.

A diffusely enlarged gland should regress in 6 to 12 months, but long-standing multinodular goiter may take several years to respond. Therapy may be continued indefinitely or terminated when appropriate. Permanent loss of TSH secretion never occurs, even after years of T_4 suppression. Recovery will take place within six to eight weeks following the withdrawal of therapy. Goiters that fail to suppress, that are associated with pressure features, or that are large enough to be cosmetically embarrassing should be surgically removed.

The Solitary Thyroid Nodule

Thyroid nodules occur in approximately 5 per cent of the population. A nodule is a focal area of gland enlargement. It can be caused by a number of factors, but solitary nodules are predominantly

TABLE 68–6. PATHOGENESIS OF THYROID NODULES

LESIONS*	PREVALENCE (%)
Benign thyroid nodule	40
Multinodular goiter	20
Cyst	12
Thyroiditis	10
Follicular adenoma	12
Carcinoma	6

* Data are representative of findings on fine needle aspiration followed by surgical excision in indicated cases.

adenomatous and benign (Table 68–6). Since a small percentage are carcinomatous, a practical clinical approach must be pursued to detect these patients. A number of factors from the clinical history, examination, and specific evaluations are helpful in the differentiation of benign from malignant lesions (Table 68–7). These relate to patient age and sex and whether the nodule is single or part of a multinodular gland. A young man presenting with a single dominant nodule associated with hoarseness and lymph node enlargement has a high possibility of malignancy. Any individual who presents with a nodule and a past history of head-neck irradiation should be referred for thyroidectomy, as these lesions are predominantly malignant (~ 30 per cent).

The traditional approach is to perform a RAIU study initially to determine the functional status of the nodule. Scanning with ^{123}I will demonstrate no accumulation ("cold nodule"), equal isotope trapping ("warm nodule"), or greater accumulation ("hot nodule") when compared with the rest of the gland. Warm and hot nodules are overwhelmingly benign (99.8 per cent). Cold nodules are also predominantly benign (90 per cent). Patients with hot nodules may be hyperthyroid. These can be treated effectively with ^{131}I therapy. Generally, however, they are not currently hyperthyroid, but they should be followed carefully, since approximately 30 per cent will eventually become hyperthyroid.

Most solitary nodules are "cold" (80 per cent). A definitive pathological diagnosis can be made in most of these subjects (80 per cent) by cytological examination of a tissue specimen obtained by fine needle aspiration biopsy (FNA). In fact, most centers now perform FNA as the initial procedure. Benign lesions (75 per cent) such as benign thyroid nodules, multinodular goiter, and thyroiditis can be identified by the expert cytologist. In addition, malignant lesions (5 per cent), such as papillary, anaplastic, and medullary carcinoma, can be specifically diagnosed. Follicular neoplasms (20 per cent), however, cannot be identified as benign or malignant by this technique and require examination of tissue specimens obtained by surgical excision. Despite the lack of sensitivity in the analysis of the follicular neoplasm, FNA has proved to be a powerful diagnostic procedure in the evaluation of the thyroid nodule. The ability to make a definitive diagnosis through the application of this safe and simple technique has markedly reduced the need for diagnostic thyroid surgery. The therapy for a malignant nodule is considered in the section on thyroid carcinoma. Benign lesions are treated with T_4 suppression therapy. Regression of the nodule may occur during a six-month course. Generally, long-standing nodules remain stable and do not progress. Should the nodule increase in size, it should be re-evaluated and the appropriate therapy instituted.

THYROID CARCINOMA

Thyroid cancer is a relatively rare disorder (4 in 100,000). Furthermore, most varieties of thyroid cancer are of low-grade malignancy. Papillary or follicular carcinomas constitute about 90 per cent of all thyroid cancers. Anaplastic and medullary carcinoma accounts for the remainder.

Papillary carcinoma generally presents as a thyroid nodule that may be associated with local invasion and lymph node spread. The size of the initial lesion (>2.5 cm) and the presence of lymph node involvement adversely influence the recurrence rate and long-term prognosis. Follicular carcinoma is more aggressive and frequently presents with metastases, especially to the lung, bone, or brain. The size of the initial lesion does not influence prognosis. In many cases the small thyroid primary is overlooked and is diagnosed in retrospect following examination of the metastatic tissue. Both of these cancers have a low recurrence rate and a relatively good prognosis.

Primary therapy entails total thyroidectomy with nodal dissection followed in most cases (six weeks postoperatively) by ^{131}I ablative therapy for any remnant tissue. Irradiation is probably not indicated for small (<2.5 cm), noninvasive papillary lesions. Both surgical and radioactive ablative therapies are followed with T_4 suppression of TSH. Measurement of serum thyroglobulin has no pretherapeutic diagnostic value. It is, however, an excellent way to determine the effect of treatment and to monitor for recurrence.

Anaplastic carcinoma predominantly affects older individuals (>50 years). It is very aggressive and rapidly induces pain and symptoms related to local pressure (dysphagia, hoarseness). Death generally occurs within 12 months, but surgically resectable disease may have a better prognosis, with a five-year survival of approximately 30 per cent.

Medullary carcinoma, which develops in the parafollicular cells (C cells), may be sporadic or familial (autosomal dominant). When familial, it is frequently a component of a multiple endocrine neoplasia syndrome (MEN Type II). This tumor produces calcitonin; measurement of basal serum calcitonin can substantiate its presence. Provocative testing with calcium or pentagastin (calcitonin response) may detect early C-cell hyperplasia in subjects at risk (MEN Type II families). Surgical excision of the primary lesion in the ab-

TABLE 68–7. HIGH RISK FACTORS FOR CANCER IN A THYROID NODULE

History	Childhood therapeutic irradiations (low dose <500 rads) of head or neck
	Hoarseness
	Rapid growth
	Pain
Clinical Features	Children, young adults, men
	Solitary, firm, dominant nodule
	Associated lymphadenopathy
	Vocal cord paralysis
	Distant metastasis
Serum Factors	Elevated serum calcitonin
Scanning Techniques	
Pattern on [123]I	"Cold" nodule
ECHO scan	Solid lesion
Thyroxine Therapy	No regression

sence of nodal involvement produces an excellent prognosis (90 per cent survival at 10 years). In contrast, patients with nodal disease have only a 40 per cent survival at 10 years.

One of the most important factors in the evaluation of a patient with suspected thyroid cancer (thyroid nodule) is a history of low-dose irradiation (<500 rads) to the head or neck area during childhood. Such individuals are at high risk for thyroid cancer. Careful investigation of such patients will detect follicular or papillary carcinoma in about 30 per cent of cases. It is now recommended that irradiated patients have a thyroid (clinical) examination at two-year intervals. In the absence of palpable disease, laboratory evaluation is not warranted. Postirradiated patients with a palpable dominant nodule should receive total thyroidectomy with removal of nodes if there is metastatic disease. If invasive carcinoma is present, postoperative remnant ablation with ^{131}I should be carried out at six weeks. Suppressive therapy with T_4 will be necessary for life.

THYROIDITIS

In subacute granulomatous (de Quervain's) thyroiditis, a common disorder, the thyroid gland is painful and tender, and symptoms may be preceded by or associated with fever. Clinical hyperthyroidism may occur during the early phase, followed by transient hypothyroidism and then eventual recovery. The elevated serum total and free T_4 values are associated with a depressed RAIU test. Antithyroid antibodies are rarely detected. The erythrocyte sedimentation rate is characteristically high.

Therapy is symptomatic; the symptoms of thyroid pain and tenderness generally respond to aspirin. However, a small percentage of patients may need a short course of prednisone (20 mg b.i.d.) for relief. Symptomatic hyperthyroidism should be treated with propranolol (40 mg t.i.d.). Since both the hyper- and hypothyroid phases are self-limiting (total disease course 8 to 12 weeks), patient reassurance is generally all that is needed.

Subacute lymphocytic thyroiditis (silent thyroiditis) is currently considered to be an autoimmune disorder that is responsible for 20 to 30 per cent of all cases of thyrotoxicosis. This condition was discussed in the section on hyperthyroidism. Chronic lymphocytic thyroiditis (Hashimoto's disease) is probably the most common cause of goiter in the western world. High titers of antithyroid antibodies are present in 90 per cent of cases. It is frequently complicated by hypothyroidism and was discussed in that section. Acute suppurative thyroiditis, an unusual disorder, generally follows bacteremia rather than being a primary infection.

REFERENCES

Borst GC, Eil C, and Burman KD: Euthyroid hyperthyroxinemia. Ann Intern Med 98:366–378, 1983.

Chopra IJ, Hershman JM, Pardridge WM, and Nicoloff JT: Thyroid function in nonthyroidal illness. Ann Intern Med 98:946–957, 1983.

Cooper DS: Antithyroid drugs. N Engl J Med 311(21):1353–1362, 1984.

Larsen PR: The thyroid. In Wyngaarden JB, and Smith LH Jr (eds): Cecil Textbook of Medicine. 17th ed, Philadelphia, WB Saunders Co, 1985, pp. 1275–1299.

Nikolai TF, Brosseau J, Kettrick M, Roberts R, and Beltaos E: Lymphocytic thyroiditis with spontaneously resolving hyperthyroidism (silent thyroiditis). Arch Intern Med 140:478–481, 1980.

Tachmann ML, and Guthrie GB: Hypothyroidism: Diversity of presentation. Endocr Rev 5:456–465, 1984.

Van Herle AJ, Rich P, Ljung BM, Ashcraft MW, Solomon DH, and Keeler EB: The thyroid nodule. Ann Intern Med 96:221–232, 1982.

Weetman AP, and McGregor AM: Autoimmune thyroid disease: Developments in our understanding. Endocr Rev 5:309–354, 1984.

69 ADRENAL GLAND

The adrenal glands, paired structures located retroperitoneally at the upper pole of each kidney, include two distinct endocrine organs: an outer cortex that secretes steroid hormones and an inner medulla that, as part of the sympathetic nervous system, secretes catecholamines. The cortex consists of three zones: the outer zona glomerulosa, which secretes a potent mineralocorticoid hormone, and the inner zonae fasciculata and reticularis, which secrete glucocorticoids, androgens, and small quantities of estrogens. Each of these steroid hormones as well as the catecholamines (epinephrine and norepinephrine) causes striking effects when produced in excess. In contrast, only glucocorticoid and mineralocorticoid hormones, which are secreted exclusively by the adrenal gland, are physiologically important products. Presumably the gonadal production of androgens and estrogens and secretion of norepinephrine by sympathetic ganglia are quantitatively more important sources of these hormones and neurotransmitters.

MAJOR HORMONES OF THE ADRENAL GLAND

Cortisol is the major glucocorticoid secreted by the adrenal cortex. Glucocorticoids are involved in multiple biological processes, affecting carbohydrate, protein, lipid, and water metabolism. Cortisol secretion is under the control of adrenocorticotropin (ACTH), which in turn is regulated by the secretion of corticotropin-releasing hormone (CRF) (Fig. 69–1A). Secretion of ACTH and cortisol is pulsatile, manifests a diurnal circadian rhythm, and is under negative feedback control. Stress in a variety of forms can override the diurnal rhythm as well as the negative feedback relationship of the system.

Aldosterone is the principal mineralocorticoid hormone secreted by the adrenal cortex. Normally, the renin-angiotensin system is the major factor controlling aldosterone secretion (Fig. 69–2). Renin is released from the juxtaglomerular cells of the kidney in response to a reduction in renal perfusion pressure or a decrease in effective circulating volume, or both. Renin enzymatically cleaves the hepatic alpha-2 globulin renin substrate to liberate a decapeptide, angiotensin I. Removal of the carboxy terminal dipeptide by an endothelial converting enzyme produces the octapeptide angiotensin II. Angiotensin II stimulates the zona glomerulosa of the adrenal gland directly to increase aldosterone secretion. Aldosterone increases transepithelial transport of sodium by the kidney, and the resultant sodium retention tends to ameliorate the initial stimulus for renin secretion. Increases in plasma K^+ concentration normally increase aldosterone secretion, whereas hypokalemia suppresses it. Inasmuch as aldosterone promotes K^+ secretion by the kidney, this provides a second feedback mechanism regulating aldosterone secretion. When stimulation by the renin-angiotensin system is reduced during periods of recumbency, plasma aldosterone concentration correlates with the pulsatile release of cortisol, implying that ACTH also plays a role in the physiological regulation of aldosterone secretion.

The clinical disorders of the adrenal glands discussed in this chapter are relatively uncommon but, when present, result in some of the most striking syndromes in clinical medicine. When suspected, the diagnosis can be established using biochemical measurements that are readily available in clinical laboratories and, in most instances, the response to appropriate therapy is dramatic and rewarding.

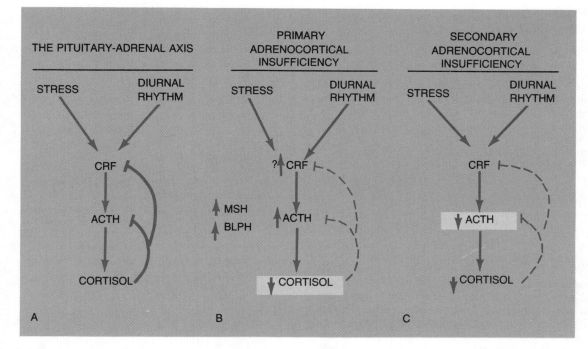

FIGURE 69–1. The hypothalamic-pituitary-adrenal axis. Secretion of corticotropin-releasing hormone (CRF) normally regulates secretion of ACTH, which in turn controls cortisol production (*A*). The system is subject to negative feedback control: Reduced levels of cortisol result in diminished feedback regulation (dashed lines) and marked increases in ACTH levels as in primary adrenocortical insufficiency (*B*). Hypothalamic-pituitary disorders that diminish ACTH secretion result in secondary adrenocortical insufficiency (*C*).

FIGURE 69–2. The renin-angiotensin-aldosterone system. Aldosterone secretion is principally regulated by the renin-angiotensin system. Potassium (K^+) and ACTH also stimulate aldosterone secretion, whereas sodium and dopamine (not shown) may inhibit it. Negative feedback control occurs by virtue of mineralocorticoid-induced kaliuresis and sodium retention, which reduce levels of K^+ and angiotensin II (AII), respectively.

SYNDROMES OF ADRENOCORTICAL HYPOFUNCTION (Table 69–1)

Hypofunction of the adrenal cortex can occur either from a primary adrenal disorder or from an alteration in the regulatory factors that control adrenal steroid biosynthesis. The major manifestations vary depending upon the relative involvement of mineralocorticoid, glucocorticoid, or androgen/estrogen secretion by the gland.

GENERALIZED ADRENOCORTICAL INSUFFICIENCY

Pathophysiology

Generalized adrenocortical insufficiency (Addison's disease) occurs when destruction of adrenocortical tissue reduces secretory rates of both mineralocorticoid and glucocorticoid hormones below the physiological needs of the organism. This combined deficiency is usually fatal if untreated. A similar combined hormonal deficiency results from surgical removal of both adrenal glands and from certain inherited disorders of steroid biosynthesis.

Cortisol deficiency results in anorexia, weight

loss, weakness, apathy, and a general inability to withstand "stress." Cortisol normally inhibits ACTH secretion so that markedly elevated levels of ACTH are characteristic of Addison's disease (see Fig. 69–1B). Hyperpigmentation results from the increased levels of ACTH or related proopiomelanocortin-derived peptides (lipotropin, melanocortin). Mineralocorticoid deficiency results in impaired renal Na^+ conservation as well as impaired K^+ and H^+ secretion in the distal nephron. If the Na^+ intake is sufficiently large, extracellular fluid volume and plasma K^+ and bicarbonate levels can be maintained at normal or nearly normal levels. If the Na^+ intake is low, however, or if extrarenal losses of Na^+ occur, the inability to conserve Na^+ maximally results in marked Na^+ deficits, hyponatremia, hyperkalemia, acidosis, hypovolemia, and increased plasma renin levels. Glucocorticoid deficiency may add to the severity of the hypovolemia by redistributing fluid between vascular and extravascular compartments and of the hyponatremia by impairing renal diluting ability.

Etiology

Generalized adrenocortical insufficiency may result from tuberculosis, histoplasmosis and other fungal diseases, metastatic carcinoma, amyloidosis, and bilateral adrenal hemorrhage secondary to anticoagulant therapy. Currently, Addison's disease results most frequently from autoimmune injury that causes selective atrophy of the adrenal cortex ("idiopathic" adrenal insufficiency), usually sparing the adrenal medulla. Patients so affected often manifest evidence of other autoimmune processes affecting the thyroid, islet cells, gonads, and other tissues.

Adrenocortical Insufficiency in Congenital Adrenal Hyperplasia. Combined glucocorticoid and mineralocorticoid deficiency also occurs in several congenital disorders of the adrenal gland characterized pathologically by diffuse bilateral enlargement of the adrenal cortex and collectively referred to as congenital adrenal hyperplasia. These disorders result from inherited defects in adrenal steroid biosynthesis inferred to result from adrenal enzyme defects. The reduced secretion of steroids by the adrenal gland leads to supernormal circulating levels of adrenocorticotropic hormones (ACTH and/or angiotensin), which attempt to increase the rate of secretion of the steroids by the defective gland and thereby induce adrenal hyperplasia. The commonest form of congenital adrenal hyperplasia results from defective 21-hydroxylation in the zona fasciculata and in some, but possibly not all, patients in the zona glomerulosa as well. Secretion by the zona fasciculata of all glucocorticoid and mineralocorticoid hormones (21-hydroxylated steroids) is subnormal, whereas secretion of progesterone and 17-hydroxyprogesterone (the normal substrates for 21-hydroxylation) is increased. Signs and symptoms of combined glucocorticoid and mineralocorticoid deficiency are commonly but not invariably present. The increased levels of 17-hy-

---

TABLE 69–1. SYNDROMES OF ADRENOCORTICAL HYPOFUNCTION

I. **Primary Adrenal Disorders**
   A. Combined Mineralocorticoid and Glucocorticoid Deficiency
      1. Addison's disease
         Autoimmune
         Tuberculosis, fungal, sarcoid, hemochromatosis
         Metastatic carcinoma, lymphoma
         Bilateral adrenal hemorrhage
      2. Bilateral adrenalectomy
      3. Adrenal enzyme deficiency states
         21-hydroxylase deficiency
         3β-ol dehydrogenase deficiency
         Desmolase deficiency
   B. Aldosterone Deficiency Without Glucocorticoid Deficiency
      1. Corticosterone methyl oxidase deficiency, types I and II
      2. Isolated zona glomerulosa defect
      3. Critically ill patients
      4. Heparin therapy
      5. Converting enzyme inhibitors
II. **Secondary Adrenal Disorders**
   A. Secondary Adrenal Insufficiency
      1. Panhypopituitarism
      2. Selective deficiency of ACTH
      3. Exogenous glucocorticoids
   B. Hyporeninemic Hypoaldosteronism
      1. Diffuse, histologically evident renal disease
         Diabetic nephropathy
         Tubulointerstitial diseases
         Obstructive uropathy
      2. Autonomic neuropathy
      3. Extracellular volume expansion
      4. Impaired conversion of prorenin to active renin
      5. Impaired renal prostaglandin production
         Nonsteroidal anti-inflammatory drugs

droxyprogesterone in the fasciculata cells result in overproduction of adrenal androgens, causing clinical virilization (female pseudohermaphroditism, male precocious puberty), differing greatly in severity among patients. The increased levels of 17-hydroxyprogesterone and progesterone in the peripheral circulation contribute to the clinical manifestations of mineralocorticoid insufficiency, inasmuch as these steroids are mineralocorticoid receptor antagonists that inhibit the renal action of aldosterone.

Clinical Manifestations

The clinical manifestations of Addison's disease have largely been described under the section on pathophysiology and are summarized in Table 69–2.

Diagnosis and Treatment

The diagnosis of generalized adrenocortical insufficiency is confirmed by the finding of subnormal plasma levels of cortisol and aldosterone and by reduced urinary excretion of their major metabolites, the urinary 17-hydroxycorticoids and aldosterone-18-glucuronide, respectively. The primary abnormality resides in the adrenal cortex; plasma levels of ACTH and renin are elevated concomitantly. Inasmuch as plasma ACTH levels are not available in all laboratories and special precautions are required for handling such samples, the primary nature of the adrenal disorder is frequently demonstrated by measurement of cortisol levels following either acute or chronic stimulation by exogenously administered ACTH. Subnormal levels of cortisol that fail to increase in response to ACTH point to a primary abnormality of cortisol secretion. Aldosterone levels will also fail to increase normally in such patients. Prolonged administration of ACTH may be required in certain circumstances to distinguish primary from secondary syndromes of adrenocortical deficiency.

Generalized adrenocortical insufficiency often

TABLE 69–2. CLINICAL FEATURES OF CHRONIC PRIMARY ADRENOCORTICAL INSUFFICIENCY

SIGNS AND SYMPTOMS	PER CENT
Weakness and fatigue	100
Weight loss	100
Anorexia	100
Hyperpigmentation	92
Hypotension	88
Gastrointestinal symptoms	56
Salt craving	19
Postural symptoms	12

Adapted from Baxter JD, and Tyrrell JB: The adrenal cortex. In Felig P, Baxter JD, Broadus AH, and Frohman LA (eds): Endocrinology and Metabolism. New York, McGraw-Hill Book Co, 1981, p 453.

presents as a medical emergency; therapy should never be withheld pending laboratory results that establish the diagnosis. When the diagnosis of adrenal insufficiency is suspected in a critically ill patient, it is prudent to obtain plasma samples in which cortisol, aldosterone, ACTH, and renin activity can be measured subsequently. Intravenous administration of β^{1-24} ACTH (Cortrosyn, 25 U) given as a bolus followed by a second plasma sample one hour later, is an additional useful step in diagnosis. If delay of therapy for even one hour is deemed inadvisable, glucocorticoid therapy can be initiated with dexamethasone, a potent synthetic glucocorticoid that will not be reflected in the subsequent plasma cortisol measurement. In adrenal crisis, glucocorticoids should be administered in doses that reflect the levels normally secreted by the adrenal cortex under maximal stress, usually 200 to 300 mg of hydrocortisone per day or its equivalent. The manifestations of associated mineralocorticoid deficiency are best treated in such circumstances with parenteral fluids and salt replacement rather than with mineralocorticoid hormones.

Treatment with hydrocortisone or an equivalent glucocorticoid is required on a lifelong basis. The usual doses are 20 to 30 mg daily with one half to two thirds being given on arising and the remainder in early evening. Doses should be increased at times of stress such as occurs with surgical procedures or severe medical illnesses. Because aldosterone production is also decreased, mineralocorticoid replacement is added frequently, but many patients can be maintained on a high sodium intake without mineralocorticoid. The need for mineralocorticoid replacement therapy can be assessed by measurement of plasma renin activity, a sensitive index of extracellular volume in patients with Addison's disease. The usual mineralocorticoid steroid administered therapeutically is fludrocortisone, which is effective orally. Although 50 to 150 μg fludrocortisone per day is the usual recommended dose range, such doses may be suboptimal; doses in the range of 200 to 300 μg per day may be required to reduce renin levels into the normal range. At these doses, however, blood pressure levels may increase substantially and frank hypertension may occur. Thus, careful monitoring for evidence of hypertension or congestive heart failure must be done along with determination of plasma renin levels in order to determine the optimal replacement dose in individual patients. The patient should wear a Medic Alert bracelet.

ALDOSTERONE DEFICIENCY WITHOUT GLUCOCORTICOID DEFICIENCY

Aldosterone deficiency in the absence of glucocorticoid deficiency is most commonly the result of deficient secretion of renin, so-called hyporeninemic hypoaldosteronism (see below). Rarely, isolated deficiency of aldosterone may result from a primary abnormality of the adrenal cortex, either as a consequence of an inherited deficiency of the enzyme complex responsible for the final step of aldosterone biosynthesis (corticosterone methyloxidase) or as a manifestation of rare acquired disorders that selectively impair zona glomerulosa function. Such syndromes of primary isolated aldosterone deficiency are characterized by elevated levels of plasma renin activity in contrast to hyporeninemic hypoaldosteronism (Fig. 69–3).

Acquired lesions that selectively destroy the zona glomerulosa include a chronic autoimmune process in which antibodies are directed only against cells of the zona glomerulosa and the initial phase of a pathologic process that eventually leads to generalized adrenocortical insufficiency. Mineralocorticoid replacement is given as in other primary adrenal disorders. Hypoaldosteronism that occurs in critically ill patients or in those on heparin therapy rarely results in clinically significant electrolyte disorders, and thus mineralocorticoid therapy may not be indicated. Administration of converting enzyme inhibitors (that block the synthesis of angiotensin II) may cause significant hyperkalemia, particularly in patients with underlying renal insufficiency. In such patients hyper-reninemic hypoaldosteronism is present as a consequence of reduced angiotensin II levels and does not imply the presence of a primary adrenal abnormality. Mineralocorticoid therapy will correct the electrolyte abnormalities, but the usual approach is to discontinue the agent.

SECONDARY ADRENAL INSUFFICIENCY

Secondary adrenal insufficiency refers to glucocorticoid deficiency that results from inadequate stimulation of the adrenal cortex by ACTH. This can occur as a consequence of destructive lesions in the hypothalamic-pituitary axis, from an isolated defect in ACTH secretion, or as a consequence of prolonged suppression of the pituitary-adrenal axis by exogenously administered

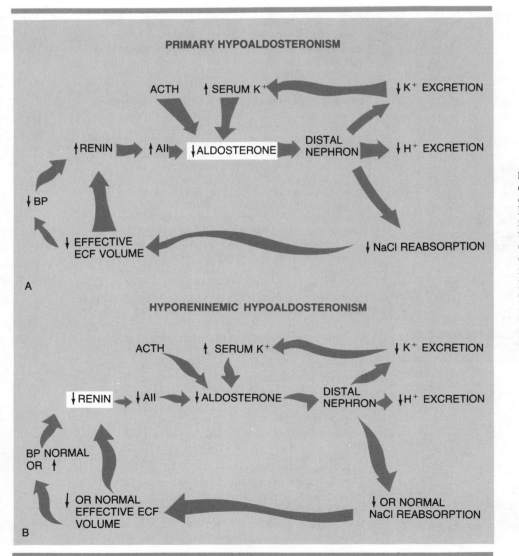

FIGURE 69–3. Pertubations of the renin-angiotensin-aldosterone system in primary hypoaldosteronism (A) and in hyporeninemic hypoaldosteronism (B). Hypoaldosteronism in primary adrenal disorders can occur as an isolated defect or as a component of generalized adrenocortical deficiency. In the latter, ACTH levels are also increased as a consequence of cortisol deficiency (see Fig. 69–1B).

glucocorticoid hormones. Inasmuch as aldosterone secretion is primarily regulated by the renin-angiotensin system and not chronically by ACTH, mineralocorticoid deficiency is rare in such circumstances.

The clinical findings are similar to those that occur in primary glucocorticoid deficiency with several important differences. Inasmuch as plasma levels of ACTH and related proopiomelanocortin-derived peptides are reduced, hyperpigmentation is absent (Fig. 69–1C). Because mineralocorticoid levels are normal, hyperkalemia and metabolic acidosis are also not evident, but patients may develop hyponatremia as a consequence of the impaired water excretion that accompanies glucocorticoid deficiency. Primary diseases of the pituitary may result in the reduction of other trophic hormones, and the clinical manifestations of secondary adrenocortical insufficiency may be complicated by those of secondary hypothyroidism and hypogonadism (see Chapter 68).

Secondary adrenocortical insufficiency commonly results from prior administration of glucocorticoids. Glucocorticoid suppression of the hypothalamic-pituitary axis occurs rapidly, with a degree that depends upon the duration and dose of the therapy, and can be minimized by the use of alternate-day therapy when this is feasible. Three potential problems occur when glucocorticoids are withdrawn: (1) exacerbation of the underlying inflammatory disease for which the agent was being given; (2) a steroid withdrawal syndrome in which clinical manifestations suggesting adrenal insufficiency occur despite the fact that glucocorticoid levels may still be in the normal range; and (3) a true adrenal insufficiency that occurs when the doses of glucocorticoids are reduced below maintenance levels. Recovery of normal function may take up to a year, during which time resumption of normal ACTH secretion must precede the eventual recovery of adrenal function. The recovery process can be accelerated if the patient can tolerate total withdrawal of glucocorticoid therapy, although there should be no hesitancy to provide such medication in the case of an intercurrent medical or surgical illness.

HYPORENINEMIC HYPOALDOSTERONISM

Pathophysiology

In adults, mineralocorticoid deficiency occurs in numerous renal and extrarenal disorders that cause diminished renal secretion of renin. Under ordinary physiological conditions in healthy subjects, the product of renin's action, angiotensin II, provides the major tonic stimulatory effect on aldosterone secretion. Hypoangiotensinemia secondary to diminished renin secretion leads to a clinically significant state of mineralocorticoid deficiency, so-called hyporeninemic hypoaldosteronism. Diabetes mellitus and chronic tubulointerstitial diseases of the kidney are the most common underlying disorders that result in inability of the kidney to secrete sufficient renin.

In affected patients, mineralocorticoid deficiency is usually manifested as hyperkalemia and commonly as hyperchloremic metabolic acidosis. Sodium depletion and renal sodium wasting, however, are not invariably present. In some patients, total body sodium and extracellular fluid volume are supernormal, suggesting that in such patients deficient renin secretion is a functional consequence of reduced renal clearance of sodium chloride.

The pathophysiology of the hyporeninemia is probably multifactorial. Sclerosis of the juxtaglomerular apparatus and functional disorders including impairment of normal stimulation by the sympathetic nervous system (such as might occur in autonomic insufficiency in diabetic subjects) interfere with renin secretion. Impaired conversion of prorenin to active renin also occurs in some affected individuals. Administration of certain pharmacologic agents such as nonsteroidal anti-inflammatory agents, inhibitors of angiotensin converting enzyme, and beta-adrenergic receptor antagonists can produce a clinical syndrome similar to that which occurs spontaneously.

Treatment

Patients with this syndrome are usually asymptomatic. Nevertheless, life-threatening arrhythmias can occur from markedly elevated serum potassium levels, and protracted metabolic acidosis can adversely affect bone mineralization and other cellular functions. Administration of fludrocortisone in doses from 100 to 300 μg per day generally results in a prompt increase in renal potassium and hydrogen ion excretion and amelioration of hyperkalemia and metabolic acidosis. Patients with hyporeninemic hypoaldosteronism may respond less to the renal effect of mineralocorticoids because of their underlying renal insufficiency.

Treatment of hyperkalemia and acidosis with fludrocortisone, however, is not always effective and safe, particularly in those patients who are hypertensive and have measured pretreatment increases in extracellular fluid volume and total exchangeable sodium. Treatment with fludrocortisone increases renal tubular reabsorption of sodium chloride and might exacerbate hypertension and lead to other deleterious consequences of extracellular fluid volume expansion. Furosemide, in doses of 40 to 120 mg daily, increases potassium and net acid excretion and ameliorates the hyperkalemia and metabolic acidosis in such patients. With more severe degrees of hypoaldosteronism, the ameliorative effect of furosemide is enhanced by pretreatment with small doses of fludrocortisone. The combination of fludrocortisone and furosemide offers the advantages of mutual potentiation of kaliuretic and acid-excretory effects and countervailing natriuretic and chloruretic effects. This combination reduces hyperkalemia and acidosis and concomitantly, by adjustment of the relative dose of the two agents, allows control of body content of sodium chloride.

TABLE 69–3. SYNDROMES OF ADRENOCORTICAL HYPERFUNCTION

I. **Syndromes of Glucocorticoid Excess (Cushing's Syndrome)**
  A. Secondary to Increased ACTH Stimulation
    1. Hypothalamic-pituitary abnormality (Cushing's disease)
       Pituitary microadenoma
       Corticotropin-releasing hormone (?)
    2. Ectopic ACTH secretion
       Small cell carcinoma of the lung
       Islet cell tumor
       Thymoma
  B. Primary Adrenal Abnormality
    1. Adenoma
    2. Carcinoma
  C. Exogenous Glucocorticoid Therapy
II. **Syndromes of Mineralocorticoid Excess**
  A. Primary Aldosteronism
    1. Aldosterone-producing adenoma
    2. Bilateral adrenal hyperplasia (idiopathic hyperaldosteronism)
    3. Adrenal carcinoma
    4. Glucocorticoid-remediable hyperaldosteronism
  B. Adrenal Enzyme Defects
    1. 11β-hydroxylase deficiency
    2. 17α-hydroxylase deficiency
  C. Exogenous Mineralocorticoids
    1. Licorice
    2. Carbenoxolone
  D. Secondary Aldosteronism
    1. Nonhypertensive disorders
       Sodium depletion, hemorrhage
       Pregnancy
       Edematous states
       Renal tubular acidosis
       Bartter's syndrome
       Diuretic therapy
    2. Hypertensive disorders
       Accelerated and renovascular hypertension
       Renin-secreting tumors
       Necrotizing vasculitis
       Estrogen therapy

SYNDROMES OF ADRENOCORTICAL HYPERFUNCTION (Table 69–3)

The major clinical manifestations of adrenocortical hyperfunction vary depending upon the predominant steroid produced in excess. Hypersecretion of glucocorticoid hormone results in Cushing's syndrome, a metabolic disorder affecting carbohydrate, protein, and lipid metabolism. Hypersecretion of aldosterone and related mineralocorticoid hormones results in a disturbance of electrolyte and blood pressure homeostasis.

CUSHING'S SYNDROME

Pathophysiology

Cushing's syndrome, the consequence of chronic exposure to excessive amounts of glucocorticoid hormone, can occur as a consequence of increased endogenous production of cortisol (Fig. 69–4) or, more commonly, as the result of prolonged exposure to glucocorticoid therapy administered in superphysiological doses. Of the endogenous causes, the most common in adults is bilateral adrenal hyperplasia due to excessive pituitary secretion of ACTH, a condition referred to as Cushing's disease (Fig. 69–4A). Bilateral adrenal hyperplasia can also result from ectopic production of ACTH by a variety of neoplasms (Fig. 69–4B). Primary adrenal tumors, either adenomas or carcinomas, account for the remaining cases (Fig. 69–4C).

In Cushing's disease the hypersecretion of ACTH by the pituitary gland appears to be due to the presence of an adenoma in approximately 90 per cent of cases. These are frequently small (mi-

FIGURE 69–4. Pertubations of the hypothalamic-pituitary-adrenal axis that result in Cushing's syndrome.

croadenomas) and basophilic. Whether such an adenoma arises spontaneously or as a secondary consequence of excessive secretion of corticotropin-releasing hormone has not been resolved. This disorder is much more common in women (female to male ratio, 5:1), typically occurs during the childbearing years and, as a consequence of an insidious onset, may go undetected for many years.

In patients with bilateral adrenal hyperplasia due to ectopic ACTH secretion, the level of cortisol may be several times higher than in Cushing's disease, yet the clinical manifestations are often less striking. This difference is presumably due to the more rapid progression of the disease, as a consequence of the underlying neoplasm. In addition to marked increases in cortisol production, such patients may have greatly increased levels of deoxycorticosterone (DOC), a potent mineralocorticoid that can result in severe hypertension and hypokalemic metabolic alkalosis. Small cell carcinoma of the lung, bronchial carcinoid, and medullary carcinoma of the thyroid are among the neoplasms reported to secrete ACTH ectopically. Ectopic ACTH syndrome occurs more frequently in men, and the age of onset is typically later than in Cushing's disease.

The primary adrenal neoplasms that result in Cushing's syndrome may also be associated with severe hypokalemic metabolic alkalosis and hypertension as a consequence of marked increases in mineralocorticoid hormone secretion. Such tumors may also present with findings reflecting predominant secretion of androgens or estrogens, causing virilization or feminization in women and men, respectively. Adrenal carcinomas are the most frequent cause of Cushing's syndrome in children.

Clinical Manifestations

The clinical manifestations of Cushing's disease are very diverse (Table 69–4). Regardless of the etiology, hypercortisolism results in obesity, carbohydrate intolerance, muscle wasting, and osteoporosis. Obesity is centripedal, manifested typically by a "buffalo hump," increased supraclavicular fat pads, and moon facies. Easy bruisability and abdominal striae may be noted. Mild hypertension is common. Mental changes also occur commonly. An increase in adrenal androgen production can result in hirsutism, acne, and menstrual disorders in women. Men may complain of impotence and loss of libido.

Diagnosis

The diagnostic approach in patients who are suspected of having Cushing's syndrome consists of two phases. In the first, the presence of hypercortisolism is established to separate those with Cushing's syndrome from patients who may have certain clinical features that suggest the diagnosis but in whom glucocorticoid excess is not present. Once hypercortisolism is established, the challenge is to differentiate among the causes discussed above.

TABLE 69–4. INCIDENCE OF CLINICAL FEATURES OF CUSHING'S SYNDROME

FEATURE	PER CENT
Obesity	94
Facial plethora	84
Hirsutism	82
Menstrual disorders	76
Hypertension	72
Muscular weakness	58
Back pain	58
Striae	52
Acne	40
Psychological symptoms	40
Bruising	36
Congestive heart failure	22
Edema	18
Renal calculi	16
Headache	14
Polyuria/polydipsia	10
Hyperpigmentation	6

Modified from Plotz CM, et al: Am J Med 13:597, 1952, and Ross EJ, et al: Q J Med 35:149, 1966, and reprinted from Baxter JD, and Tyrrell JB: The adrenal cortex. In Felig P, Baxter JD, Broadus AE, and Frohman LA (eds): Endocrinology and Metabolism. New York, McGraw-Hill Book Co, 1981, p 472.

Does the patient have Cushing's syndrome? Although surreptitious administration of glucocorticoids may occur rarely, one is generally able to exclude an exogenous cause of Cushing's syndrome by the medical history. Endogenous Cushing's syndrome is relatively uncommon. In view of the severity of the untreated illness, the diagnosis should be considered in all patients who manifest typical clinical features. Since many of these abnormalities (e.g., obesity, hirsutism, hypertension, acne) occur in patients who do not have Cushing's syndrome, a reliable means of differentiating among such individuals is necessary.

Endogenous Cushing's syndrome is characterized by varying degrees of autonomous production of cortisol, resulting in an overall net increase in steroid production. Inasmuch as cortisol secretion is normally pulsatile, only distinctly elevated random measurements of plasma cortisol help in establishing the diagnosis. A more reliable index of the integrated plasma concentration can be obtained by demonstration of the loss of diurnal rhythm by comparing plasma cortisol levels in the early morning and late afternoon as well as by measurements of the 24-hour urinary excretion of cortisol. Measurement of a urinary metabolite of cortisol (such as 17-hydroxycorticoids) can also be performed, but values often overlap normal levels, limiting the usefulness of this procedure.

One of the most reliable means of detecting Cushing's syndrome is the overnight dexamethasone suppression test. Dexamethasone, 1 mg, is administered orally between 11:00 PM and midnight and the plasma cortisol is obtained at approximately 8:00 AM the following morning. A value of plasma cortisol of less than 5 μg/dl excludes the diagnosis of Cushing's syndrome. False-negative results are unusual. False-positive results can occur in patients with depression or other stressful situations and with ingestion of drugs such as phenytoin and estrogens. In patients in whom this screening test suggests the diagnosis of Cushing's syndrome, confirmation should be sought by other means, such as measurement of urinary free cortisol.

If Cushing's syndrome is present, what is its cause? Once the diagnosis of Cushing's syndrome is established, additional procedures are required to identify the underlying etiology (see Table 69–3). The high-dose dexamethasone suppression test should distinguish between patients with Cushing's disease and those with ectopic ACTH secretion or a primary adrenal neoplasm. In this test dexamethasone, 2 mg q6h, is administered orally for two consecutive days. Suppressibility of endogenous cortisol production is evaluated either by a plasma cortisol measurement at the end of this period or by measurement of urinary free cortisol or 17-hydroxycorticoid excretion on the second day of dexamethasone administration. Patients with Cushing's disease, in whom cortisol production is not entirely autonomous, will usually manifest a 50 per cent or greater suppression of cortisol levels in response to these large doses of dexamethasone. In contrast, cortisol production in patients with adrenal neoplasms or ectopic ACTH syndrome is usually more autonomous, so that little or no change in the cortisol level occurs during this procedure. Some patients with ectopic tumors, however, particularly those with a bronchial carcinoid or an adenoma, will undergo at least partial suppression and may appear therefore to have Cushing's disease. Also, some patients with Cushing's disease do not adequately suppress with dexamethasone. Despite these relatively uncommon exceptions, the high-dose dexamethasone suppression test remains one of the most reliable means of distinguishing among the causes of Cushing's syndrome.

Measurement of the plasma ACTH level, when available, is also helpful in differentiating among subtypes of Cushing's syndrome. Plasma ACTH levels are normal to only modestly increased in patients with Cushing's disease, are usually markedly elevated in those with ectopic ACTH secretion, and are generally undetectable in patients with primary adrenal neoplasms. Additional procedures that can help to localize the primary abnormality and to confirm the etiologic diagnosis include high-resolution contrast-enhanced CT scans of the pituitary and CT scans of the adrenal to localize a primary adrenal neoplasm. A normal CT scan of the pituitary fossa does not exclude an adenoma, however, since these tumors are frequently small and may be detected only at the time of surgery.

Treatment

Treatment of Cushing's syndrome depends on its cause. Pituitary microsurgery employing the transsphenoidal approach is now the treatment of choice for patients with suspected pituitary adenomas. In experienced hands an adenoma may be localized in some 90 per cent of patients and removed with a low morbidity. This approach has the advantage of preserving the surrounding pituitary tissue so that hypopituitarism is a rare complication. Pituitary irradiation using either conventional sources or heavy particle beams is also successful in many cases, but the incidence of hypopituitarism is higher than with transsphenoidal hypophysectomy. This may be an important consideration in women in the child-bearing years or in children who have not yet achieved adult height. Bilateral adrenalectomy, once performed commonly, is associated with a high incidence of subsequent enlargement of the pituitary neoplasm and hyperpigmentation (Nelson's syndrome) and should be reserved for patients who do not respond to the other approaches. Treatment of patients with primary adrenal neoplasms generally consists of surgical removal of the affected adrenal gland. Even those with carcinoma in whom cure is rare should have the tumor removed in an effort to control the hypercortisolism. Surgery is also recommended in patients with ectopic ACTH syndrome due to well localized ACTH-secreting tumors. In those with benign ACTH-secreting tumors such as bronchial carcinoid, pheochromocytoma, or thymoma, such an operation is frequently curative. In patients with ectopic malignancies that are already metastatic as well as in those who have inoperable adrenal carcinoma, medical inhibition of adrenal cortisol secretion by drugs such as mitotane, aminoglutethimide, and metyrapone, may be helpful.

PRIMARY ALDOSTERONISM

Pathophysiology

Hypersecretion of aldosterone can occur as a primary adrenal disorder or in response to increased stimulation by the renin-angiotensin system or ACTH. Primary aldosteronism is an adrenal disorder characterized by autonomous production of mineralocorticoid hormone (Fig. 69–5). Secondary aldosteronism results from the overstimulation of an otherwise normal adrenal gland by the renin-angiotensin system. The latter disorders are pathophysiologically and clinically distinct from primary aldosteronism and will be considered in a separate section.

Primary overproduction of aldosterone results in increased sodium reabsorption in the distal nephron. As a consequence, the extracellular fluid volume is expanded until approximately 1.5 to 2.5 kg of excess fluid has been retained. At this point, proximal tubular sodium reabsorption becomes markedly reduced. The resultant increased delivery of sodium to the distal tubule overwhelms the increased capacity for distal sodium reabsorption so that a new steady state of sodium balance is achieved. This phenomenon is referred to as "mineralocorticoid escape." Further expansion of extracellular fluid volume does not occur despite continued hypersecretion of mineralocorticoid hormone. Affected subjects actually excrete an administered sodium load more rapidly than

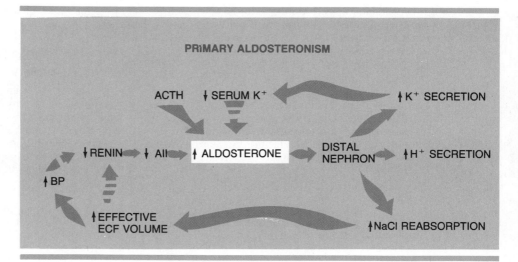

FIGURE 69–5. Pertubations of the renin-angiotensin-aldosterone system in primary aldosteronism. The dashed arrows indicate diminished stimulation of aldosterone secretion (as a consequence of hypokalemia) and of renin secretion (as a consequence of increased effective ECF volume).

do normals. Two of the cardinal findings of the syndrome of primary aldosteronism, hypertension and suppressed plasma renin activity, probably result from this expansion of extracellular fluid volume.

The mineralocorticoid hormone-enhanced sodium reabsorption in the distal tubule and collecting duct results in increased secretion of potassium and hydrogen ion in these portions of the nephron. Even when the renal escape mechanism allows a new steady state of sodium balance to develop, mineralocorticoid-dependent potassium secretion and hydrogen ion secretion continue. The increased delivery of sodium to the distal nephron may actually augment the potassium secretion.

In the syndrome of primary aldosteronism, autonomous overproduction of aldosterone by the adrenal gland can be due to a benign adenoma, a carcinoma, or diffuse bilateral nodular hyperplasia, with adenomas accounting for 75 to 85 per cent of cases. Less than 1 per cent are due to a functioning carcinoma, and the remaining 15 to 25 per cent result from bilateral hyperplasia. The extremely rare cases of so-called glucocorticoid-remediable hyperaldosteronism are believed to result from excessive stimulation of the adrenal cortex by ACTH. The patterns of mineralocorticoid secretion and the degree of autonomy from the renin-angiotensin system vary between the different entities.

Clinical Manifestations

The major clinical manifestation of primary aldosteronism is that of hypertension. In addition, hypernatremia, hypokalemia, and metabolic alkalosis are characteristically found. A dilute urine may be present because hypokalemia impairs the renal concentrating mechanism. Most presenting symptoms relate to hypokalemia, with a presence and severity that depend on the degree of potassium depletion. Mildly hypokalemic patients complain of muscle weakness, polyuria (especially nocturia), polydipsia, and paresthesias. Pa-

tients with more severe hypokalemia experience intermittent paralysis of the legs and arms or even tetany. Patients with marked hypokalemia sometimes experience autonomic dysfunction with orthostatic hypotension occurring without reflex tachycardia.

Diagnosis and Treatment

Recognition of primary aldosteronism, usually during evaluation of hypertension, is important because it is a potentially curable form of hypertension. Less than 1 per cent of unselected hypertensive patients have this disorder, which is found in women more often than in men by a 2:1 margin. The patients are usually between 30 and 50 years of age.

Hyperaldosteronism can be documented by showing an increased secretion rate, an increased excretion rate, or an elevated plasma concentration of the hormone. Single measurements of plasma aldosterone concentration may be misleading because even patients with markedly increased secretion rates show diurnal variations in plasma levels that can obscure recognition of hyperaldosteronism. The measurement of the 24-hour urinary excretion of the 18-glucuronide metabolite of aldosterone has been shown to reflect aldosterone production accurately. The urine should be collected while the patient consumes a normal sodium intake (120 to 180 mEq/day).

Demonstration of suppressed and nonstimulable plasma renin activity in a patient with elevated plasma or urinary aldosterone levels establishes the diagnosis of primary aldosteronism. Autonomy of aldosterone production can be confirmed by demonstrating failure of suppression of the hormone levels by maneuvers that normally suppress the renin-angiotensin-aldosterone system, such as administration of mineralocorticoid hormones (DOCA, fludrocortisone) or intravenous infusion of normal saline.

The principal reason for attempting to differentiate between aldosterone-producing adenoma and bilateral hyperplasia is to select the most appropriate therapy. Unilateral adrenalectomy cures approximately 70 per cent of cases due to an adenoma, whereas even bilateral adrenalectomy in most cases of hyperplasia does not ameliorate the hypertension. Several biochemical determinations have been proposed to differentiate adenoma from hyperplasia. Patients with an adenoma generally have lower plasma renin activity values and plasma potassium concentrations with higher basal plasma aldosterone concentrations than patients with hyperplasia. Plasma aldosterone levels in patients with adenoma fail to increase with upright posture, in contrast to a two- to three-fold increase in those with hyperplasia. Specific techniques for localizing an adenoma (iodocholesterol scan, CT scan, adrenal venous catheterization) also aid in differentiating those with tumor from those with bilateral hyperplasia.

ADRENAL ENZYME DEFECTS

Genetically transmitted deficiencies of the enzymes required for adrenal steroid biosynthesis lead to distinct clinical syndromes of disturbed mineralocorticoid production. In two such enzyme deficiency states, 11β- and 17α-hydroxylase deficiency, impaired cortisol production results in increased ACTH secretion and secondary increased production of DOC, which produces a typical syndrome of mineralocorticoid excess. In 11β-hydroxylase deficiency, conversion of DOC to corticosterone and its derivatives is impaired, and thus corticosterone, 18-hydroxycorticosterone, and/or aldosterone may be deficient. In 17α-hydroxylase deficiency, conversion of DOC to its derivatives is not enzymatically blocked; hence corticosterone levels are markedly elevated and may contribute to the hypermineralocorticoid state. Despite the intact enzymatic pathway to aldosterone, aldosterone production is generally subnormal, presumably as a consequence of the reduced plasma renin activity and the hypokalemia that occur due to the hypermineralocorticoid state.

These two syndromes may be readily distinguished clinically by their different effects on sexual development. In the 17α-hydroxylase deficiency syndrome, biosynthesis of adrenal and gonadal androgen and estrogen is impaired, inhibiting normal sexual maturation. Genotypic female patients fail to undergo menarchy or to develop secondary sexual characteristics. Genotypic male patients become pseudohermaphrodites as a consequence of androgen deficiency in utero. In the 11β-hydroxylase deficiency syndrome, the enzymatic steps required for the synthesis of adrenal sex steroids are unimpaired. The increased ACTH level stimulates increased production of adrenal androgen, frequently causing virilism. In both syndromes, glucocorticoid hormone replacement therapy inhibits both ACTH secretion and the resultant excess mineralocorticoid production and therefore ameliorates the hypermineralocorticoid state. In treated patients with the 11β-hydroxylase deficiency syndrome, androgen production diminishes and signs of virilization tend to disappear.

SECONDARY ALDOSTERONISM (Table 69–3)

Increased aldosterone secretion occurs as a physiological response to reduced effective arterial blood volume owing to activation of the renin-angiotensin system. The resultant increase in plasma aldosterone concentration stimulates renal tubular reabsorption of Na^+ and Cl^- and thereby tends to restore normal "effective" blood volume. When hypovolemia is of extrarenal origin (vomiting, diarrhea, and hemorrhage) and renal tubular reabsorption of Na^+ and Cl^- is not specifically impaired, the Na^+-retaining effect of hypermineralocorticoidism is manifested by reduced urinary excretion rates of Na^+ that persist until effective arterial blood volume is restored. Provision of adequate amounts of dietary NaCl may normalize the effective arterial blood volume. The Na^+-retaining effect of hypermineralocorticoidism does not reduce excretion rates of Na^+ when hypovolemia is caused predominantly by impaired renal tubular reabsorption of Na^+ and Cl^- (e.g., diuretic administration, Bartter's syndrome, and some types of renal tubular acidosis). When the reduction in effective arterial blood volume is due to congestive heart failure, cirrhosis, or the nephrotic syndrome, provision of dietary NaCl leads to progressive expansion of extracellular fluid volume and edema without restoration of effective blood volume.

Hyperaldosteronism secondary to activation of the renin-angiotensin system also occurs in patients with accelerated hypertension, renovascular or segmental renal lesions, and, rarely, renin-secreting neoplasms. Activation of the renin-angiotensin-aldosterone system in the absence of hypovolemia results in hypertension.

The exact contribution of excess mineralocorticoid production to the pathophysiology observed in states of secondary hyperaldosteronism is not always clear. Hypertension persists despite adrenalectomy in patients with a renin-secreting tumor and in animals with experimental renovascular hypertension. Reduction of Na^+ excretion and edema formation can occur in patients with cardiac, renal, or hepatic disease without increased aldosterone secretion. Potassium wasting persists despite sustained correction of secondary hyperaldosteronism in some patients with type 1 renal tubular acidosis and in some patients with Bartter's syndrome. In these disorders, it seems likely that the secondary aldosteronism serves to amplify the consequences of the primary defect causing renal potassium wasting.

ADRENAL MEDULLARY HYPERFUNCTION

The adrenal medulla synthesizes and releases biologically active amines derived from the amino acid tyrosine. Norepinephrine, the major product of this biosynthetic pathway, is also synthesized in the central nervous system and sympathetic postganglionic neurons, whereas epinephrine originates nearly entirely from the adrenal gland. A third catecholamine, dopamine, which acts as a neurotransmitter in the central nervous system, has a less clearly defined role as a circulating hormone, although recent studies suggest that dopamine may normally inhibit aldosterone secretion.

Catecholamines have a variety of potent hemodynamic and metabolic effects depending upon their relative abilities to serve as agonists for the alpha- and beta-adrenergic receptors. Epinephrine acts chiefly on beta receptors, having a positive chronotropic and inotropic effect on the heart and producing vasodilatation in most vascular beds. Epinephrine also increases plasma glucose concentration by inhibiting insulin secretion and stimulating glycogenolysis in the liver. Epinephrine is released from the medulla in response to a variety of stresses, including hypoglycemia. Norepinephrine has predominant alpha-agonist effects, causing vasoconstriction with relatively little metabolic action. Inasmuch as norepinephrine is secreted widely throughout the sympathetic nervous system, the contribution by the adrenal medulla is relatively small. Bilateral adrenalectomy results in little if any measurable change in the levels of norepinephrine, although epinephrine levels are markedly reduced. Thus, adrenal medullary hypofunction has little or no physiological impact, whereas hypersecretion of catecholamines produces a dramatic clinical syndrome, namely pheochromocytoma.

PHEOCHROMOCYTOMA

Pathophysiology

Pheochromocytoma, an uncommon but important tumor, arises from chromaffin cells and can occur in any sympathetic ganglion in the body. More than 90 per cent of such tumors, however, arise from the adrenal medulla. The majority of extra-adrenal pheochromocytomas are associated with sympathetic ganglia in the mediastinum or abdomen. Bilateral adrenal pheochromocytomas or multiple tumors may be present in 5 to 10 per cent of cases. Such patients may also have medullary carcinoma of the thyroid and other manifestations of the multiple endocrine neoplasia syndrome, type 2 (Sipple's syndrome). Pheochromocytoma should always be considered in patients with this syndrome, in which there is also a familial tendency to develop tumors of the C cells of the thyroid (medullary carcinoma) and of the parathyroid glands.

Clinical Manifestations

The clinical manifestations of pheochromocytoma depend upon the predominant catecholamine secreted by the tumor. Since the vast majority of tumors secrete norepinephrine as the principal product, hypertension is one of the most common findings. Superimposed on sustained hypertension are classic paroxysms in which a sudden release of catecholamines results in exacerbation of hypertension, accompanied by palpitation, headache, pallor, sweating, flushing, and anxiety. Such attacks can be provoked by ingestion of tyramine-containing foods, particularly in patients taking monoamine oxidase inhibitors. Occasionally, patients with pheochromocytoma may not exhibit hypertension at all and in fact may become hypotensive during paroxysms. Such patients usually have epinephrine-secreting tumors or tumors whose principal product is dopamine. Orthostatic hypotension is common in patients with pheochromocytoma even in those who have sustained supine hypertension.

Diagnosis and Treatment

The diagnosis of pheochromocytoma can be difficult, since the symptoms are relatively nonspecific, often resembling those of simple anxiety. In addition, because secretion may be episodic in some patients, plasma and urinary levels of catecholamines may be intermittently normal. The diagnosis should be established on biochemical grounds by demonstrating increased plasma levels or urinary excretion of catecholamines or their major metabolites, the metanephrines and vanillylmandelic acid (VMA). Of these, urinary metanephrines are said to be the most sensitive index, although all of the major metabolites are usually elevated in patients with an actively secreting tumor. Since the enzyme required for conversion of norepinephrine to epinephrine is only present in the adrenal medulla and organ of Zuckerkandl, norepinephrine is the sole product of tumors arising in sympathetic ganglia outside of these sites. In addition, norepinephrine is the major secretory product of adrenal pheochromocytoma. Plasma measurements of catecholamines are being used with greater frequency in the diagnosis of pheochromocytoma, but meticulous attention must be given to the technique of specimen collection and caution must be exercised in interpreting borderline elevated levels in stressed individuals. Administration of clonidine, which suppresses catecholamine levels in normal subjects, fails to do so in patients with pheochromocytoma, suggesting a promising future as a means of evaluating patients with only borderline biochemical abnormalities.

Pharmacologic tests using blood pressure responses to detect the presence of pheochromocytoma are dangerous and have little place in current diagnosis. Occasionally it may be reasonable to attempt to provoke secretion of catecholamines once the patient has received adequate amounts of adrenergic blockade to prevent a hypertensive crisis. Glucagon, 1 mg intravenously, will provoke marked increases in catecholamine levels and may be useful in confirming the diagnosis or in evaluating the adequacy of alpha-adrenergic blockade preoperatively.

Pheochromocytomas, particularly those arising from the adrenal medulla, are usually several centimeters in diameter by the time symptoms develop and can be readily visualized on abdominal CT scans. In the absence of an obvious adrenal tumor, localization of the tumor in the sympathetic ganglia may be difficult. Catheterization of the inferior vena cava with sampling of multiple sites for catecholamine measurements may help to localize the tumor preoperatively. Recently, an isotope scan technique utilizing ^{131}I-metaiodo-benzylguanidine has been demonstrated to localize small neoplasms effectively. The possibility of multiple pheochromocytomas should be considered, particularly in patients with family histories of other endocrine neoplasms.

The treatment of pheochromocytoma is surgical if the lesion can be located and removed. Preoperative adrenergic blockade has markedly improved the once formidable surgical morbidity and mortality. Alpha blockade using either phenoxybenzamine, dibenzyline, or prazosin in sufficient doses and for a sufficient period of time to prevent episodes of hypertension and to allow expansion of the effective extracellular fluid volume is the mainstay of therapy in patients with norepinephrine-secreting lesions. Beta-adrenergic blockade may also be useful, particularly in those who develop tachycardia on alpha blockers. Careful preoperative planning among an experienced anesthesiologist, an endocrinologist, and a surgeon usually assures a good outcome.

In patients with inoperable tumors or with metastatic pheochromocytoma, pharmacologic therapy may be continued on a chronic basis. In addition, alpha-methyltyrosine has been shown to be of some benefit in reducing catecholamine secretion by the neoplastic tissue.

REFERENCES

Biglieri EG, and Baxter JD: The endocrinology of hypertension. In Felig P, Baxter JD, Broadus A, and Frohman L (eds): Endocrinology and Metabolism. New York, McGraw-Hill Book Co, 1981, pp 551–598.

Crapo L: Cushing's syndrome: A review of diagnostic tests. Metabolism 28:955–977, 1979.

DeFronzo RA: Hyperkalemia and hyporeninemic hypoaldosteronism. Kidney Int 17:118–134, 1980.

Engleman K: Pheochromocytoma. In Landsberg L (ed): Clinics in Endocrinology and Metabolism—Catecholamines. Philadelphia, WB Saunders Co, 1977, Vol 6, p 767.

Gold EM: The Cushing syndromes: Changing views of diagnosis and treatment. Ann Intern Med 90:829–844, 1979.

Schambelan M, Sebastian A, and Biglieri EG: Prevalence, pathogenesis, and functional significance of aldosterone deficiency in hyperkalemic patients with chronic renal insufficiency. Kidney Int 17:89–101, 1980.

Tyrrell JB, and Baxter JD: Disorders of the adrenal cortex. In Wyngaarden JB, and Smith LH Jr (eds): Cecil Textbook of Medicine. 17th ed. Philadelphia, WB Saunders Co, 1985, pp 1300–1320.

70 FEMALE ENDOCRINOLOGY

The adult ovaries measure approximately 4 × 3 × 1 cm. Each ovary is attached to the lateral pelvic wall and to the uterus by the ovarian ligament. The follicle in its different stages of maturation is the critical structural and functional component of the ovary. Both steroidogenesis and gametogenesis depend on the follicle complex. The primary components of the follicle are the oocyte, granulosa cells, and interstitial cells (theca cells) (Fig. 70–1).

SEXUAL DEVELOPMENT AND DIFFERENTIATION

Normal sexual development and differentiation depend on a full complex of sex and autosomal chromosomes. The genital ridge develops at approximately three weeks' gestation. Subsequently germ cells migrate to the genital ridge from the yolk sac. Undifferentiated gonads consisting of both müllerian and wolffian ducts are present by six weeks' gestation. Differentiation of the female gonad proceeds in the absence of müllerian-inhibiting factor and androgens, facilitating the development of female ducts and the regression of male ducts. Appropriate female genitalia develop consequent to the lack of androgen secretion. The genes determining ovarian formation have not been identified.

Normal ovarian function requires the integrated action of the hypothalamic-pituitary-ovarian axis (Fig. 70–2). Follicular growth, steroid hormone production (secretion), ovulation, and atresia are gonadotropin-dependent (follicle stimulating hormone, FSH; luteinizing hormone, LH). Subsequent to synthesis (Fig. 70–3) and secretion, ovarian sex steroid hormones (estrogens, androgens, progestins) mediate their effects locally on the ovary and the genital tract (uterus, cervix, and vagina) and systemically to coordinate functions of the hypothalamic-pituitary complex. Measurement of serum estradiol, progesterone, FSH, and LH levels with specific radioimmunoassays provides accurate information on the integrity of the hypothalamic-pituitary-ovarian axis in health and disease. In addition, the biological activity of the sex steroids on target organs can be reliably evaluated by analyzing cellular morphology and mucus characteristics. Estrogens increase the quantity, viscosity, and elasticity ("spinnbarkeit") of the cervical mucus as well as the ten-

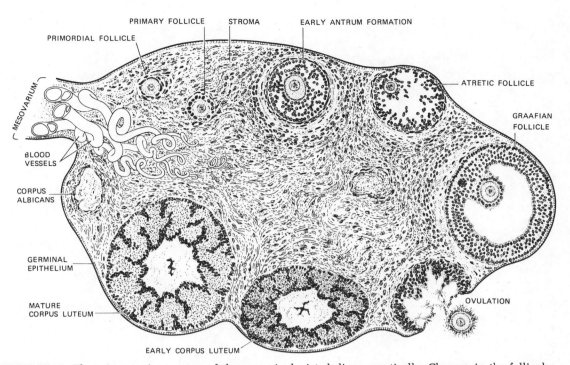

FIGURE 70–1. The microscopic anatomy of the ovary is depicted diagrammatically. Changes in the follicular complex occurring during atresia and ovulation are shown progressively clockwise from primordial follicle (upper left) to a corpus albicans (lower left). (Modified from Ross GT, and Schreiber JR: The ovary. In Yen SSC, and Jaffe RB (eds): Reproductive Endocrinology: Physiology, Pathophysiology and Clinical Management. Philadelphia, WB Saunders Co, 1978, p 64.)

dency of the electrolytes to crystallize in a "ferning" pattern. Progesterone inhibits these changes in mucus.

ABNORMAL SEXUAL DIFFERENTIATION

Chromosomal

Turner's syndrome, the most common disorder of gonadal differentiation in the female, results from a 45XO chromosomal abnormality. It has an incidence of 1 in 3000 newborn females. These patients have nonfunctioning streak gonads (gonadal dysgenesis) and unambiguous female external genitalia and internal ducts and may exhibit many or all of the following abnormalities: sexual infantilism, short stature, musculoskeletal abnormalities (webbed neck, low hairline, shield chest, cubitus valgus, short digits), hypertension, coarctation of the aorta, renal disorders, and deafness. Patients with a mosaic karyotype present fewer stigmata, and gonadal function may be normal. The short stature can be treated with anabolic steroids between 10 and 14 years. Feminization can be induced with estrogen replacement.

Enzymatic

Pseudohermaphodites are females with a normal 46XX karyotype and internal sexual organs but masculinized external genitalia (male phenotype) due to excess androgens. The extent of the virilization and the degree of ambiguity in genital development depend on the timing and severity of the androgen exposure. The most common cause of female pseudohermaphroditism is *congenital adrenal hyperplasia* (CAH). This syndrome has a wide spectrum of clinical presentations due to the variable involvement of specific enzymes necessary for cortisol synthesis by the adrenal cortex (Fig. 70–3). This syndrome complex is inherited in an autosomal recessive manner and expresses itself only in the homozygous offspring. It has a prevalence of 1 per 60,000 births. The cortisol deficiency results in increased ACTH secretion and consequent adrenal hyperplasia. The most frequent lesion involves a deficiency of 21-hydroxylase. The hyperplastic glands secrete androgens in excess, which masculinize the female fetus. Furthermore, the excess secretion of 17-hydroxyprogesterone causes salt wasting. In the 11-hydroxylase form, masculinization also occurs, but salt retention and hypertension develop because of the excess production of 11-deoxycorticosterone. Congenital adrenal hyperplasia can be successfully treated with a glucocorticoid (hydrocortisone); this is supplemented with a mineralocorticoid (deoxycorticosterone acetate) in the salt-wasting form of the syndrome. Surgical correction of the external genitalia should be performed before the age of three years.

PUBERTY

The adolescent or pubescent phase of development provides the individual with reproduc-

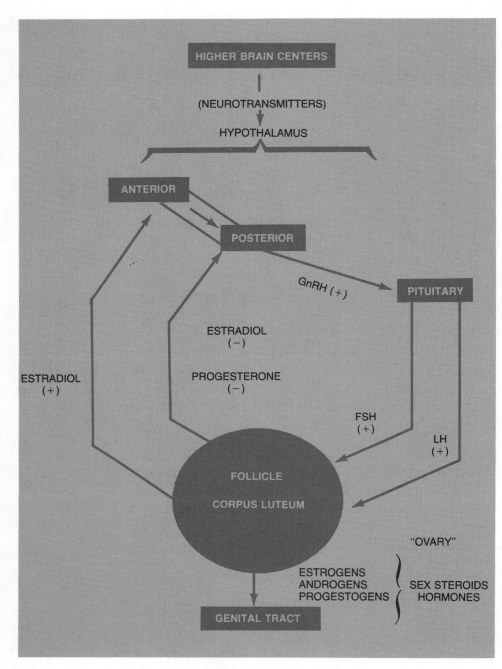

FIGURE 70–2. Hypothalamic-pituitary-ovarian axis. Gonadotropin-releasing hormone (GnRH) stimulates the pituitary gland to synthesize and secrete the gonadotropins FSH (follicle-stimulating hormone) and LH (luteinizing hormone). These hormones stimulate sequential ovarian follicle development and differentiation. The sex steroid hormones secreted by the ovary regulate genital tract changes and modulate hypothalamic GnRH secretion.

tive capacity. In the female characteristically somatic growth accelerates, the breasts develop (thelarche), pubic hair appears (pubarche), and finally the menarche occurs. This process generally begins between 8 and 14 years of age with full development over a three-year period. The order of appearance of pubertal features varies greatly.

The age of onset of puberty is variable and influenced by genetic factors, socioeconomic conditions, and general health. Prepubertal girls have low serum levels of gonadotropins and sex steroid hormones. During the progression of puberty the characteristic inhibitory effect of estrogens on gonadotropin (FSH, LH) secretion declines and in the case of LH a positive feedback process develops (see Fig. 70–2). An early feature of the pu-

bescent girl is the nocturnal pulsatile secretion of LH. Enhanced LH activity stimulates the ovary to secrete increasing amounts of estrogens, and secondary sex characteristics subsequently develop.

PRECOCIOUS PUBERTY

Isosexual precocious puberty relates to the premature (less than age eight years) development of adult genitalia consistent with the chromosomal sex of the child. In girls the majority of cases (80 per cent) are idiopathic, with both gonadotropins (FSH and LH) and sex steroid hormones (estradiol and progesterone) in the normal adult range. Isosexual precocious puberty also occurs in the McCune-Albright syndrome (polyostotic fibrous

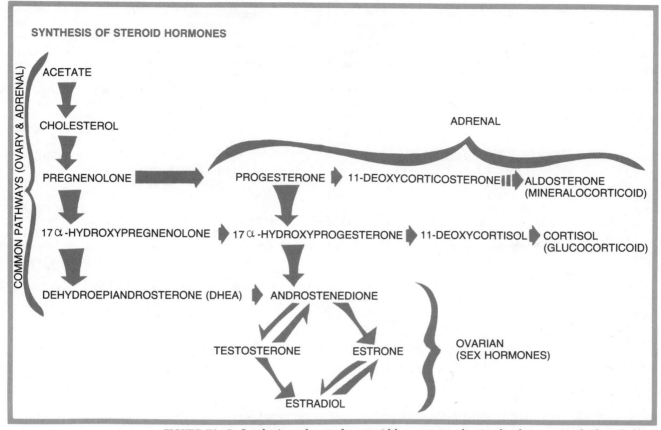

FIGURE 70–3. Synthetic pathways for steroid hormone production by the ovary and adrenal gland.

dysplasia). High gonadotropin levels should suggest an intracranial lesion or a human chorionic gonadotropin (HCG) secreting tumor. Hypothyroidism can also be associated with precocious puberty due to increased secretion of gonadotropins. Precocious puberty associated with low levels of gonadotropins should suggest an ovarian or adrenal tumor. Adrenal tumors generally secrete large amounts of steroids that can be detected as urinary 17-ketosteroids. Ovarian tumors can usually be detected on physical examination.

In heterosexual precocious puberty, pubertal changes occur that are consistent with the opposite sex of the child. This occurs most frequently in congenital adrenal hyperplasia (CAH) or due to androgen-secreting tumors of the adrenal cortex or ovary. High serum levels of 17-hydroxyprogesterone are typically found in congenital adrenal hyperplasia.

Treatment. Gonadal and adrenocortical tumors should be removed surgically. Intracranial tumors may be treated surgically, by radiation, and/or by chemotherapy. The progression of idiopathic precocious puberty can be delayed by medical intervention. This avoids psychosocial problems in the young child and may avoid premature closure of the epiphyses with permanent short stature. Depomedroxyprogesterone acetate (200 to 300 mg IM weekly) will stop breast development and menstruation. However, adult short stature may

remain a problem. Analogues of GnRH will also effectively stop the progression of precocious puberty. Currently this approach is not standard practice owing to the lack of availability of these preparations. Patients with congenital adrenal hyperplasia must receive replacement therapy with a glucocorticoid preparation.

Incomplete Sexual Precocity

Isolated premature breast development (thelarche) and pubic hair growth (pubarche or adrenarche) are benign conditions that rarely warrant specific therapy. Bone age may be slightly advanced in association with either of these forms of incomplete precocious puberty.

DELAYED PUBERTY

Girls who have not displayed breast growth by age 14 years are considered delayed developers. The majority of these cases are constitutional and will eventually undergo puberty spontaneously. Understandably these delays create psychological problems and parental anxiety. Thus reassurance can only be provided once other lesions have been excluded. Delayed puberty is also associated with nutritional disorders such as anorexia nervosa, chronic systemic illnesses (especially those involving the gastrointestinal tract), and hypothyroidism. Rarely, delayed puberty is due to hypogonadotropic hypogonadism (hypothalamic-pituitary disorders) or primary gonadal failure (gonadal dysgenesis), with increased levels of gonadotropins. If indicated, secondary sexual characteristics can be induced with estrogens (e.g., ethinylestradiol 20 μg P.O. daily) over a six-month period. Spontaneous progression of puberty frequently develops during or subsequent to therapy.

MENSTRUAL CYCLE

The onset of menarche (initiation of regular menstrual cycles) indicates the completion of normal sexual development. Menarche occurs at a mean age of 12.6 years, with a standard deviation of 1.2 years. The current age range of menarche in the United States is 9 to 16 years. Early (<9 years) and delayed (>16 years) menarche warrants evaluation.

The menstrual cycle is conveniently divided into three phases—the follicular, the ovulatory, and the luteal phases (Fig. 70–4). Menstruation conventionally marks the beginning of a new cycle. Plasma FSH increases at the completion of the luteal phase of the previous cycle and initiates maturation of the follicle. During this phase the developing follicle secretes increasing amounts of estradiol, reaching a peak secretion about 12 hours before the LH ovulatory surge. This sudden increase in estradiol triggers the LH/FSH spike through a positive feedback process on the anterior hypothalamus. The mid-cycle surge in gonadotropins induces ovulation. Following ovulation the ruptured follicle is transformed into the corpus luteum (see Fig. 70–1). A rapid decrease in serum estradiol and increase in serum progesterone occur during the early part of the luteal phase. Subsequently the developing corpus luteum secretes increasing amounts of progesterone and estradiol and serum levels peak at about seven days postovulation. The corpus luteum then regresses, with a consequent decrease in

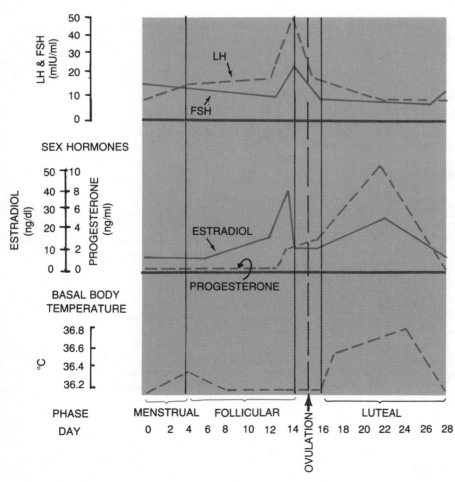

FIGURE 70–4. Normal menstrual cycle. The sequential changes that occur in serum gonadotropins (LH and FSH), estradiol, and progesterone during the various phases of the cycle are outlined. Day 0 correlates to the first day of menstruation. A typical basal body temperature chart is also depicted.

serum hormone levels. At day 28 of the cycle, serum estradiol and progesterone are at their nadir, menstruation occurs, and a new cycle begins.

THE PREMENSTRUAL SYNDROME

This common clinical entity affects about 70 per cent of women. Many women will experience some of the following symptoms before menses—bloating and weight gain, emotional lability, headaches (migraine), breast congestion, acne, and arthralgias. For most women these symptoms are merely a nuisance; about 20 per cent of patients, however, may experience severe problems from the time of ovulation to menstruation such that normal daily activities may be interrupted.

The cause of the premenstrual syndrome is not understood. Water retention, estrogen excess, and possibly central nervous system dopamine deficiency have been postulated as pathogenetic factors. These patients should be advised to restrict salt intake and exercise regularly to decrease fluid retention. Women with severe symptoms may benefit from diuretic therapy during the second half of the menstrual cycle. Oral pyridoxine (500 mg orally daily) may be effective in some patients with a severe premenstrual syndrome. Pyridoxine is a cofactor in dopamine synthesis.

AMENORRHEA

Absence of menses for three months or longer defines amenorrhea. Failure of menarche to occur during adolescent development is primary amenorrhea, whereas the discontinuation of menses after the onset of menarche is secondary amenorrhea. Physiological amenorrhea occurs during pregnancy and after menopause. Approximately 5 per cent of women suffer from nonphysiological amenorrhea.

Primary Amenorrhea

Primary amenorrhea always calls for a detailed history and physical examination. It may occur in association with normal, decreased, or increased sex steroid hormone production (Table 70–1). Women with normal secondary sex characteristics may have an abnormality of the outflow tract (vaginal aplasia or imperforate hymen) and retain the menstrual effluent. This may lead to endometriosis and cyclic abdominal pain but absent menstruation.

Incorrect gender assignment to genetic males (male pseudohermaphroditism) in the neonatal period accounts for about 50 per cent of cases of primary amenorrhea. The phenotypic females develop consequent to deficient testosterone synthesis and various androgen-resistant syndromes.

A spectrum of sexual immaturity may occur consequent to hypofunction of the hypothalamic-pituitary complex (hypogonadotropic hypogonadism). Secondary sexual characteristics do not develop and menses do not occur. Kallman's syndrome is a familial disorder characterized by an-

TABLE 70–1. CAUSES OF PRIMARY AMENORRHEA

1. Normal Sex Hormone Production
      Müllerian dysgenesis
      Amenorrhea traumatica
2. Decreased Sex Hormone Production
      Male pseudohermaphroditism due to an absolute or relative deficiency of testosterone
          Enzymatic defect in synthesis
          Impaired activation (5α-reductase deficiency)
          Androgen resistant states
      Gonadal dysgenesis (Turner's syndrome)
      Hypothalamic-pituitary disease
          Familial hypogonadotropic hypogonadism (Kallman's syndrome)
          Pituitary and parapituitary tumors
          Anorexia nervosa
      Systemic diseases
3. Increased Sex Hormone Production
      Congenital adrenal hyperplasia
      Polycystic ovarian disease (Stein-Leventhal syndrome)
      Androgen-secreting ovarian and adrenal tumors

osmia or hyposmia, various midline defects (hair lip, cleft palate) and sexual immaturity due to low gonadotropin levels. Acquired forms may result from pituitary tumors, craniopharyngiomas and other parapituitary lesions. Psychogenic and stressful systemic disorders may also interfere with hypothalamic-pituitary function and delay sexual maturation and menarche.

A relatively common cause of primary amenorrhea without secondary sexual characteristics is gonadal dysgenesis (Turner's syndrome). This syndrome, characterized by streak gonads, elevated serum gonadotropin levels, short stature, and various other abnormalities, was described earlier.

Congenital adrenal hyperplasia (adrenogenital syndrome) may cause primary amenorrhea if not detected and treated. Mild forms with minimal genital ambiguity are often not detected until puberty. These patients are usually of short stature owing to androgen-induced premature closure of epiphyses. Primary amenorrhea can rarely be associated with polycystic ovaries or with androgen-secreting tumors.

Secondary Amenorrhea

Secondary amenorrhea is not a disease entity but a signal that function has been compromised at some level in the hypothalamic-pituitary-ovarian-uterine axis. Absence of menses for three to six months in a previously normally menstruating woman establishes the diagnosis of secondary amenorrhea. The most common cause of secondary amenorrhea is pregnancy. Thus such a patient should be considered pregnant until proven otherwise with a sensitive pregnancy test.

Secondary amenorrhea also occurs in association with normal, decreased, or increased sex steroid hormone production (Table 70–2). Amenorrhea associated with normal cyclic changes in the secretion of ovarian steroid hormones is a frequent finding in women with damaged endometrium. This may occur consequent to repeated uterine curettage following delivery or abortion or

TABLE 70–2. CAUSES OF SECONDARY AMENORRHEA

1. Normal Sex Hormone Production
    Amenorrhea traumatica
        Postinfectious
        Postoperative
2. Decreased Sex Hormone Production
    A. Primary ovarian failure (high serum gonadotropins)
        Postsurgery, irradiation, chemotherapy, or toxins
        Autoimmune premature ovarian failure
        Gonadal dysgenesis
    B. Secondary ovarian failure (low serum gonadotropins)
        Hypothalamic-pituitary dysfunction
        Postsurgery, irradiation, infection, infarction
        Pituitary tumor with normal prolactin
        Empty sella syndrome
        Pituitary tumor with hyperprolactinemia
        Postpartum or postpill amenorrhea
        Psychogenic
        Anorexia nervosa
        Endocrine disorders—thyroid, adrenal, diabetes
        Systemic disorders
3. Increased Sex Hormone Production
    A. Polycystic ovarian disease
    B. Androgen-secreting ovarian or adrenal tumor

following infection (e.g., tuberculosis). Surgical or medical correction of these lesions generally leads to a resumption of menses.

Primary ovarian failure may develop following abdominal irradiation, chemotherapy, or surgery. However, premature ovarian failure probably occurs most commonly secondary to autoimmune injury. Serum gonadotropin levels are high. Destructive lesions of the hypothalamus and pituitary, such as surgery, irradiation, chemotherapy, infection, infarction, or tumor, may result in secondary ovarian failure. Pituitary tumors secreting prolactin account for about 30 per cent of cases with secondary amenorrhea. Most of these lesions can be detected by CT scanning. These patients have high serum prolactin levels and low serum levels of gonadotropins. Many cases of secondary amenorrhea are due to hypothalamic-pituitary dysfunction resulting from severe emotional stress or systemic disease. Thus amenorrhea may occur in association with anorexia nervosa, intensive exercise, endocrine disease (thyroid, adrenal, diabetes), and medications (postpill amenorrhea). Ovarian tumors may produce excess sex steroids (androgens), which suppress gonadotropins and cause amenorrhea. A frequent cause of secondary amenorrhea consequent to increased ovarian production of androgens (androstenedione) is polycystic ovaries (Stein-Leventhal syndrome). An elevated LH/FSH ratio is very characteristic of this disorder. The etiology of polycystic ovaries is not known in most cases, although recent data suggest it may be hypothalamic in origin. These patients present with amenorrhea (anovulation), hirsutism, obesity, and bilaterally enlarged ovaries.

DIAGNOSIS AND TREATMENT

In a patient with amenorrhea the physician should first exclude pregnancy, pituitary tumor, and premature menopause. Pregnancy can be easily detected by measuring the serum level of the beta subunit of human chorionic gonadotropin. A normal serum FSH level rules out premature menopause. Pituitary microadenoma can generally be detected by sella turcica CT scanning. A positive finding in conjunction with high serum prolactin and low gonadotropin levels documents the presence of a pituitary tumor (see Chapter 67). Additional studies should focus on specific disorders of the central nervous system, thyroid, adrenal, pancreas (diabetes), ovary, uterus, and vagina.

In the absence of clinically detectable disease, very valuable information concerning the cause of amenorrhea can be obtained by proceeding through the following diagnostic steps. In most cases the need for expensive laboratory tests can be avoided.

A normal estrogen effect (sex steroid hormone production) can generally be deduced from a healthy vaginal mucosa and copious amounts of clear cervical mucus. A progesterone withdrawal (medroxyprogesterone acetate 10 mg daily for five days) screening test may be performed to test the integrity of the reproductive axis. Menstrual bleeding following this short course of progesterone indicates that the axis is functional and that the amenorrhea most likely is due to anovulation. If bleeding does not occur, a course of conjugated estrogens (Premarin 1.25 mg daily for 21 days) should be administered and followed by the progesterone withdrawal test. Failure to bleed following this regimen indicates target organ (endometrium) or outflow tract failure. The patient should be referred to a gynecologist for further investigations. A positive withdrawal test should be followed by measurement of gonadotropins and prolactin levels. High gonadotropin levels are consistent with primary ovarian disease, whereas low values indicate hypothalamic-pituitary dysfunction or failure. Individuals with high levels should have a karyotype performed to detect Turner's syndrome (XO) or male pseudohermaphroditism (female phenotype).

The approach to therapy for each specific cause of amenorrhea should be dictated by the lesion and the patient's wishes. If no clearly detectable lesion is evident, reassurance and follow-up are appropriate. A desire for regular menstrual cycles can be fulfilled by medication with a cyclic estrogen-progesterone preparation.

Amenorrhea associated with hyperprolactinemia can be treated surgically or medically, depending on the size of the pituitary tumor. Pituitary microadenomas (less than 10 mm) can be treated with bromocriptine (orally 2.5 mg b.i.d.). This restores regular cycles and fertility in the majority of patients. Premature ovarian failure should usually be treated with estrogen replacement (e.g., Premarin 0.625–1.25 mg daily).

DYSFUNCTIONAL UTERINE BLEEDING

Dysfunctional uterine bleeding is defined as abnormal uterine bleeding that cannot be attributed to an organic lesion. The majority of these cases are associated with anovulation and occur at each end of the reproductive years, as postmenarcheal adolescent bleeding secondary to hypothalamic immaturity or as premenopausal bleeding consequent to imminent ovarian failure. Most cases of anovulatory bleeding are examples of estrogen withdrawal or estrogen breakthrough bleeding. Unopposed estrogen induces a progressive endometrial hyperplasia. In the absence of growth-limiting progesterone and natural periodic menstruation, the endometrium achieves an abnormal height without the necessary structural support. This fragile tissue will intermittently undergo spontaneous necrosis, and bleeding results. The classic presentation is one of a pale, frightened teenager who has bled excessively for weeks or an older women with prolonged bleeding who is concerned about the development of a possible neoplasm.

Therapy attempts to control the acute bleeding and to prevent recurrent bleeding. Acute hemostasis can be accomplished rapidly (less than 24 hours) with a high dose of a progesterone-estrogen combination birth control pill. Therapy is administered as one pill q.i.d. for seven days. These patients must be warned that a heavy flow associated with severe cramping will probably occur two to four days after stopping therapy. This initial withdrawal bleeding should be followed with three cycles of therapy using a low-dose combined contraceptive pill. The three months of therapy will restore the endometrium to its normal height. Each patient should subsequently be followed closely in order to document normal ovulatory cycles.

HIRSUTISM

Excessive growth of body hair in women is called hirsutism. An abnormal pattern of body hair growth, such as terminal hair on the upper abdomen, shoulders, back, and face, may be a sign of disease. In the majority of patients, however, no underlying disease can be found.

Hirsutism is predominantly an androgen-dependent process, except when associated with specific drugs (phenytoin, steroids, minoxidil), malnutrition (anorexia nervosa), or rare genetic disorders. Because androgens in women are secreted only by the ovaries or adrenal glands, a disorder of one or the other must be the source of any excess androgens (Table 70–3). Thus excessive secretion of testosterone or of its immediate precursors androstenedione and dehydroepiandrosterone, which are subsequently converted to testosterone in peripheral tissues, can cause abnormal terminal hair growth.

Clinical hirsutism is generally associated with acne, temporal balding, increased muscle strength, altered libido, and, in virilized patients, clitoral enlargement and deepening of the voice. There is generally defeminization with amenorrhea, decrease in breast size, and an alteration in the female body habitus. However, the two most common causes of hirsutism, idiopathic hirsutism and polycystic ovarian disease, are rarely associated with virilization or deepening of the voice. The hair growth is generally first noted in the peripubertal period and tends to stabilize after progressing for a few years. Adrenal and ovarian tumors generally present in adults. Most ovarian tumors are palpable on physical examination. Overt virilization occurs with most of the androgen-secreting ovarian tumors but rarely consequent to the weak androgens secreted by adrenal tumors. Congenital adrenal hyperplasia usually becomes clinically apparent at birth or during childhood. It is characterized by rapid growth, heterosexual precocious puberty in girls, and occasionally hypertension.

The etiology of most cases of hirsutism can be determined by measuring serum total testosterone and dehydroepiandrosterone sulfate (DHEA sulfate). Increased levels of plasma testosterone (values in excess of 200 ng/dl) are rarely associated with idiopathic hirsutism or polycystic ovarian syndrome but are frequently present in patients with ovarian tumors. Adrenal lesions (CAH or tumor) will have high plasma DHEA sulfate levels. In the benign process (CAH) DHEA sulfate will suppress after three days of dexamethasone (0.5 mg q.i.d.), whereas the secretion of DHEA sulfate will not suppress in cases with tumor. Furthermore, the high testosterone level associated with the polycystic ovarian syndrome will normalize on a ''pill'' (estrogen-progesterone) suppression test, in contrast to the lack of suppression in a patient with an ovarian tumor.

Ovarian and adrenal tumors are treated surgically. Congenital adrenal hyperplasia is suppressed with glucocorticoid replacement. Hirsutism associated with idopathic hirsutism and polycystic ovarian disease is generally stable and rarely progresses to virilization. Thus, the abnormal hair growth is primarily a cosmetic and psychological problem. In this group, which consists of the majority of cases of hirsutism, the risks of suppressive therapy with either contraceptives, glucocorticoids, or antiandrogens (cyproterone) and spironolactone must be carefully evaluated. These hormonal approaches have had mixed success.

TABLE 70–3. HIRSUTISM

1. Ovarian Causes
    Idiopathic hirsutism
    Polycystic ovarian disease
    Ovarian tumors secreting excess androgens
2. Adrenal Disorders
    Congenital adrenal hyperplasia
    Virilizing adrenal tumors
3. Medications
    Minoxidil, phenytoin, diazoxide
    Androgens, glucocorticoids

GALACTORRHEA

Nonpuerperal lactation (galactorrhea) is of benign significance in about 30 per cent of patients.

TABLE 70–4. GALACTORRHEA

CAUSES	FREQUENCY
Idiopathic with menses	32%
Idiopathic with amenorrhea	9%
Pituitary tumor	18%
Postpartum or postabortion	8%
Postpill or pill-related	10%
Drugs (phenothiazides, etc.)	8%
Hypothyroidism	4%
Empty sella syndrome	2%
Miscellaneous	9%
	100%

This is termed idiopathic and is associated with regular menses. If associated with amenorrhea, however, galactorrhea often indicates the presence of a serious condition such as a pituitary tumor (30 per cent). Table 70–4 outlines the relative frequency of disorders causing galactorrhea. The measurement of serum prolactin is very helpful in the evaluation of a patient with galactorrhea. The serum prolactin level is normal in the majority (85 per cent) of patients with idiopathic galactorrhea associated with continued menstruation. Thus a normal prolactin level generally indicates a benign disorder. Hyperprolactinemia is present in most (70 per cent) patients with galactorrhea associated with amenorrhea. This is the most common presentation of a pituitary tumor secreting prolactin in women. A patient presenting with a serum prolactin greater than 300 ng/ml invariably has a prolactinoma. The prolactin response to thyrotropin-releasing hormone (TRH) may be a useful screening test for differentiation of cases with hyperprolactinemia (less than 300 ng/ml) due to tumor from other causes. Patients with tumor demonstrate a flat or blunted prolactin response to TRH (TRH 500 μg intravenously) in contrast to nontumor cases, which show normal response. Galactorrhea in this latter group may be idiopathic (with amenorrhea), postpartum, postpill, or associated with endocrine disease (hypothyroidism, acromegaly, Cushing's syndrome) or drug therapy (phenothiazines, benzodiazepines, alpha methyldopa, reserpine). Rarely galactorrhea may be due to the empty sella syndrome or hypothalamic disease.

The suspected presence of a pituitary tumor can generally be documented by a plain skull radiograph of the sella turcica (macroadenoma, serum prolactin greater than 300 ng/ml) or a CT scan of the sella for a microadenoma (tumor less than 10 mm).

Treatment of galactorrhea depends upon the primary disorder. Hypothyroidism, acromegaly, and Cushing's syndrome can be effectively corrected. Offending drugs should be stopped. Hyperprolactinemia due to a pituitary microadenoma or idiopathic hyperprolactinemia can be successfully treated with bromocryptine, a dopamine agonist. Macroadenomas may also respond successfully to bromocryptine therapy, and this is an acceptable form of treatment in the absence of local pituitary erosion or suprasellar extension. Large sellar tumors are generally treated definitively by transsphenoidal surgery and/or radiotherapy.

MENOPAUSE

The menopause refers to the cessation of menses. The mean age of spontaneous menopause is currently 50 years, although generally there is a transitional phase of ovarian failure over 6 to 18 months during the perimenopausal period. Pituitary gonadotropins are secreted excessively as progressive ovarian (follicular) failure reduces estrogen secretion. Measurement of serum follicle-stimulating hormone (FSH) is the single best test to detect ovarian failure (FSH > 50 mIU/ml).

The majority (85 per cent) of women experience some feature of estrogen deficiency at menopause. Breasts atrophy, thermoregulatory dysfunction begins (hot flushes, sweats), vaginal epithelium thins, vaginal and cervical secretions decline (dyspareunia may be experienced), the endometrium atrophies, and osteoporotic changes in bone accelerate (see Chapter 77). These alterations become sufficiently severe to warrant estrogen replacement in about 25 per cent of postmenopausal women.

Estrogen replacement will generally control hot flushes. The minimal effective dose should be given for as short a time as required for the relief of symptoms. Relief of symptoms can usually be achieved by sub-bleeding (withdrawal) doses of estrogen. The generally effective dose of conjugated estrogens (Premarin) ranges from 0.625 to 1.25 mg per day. These preparations are administered on a cyclic basis, e.g., three weeks on, one week off. Local estrogen creams may be used to treat vaginal atrophy and the frequently associated dyspareunia. These estrogens are absorbed systemically, however, and the accepted contraindications to estrogen use also apply to such preparations. Long-term estrogen use at low doses will retard the accelerated bone loss associated with menopause and may possibly prevent the related fractures (see Chapter 77).

Estrogen use is contraindicated in patients with a history of thromboembolic disorders and vascular problems, including thrombophlebitis, cerebral vascular disorders, myocardial infarction and coronary artery disease, and hypertension. Estrogens should not be prescribed for patients with known or suspected breast carcinoma or other estrogen-dependent neoplasias such as endometrial cancer. The presence of significant diffuse liver disease or benign or malignant liver tumors also prohibits the use of estrogens. Obviously all women taking estrogen preparations need constant surveillance to detect the onset of these disorders.

BREAST, OVARIAN, AND UTERINE NEOPLASMS

BREAST CANCER

One of eight women will develop breast cancer, the second leading cause of cancer death in

TABLE 70–5. TNM CLASSIFICATION OF BREAST CANCER

CLINICAL STAGE		TREATMENT OPTIONS	FIVE-YEAR SURVIVAL
Stage I	Tumor <2 cm Negative nodes No distant metastases	Modified radical mastectomy and axillary node dissection or "Lumpectomy" with axillary node dissection and postoperative radiation therapy	85%
Stage II	Tumor <5 cm Positive nodes, not fixed No distant metastases	Modified radical mastectomy and axillary node dissection	65%
Stage III	Tumor > 5 cm or skin or chest wall involvement Positive supraclavicular nodes No distant metastases	Hormonal manipulation or Combination chemotherapy	40%
Stage IV	Distant metastases	Hormonal manipulation or Combination chemotherapy Palliative radiation therapy	10%

women. Unopposed estrogen activity is probably an important pathogenic factor; the other identified risk factors include nulliparity, early menarche, late menopause, a family history of breast cancer, middle age, and prior breast cancer.

Breast cancer usually presents as a painless lump, alone or with associated nipple discharge and skin retraction. Other symptoms are generally due to metastases to bone, brain, lungs, and liver. Early diagnosis is aided by monthly self-exams. Mammography has proven benefit in early detection in women over 40 and is useful for younger women with known risk factors or for those with difficult breast exams.

Breast carcinoma originates either in ducts (90 per cent) or in lobules (10 per cent). Of the ductal carcinomas, an infiltrating ductal pathology is seen in 75 per cent of the cases. Breast cancer is staged by the TNM (Tumor-Node-Metastasis) classification scheme, useful for both prognosis and treatment guidelines (Table 70–5).

Treatment, which is currently in evolution, varies with the disease stage. Table 70–5 presents an algorithm for currently held therapies for various stages of disease. It is essential to assay tumor material for estrogen receptors, since their presence indicates a high probability of tumor regression with hormonal manipulation.

OVARIAN CANCER

Ovarian carcinoma is the leading cause of death from reproductive tract tumors in women. The incidence is rising in industrialized countries and is more common in women with prior breast or uterine cancer. Ovarian tumors are commonly classified according to their histologic features (Table 70–6). For practical purposes, ovarian masses that are cystic tend to be benign; solid masses are generally malignant.

Ovarian tumors are commonly asymptomatic. In later stages, presenting symptoms include vague abdominal pain, often with an associated mass or ascites. Granulosa cell tumors can present with precocious puberty, and Sertoli-Leydig tumors (arrhenoblastoma) with masculinization.

CT scanning is beneficial in defining mass size and metastatic lesions; laparotomy is mandatory for tissue diagnosis and direct examination of the extent of disease. The minimal surgical resection is a hysterectomy with bilateral salpingo-oophorectomy. Whenever possible, all tumor should be "debulked," since reducing the tumor load to less than 2 cm improves survival. Adjuvant chemotherapy with an alkylating agent and a later "second-look operation" are recommended to assess tumor response to chemotherapy and to debulk recurrent disease.

CANCER OF THE UTERINE CORPUS AND CERVIX

Risk factors for the development of uterine adenocarcinoma appear to be related to unopposed estrogen exposure, for example, exogenous estrogens or the Stein-Leventhal syndrome. Patients usually present with abnormal vaginal bleeding.

TABLE 70–6. OVARIAN TUMOR HISTOLOGY

EPITHELIAL (85%)	GONADAL STROMAL TUMORS (10%)	GERM CELL TUMORS (5%)
Serous cystadenocarcinoma (40%) Endometroid carcinoma (15%) Mucinous cystadenocarcinoma (12%) Clear cell (13%) Undifferentiated (5%)	Sertoli-Leydig cell Granulosa-stromal cell Androblastoma	Dysgerminoma Endodermal sinus Embryonal carcinoma Choriocarcinoma Teratoma

Fractional curettage is the diagnostic method of choice; hysterectomy with bilateral salpingo-oophorectomy is indicated for early disease. Radiation therapy is added in the presence of more progressive disease. Chemotherapy is of little benefit; hormonal therapy with progestational agents may be palliative.

Cancer of the cervix has an extremely high cure rate owing to early detection with routine cytopathologic (PAP) smears. The risk factors include early age at first coitus, early pregnancy, multiple sexual partners, and venereal disease. Serologic and cytohistopathologic evidence supports a role for herpes simplex type 2 virus as a possible etiologic agent. Surgical treatment ranges from conization with early disease to radical abdominal hysterectomy with bilateral deep pelvic node dissection in advanced disease. There is no role for hormonal therapy or chemotherapy; radiation therapy is used with invasive disease.

REFERENCES

Frantz AG: Prolactin. N Engl J Med 298:201, 1978.
Judd H, Meldrum D, Deftos L, and Henderson B: Estrogen replacement therapy: Indications and complications. Ann Intern Med 98:195, 1983.
Ross GT: The ovaries. In Wyngaarden JB, and Smith LH Jr (eds): Cecil Textbook of Medicine. 17th ed. Philadelphia, WB Saunders Co, 1985, p 1379.
Speroff L, Glass RH, and Kase NG (eds): Clinical Gynecologic Endocrinology and Infertility. 3rd ed. Baltimore, Williams and Wilkins, 1983.
Styne DM, and Grumbach MM: Puberty in male and female: Its physiology and disorders. In Yen SSC, and Jaffe RB (eds): Reproductive Endocrinology. Philadelphia, WB Saunders Co, 1978, p 189.
Zumoff B, Freeman R, Coupey S, Saenger P, Markowitz M, and Kream J: A chronologic abnormality of luteinizing hormone secretion in teenage girls with the polycystic ovary syndrome. N Engl J Med 309:1206, 1983.

TESTICULAR AND BREAST DISORDERS IN MALES

Hypogonadism can refer to either (1) the failure of the testes to produce adequate testosterone, resulting in the signs and symptoms of androgen deficiency, or (2) impaired spermatogenesis, resulting in infertility. Impaired spermatogenesis and infertility may be present with normal testosterone production, but testosterone production is necessary for normal spermatogenesis. Normal

TABLE 71–1. CLASSIFICATION OF THE CAUSES OF ABNORMALITIES IN TESTICULAR FUNCTION

	ANDROGEN DEFICIENCY AND INFERTILITY	INFERTILITY ONLY
Primary Hypogonadism		
1. Developmental and genetic disorders	Klinefelter's syndrome	Sertoli cell only syndrome
		Kartagener's syndrome
		Cryptorchidism
2. Structural defects	Anorchia	Varicocele
3. Acquired defects	Viral or bacterial orchitis	Radiation
	Trauma	Drugs—alkylating agents
	Radiation	and antimetabolites
	Polyendocrine autoimmune failure	
	Granulomatous disease	
	Drugs—spironolactone, alcohol, marijuana	
	Ischemia (torsion)	
4. Associated with systemic disease	Liver disease	Myotonic dystrophy
	Renal disease	Paraplegia
	Sickle cell disease	Febrile illness
Secondary Hypogonadism	Panhypopituitarism	Isolated FSH deficiency
	Hyperprolactinemia	Congenital adrenal hyperplasia
	Kallman's syndrome	Exogenous sex steroid use
	Malnutrition	
	Cushing's syndrome	
Other	Androgen resistance	Absence or obstruction of the vas deferans (cystic fibrosis)

adult males produce approximately 7 mg of testosterone per day and normal serum plasma concentrations are 0.3 to 1.2 µg/dl. As illustrated in Figure 71–1, testosterone production is dependent on an intact hypothalamus, pituitary gland, and Leydig cells in the testis. Spermatogenesis requires both intact pituitary and Leydig cell function. The 5 α-reduced derivative of testosterone, 5 α-dihydrotestosterone, is the active form of the hormone and is responsible for inducing growth and differentiation of the male secondary sex structures.

The causes of hypogonadism can be divided into two major categories (Table 71–1): (1) *Primary hypogonadism* is due to testicular disorders and is associated with elevated serum gonadotropin levels. (2) *Secondary hypogonadism* results from hypothalamic pituitary disease and is associated with low or low-normal serum gonadotropin levels. In primary hypogonadism when testosterone levels are low, serum LH levels are increased, and when spermatogenesis is impaired, serum FSH levels are elevated.

ANDROGEN DEFICIENCY

The signs and symptoms of androgen deficiency depend upon the age of onset and the severity of the deficiency. If androgen deficiency occurs prior to puberty, the usual changes associated with puberty do not occur and the patient will develop the features of eunuchoidism (Table 71–2). Disproportionate growth of long bones occurs due to the delay in epiphyseal closure. If testosterone secretion fails after sexual maturity, the signs of androgen deficiency are much less overt (Table 71–2). The most common symptoms and signs are a reduction in prostate size, decreased rate of growth of beard and body hair, the appearance of fine wrinkles around the eyes, decreased semen volume, decreased libido, and impotence. Occasionally libido and potency will persist despite androgen deficiency.

When androgen deficiency is suspected, serum testosterone levels should be measured. If the serum testosterone concentration is low, serum LH and FSH levels should be determined next. Elevated LH and FSH concentrations indicate primary hypogonadism, whereas low or normal LH and FSH levels are most consistent with secondary hypogonadism.

Androgen deficiency regardless of etiology is treated by administering testosterone. Testosterone may be given orally, sublingually, buccally, or intramuscularly via injections. In general, androgen replacement is most effective when long-acting testosterone preparations are administered intramuscularly. Undesirable effects of androgen replacement include edema secondary to sodium retention, erythremia, acne, gynecomastia, and premature closure of the epiphyses (if given during or before puberty). Methyltestosterone and other oral androgens will occasionally cause intrahepatic cholestatic jaundice. Androgen therapy is contraindicated in patients with prostatic car-

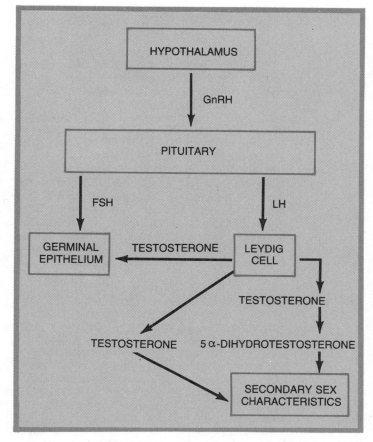

FIGURE 71–1. Pathway of production of testosterone.

cinoma and on occasion can precipitate urinary retention secondary to prostatic hypertrophy. Exogenous androgen therapy will not restore fertility.

INFERTILITY

About 15 per cent of married couples have fertility problems and in 30 per cent of these cases the male is the major cause of the infertility. The initial diagnostic procedure in evaluating a male for the many possible causes of infertility is a semen analysis. The test is considered abnormal if (1) the total sperm count is less than 60 million,

TABLE 71–2. CLINICAL FEATURES OF EUNUCHOIDISM AND HYPOGONADISM

Eunuchoidism
Increased height and a span more than 2 inches greater than height
Lack of adult hair distribution
High-pitched voice
Small penis, testes, and scrotum
Decreased muscle mass
Hypogonadism Beginning After Puberty
Decreased prostate size
Diminished rate of growth of beard and body hair
Fine wrinkles around eyes
Decreased potency and libido

(2) less than 60 per cent of the sperm are actively motile, or (3) more than 40 per cent of the sperm have an abnormal morphology. There is considerable variability in the sperm count for a given individual, so several counts over a period of time should be done if the count is borderline. Abnormalities in semen do not preclude fertility; many men with low sperm counts have fathered children. Fertility in the male is dependent on his female partner's fertility; i.e., a male with a relatively low sperm count may father a child with a partner of relatively high fertility.

If the semen analysis is abnormal, serum testosterone and FSH levels should be measured next. If a patient has azoospermia with a normal testosterone and FSH level, an obstructive disorder is a likely diagnostic possibility. Normal testosterone levels and elevated FSH concentrations indicate a primary testicular disorder of spermatogenesis as the basis for the infertility.

PRIMARY HYPOGONADISM

Klinefelter's Syndrome. Klinefelter's syndrome and its variants are important causes of male infertility and occur in approximately 1 in 500 newborn males. This syndrome is characterized by more than one X chromosome, most commonly a 47XXY karyotype, but occasionally 48XXYY, 48XXXY, or 49XXXXY karyotype has been described.

The classic features of this disorder are small, firm testes (usually less than 2 cm in length), azoospermia, gynecomastia, decreased signs of androgenicity, and elevated gonadotropin levels. Patients with this disorder are often tall, but the span-to-height ratio is frequently less than 1, suggesting that the increased height is not simply due to eunuchoidism. In some patients a mild degree of mental retardation is present, and poor social adaptation is not uncommon. Chronic pulmonary disease and varicose veins have been described as being more common in patients with Klinefelter's syndrome.

The manifestations of Klinefelter's syndrome may vary and may be minimal in some patients. Sex chromosome mosaicism, in which at least two populations of cells have different chromosomal complexes (example XY in one cell type and XXY in another), perhaps accounts for this remarkable variability in severity. In fact, fertility has been documented in rare individuals with this disorder.

Serum testosterone levels in patients with Klinefelter's syndrome vary from very low to low-normal. FSH levels are invariably elevated, but LH levels may be within the normal range, especially in those individuals with adequte testosterone levels. Buccal smears will frequently detect the condensed X chromosome (Barr bodies), but karyotyping of various cell types is the most definitive diagnostic procedure.

The treatment of this disorder is by testosterone replacement if there is evidence of androgen deficiency.

Myotonic Muscular Dystrophy. This syndrome is characterized by muscle wasting, myotonia, frontal baldness, cataracts, diabetes, and testicular atrophy, which occurs in the third to fourth decade. Androgen deficiency and gynecomastia occur in only a small percentage of these patients.

Sertoli Cell Only Syndrome (Germ Cell Aplasia). This syndrome is characterized by fully developed secondary sex characteristics and azoospermia. FSH levels are increased, and testosterone and LH levels are within the normal range. Testicular biopsy reveals seminiferous tubules that do not contain germinal cells and are lined only with Sertoli cells.

Kartagener's Syndrome. This genetic syndrome includes situs inversus, chronic sinusitis, bronchiectasis, and infertility secondary to nonmotile sperm. The immotility of the sperm and the respiratory difficulties are due to the absence of the protein dynein, a constituent of both the tail of the sperm and the cilia of the respiratory tract mucosa.

Anorchia. Absence of both testes in a phenotypically normal male is very rare. It is important to distinguish bilateral abdominal cryptorchidism from anorchia because of the increased incidence of malignancy in cryptorchidism. Low testosterone levels that fail to rise following HCG stimulation suggest anorchia, but the final diagnosis depends on surgical exploration. Unilateral anorchia is more common and may result from developmental disturbances or following surgical procedures such as orchiopexy or herniorrhaphy.

Acquired Hypogonadism. Numerous chemical and physical factors can affect gonadal function and result in either transient or permanent dysfunction. Germ cells are sensitive to ischemia, and testicular torsion if not rapidly corrected can irreversibly damage the testes. In adults, mumps is complicated by orchitis in 15 to 25 per cent of patients, and the affected testes may sustain permanent damage. Mumps orchitis is usually unilateral and typically does not affect testosterone production. Other viruses and bacterial infections can also cause orchitis and result in hypogonadism. Many chemicals and drugs are directly toxic to spermatogenesis or affect the androgen-to-estrogen ratio and thus may result in oligospermia or azoospermia. Many of the alkylating agents and antimetabolites that are commonly used in cancer chemotherapy adversely affect spermatogenesis. Ionizing radiation primarily inhibits spermatogenesis. Testicular failure occurs rarely as part of the polyendocrine failure syndrome secondary to an autoimmune process. Lastly, systemic disorders such as hepatic or renal failure can result in hypogonadism.

SECONDARY HYPOGONADISM

Secondary hypogonadism, due to the decreased secretion of gonadotropins by the pituitary gland, may result from any disorder that adversely affects pituitary or hypothalamic function (see

Table 71–1). Gonadotropins may be decreased as an isolated deficiency or in association with deficiency of other pituitary hormones. A functional and reversible suppression of gonadotropin secretion occurs in malnutrition and in disorders that cause hyperprolactinemia. High serum concentrations of either androgens or estrogens can also inhibit gonadotropin secretion. The hypogonadism that occurs in patients with liver disease, for example, is partially due to increased levels of estrogen. Exogenous sex steroid intake by athletes also will lead to infertility.

Kallmann's syndrome is a familial disorder that is characterized by hypogonadotropic hypogonadism that occurs in association with anosmia or hyposmia. The hypogonadism is due to an abnormality in the secretion of gonadotropin-releasing factor by the hypothalamus.

Fertility can occasionally be restored in individuals with secondary hypogonadism by treatment with Pergonal (FSH activity) and human chorionic gonadotropin (LH activity).

CRYPTORCHIDISM

Cryptorchidism refers to a testes that has never descended into the scrotum. Unilateral cryptorchidism is approximately four times as common as bilateral cryptorchidism. Undescended testes are found at birth in 3 to 4 per cent of male infants but by one year of age only 0.5 per cent of male infants have an undescended testes. In adult males approximately 0.2 to 0.4 per cent have either unilateral or bilateral cryptorchidism.

It is important to distinguish an undescended testis from the more common retractile testes of childhood. Repeated examinations in a warm room with the patient standing, squatting, recumbent, or performing a Valsalva maneuver are necessary. Careful questioning to determine if the testis has ever been in the scrotum is mandatory. Absence of the testis in the scrotum historically and on repeated physical examination suggests that the testis is truly undescended.

Adult men with bilateral cryptorchidism are sterile. However, the age at which these testes become infertile is uncertain. Abnormalities in testicular histology have been noted as early as six years of age, but the significance of these changes is uncertain. After puberty the undescended testis shows degenerative changes that eventually progress to atrophy. Even when cryptorchid testes are placed in the scrotum degenerative changes occur in approximately 50 per cent, suggesting that intrinsic abnormalities of the organ account for the failure of normal descent. Even when unilateral cryptorchidism is corrected many patients have abnormal spermatogenesis, suggesting that the testicular abnormality is bilateral. Thus in many cases the degenerative changes are due to a testicular abnormality that orchiopexy will not correct. The incidence of malignancy in an undescended testis is 30 to 50 times greater than in the normal testis.

Cyptorchidism is treated by orchiopexy, although some clinicians first administer HCG followed by orchiopexy if the testis does not descend. The age when therapy should be initiated is uncertain, but it certainly should be prior to the onset of puberty. Many experts recommend treatment between five and seven years of age.

IMPOTENCE

Impotence is a common problem that can occur secondary to a wide variety of causes (Table 71–3). While impotence that is psychogenic in origin is not uncommon, a specific etiology can frequently be identified. Patients with psychogenic impotence have morning erections and/or erections that are associated with REM sleep, whereas in patients with physiological impotence erections at these times are either impaired or absent. The measurement of nocturnal penile tumescence by a variety of different procedures can therefore be helpful in the evaluation of impotent men. A very careful drug history is also indicated in all patients. The physical examination should search thoroughly for the signs of peripheral vascular disease or neuropathies. On occasion hyperprolactinemia may be the cause of the impotence, and lowering the prolactin level can restore potency. If the cause of the impotence cannot be corrected, many men will benefit by the implantation of a penile prosthesis.

GYNECOMASTIA

Gynecomastia, the enlargement of the male breast, may occur unilaterally or bilaterally. Gynecomastia is very commonly observed during the newborn period and puberty and in senescence. For example, approximately 50 per cent of normal

TABLE 71–3. CLASSIFICATION OF THE CAUSES OF IMPOTENCE

Psychogenic
Endocrine
   Hypogonadism
   Hyperprolactinemia
Neurologic
   Spinal cord lesions
   Diabetes mellitus
   Tabes dorsalis
   Polyneuropathies
   Parasympathetic nerve damage following surgical procedure such as prostatectomy, aortic bypass, or rectosigmoid operation
Vascular Disease
Drugs
   Antihypertensives—clonidine, methyldopa, propranolol, reserpine, spironolactone, thiazides
   Antihistamines—cimetidine, diphenhydramine
   Antidepressants—doxepin, amitriptyline
   Antipsychotics—chlorpromazine, haloperidol
   Tranquilizers—diazepam, barbiturates, chlordiazepoxide
   Anticholinergics
   Addicting drugs—alcohol, heroin, methadone
Penile Disease
   Priapism
   Peyronie's disease

boys at puberty and 40 per cent of elderly men have been noted to have gynecomastia. If gynecomastia develops between late puberty and male senescence, one should search carefully for an underlying disorder that can account for the breast enlargement (Table 71–4).

Estrogens stimulate while androgens inhibit breast development, and therefore disorders that alter the usual ratio of estrogens to androgens can result in gynecomastia. Increased estrogen production secondary to adrenal carcinoma, testicular tumors, and some types of congenital adrenal hyperplasia will lead to breast development. Similarly, the increased conversion of androgens to estrogens which occurs in liver disease, thyrotoxicosis, obesity, and refeeding after starvation will also result in gynecomastia. Conversely the decreased production of androgens in primary or secondary testicular failure or insensitivity to the cellular effects of testosterone can also result in breast enlargement. Lastly, gynecomastia occurs in association with the use of a wide variety of drugs. Estrogen treatment will lead to gynecomastia; androgen administration may also on occasion result in breast development because of the biotransformation of androgens to estrogens. Some drugs, such as HCG, will increase endogenous estrogen production and other drugs such as digitalis or marijuana have an estrogen-like effect.

TABLE 71–4. CLASSIFICATION OF THE CAUSES OF GYNECOMASTIA

Physiological—Newborn, Puberty, Senescence
Pathological
  Increased Estrogen Secretion
    Adrenal carcinoma
    Testicular tumors
    HCG secreting tumors (lung, liver, etc.)
    Congenital adrenal hyperplasia
    Hermaphroditism
  Increased Conversion of Androgens to Estrogens
    Liver disease
    Adrenal disease
    Nutritional (refeeding after starvation)
    Thyrotoxicosis
  Decreased Androgen Secretion
    Primary hypogonadism
    Secondary hypogonadism
  Androgen Resistance
    Testicular feminization
    Reifenstein's syndrome
Drugs
  Hormones—estrogens, androgens, HCG
  Antihypertensives—reserpine, methyldopa, spironolactone
  Psychotropics—phenothiazine, butyrophenone, marijuana, methadone, heroin, tricyclic antidepressants, diazepam
  Cardiac—digitalis
  Gastrointestinal—cimetidine, metoclopramide
  Cytotoxic—cyclophosphamide, vincristine, mitotane
  Miscellaneous—penicillamine

Additionally, drugs can block testosterone synthesis (chemotherapeutic agents, high doses of spironolactone) or interfere with the action of testosterone (cyproterone, low doses of spironolactone), resulting in gynecomastia.

It is essential to be sure that "true" gynecomastia is present. The most frequent error is to confuse the fatty breast of the obese patient, which lacks the glandular elements, with gynecomastia. The diagnosis of gynecomastia is based on the palpation of subareolar glandular tissue. Particular attention should be paid to the testes, as either small testes or a testicular mass will suggest the likely mechanism for the gynecomastia. Additionally, a careful search for signs of liver disease, thyrotoxicosis, other evidence of feminization, and galactorrhea is indicated. Lastly, in all patients with gynecomastia a complete drug history (including illicit drugs) is essential.

Many laboratory studies can be useful in the evaluation of gynecomastia when judiciously selected on the basis of history and physical examination. In the pubertal boy, for example, laboratory studies are not usually indicated. Liver function tests, serum estrogen, testosterone, LH and HCG concentrations, and urinary ketosteroids are sometimes useful in the evaluation of patients with gynecomastia.

Regression or significant improvement in gynecomastia occurs in a substantial number of patients. Gynecomastia usually improves after stopping an offending drug or after correcting a hormonal deficiency or excess. Pubertal gynecomastia will spontaneously regress and drug therapy is not indicated. Long-standing cases of gynecomastia or large breasts will rarely regress entirely after the causal disorder has been corrected. In these instances cosmetic mastectomy may be very helpful. The risk of breast cancer in men is proportional to the amount of breast tissue present and therefore is increased in patients with substantial gynecomastia.

REFERENCES

Lipsett MB: Physiology and pathology of the Leydig cell. N Engl J Med 303:682, 1980.
Lipsett MB: The testis. In Wyngaarden JB, and Smith LH Jr (eds): Cecil Textbook of Medicine. 17th ed. Philadelphia, WB Saunders Co, 1985, pp 1365–1375.
Odell WD, and Swerdloff RD: Male hypogonadism. West J Med 124:446, 1976.
Schiavi RC: Male erectile disorders. Annu Rev Med 32:509, 1981.
Tolis G: Nonmalignant diseases of the breast. In Wyngaarden JB, and Smith LH Jr (eds): Cecil Textbook of Medicine. 17th ed. Philadelphia, WB Saunders Co, 1985, pp 1398–1401.
Wilson JD, Himan J, and MacDonald PC: The pathogenesis of gynecomastia. Adv Intern Med 25:1, 1980.

DIABETES MELLITUS

72

Diabetes mellitus is a very common disorder with an estimated prevalence between 2 and 4 per cent in the United States. The complications of diabetes account for 25 per cent of all new cases of end-stage renal failure and 50 per cent of all lower extremity amputations, and diabetes is the leading cause of blindness, with approximately 5,000 new cases per year. Additionally, diabetic patients account for 10 per cent of all acute care hospital days.

DIAGNOSIS

A patient is considered to have diabetes mellitus if any of the three criteria shown in Table 72–1 are met. Nearly all patients who are diabetic according to oral glucose tolerance test criteria also have fasting plasma glucose levels greater than 140 mg/dl. Routine screening of patients with glucose tolerance tests is therefore not usually indicated. An oral glucose tolerance test may be indicated in individuals with normal fasting blood glucose levels if there is a strong suspicion of diabetes, such as the presence of complications possibly secondary to diabetes, extensive family histories of diabetes, or certain genetic syndromes. In general, the diagnosis of diabetes mellitus should rarely be made in the absence of fasting hyperglycemia.

"Impaired glucose tolerance" exists if the fasting plasma glucose is less than 140 mg/dl and during glucose tolerance testing, the 30-, 60-, or 90-minute plasma glucose level exceeds 200 mg/dl, with a two-hour value beteen 140 and 200 mg/dl. The majority of individuals with impaired glucose tolerance do not progress to diabetes and the specific microvascular complications associated with diabetes rarely occur. The clinical significance of impaired glucose tolerance is unclear.

CLASSIFICATION OF DIABETES
(Tables 72–2 and 72–3)

Type I Insulin-dependent Diabetes Mellitus (IDDM)

Type I diabetes is characterized by little or no endogenous insulin secretion. Because of the marked hypoinsulinemia, patients with this disorder usually present with the acute complications of diabetes mellitus such as polyuria, polydipsia, polyphagia, and ketoacidosis. In order to prevent ketoacidosis and death, these patients require exogenous insulin replacement. After the onset of diabetes, patients occasionally enter a "honeymoon phase" that may last several weeks or months during which time endogenous insulin secretion is restored and glucose metabolism is normal. Unfortunately, the disease invariably relapses and lifelong insulin therapy is required.

The peak age of onset of IDDM is between 11

and 13 years, coinciding with the onset of puberty, but Type I diabetes can begin at any age, including in the elderly. Patients with this disorder are usually of normal weight or thin. Specific HLA phenotypes (DR3, DR4) occur at a much greater frequency in patients with IDDM than in the general population. There is only a 50 per cent concordance rate for diabetes in identical twins with IDDM (i.e., only 50 per cent of identical twins

TABLE 72–1. CRITERIA FOR THE DIAGNOSIS OF DIABETES IN NONPREGNANT ADULTS

Any one of the following are considered diagnostic of diabetes:
  A. Presence of the classic symptoms of diabetes, such as polyuria, polydipsia, ketonuria, and rapid weight loss, together with gross and unequivocal elevation of plasma glucose.
  B. Elevated fasting glucose concentration on more than one occasion, venous plasma glucose ≥ 140 mg/dl (7.8 mmol/L).
  C. Fasting glucose concentration less than that which is diagnostic of diabetes (B), but sustained elevation of glucose concentration during the oral glucose tolerance test* on more than one occasion. Both the two-hour sample and some other sample taken between the administration of the oral 75-gram glucose dose and the two-hour sample must meet the following criteria, venous plasma glucose ≥ 200 mg/dl (11.1 mmol/L).

* O.G.T.T. should be performed in the morning after at least three days of unrestricted diet (≥150 grams carbohydrate) and physical activity. The subject should have fasted at least 10 hours and should remain seated throughout the study. (These guidelines were taken from the National Diabetes Data Group. Diabetes 28:1039, 1979.)

TABLE 72–2. CLASSIFICATION OF DIABETES

Type I—Insulin-Dependent Diabetes
Type II—Non–Insulin-Dependent Diabetes
Secondary Diabetes
    Pancreatic disease
    Hormonal
    Drug-induced
    Insulin receptor abnormalities
    Specific genetic syndromes

TABLE 72–3. COMPARISON OF TYPE I AND TYPE II DIABETES

	TYPE I	TYPE II
Synonym	IDDM	NIDDM
	Juvenile onset	Adult onset
Age of onset	Usually <30	Usually >40
Ketosis	Common	Uncommon
Body weight	Nonobese	Obese (50–90%)
Endogenous insulin secretion	Severe deficiency	Moderate deficiency
Insulin resistance	Ocassional	Almost always
HLA association	DR3, DR4	None
Identical twins	50% concordant	Almost 100% concordant
Islet cell antibodies	Frequently present	Absent
Association with other autoimmune disease	Yes	No
Treatment with insulin	Always necessary	Usually not required

both have diabetes), suggesting the importance of both genetic and environmental factors.

The etiology of IDDM is unknown. A leading hypothesis is that a viral illness or another yet unspecified initiating event may damage the beta cells of the pancreas, followed by a slow autoimmune destruction of the remaining beta cells in susceptible individuals. Anti–islet cell antibodies may be detected in some individuals several years prior to the onset of diabetes, followed by a slow deterioration in glucose tolerance which finally results in the abrupt onset of clinical diabetes. Soon after the onset of the disease, antibodies against the islet cells of the pancreas are present in as high as 90 per cent of Type I diabetic patients, but they diminish in frequency to 5 to 10 per cent after 20 years. This autoimmune hypothesis would also account for the increased risk of developing diabetes in individuals with certain HLA genes, because the genes that control the immune response are located on the sixth chromosome close to the HLA loci.

Type II Non–Insulin-dependent Diabetes Mellitus (NIDDM)

Type II diabetes is much more common than IDDM (approximately 10 cases of Type II diabetes for every case of Type I) and usually has its onset after age 40. Between 50 and 90 per cent of the patients with NIDDM are overweight. Some patients are asymptomatic and an elevated plasma glucose is noted on routine laboratory study. In other patients, polyuria, polydipsia, weakness, fatigue, or weight loss brings the patient to the attention of the physician. More rarely, patients with NIDDM first seek medical care because of the complications of long-standing diabetes.

Plasma insulin levels are decreased in patients with NIDDM but are not as severely reduced as in Type I diabetics. In some individuals, plasma insulin levels may be within the normal range. Patients with NIDDM almost always secrete decreased amounts of insulin, however, following oral glucose challenge. Because insulin deficiency is not marked, ketoacidosis does not occur in NIDDM unless a stressful event such as a myocardial infarction or infection is superimposed.

In addition to the abnormalities of insulin secretion, patients with NIDDM are also resistant to the action of insulin. This insulin resistance is due both to a decrease in insulin binding to its plasma membrane receptor and to postreceptor defects in insulin action. Thus, both a decrease in insulin secretion and impaired insulin action contribute to the hyperglycemia observed in NIDDM. At this time, the relative importance of these abnormalities in producing the impaired glucose metabolism is unclear.

Identical twins are almost 100 per cent concordant for NIDDM, suggesting a very strong genetic component to this disorder.

While this classification is convenient and useful, there are some patients who are difficult to place in a specific category. Additionally, patients will, on occasion, progress from a Type II form of diabetes to a Type I. It is likely that within each category, there are multiple subtypes that have not yet been recognized and defined.

Secondary Diabetes

Diabetes that is secondary to an identifiable condition is comparatively rare. For example, destruction of the pancreas secondary to pancreatitis will impair insulin secretion and result in diabetes. In certain endocrine disorders such as Cushing's syndrome, acromegaly, pheochromocytoma, and glucagonoma, the increased secretion of hormones that counteract the effect of insulin can also result in hyperglycemia. By a variety of mechanisms, a number of commonly used drugs such as diuretics, corticosteroids, propranolol, phenytoin, and adrenergic agents also cause or exacerbate diabetes.

Acanthosis nigricans may be associated with severe insulin resistance, resulting in diabetes by two distinct mechanisms: (1) Type A—the insulin resistance is due to a marked decrease in the number of cellular insulin receptors. These patients are usually young females with hirsutism and polycystic ovaries. (2) Type B—the insulin resistance is due to autoantibodies against the insulin receptor as part of a more generalized autoimmune process manifested by proteinuria, leukopenia, and antinuclear antibodies.

GENETICS

Diabetes has a strong familial tendency. Genetic factors are clearly important in the development of both Type I and Type II diabetes, but the mode of inheritance of both disorders is unknown. The direct transmission of clinical diabetes from a single parent with the disorder to offspring is relatively low: only 2 to 5 per cent for IDDM and 10 to 15 per cent for NIDDM. If a nonidentical sibling has either IDDM or NIDDM, the chance of an individual having diabetes is only approximately 10 per cent. However, in IDDM, if the siblings are identical for HLA phenotypes, the chances of being concordant for diabetes are greatly increased, whereas if all HLA phenotypes are different, the chances of concordance are greatly reduced. Recognizing these low rates of transmission from parent to sibling and the low incidence of concordance between siblings is important in counseling and reassuring patients.

ACUTE SYMPTOMS OF DIABETES

Hyperglycemia can result in a wide variety of symptoms (Table 72–4). When plasma glucose concentration exceeds the renal threshold for glucose reabsorption (approximately 180 mg/dl plasma glucose), glycosuria occurs and results in an osmotic diuresis. The resulting symptoms of nocturia and polyuria are directly attributed to this osmotic diuresis. The osmotic diuresis tends to lead to dehydration and hyperosmolality,

TABLE 72–4. ACUTE SYMPTOMS OF HYPERGLYCEMIA

Polyuria
Polydipsia
Polyphagia
Weight loss
Fatigue
Candida infections
Blurred vision

which stimulate thirst and polydipsia. Each gram of urinary glucose represents approximately 4.5 calories. A poorly controlled diabetic who spills one hundred grams of glucose per day in the urine, for example, loses 450 calories per day, enough to result in weight loss and stimulation of food intake (polyphagia). Thus, the polyuria, polyphagia, polydipsia, and weight loss, which are the cardinal signs of poorly controlled diabetics, are all attributable to increased urinary loss of glucose.

In addition to the above symptoms, transient visual blurring secondary to osmotic swelling of the lens is a common complaint of a poorly controlled diabetic and should not be confused with diabetic retinopathy. *Candida* vaginitis, thrush, or balanitis are occasionally observed and frequently do not respond to appropriate antibiotics until the plasma glucose concentration is lowered. Lastly, generalized fatigue is a common complaint in diabetic patients with persistent hyperglycemia.

THERAPY

GENERAL PRINCIPLES

The initial goal of treatment in all diabetic patients is the elimination of the symptoms that occur secondary to hyperglycemia. A second goal of therapy is the prevention of the long-term complications of diabetes. At this time, there is no *definitive* evidence that a reduction in blood glucose levels will prevent the long-term complications of diabetes. Nevertheless, there is substantial clinical and experimental evidence that elevated blood glucose levels may be detrimental. It seems worthwhile, therefore, to attempt to normalize blood glucose levels in diabetic patients. Hypoglycemia is a serious and potentially fatal complication of therapy, and therefore the physician must balance the possible benefits of "tight" glucose control with the risks of inducing hypoglycemia.

Factors that predispose to serious hypoglycemia, such as end-stage liver or kidney disease, adrenal or pituitary insufficiency, autonomic insufficiency, ethanol abuse, and psychiatric disturbances, are strong contraindications to "tight" control (Table 72–5).

In patients with cerebral vascular disease or coronary artery disease, the potential complications of hypoglycemia are more severe, and there-

fore aggressive therapy should also not be undertaken lightly. The goal of "tight" metabolic control is to prevent complications; if a patient already has severe diabetic complications, there is little evidence to suggest that aggressive therapy will be beneficial. The complications of diabetes usually take 10 to 20 years to develop and therefore in a patient whose life expectancy is greatly reduced due to other medical disorders, "tight" control is not usually indicated. Success in normalizing blood glucose levels requires a patient who is willing and able to undertake the responsibility of extensive self care.

In a patient who is capable of undertaking the responsibilities of extensive self care and who has no contraindications to aggressive metabolic control, an attempt should be made to control blood glucose in the range of a fasting plasma glucose concentration between 100 to 140 mg/dl and a two-hour postprandial plasma glucose level between 100 to 200 mg/dl.

TREATMENT OF TYPE I DIABETES

By definition, Type I diabetics require insulin therapy. Nevertheless, dietary treatment is also an important part of the management of IDDM.

Diet

Dietary therapy for Type I diabetics attempts to maintain consistency in the timing and caloric content of meals and to furnish a diet that will diminish the risks of vascular disease. In patients treated with intermediate or long-acting insulin, the timing of meals must be coordinated with the action of insulin. If meals are delayed or missed or are substantially smaller than usual, the chances of hypoglycemia are increased. Conversely, meals much larger than usual can result in hyperglycemia. Consistency in the timing and caloric content of meals allows an insulin regimen to be tailored to suit the particular patient's lifestyle. If consistency in meal patterns is impossible, the goal of good control will not be achievable using intermediate or long-acting insulins.

TABLE 72–5. CONTRAINDICATIONS TO AGGRESSIVE INSULIN THERAPY

Factors that Predispose to Hypoglycemia
Pituitary insufficiency
Adrenal insufficiency
End-stage liver or kidney disease
Autonomic insufficiency
Ethanol abuse
Psychiatric disturbance
Use of high doses of beta-blocking drugs
Inability of patient to self-monitor glucose
Increased Risk from Hypoglycemic Episode
Coronary artery disease
Cerebrovascular disease
Living alone
Reduced Benefits from Good Control
Severe microvascular disease
Short life expectancy

To diminish the risk of vascular disease, all diabetic patients should be placed on a diet low in fat (less then 30 per cent of the total caloric content should be lipids) with a polyunsaturated-to-saturated fat ratio of at least 1:1 and with a low cholesterol content (less than 350 mg/day). Therefore, the recommended "diabetic" diet is between 25 and 30 per cent lipid, 50 and 60 per cent carbohydrate, and 10 and 20 per cent protein. Diets containing this percentage of carbohydrate are no longer believed to be detrimental to diabetic control. It is hoped that such a diet will reduce blood lipid levels and thereby decrease the risk of macrovascular disease.

The role of dietary fiber in the diabetic diet is unresolved. Large quantities of dietary fiber tend to slow the rate of carbohydrate absorption and lower serum lipid levels. Patients should be encouraged, therefore, to incorporate foods with a high fiber content into their diets.

The effect of simple sugars and complex carbohydrates on blood glucose levels is currently being re-evaluated. Simple sugars ingested with meals do not, as previously thought, adversely affect blood glucose levels. All complex carbohydrates cannot be grouped together, because the glycemic response to different starches varies greatly. When incorporated into meals, various complex carbohydrates may also have significantly different effects on blood glucose levels. As a result, definitive recommendations regarding simple and complex carbohydrates must await further data.

Insulin

The various insulins currently in use differ in their time course of action, degree of purity, and source (Table 72–6). The time of the peak effect of insulin and the duration of action of insulin may vary a great deal from patient to patient. Even in a particular patient the absorption of subcutaneous insulin can vary from site to site and from day to day. For example, exercise of an extremity injected with insulin can increase the speed of insulin absorption and contribute to exercise-induced hypoglycemia. Most insulin-dependent patients require between 20 and 60 units of insulin per day. A requirement of greater than 200 units

of insulin per day indicates insulin resistance, which can be due to a variety of factors, including circulating antibodies that bind insulin.

The indications for highly purified insulins or human insulin in the treatment of diabetes are currently unresolved. Insulin resistance secondary to antibodies, allergic reactions to insulin, and lipodystrophy should be treated with either highly purified pork insulin or human insulin. Some physicians believe that all patients who are going to be intermittently treated with insulin should be treated with human insulin to decrease the possibility of the future development of antibodies. Additionally, some physicians start all new patients on either human or purified pork insulin, but the clinical advantage for this practice has not yet been shown.

Rather than using rigid recipes, it is far better to tailor the insulin regimen for each individual patient. The degree of glycemic control desired, the time of insulin action, the timing and size of meals, and the preferences of the individual patient are all factors that will determine the appropriate insulin regimen.

As one approach, patients of normal weight who have IDDM can be started on a single morning dose of intermediate insulin (approximately 20 to 25 units) with close following of their plasma glucose levels. If glucose values are uniformly elevated, the morning insulin dose can be slowly increased (approximately 5 units every other day) until glucose levels are lowered. In the occasional patient in whom plasma glucose levels measured at 7 AM, 11 AM, 4 PM and 9 PM are all within an acceptable range, this single daily dose of intermediate insulin suffices. More commonly, glucose levels are decreased only for a particular portion of the day and more complex insulin regimens are required. If glucose levels are high early in the day but are in an acceptable range later in the day (late-acting insulin), a short-acting insulin should be added in the morning. Conversely, if control is reasonable early in the day but glucose levels are not acceptable later in the day (early-acting insulin), a second injection of intermediate insulin is indicated in the afternoon. Further refinements in the insulin regimen can be carried out based on additional glucose measurements.

The type, dose, and timing of the insulin given should be based on the patient's response and not on a preconceived ideal. Furthermore, an insulin regimen established for a particular patient is not fixed and will in all likelihood need adjustments with time. Changes in physical activity, growth status, or meal content and the use of other drugs or the advent of intercurrent illnesses or stresses will require adjustments in the insulin regimen. The physician and patient must constantly monitor the diabetic control and be prepared to make changes as indicated.

In recent years, there has been an increasing use of intensive insulin treatment programs. The administration of regular insulin delivered via an insulin pump in carefully selected patients has resulted in excellent control. In this regimen, continuous regular insulin is given subcutaneously at

TABLE 72–6. INSULIN PREPARATIONS

TYPE	PROTEIN ADDITIVE	PEAK ACTION (hours)	DURATION OF ACTION (hours)
Rapid			
Regular	None	2–4	6–8
Semilente	None	2–6	10–12
Intermediate			
NPH	Protamine	6–12	18–24
Lente	None	6–12	18–24
Long-acting			
Protamine zinc	Protamine	14–24	36
Ultralente	None	18–24	36

a basal rate, supplemented by an additional bolus of regular insulin prior to meals. Another intensive treatment regimen involves the use of very long-acting ultralente insulin (basal insulin delivery) and injections of regular insulin prior to each meal. This regimen can also result in the normalization of blood glucose levels. Success with either of these regimens requires a highly motivated and educated patient who is dedicated to the achievement of excellent control.

Complications of Insulin Therapy. The major complication of insulin therapy is hypoglycemia. The symptoms and signs of hypoglycemia are listed in Table 73–1. Occasional mild episodes of hypoglycemia, especially if due to an identifiable cause such as increased exercise or delaying a meal, are not indications for altering the insulin regimen. However, frequent mild hypoglycemic reactions or a severe reaction are unacceptable and require an alteration in insulin treatment. The ability of some diabetics to recover from hypoglycemia is seriously impaired. In normal individuals, the secretion of glucagon is chiefly responsible for the recovery from hypoglycemia. In the absence of glucagon the secretion of epinephrine can result in a relatively normal recovery. In some diabetics, especially those with long-standing diabetes and autonomic insufficiency, the release of these two counter-regulatory hormones is impaired and recovery from hypoglycemia is absent or sluggish.

Hypoglycemia will occasionally result in rebound hyperglycemia, perhaps due to excessive secretion of counter-regulatory hormones (the Somogyi phenomenon). Characteristically, unrecognized nocturnal hypoglycemia results in morning hyperglycemia. If the insulin dose is increased, the frequency of hypoglycemia is increased, resulting in a paradoxical worsening of the morning hyperglycemia. The appropriate therapy is to decrease the insulin dose. The Somogyi phenomenon should always be considered in a poorly controlled diabetic.

A variety of local and systemic allergic reactions occur occasionally with insulin administration, but the frequency of these reactions has decreased with the use of purified insulins. Similarly, lipoatrophy at the injection site is only rarely observed with purified insulin. Lipohypertrophy secondary to the lipogenic effects of insulin occasionally occurs, but it can be prevented by rotating injection sites.

TREATMENT OF TYPE II DIABETES

In patients with NIDDM, diet therapy is of greatest importance. If diet does not satisfactorily control blood glucose levels, the use of oral hypoglycemic agents or insulin is indicated. The choice of an oral hypoglycemic drug or insulin will depend on many factors, including the degree of hyperglycemia, the social and economic situation, the relative risks and dangers of hypoglycemia, and the personal preferences of the patient and physician.

Diet

The majority of Type II patients are obese; the main goal of diet therapy is therefore weight loss. A diet restricted in calories frequently results in a marked amelioration of the patient's hyperglycemia. This effect on blood glucose levels can occur even before significant weight loss is achieved. In some cases, a reduction in caloric intake will result in a normalization of fasting plasma glucose concentrations.

A wide variety of different diets has been advocated for inducing weight loss. The success rate of long-term weight loss is very poor in both the general population and in patients with NIDDM. It is crucial that the physician stress to the patient the important relationship between food intake and diabetic control. Occasionally, a short hospitalization with strict dietary supervision will convince the patient that caloric restriction can greatly improve their metabolic control. In thin, Type II patients calories should not be restricted. The diet of all patients with NIDDM should be limited in fat and cholesterol with an increased ratio of polyunsaturated to saturated fats.

Oral Hypoglycemic Drugs

A substantial number of patients with Type II diabetes do not attain successful metabolic control with dietary therapy alone. In these patients, the use of an oral hypoglycemic agent in conjunction with diet is the next therapeutic step. There are several different oral hypoglycemic agents available in this country (Table 72–7). The main difference between these sulfonylureas is their duration of action and the mode by which they are metabolized and excreted. While they exhibit a wide range of potency, no specific sulfonylurea, including the "second generation" drugs, has been shown to be any more effective in low-

TABLE 72–7. ORAL HYPOGLYCEMIC DRUGS

GENERIC NAME	BRAND NAME	DAILY DOSE (mg)	DOSES/DAY	DURATION OF EFFECT (hours)
Tolbutamide	Orinase	500–3000	2–3	6–12
Chlorpropamide	Diabinase	100–500	1	60
Acetohexamide	Dymelor	250–1500	1–2	12–24
Tolazamide	Tolinase	100–1000	1–2	10–18
Glyburide	Micronase Diabeta	2.5–20	1–2	10–30
Glipizide	Glucotrol	5–40	1–2	18–30

ering blood glucose levels. The sulfonylureas lower blood glucose levels by enhancing insulin secretion by the beta cells of the pancreas and/or by increasing the sensitivity of tissues to the metabolic effects of insulin.

The major complication of oral hypoglycemic drug therapy is hypoglycemia, most frequently observed with long-acting agents such as chlorpropamide. Elderly patients, those who abuse ethanol, and those with either renal or hepatic disease are most likely to become hypoglycemic. Some diabetics, especially those receiving chlorpropamide, develop an antabuse–like intolerance to alcohol, with flushing. Idiosyncratic reactions may occur with gastrointestinal symptoms, diffuse skin rashes, cholestatic jaundice, agranulocytosis, and aplastic anemia, but these adverse reactions are very rare. Chlorpropamide potentiates the secretion and/or the action of ADH and therefore can result in water retention and hyponatremia, especially in patients with congestive heart failure or cirrhosis.

Insulin

Some patients with NIDDM require insulin therapy. Acceptable metabolic control may not be achievable with oral hypoglycemic agents (primary failure) or a patient who initially responded to oral agents may, with time, no longer achieve adequate control (secondary failure). Additionally, in some Type II diabetic patients who are thin and have had very high blood glucose levels, it may be preferable to treat initially with insulin because these patients, in general, do not do well with other treatments.

The use of insulin in Type II diabetes is similar to that described in Type I patients above, except that because of the presence of insulin resistance, higher doses of insulin are frequently required. Additionally, because of some residual endogenous insulin secretion, NIDDM patients are more likely to be well-controlled on simpler regimens, such as a single daily dose of an intermediate insulin, than are patients with IDDM.

MONITORING DIABETIC CONTROL

Traditionally, diabetic control has been monitored by measuring urine glucose concentration at various times throughout the day. The concentration of glucose in the urine is dependent on the renal threshold for glucose excretion (quite variable in the diabetic patient), the renal blood flow, and the urine volume. As a result, the correlation between urine glucose values and blood glucose measurements has generally been poor. Additionally, because the renal threshold for plasma glucose is approximately 180 mg/dl, urinary glucose measurements are negative when the plasma glucose is less than 180 mg/dl and, therefore, one cannot determine the degree of control in the glucose range that is most important.

Home blood glucose monitoring, employing a variety of different techniques, is the method of choice for monitoring diabetic control. Patients are instructed to measure their blood glucose levels at various times throughout the day as a basis for therapy. The accurate and routine measurement of home blood glucose levels is an essential ingredient in any intensive treatment regimen.

The measurement of glycosylated hemoglobin is very useful in assessing the degree of control over the preceding several months. Nonenzymatic glycosylation of hemoglobin is proportional to and therefore reflects average blood glucose experienced by the red blood cell during its lifespan. In normals, approximately 5 to 8 per cent of the hemoglobin is glycosylated, whereas in diabetics, as much as 20 per cent is in the glycosylated form. With tight control, the percentage of hemoglobin that is glycosylated will decrease and approach that in normal subjects. Glycosylated hemoglobin measurements, while useful in giving an overall picture of metabolic control, are not helpful in making specific adjustments in insulin therapy.

Lastly, quantitative measurement of glucose in 24-hour urine samples has been used to assess diabetic control. The excretion of less than 10 grams of glucose per day is indicative of excellent control.

ACUTE COMPLICATIONS

Diabetic Ketoacidosis

Diabetic ketoacidosis is characterized by hyperglycemia, acidosis (pH < 7.2, HCO_3^- < 15 mEq/L), and elevated plasma ketone concentrations. The hyperglycemia is secondary to insulin deficiency, which leads to both an increase in hepatic glucose production and a decrease in peripheral glucose utilization. Hyperglycemia produces an osmotic diuresis that can result in volume depletion and urinary loss of electrolytes.

Plasma ketone levels rise because of their overproduction by the liver. In the insulin-deficient state, especially if there is an increased secretion of catecholamines, excessive amounts of free fatty acids are released from the adipose tissue and transported to the liver. In the liver, free fatty acids can either be re-esterified or enter the mitochondria and be oxidized to ketones. In patients with hypoinsulinemia and hyperglucagonemia, fatty acids preferentially enter the mitochondria at an accelerated rate, resulting in an increased production of ketones. Thus, ketosis requires both an increased delivery of free fatty acids to the liver and a liver that is primed to transport them into the mitochondria. Low plasma insulin levels, in conjunction with elevations in glucagon and other hormones, can result in both of these conditions and thus account for the ketosis. The accompanying acidosis results from the accumulation of the keto acids, β-hydroxybutyrate and acetoacetate, and is associated with low serum bicarbonate levels and an anion gap.

Patients with diabetic ketoacidosis usually present after several days of polyuria and polydipsia with associated nausea, vomiting, anorexia, and occasionally abdominal pain. The abdominal pain can sometimes mimic an acute abdominal condition. Diabetic ketoacidosis occurs in both young and old diabetic patients and may be the presenting manifestation of the disease. Infections, trauma, cardiovascular events, emotional stress, and omission of insulin are common precipitating causes, but in some cases, there is no obvious etiology for the diabetic ketoacidosis. In all patients with diabetic ketoacidosis a careful search for the precipitating factor is required.

Patients with diabetic ketoacidosis typically exhibit tachypnea, dehydration, acetone halitosis (a fruity odor on the breath), and an altered mental status ranging from disorientation to coma. The alteration in mental status correlates directly with elevations in the serum osmolality. Kussmaul respirations are usually present when the acidosis is severe.

The clinical diagnosis of diabetic ketoacidosis should be confirmed by demonstrating elevations in blood glucose levels, ketones in the blood or urine, and acidosis. The blood glucose levels can be quite variable, ranging from 200 mg/dl to values greater than 1000 mg/dl. Blood and urine ketones are usually measured semiquantitatively by using Keto-Diastix or Acetest tablets. Both of these methods detect primarily acetoacetate (the nitroprusside reaction). In ketoacidosis, β-hydroxybutyrate levels are usually higher than the acetoacetate levels, and thus the actual degree of ketosis is not accurately measured by the nitroprusside reaction. In patients with concomitant lactic acidosis or ethanol intake, β-hydroxybutyrate levels are much higher than acetoacetate levels, and the routine tests for ketosis can be falsely low. Additionally, during the course of treatment of diabetic ketoacidosis, β-hydroxybutyrate may be converted to acetoacetate, giving the false impression that the diabetic ketoacidosis is worsening.

In the treatment of diabetic ketoacidosis the clinical status must be frequently and carefully assessed. A complete flow sheet, including fluids, electrolytes, and insulin administered, as well as laboratory data, is extremely helpful in monitoring therapy.

Many insulin regimens have been successfully used in the treatment of diabetic ketoacidosis, varying from continuous intravenous insulin to intermittent boluses of intramuscular or subcutaneous insulin. In the majority of patients, 5 to 10 units of regular insulin/hour given intravenously, intramuscularly, or subcutaneously are adequate to correct the metabolic disturbance. In patients who are hypotensive, intravenous administration of the insulin is desirable because the absorption of the insulin may be impaired due to poor tissue perfusion. Regardless of the route of administration and dosage, it is important to follow closely the decline in blood glucose levels. If the blood glucose concentrations are not decreasing, one should increase the insulin dosage and strongly consider employing the intravenous route.

Patients with diabetic ketoacidosis are usually dehydrated and hypovolemic. The average fluid deficit in adults is approximately 6 liters. Rapid volume expansion is usually required; this is best begun by administering normal saline at a rate of 1 liter/hour. In patients with cardiovascular or renal disease, slower rates of administration may be necessary. After the delivery of 2 liters of normal saline, if there are no signs of orthostatic hypotension, the rate of fluid administration can be decreased and the solution switched to half-normal saline. The remainder of the fluid deficit should be replaced over the next 12 to 24 hours.

On initial evaluation, many patients with diabetic ketoacidosis are hyperkalemic because of acidosis, dehydration, and hypoinsulinemia, but total body potassium stores are usually depleted. With correction of the acidosis and dehydration and the administration of insulin, plasma potassium concentrations will decrease. To prevent hypokalemia, it is very important to administer potassium in the intravenous fluids (20 to 40 mEq KCl per liter) as soon as urine flow is established and renal function is adequate.

Phosphate depletion also occurs in diabetic ketoacidosis, but its replacement has not been shown to have a beneficial clinical effect. Therefore, the routine administration of phosphate is not indicated unless an additional disorder that also depletes body phosphate stores is present. Bicarbonate replacement also should not routinely be administered to patients with diabetic ketoacidosis unless the patient is severely acidotic (pH < 6.9).

Once the plasma glucose is in the range of 250 mg/dl, glucose should be included in the intravenous fluids to prevent hypoglycemia. Insulin administration should not be discontinued when the glucose falls because this will result in the recurrence of diabetic ketoacidosis. When the acidosis has cleared, the dehydration has been corrected, and the patient is eating, it is possible to return to the usual diabetic treatment schedules.

The major complications of the treatment of diabetic ketoacidosis are (1) hypoglycemia, (2) hypokalemia, and (3) cerebral edema. Both the hypoglycemia and hypokalemia can be prevented by careful management. Cerebral edema is very rare, is usually observed in children, and may occur because of the too-rapid correction of the metabolic disturbance.

Nonketotic Hyperosmolar Syndrome

This disorder primarily occurs in Type II diabetics who present with dehydration, hypovolemia, and cerebral symptoms ranging from confusion to coma. Blood glucose levels are markedly elevated (600 to 2000 mg/dl), but ketosis and acidosis are not present. The absence of ketones may be secondary to residual insulin secretion sufficient to suppress lipolysis. The symptoms of poorly controlled diabetes have frequently been present for several days to weeks prior to presentation, and the acute decompensation is often secondary to an inability to consume adequate quantities of water, which may be precipitated by infection, stroke, myocardial infarction, abdominal disorder, etc. In the absence of sufficient water replacement, the hyperglycemia-induced osmotic diuresis results in dehydration, hypovolemia, impaired renal function, and decreased renal glucose excretion, which further increases plasma glucose levels.

Similar to diabetic ketoacidosis, the alterations in mental status are believed to be secondary to the high serum osmolality. Stupor and coma occur only when the effective serum osmolality is greater than 340 mOsm/liter [effective serum osmolality = $2(Na + K) + glucose/18$]. If the effective serum osmolality is not in this range, another etiology for the change in mental status should be sought.

The therapy of the hyperosmolar syndrome is very similar to that for diabetic ketoacidosis, with the administration of insulin, fluids, and potassium being the chief priorities. Patients with the hyperosmolar syndrome have a substantial mortality that is usually secondary to concomitant medical disorders such as myocardial infarction, stroke, infection, pulmonary emboli, etc.

CHRONIC COMPLICATIONS (Table 72–8)

The chronic complications of diabetes can be divided into three main categories: (1) Microvascular disease, which is specific for diabetes, involves small blood vessels and is clinically manifested by eye and kidney disease. (2) Macrovascular disease, which involves the large blood vessels and is clinically manifested by coronary, cerebral, and peripheral vascular disease. The macrovascular disease is similar to that observed in nondiabetics. (3) Neuropathy, which can affect motor, sensory, cranial, and autonomic nerves. The diabetic is also particularly susceptible to develop foot ulcers as well as certain skin lesions especially of the legs, known as necrobiosis lipoidica diabeticorum, and diabetic dermopathy.

DIABETIC MICROANGIOPATHY

Eye

Diabetic retinopathy can be classified as *nonproliferative retinopathy* (background) or *proliferative retinopathy*. Nonproliferative retinopathy is characterized by microaneurysms, hard waxy exudates, cotton-wool or soft exudates, and retinal hemorrhages. Nonproliferative retinopathy is

TABLE 72–8. CHRONIC COMPLICATIONS OF DIABETES

Microvascular Disease
  Retinopathy
  Nephropathy
Macrovascular Disease
  Coronary artery disease
  Cerebrovascular disease
  Peripheral vascular disease
Neuropathic
  Peripheral symmetrical polyneuropathy
  Mononeuropathies
  Autonomic neuropathies
  Diabetic amyotrophy
Foot Ulcers
Dermopathies

very common, and its frequency increases with the duration of diabetes. By 10 years, approximately 50 per cent and by 20 years, approximately 90 per cent of diabetics have nonproliferative retinopathy. Nonproliferative retinopathy usually does not impair vision and, in many diabetics, remains relatively stable.

In a small percentage of diabetics, nonproliferative retinopathy progresses to proliferative retinopathy. Proliferative retinopathy is characterized by neovascularization (new vessel formation), which can result in vitreous hemorrhages and traction retinal detachments that lead to severe visual loss or blindness. The incidence of proliferative retinopathy increases with the duration of diabetes. Approximately 25 per cent of Type I diabetics develop proliferative retinopathy after 20 years of disease. Laser photocoagulation, the main treatment of proliferative retinopathy, can greatly decrease the incidence of visual loss.

Macular edema, which is due to the accumulation of intraretinal fluid secondary to breakdown of the blood/brain barrier, can result in a marked impairment of central vision. Macular edema is a common cause of visual loss in elderly diabetics. Laser therapy may also be beneficial in the treatment of this type of diabetic eye disease.

Other nonmicroangiopathic disorders, such as cataracts and glaucoma, occur more frequently in patients with diabetes and can adversely affect visual acuity.

Kidney Disease

The first major clinical manifestation of diabetic nephropathy is persistent proteinuria (> 500 mg/24 hr) which usually occurs between 15 and 20 years after the onset of diabetes in approximately 50 per cent of Type I diabetics. Microproteinuria may be seen many years earlier and is thought to be predictive of the eventual development of significant renal disease. The proteinuria, if of significant magnitude, can cause all of the classic features of the nephrotic syndrome. Hypertension is also present in most patients with renal dysfunction, and treatment of the hypertension is thought to slow the progression of renal disease. In addition to proteinuria, a slow but persistent decrease in glomerular filtration rate occurs, eventually resulting in azotemia. On the average, azotemia occurs three years after the onset of persistent proteinuria, and end-stage renal failure develops three years after the azotemia. The rate of loss of renal function is quite variable among diabetic patients, but for any individual patient, the loss occurs at a predictable rate. There is a linear inverse relationship between serum creatinine concentration and time which allows one to predict the progression of dysfunction by plotting serial laboratory values.

The diagnosis of diabetic nephropathy is usually obvious; renal biopsy is rarely required. An active urinary sediment, the absence of retinopathy or an atypical clinical course are indications for renal biopsy. Contrast studies, such as intravenous pyelography, should not be routinely conducted without clear indications, since rapid deterioration of renal function has been observed in azotemic diabetic patients following such studies. When a contrast study is necessary, diabetic patients should be well-hydrated prior to the procedure.

In any diabetic with renal failure, it is important to consider other factors that could be contributing to the renal dysfunction. The possibility of a neurogenic bladder secondary to diabetic neuropathy, urinary tract infections, uncontrolled hypertension, or renal papillary necrosis needs to be considered. Renal failure, regardless of etiology, tends to decrease the daily insulin requirement, and therefore the treatment regimen may need to be adjusted.

Diabetic patients with renal failure are treated with either hemodialysis, peritoneal dialysis, or renal transplantation. In general, the death rate of diabetic patients on dialysis is greater than that observed in nondiabetic patients. Additionally, because of the progression of retinopathy, neuropathy, and vascular disease, the functional status of diabetic patients on hemodialysis is generally poor. The results of renal transplantation in a select group of diabetic patients have been encouraging, with survival rates in the diabetics approaching those observed in nondiabetics.

MACROVASCULAR DISEASE

Arteriosclerosis is a common problem in diabetics and occurs more extensively and earlier than in the general population. The etiology of the accelerated atherosclerosis in diabetics is unknown, but the causes are probably multifactorial. Because of the high risk of atherosclerosis, the usual risk factors for vascular disease must be aggressively treated. Diabetic patients should be strongly encouraged to stop smoking, and hypertension, if present, should be carefully treated. Elevated plasma lipid levels are frequently observed in diabetic patients, and efforts should be made to reduce them. Plasma lipid levels will frequently improve with control of the hyperglycemia. In populations such as Japan, with a low incidence of atherosclerosis, the incidence of vascular disease in diabetic patients is much lower than in the United States, suggesting that the amelioration of other risk factors will be very beneficial.

Atherosclerotic vascular disease in diabetic patients affects the coronary, cerebral, and peripheral vessels, and the manifestations of vascular disease are similar to those observed in nondiabetics. There is a tendency for the vascular disease to be more diffuse in diabetics, making vascular reconstructive surgery more difficult. Nevertheless, the indications for vascular surgery and the success of vascular surgery are not significantly different than in the nondiabetic population.

NEUROPATHY

Diabetic neuropathy is a common disabling complication of diabetes, resulting in a great deal of morbidity and a reduced quality of life. Diabetic neuropathy may be classified into four main categories:

Symmetrical Distal Polyneuropathy

This form of neuropathy usually presents with a loss of sensation in a "stocking-glove" distribution that is most commonly observed bilaterally in the distal lower extremities but can also affect the upper extremities. The decreased sensory perception may result in neuropathic foot ulcers or Charcot joints. Frequently, in addition to the lack of sensation, there is associated numbness, tingling, a "pins-and-needles" sensation, burning, cramping, or shooting pains. The pain and discomfort that occur in association with diabetic neuropathy can be very disabling and are often worse at night. In many instances, the pain spontaneously disappears in six months to one year. The pain associated with neuropathy has been treated with variable success with phenytoin, carbamazepine, or a combination of amitriptyline and fluphenazine. In addition to sensory nerve dysfunction, symmetrical motor nerve abnormalities can occur and are often manifested by bilateral wasting of the interosseous muscles of the hand. This polyneuropathy and the autonomic neuropathies described below are thought by some to be secondary to the metabolic abnormalities of diabetes.

Asymmetrical Neuropathy

Diabetic mononeuropathies can involve cranial nerves 3, 4, or 6, resulting in extraocular muscle paralysis with diplopia. The most common syndrome is a third nerve palsy with sparing of the pupillary reflex. The onset is usually abrupt, and pain around the eye frequently occurs. Findings are occasionally bilateral, and more than one cranial nerve can be involved. Spontaneous recovery generally occurs in 3 to 12 months, but recurrences are not uncommon.

Peripheral nerve mononeuropathies usually occur at sites of external pressure and can result in wrist or foot drop. Mononeuropathies can also affect sensory nerves and result in painful dysesthesias and hypesthesias localized to the anatomical distribution of the nerve. Similar to the mononeuropathies affecting the cranial nerves, these neuropathies frequently remit spontaneously in several weeks to months. These mononeuropathies are thought to be due to a vascular insult.

Autonomic Neuropathy

Diabetic autonomic neuropathy has a wide variety of clinical manifestations affecting a number of different organs. Most patients with significant autonomic neuropathies also have symmetrical distal polyneuropathies.

Impotence is a common manifestation of autonomic neuropathy but, of course, is often due to other etiologies, such as vascular insufficiency, psychological causes, or endocrinological dysfunction. A neurogenic bladder with associated urinary retention and urinary tract infections is another very troublesome complication. Orthostatic hypotension occurs secondary to autonomic neuropathies and can be disabling if severe. The entire gastrointestinal tract can be affected by autonomic nerve dysfunction, resulting in dysphagia, gastroparesis, intermittent diarrhea, especially with postprandial and nocturnal discharge, constipation, and anal incontinence. Gastroparesis can result in poor diabetic control because of the erratic food absorption. Abnormal sweating, manifested by anhidrosis or hyperhidrosis, is also sometimes observed.

Diabetic Amyotrophy

Diabetic amyotrophy is a type of neuropathy that occurs mainly in elderly men and most commonly presents with unilateral atrophy and weakness of the large muscle groups of the upper leg and pelvic girdle. The neuropathy on occasion can be bilateral and/or affect the upper extremity. In addition to the neuropathy, marked weight loss and depression are frequently observed. In the majority of cases, recovery occurs spontaneously in 6 to 12 months.

FOOT ULCERS

Foot ulcers can occur in diabetic patients secondary to large vessel atherosclerosis, microangiopathy, neuropathy, or a combination of these factors. Ulcers secondary to large vessel disease characteristically occur on the tip of the toes, whereas those secondary to neuropathy occur in areas of weight-bearing and pressure (plantar surface).

The best therapy of diabetic foot ulcers is prevention. Patients with diabetes should be instructed to examine their feet daily for calluses, blisters, or inflammation, and their feet should be kept clean and dry. In addition, the shoes of a diabetic should be properly fitted and patients should be instructed to wear new shoes for short periods of time until well broken-in. Walking barefoot is dangerous and should be strongly discouraged. Meticulous foot care can decrease the incidence of ulcers and gangrene and prevent amputations.

REFERENCES

Bradley WE (ed): Aspects of diabetic autonomic neuropathy. Ann Intern Med 92 (2 Suppl, Part 2):289, 1980.

Cahill GF Jr, and McDevitt HO: Insulin dependent diabetes mellitus: The initial lesion. N Engl J Med 304:1454, 1981.

Feingold KR: Hypoglycemia: A pitfall of insulin therapy. West J Med 139:688, 1983.

Foster DW, and McGarry JD: The metabolic derangements and treatment of diabetic ketoacidosis. N Engl J Med 309:159, 1983.

Ganda OP: Pathogenesis of macrovascular disease in the human diabetic. Diabetes 29:931, 1980.

Health and Public Policy Committee, American College of Physicians: Glycosylated hemoglobin assays in the management and diagnosis of diabetes mellitus. Ann Intern Med 101:710, 1984.

Kohner EM, and Barry PJ: Prevention of blindness in diabetic retinopathy. Diabetologia 26:173, 1984.

LoGerfo FW, and Coffman JD: Current concepts: Vascular and microvascular disease of the foot in diabetes: Implications for foot care. N Engl J Med 311:1615, 1984.

National Diabetes Data Group. Classification and diagnosis of diabetes mellitus and other categories of glucose intolerance. Diabetes 28:1039, 1979.

Nutall FQ: Diet and the diabetic patient. Diabetes Care 6:197, 1983.

Olefsky JM: Diabetes mellitus. In Wyngaarden JB, and Smith LH Jr (eds): Cecil Textbook of Medicine. 17th ed. Philadelphia, WB Saunders Co, 1985, pp 1320–1341.

Symposium on home blood glucose monitoring. Diabetes Care, 3:57, 1980.

73 HYPOGLYCEMIA

The diagnosis of hypoglycemia is based on the presence of the triad of a low plasma glucose concentration, symptoms consistent with hypoglycemia, and the improvement of these symptoms following an increase in plasma glucose levels. Hypoglycemia has often arbitrarily been defined as a plasma glucose level less than 50 mg/dl, but plasma glucose levels below 50 mg/dl may occur in normal subjects, especially during oral glucose tolerance tests. Furthermore, in a significant percentage of healthy young women (but rarely in men) a 24-hour fast also results in a plasma glucose level below 50 mg/dl. Therefore, in men a fasting plasma glucose less than 45 to 50 mg/dl is highly suspicious of significant hypoglycemia, whereas in women the fasting plasma glucose must be below 35 to 40 mg/dl to be abnormal.

Plasma glucose levels should be interpreted in relation to a patient's symptoms. During a 5-hour oral glucose tolerance test at least 10 per cent of normal individuals have plasma glucose levels less than 50 mg/dl, but few are symptomatic. Conversely, many patients have symptoms resembling those observed with hypoglycemia, even though the plasma glucose level is not below the "normal" range. Additionally, it is important to

TABLE 73–1. SYMPTOMS AND SIGNS OF HYPOGLYCEMIA

Secondary to Catecholamine Release (Adrenergic)
- Sweating
- Shakiness
- Anxiety
- Palpitations
- Weakness
- Tremor
- Hunger
- Faintness
- Tachycardia

Secondary to CNS Dysfunction (Neuroglucopenic)
- Confusion
- Irritability
- Headaches
- Abnormal behavior
- Weakness
- Diplopia
- Inappropriate affect
- Motor incoordination
- Convulsions
- Coma

Nocturnal Hypoglycemia (usually due to excessive insulin therapy)
- Morning headaches
- Lassitude
- Night sweats
- Nightmares
- Difficulty in waking
- Psychological changes
- Restlessness during sleep
- Loud respirations
- Symptoms do not usually awaken the patient.

demonstrate that the symptoms, presumed to be secondary to hypoglycemia, improve or disappear with increases in plasma glucose following carbohydrate ingestion. Therefore *the triad of a low plasma glucose, symptoms consistent with hypoglycemia, and the improvement of these symptoms following an increase of plasma glucose concentration is necessary to confirm the diagnosis of hypoglycemia (Whipple's triad).*

CLINICAL MANIFESTATIONS

The symptoms of hypoglycemia result from catecholamine release or from impaired CNS function (Table 73–1). The degree of hypoglycemia that produces symptoms and the clinical manifestations produced are quite variable from individual to individual. In a particular individual, the symptoms induced by hypoglycemia tend to be reproducible. The adrenergic symptoms predominate when plasma glucose concentrations fall rapidly, whereas the cerebral manifestations of hypoglycemia may appear without the adrenergic warning when the decrease in plasma glucose levels occurs slowly or when hypoglycemia is a chronic problem. The symptoms and signs of hypoglycemia usually are rapidly reversible with treatment, but permanent brain damage can result from prolonged severe hypoglycemia.

CAUSES OF HYPOGLYCEMIA
(Table 73–2)

The classification of the causes of hypoglycemia is based on whether symptoms occur in the fasting state or following food intake (postprandial). Occasionally patients with fasting hypoglycemia, especially if it is due to an insulinoma, can have postprandial hypoglycemia as well. An approach to the evaluation of patients suspected of having hypoglycemia is shown in Figure 73–1.

FASTING HYPOGLYCEMIA

Insulinoma

Insulinomas are relatively rare tumors that occur most commonly between the ages of 40 and 70 years and in approximately equal frequency in men and women. Between 5 and 10 per cent of insulinomas are malignant; in 10 per cent of cases multiple benign tumors are present. In patients with the multiple endocrine neoplasia Type I (MEN I) syndrome, insulinomas occur at an earlier age and multiple benign tumors are very common.

The symptoms of hypoglycemia may be present for many years prior to the diagnosis of an insulinoma because the symptoms of chronic hypoglycemia are nonspecific and not initially attributed to hypoglycemia. Often the patients are thought to have a psychiatric or neurological disorder prior to the correct diagnosis. Patients sometimes increase their food consumption to prevent symptoms and, therefore, obesity is occasionally observed.

The diagnosis of an insulinoma is based on the demonstration of a low plasma glucose level in the presence of an inappropriately high plasma insulin concentration. The most reliable test is a prolonged *supervised fast*. In normal individuals, fasting results in a decline in both plasma glucose and insulin levels. In the majority of patients with an insulinoma hypoglycemia occurs within 24

TABLE 73–2. CAUSES OF HYPOGLYCEMIA

Fasting
- Insulinoma
- Extrapancreatic tumors
- Hormonal deficiency—glucocorticoids, growth hormone, glucagon, and epinephrine
- Chronic renal failure
- Extensive hepatic dysfunction
- Starvation
- Drugs—insulin, oral hypoglycemic agents, ethanol, salicylates, propranolol, pentamidine, disopyramide, and quinine when used to treat malaria
- Disorders of childhood—glycogen storage diseases
- Immune disease with insulin antibodies

Postprandial
- Alimentary hypoglycemia
- Idiopathic reactive hypoglycemia
- Leucine intolerance
- Genetic disorders—galactosemia, fructose intolerance

Artifactual
- Leukemia
- Polycythemia

hours, but in a small number of patients a fast lasting 72 hours with or without exercise will be required to induce hypoglycemia. Plasma for insulin measurements should be obtained at the time the patient is hypoglycemic. In patients with an insulinoma, plasma insulin levels are inappropriately elevated. During the fast a patient suspected of harboring an insulinoma must be closely observed for symptoms of hypoglycemia, and if symptoms occur the plasma glucose must be rapidly determined and the fast terminated if the patient is hypoglycemic. Additionally, it is important to measure plasma glucose levels every four to six hours because patients with significant hypoglycemia may at times be asymptomatic.

In addition to determining plasma insulin levels, it is also helpful to measure plasma C-peptide concentrations during the fast to eliminate the possibility of self administration of insulin as the etiology of the hypoglycemia. In individuals who surreptitiously administer insulin, plasma C-peptide levels will be very low; in patients with an insulinoma, plasma C-peptide levels are elevated

in parallel with insulin, reflecting its rate of secretion.

In the past many provocative maneuvers such as the use of glucagon, tolbutamide, leucine, or calcium were employed to diagnose patients with insulinomas. Currently, because of the high frequency of false-positive and false-negative results, these tests are only rarely used for this purpose.

Once the diagnosis of an insulinoma is firmly established, additional studies may be helpful in localizing the tumor within the pancreas. CT scans and ultrasonography detect only relatively large tumors. Celiac or superior mesenteric arteriography may detect smaller tumors as vascular masses. Nevertheless, in a significant number of patients with insulinomas radiographic studies do not localize the insulinoma. In some centers percutaneous transhepatic portal venography with selective blood sampling for insulin measurement may be useful in the localization of insulinomas. However, failure to localize an insulinoma should not obviate surgery, since experienced surgeons

FIGURE 73–1. Evaluation of hypoglycemic disorders. (From Service FJ: Hypoglycemic disorders. In Wyngaarden JB, and Smith LH Jr (eds): Cecil Textbook of Medicine. 17th ed. Philadelphia, WB Saunders Co, 1985, p 1343.)

are very often successful in localizing the tumor intraoperatively. Serum levels of HCG or one of its subunits are elevated in approximately two thirds of patients with a malignant insulinoma, but not in individuals with benign insulinomas.

The treatment of an insulinoma is the surgical removal of the tumor, which will usually restore normal glycemia. In approximately 5 to 10 per cent of individuals, hypoglycemia will persist following surgery, owing to metastatic insulinomas, islet cell hypertrophy, or a tumor that could not be located during surgery. These patients will require medical therapy to prevent hypoglycemic episodes. Initial treatment should include frequent high carbohydrate feedings. If this is not successful, diazoxide, a drug that inhibits insulin secretion, can be administered. Other drugs that are occasionally beneficial in the medical treatment of insulinomas include phenytoin and propranolol. Streptozotocin with or without 5-fluorouracil is useful in the treatment of malignant insulinomas that cannot be surgically removed.

Extrapancreatic Tumors

Hypoglycemia also occurs secondary to a wide variety of neoplasms. Mesenchymal tumors or sarcomas located in the retroperitoneal spaces of the chest and abdomen are the tumors most commonly implicated and are usually very large and easily detectable. Hypoglycemia has also been described in association with hematologic malignancies, hepatomas, and adrenocortical, gastrointestinal, bronchial, and pancreatic carcinomas.

The mechanism by which tumors cause hypoglycemia is unresolved and probably varies depending upon tumor type. Plasma insulin levels are low during hypoglycemia, indicating that ectopic insulin production by the tumor is not the cause of the hypoglycemia. In some instances, elevated levels of a substance that resembles nonsuppressible insulin-like activity (insulin-like growth factors) have been found, and it is possible that the production by the tumor of such hormones could account for the hypoglycemia. Other possible mechanisms for tumor-induced hypoglycemia include increased utilization of glucose by the tumor; metastatic destruction of the liver, adrenals, or pituitary glands; the production of substances that inhibit hepatic glycogenesis; and generalized cachexia. Total or partial surgical removal of the tumor is the ideal treatment and usually results in the amelioration of the hypoglycemia. However, most of the tumors associated with hypoglycemia cannot be resected and, therefore, management must be directed toward increasing plasma glucose levels through frequent feedings, glucose infusions, and prednisone therapy.

Hepatic, Renal, and Endocrine Disease

Hypoglycemia secondary to liver disease, other than that due to hepatomas, is rare and is usually associated with massive hepatic necrosis. In order for hypoglycemia to occur as a result of liver disease, approximately 80 to 90 per cent of the liver must be destroyed, and therefore the hypoglycemia is frequently a premorbid event. Hypoglycemia that occurs in the setting of cirrhosis is most commonly due to ethanol ingestion.

In patients with Addison's disease hypoglycemia will occur with prolonged fasting. Adequate cortisol replacement prevents the hypoglycemia. Hypopituitarism, regardless of etiology, may also result in hypoglycemia because of low cortisol levels and impaired growth hormone production. Cortisol replacement prevents symptomatic hypoglycemia in adults, but in children hypoglycemia can still occur despite adequate cortisol replacement.

Occasional patients with chronic renal failure develop hypoglycemia; this complication is observed most commonly in cachectic individuals.

Drug-Induced Hypoglycemia

Insulin. Insulin-induced hypoglycemia is a frequent occurrence in insulin-requiring diabetics. Most of these hypoglycemic reactions are mild and rapidly relieved by food ingestion. However, severe hypoglycemia requiring admission to the hospital is not infrequent. Moreover, death due to hypoglycemia occurs in approximately 2 to 7 per cent of insulin-dependent diabetics.

On rare occasions, a nondiabetic will surreptitiously take insulin and induce hypoglycemia. Most of these individuals are women who have been associated with the health professions. The presence of insulin antibodies in the plasma of a nondiabetic patient being evaluated for hypoglycemia is very suggestive of surreptitious insulin usage. The presence of antibodies to insulin will result in an artifactual elevation in plasma insulin levels when assayed in most radioimmunoassays. Additionally, as discussed earlier, the presence of hypoglycemia, high insulin levels, and a low C-peptide level indicates exogenous insulin administration as the etiology of hypoglycemia.

Oral Hypoglycemic Drugs. Hypoglycemia in diabetics on oral hypoglycemic drugs is much less common than in insulin-treated diabetic patients. Long-acting oral hypoglycemic agents such as chlorpropamide are more frequently associated with hypoglycemia than are short-acting agents such as tolbutamide. Severe hypoglycemia secondary to oral hypoglycemic agents occurs most commonly in patients who abuse ethanol or have renal or hepatic disease.

The surreptitious use of oral hypoglycemic agents can induce hypoglycemia in nondiabetics. In these cases, the insulin and C-peptide measurements are identical to those seen in patients with insulinomas. When oral agents are suspected as the cause of hypoglycemia in nondiabetics, either blood or urine should be assayed for the presence of these drugs.

Ethanol Ingestion. The syndrome of ethanol-induced hypoglycemia is most prevalent in chronically malnourished alcoholic males and occurs because ethanol inhibits hepatic gluconeogenesis. Nonalcoholics are also susceptible to ethanol-induced fasting hypoglycemia, which can occur with moderate ethanol intake in individuals who have missed one or two meals. Diabetics using insulin or oral hypoglycemics are particularly at risk for ethanol-induced hypoglycemia.

POSTPRANDIAL HYPOGLYCEMIA
(Reactive Hypoglycemia)

True postprandial hypoglycemia is most commonly observed in patients who have undergone gastric surgery (alimentary hypoglycemia). In these individuals rapid gastric emptying with brisk glucose absorption and secretion of gastrointestinal hormones leads to excessive insulin release. Glucose is metabolized rapidly, but the insulin levels remain high, resulting in hypoglycemia approximately one to two hours postprandially. Very rarely alimentary hypoglycemia is present in patients who have not undergone gastric surgery. The elimination of simple sugars, especially beverages, from the diet usually results in an improvement of symptoms.

Diabetes mellitus in its earliest phases is frequently listed as a cause of reactive hypoglycemia, but this is not well-documented. Symptomatic hypoglycemia as a premonitory symptom of diabetes occurs very rarely, if at all.

Idiopathic postprandial hypoglycemia is a rare syndrome whose mechanism is unknown. Much more common are patients with "nonhypoglycemia," who have a wide variety of nonspecific symptoms that occur two to five hours after a meal. The lay press and misinformed physicians have often attributed these nonspecific symptoms to hypoglycemia. In some of these patients, oral glucose tolerance tests are performed and, just as in normal individuals without symptoms, occasionally low blood glucose levels are observed. Because of the high frequency in normal individuals of plasma glucose concentrations below 50 mg/dl during oral glucose tolerance tests, this procedure is not very helpful in attempting to diagnose postprandial hypoglycemia. It is far better to measure plasma glucose levels after meals that are similar to those that caused the symptoms in the individual under study. After these more typical test meals, hypoglycemia is not consistently observed in the vast majority of patients. Occasionally, one will observe a patient in whom both symptoms and low plasma glucose levels occur simultaneously and consistently after a test meal. In these individuals idiopathic postprandial hypoglycemia is a reasonable diagnosis, and they should be treated with frequent small meals that are low in carbohydrate and high in protein. Much more commonly the symptoms attributed to hypoglycemia occur after the test meal but the plasma glucose levels are within the normal range. The explanation for these patients' symptoms may be related to adrenergic stimulation, but the symptoms should not be attributed to hypoglycemia.

TREATMENT OF SEVERE HYPOGLYCEMIA

The initial treatment of a confused or comatose patient with hypoglycemia is to infuse a bolus of 50 ml of 50 per cent glucose intravenously. In every unconscious patient hypoglycemia should be considered and a bolus of glucose administered as soon as possible. The bolus of glucose should be followed by the continuous infusion of 10 per cent glucose at a rate sufficient to keep the plasma glucose greater than 100 mg/dl. When the patient is capable of eating, a diet with a minimum of 300 grams/day of carbohydrates should be supplied. In many situations, especially following long-acting insulin or oral hypoglycemic drugs, the hypoglycemia will last for an extended period of time. It is very important to continue treatment and close observation for an extended period to prevent a relapse.

REFERENCES

Fajans SS, and Floyd JC Jr: Fasting hypoglycemia in adults. N Engl J Med 294:766, 1976.

Fajans SS, and Floyd JC Jr: Diagnosis and medical management of insulinomas. Annu Rev Med 30:313, 1979.

Gastineau CF: Is reactive hypoglycemia a clinical entity? Mayo Clin Proc 58:545, 1983.

Merimee TJ: Spontaneous hypoglycemia in man. Adv Intern Med 22:301, 1977.

Seltzer HS: Severe drug induced hypoglycemia: A review. Comp Ther 5:21, 1979.

Service FJ: Hypoglycemic disorders. In Wyngaarden JB, and Smith LH Jr (eds): Cecil Textbook of Medicine. 17th ed. Philadelphia, WB Saunders Co, 1985, pp 1341–1348.

Yager J, and Young RT: Nonhypoglycemia is an epidemic condition. N Engl J Med 291:907, 1974.

DISEASES OF BONE AND BONE MINERAL METABOLISM

74

NORMAL PHYSIOLOGY OF BONE AND BONE MINERALS

BONE STRUCTURE AND METABOLISM

One of the largest organs in the body, bone is a living tissue that is superbly constructed to carry out the following vital functions: (1) to provide the necessary support to maintain the structures of the body, including the integrity of such specialized "containers" as the thorax and the cranium; (2) to allow for movement by providing levers, articulations, and points of attachment for muscles; (3) to provide a reservoir of simple but essential elements such as calcium, magnesium, phosphorus, and sodium; (4) to surround and protect the hematopoietic system.

Bone is about two thirds mineral, largely hydroxyapatite with the approximate formula $Ca_{10}(PO_4)_6(OH)_2$. This mineral phase is deposited with high specificity at certain sites in Type I collagen, the major organic component of bone. In addition, bone contains water, various proteoglycans, and other noncollagenous proteins including osteocalcin, which contains a distinctive calcium-binding amino acid, γ-carboxyglutamic acid.

Bone Cells. At least three specialized cells in bone are necessary for the synthesis, modeling, and remodeling of this largely extracellular tissue:

OSTEOBLASTS. These mesenchymal cells secrete the three chains that make up Type I collagen to form osteoid, the uncalcified precursor of bone, at the surface sites of growth or remodeling. It is probable that osteoblasts also influence the local availability of calcium and/or phosphate necessary for mineralization. Osteoblasts contain alkaline phosphatase, the function of which is not clear. It may serve to hydrolyze pyrophosphate locally, a potent inhibitor of mineralization. With increased activity of osteoblasts the level of serum alkaline phosphatase rises; the increase of this isozyme of alkaline phosphatase is used clinically as a marker for osteoblastic activity.

OSTEOCYTES. Osteocytes are thought to be relatively quiescent osteoblasts that have become entrapped within the structure of bone. They appear to communicate with one another and with surface osteoblasts as a network through bone canaliculi. They probably play a role in mobilizing bone minerals, although the mechanisms involved are obscure.

OSTEOCLASTS. These multinucleated giant cells, derived from mononuclear phagocytic cells of hematopoietic origin, destroy bone as part of its continuous remodeling process. This complex process of destruction requires the removal of bone minerals followed by the action of collagenases and other proteolytic enzymes. Osteoclastic function is normally stimulated by parathyroid hormone (PTH) and probably by other factors as well: e.g., lymphokines (osteoclast-activating factor), growth factors, and prostaglandins of the E series.

Heparin can also stimulate osteoclasts. Deficiency of osteoclastic activity results in osteopetrosis (marble bone disease), a serious disorder of increased bone density.

Types of Bone. Bone is complex and heterogeneous in structure and is designed to give maximal strength with minimal mass (Fig. 74–1). In general there are two kinds of bone in the adult. *Cortical bone* is densely packed with concentric parallel layers of mineralized collagen surrounding its central vascular supply to form a unit known as an osteon or a haversian system. This type of bone is predominant in the cortex of long bones. Cortical bone serves principally for support. *Trabecular bone*, also called cancellous bone, forms a more open, spongy pattern and is predominant in the axial skeleton.

This type of bone serves as a calcium buffer for calcium homeostasis.

Bone Turnover. Even in the adult, bone is constantly being shaped and remodeled at its surfaces owing to the coordinated activities of osteoblasts, osteoclasts, and osteocytes, acting presumably under the influence of a number of exogenous factors, both known and unknown. As much as one fifth of bone calcium turns over annually, yet the destruction and formation of bone are normally closely coordinated. Bone biopsies demonstrate that in remodeling destruction and synthesis occur simultaneously but at distinct sites within the examined section. The balance between bone destruction and synthesis, which determines bone density, is influenced by stress on the bone through unknown mechanisms as well as by hormones.

Clinical Studies. Several techniques are available to study patients suspected of having generalized (metabolic) bone diseases:

1. Measurement of serum calcium, phosphorus, and alkaline phosphatase. The patterns of abnormalities discovered may give considerable information about the type of disorder, as will be documented later in the discussion of specific entities.

2. Measurement of parathyroid hormone and/or vitamin D, usually 25-OH-D. These measurements are usually obtained if abnormalities are noted in the tests mentioned above.

3. Studies of bone density. Routine radiographs of bone are notoriously insensitive for detecting generalized osteopenia but may demonstrate vertebral compression fractures in osteoporosis or pseudofractures (see below) in osteomalacia. Recently more accurate methods have become available to measure bone density: quantitative CT scans of vertebral trabecular bone, dual photon absorptiometry (used primarily for axial skeleton), and single photon absorptiometry (used primarily for the study of peripheral cortical bone).

4. Studies of bone turnover. Examination of sections of undemineralized bone obtained by trans-

FIGURE 74–1. Diagram of some of the main features of the microstructure of mature bone seen in both transverse (top) and longitudinal sections. Areas of cortical (compact) and trabecular (cancellous) bone are included. The central area in the transverse section simulates a microradiograph, with the differences in density reflecting variations in mineralization. Note the general construction of the osteons, the distribution of the osteocyte lacunae, the haversian systems, resorption spaces, and the different views of the structural basis of bone lamellation. (Adapted from Warwick R, Williams PL [eds.]: Gray's Anatomy. 35th ed. Edinburgh, Churchill Livingstone, 1973, p 217.)

iliac biopsy may demonstrate the relative activities of bone formation and destruction, especially when combined with the use of tetracycline given orally in advance at timed intervals. Tetracycline binds to recently mineralized bone, so the distance between bands is an indication of the rate of osteogenesis. As a research technique bone turnover can also be studied with isotopes such as $^{47}Ca^{++}$.

CALCIUM METABOLISM

A normal adult usually has 20 to 25 grams of calcium/kg of body weight, over 98 per cent of which is in the skeleton. Although our emphasis in this discussion is on bone formation, ionized calcium is also of great importance in many other functions, such as neuromuscular excitability, blood coagulation, and integrity of membranes, and as an intracellular second messenger for hormone action. Because of these various and important functions, the level of ionized calcium in extracellular fluid is carefully maintained in homeostasis.

Normal Plasma Calcium. Calcium circulates in plasma in three forms: (a) ionized as Ca^{++}, ap-proximately 46 per cent, (b) protein-bound (80 per cent to albumin), approximately 46 per cent, (c) diffusible but complexed, approximately 8 per cent (Fig. 74–2). Serum calcium is usually reported in the United States as its total concentration with a normal range of 8.9 to 10.1 mg/dl, rather than as a measurement of its biologically active ionized fraction. The bound fraction will vary as a percentage of total serum calcium based on the protein concentration and is often estimated as:

Per cent protein-bound calcium = 8 × albumin (grams/dl) + 2 × globulin (grams/dl) + 3

As a short-hand estimate, the serum calcium can be adjusted downward by 0.8 mg/dl for each 1 gram/dl decrease in serum albumin.

Absorption of Dietary Calcium. The average diet of an adult in the United States contains 600 to 1000 mg of calcium, in considerable measure derived from dairy products (milk has approximately 1 mg/ml). Usually there is a net absorption of 150 to 300 mg of calcium per day, in part by active transport in the proximal small intestine stimulated by 1,25-dihydroxycholecalciferol (Fig. 74–3). Calcium is present in all intestinal secre-

NORMAL RANGES			
	mg/dl	mmol/L	
TOTAL	8.9-10.1	2.2-2.5	
PROTEIN	4.1-4.7	1.0-1.2	46%
IONIZED	4.1-4.7	1.0-1.2	46% TOTAL PLASMA CALCIUM
COMPLEXED	0.7-0.8	0.18-0.2	8%
TOTAL	2.5-4.5	0.8-1.4	
PROTEIN BOUND	0.4-0.7	0.12-0.2	15%
FREE	2.1-3.8	0.68-1.2	85% TOTAL PLASMA PHOSPHORUS

$85\% = HPO_4^{2-} + NaHPO_4^-$
$15\% = H_2PO_4^-$

FIGURE 74–2. Distribution and normal ranges of calcium and phosphorus in the plasma. (From Arnaud CD: Mineral and bone homeostasis. In Wyngaarden JB, and Smith LH Jr (eds): Cecil Textbook of Medicine. 17th ed. Philadelphia, WB Saunders Co, 1985, p 1417.)

tions (bile, pancreatic and gastric juices, succus entericus), so that there is a fecal loss of about 100 mg of endogenous calcium per day. In general, calcium absorption is diminished in many generalized malabsorptive states (see Chapter 36C) as well as by hypovitaminosis D and dietary phytates or phosphate. Absorption is increased by 1,25-dihydroxycholecalciferol, with excessive calcium ingestion (the "milk-alkali syndrome"), and in absorptive idiopathic hypercalciuria.

Excretion of Calcium. As noted, some endogenous calcium is secreted into the gut with a net fecal loss of about 100 mg. The primary route of excretion, however, is via the kidney. Over 50 per cent of plasma calcium (that fraction not bound to protein) is filterable by the glomerulus, representing 7 to 10 grams in the glomerular filtrate per day. Only 100 to 250 mg of calcium are normally excreted in the urine, less than 4 mg/kg/24 hours, reflecting a net tubular reabsorption of about 98 per cent. Renal tubular reabsorption is enhanced by PTH, phosphate, metabolic alkalosis, thiazide diuretics, and enhanced reabsorption of sodium. Hypercalciuria may be caused by reduced PTH, metabolic acidosis, hypermagnesemia, and saline diuresis.

Calcium Balance. The level of ionized calcium in the extracellular fluid and the integrity of bone mineral content are homeostatically maintained over years of varied calcium ingestion by an effective balance of bone formation, bone destruc-

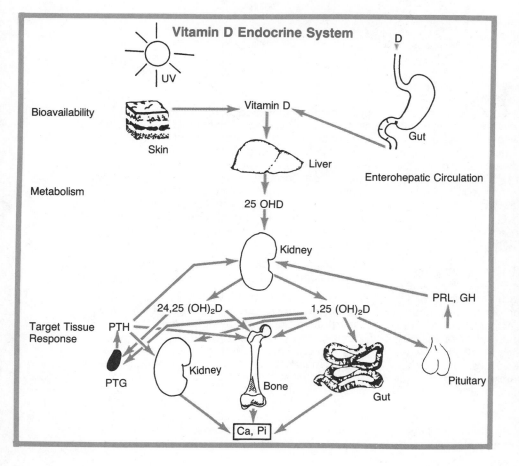

FIGURE 74–3. The vitamin D endocrine system. Vitamin D is made available to the body by photogenesis in the skin and absorption from the intestine. Vitamin D is then hydroxylated in the liver to 25OHD, then in the kidney to 1,25(OH)₂D and 24,25(OH)₂D. The active vitamin D metabolites act on different tissues to produce a variety of responses. The three target tissues principally responsible for calcium (Ca) and phosphate (Pi) homeostasis are kidney, bone, and intestine. Endocrine tissues such as the parathyroid gland (PTG) and anterior pituitary are also target tissues. Their hormones, parathyroid hormone (PTH), prolactin (PRL), and growth hormone (GH), help regulate vitamin D metabolism in the kidney. In addition, PTH has a direct effect on bone and kidney regulation of calcium and phosphate homeostasis. (Reproduced with permission from Bikle DD: The vitamin D endocrine system. In Stollerman GH, et al (eds): Advances in Internal Medicine, Volume 27. Copyright © 1982 by Year Book Medical Publishers, Inc., Chicago.)

tion, calcium absorption, and calcium excretion (Fig. 74–3). Some of the control mechanisms are known and will be described briefly below in separate sections (PTH, vitamin D, calcitonin); others are not. For convenience the symptoms and signs of hypercalcemia and hypocalcemia will be described in the chapter on the parathyroid glands (Chapter 75).

PHOSPHORUS METABOLISM

A normal adult usually has about 10 to 13 grams of phosphorus/kg of body weight (700 to 900 grams), of which about 80 to 85 per cent is in the skeleton and 10 per cent is in muscle. Phosphorus in the form of phosphate is necessary for a wide variety of structural and metabolic functions in addition to its role in bone mineralization: e.g., phospholipids in internal and external cell membranes, high-energy phosphate in energy capture and transfer ($\sim$P), as a second messenger in the endocrine system (cAMP), and as the backbone of DNA and RNA. Abnormalities of phosphorus metabolism can therefore lead to many manifestations.

Normal Plasma Phosphorus. In plasma the normal concentration of phosphorus is 2.5 to 4.5 mg/dl (0.8 to 1.4 mM). This is conventionally expressed as elemental P because the amount of P in its different forms ($H_2PO_4^-$, $HPO_4^=$) varies with pH. In contrast to calcium, 85 per cent is free and only 15 per cent is protein-bound (Fig. 74–2). The normal range of plasma P varies much more than that of calcium, including variation with age (higher in children). Plasma P is transiently reduced following carbohydrate ingestion; by insulin (because of the formation of intracellular phosphate esters); and by acute respiratory alkalosis.

Absorption of Dietary Phosphate. The average diet of an adult in the United States contains about 1000 mg of P, most of which (70 to 90 per cent) is absorbed by active transport. Deficiency of dietary phosphate or of absorption is rarely a cause of phosphate deficiency except in alcoholics or in patients taking large amounts of antacids, such as aluminum hydroxide, which bind phosphate in the intestine and prevent its absorption. The control of phosphate balance is largely in its excretion.

Excretion of Phosphate. Being non–protein-bound, most plasma phosphate is filtered by the glomerulus, following which about 70 to 90 per cent is actively reabsorbed, largely in the proximal tubule. Proximal tubular reabsorption of phosphate is increased by phosphate depletion, hypoparathyroidism, volume contraction, growth hormone, and hypocalcemia. Reabsorption is diminished (and renal clearance therefore increased) by phosphate loading, PTH, volume expansion, hypercalcemia, and carbonic anhydrase inhibitors, including thiazides and furosemide.

Hyperphosphatemia. Except for the condition of excessively rapid infusion of phosphate-containing solutions, hyperphosphatemia is encoun-

tered only in renal insufficiency (acute or chronic), hypoparathyroidism, acromegaly, rhabdomyolysis, or acute tumor lysis (e.g., chemotherapy of lymphoma). As noted, serum P is normally elevated over the usual adult range in growing children. The acute effects of elevating serum P are usually those of secondary hypocalcemia with tetany and/or seizures. Acute or chronic elevation of serum P may be associated with metastatic calcification.

Hypophosphatemia. The causes of hypophosphatemia most frequently encountered clinically are listed in Table 74–1. The long-term effects of phosphate depletion are commonly those of osteomalacia or rickets, to be described later (see Chapter 76). The acute effects are more likely to be metabolic (Table 74–2). Phosphate depletion may be associated with a reduction in erythro-

TABLE 74–1. CAUSES OF HYPOPHOSPHATEMIA*

Moderate hypophosphatemia (P 1.0 to 2.5 mg/dl)
  Hyperparathyroidism
  Osteomalacia (usually with hyperparathyroidism), malabsorption, deficiency of vitamin D, familial hypophosphatemic rickets, vitamin D–dependent rickets, oncogenic rickets
  Carbohydrate administration or ingestion or enhanced metabolism—glucose, fructose, glycerol, lactate, insulin administration
  Hypomagnesemia
  ECF volume expansion
  Acute alkalosis—bicarbonate infusion or moderate hyperventilation
  Hemodialysis
Severe hypophosphatemia (P less than 1.0 mg/dl)
  Chronic alcoholism and alcoholic withdrawal
  Diabetic ketoacidosis, recovery phase
  Enteric phosphate binding—excessive use of agents binding phosphate in the gut
  Hyperalimentation
  Nutritional recovery syndrome

* From Smith LH Jr: Phosphorus deficiency and hypophosphatemia. In Wyngaarden JB, and Smith LH Jr (eds): Cecil Textbook of Medicine. 17th ed. Philadelphia, WB Saunders Co, 1985, p 1164. Modified from Knochel JP: West J Med 134:15, 1981.

TABLE 74–2. CONSEQUENCES OF SEVERE HYPOPHOSPHATEMIA*

Acute—"metabolic"
  Hematologic
    Red cell dysfunction and hemolysis
    Leukocyte dysfunction
    Platelet dysfunction
  Muscle
    Weakness
    Rhabdomyolysis
    Myocardial dysfunction
  Central nervous system dysfunction
  Hepatic dysfunction
Chronic—"structural"
  Osteomalacia or rickets

* From Smith LH Jr: Phosphorus deficiency and hypophosphatemia. In Wyngaarden JB, and Smith LH Jr (eds): Cecil Textbook of Medicine. 17th ed. Philadelphia, WB Saunders Co, 1985, p 1164.

TABLE 74–3. CAUSES OF HYPOMAGNESEMIA (SEEN MOST FREQUENTLY CLINICALLY IN ALCOHOLISM AND MALABSORPTION)*

Decreased absorption from dietary sources
    Diet poor in magnesium
    Parenteral feeding without magnesium
    Ethanol effect on absorption
    Malabsorption syndromes
    Uremia
    Selective intestinal defect for magnesium absorption (rare)
Increased loss of magnesium from the body
    Gastrointestinal tract
    Kidney
        Primary renal tubular defects
        Secondary—diuretics, Ca^{++}, ethanol, expansion of ECF, diabetes mellitus, treatment with gentamicin, cis-platinum, or amphotericin
    Breast—lactation hypomagnesemia (mostly in cattle, rarely in humans)
Increased loss into bone ("hungry bone syndrome")

*From Smith LH Jr: Disorders of magnesium metabolism. In Wyngaarden JB, and Smith LH Jr (eds): Cecil Textbook of Medicine. 17th ed. Philadelphia, WB Saunders Co, 1985, p 1166.

cytic 2,3-diphosphoglycerate (2,3-DPG), a molecule that normally affects the dissociation curve of oxyhemoglobin to enhance tissue availability of oxygen. In phosphate deficiency, therefore, tissue delivery of oxygen may be impaired. In very severe phosphate deficiency (P < 1.0 mg/dl), erythrocytic ATP may be reduced low enough that the integrity of the cell membrane cannot be maintained, with resulting hemolytic anemia. Leukocyte and platelet dysfunction are less well-established. Patients may be generally weak; severe phosphate deficiency may lead to rhabdomyolysis, perhaps comparable in mechanism to hemolytic anemia. Central nervous system function may be impaired, with symptoms varying from fatigue and irritability to metabolic encephalopathy with coma. The metabolic abnormalities associated with hypophosphatemia and phosphate depletion are rapidly reversible with phosphate therapy. The structural changes in bone, as noted in Chapter 76, require months or even years of replacement therapy.

TABLE 74–4. CONSEQUENCES OF MAGNESIUM DEFICIENCY*

Neuromuscular
    Lethargy, weakness, fatigue, decreased mentation
    Neuromuscular irritability, in part due to associated hypocalcemia
    Hyaline and vacuolar degeneration of myofibers with segmental necrosis
Gastrointestinal
    Anorexia, nausea, vomiting
    Paralytic ileus
Cardiovascular
    Increased sensitivity to digitalis glycosides
    Possible cause of tachyarrhythmias
Metabolic
    Hypocalcemia—probably due to the combined result of decreased PTH secretion and decreased end organ responsiveness to PTH
    Hypokalemia—tendency toward renal potassium wasting

*From Smith LH Jr: Disorders of magnesium metabolism. In Wyngaarden JB, and Smith LH Jr (eds): Cecil Textbook of Medicine. 17th ed. Philadelphia, WB Saunders Co, 1985, p 1166.

MAGNESIUM METABOLISM

An adult normally has about 0.35 gram of magnesium/kg of body weight (a total of 25 grams or 100 mmol), of which about 50 to 60 per cent is in bone. In addition to its structural role in bone crystals, magnesium is an important cofactor in a large number of enzymatic reactions, especially those involving ATP. It also plays an obligate role in the function of chlorophyll.

Magnesium Balance. The normal serum level of magnesium is 1.6 to 2.1 mEq/L, of which about 30 per cent is protein-bound. About one third of ingested magnesium (the average diet contains about 500 mg) is absorbed in the intestine. This is balanced by its renal excretion, which reflects both filtration and active tubular reabsorption. Magnesium metabolism has a close interaction with that of calcium: (1) these cations are competitive for renal tubular reabsorption; (2) magnesium and calcium are physiological antagonists in the central nervous system; (3) magnesium is necessary for the release of parathyroid hormone by the parathyroid glands and for the action of the hormone on its target tissues. Magnesium balance is usually assessed by its serum level, although this may not parallel tissue levels precisely. This assessment can be extended by measuring the amount of Mg excreted in the urine after its intravenous infusion (the Thoren test). Retention is presumed to reflect depleted stores. When dietary Mg is restricted, the normal kidney can reduce urinary loss to less than 1 mEq/day.

Hypomagnesemia. The most common causes of hypomagnesemia are summarized in Table 74–3. In clinical practice magnesium deficiency is encountered most frequently in alcoholics (poor dietary intake, vomiting, diminished absorption, increased renal excretion) and in patients with malabsorption. Significant depletion of magnesium may result in any or all of the abnormalities listed in Table 74–4. Many of these manifestations are relatively nonspecific, and magnesium deficiency rarely occurs as a pure entity without other nutritional and metabolic abnormalities. Its most characteristic presentation is that of hypocalcemia (irritability, tetany, positive Chvostek and Trousseau signs) because of the failure of normal secretion and action of parathyroid hormone. In effect Mg deficiency leads to a combination of functional hypoparathyroidism and pseudohypoparathyroidism (see Chapter 75). This form of hypocalcemia responds rapidly to Mg replacement therapy. Mg deficiency is not a recognized cause of metabolic bone disease. Treatment of magnesium deficiency is rarely an emergency. When it is urgent, approximately 1 mEq/kg/24 hr can be given by intravenous infusion. Long-term oral replacement can be carried out with various magnesium preparations, with careful attention to dosage in order not to induce diarrhea.

Hypermagnesemia. Hypermagnesemia rarely occurs. With normal renal function excess Mg is readily excreted. In a patient with impaired renal function the use of magnesium-containing antacids may rarely produce hypermagnesemia, or it may occur with injudicious use of intravenous Mg in the acute treatment of hypertension. Hypermagnesemia may result in depression of central nervous system function, vasodilatation with hypotension and depression of the cardiac conduction system, ultimately leading to cardiac arrest in diastole. Discontinuation of magnesium infusion or ingestion usually suffices for treatment. Calcium is an antagonist of Mg in the central nervous system and can be used by intravenous injection if magnesium toxicity is acute.

VITAMIN D

Vitamin D may be considered to be misnamed in that it is more properly a hormone than a vitamin: (1) When there is sufficient exposure to ultraviolet light no dietary source is required. (2) "Vitamin" D undergoes successive modifications in the body under hormonal and metabolic control, and then functions as a hormone-like agent in the metabolism of bone and bone salts.

Synthesis of Vitamin D (Fig. 74–3). The active form of vitamin D is synthesized in three sequential steps: (1) the dermal phase, (2) the hepatic phase, and (3) the renal phase. Ultraviolet light (approximately 290 to 320 nm wavelength) converts epidermal 7-dehydrocholesterol to an unstable previtamin D_3. The latter slowly converts nonenzymatically to vitamin D_3 (cholecalciferol) by a molecular rearrangement over the subsequent 24 to 48 hours. Vitamin D_3, bound to a specific vitamin D–binding protein (DBP), is then transported to the liver, where it is enzymatically hydroxylated to 25-hydroxyvitamin D (25-OH-D). This activation step, catalyzed by a cytochrome P450 mixed function oxidase in hepatocytes, is not under tight homeostatic control. The product, 25-OH-D (also called calcifediol), is not the most biologically potent form of vitamin D, but its circulating level furnishes a good index of the bioavailability.

25-OH-D, bound to DBP, is then transported to the kidney. In the renal parenchyma it may undergo one of two competing metabolic transformations:

1. FORMATION OF 1,25-DIHYDROXYCHOLECALCIFEROL (CALCITRIOL). The 25-OH-D from the liver is further hydroxylated enzymatically at the 1 position to yield $1\alpha,25\text{-}(OH)_2D$, the most active hormonal form of the vitamin. This hydroxylation, which is normally highly specific for the kidney and the placenta, is under tight metabolic control. Activity of this 1-hydroxylase is increased by PTH, hypocalcemia, hypophosphatemia, and low levels of $1,25\text{-}(OH)_2D$. Conversely, synthesis of $1,25\text{-}(OH)_2D$ is diminished by reductions in PTH, hypercalcemia (independent of PTH), hyperphosphatemia, high levels of $1,25\text{-}(OH)_2D$, and severe renal diseases.

2. FORMATION OF 24,25-DIHYDROXYCHOLECALCIFEROL. The kidney may alternatively hydroxylate 25-OH-D in the 24 position, catalyzed by a separate hydroxylase, to produce $24,25\text{-}(OH)_2D$. Less is known about the control or purpose of this pathway, but high levels of $1,25\text{-}(OH)_2D$ calcium and phosphate tend to divert 25-OH-D into the $24,25\text{-}(OH)_2D$ pathway.

Other pathways of vitamin D metabolism have been described, but their physiological roles, if any, remain to be demonstrated.

Absorption of Vitamin D. Ingested vitamin D bypasses the dermal step in the activation process. The usual dietary source is vitamin D_2 (ergocalciferol) formed from the irradiation of ergosterol, a plant sterol. This differs in the structure of the side chain from vitamin D_3 (cholecalciferol) but is equal in potency, undergoes the same biotransformations, and is measured by the same commonly employed competitive protein-binding assays.

The dietary requirement of vitamin D is difficult to establish owing to the vagaries of endogenous synthesis. In the absence of better information, the suggested dietary requirement for an adult in the United States is about 10 μg (400 International Units) of vitamin D_2 or vitamin D_3 daily. As a fat-soluble molecule, vitamin D depends for its absorption on the complex series of events described for the absorption of fat in Chapter 36C. Chronic malabsorption of fat in the absence of adequate exposure to ultraviolet light can lead to hypovitaminosis D.

Assessment of Vitamin D Metabolism. In the past it was not possible to measure vitamin D or its metabolites. One was dependent on the demonstration of rickets or osteomalacia for which no other cause was apparent and which was responsive to vitamin D for diagnosis of hypovitaminosis D; or on hypercalcemia, with a history of excessive ingestion of the vitamin, for the diagnosis of hypervitaminosis D. Currently assay methods are available using natural binding proteins, immunoassays, or a bioassay based on resorption of cultured bone in vitro. Values vary from laboratory to laboratory, but the most frequently measured products are 25-OH-D, 10–50 ng/ml, and $1,25\text{-}(OH)_2D$, 15–55 pg/ml.

Function of Vitamin D. Vitamin D acts with PTH to maintain the level of ionized calcium in extracellular fluid and to enhance calcification of osteoid by actions on the intestine, on bone and, to a lesser extent, on the kidney.

In its best known effect vitamin D, largely as $1,25\text{-}(OH)_2D$, enhances the intestinal absorption of calcium through complex mechanisms, including the synthesis of a cytosolic calcium-binding protein. It also enhances phosphate absorption. In its effect on the absorption of calcium and phosphate it enhances the mineralization potential of extracellular fluid (the calcium × phosphate product). In its direct action on bone, $1,25\text{-}(OH)_2D$ is synergistic with PTH in enhancing bone resorption. There is some evidence, however, that $24,25\text{-}(OH)_2D$ may stimulate bone formation rather than bone resorption. Vitamin D may enhance renal tubular reabsorption of calcium, but such a direct effect has been difficult to separate from its interaction with PTH and phosphate.

Hypervitaminosis D. Hypervitaminosis D occurs from the excessive ingestion of vitamin D or one of its active metabolites or from the abnormal conversion of 25-OH-D to 1,25-$(OH)_2$D at sites not subject to tight metabolic regulation. The former occurs usually in the therapy of hypoparathyroidism, osteomalacia, or osteoporosis. The latter occurs in certain granulomatous diseases, notably sarcoidosis, in which the 1-hydroxylase is pathologically expressed in the abnormal tissue.

The clinical picture of hypervitaminosis D is that of hypercalcemia (see Chapter 75) and metastatic calcification. For a given level of serum calcium, patients with this syndrome are more likely to have metastatic calcification (especially calcium nephropathy, band keratopathy, and calcifications in bursae and around joints) than are patients with hyperparathyroidism, since the level of PTH is suppressed and serum phosphate levels are higher. Treatment is by discontinuation of vitamin D, the usual acute treatment of hypercalcemia if indicated (Chapter 75), and the use of prednisone.

Hypovitaminosis D. The clinical picture of hypovitaminosis D is that of rickets or osteomalacia, to be described in Chapter 76. Hypovitaminosis D is also one component of the complex entity, renal osteodystrophy (Chapter 79).

CALCITONIN

Calcitonin is a small polypeptide hormone that is secreted by the parafollicular C cells in the thyroid gland in response to a rise in the level of ionized calcium. As a physiological antagonist of parathyroid hormone, calcitonin inhibits bone resorption and increases the renal excretion of calcium and phosphate, tending to return the level of calcium toward normal. Calcitonin secretion can also be enhanced by gastrin, glucagon, alcohol, and beta-adrenergic agonists, but these agents may not play any physiological or even pharmacological role in the control of its secretion.

Hypocalcitoninemia. No deficiency syndrome for calcitonin has been clearly established. Patients with total thyroidectomy do not require replacement with this hormone and do not develop hypercalcemia. Calcitonin secretion normally declines with age, especially in women. It is speculated that this may contribute to involutional osteoporosis, since secretion of PTH remains and is less opposed in its action.

Hypercalcitoninemia. Excessive secretion of calcitonin usually reflects a medullary carcinoma of the thyroid gland, a malignancy of the parafollicular cells. Elevated serum levels of calcitonin may also be found with its ectopic secretion by other tumors and in uremia and pregnancy.

The excessive secretion of calcitonin by medullary carcinomas does not usually lead to any bone disease or to any change in the serum calcium, phosphorus, or alkaline phosphatase. Sporadic medullary carcinoma usually presents with a hard thyroid mass. Familial medullary carcinoma may present with some other features of the associated polyendocrine syndrome. These tumors are often versatile in their secretory capabilities, producing ACTH (with Cushing's syndrome), prostaglandins, nerve growth factor, serotonin, histaminase, vasoactive intestinal peptide, and prolactin. About 20 per cent have an associated secretory diarrhea that remits with the removal of the tumor.

Familial Medullary Carcinoma. Medullary carcinoma may occur sporadically; it is also found in two distinct patterns of familial multiple endocrine neoplasia (MEN) syndrome, both of which are transmitted as autosomal, dominant traits:

MEN Type II (also called IIA) (Sipple's syndrome). In this syndrome familial parafollicular C-cell hyperplasia evolving into medullary carcinoma is linked with pheochromocytomas (20 to 30 per cent) and chief cell hyperplasia of the parathyroid glands (20 to 30 per cent). The pheochromocytomas tend to be bilateral and benign. Only about 10 per cent of patients exhibit hypercalcemia with its associated symptoms.

MEN Type III (also called Type IIB). This syndrome resembles Type II in the linkage of medullary carcinoma and pheochromocyomas but differs in that the parathyroid glands are rarely involved. In addition there tends to be a distinct body habitus resembling the Marfan syndrome, and patients develop visible, sometimes disfiguring, benign neuromas of the lips, tongue, and buccal mucosa.

In addition, medullary carcinoma can occur as a familial disorder without being associated with other endocrine disorders. In all about 10 per cent of medullary carcinomas are familial and approximately 5 to 10 per cent of all thyroid carcinomas are medullary.

DIAGNOSIS AND TREATMENT. The diagnosis of medullary carcinoma (or of familial C-cell hyperplasia) is best established by measuring serum immunoreactive calcitonin before and after a provocative test with the infusion of calcium or of pentagastrin. Treatment is total thyroidectomy for familial cases, since the tumor is usually multicentric.

REFERENCES

Bone

Arnaud CD: Mineral and bone homeostasis. In Wyngaarden JB, and Smith LH Jr (eds): Cecil Textbook of Medicine. 17th ed. Philadelphia, WB Saunders Co, 1985, p 1415.

Avioli L, and Raisz L: Bone metabolism and disease. In Bondy PK, and Rosenberg LE (eds): Metabolic Control and Disease. Philadelphia, WB Saunders Co, 1980, p 1709.

Krane SM, and Neer RM: Connective tissue. In Smith LH Jr, and Thier SO (eds): Pathophysiology, The Biological Principles of Disease. 2nd ed. Philadelphia, WB Saunders Co, 1985, p 611.

Sledge CB: Formation and resorption of bone. In Kelley WN, Harris ED Jr, Ruddy S, et al (eds): Textbook of Rheumatology. 2nd ed. Philadelphia, WB Saunders Co, 1985, p 271.

Calcium

Agus ZS, Goldfarb S, and Wasserstein A: Disorders of calcium and phosphate balance. In Brenner BM, and Rector FC Jr (eds): The Kidney. 2nd ed. Philadelphia, WB Saunders Co, 1981, p 940.

Bikle DD: Calcium absorption and vitamin D metabolism. Clin Gastroenterol 12:379, 1983.

Lee DBN, Zawada ET, and Kleeman CR: The pathophysiology and clinical aspects of hypercalcemic disorders. West J Med 129:278, 1978.

Phosphorus

Fitzgerald FT: Hypophosphatemia. Adv Intern Med 23:137, 1978.

Knochel JP: The clinical status of hypophosphatemia: An update. N Engl J Med 313:447, 1985.

Smith LH Jr: Phosphorus deficiency and hypophosphatemia. In Wyngaarden JB, and Smith LH Jr (eds): Cecil Textbook of Medicine. 17th ed. Philadelphia, WB Saunders Co, 1985, p 1163.

Magnesium

Cronin RE, and Knochel JP: Magnesium deficiency. Adv Intern Med 28:509, 1983.

Levine BS, and Coburn JW: Magnesium, the mimic/antagonist of calcium. N Engl J Med 310:1253, 1984.

Smith LH Jr: Disorders of magnesium metabolism. In Wyngaarden JB, and Smith LH Jr (eds): Cecil Textbook of Medicine. 17th ed. Philadelphia, WB Saunders Co, 1985, p 1165.

Vitamin D

Audran M, and Kumar R: The physiology and pathophysiology of vitamin D. Mayo Clin Proc, 1985 (in press).

Avioli LV, and Haddad JG: The vitamin D family revisited. N Engl J Med 311:47, 1984.

Bikle DD: Vitamin D. In Wyngaarden JB, and Smith LH Jr (eds): Cecil Textbook of Medicine. 17th ed. Philadelphia, WB Saunders Co, 1985, p 1423.

Bikle DD: The vitamin D endocrine system. Adv Intern Med 27:45, 1982

Fraser DR: Regulation of the metabolism of vitamin D. Physiol Rev 60:551, 1980.

Calcitonin

Arnaud CD: The ultimobranchial cells and calcitonin. In Wyngaarden JB, and Smith LH Jr (eds): Cecil Textbook of Medicine. 17th ed. Philadelphia, WB Saunders Co, 1985, p 1451.

Austin L, and Heath H III: Calcitonin: Physiology and pathophysiology. N Engl J Med 304:269, 1981.

Loeb JN: Polyglandular disorders. In Wyngaarden JB, and Smith LH Jr (eds): Cecil Textbook of Medicine. 17th ed. Philadelphia, WB Saunders Co, 1985, p 1405.

THE PARATHYROID GLANDS, HYPERCALCEMIA, AND HYPOCALCEMIA

75

NORMAL PHYSIOLOGY

The parathyroid glands, usually four in number, normally weigh only about 120 mg. They are usually found in close association with the thyroid gland, but not infrequently one or both of the lower glands may be found in the superior mediastinum.

Secretion of PTH. Parathyroid hormone (PTH) is an 84-amino acid linear polypeptide (molecular weight 9500) whose main function is the control of the level of ionized calcium in extracellular fluid. When the level of ionized calcium falls, PTH secretion is stimulated; when ionized calcium rises above the normal set point, the secretion of PTH is suppressed. When ionized calcium is reduced over long periods of time, as for example in uremia, the parathyroid glands are capable of undergoing massive hyperplasia in order to enhance their secretory capacity. A normal or nearly normal level of ionized magnesium in extracellular fluid is necessary for normal secretion of PTH.

Actions of PTH (Fig. 75–1). The main function of PTH is to defend against hypocalcemia. In this defense it acts in a number of ways, both direct and indirect. All of these actions depend upon binding to specific receptors on the cell membrane and probably upon the subsequent intracellular release of cyclic AMP.

1. PTH stimulates osteolysis by osteoclasts that release calcium and phosphate into extracellular fluid. This action on bone, through mechanisms that are not well understood, is partially impaired when there is deficiency of calcitriol or of extracellular magnesium.

2. PTH *increases* the renal tubular reabsorption of calcium (and magnesium), reducing urinary loss of that which has been filtered.

3. PTH *decreases* the renal tubular reabsorption of phosphate and of bicarbonate, enhancing their urinary loss. This helps to get rid of the phos-

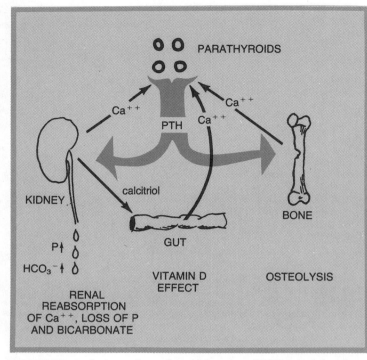

FIGURE 75–1. Actions of parathyroid hormone (PTH) in calcium homeostasis.

phate released from bone, which might otherwise tend to reduce ionized calcium. The loss of bicarbonate produces a form of renal tubular acidosis that tends to diminish protein binding of calcium.

4. PTH increases the synthesis of the active form of vitamin D, calcitriol, from 25-OH-D through activation of the specific 1-hydroxylase in the kidney (see Chapter 74). It therefore indirectly enhances the intestinal absorption of calcium.

Many of the actions of PTH are upon the kidney. This is indirectly reflected in the amount of cyclic AMP of nephrogenous origin excreted in the urine.

Measurement of PTH. PTH can be measured directly using radioimmunoassay procedures. There are inherent difficulties with the current assays, however, because of two variables: (1) "Immunoreactive PTH" (iPTH) does not circulate as a single entity. In plasma there are a number of fragments of the active hormone. Most of the immunological activity measured by assay is not in fact the active hormone. (2) The antibodies used are multivalent and heterogeneous, recognizing different parts of the PTH linear peptide. In the future, monoclonal antibodies specific for the active site (the amino end) of PTH may become more available. In the interim interpretations must be made in light of the specific test being employed.

Because of these current limitations with the immunoassays available, new approaches are being made with in vitro cytochemical assays for active PTH. Measurement of the excretion of nephrogenous cAMP can also be used to reflect PTH action on the kidney.

PRIMARY HYPERPARATHYROIDISM

Primary hyperparathyroidism is a relatively common endocrine disorder in which PTH continues to be secreted inappropriately despite an elevation in the level of ionized calcium in extracellular fluid. The disorder is more common in women than in men (two to four times greater), is very rare before the age of puberty, and increases in incidence with age. Population surveys have found the prevalence of primary hyperparathyroidism in adults to be as high as 1 in 200 to 1 in 800.

Etiology. Primary hyperparathyroidism results from the development through unknown mechanisms of autonomous parathyroid tissue. In fact there may not be complete autonomy, since PTH secretion may be partially suppressed at higher levels of ionized calcium. A single parathyroid adenoma accounts for 80 to 85 per cent of cases; most other patients with primary hyperparathyroidism have hyperplasia of all four glands. Carcinoma of the parathyroids is rare (less than 2 per cent of cases) and is usually not very malignant. Although most patients represent sporadic cases, primary hyperparathyroidism can occur in various patterns as a familial disorder, usually with hyperplasia and with a dominant mode of transmission: (1) familial hyperparathyroidism alone; (2) multiple endocrine neoplasia Type I (Werner's syndrome)—hyperparathyroidism, islet cell tumors, pituitary tumors; (3) multiple endocrine neoplasia Type II (Sipple's syndrome)—medullary carcinoma of the thyroid, pheochromocytoma, hyperparathyroidism. Hyperparathyroidism is rare in multiple endocrine neoplasia Type IIB or III—medullary carcinoma of the thyroid, pheochromocytoma, mucosal neuromas, and marfanoid body habitus.

Symptoms and Signs. Many patients are now discovered by measurement of serum calcium to have hyperparathyroidism when they are asymptomatic. When symptoms do occur, they most frequently result from hypercalcemia (Table 75–1). They may vary from easy fatigability to coma, but generally hypercalcemia is modest (11.0 to 12.5 mg/dl) and symptoms are mild. Symptoms may also result from hypercalciuria, since kidney stones occur in about 10 per cent of patients with hyperparathyroidism. Approximately 5 per cent of patients with kidney stones are found to have hyperparathyroidism. More rarely bone pain due to osteitis fibrosa cystica (the bony lesion caused by excess PTH) may dominate the symptomatology, and very rarely there may be a pathological fracture at the site of a bone cyst. Physical findings of hyperparathyroidism are usually absent. A nodule felt in the neck is more likely to be in the thyroid gland than to be the offending parathyroid adenoma.

Laboratory and Radiographic Manifestations. Serum calcium levels are elevated and serum phosphorus levels tend to be low in primary hyperparathyroidism. Occasionally the total serum calcium is at the upper normal range but with ionized calcium increased. Serum alkaline phosphatase is elevated in the minority of patients in whom there is significant osteitis fibrosa cystica; its elevation reflects reparative osteoblastic activity. Urinary calcium may be normal or elevated and its measurement is of use only in the diagnosis of benign familial hypercalcemia (see below). Because of the effect of PTH on bicarbonate excretion, the serum chloride is often elevated (> 105 mEq/L) and the serum bicarbonate somewhat reduced. Immunoassay of PTH should show an inappropriately high level of the hormone (and its related peptides) for the level of serum calcium (Fig. 75–2).

Most patients with primary hyperparathyroidism show no radiographic evidence of bone disease. When bone disease is found, it is most readily demonstrated as subperiosteal resorption of the cortex in the phalanges (Fig. 75–3). In addition, there may be generalized osteopenia and, in more advanced cases, resorption of the distal ends of the clavicle and of distal phalangeal tufts and a characteristic "salt-and-pepper" mottling of the skull.

Diagnosis. The diagnosis of primary hyperparathyroidism in the past was primarily based on finding hypercalcemia, usually with hypophosphatemia, in the absence of any other detectable cause of this abnormality (Table 75–2). That same differential diagnosis exists today, but the diagnosis can now be made with greater assurance using an immunoassay (or cytochemical bioassay) for PTH (Fig. 75–2). In all other causes of hypercalcemia the level of PTH should be suppressed by an elevation of ionized calcium. Most of the other causes of hypercalcemia listed in Table 75–2 can be readily identified by other clinical manifestations or by laboratory studies. Two entities continue to be troublesome in the differential diagnosis:

1. **Hypercalcemia of Malignancy.** Hypercalcemia occurs frequently with malignant tumors with or without metastases to bone. Osteolytic factors associated with malignant tumors include osteoclast-activating factor (especially with multiple myeloma), prostaglandins of the E_2 series, PTH, and other "PTH-like factors." Tumors may rarely secrete actual PTH ("pseudohyperparathyroidism") as opposed to other factors with similar biological activity, but newer evidence tends to support the latter as more frequently implicated in the hypercalcemia of malignancy. Clearly, the level of immunoreactive PTH tends to be lower for the level of serum calcium in malignancy than in primary hyperparathyroidism (Fig. 75–2).

2. **Benign Familial Hypercalcemia** (also called familial hypocalciuric hypercalcemia). This genetic disorder, transmitted as a dominant trait, is characterized by modest hypercalcemia, a definite hypocalciuria, and no symptoms. There is no evidence of bone disease and, as expected, no stone diathesis. The PTH levels by immunoassay are usually normal. The diagnosis is important, since surgery is contraindicated. To rule out this

TABLE 75–1. SYMPTOMS AND SIGNS OF PRIMARY HYPERPARATHYROIDISM

Related to hypercalcemia per se
Central nervous system
 lethargy
 drowsiness
 depression
 stupor
 coma
Neuromuscular
 fatigue
 weakness
 proximal myopathy
 hypotonia
Cardiovascular
 hypertension
 bradycardia
 short Q-T interval
 potentiation of digitalis intoxication
Renal
 polyuria
 calcium nephropathy—nephrocalcinosis
Gastrointestinal
 nausea
 vomiting
 constipation
 dyspepsia
 increased peptic ulcer ?
 pancreatitis
Metastatic calcification (usually requires P to be elevated as well)
 band keratopathy
 pruritus
Related to hypercalciuria
Kidney stone diathesis (10 per cent)
Related to PTH effect on bone and joints
Bone pain from osteitis fibrosa cystica
Bone cysts—rarely with fracture
Epulis—a brown tumor (osteoclastic) of the jaw
Arthralgias
Increased incidence of gout and pseudogout

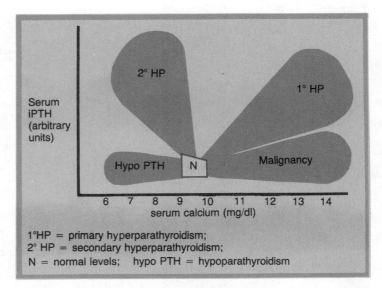

FIGURE 75–2. Relation of iPTH and serum calcium in various disorders.

TABLE 75–2. DIFFERENTIAL DIAGNOSIS OF HYPERCALCEMIA

Due to increased PTH
Primary hyperparathyroidism
Hypercalcemia of malignancy (probably few)
Without increased PTH (PTH usually suppressed)
Hypercalcemia of malignancy
    malignant hematologic disorders (especially multiple myeloma)—often due to OAF
    nonhematologic malignancies—PTH-like factors, PGE_2, possibly other factors
Vitamin D excess
    excessive ingestion
    excessive activation—sarcoidosis, berylliosis
Milk-alkali syndrome—excessive ingestion
Use of thiazide diuretics
Benign familial hypercalcemia (familial hypocalciuric hypercalcemia)
Immobilization (especially with Paget's disease or paraplegia)
Hyperthyroidism
Miscellaneous—Addison's disease, vitamin A excess, hyperproteinemia states (increased bound calcium), idiopathic hypercalcemia of infancy

recently discovered disorder, urine calcium should be measured in patients with asymptomatic hypercalcemia, and serum calcium levels should be measured in the relatives of those with hypocalciuria.

The diagnosis of hyperparathyroidism can also be strengthened if subperiosteal bone reabsorption is present (Fig. 75–3), if nephrogenous cAMP is elevated in the urine, and if an enlarged parathyroid gland is found by ultrasonography.

Treatment. The treatment of choice for primary hyperparathyroidism is surgical removal of the abnormal gland or glands. With hyperplasia subtotal ($3\frac{1}{2}$ glands) parathyroidectomy is carried out. In some patients with slight elevations of serum calcium (<11.0 mg/dl) or in those with contraindications to surgery, it is justifiable to follow the patient medically, maintaining adequate hydration and increased phosphate intake (if there is hypophosphatemia) and withholding thiazide diuretics or excessive dietary calcium.

HYPERCALCEMIA

Normal calcium metabolism was discussed in Chapter 74. For convenience hypercalcemia is being considered with the discussion of primary hyperparathyroidism.

Clinical Manifestations. The clinical manifestations of hypercalcemia are summarized in Table 75–1. In general, the severity of these manifestations tends to parallel the level of ionized calcium in extracellular fluid, but there are wide variations in the manner in which individual patients exhibit these various symptoms. Most frequently now elevations of serum calcium are found on routine chemical determinations. These tests should be repeated several times, since false elevations may be reported.

Differential Diagnosis. The differential diagnosis of hypercalcemia is presented in Table 75–2. These specific entities will not be discussed further here.

Treatment. Obviously the treatment of hypercalcemia should be directed toward reversal of the pathogenetic mechanisms responsible for it whenever possible. For example, primary hyperparathyroidism is usually treated by surgery. Successful treatment of malignancy may reverse or diminish its associated hypercalcemia, at least temporarily. The slight hypercalcemia found with hyperthyroidism or with Addison's disease is readily reversed by the treatment of those endocrine disorders. We shall discuss here the medical treatment of acute severe hypercalcemia (>13 to 14 mg/dl). The following approaches, presented briefly, are available and may be used in se-

FIGURE 75–3. Magnified x-ray of an index finger on fine-grain industrial film, showing classic subperiosteal resorption in a patient with severe primary hyperparathyroidism. (Courtesy of Professor H. Genant, University of California, San Francisco, Department of Radiology.) (From Arnaud CD: The parathyroid glands, hypercalcemia, and hypocalcemia. In Wyngaarden JB, and Smith LH Jr (eds): Cecil Textbook of Medicine. 17th ed. Philadelphia, WB Saunders Co, 1985, p 1437.)

quence, or many of them can be used concurrently if indicated by the severity of the patient's illness:

HYDRATION. Urinary excretion of calcium tends to parallel that of sodium. Patients should be vigorously hydrated, usually with normal saline, in order to enhance excretion.

FUROSEMIDE (OR ETHACRYNIC ACID). Large doses of furosemide increase further the urinary excretion of calcium. Since excretion of potassium and magnesium is also increased, their serum levels must be closely followed and the amount lost in the urine replaced.

GLUCOCORTICOIDS. High doses of glucocorticoids (prednisone 50 to 100 mg per day or the equivalent of another agent) may lower serum calcium, especially in sarcoidosis, vitamin D poisoning, multiple myeloma, or other hematopoietic malignancies.

CALCITONIN. Calcitonin (usually as salmon calcitonin) given intravenously may diminish the release of calcium from bone (see Chapter 76).

MITHRAMYCIN. This agent diminishes osteoclastic activity when given intravenously (25 μg/kg body weight).

PHOSPHATE. Orthophosphate must be given with great care in the treatment of severe hypercalcemia because of the danger of metastatic calcification. In the presence of hypophosphatemia and good renal function, intravenous or preferably oral phosphate can be given in amounts sufficient to return its serum level to normal.

DIALYSIS. Very rarely, especially when there is acute hypercalcemia and renal insufficiency, dialysis may be required for the treatment of hypercalcemia.

These measures are usually successful in controlling acute hypercalcemia. The most difficult problems usually arise in the long-term treatment of the hypercalcemia of inoperable malignancy.

SECONDARY HYPERPARATHYROIDISM

Whenever the level of ionized calcium in extracellular fluid falls, the parathyroid glands are stimulated to secrete PTH. If the tendency toward hypocalcemia is sustained, the glands become hyperplastic and secrete increasing amounts of PTH, a condition known as secondary hyperparathyroidism. By definition the serum calcium level is low-normal or low in secondary hyperparathyroidism, since this is the driving force for hyperplasia and hypersecretion. The serum phosphorus will usually be low if renal function is intact. Osteitis fibrosa cystica may be present as noted by bone pain, subperiosteal bone resorption (Fig. 75–3), or elevation of serum alkaline phosphatase. The most frequent causes of secondary hyperparathyroidism, to be described below, are chronic renal failure (renal osteodystrophy), malabsorption of calcium (rickets, osteomalacia), and pseudohypoparathyroidism. The term "tertiary hyperparathyroidism" is sometimes used to describe hypercalcemia arising in the setting of severe secondary hyperparathyroidism in which chronic stimulation is thought to produce relatively autonomous parathyroid tissue.

TABLE 75–3. ETIOLOGY OF HYPOPARATHYROIDISM

Surgical removal of the parathyroids
Radiation injury to parathyroids
Impaired secretion of PTH—Mg deficiency
Inherited forms of hypoparathyroidism
  DiGeorge's syndrome—congenital absence of parathyroids and thymus
  Multiple endocrine deficiency—autoimmune—candidiasis (MEDAC) syndrome
Sporadic, idiopathic hypoparathyroidism
Pseudohypoparathyroidism—target organ resistance
  acquired—Mg deficiency
  inherited—various subtypes noted

HYPOPARATHYROIDISM

In contrast to hyperparathyroidism, hypoparathyroidism is rare. In this section hypocalcemia in general will be discussed.

Etiology. The causes of hypoparathyroidism are listed in Table 75–3. They range from surgical removal of the glands to resistance to the action of PTH at the tissue level. Magnesium deficiency was discussed in Chapter 74, and pseudohypoparathyroidism will be discussed subsequently. DiGeorge's syndrome is a very rare congenital abnormality representing absence of embryological formation of the parathyroids and of the thymus, both products of the third and fourth branchial clefts. These children usually die of immunodeficiency (T-cell dysfunction) in early life. The MEDAC syndrome (Table 75–3) is characterized by chronic mucocutaneous candidiasis and autoimmune injury of various endocrine glands, especially of the parathyroids and the adrenal cortex (producing Addison's disease).

Symptoms and Signs (Table 75–4). Symptomatology varies not only with the level of ionized calcium but also with the rate at which hypocalcemia has developed and its total duration. A rapid fall in ionized calcium is more likely to produce symptoms. The symptoms associated with hypoparathyroidism largely relate to the neuromuscular consequences of hypocalcemia. They can vary from a vague sense of anxiety with paresthesias to recurrent grand mal seizures, erroneously treated with phenytoin. Most of the other symptoms and signs listed in Table 75–4 occur only after years of hypocalcemia. Physical findings are those of neuromuscular irritability (positive Chvostek's and/or Trousseau's sign) and

TABLE 75–4. SYMPTOMS AND SIGNS OF HYPOCALCEMIA

Enhanced neuromuscular irritability
  Paresthesias (numbness, tingling), especially around mouth and tips of fingers
  Tetany—positive Chvostek's and Trousseau's sign
  Grand mal seizures
Lenticular cataracts—decreased vision
Basal ganglia calcification—rarely extrapyramidal abnormalities
Papilledema and increased intracranial pressure
Intestinal malabsorption (which may further exacerbate hypocalcemia)
Trophic changes in skin, fingernails, and developing teeth
Prolonged Q-T interval; rarely heart block and congestive heart failure

sometimes cataracts, basal ganglia signs, dry dystrophic skin and nails, or rarely associated findings such as candidiasis, signs of Addison's disease, a scar from a previous thyroidectomy, or the physical findings of pseudohypoparathyroidism to be noted below.

Laboratory and Radiographic Manifestations. Hypoparathyroidism is characterized by hypocalcemia and hyperphosphatemia, a combination that is diagnostic in the absence of renal insufficiency or the acute infusion of phosphate. Serum bicarbonate tends to be slightly elevated and serum iPTH is undetectable or markedly reduced, except in pseudohypoparathyroidism. There are no radiographic changes in bone, but calcification of basal ganglia may be noted. Skeletal changes of pseudohypoparathyroidism are noted below. The ECG usually shows a long Q-T interval and may exhibit heart block.

Diagnosis. The diagnosis of hypoparathyroidism is relatively simple once it is considered or when hypocalcemia is discovered. The triad of hypocalcemia, hyperphosphatemia, and normal renal function is virtually diagnostic of the disorder. Hypomagnesemia should be ruled out. Measurement of iPTH should readily confirm the diagnosis and rule out pseudohypoparathyroidism (in which condition it should be elevated). Urinary excretion of cAMP in response to intravenous PTH can be used to test end-organ responsiveness.

Other causes of hypocalcemia are readily excluded: hypoproteinemia, acute pancreatitis, azotemia, and malabsorption of calcium. In the latter condition there is secondary hyperparathyroidism, so that the serum phosphorus should be low and the level of iPTH high.

Treatment. Replacement therapy with PTH is not currently practicable owing to the necessity for its parenteral administration and its cost. Patients are usually treated, therefore, with a regimen of a high calcium diet and a vitamin D preparation along with phosphate binders ($Al(OH)_3$). Dihydrotachysterol has been used most frequently, but calcitriol has some theoretical advantages. Care must be taken to avoid hypercalcemia, since metastatic calcification and calcium nephropathy are special dangers with elevated levels of serum P. In the absence of PTH, normocalcemic hypercalciuria may increase the tendency to kidney stone formation. Acute tetany may require use of an intravenous preparation of calcium, such as calcium gluconate, to raise levels of ionized calcium to the normal level.

PSEUDOHYPOPARATHYROIDISM

This rare group of disorders has elicited more interest than its prevalence would warrant, in considerable measure because pseudohypoparathyroidism was the first clear-cut demonstration of an endocrine deficiency syndrome caused by unresponsiveness of a target organ (Albright and his colleagues, 1942). As would be expected, the clinical manifestations of hypocalcemia are the same in these patients as in those with other forms of hypoparathyroidism (Table 75–4). The laboratory findings are also similar except for the fact that the serum level of iPTH is elevated, since the persistent hypocalcemia tends to drive parathyroid secretion. Pseudohypoparathyroidism differs from other forms of hypoparathyroidism in two general ways:

1. There are a number of dominantly inherited developmental and skeletal abnormalities that may be associated with the disorder. These include short stature, shortening of the metacarpal and metatarsal bones (especially the fourth and fifth bones), thickening of the calvarium, exostoses, and frequently mental deficiency. The appearance is often typical, with short stature, a round face, obesity, and a short neck, together with the bony abnormalities above. When these findings occur in the absence of hypoparathyroidism, the condition is termed "pseudopseudohypoparathyroidism."

2. End-organ resistance to PTH can be demonstrated in a number of ways and occurs in various patterns. For patients with the skeletal anomalies described above, the molecular defect thought to cause PTH resistance is a 50 per cent decrease in the membrane protein that couples the PTH receptor to adenylate cyclase. Other possibilities for end-organ resistance include a structurally abnormal hormone or an inhibitor of hormone action. Resistance is usually demonstrated by an impaired effect of administered PTH on the kidney, as judged by phosphaturia or nephrogenous cAMP. Rarely cAMP may be elevated but no phosphaturia results. Rarely PTH may be effective on bone but not on the kidney, producing osteitis fibrosa cystica in the presence of hypoparathyroidism.

Treatment of pseudohypoparathyroidism is similar to that for other forms of hypoparathyroidism.

REFERENCES

Arnaud C: The parathyroid glands, hypercalcemia, and hypocalcemia. In Wyngaarden JB, and Smith LH Jr (eds): Cecil Textbook of Medicine. 17th ed. Philadelphia, WB Saunders Co, 1985, p 1431.

Bilezikian JP: Surgery or no surgery for primary hyperparathyroidism. Ann Intern Med 102:402, 1985.

Farfel Z, Brickman AS, Kaslow HR, et al: Defect of receptor-cyclase coupling protein in pseudohypoparathyroidism. N Engl J Med 303:237, 1980.

Habener JF, and Potts JT Jr: Clinical features of primary hyperparathyroidism. In DeGroot LJ, et al (eds): Endocrinology. New York, Grune & Stratton, 1979, p 693.

Heath H III, Hodgson SF, and Kennedy MA: Primary hyperparathyroidism: Incidence, morbidity and potential economic impact in a community. N Engl J Med 302:189, 1980.

Juan D: Hypocalcemia: Differential diagnosis and mechanisms. Arch Intern Med 139:1166, 1979.

Mundy GR, and Martin TJ: The hypercalcemia of malignancy: Pathogenesis and management. Metabolism 31:1247, 1982.

Osteomalacia and rickets represent the same metabolic bone disease characterized by inadequate calcification of osteoid on trabecular surfaces or in newly formed haversian systems. In rickets there is also an abnormality in the zone of provisional calcification related to endochondral skeletal growth at the open epiphyses.

Pathogenesis

The normal structure of bone was reviewed briefly in Chapter 74 (see Fig. 74–1). In the process of new bone formation in growth or in remodeling, osteoid is laid down in an appositional fashion by the osteoblasts. Soon thereafter bone salts are deposited in the osteoid to form bone, a process of mineralization that is still incompletely understood but that depends on a normal ion product of ionized calcium and phosphate, on alkaline phosphatase (probably necessary to remove the inhibitor pyrophosphate), and probably on several of the metabolites ($1,25\text{-}(OH)_2D$ and $24,25\text{-}(OH)_2D$) of vitamin D. Other factors may normally influence this process; mineralization can be impeded by inhibitors such as aluminum or diphosphonates.

In osteomalacia and in rickets, mineralization of osteoid (and of cartilage in rickets) does not keep pace with osteoid formation. As a result the osteoid seams are much wider and are found more extensively throughout bone. The bones are therefore weaker (osteomalacia means bone softening); in children the epiphyseal plate is widened, flared, and irregular. These changes are potentially reversible as normal mineralization is restored.

Specific Causes

The conditions in which osteomalacia and rickets are most frequently found are listed in Table 76–1. It has not been firmly established whether a pure deficiency of calcium results in osteomalacia. The major categories are those of inadequate bioavailability of the active metabolites of vitamin D, chronic phosphate depletion, abnormal inhibition of mineralization, and hypophosphatasia. These will be commented upon very briefly. A full discussion of these entities is beyond the scope of this introductory book.

Reduced Bioavailability of Active Forms of Vitamin D. The metabolic cycle in which vitamin D is successively converted to its active hormonal form is described in Chapter 74 and illustrated in Figure 74–3. As might be expected, and as summarized in Table 76–1, a wide variety of disorders may interfere with the formation of sufficient $1,25\text{-}(OH)_2D$ for its action on the gut and its action (or that of $24,25\text{-}(OH)_2D$) on bone. These vary from malabsorption of the vitamin, especially if there is inadequate sunlight for endogenous synthesis of precursors, impaired activation in the liver and kidney, increased catabolism or excretion, and failure of tissue responsiveness (diffuse disease or shortening of the bowel; vitamin D–dependent

rickets Type II, in which there do not seem to be normal receptors for $1,25\text{-}(OH)_2D$.

Chronic Depletion of Phosphate. Normal metabolism of phosphate and the metabolic consequences of phosphate depletion are summarized in Chapter 74 (see Tables 74–1 and 74–2). In chronic phosphate depletion there is likely to be osteomalacia or rickets, depending upon the patient's age. As noted, the causes of hypophosphatemia are many and range from enteric binding of phosphate with antacids to renal tubular wasting of phosphate (e.g., as a specific renal tubular disorder, due to secondary hyperparathyroidism, or as part of the Fanconi syndrome). Whatever the cause, the resulting hypophosphatemia may reduce the mineralization potential of bone salts below the critical level for normal deposition in osteoid.

Inhibitors of Mineralization. The use of aluminum-containing antacids in the presence of azotemia or the use of dialysis fluid high in aluminum may result in aluminum levels sufficient to inhibit mineralization, as may the use of diphosphonates in the treatment of Paget's disease. Chronic renal failure itself may inhibit normal mineralization (see Chapter 79).

Hypophosphatasia. This is a rare genetic dis-

TABLE 76–1. CAUSES OF OSTEOMALACIA OR RICKETS OR BOTH*

1. Vitamin D deficiency—dietary lack, too little sunshine, neonatal rickets
2. Vitamin D malabsorption—sprue, postgastrectomy, bile salt deficiency, pancreatic insufficiency, small bowel disease, bypass or resection
3. Impaired activation of vitamin D
   a. 25-Hydroxylation (liver)—immaturity, cirrhosis of liver ± alcoholism
   b. 1-Hydroxylation (kidney)—chronic renal failure, genetic enzyme defect (vitamin D dependency), parathyroid hormone deficiency or "resistance," ? hyperphosphatemia
4. Increased catabolism or excretion of vitamin D and its metabolites
   a. Hepatic microsomal enzyme induction—anticonvulsants (phenytoin, barbiturates)
   b. Renal excretion—nephrotic syndrome, biliary cirrhosis
5. Phosphate depletion and hypophosphatemia
   a. Complicating 1 through 4 above owing to PTH excess or lack of vitamin D metabolites or both
   b. Negative phosphate balance—malabsorption, phosphate-binding antacids, hemodialysis
   c. Primary hypophosphatemia (vitamin D refractory)—vitamin D-resistant rickets (VDRR), several types; oncogenic rickets and osteomalacia, neurofibromatosis
   d. Metabolic acidosis—distal renal tubular acidosis, ureterocolostomy
   e. Fanconi's syndrome—cystinosis, Wilson's disease, etc.
6. Inhibitors of mineralization—diphosphonates, fluoride, chronic renal failure, aluminum
7. Miscellaneous or unclassified—hypophosphatasia, "axial" osteomalacia, fibrogenesis imperfecta ossium

* From Avioli LV: Osteomalacia and rickets. In Wyngaarden JB, and Smith LH Jr (eds): Cecil Textbook of Medicine. 16th ed. Philadelphia, WB Saunders Co, 1982, p 1337. Modified from Frame B, and Parfitt AM: Osteomalacia: Current concepts. Ann Intern Med 89:966, 1978.

A   B

FIGURE 76–1. The clinical (A) and radiologic (B) appearance of a young boy with X-linked hypophosphatemic rickets. The most striking abnormalities are the bowing of the legs, apparent in both femora and tibiae, with flaring of the ends of these bones at the knee. (Photographs courtesy of Dr. Sara B. Arnaud.) (From Bikle DD: Osteomalacia and rickets. In Wyngaarden JB, and Smith LH Jr (eds): Cecil Textbook of Medicine. 17th ed. Philadelphia, WB Saunders Co, 1985, p 1429.)

order, transmitted as an autosomal recessive trait, in which there are low tissue and serum levels of alkaline phosphatase. The disease varies in severity from severe, deforming rickets to mild osteomalacia in adults.

FIGURE 76–2. Radiographic evidence of osteomalacia is shown by an incomplete fracture (Looser's zone) of the lateral scapular border. (From Avioli LV: Osteomalacia and rickets. In Wyngaarden JB, and Smith LH Jr (eds): Cecil Textbook of Medicine. 16th ed. Philadelphia, WB Saunders Co, 1982, p 1338.)

Clinical Manifestations

In the adult the manifestations of osteomalacia are often subtle. They may consist of aching in bones, tenderness over bones, and muscle weakness, especially of proximal and pelvic girdle muscles. As a result there may be a waddling gait. Bones may fracture more easily than normal.

The clinical manifestations of rickets are more striking and characteristic (Fig. 76–1). The child is usually listless and hypotonic and fails to grow normally. The epiphyses are enlarged and tender, and the long bones are often bowed. The chondrocostal junctions are enlarged and prominent to produce the "rachitic rosary." The pull of the diaphragm on the softened rib cage may produce an indentation known as a Harrison's groove. Rachitic bones are easily fractured. Dentition is delayed and poor.

Laboratory and Radiographic Abnormalities

The laboratory findings depend to a considerable degree on the specific cause of the defect in mineralization (Table 76–1). In the absence of renal failure the most typical finding would be slight hypocalcemia, more significant hypophosphatemia, an elevated serum alkaline phosphatase, and an elevated level of iPTH, representing secondary hyperparathyroidism. Osteomalacia can exist in the absence of any of these findings, however.

The radiographic findings in osteomalacia are most often nonspecific and show only osteopenia, which cannot readily be differentiated from osteoporosis. Pseudofractures (also known as Looser's zones) occasionally occur and when found are virtually pathognomonic for osteomalacia or rickets. These appear as ribbon-like clear zones, often bilaterally and symmetrically, and most characteristically in the pubic and ischial rami, the femoral neck, the ribs, and the axillary margins of the scapulae (Fig. 76–2). The radiographic abnormalities in rickets are more characteristic and are shown in Figure 76–1.

Diagnosis

The diagnosis of rickets is rarely difficult because of the characteristic clinical and radiographic findings. The diagnosis of osteomalacia may be more difficult, especially if there are no demonstrable pseudofractures. The diagnosis is best established by use of a transcortical bone biopsy (most frequently taken from the iliac crest) with careful histological study of the undecalcified specimen for widened osteoid seams. The biopsy is more definitive when it follows the use of timed tetracycline to determine the rate of bone formation (depressed in osteomalacia), as noted in Chapter 74.

Treatment

It is difficult to generalize about the treatment of a condition with such diverse pathogenetic mechanisms. Most frequently calcium and vitamin D are given; in some patients large supplements of phosphate may be required as well (e.g.,

X-linked hypophosphatemia). The reader is referred to discussions of the specific disorders in Table 76–1 for a summary of their respective modes of therapy.

REFERENCES

Bikle DD: Calcium absorption and vitamin D metabolism. Clin Gastroenterol 12:379, 1983.

Bikle DD: Osteomalacia and rickets. In Wyngaarden JB, and Smith LH Jr (eds): Cecil Textbook of Medicine. 17th ed. Philadelphia, WB Saunders Co, 1985, p 1425.

Frame B, and Parfitt AM: Osteomalacia: Current concepts. Ann Intern Med 89:966, 1978.

Krane SM, and Neer RM: Connective tissue. In Smith LH Jr, and Thier SO (eds): Pathophysiology, The Biological Principles of Disease, 2nd ed. Philadelphia, WB Saunders Co, 1985, p 611.

Mankin HJ: Rickets, osteomalacia, and renal osteodystrophy. J Bone Joint Surg 56A:101, 352, 1974.

Tieder M, Modai D, Samuel R, et al: Hereditary hypophosphatemic rickets with hypercalciuria. N Engl J Med 312:611, 1985.

OSTEOPOROSIS 77

Osteoporosis, a common type of metabolic bone disease, is characterized by a diffuse reduction in the amount of bone (osteopenia), with the residual bone being of normal composition. A reduction in the amount of bone occurs normally with aging; the frontier between this bone loss and the pathological entity of osteoporosis is not always clear. Osteoporosis is a major health problem in the elderly, particularly in elderly women, with increased susceptibility to serious fractures, disability, and death.

Pathology

In osteoporosis there is too little bone, but that which is present is normally composed of osteoid and bone minerals. Osteoporosis can be localized to the bones of one extremity, as in disuse atrophy with immobilization in a cast, but usually it is generalized. Different types may be most markedly manifested in the trabecular bone of the axial skeleton or in both trabecular and cortical bone.

Etiology and Pathogenesis

As noted in Chapter 74, bone is a living tissue that undergoes remodeling throughout life, with balanced processes of destruction (osteolysis) and repair (osteogenesis). Osteopenia must result from increased destruction, decreased formation, or a combination of the two. Although all combinations of these factors have been described in the osteoporotic syndromes, a relative increase in the rate of destruction is most commonly found in the osteoporosis of the elderly. It is not always possible to determine a specific cause of osteoporosis in a given individual. In this brief discussion certain general risk factors will be described, as well as a listing of the clinical conditions in which osteoporosis is most frequently manifested. The risk factors include the following:

Decreased Estrogen. Osteoporosis, more common by far in women than in men, occurs most frequently in the postmenopausal period. Bone loss is accelerated with reduction of ovarian function by either spontaneous or surgically induced menopause. The rate of bone loss varies markedly among women, but bone loss can largely be prevented by the continued administration of exogenous estrogens. The link between estrogen deficiency and increased bone destruction is not clear. Possibly there is both enhanced sensitivity to parathyroid hormone and reduced secretion of calcitonin. This type of involutional osteoporosis is sometimes described as "Type I," or postmenopausal, and is most marked in trabecular bone, resulting in vertebral fractures.

Starting Level of Bone Density. Over a normal life span a woman loses about half of her bone mass and a man about a quarter of his bone mass from that present in young adulthood. Whether the residual level is reduced enough to be considered pathological osteoporosis with enhanced danger of fracture depends in part on the starting level. Blacks, for example, in general have more initial bone and therefore rarely develop clinical osteoporosis. Small, slender women of northern European extraction have lighter bones and are more prone to develop osteoporosis.

Ingestion and Absorption of Calcium. If absorbed calcium is insufficient to replace its obligatory loss in urine and stool (150 to 250 mg per day), it will be mobilized from the skeleton under the influence of PTH. Since dietary calcium is often marginal, particularly so with the decreased efficiency of its absorption in the aged, this may contribute to loss of bone mass.

Aging. Beyond the hormonal effects of estrogen deficiency, there is age-related loss of bone in both men and women, especially after the age of 75, sometimes referred to as "Type II" involutional osteoporosis. There is usually a balanced loss of both trabecular and cortical bone, and therefore fractures occur in the hip, pelvis, and long bones as well as in the trabecular bone of the vertebral bodies. Type II osteoporosis is thought to result from decreased bone formation as well as from a secondary increase in PTH secretion because of reduced calcium absorption.

Other risk factors are known, as shown in Table

TABLE 77–1. CLASSIFICATION OF CAUSES OF OSTEOPOROSIS*

Primary osteoporosis	Bone marrow disorders
Juvenile	Multiple myeloma and related
Idiopathic (young adults)	disorders
Involutional osteoporosis	Systemic mastocytosis
Endocrine diseases	Disseminated carcinoma
Hypogonadism	Connective tissue diseases
Ovarian agenesis	Osteogenesis imperfecta
Hyperadrenocortisolism	Homocystinuria
Hyperthyroidism	Ehlers-Danlos syndrome
Hyperparathyroidism	Marfan's syndrome
Diabetes mellitus (?)	Miscellaneous causes
Gastrointestinal diseases	Immobilization
Subtotal gastrectomy	Chronic obstructive pulmonary
Malabsorption syndromes	disease
Chronic obstructive jaundice	Chronic alcoholism
Primary biliary cirrhosis	Chronic heparin administration
Severe malnutrition	Rheumatoid arthritis (?)
Alactasia	

* From Riggs BL: Osteoporosis. In Wyngaarden JB, and Smith LH Jr (eds): Cecil Textbook of Medicine. 17th ed. Philadelphia, WB Saunders Co, 1985, p 1457.

77–1, such as excess glucocorticoids, alcoholism, immobilization, certain rare genetic abnormalities of connective tissue, heparin (either administered or associated with mastocytosis), multiple myeloma, and a number of gastrointestinal disorders associated with impaired bioavailability of calcium. In addition, severe transient osteoporosis of unknown cause may occur in children or young adults.

Clinical Manifestations

Osteoporosis is usually asymptomatic unless it results in a fracture—a vertebral compression fracture or a fracture of the hip, pelvis, humerus, or any other bone. The most typical symptom is the sudden onset of back pain associated with vertebral compression caused by a modest stress (e.g., picking up an object, leaning over). This may be associated with muscle spasms and ileus but usually improves over some weeks. With a series of such axial fractures, usually with anterior wedging, there is telescoping with loss of height and the development of kyphosis. Compression of the vertebral bodies may occur gradually without acute episodes of pain and produce the characteristic dorsal kyphosis with cervical lordosis, sometimes known as the "dowager's hump." Fractures of the hip may occur with modest trauma or even spontaneously and carry a mortality rate of 15 per cent as well as resulting in severe disability and long-term care for many of those who survive.

Diagnosis

The diagnosis of osteoporosis can usually be established by the presence of typical radiographic changes (see below) in a patient in whom the disease might be anticipated (e.g., a white woman 10 to 20 years postmenopausal) and in the absence of evidence for any other cause of diffuse osteopenia. Serum calcium, phosphorus, and alkaline phosphatase levels are usually normal, although the alkaline phosphatase level may rise slightly after a fracture. The conditions in Table 77–1 should be carefully considered. It is especially important to rule out by laboratory methods multiple myeloma, which can closely mimic involutional osteoporosis. If osteomalacia is considered to be a possibility, a bone biopsy may be warranted, since the therapy would be very different (see Chapter 76).

Radiographic Findings

The most characteristic radiographic findings of osteoporosis are in the spine, illustrated diagrammatically in Figure 77–1. With the loss of trabecular bone, the end plates of the vertebral bodies stand out, and the washed-out radiolucent bodies tend to show fine vertical striations because of preferential loss of horizontal trabeculae. The intervertebral discs expand into concavities within the vertebral bodies and may rupture into the body (Schmorl's nodules). There is loss of height with compression fractures producing anterior wedging.

Treatment

The treatment of osteoporosis will depend on its cause and the stage of the illness. For example, if there is Cushing's syndrome, multiple myeloma, or thyrotoxicosis, the treatment differs from that of either Type I or Type II involutional os-

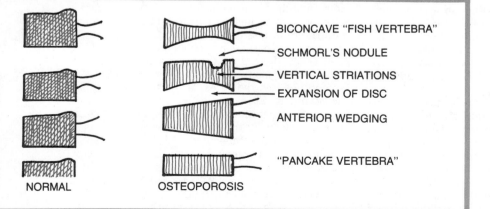

FIGURE 77–1. Vertebral changes in osteoporosis.

teoporosis. During the acute phase of a vertebral compression, attention is directed toward relief of pain (analgesics, heat, massage, rest), but early ambulation and careful exercises of back muscles should be encouraged. Most patients with symptomatic osteoporosis are elderly woman. An approach to the treatment of this group of patients is directed toward the prevention of further loss of bone.

Estrogens. Small doses of estrogens (the equivalent of 0.625 to 1.25 mg of estrone sulfate daily) can reduce the loss of bone in postmenopausal women. This should be given with a progestin during the last 10 days of the cycle to reduce the danger of endometrial carcinoma.

Calcium. Supplement of the diet by 1.0 to 1.5 grams of calcium may enhance absorption sufficiently to reduce bone loss, particularly by reducing secondary hyperparathyroidism. If the patient has a malabsorptive syndrome, supplementary vitamin D may also be useful, but it should be used cautiously in order to prevent hypercalcemia.

Experimental forms of therapy include the use of calcitonin to reduce bone destruction and the use of sodium fluoride (together with calcium supplementation) to stimulate osteoblastic formation of trabecular bone in the axial skeleton. Response to all forms of treatment can be followed by careful measurement of the patient's height over time as an index of compression of vertebral bones or more accurately and expensively by use of quantitative computed tomography of the vertebral bodies or photon absorptiometry of peripheral cortical bone.

REFERENCES

Avioli LV: Osteoporosis: Pathogenesis and therapy. In Avioli LV, and Krane SM (eds): Metabolic Bone Disease. Vol. 1. New York, Academic Press, 1977, p 307.

Ettinger B, Genant HK, and Cann CE: Long-term estrogen replacement therapy prevents bone loss and fractures. Ann Intern Med 102:319, 1985.

Genant HK, Gordan GS, and Hoffman PG Jr: Osteoporosis. Medical Staff Conference, University of California, San Francisco. West J Med 139:75, 204, 1983.

Haber RJ: Should postmenopausal women be given estrogen? Medical Staff Conference, University of California, San Francisco. West J Med 142:672, 1985.

Riggs BL: Osteoporosis. In Wyngaarden JB, and Smith LH Jr (eds): Cecil Textbook of Medicine. 17th ed. Philadelphia, WB Saunders Co, 1985, p 1456.

PAGET'S DISEASE OF BONE 78

Paget's disease of bone, also called osteitis deformans, is characterized by chronic, localized areas of bone destruction complicated by concurrent exuberant bone repair. Approximately 3 per cent of adults over age 40 have histological evidence of Paget's disease at autopsy, the prevalence increasing with age. Less than 1 per cent have radiographic evidence of the disease.

Etiology

The etiology of Paget's disease has not been established. Strictly speaking it is not a metabolic bone disease, since it is localized (although many bones may be involved); a primary abnormality of endocrine function or of mineral metabolism seems highly unlikely. It is provocative that inclusion bodies resembling certain viral nucleocapsids can be demonstrated in pagetic osteoclasts, and these inclusions have shown immunological reactivity to antisera to the measles virus and to the syncytial virus.

Pathology and Pathophysiology

The primary process in Paget's disease is localized osteolysis, which seems to result from an enhanced number and activity of osteoclasts. This chronic destructive process occurs in the setting of continued reparative osteogenesis by osteoblasts, the products of which may also undergo simultaneous or subsequent destruction. The result is usually thickened but weakened bone without the normal pattern of cortical or trabecular bone. The resulting random mix of cement lines is generally described as a "mosaic pattern." The weakened bone may fracture or bend under stress. For example, the base of the skull may flatten with basilar invagination (platybasia); cortical infractions may occur on the convex surfaces of bowed long bones, particularly with the characteristic lateral bowing of the femur and anterior bowing of the tibia.

Repair usually matches destruction, so that serum calcium and phosphorus are usually normal despite a remarkably enhanced bone turnover rate. Serum alkaline phosphatase may be markedly elevated, reflecting osteoblastic activity, and urinary hydroxyproline is usually increased, reflecting increased osteoclastic activity.

Clinical Picture (Table 78–1)

Most patients with Paget's disease have no symptoms, the disorder being discovered by radiographs taken for some other purpose or during investigation of the source of an elevated alkaline phosphatase. The most common symptom is pain in the area of bone involvement, which occurs most frequently in the sacrum, pelvis, and spine. Sudden onset of pain may result from a fracture or an infraction of a long bone. More rarely the patient may note painless deformity of the skull

FIGURE 78–1. "Cottonwool" appearance of the skull in the osteoblastic phase of Paget's disease. (From Kelley WN, Harris ED Jr, Ruddy S, and Sledge CB (eds): Textbook of Rheumatology. 2nd ed. Philadelphia, WB Saunders Co, 1985, p 1677.)

or of the long bones of the leg. Involvement of the skull may result in headaches, deafness, tinnitus, or vertigo. With platybasia, compression of the spinal cord and brain stem may result in serious neurological complications. Osteogenic sarcoma occurs in a small number of pagetic patients, especially those with polyostotic involvement of long duration.

The physical examination may show an enlarged skull, typical bowing of the long bones of the legs, redness and heat from vasodilatation over the areas of bone involvement, and angioid streaks in the optic fundi. Very rarely the increased cardiac output to the involved bone may result in high-output congestive failure. Other clinical and laboratory findings are listed in Table 78–1.

Diagnosis

The diagnosis can usually be established by the clinical picture and the characteristic radiographic findings (Fig. 78–1). Very rarely bone biopsy may be indicated to exclude the presence of osteoblastic metastases.

Treatment

Most patients do not require therapy, or else they respond adequately to full doses of salicylates or indomethacin. If symptoms persist, three approaches have been used with some success in reducing the activity of the disease, as measured by serum alkaline phosphatase or by the urinary excretion of hydroxyproline-containing (collagen-derived) peptides:

Calcitonin. This hormone is given parenterally, usually as salmon calcitonin, to inhibit osteoclastic activity.

Diphosphonates. Oral disodium etidronate may be effective in inhibiting bone resorption but in large doses may inhibit mineralization as well, producing osteomalacia.

Mithramycin. This potent cytotoxic agent seems to have particular activity against the osteoclast, and its use parenterally may cause a remission of disease activity.

In addition, patients may benefit from orthopedic surgery to reduce deformities, replace a degenerative hip, or relieve neurological compression.

TABLE 78–1.   CLINICAL MANIFESTATIONS OF PAGET'S DISEASE

Musculoskeletal pain
Skeletal deformity
Pathological fractures
Enlarged skull
   leontiasis ossea
   deafness, tinnitus
Platybasia—spinal cord and brain stem compression
Erythema and heat over pagetic areas
Increased cardiac output—rarely congestive failure
Angioid streaks in retina
Osteogenic sarcoma
Reparative granuloma
Characteristic radiographs
Serum alkaline phosphatase increased
Urinary hydroxyproline increased
Hypercalciuria and hypercalcemia during immobilization (decreased reparative osteogenesis)
Hyperuricemia—not uncommon, sometimes with gout

REFERENCES

Nagant De Deuxchaisnes C, and Krane SM: Paget's disease of bone; Clinical and metabolic observations. Medicine 43:233, 1964.

Singer FR: Paget's Disease of Bone. New York, Plenum Press, 1977.

Singer FR: Paget's disease of bone (osteitis deformans). In Wyngaarden JB, and Smith LH Jr (eds): Cecil Textbook of Medicine. 17th ed. Philadelphia, WB Saunders Co, 1985, p 1461.

Renal osteodystrophy refers to the complex form of bone disease that occurs with varying degrees of severity in almost all patients with chronic renal failure and azotemia. Although the various components may differ in degree, four types of metabolic bone disease may coexist: osteitis fibrosa cystica, osteomalacia (rickets in children), osteosclerosis, and osteoporosis. These entities have been described in other chapters, so they will be discussed only briefly here.

Osteitis Fibrosa Cystica

Renal failure is the commonest cause of severe secondary hyperparathyroidism (see Chapter 75). The rise in extracellular phosphate tends to reduce the level of ionized calcium and also to diminish the synthesis of 1,25-dihydroxycholecalciferol (calcitriol) in the proximal renal tubule (see Chapter 74). Furthermore, renal disease per se impairs the enzymatic capacity of the kidney to carry out this synthesis and therefore indirectly reduces calcium absorption. The parathyroid glands respond by increasing the secretion of PTH and also by undergoing chief cell hyperplasia to increase total secretory capacity. The highest levels of circulating iPTH are those measured in the severe secondary hyperparathyroidism of renal insufficiency, although in part these levels are artifactually elevated, since biologically inactive but immunologically reactive fragments of PTH circulate longer in this condition.

PTH markedly increases osteoclastic activity but is usually unable to reduce extracellular phosphate to normal because of disease of the target organ, the kidney. The resulting osteitis fibrosa cystica is sometimes radiographically apparent as subperiosteal bone resorption (see Fig. 75–3) and is the source of distressing symptoms. Histological evidence of this characteristic lesion of hyperparathyroidism is evident in most patients with chronic renal failure in whom the rise in serum P has not been prevented.

Osteomalacia (See Chapter 76)

In osteomalacia bone is weakened because of inadequate rates of mineralization of newly formed osteoid. The mechanism of this defective deposition of bone salts into osteoid in uremia is only partially understood. The alterations in the metabolism of vitamin D have been noted above. A lack of active metabolites of vitamin D may contribute directly through loss of a proposed effect on mineralization per se as well as indirectly through a reduced absorption of dietary calcium. The ion product (Ca × P) at the site of mineralization may therefore be inadequate. In uremia there may be retention of other inhibitors of mineralization as well, such as pyrophosphate, and uremic acidosis may adversely affect bone formation. In a minority of patients osteomalacia resistant to vitamin D therapy may develop because of aluminum accumulation. This occurs in the setting of excessive use of aluminum-containing antacids or use of dialysis water high in aluminum in uremic patients.

As noted in Chapter 76, osteomalacia generally presents only as a nonspecific osteopenia, unless the characteristic pseudofractures (Looser's zones) are seen (see Fig. 76–2). The diagnosis otherwise requires a bone biopsy with examination of an undecalcified specimen, preferably after the use of oral tetracycline for labeling the mineralization front.

Osteosclerosis

In uremia an increased density of woven bone in a bandlike pattern may be noted in the spine, most commonly at the upper and lower borders of the vertebral bodies. Taken together with the decreased radiodensity between, this striped appearance has been called the "rugger-jersey" sign. These areas of osteosclerosis may be seen more rarely in the pelvis and long bones. The pathogenesis of this osteosclerosis is unclear, and there is no specific clinical correlation. Some believe that this lesion with its distinctive radiographic pattern reflects the bone's response to long-term severe hyperparathyroidism.

Osteoporosis (See Chapter 77)

Osteoporosis occurs in renal osteodystrophy, but it is rarely a significant component of the entity.

SYMPTOMS AND SIGNS

The clinical manifestations of renal osteodystrophy are those of its constituent forms of bone disease (largely osteitis fibrosa cystica and osteomalacia) and vary widely in severity. They are largely those of bone pain, bone tenderness, and muscle weakness. Occasionally these symptoms may be the main cause of disability in a uremic patient.

TREATMENT

The key to the treatment of renal osteodystrophy lies in its prevention, largely through the control of phosphate accumulation and provision of adequate calcium. This can usually be achieved by restricting dietary phosphate, including the use of phosphate-binding antacids to prevent its absorption, and the use of supplemental oral calcium, 1.0 to 2.0 grams/day, when the level of phosphate has been controlled. When osteomalacia is present, judicious vitamin D therapy may be required, preferably using calcitriol 0.5 to 1.0 µg/day, since it is the final "postrenal" product and also has a short half-life in case of resulting overshoot with hypercalcemia. Aluminum-induced osteomalacia should obviously be treated by removal of the source of excess aluminum (antacids, high-Al dialysis fluid) and possibly also by the use of deferoxamine. Very rarely parathyroidectomy may be required to reduce the total mass of functioning parathyroid tissue.

REFERENCES

Coburn JW, and Slatopolsky E: Vitamin D, parathyroid hormone and renal osteodystrophy. In Brenner BM, and Rector FC Jr (eds): The Kidney. 2nd ed. Philadelphia, WB Saunders Co, 1981, p 2213.

Slatopolsky E: Renal osteodystrophy. In Wyngaarden JB, and Smith LH Jr (eds): Cecil Textbook of Medicine. 17th ed. Philadelphia, WB Saunders Co, 1985, p 1453.

INFECTIOUS DISEASES

80 ORGANISMS THAT INFECT HUMANS

VIRUSES

Viruses produce a wide variety of clinical illnesses. A virus consists of either DNA or RNA wrapped within a protein nucleocapsid. The nucleocapsid may be covered by an envelope composed of glycoproteins and lipids. Viral genes can code for only a limited number of proteins, and viruses possess no metabolic machinery. They are entirely dependent upon host cells for protein synthesis and replication and are therefore obligate intracellular parasites. Some viruses are dependent upon other viruses to produce active infection. Such is the case with the delta agent, which produces disease only in the presence of hepatitis B infection. All must attach to "receptors" on the host cell and achieve entry into the cell through host-derived mechanisms, usually pinocytosis. Once within the cells, the virus uncoats, allowing its nucleic acid to utilize host cellular machinery to reproduce (productive infection) or to integrate into the host cell (latent infection). Viruses have developed several mechanisms of evading host defense mechanisms. By multiplying within host cells, viruses can avoid cytotoxic antibodies and other host defenses. Some viruses can spread to uninfected cells by intercellular bridges. Some viruses, especially the herpes group, are capable of persisting without multiplication within host cells for prolonged periods (latency). The influenza virus is capable of extensive gene rearrangements, resulting in significant changes in surface antigen structure. This allows new strains to evade host antibody responses to earlier strains.

Some viruses, as they exit the host cell during productive infection, may carry antigens of host cell origin, thus providing another mechanism for evading host defenses.

CHLAMYDIA

Chlamydia are also obligate intracellular parasites, but unlike viruses they contain both DNA and RNA, divide by binary fission (rather than multiplying by assembly), can synthesize proteins, and contain ribosomes. They are unable to synthesize ATP and thus depend on energy from the host cell to survive. The two chlamydial species known to cause disease in man are *Chlamydia trachomatis* and *Chlamydia psittaci*. *C. trachomatis* causes trachoma, the major cause of blindness in the developing world, and a variety of sexually transmitted genitourinary disorders including urethritis, salpingitis, and lymphogranuloma venereum. *C. psittaci*, a common infectious disease of birds, can produce a serious systemic illness, with prominent pulmonary manifestations, in man. These organisms are susceptible to tetracycline.

RICKETTSIA

Rickettsia are small bacterial organisms that, like chlamydia, are obligate intracellular parasites. Rickettsia are animal pathogens that generally produce disease in man through the bite of an insect vector such as a tick, flea, louse, or mite. The organisms specifically infect vascular endothelial cells. With the exception of Q fever, rash due to vasculitis is a prominent manifestation of these often disabling febrile illnesses. These organisms are susceptible to tetracyclines and chloramphenicol.

MYCOPLASMAS

Mycoplasmas are the smallest free-living organisms. In contrast to viruses, chlamydia, and rickettsia, mycoplasmas can grow on cell-free media and produce disease without intracellular penetration. Like other bacteria, these organisms have a membrane but, unlike other bacteria, they have no cell walls. Thus, antibiotics that are active against bacterial cell walls have no effect on mycoplasmas. Three major species of mycoplasmas cause disease in man: *Mycoplasma pneumoniae* is an agent of pharyngitis and pneumonia, whereas *Mycoplasma hominis* and *Ureaplasma urealyticum* are agents of genitourinary disease. Mycoplasmas are sensitive to erythromycin or tetracycline or both.

BACTERIA

Bacteria are a tremendously varied group of organisms that are generally capable of cell-free growth, although some produce disease as intracellular parasites. There are numerous ways of classifying bacteria, including morphology, ability to retain certain dyes, growth in different physical conditions, ability to metabolize various substrates, and antibiotic sensitivities. Although combinations of these methods are used to identify bacteria in hospital bacteriology laboratories, relatedness for taxonomic purposes is established by DNA homology.

SPIROCHETES

Spirochetes are slender, motile, spiral-shaped organisms that are not readily seen under the microscope unless stained with silver or viewed under darkfield illumination. Many of these organisms cannot yet be cultured on artificial media or in cell culture. There are four genera of spirochetes that cause disease in man. *Treponema* include the pathogens of syphilis and the nonvenereal endemic syphilis-like illnesses of yaws, pinta, and bejel. The illnesses caused by these organisms are chronic and characterized by prolonged latency in the host. Penicillin is active against *Treponema*. *Leptospira* species are the causative agents of leptospirosis, an acute or subacute febrile illness occasionally resulting in aseptic meningitis, jaundice, and (rarely) renal insufficiency. *Borrelia* species are arthropod-borne spirochetes that are the causative agents of relapsing fever. During afebrile periods, these organisms reside within host cells and emerge with modified cell surface antigens. These modifications may permit the bacterium to evade host immune responses and produce relapsing fever and recurrent bacteremia. *Spirillum minor* is one of the causative agents of rat-bite fever. A recently identified spirochete is the causative agent of Lyme disease. The organism is transmitted to humans through the bite of the small ixodid tick and produces a characteristic rash, erythema chronicum migrans, followed by an illness typified by recurrent arthritis and occasionally meningoencephalitis.

ANAEROBIC BACTERIA

Anaerobes are organisms that cannot grow in atmospheric oxygen tensions. Some are killed by very low oxygen concentrations, whereas others are relatively aerotolerant. As a general rule, anaerobes that are pathogens for man are not as sensitive to oxygen as nonpathogens. Anaerobic bacteria are primarily commensals. They inhabit the skin, gut, and mucosal surfaces of all healthy individuals. In fact, the presence of anaerobes may inhibit colonization of the gut by virulent, potentially pathogenic bacteria. Anaerobic infections generally occur in two circumstances: (1) contamination of otherwise sterile sites with anaerobe-laden contents. Examples include (a) aspiration of oral anaerobes into the bronchial tree, producing anaerobic necrotizing pneumonia; (b) peritonitis and intra-abdominal abscesses following bowel perforation; (c) fasciitis and osteomyelitis following periodontal infections or oral surgery. (2) Infections of tissue with lowered redox potential as the result of a compromised vascular supply. Examples include (a) foot infections in diabetic patients, in whom vascular disease may produce poor tissue oxygenation; and (b) infections of pressure sores, in which perianal anaerobic flora gain access to tissue whose vascular supply is compromised by pressure. The pathogenesis of anaerobic infections, i.e., soilage by a complex flora, generally results in polymicrobial infections. Thus, the demonstration of one anaerobe in an infected site generally implies the presence of others. Often facultative organisms (organisms capable of anaerobic and aerobic growths) coexist with anaerobes. Certain anaerobes such as *Clostridium* produce toxins that cause well-defined illnesses such as food poisoning, tetanus, and botulism. Other toxins may play a role in the soft tissue infections—cellulitis, fasciitis, and myonecrosis—occasionally produced by *Clostridium* species. *Bacteroides fragilis*, the most numerous bacterial pathogen in the normal human colon, has a polysaccharide capsule that inhibits phagocytosis and promotes abscess for-

mation. Clues to the presence of anaerobic infection include (a) a foul odor (the diagnosis of anaerobic pneumonia can, on occasion, be made from across the room); (b) the presence of gas, which may be seen radiographically or manifested by crepitus on examination (however, not all gas-forming infections are anaerobic); and (c) the presence of mixed gram-positive and gram-negative flora on a Gram's stain of purulent exudate, especially when there is little or no growth on plates cultured aerobically. Most anaerobes are sensitive to penicillin. Exceptions are strains of *Bacteroides fragilis* (usually sensitive to metronidazole, clindamycin, or chloramphenicol) and *Clostridium difficile*, which is sensitive to metronidazole and vancomycin. Strains of *Fusobacterium* may also be relatively resistant to penicillin. As a general rule, infections caused by anaerobes originating from sites above the diaphragm are penicillin-sensitive, whereas infections below the diaphragm are often caused by penicillin-resistant organisms.

GRAM-NEGATIVE BACTERIA

The cell walls of these bacteria, which appear pink on a properly prepared Gram's stain, contain lipopolysaccharide, a potent inducer of endogenous pyrogen release and fever. These organisms cause a wide variety of illnesses. Gram-negative bacteria are the most common cause of cystitis and pyelonephritis. Excepting *Haemophilus* species, they are uncommon causes of community-acquired pneumonia but common causes of nosocomial pneumonia. Excepting the peculiar risk of *Pseudomonas* infection in I.V. drug abusers, gram-negative organisms are rare causes of endocarditis on natural heart valves but occasional pathogens on prosthetic valves. The Enterobacteriaceae include *Escherichia coli*, *Klebsiella*, *Enterobacter*, *Serratia*, *Salmonella*, *Shigella*, and *Proteus*. These are large gram-negative rods. Except for the occasional presence of a clear space surrounding some *Klebsiella* (representing a large capsule), these organisms are not readily distinguished from each other on Gram's stain. The Enterobacteriaceae can be thought of as gut-related or genitourinary pathogens. *Salmonella*, a relatively common cause of enteritis, may occasionally infect atherosclerotic plaques or aneurysms. *Shigella* is an agent of bacterial dysentery. *Proteus* species, which split urea, are the agents associated with staghorn calculi of the ureters and urinary collecting system.

GRAM-POSITIVE BACTERIA

Although these organisms lack endotoxin, infections with gram-positive bacteria also produce fever and cannot be reliably distinguished, on clinical grounds, from infections caused by gram-negative bacteria.

GRAM-POSITIVE RODS

Infections due to gram-positive rods are relatively uncommon outside certain specific settings. Diphtheria is rare but other corynebacteria produce infections in the immunocompromised host and on prosthetic valves and shunts. Because corynebacteria are regular skin colonists, they often contaminate blood cultures; in the appropriate setting, however, they must be considered potential pathogens. *Listeria monocytogenes* resembles *Corynebacterium* on initial isolation and is an important cause of meningitis and bacteremia in the immunocompromised patient. *Bacillus cereus* is a recognized cause of food poisoning. Serious infections due to this and other *Bacillus* species occur among I.V. drug abusers. *Clostridium* species are gram-positive rods. Infections due to these organisms are discussed under anaerobes (see above).

GRAM-POSITIVE COCCI

Staphylococcus aureus is a common pathogen that produces a wide spectrum of disease in man. Staphylococci can infect any organ system. They are common causes of bacteremia and sepsis. The organism often colonizes the anterior nares, particularly among diabetics, hemodialysis patients, and I.V. drug abusers; these populations also appear to have a greater frequency of infections due to this organism. Hospital workers colonized with *Staphylococcus aureus* have also been responsible for hospital epidemics of staphylococcal disease.

Generally protected by an antiphagocytic polysaccharide capsule, staphylococci also possess catalase, which inactivates toxic hydrogen peroxide—a mediator of bacterial killing by neutrophils. Staphylococci tend to form abscesses; the low pH within an abscess cavity also limits the effectiveness of host defense cells. Staphylococci elaborate several toxins that mediate certain manifestations of disease. A staphylococcal enterotoxin is responsible for staphylococcal food poisoning. Staphylococcal toxins also mediate the scalded skin syndrome and the multisystem manifestations of toxic shock syndrome. Most staphylococci are penicillinase-producing and some are resistant to penicillinase-resistant penicillin analogues as well. Vancomycin is active against all strains. Some staphylococci are "tolerant" to cell wall–active antibiotics such as penicillins or vancomycin; such organisms are inhibited but not killed by these agents. The clinical significance of tolerance is not certain. Other staphylococci are distinguished from *Staphylococcus aureus* primarily by their inability to produce coagulase. Some of these coagulase-negative staphylococci produce urinary tract infection (*Staphylococcus saprophyticus*). Another, *Staphylococcus epidermidis*, is part of the normal skin flora and an important cause of infection on foreign bodies such as prosthetic heart valves, ventriculoatrial shunts, and intravascular catheters. Like *Corynebacterium*, *Staphylococcus epidermidis* may be a contaminant of blood cultures but in the appropriate setting should be considered a potential pathogen. *Staphylococcus saprophyticus* is sensitive to a variety of antibiotics used in the treatment of urinary

tract infection; *Staphylococcus epidermidis* is often resistant to most antimicrobials but is sensitive to vancomycin.

Streptococci are a group of organisms whose classifications humble the internist and embarrass the microbiologist. Streptococci are classified into groups according to the presence of serologically defined carbohydrate capsules (Lancefield typing). Group A streptococci produce skin infections and pharyngitis. These organisms are also associated with the immunologically mediated post-streptococcal disorders—glomerulonephritis and acute rheumatic fever. Group D streptococci include enterococci, which are unique among the streptococci in their relative resistance to penicillin. Streptococci can be classified according to the pattern of hemolysis on blood agar—alpha for incomplete hemolysis (producing a green discoloration on the agar), beta for complete hemolysis, and gamma for nonhemolytic stains. Most Lancefield group strains are beta-hemolytic. An important alpha-hemolytic strain is *Streptococcus pneumoniae* (pneumococcus), the most common cause of bacterial pneumonia and an important cause of meningitis and otitis media. A heterogenous group of streptococci, often improperly referred to as viridans streptococci (these organisms show alpha- or gamma-hemolysis) includes several species of streptococci that are common oral or gut flora and are important agents of bacterial endocarditis, abscesses, and odontogenic infections.

MYCOBACTERIA

Mycobacteria are a group of rod-shaped bacilli that stain weakly gram-positive. These organisms are rich in lipid content and are recognized in tissue specimens by their ability to retain dye after washing with acid-alcohol (acid-fast). These bacteria are fairly slow-growing (some require up to six weeks to demonstrate growth on solid media) obligate aerobes. They generally produce chronic disease and manage to survive for years as intracellular parasites of mononuclear phagocytes. Some escape intracellular killing mechanisms by inhibiting phagosome-lysosome fusion. Almost all provoke cell-mediated immune responses in the host, and clinical disease expression may be related in large part to the nature of the host immune response. Tuberculosis is caused by *Mycobacterium tuberculosis*. Other mycobacteria—nontuberculous mycobacteria—can produce diseases resembling tuberculosis. Certain rapid-growing mycobacteria cause infections following surgery or implantations of prostheses, and *Mycobacterium avium-intracellulare* has been implicated as an important cause of disseminated infection among patients with the acquired immunodeficiency syndrome. Leprosy is a mycobacterial disease caused by *M. leprae*.

"HIGHER BACTERIA"

Nocardia and *Actinomyces* are weakly gram-positive filamentous structures. *Nocardia* is acid-fast and aerobic; *Actinomyces* is anaerobic and not acid-fast. *Actinomyces* inhabits the mouth, gut, and vagina and produces cervicofacial osteomyelitis and abscess, pneumonia with empyema, and intra-abdominal and pelvic abscesses, the latter generally associated with intrauterine contraceptive devices. *Nocardia* most commonly produces pneumonia and brain abscess. Approximately half of patients with *Nocardia* infection have underlying impairments in cell-mediated immunity. Infections with both of these organisms require long-term treatment. *Actinomyces* is relatively sensitive to most antibiotics; penicillin is the treatment of choice. *Nocardia* infections are treated with high doses of sulfonamides.

FUNGI

Fungi are larger than bacteria. Unlike bacteria, they have rigid cell walls that contain chitin as well as polysaccharides. They reproduce by budding and/or by spore formation. Excepting *Candida* and related species, fungi are rarely visible on Gram's stain but can be stained with Gomori methenamine silver stain. They are also resistant to potassium hydroxide and can often be visualized on wet mounts of scrapings or secretions to which one drop of 10 per cent solution of potassium hydroxide has been added. Fungi are resistant to antibiotics used in the treatment of bacterial infections and must be treated with drugs active against their unusual cell wall. Most fungi can exist in a yeast form—round to ovoid cells that may reproduce by budding—and a mold form—a complex of tubular structures (hyphae) that grow by branching or extension.

Candida species are oval yeasts that often colonize the mouth, gastrointestinal tract, and vagina of healthy individuals. They may produce disease by overgrowth and/or invasion. *Candida* stomatitis (thrush) often occurs in individuals who are receiving antibiotic or corticosteroid therapy or who have impairments of cell-mediated immunity. Vulvovaginitis due to *Candida* may occur in these same settings but is also seen among women with no apparent predisposing factors. *Candida* can also colonize and infect the urinary tract, particularly in the presence of an indwelling urinary

catheter. Occasionally *Candida* species may gain entry into the blood stream and produce sepsis. This may occur in the setting of neutropenia and chemotherapy, where the portal of entry is the gastrointestinal tract, or in individuals receiving intravenous feedings, in whom the catheter is the source of the infection. Mucosal candidiasis can be treated with topical (clotrimazole) or systemic (ketoconazole) imidazole drugs; systemic candidiasis is generally treated with amphotericin B.

Histoplasma capsulatum is a fungus, endemic to the Ohio and Mississippi River valleys, which produces a mild febrile syndrome in most individuals and a self-limited pneumonia in some. Occasionally patients develop potentially fatal disseminated disease. Some individuals with chronic pulmonary disease may develop chronic pneumonia due to this yeast. Systemic or progressive disease is treated with amphotericin B; ketoconazole may also be effective in some cases.

Coccidioides immitis is endemic in the Southwestern United States and, like *Histoplasma capsulatum*, produces a self-limited respiratory infection or pneumonia in most individuals. Some individuals, particularly blacks and patients of Phillippine descent, may be at greater risk for fatal systemic dissemination. Amphotericin B is used for progressive or extrapulmonary disease.

Cryptococcus neoformans is a yeast with a large polysaccharide capsule. It produces a self-limited or chronic pneumonia, but the most common clinical manifestation of infection with this fungus is a chronic meningitis. Although patients with impairment in cell-mediated immunity are at risk for cryptococcal meningitis, up to half of patients with this syndrome have no identifiable immunodeficiency. Treatment is with amphotericin B.

Blastomyces dermatitidis is a yeast also endemic in the Ohio and Mississippi River basins. Acute self-limited pulmonary infection is followed rarely by disseminated disease. Skin disease is most common, but bones and genitourinary tract may be involved as well. Amphotericin B is used for systemic disease.

Aspergillus is a mold that produces several different clinical illnesses in man. Acute bronchopulmonary aspergillosis is an IgE-mediated hypersensitivity to *Aspergillus* colonization of the

TABLE 80–1. SOME PROTOZOAN DISEASES OF MAN

PROTOZOAN	CLINICAL ILLNESS	TRANSMISSION	DIAGNOSIS
Plasmodium	Malaria: fever, hemolysis	Mosquito, transfusion	Peripheral blood smear
Babesia microti	Fever, hemolysis	Tick, transfusion	Peripheral blood smear
Trichomonas vaginalis	Vaginitis	Sexual contact	Vaginal smear
Toxoplasma gondii	Fever, lymph node enlargement. Encephalitis, brain abscess in compromised host	Raw meat, cat feces	Serologies, tissue biopsy
Pneumocystis carinii	Pneumonia in immuno-compromised host	?Airborne	Lung biopsy, bronchial lavage
Entamoeba histolytica	Colitis, hepatic abscess	Fecal-oral	Stool smear, serologies
Giardia lamblia	Diarrhea, malabsorption	Fecal-oral	Stool smear, small bowel aspirate
Cryptosporidium	Diarrhea	?Fecal-oral	Sugar flotation, acid-fast stain of stool

respiratory tract. This produces wheezing and fleeting pulmonary infiltrates in patients with asthma. Occasionally, *Aspergillus* will colonize a pre-existent pulmonary cavity and produce a mycetoma or fungus ball. Hemoptysis is the most serious complication of such infection. Invasive pulmonary aspergillosis can be a chronic illness of otherwise healthy or marginally compromised hosts, but more often it is a cause of acute pneumonia in patients with neutropenia or recipients of organ transplants. Amphotericin B is the drug of choice for invasive aspergillosis.

The zygomycetes (Mucorales) are ribbon-shaped molds that produce disease in patients with poorly controlled diabetes mellitus or hematologic malignancy and among recipients of organ transplantation. Invasive disease of the palate and nasal sinuses, producing venous thrombosis and infarcts in the brain, is the most common presentation, but pneumonia may be seen as well. These infections are generally treated with surgical excision plus amphotericin B.

PROTOZOANS

In contrast to the pathogens listed above, these single-cell organisms are animals, not plants. With the exception of *Plasmodium*, the pathogens listed on Table 80–1 are all transmitted within the United States.

HELMINTHS

Diseases due to helminths are among the most prevalent diseases in the developing world but are uncommon causes of acute illness in North America.

REFERENCE

Gardner P, and Provine HT: Manual of Acute Bacterial Infections. Little, Brown & Co, 1975.

81 HOST DEFENSES AGAINST INFECTIONS

Both nonspecific and specific host defense mechanisms contribute to the prevention of infectious diseases. The integument, mucous membranes, and epithelial surfaces provide a vital mechanical barrier to infection. The indigenous flora of these surfaces prevents colonization with virulent organisms by competing for nutrients and receptor sites on host cells and producing factors, termed bacteriocins, that are toxic to other bacteria. The local milieu, chiefly the pH and redox potential, provides an additional barrier to colonization and infection with certain organisms. The normal flow of mucus and other secretions helps to eliminate pathogenic microorganisms. The mucociliary blanket, for example, transports organisms away from the lungs. In addition, locally produced and active antimicrobial substances prevent infection. Secretory IgA has a particularly important role in this respect, opsonizing organisms and thereby blocking their ability to adhere to epithelial surfaces and colonize the mucosa.

The elements comprising systemic host resistance to infection are best considered in separate categories as humoral and cellular immune mechanisms and nonspecific effector cell responses. Effective resistance requires interaction of these elements as indicated by the overlapping nature of host defenses against specific infectious agents.

HUMORAL IMMUNITY

Antibody

Initial exposure of humans to microbial antigens leads to proliferation and differentiation of B cells recognizing the antigen into antibody-forming plasma cells. T-cell help is required for responses to most antigens, although bacterial polysaccharides may directly elicit antibody production. Following the first exposure to an antigen, IgM is the main antibody class or isotype produced. An isotype switch then occurs such that IgG predominates. On any re-exposure to the antigen, production of IgG antibody is accelerated and antibody is produced in high titer and with high avidity for the antigen. Secretory IgA is found in tears, saliva, and bronchial, nasal, vaginal, prostatic, and intestinal secretions. Its primary role is to prevent organisms and antigens from breaching mucosal barriers.

IgM accounts for 10 per cent of normal immunoglobulins and is most efficient at complement fixation. IgG also fixes complement. Both IgM and IgG can neutralize the infectivity of viruses and lyse bacteria through complement fixation. Mononuclear phagocytes, neutrophils, and some lymphocytes possess surface receptors for the Fc fragment of IgG. Therefore, IgG antibody can bind to

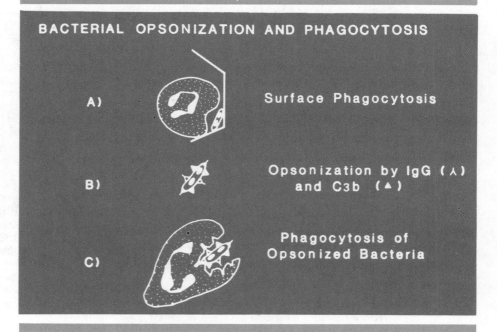

FIGURE 81–1. Ingestion of pneumococci by the neutrophil. In the absence of opsonins, the slippery pneumococcus must be forced against an alveolar surface to be ingested, the inefficient process of surface phagocytosis. Bacteria are opsonized by C3b and IgG, which interact with receptors on the neutrophil, thereby facilitating phagocytosis.

and opsonize bacteria, facilitating their phagocytosis (Fig. 81–1), and arm host effector cells for preferential destruction of selected targets by the process of antibody-dependent cellular cytotoxicity.

Complement

The complement system is of primary importance as the humoral mediator of antigen-antibody complexes. Bacterial polysaccharides can directly activate complement through the alternative pathway. Complement destroys viruses and bacteria, although the degree varies with the individual species. Complement also is important

in generation of the inflammatory response, through its chemotactically active fragments. Complement binds to bacteria, facilitating their attachment to C3b receptors on phagocytes and thus constituting the heat-labile opsonin system (Fig. 81–1).

CELL-MEDIATED IMMUNITY

The cell-mediated immune response is based on interactions between microbes, antigen-specific T lymphocytes, and the mononuclear phagocyte system (Fig. 81–2). The microbe is ingested

FIGURE 81–2. The cytokine cascade. The monocyte or other accessory cell presents antigen to T cells and produces the amplifying cytokine interleukin-1 (IL-1). T cells are activated to express surface receptors for the lymphokine interleukin-2 (IL-2) and to produce IL-2. The binding of IL-2 to its receptor leads to clonal expansion and enhances production of interferon-γ (IFN-γ). IFN-γ has major macrophage activating activity and promotes destruction of intracellular parasites such as the tubercle bacillus. IL-2 and IFN-γ also are required for the differentiation of cytotoxic T lymphocytes (not shown). IL-1, IL-2, and IFN-γ now are available in recombinant form and may prove useful in treating immunodeficiency states and refractory infectious diseases.

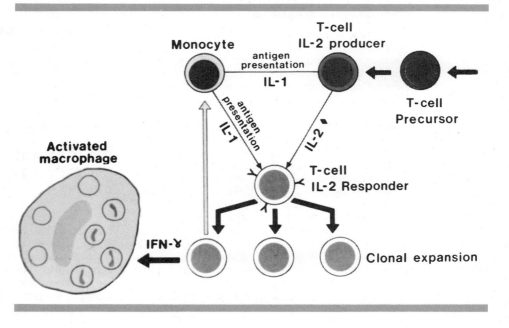

by an accessory cell (mononuclear phagocyte or dendritic cell), which presents appropriate antigens to previously sensitized T lymphocytes. T cells are activated to produce macrophage-activating factors such as interferon-γ. These lymphokines activate mononuclear phagocytes morphologically, biochemically, and functionally, enhancing phagocytosis and allowing destruction of organisms otherwise capable of intracellular persistence. Lymphokines also are important in the differentiation of cytotoxic T cells, which function in antiviral resistance. The cell-mediated immune system demonstrates the cardinal features of an immune reaction—memory, specificity, and systemic expression.

NONSPECIFIC EFFECTOR MECHANISMS

Neutrophils. The neutrophil ingests bacteria and kills them through its production of toxic oxygen metabolites and halogenation of proteins via myeloperoxidase.

Mononuclear Phagocytes. Macrophages have immunoregulatory and secretory properties in addition to their role as effector cells of cell-mediated immunity. Macrophages degrade and kill bacteria directly and in antibody-dependent reactions.

Natural Killer Cells. These cells are defined by their ability to lyse certain tumor targets. However, natural killer cells also are important in antiviral immunity; they kill virus-infected cells.

Integration of the various host defense mechanisms is apparent as one examines resistance to specific infectious agents.

RESISTANCE TO EXTRACELLULAR BACTERIA

Encapsulated Organisms

Streptococcus pneumoniae. The type-specific polysaccharide capsule is a major virulence factor because of its antiphagocytic properties. Antibody to the polysaccharide is capable, in itself, of preventing pneumococcal disease, as reflected by the efficacy of pneumococcal polysaccharide vaccines.

In the absence of immunity, pneumococci reaching the alveoli are not effectively contained by the host. Their phagocytosis by neutrophils is inefficient, since organisms must be trapped against a surface to be ingested ("surface phagocytosis"—Fig. 81–1). The pneumococcus does, however, elicit a neutrophilic inflammatory response. The organism activates complement by the alternative pathway and interactions of C-reactive protein in serum with pneumococcal C-polysaccharide. Activated complement fragments (C3a, C5a, C567) and bacterial oligopeptides are chemotactic for neutrophils. Opsonic complement fragments (C3b) coating pneumococci favor their attachment to neutrophils but are less effective in promoting phagocytosis and killing than is specific antibody. Clinical observations also directly support the primal role of antibody in immunity. It is the development of specific antibody on day five to nine of untreated pneumococcal pneumonia that produces a clinical "crisis" with dramatic resolution of symptoms.

Neisseria Meningitidis. Capsular polysaccharide also represents an important virulence factor for meningococci. In addition, pathogenic Neisseria species produce an IgA protease that dissociates the Fc fragment from the Fab portion of secretory and serum IgA, thus interfering with effector properties of the antibody molecule. Antibody-dependent complement-mediated bacterial killing is the critical host defense against meningococci. Illustrating this principle, the incidence of meningococcal meningitis during the first 12 years of life is inversely proportional to the age-related frequency of serum bactericidal antibody directed against capsular and cell wall bacterial antigens. Therefore, the presence of bactericidal antibody is associated with protection against the meningococcus. In epidemic situations, 40 per cent of individuals who become colonized with the epidemic strain, but lack bactericidal antibodies, develop disease. Protective serum antibody is elicited by colonization with (1) nonencapsulated and encapsulated strains of meningococci of low virulence sharing serotype antigens with virulent strains, and (2) E. coli and Bacillus species with cross-reacting capsular polysaccharides. The lack of bactericidal activity in susceptible adolescents and adults may be due to blocking IgA antibody. Susceptibility of patients lacking C6, C7, or C8 to meningococcal infection provides important evidence that the dominant protective mechanism against this organism involves complement-mediated bacteriolysis. Evaluation of children developing meningococcal disease in a nonepidemic setting reveals that a sizable proportion, in fact, have underlying abnormalities of the complement system.

Exotoxin-producing Organisms

Clostridium Tetani. All disease manifestations produced by this organism can be ascribed to the tetanus toxin, tetanospasmin. Antibody to toxin is protective. Survival from tetanus does not, however, lead to immunity to subsequent infection, because the toxin is sufficiently potent to cause disease at subimmunogenic concentrations.

RESISTANCE TO OBLIGATE INTRACELLULAR PARASITES: VIRUSES

The host directs several defenses against viral infection. The same humoral and cellular mechanisms that destroy bacteria serve to clear extracellular viruses. However, the host immune response also is effective against intracellular replicative stages of viruses and may destroy infected host cells with viral surface antigens. Clinical and experimental observations indicate the relative roles of humoral and cellular immunity in antiviral resistance. In Hodgkin's disease and in T lymphocyte–deficient experimental models, selective defects in cellular immunity lead to reactivation of certain Herpetoviridae: herpes simplex, varicella-zoster, and cytomegalovirus. The prominent role for cellular immunity against these agents is biologically advantageous because virions spread intercellularly via desmosomes or intercellular bridges; viruses thereby escape exposure to the antibody-rich extracellular milieu. Destruction of virus-infected cells by specific cytotoxic T cells becomes an essential first step, allowing extracellular mechanisms to mop up free viral particles.

In contrast, antibody-dependent mechanisms assume major importance against viruses that themselves lyse host cells and spread by extracellular means; for these agents, passive transfer of antibody confers protection. Nevertheless, the absence of any great susceptibility of hypogammaglobulinemic patients to measles and influenza implies continued effectiveness of cellular immunity in protection against these agents and indicates important overlap in antiviral host effector mechanisms.

The major antiviral defenses are:

Humoral Immunity

Complement-Independent Neutralization. Specific IgG, IgM, and IgA neutralize infectivity of all known viruses. The respective antibodies first combine with proteins of the virus coat. Resultant conformational changes prevent adsorption of viruses to cells and cellular penetration; sometimes antibody coating of extracellular virus interferes with subsequent intracellular events such as uncoating. Alternatively, antibody may physically aggregate viral particles.

IgA is the key defender against viruses that begin in or are confined to respiratory epithelium. For infections such as polio, measles, and rubella, which begin on a mucosal surface and then disseminate hematogenously, local IgA antibody prevents infection, whereas serum antibody prevents disease.

Complement-Facilitated Neutralization. Complement neutralizes some enveloped viruses (e.g., retroviruses) by direct or antibody-dependent steric changes or aggregation. Infected cells expressing surface virus antigens also are susceptible to lysis by mechanisms involving the alternate complement pathway and further enhanced by antibody.

Opsonization of extracellular viruses by complement and IgG antibody facilitates phagocytosis by neutrophils and macrophages. This process destroys some viruses (enteroviruses) but aids cell penetration and replication of others (arboviruses).

Enzyme Inhibition. Antibody may interfere with release of progeny influenza virus by blocking viral neuraminidase. Replication is thereby limited, although the virion is not neutralized.

Cellular Immunity

These defenses are of chief relevance for viruses that spread by intercellular means.

Cytotoxic T lymphocytes (CTL). These cells appear early in viral infection and are specific for viral antigens expressed on the surface of parasitized cells.

Antibody-Dependent Cellular Cytotoxicity (ADCC). Virus-infected cells that display surface viral antigens are opsonized by IgG antibodies and lysed by ADCC. The effector cells are lymphocytes (killer cells), macrophages, and neutrophils; all bear surface Fc receptors.

Natural Killer (NK) Cells. NK cells spontaneously lyse virally infected cells; this effector mechanism is activated by interferon.

Interferons

The antiviral action of interferon provides a major host defense against viruses. Interferons are a family of proteins produced by lymphocytes, fibroblasts, epithelial cells, and macrophages early in the course of viral infection before specific antibody develops. Exposure of cells to interferon induces their synthesis of proteins that, in turn, selectively inhibit the production of viral proteins. The immunoregulatory effects of gamma interferon also may contribute indirectly to antiviral immunity by activating effector cells.

RESISTANCE TO FACULTATIVE INTRACELLULAR PARASITES: MYCOBACTERIUM TUBERCULOSIS

Activation of host phagocytes provides the critical defense mechanism against *M. tuberculosis*. Primary infection progresses locally in the nonhypersensitive host, since ingested organisms persist and multiply within mononuclear phagocytes. The bacteria escape intracellular digestion by virtue of constituents (sulfatides, suramin, poly-D-glutamic acid) that inhibit phagolysosomal fusion. Antibody-coated mycobacteria do not evade phagolysosomal fusion but nonetheless resist degradation, probably because of shielding provided by their rich lipid content. The development of cellular immunity leads to T lymphocyte–dependent macrophage activation and to the killing of the intracellular tubercle bacillus organism. The lesions of primary tuberculosis regress. However, latent foci persist, and delayed reactivation remains a threat throughout the lifetime of the host.

REFERENCE

Stites DP, Stobo JD, Fudenberg HH, and Wells JV: Basic and clinical immunology. Los Altos, CA, Lange Medical Publications, 1984.

82 LABORATORY DIAGNOSIS OF INFECTIOUS DISEASES

Four basic laboratory techniques can be used in the diagnosis of infectious diseases: (1) direct visualization of the organism; (2) detection of microbial antigen; (3) a search for "clues" produced by the host immune response to specific microorganisms; and (4) isolation of the organism in culture. Each technique has its use and each its pitfalls. The laboratory can usually provide the clinician with prompt, accurate and, if used judiciously, inexpensive diagnosis.

DIAGNOSIS BY DIRECT VISUALIZATION OF THE ORGANISM

In many infectious diseases, pathogenic organisms can be directly visualized by microscopic examination of readily available tissue such as sputum, urine, pus, and pleural, peritoneal, or cerebrospinal fluid. Using Gram's or acid-fast stains, bacteria, mycobacteria, and *Candida* can be readily identified. An India ink preparation can often identify *Cryptococcus*, and potassium hydroxide (KOH) preparations can occasionally identify other fungal pathogens.

Preparation of Specimens for Staining

Sputum and pus are often thick, and thinning is necessary to obtain a helpful preparation. A drop of sputum or pus is placed on a clean glass slide and another slide is pressed on top of the specimen and pulled away. This step can be repeated as often as necessary (using a clean slide each time) until the specimen has been thinned sufficiently to allow newsprint to be read through it. Unless grossly purulent, fluids such as cere-brospinal fluid (CSF) must be centrifuged to concentrate the organisms and the pellet used for staining. Grossly purulent material may be stained unspun *immediately* to save time. In examining unspun CSF, if no organisms are seen, the pellet must then be examined. To prevent the specimen from washing away during the staining procedure, a drop of CSF may be mixed with a drop of fresh serum or other protein source. The specimen is allowed to air dry and is then gently fixed by passing it quickly through a flame.

Gram's Stain
1. Flood the slide with crystal violet—15 sec.
2. Rinse with water.
3. Flood with Gram's iodine—15 sec.
4. Rinse with water.
5. Decolorize with 95 per cent ethyl alcohol. This step is critical. Rinse with alcohol until blue stain just disappears from the rinse.
6. Immediately rinse with water.
7. Flood with safranin—15 sec.
8. Rinse with water.
9. Air dry.
10. Examine using oil immersion lens.

Proper decolorization is crucial. A good Gram's stain should show neutrophil nuclei as deep pink in all but the most dense regions, where they may have a touch of blue.

Acid-Fast Stain
1. Flood slide with Kinyoun carbol fuchsin—5 min.
2. Wash repeatedly with acid alcohol until wash is clear.
3. Rinse with water.
4. Counterstain with brilliant green or methylene blue—1 min.

Examine for at least 10 minutes using oil immersion lens. Mycobacteria will appear pink, often beaded, and slightly curved. Other bacteria will not retain pink dye. (Exceptions: *Nocardia* and the Pittsburgh agent [*Legionella micdadii*] may also appear acid-fast.)

India Ink Preparation. A drop of centrifuged cerebrospinal fluid is placed on a microscope slide next to a drop of artist's India ink. A coverslip is placed over the drops, and the interface between the CSF and India ink is examined at 100× magnification. Cryptococci are identified by their large capsules that exclude the India ink (Fig. 82–1). The entire slide should be examined.

KOH Preparation. A drop of sputum or skin scraping is placed on a slide together with one drop of 5 to 40 per cent KOH. A coverslip is placed on the specimen and the slide is heated for a few seconds above a flame. The condenser of the microscope is lowered and the specimen is examined at 100× magnification when searching for elastin fibers (whose presence in sputum suggests a necrotizing pneumonia) or 400× when looking

FIGURE 82–1. India ink preparation of cerebrospinal fluid revealing encapsulated cryptococci. Note the large capsules surrounding the smaller organisms.

for fungal forms. The KOH will dissolve host cells and bacteria, sparing fungi and elastin fibers (Fig. 82–2).

These simple bedside techniques can provide rapid and inexpensive diagnosis of many infectious disease processes. There are other techniques that directly visualize pathogens, but they require more sophisticated techniques. Silver staining using the Gomori methenamine technique can identify most fungi and *Pneumocystis carinii*. Immunofluorescence techniques using antibodies directed against the organisms rapidly identify pathogens such as *Legionella pneumophila* and *Bordetella pertussis* in clinical specimens. Darkfield microscopy can identify *Treponema pallidum*, and electron microscopy can often detect viral particles in infected cells.

DIAGNOSIS BY DETECTION OF MICROBIAL ANTIGENS

Certain pathogens can be detected by examination of specimens for microbial antigens (Table 82–1). These studies can be performed rapidly—often within one hour. The diagnosis of meningitis due to *Pneumococcus*, *Haemophilus*, some strains of *Meningococcus*, and *Cryptococcus* can be made rapidly by detection of specific polysaccharide antigen in the cerebrospinal fluid using counterimmunoelectrophoresis (CIE) or latex agglutination. The demonstration of hepatitis B surface antigen in blood establishes the presence of infection by this virus. Cultures of blood of immunocompromised patients with disseminated candidiasis or aspergillosis are often negative. Detection of fungal antigens in blood is still experimental.

DIAGNOSIS BY EXAMINATION OF HOST IMMUNE OR INFLAMMATORY RESPONSES

Histopathologic examination of biopsied or excised tissue often reveals patterns of the host inflammatory response that can narrow down diagnostic possibilities. As a general rule, a polymorphonuclear leukocytic infiltrate is compatible with acute infection and suggests a bacterial process. A lymphocytic infiltrate is compatible with a more chronic process and is seen in viral, fungal, and other nonbacterial infections. Eosinophilia is often seen in parasitic infestations. Granuloma formation suggests mycobacterial and certain fungal infections. Some diseases such as syphilis, cat-scratch disease, and lymphogranuloma venereum have fairly characteristic histological features. Several viral infections produce characteristic changes in host cells; these may be detected by cytological examination. Skin or respiratory infection due to herpesviruses, or pneumonia due to cytomegalovirus or measles virus, for example, can be diagnosed with reasonable accuracy by cytological examination. Similarly, examination of cells and chemistries in in-

FIGURE 82–2. KOH preparation revealing elastin fibers (×400). (Reprinted from Shlaes DM, Lederman M, Chmielewski R, Tweardy D, and Wolinsky E: Elastin fibers in the sputum of patients with necrotizing pneumonia. Chest 83:885, 1983, with permission.)

fected fluids such as cerebrospinal fluid will provide clues to the etiology of the infection. Bacterial infections generally provoke a polymorphonuclear leukocytosis with elevated protein and depressed glucose concentrations. Viral infections most often provoke a lymphocytic pleocytosis; protein elevations are less marked and glucose levels are usually but not always normal.

Host cell-mediated immune responses can be used to help make certain diagnoses. A positive skin test for delayed-type hypersensitivity to mycobacterial or fungal antigens indicates active or previous infection with these agents. A negative skin test may be seen despite active infection in anergic patients. Therefore, control skin tests using commonly encountered antigens (e.g., mumps, *Trichophyton*) must also be applied to ascertain if the patient can mount a delayed-type hypersensitivity response.

Host humoral responses may be used to diagnose certain infections, particularly those due to organisms whose cultivation is difficult or expensive to perform or hazardous to laboratory personnel (Table 82–2). In general, two sera are obtained at intervals of at least two weeks. A fourfold or greater rise (or fall) in antibody titer generally suggests a recent infection. Antibodies of the IgM class also suggest recent infection.

TABLE 82–1. DISEASES OFTEN DIAGNOSED BY DETECTION OF MICROBIAL ANTIGENS

DISEASE	ASSAY
Meningitis	
Pneumococcus	CIE*, latex agglutination
Haemophilus	CIE, latex agglutination
Meningococcus	CIE, latex agglutination
Cryptococcus	Latex agglutination
Hepatitis B	Hepatitis B surface antigen (radioimmunoassay)

*Counterimmunoelectrophoresis

TABLE 82–2. DISEASES OFTEN DIAGNOSED BY MEASUREMENT OF HOST HUMORAL RESPONSES (ANTIBODY LEVELS)

Many viral infections	Rheumatic fever
Mycoplasma pneumonia	Legionnaire's disease
Rickettsial infections	Tularemia
Chlamydial infections	Brucellosis
Lyme disease	Histoplasmosis
Syphilis	Coccidioidomycosis
Leptospirosis	Amebiasis

DIAGNOSIS BY ISOLATION OF THE ORGANISM IN CULTURE

Isolation of a single microbe from an infected site is generally considered evidence that the infection is due to this organism. Information obtained from the culture must, however, be interpreted according to the clinical setting. For example, cultures obtained from ordinarily contaminated sites (e.g., vagina, pharynx) may be overgrown with nonpathogenic commensals, and fastidious organisms such as *Neisseria gonorrhoeae* will be difficult to recognize unless cultured on medium that selects for their growth. Similarly, cultures of expectorated "sputum" may also be uninterpretable if heavily contaminated with saliva. The culture of an organism from an infected but ordinarily sterile site is reasonable evidence for infection due to that organism. On the other hand, the failure to culture an organism may simply result from inadequate culture conditions (e.g., "sterile" pus from brain abscess cultured only on aerobic media. Most brain abscesses are caused by anaerobic bacteria that do not grow under the aerobic conditions most commonly utilized.) Thus, when submitting samples for culture, the physician must alert the laboratory to likely pathogens.

Gram's stains of specimens submitted for culture are often invaluable aids to the interpretation of culture results. A Gram's stain of "sputum" will readily detect contamination by saliva if squamous epithelial cells are seen. On the other hand, a Gram's stain revealing bacteria despite negative cultures suggests infection by fastidious organisms.

Viral Isolation. Since all viral pathogens that can be cultured require eukaryotic cells in which to grow, virus isolation is expensive and often laborious. Throat washings, stool samples, or cultures of infected sites should be transported immediately to the laboratory, or if this is not possible, placed in virus transport medium—usually an isotonic salt solution containing antibiotics and protein—and refrigerated overnight until they can be cultured in the laboratory. Notifying the laboratory of the suspected pathogens allows selection of the best cell lines for culture. The clinician must be aware of the viruses that the hospital's laboratory can isolate. In most instances, the expense of virus isolation and the limited therapeutic options available for most viral infections severely limit the usefulness of viral studies.

Isolation of Rickettsia, Chlamydia, and Mycoplasma. Rickettsia are cultivated primarily in reference laboratories. Diagnosis of rickettsial illness is generally made on clinical grounds and confirmed serologically. Chlamydia can be propagated in cell cultures used in most hospital virology laboratories. Mycoplasma will grow on selective media; the prolonged period of incubation required results in little advantage over serologic diagnosis.

Bacterial Isolation. Isolation of common bacterial pathogens is achieved readily by most hospital laboratories. Specimens should be carried promptly to the laboratory or, in certain instances, placed directly onto the culture medium with careful attention to sterile technique. The specimen is placed onto the culture plate. A loop is sterilized in a flame until it is red, then allowed to cool. The specimen is then streaked as shown in Figure 82–3. This allows separation of different bacterial colonies and rough quantitation of bacterial growth. Choice of agar plates and culture conditions for bedside culture are shown in Table 82–3.

Isolation of anaerobic bacteria is often critically important for clinical diagnosis. When anaerobes are suspected, the specimen, if pus or liquid, can be drawn into a syringe, the air expelled, and the needle capped before transport to the laboratory. Otherwise, specimens must be taken immediately to the laboratory or placed in an anaerobic transport medium appropriate for survival of pathogens. Alternatively, the specimen may be placed in a vial containing thioglycollate broth. This will

FIGURE 82–3. Streaking a bacteriologic plate. The specimen is streaked on the plate. The loop is then heated until red, allowed to cool, then passed through one end of the primary streak as shown, spreading the bacteria to another segment of the plate. This process is repeated, resulting in the pattern shown.

permit anaerobic growth but will not allow quantification of growth. Because of contamination by oral anaerobes, sputum should not be cultured anaerobically unless the sample was obtained by transtracheal or percutaneous lung aspiration.

Isolation of Fungi and Mycobacteria. Specimens for fungal and mycobacterial culture must be processed and cultured by the microbiology laboratory. Although some fungi and mycobacteria will grow readily on standard agars used for routine isolation of bacteria, others must be cultured on special media for as long as several weeks.

REFERENCES

Finegold SM, Martin WJ, and Scott EG (eds): Bailey & Scott's Diagnostic Microbiology. 1978. St. Louis. The C. V. Mosby Co, 1978.

Menegus MA, and Douglas RG: Viruses, rickettsia, chlamydia and mycoplasmas. In Mandell GL, Douglas RG, and Bennett JE (eds): Principles and Practice of Infectious Diseases. 2nd ed. New York, John Wiley & Sons, 1984.

Washington JA: Bacteria, fungi and parasites. In Mandell GL, Douglas RG, and Bennett JE (eds): Principles and Practice of Infectious Diseases. 2nd ed. New York, John Wiley & Sons, 1984.

TABLE 82–3. CHOICE OF MEDIA FOR BEDSIDE BACTERIAL CULTURES

SOURCE	PLATE	CONDITIONS
Throat	BAP[1]	37°C candle jar
Sputum	BAP + CHOC	37°C candle jar
CSF	BAP + CHOC	37°C candle jar
Urine	BAP + EMB or MAC	37°C
Suspected gonorrhea	TM[3]	37°C candle jar
Pus	BAP + EMB or MAC[4]	37°C[4]
Stool[2]		

[1]BAP = blood agar; CHOC = chocolate agar; EMB = eosin methylene blue; MAC = MacConkey; TM = Thayer Martin. EMB and MAC plates inhibit growth of gram-positive bacteria and have an indicator that detects lactose-fermenting bacteria. TM contains antibiotics that inhibit growth of most bacteria except pathogenic *Neisseria*.

[2]Stool cultures should be processed by the clinical laboratory immediately because of the variety of media and conditions needed to isolate stool pathogens.

[3]TM should be used only when culturing contaminated sites (e.g., pharynx, urethra, rectum, cervix). When *N. gonorrhoeae* is suspected elsewhere (e.g., joint space), the specimen should be placed on chocolate agar. This is because TM will also inhibit the growth of 3 per cent of pathogenic *Neisseria*.

[4]Use CHOC plus candle jar if respiratory pathogens suspected. Pus also should be cultured anaerobically (see text).

Note: A candle jar provides increased tension of carbon dioxide but does not provide anaerobic conditions.

FEVER AND THE FEBRILE PATIENT 83

REGULATION OF BODY TEMPERATURE

Although "normal" body temperature ranges vary considerably, oral temperature readings in excess of 37.8°C (100.2°F) are generally abnormal. In healthy humans, core body temperature is maintained within a narrow range so that for each individual, daily temperature variations greater than 1 to 1.5°C are distinctly unusual. This homeostasis is controlled by hypothalamic nuclei that establish "set points" for body temperature. This is effected by a complex balance between heat generating and conserving mechanisms that raise body temperature on the one hand, and mechanisms that dissipate heat and lower body temperature on the other (Table 83–1). Heat is regularly generated as a by-product of obligate energy utilization (e.g., cellular metabolism, myocardial contraction, breathing). When an increase in body temperature is needed, shivering—nondirected muscular contraction—generates large amounts

of heat. Peripheral vessels vasoconstrict to diminish heat lost to the environment. At the same time, the person *feels* cold; this heat preference promotes heat-conserving behavior such as wrapping up in a blanket.

TABLE 83–1. MECHANISMS OF HEAT REGULATION

To raise body temperature
  Heat generation
    Obligate heat production
    Muscular work
    Shivering
  Heat conservation
    Vasoconstriction
    Heat preference
To lower body temperature
  Heat loss
    Obligate heat loss
    Vasodilatation
    Sweating
    Cold preference

Obligate heat loss to the environment occurs through the skin and by evaporation of water through sweat and respiration. When the body must cool down, heat loss is promoted. Vasodilatation flushes the skin capillaries, temporarily raising skin temperature but ultimately lowering core body temperature by increasing heat loss through the skin to the cooler environment. Sweating promotes rapid heat loss via evaporation and, at the same time, the subject *feels* warm and will shed blankets to promote heat loss.

FEVER AND HYPERTHERMIA

Fever is an elevated body temperature that is mediated by an increase in the hypothalamic heat-regulating set point. Thus, although fever may be precipitated by exogenous substances such as bacterial products, the increase in body temperature is achieved through physiological mechanisms. In contrast, hyperthermia is an increase in body temperature that overrides or bypasses the normal homeostatic mechanisms. As a general rule, body temperatures in excess of 41°C are rarely physiologically mediated and suggest hyperthermia. Hyperthermia may be seen after *vigorous exercise*, in patients with *heatstroke*, as a heritable reaction to anesthetics (*malignant hyperthermia*), as a response to phenothiazines (*neuroleptic malignant syndrome*), and occasionally in patients with *central nervous system disorders*.

Fever usually is a physiological response to infection or inflammation. Monocytes or tissue macrophages are activated by various stimuli to liberate a peptide called endogenous pyrogen (Fig. 83–1). Endogenous pyrogen has multiple other biological activities. For example, it is identical to interleukin-1 (an essential cofactor in initiation of the immune response, see Chapter 81). Endogenous pyrogen activates the anterior preoptic nuclei of the hypothalamus to raise the set point for body temperature by the mechanisms shown in Table 83–1. A list of classes of disorders that can cause fever is shown on Table 83–2. Infection by all types of microorganisms can be associated with fever. Tissue injury with resultant inflammation, such as seen in myocardial or pul-

TABLE 83–2. CAUSES OF FEVER

Infection
Tissue injury—infarction, trauma
Malignancy
Immune-mediated disorders
Drugs
Other inflammatory disorders
Endocrine disorders

monary infarction or after trauma, can produce fever. Certain malignancies such as lymphoma, renal carcinoma, and hepatic carcinoma are also associated with fever; in some instances this is related to liberation of endogenous pyrogen by monocytes in the inflammatory response surrounding the tumor; in other cases, the malignant cell may release endogenous pyrogen. Many immunologically mediated disorders such as connective tissue diseases, serum sickness, and some drug reactions are characterized by fever. In some cases of drug-induced fevers, the mechanisms of fever are unknown. Virtually any disorder associated with an inflammatory response (for example, crystal-induced arthritis due to gout) can be associated with fever. Certain endocrine disorders such as thyrotoxicosis, adrenal insufficiency, and pheochromocytoma can also produce fever.

The association of fever with infections or inflammatory disorders raises the question of whether fever is beneficial to the host. Although interleukin-1 (endogenous pyrogen) is critical for initiation of the immune response, certain in vitro immune responses are marginally enhanced by elevated temperatures, and some organisms prefer cooler temperatures, it is not certain that fever is helpful to the host in any infectious disease (with the possible exception of neurosyphilis). Fever is deleterious in certain situations. Among individuals with underlying brain disease such as dementia or even in the healthy elderly, fever can produce disorientation and confusion. In young children, fever can result in seizures. Fever should be controlled if the patient is particularly uncomfortable or whenever it poses a specific risk to the patient. Children with a history of febrile seizures and patients with severe congestive heart

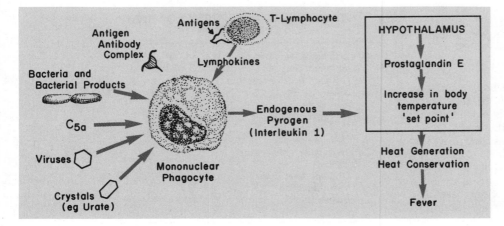

FIGURE 83–1. Pathogenesis of fever.

failure or recent myocardial infarction should have fever treated with antipyretics such as salicylates or acetaminophen. Acetaminophen is preferred for children because of the association of salicylates with Reye's syndrome.

Fever Patterns. The normal diurnal variation in body temperature results in a peak temperature in the late afternoon or early evening. This variation often persists when patients have fever. In certain instances, fever patterns may be helpful in suggesting the cause of fever. Rigors—true shaking chills—often herald a bacterial infection, although they may on occasion be seen in cases of viral infection, as well as in drug or transfusion reactions. Hectic fevers characterized by wide swings in temperature may indicate the presence of an abscess. Patients with malaria may have a relapsing fever with episodes of shaking chills and high fevers, separated by one to three days of normal body temperature and relative well-being. Patients with tuberculosis may be relatively comfortable and unaware of a markedly elevated body temperature. Patients with uremia or diabetic ketoacidosis generally have a lower body temperature, and "normal" temperature readings in these settings may indicate infection. Similarly, elderly patients with infection often fail to mount a febrile response and may present instead with loss of appetite, confusion, or even hypotension without fever.

Approach to the Patient with Fever. In most instances of fever, readily apparent localizing signs or symptoms indicate the likely etiology of the fever. Signs or symptoms of upper respiratory or genitourinary tract infection are the most common presenting complaints in ambulatory practice. On occasion, the etiology of the fever is obscure on initial presentation. Careful history and physical examination often clarify the problem. Among young children in industrialized nations, infections—often viral—account for the majority of febrile illnesses; a history of contact with school-age children should be sought among adults presenting with febrile illnesses. A good travel history—local and international—may reveal recent exposure to areas where regionally circumscribed illnesses are endemic (e.g., plague in New Mexico). Occupational history may reveal exposure to potentially pyrogenic materials such as molds or fumes. Dietary history may reveal ingestion of unpasteurized dairy or undercooked meat products or seafoods, which have been associated with febrile illnesses such as brucellosis, intestinal tuberculosis (dairy products), toxoplasmosis or trichinosis (inadequately cooked meat), hepatitis, or *Vibrio* infection (seafood). History of exposure to wild or domestic animals should be sought and may suggest the diagnosis of zoonoses such as tularemia (rabbits), toxoplasmosis (cats), or psittacosis (birds). A recent tick bite may suggest the possibility of a rickettsial illness or Lyme disease. A history of recent medication may suggest the possibility of drug fever. Although drug fever can occur at any time in the course of treatment, a typical febrile reaction develops after 7 to 10 days of treatment. A history of alcohol abuse places the patient at risk for alcoholic hepatitis or bacterial pneumonia. Intravascular infection such as septic phlebitis or endocarditis is a common problem in I.V. drug users who present with fever. History of an underlying disease may suggest a complication such as bacterial endocarditis in the setting of pre-existent valvular heart disease.

Careful physical exam often provides specific clues to the cause of fever. Inflammation of the conjunctivae is common in viral infection. The fundi may reveal infarcts suggestive of bacterial endocarditis or vasculitis or the choroid tubercles of miliary tuberculosis. Careful examination of the skin and mucous membranes may reveal a rash suggestive of drug reactions, viral or bacterial infection, or another systemic febrile disease. Local lymph node enlargement may be seen with local infection or tumor; generalized lymph node enlargement may occur in patients with viral infections such as infectious mononucleosis, cytomegalovirus or AIDS-related diseases, or other systemic illnesses such as lymphoma, systemic lupus erythematosus, or sarcoidosis.

An elevated white blood cell count is common in febrile patients; a marked shift to the left suggests bacterial infection but may be seen as well in drug reactions and viral infections. Elderly patients may fail to mount a leukocytosis in the presence of infection. The presence of vacuoles within neutrophils on peripheral blood smears suggests a bacterial cause. Toxic granulations and Döhle bodies also suggest bacterial infection but are less specific.

Uncommon presentations of common diseases are more frequent than "classic" presentations of rare diseases. In the United States, most mild undiagnosed febrile illnesses of short duration are, in all likelihood, viral in origin, and the expense of attempts at diagnosis are, in these instances, simply not warranted (see Chapter 85).

Fever of Undetermined Origin. Fever of undetermined origin is the term applied to febrile illnesses (where temperatures exceed 101°F) that are of at least three weeks' duration and remain undiagnosed after one week in hospital. The evaluation of an FUO remains among the most challenging problems facing the physician. The majority of illnesses that cause FUO are treatable, making pursuit of the diagnosis particularly rewarding. There is no substitute for a meticulous history and physical examination. These should be repeated frequently during the patient's hospital course, as frequent and patient questioning may jar an important historical clue from the patient, and important physical findings may develop while the patient is in the hospital. These clues may direct the next series of diagnostic studies. Directed biopsies of lesions should be stained and cultured for pathogenic microbes. In many instances, however, localizing clues are not present or fail to yield rewarding information. In these cases, bone marrow biopsy can reveal granulomatous or neoplastic disease, even in the absence of clinical evidence of bone marrow in-

TABLE 83–3. FEVER OF UNDETERMINED ORIGIN*

Infections		
Intra-abdominal abscesses	11	
Subphrenic		3
Splenic		2
Diverticular		2
Liver and biliary tract		3
Pelvic		1
Mycobacterial	5	
Cytomegalovirus	4	
Infection of the urinary tract	3	
Sinusitis	2	
Osteomyelitis	2	
Catheter infections	2	
Other infections	3	
TOTAL	32	
Neoplastic diseases		
Hematologic neoplasms	22	
Non-Hodgkin's lymphoma		7
Leukemia		5
Hodgkin's disease		4
Other		6
Solid tumors	11	
TOTAL	33	
Collagen diseases	9	
Granulomatous diseases	8	
Miscellaneous	7	
Factitious fever	3	
Undiagnosed	13	
GRAND TOTAL	105	

*Adapted from Larson EB, Featherstone HJ, and Petersdorf RG: Fever of undetermined origin: Diagnosis and follow-up of 105 cases, 1970–1980. Medicine 61:269–292, 1982.

volvement. Similarly, liver biopsy may also reveal the etiology of an FUO, but seldom in the absence of any clinical or laboratory evidence of liver disease. Exploratory laparotomy is generally not helpful unless signs or symptoms point to intra-abdominal pathology. Recent refinements in computerized tomography may assist in determining the need for laparotomy in the cases of FUO. If tuberculosis remains a diagnostic possibility after careful work-up fails to establish a diagnosis, an empirical trial of antituberculous drugs may be initiated while awaiting results of bone marrow, liver, and urine cultures.

Shown in Table 83–3 are the final diagnoses of 105 cases fulfilling criteria for FUO seen between 1970 and 1980. Infectious diseases were the cause of about one third of these cases; another third were due to neoplasms; the remainder were due to connective tissue disorders, granulomatous diseases, and other illnesses. Twelve per cent of cases remained undiagnosed. Half of all infections causing FUO were intra-abdominal abscesses or tuberculosis. Computerized tomography (CT) is helpful in the diagnosis of intra-abdominal abscesses. Even large abscesses, however, particularly pericolonic abscesses, can be missed by CT. Genitourinary tuberculosis is suggested by the presence of sterile pyuria. Disseminated tuberculosis may be subtle; careful attention to chest radiography may reveal a subtle miliary pattern

suggestive of the diagnosis. In this case, lung biopsy is indicated; otherwise, diagnosis can be made by biopsy of bone marrow or liver.

Hematologic neoplasms such as leukemia and lymphomas are far more often associated with fever than solid tumors. Careful review of a peripheral blood smear may reveal clues to a leukemia or preleukemic state. Lymph node enlargement, sometimes restricted to visceral nodes, may suggest the presence of lymphoma. Biopsy of bone marrow may be helpful in both instances; directed biopsy of enlarged nodes may establish the diagnosis of lymphoma.

Collagen diseases that present as FUO are often difficult to diagnose. Nonspecific aches, pains, fevers, elevated sedimentation rate, leukocytosis, and anemia in an elderly patient should raise suspicion of giant cell arteritis. The diagnosis is established by temporal artery biopsy. Still's disease (juvenile rheumatoid arthritis) should be suspected in a younger patient with high fevers, myalgias, arthralgias, sore throat, evanescent rash, lymph node enlargement, and marked leukocytosis. The diagnosis of Still's disease is one of exclusion. Multisystem disease involving the kidney should suggest polyarteritis; the diagnosis can often be made by muscle biopsy or renal angiogram.

Granulomatous hepatitis is an ill-defined entity producing prolonged febrile illnesses and variable abnormalities of liver function (especially an elevated alkaline phosphatase). Diagnosis is made by demonstration of hepatic granulomas without defined etiology. Crohn's disease can rarely present as an FUO without significant gastrointestinal complaints.

Factitious or Self-Induced Fever. Patients with factitious or self-induced illness present unique ethical and therapeutic problems. Once the possibility of factitious or self-induced illness is considered, the doctor-patient relationship is changed. Typically, the physician can rely on the good faith of the patient's history. In the case of factitious or self-induced illness, the physician must assume a more detached role in order to establish the diagnosis. Patients with factitious or self-induced fever are typically young, often women. Many have been or are employed in health-related professions. Usually articulate and well-educated, these patients are adept at manipulating their family, friends, and physicians. In these instances, a consultant new to the patient may provide a detached and helpful perspective on the problem.

Clues to factitious fever include the absence of a toxic appearance despite high temperature readings, lack of an appropriate rise in pulse rate with fever, and absence of the physiological diurnal variation in temperature. Suspected factitious readings can be evaluated by immediately repeating the reading with the nurse or physician in attendance. Use of electronic thermometers in instances of suspected factitious fevers will allow rapid and accurate recording of a patient's temperature.

Self-injection of pyrogen-containing substances, usually bacteria-laden culture medium, urine, or feces, can produce bacteremia and high fever; usually these bacteremic episodes are polymicrobial and intermittent, often suggesting a diagnosis of intra-abdominal abscess. However, patients with self-induced bacteremia may appear remarkably well between episodes of fever, in contrast to most patients with abscesses. Illicit ingestion of medications known by the patient to produce fever can also present a very difficult diagnostic problem. Clues to the presence of self-induced illness are subtle. The patients are often emotionally immature; some will exaggerate their importance and fabricate unrelated aspects of their history. Some are surprisingly stoic about the apparent seriousness of their illness and the procedures employed to diagnose or treat them. In some instances, interview of family members can elicit clues to the possibility of factitious or

self-induced illness. These patients rarely form close friendships. Confirming the diagnosis is crucial and, in many instances, requires search of the patient's hospital room. Although most will deny their role in inducing or feigning illness, the diagnosis must be explained, and psychiatric care is essential. These complicated patients are at risk for inducing life-threatening disease; some respond to psychiatric counseling.

REFERENCES

Aduan RP, Fauci AS, Dale DC, et al: Factitious fever and self-induced infection. A report of 32 cases and review of the literature. Ann Intern Med 90:230–242, 1979.
Dinarello CA, and Wolff SM: Molecular basis of fever in humans. Am J Med 72:799–819, 1982.
Larson EB, Featherstone HJ, and Petersdorf RG: Fever of undetermined origin: Diagnosis and follow-up of 105 cases, 1970–1980. Medicine 61:269–292, 1982.

BACTEREMIA AND SEPSIS 84

The presence of bacteria in the blood indicates that the rate of entrance of organisms from a local infection into the circulation exceeds the capacity of the clearance mechanisms of the reticuloendothelial system and the capillary beds. The bacteremia may be low-grade, intermittent, and of little consequence. As the intensity of infection increases, however, high-grade bacteremia itself causes symptoms and signs, justifying the designation septicemia. In pneumococcal bacteremia, mortality increases when over 1000 colony-forming units of pneumococci are present per milliliter of blood. Quantitative blood cultures rarely are performed, however, so that the intensity and significance of bacteremia must be judged on clinical grounds.

The clinical syndromes of sepsis and septic shock are due to circulating microbial products. These syndromes may occur without demonstrable bacteremia. Sometimes earlier or concurrent administration of antibiotics renders blood cultures negative. Alternatively, a severe local infection, often with mixtures of aerobes and anaerobes, may produce the clinical syndrome of sepsis with negative blood cultures. The difficulty in culturing fastidious organisms from the blood is yet another factor contributing to negative blood cultures in clinically septic patients.

EPIDEMIOLOGY

Septicemia due to gram-negative enteric organisms is the most serious infectious disease of medical progress. Only 100 cases of gram-negative

bacteremia were reported before 1920. Bacteremias among the Enterobacteriaceae were virtually restricted to Escherichia coli and Salmonella species. Antibiotic usage has been associated with a dramatic increase in incidence of gram-negative rod bacteremia, a broadening of the spectrum of causative agents to include Klebsiella, Pseudomonas, Serratia, Enterobacter, and Proteus, and an increase in the fraction of bacteremic episodes resulting from hospital-acquired infections. Other factors that contribute to the upsurge in frequency of gram-negative sepsis are use of invasive mon-

TABLE 84–1. RISK FACTORS FOR SEPSIS

Underlying Disease or Condition
  Immunodeficiency—hypogammaglobulinemic states, neutropenia
  Immunosuppression—corticosteroid and cytotoxic drug treatment, e.g., renal allograft recipients
  Leukemia and lymphoma
  Advanced solid tumors
  Metabolic diseases—uremia, chronic liver disease, diabetes mellitus
  Neurologic diseases—paraplegia
  Intravenous drug abuse
Invasive Medical Devices/Instrumentation
  Indwelling urinary catheter
  Plastic intravenous cannula
  Monitoring devices (arterial line, Swan-Ganz catheter)
  Genitourinary instrumentation
Therapeutic Procedures
  Hemodialysis
  Post genitourinary or abdominal surgery
  Post splenectomy

itoring devices, indwelling catheters, extensive surgical procedures, and the growing number of immunosuppressed patients. Patient groups at particular risk of sepsis are shown in Table 84–1. Overall, an estimated 100,000 to 300,000 cases of gram-negative bacteremia occur in the United States each year.

Gram-negative septicemia may occur without a recognized tissue site of origin; however, more commonly it is secondary to infection in the urinary tract, lungs, peritoneal cavity, biliary tract, soft tissue, or wounds.

Gram-positive bacteremia, particularly caused by *Staphylococcus aureus*, also has become an increasing problem due to the abuse of intravenous drugs and the therapeutic placement of chronic venous access sites.

PATHOGENESIS

Toxic bacterial products account for the cardiovascular and ventilatory derangements characterizing septic shock, as depicted in Figure 84–1.

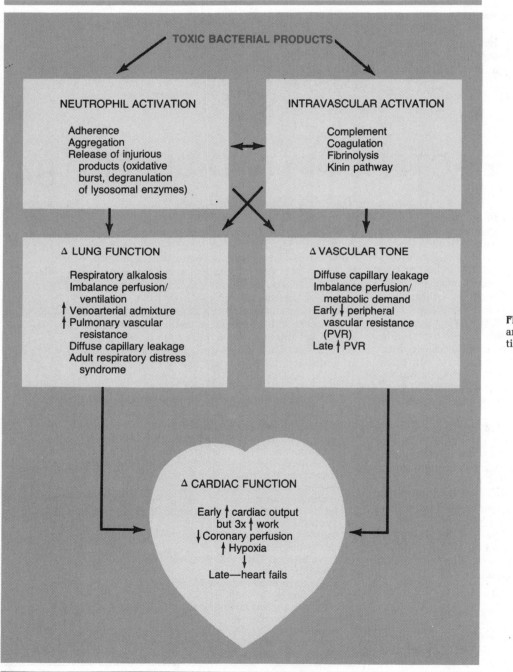

FIGURE 84–1. Pathogenesis and pathophysiology of septic shock.

CLINICAL FINDINGS

The history and physical examination usually indicate the site of origin of the bacteremia. The findings attributable to septic shock depend on whether the patient is evaluated early or late in the course. Shaking chills, often accompanied by nausea, vomiting, and diarrhea, mark the early toxic state characteristic of "warm shock." Patients appear hot, dry, flushed, and animated. Hyperventilation, and apprehension, or lethargy, and obtundation are apparent. In "cold shock," patients are cold, clammy, hypotensive, and lethargic. At this stage, findings of end-organ dysfunction due to hypoperfusion may predominate. These include a bleeding diathesis, jaundice, cyanosis, congestive heart failure, oliguria, and acidosis.

Skin lesions when present are particularly helpful, since they not only suggest sepsis but may provide a clue to the specific etiology. Ecthyma gangrenosum is a round or oval lesion 1 to 5 cm in diameter, with a central vesicle that evolves into a necrotic ulcer, set on an erythematous, indurated base (Fig. 84-2). The typical lesion is caused by *Pseudomonas* species septicemia in neutropenic hosts and results from direct infection of blood vessel walls by bacteria. Other Enterobacteriaceae, particularly *Aeromonas* and *Serratia* species, cause similar lesions on occasion. Vesiculobullous and petechial skin lesions, cellulitis, and diffuse erythema also may appear in the septic patient. Biopsy and aspiration of skin lesions sometimes allow rapid etiologic diagnosis. For example, smears of material expressed from purpuric lesions have a high diagnostic yield (>80 per cent) in meningococcemia.

LABORATORY FINDINGS

The white blood cell count is increased or decreased with an increased proportion of circulating immature neutrophils (band forms). Vacuolization of circulating neutrophils is a useful finding, since it suggests bacterial infection with a high probability of bacteremia. Such changes as toxic granulations and Döhle bodies (pale intracytoplasmic inclusions), on the other hand, merely are indicative of neutrophil immaturity. The platelet count may be decreased in sepsis, the prothrombin and partial thromboplastin times prolonged, and the bilirubin and blood urea nitrogen increased. Sometimes laboratory abnormalities relating to specific end-organ damage are so striking that misdiagnosis or faulty localization of the site of infection may ensue. An example is the disseminated coagulopathy of sepsis that may be suggestive of a primary hematologic disease.

Bacteriologic diagnosis is, of course, essential. Gram's stained preparations should be prepared from urine, sputum, and pus. The Gram's stain not only allows rapid diagnosis but also may indicate organisms that are not easily cultured (fastidious, slow-growing bacteria or anaerobes, for example). Gram's and Wright's stains of a buffy coat smear

FIGURE 84-2. Typical appearance of ecthyma gangrenosum.

also may be extremely helpful, as intracellular organisms, particularly gram-positive cocci and meningococci, are present in over one third of cases of sustained bacteremia. Three sets of blood cultures should be obtained, each from a different venipuncture site.

TREATMENT AND OUTCOME

The mortality of bacteremic shock remains in the range of 40 to 60 per cent despite rapid institution of what should be effective antibiotics. In large part, the adverse outcome reflects a lethal bacterial load at the time of diagnosis and/or a serious underlying disease.

Management of the infection dictates removal of such potential infective foci as intravenous catheters, surgical drainage of accessible abscesses, and administration of appropriate antibiotics. The possibility of infected intravenous catheters or intravenous infusates should be considered at the first suggestion of sepsis. The infusate should be cultured and the catheter removed and 2-inch segments rolled on a blood agar plate to provide semiquantification of infection. The decision to drain a deep-seated focus of infection is difficult in the patient already in extremis because of sepsis. However, stabilization and survival may depend on interrupting the vicious circle that culminates in septic shock.

Appropriate antibiotics should be administered immediately. The selection of antibiotics depends on a number of factors indicated in Table 84-2. Two antibiotics with overlapping activities

TABLE 84-2. FACTORS AFFECTING SELECTION OF ANTIBIOTICS IN THE PATIENT WITH PRESUMED SEPSIS

Community or hospital acquisition of infection
Underlying disease of the host, particularly the presence of neutropenia
Likely source of bacteremia
Organisms suspected on clinical grounds
Results of previous cultures from the patient
Prevailing sensitivities of bacteria in the hospital, particularly patterns of aminoglycoside resistance and prevalence of methicillin-resistant staphylococci

TABLE 84–3. ANTIBIOTIC REGIMENS FOR THE SEPTIC PATIENT

CLINICAL SETTING	LIKELY BACTERIA	ANTIBIOTICS
Uncertain source	Enterobacteriaceae	Gentamicin[a] or tobramycin
	Staphylococcus	+ nafcillin
Abdominal or pelvic source likely	Enterobacteriaceae Enterococcus Bacteroides fragilis	Gentamicin or tobramycin + ampicillin + clindamycin[b] or metronidazole
Neutropenic patient	Pseudomonas species Enterobacteriaceae Staphylococcus species	Tobramycin + ticarcillin + nafcillin[a]

[a]Selection of an aminoglycoside and an antistaphylococcal drug depends on patterns of bacterial sensitivity in the individual hospital.

[b]Avoid clindamycin if potential gastrointestinal side effects would be difficult to recognize (e.g., patient with abdominal pain or ileus).

clearly are necessary to treat *Pseudomonas* species infection in neutropenic patients and probably in patients with severe burns. In general, the administration of synergistic combinations of antibiotics also appears to be associated with improved outcome in patients with severe underlying disease. An additional rationale for two-drug regimens stems from the use of aminoglycosides in most septic patients. Use of a second effective agent is particularly important while aminoglycoside pharmacokinetics are being assessed and dosage schedules optimized in the individual patient. In addition, aminoglycosides are ineffective when the pH is low, as may occur in pulmonary infection. Initial antibiotic regimens suggested for patients with sepsis are presented in Table 84–3. If blood cultures are negative at 48 hours and there is no evidence of serious local infection, consideration should be given to stopping the antibiotics.

Hemodynamic stabilization of the patient with septic shock requires assessment of cardiac function. This usually necessitates monitoring with a central venous or a Swan-Ganz catheter. In the warm stage of shock, peripheral vascular resistance and left ventricular end-diastolic pressure (LVEDP) are decreased; isotonic intravenous fluids are needed, sometimes in massive volume. Pressors may be necessary as well. Dopamine is the inotropic agent of choice, since it increases cerebral, coronary, renal, and mesenteric perfusion when used at low doses. Some patients require intubation and mechanical ventilation, including positive end-expiratory pressure to maintain acceptable oxygenation. In the cold state of shock, congestive heart failure with increased LVEDP limits the use of fluids. Afterload reduction with agents such as nitroprusside is a rational form of therapy but usually requires concomitant administration of pressor agents.

Corticosteroids block complement-mediated neutrophil aggregation and endothelial damage. Initial stabilization of patients can be achieved with corticosteroids, although overall mortality is not reduced. A promising new approach to the management of septic shock is to detoxify bacterial products. Antibody to the lipopolysaccharide core improves the survival of patients in profound septic shock. The use of monoclonal antibodies directed against bacterial toxins ultimately may revolutionize management.

The optimal use of preventive measures would have the greatest impact on the morbidity and mortality of septic shock. The pneumococcal polysaccharide vaccine, for example, is effective and available but tremendously underutilized. Antibiotics should be used only when indicated and then in narrow spectrum and for appropriately short intervals. Intravenous catheters and indwelling urinary catheters should be used only when unavoidable; when necessary, they should be inserted and maintained by experienced personnel, preferably organized in special teams.

REFERENCES

Sheagren JN: Shock syndromes related to sepsis. In Wyngaarden JB, and Smith LH Jr (eds): Cecil Textbook of Medicine. 17th ed. Philadelphia, WB Saunders Co, 1985, pp 1473–1477.

Young LS, Martin WJ, Meyer RD, et al: Gram-negative rod bacteremia: Microbiologic, immunologic and therapeutic considerations. Ann Intern Med 86:456, 1977.

85 ACUTE FEBRILE SYNDROMES

Fever is one of the most common complaints that bring patients to a physician. The challenge is in discerning the few individuals who require specific therapy among the many with self-limited benign illness. The approach is simplified by considering patients in three groups: (a) fever without localizing symptoms and signs, (b) fever and rash, and (c) fever and lymphadenopathy.

FEVER ONLY

Most patients with fever as their sole complaint defervesce spontaneously or present with localizing clinical or laboratory findings within two or three weeks of illness (Table 85–1). Beyond three weeks, the patient can be considered to have a true fever of unexplained origin, a designation with its

TABLE 85–1. INFECTIONS PRESENTING AS FEVER WITHOUT LOCALIZING SIGNS OR SYMPTOMS

INFECTIOUS AGENT	EPIDEMIOLOGY/EXPOSURE HISTORY	DISTINCTIVE CLINICAL AND LABORATORY FINDINGS	DIAGNOSIS
VIRAL			
Rhinovirus, adenovirus, parainfluenzae	None (adenovirus in epidemics)	Often URI symptoms	Throat and rectal cultures, serologies
Enterovirus, ECHO virus	Summer, epidemic	Occas. aseptic meningitis, rash, pleurodynia, herpangina	Throat and rectal cultures, serologies
Arbovirus	Summer	None	Serologies
Influenza	Winter, epidemic	Headache, myalgias, arthralgias	Throat cultures, serologies
Epstein-Barr virus, cytomegalovirus	(see below)		
Colorado tick fever	Southwest, Northwest, tick exposure	Biphasic illness, leukopenia	Blood, CSF cultures, erythrocyte-associated viral antigen (indirect immunofluorescence)
BACTERIAL			
Staphylococcus aureus	I.V. drug users, patients with intravenous plastic cannulas, hemodialysis, dermatitis	Must exclude endocarditis	Blood cultures
Listeria monocytogenes	Depressed cell-mediated immunity	One half have meningitis	Blood, CSF cultures
Salmonella typhi, S. paratyphi	Food or water contaminated by carrier or patient	Headache, myalgias, diarrhea or constipation, transient rose spots	Early blood, bone marrow cultures; late stool culture
FEVER POST—ANIMAL EXPOSURE			
Coxiella burnetti (Q fever)	Infected livestock	Retrobulbar headache, occas. pneumonitis, hepatitis. Culture-negative endocarditis	Serologies
Leptospires	Water contaminated by urine from dogs, cats, rodents, small mammals	Headache, myalgias, conjunctival suffusion. Biphasic illness. Aseptic meningitis	Serologies
Brucella sp.	Exposure to cattle or contaminated dairy products	Occas. epididymitis	Blood cultures, serologies
GRANULOMATOUS INFECTION			
Mycobacterium tuberculosis	Exposure to patient with tuberculosis, known positive tuberculin skin test	Back pain, sterile pyuria or hematuria suggest vertebral, renal infection	Liver, bone marrow histology, cultures
Histoplasma capsulatum	Mississippi and Ohio River valley	Pneumonitis, oropharyngeal lesions	Serologies. Liver, bone marrow, oral lesions histology, cultures

own circumscribed group of management considerations, as discussed in Chapter 83.

VIRAL INFECTION

In young healthy individuals, acute febrile illnesses generally represent viral infections. The causative agent is rarely established. Rhinovirus, parainfluenza, or adenovirus infections usually, but not invariably, are associated with symptoms of coryza or upper respiratory tract infection (rhinorrhea, sore throat, cough, hoarseness). Enterovirus and ECHO virus infections occur predominantly in summer, usually in an epidemic setting. Undifferentiated febrile syndromes account for the majority of enteroviral infections, but the etiology is more likely to be established definitively when macular rash, aseptic meningitis, or a characteristic syndrome, such as herpangina (vesicular pharyngitis due to Coxsackie A) or acute pleurodynia (fever, chest wall pain and tenderness) are present. Serologic surveys also indicate that many arthropod-borne viruses (California encephalitis virus, Eastern, Western and Venezuelan equine encephalitis, St. Louis encephalitis) usually produce mild, self-limited, febrile illnesses. Influenza causes myalgias, arthralgias, and headache in addition to fever. It is unusual, however, for fever to persist beyond five days in uncomplicated influenza.

The mononucleosis syndromes caused by Epstein-Barr virus, cytomegalovirus, and *Toxoplasma gondii* may present in a typhoidal manner—that is, with fever, but little or no lymphadenopathy. Diagnosis and management will be discussed below under "Fever with Generalized Lymphadenopathy," the more typical presentation of these processes.

Colorado tick fever is a disease caused by arbovirus and transmitted by tick bite. Viremia is prolonged, lasting about four weeks. The illness is biphasic—two to three days of fever followed by a similar period of remission, then a second febrile episode. Some patients will have rash, pericarditis, or aseptic meningitis.

The above syndromes are self-limited and untreatable. The impetus for establishing a specific diagnosis, therefore, is small. The differentiation between viral and other causes of febrile illnesses is, on the other hand, of critical importance. Some of the features that distinguish viral and bacterial infection are shown in Table 85–2. Viral cultures of throat and rectal swabs and virus-specific antibodies in acute and convalescent serum samples may allow retrospective diagnosis of viral etiology. Usually, however, the fever is gone long before results of serologies become available.

BACTERIAL INFECTIONS

Bacterial disease may cause septicemia, which dominates the clinical presentation (see Chapter 84). *Staphylococcus aureus* and *Listeria monocytogenes* frequently cause sepsis without an obvious primary site of infection. *S. aureus* sepsis should be a consideration in patients undergoing intravenous therapy with a plastic cannula, hemodialysis patients, intravenous drug users, and patients with severe chronic dermatosis. In the patient with *S. aureus* bacteremia, the question of whether intravascular infection exists is key in determining length of therapy. The following are more typical of an intravascular focus: community-acquired infection, long duration of symptoms, absence of removable focus of infection, (e.g., I.V. cannula), metastatic sites of infection (e.g., septic pulmonary emboli, arthritis, meningitis), and new heart murmur. *Listeria monocytogenes* septicemia is seen predominantly in patients with depressed cell-mediated immunity. One half of patients with *Listeria* sepsis have meningitis. Occasionally a relatively indolent clinical syndrome belies the bacterial etiology of *S. aureus* and *L. monocytogenes* bacteremia.

Enteric fevers also may present in a subacute fashion despite the presence of bacteremia. The major species producing this syndrome are *Salmonella typhi*, which has a human reservoir, and *S. paratyphi* A, B (*S. schottmuelleri*), and C (*S. hirshfeldii*). The paratyphoid strains have their major reservoir in humans as well and produce less severe disease than *S. typhi*. *S. typhi* is acquired by ingestion of food or water contaminated with fecal material from a chronic carrier or patient with typhoid fever. A large number of bacteria (10^6 to 10^8) must be ingested to cause disease in the normal host. Major host risk factors are achlorhydria, malnutrition, malignancy (particularly lymphomas and leukemias), sickle cell anemia, and other defects in cellular and humoral immunity. Major protective mechanisms are gastric acidity and fatty acid products of bacteria comprising the normal gut flora. *Salmonella typhi* penetrates the gut wall and enters the lymphoid follicles where it multiplies within mononuclear phagocytes and produces local ulceration. Primary bacteremia occurs with spread to the reticuloendothelial system (liver, spleen, and bone marrow). After further multiplication at those sites, a secondary bacteremia occurs which can localize to tumors, aneurysms, bone infarcts, etc. Infection of the gallbladder and bile, particularly in the presence of gallstones, leads to the chronic carrier state. Approximately two weeks after exposure, patients develop prolonged fever with chills, headache, and myalgias. Diarrhea or constipation may be present but does not dominate the clinical picture. Crops of rose spots (2 to 4 mm erythematous maculopapular lesions) appear on the upper abdomen but are evanescent. Untreated, typhoid fever usually resolves in about one month. However, complication rates are high owing to bowel perforation, metastatic infection, and general debility of patients. *Salmonella typhi* must be isolated from blood or stool to confirm the diagnosis. Culture of the bone marrow is often positive early in the course of disease. Typhoid fever should be treated with chloramphenicol 50 mg/kg/day intravenously or orally for two weeks. Chloramphenicol-resistant strains of *S. typhi* have appeared in Mexico, India, and Vietnam and should be treated with ampicillin 100 mg/kg/day intravenously or orally, or trimethoprim 320 to 640 mg/sulfamethoxazole 1600 to 3200 mg per day. Ampicillin becomes the drug of choice in endocarditis or infected aneurysms (because of its bactericidal activity) and in patients with sickle cell anemia in whom the dose-related hematologic toxicity of chloramphenicol is unacceptable.

TABLE 85–2. FEATURES HELPFUL IN DISTINGUISHING VIRAL AND BACTERIAL INFECTION

	VIRAL	BACTERIAL
Epidemiology	During epidemic, close contacts with similar illness	Sporadic. Often elderly, significant underlying disease(s)
Symptoms	Associated coryza, upper respiratory tract infection	Shaking chills, fever
Signs	Relatively well appearing	Toxic appearing, confused
	Temperature-pulse dissociation	Tachycardia, tachypnea
Laboratory	Leukopenia or slight leukocytosis	Leukocytosis, shift to left (immature neutrophils), vacuolated neutrophils

Localized bacterial infection can be clinically occult and present as an undifferentiated febrile syndrome. Intra-abdominal abscess, vertebral osteomyelitis due to *Staphylococcus aureus* or *Pseudomonas aeruginosa*, streptococcal pharyngitis, urinary tract infection, infective endocarditis, and early pneumonia can cause fever and surprisingly few clinical clues to the localization of the infectious process. Therefore, urinalysis, throat and blood cultures, and a chest x-ray should be performed in the febrile patient presenting with features suggestive of a bacterial infection (Table 85–2).

FEBRILE SYNDROMES ASSOCIATED WITH ANIMAL EXPOSURE

Q fever, brucellosis, and leptospirosis are diseases associated with exposure to fluids from infected animals and may have similar clinical presentations.

Q Fever. Q fever is an underrecognized cause of acute febrile illness. *Coxiella burnetti*, the causative agent, produces mild infection in livestock. Humans are infected by inhalation of aerosolized particles or by contact with placental and amniotic fluids from infected animals. The source of animal exposure may go unnoticed. For example, in an outbreak of Q fever at the University of Colorado Medical School, 70 per cent of infected individuals lacked direct exposure to infected sheep.

Q fever characteristically begins explosively with severe, often retrobulbar headache, high fever, chills, and myalgias. Pneumonitis and hepatitis may occur but are seldom severe. Diagnosis usually is based on a four-fold rise in titer of complement-fixing antibodies. Untreated, Q fever lasts 2 to 14 days. *Coxiella burnetti* is sensitive to tetracycline, which should be used in its treatment (2 gm/day orally for 14 days). Q fever may cause endocarditis, apparently as a form of reactivation of infection. The occurrence of hepatomegaly and thrombocytopenia in a patient with apparently culture-negative endocarditis may be a clue to this diagnosis.

Leptospirosis. Humans are infected with leptospires by exposure to urine from infected dogs, cats, wild mammals, and rodents. Exposure on the farm, in the slaughterhouse, on camping trips, or during swims in contaminated water is frequent. After an incubation period of about one week, patients develop chills, high fever, headache, and myalgias. The illness often pursues a biphasic course. During the second phase of illness, fever is less prominent, but headache and myalgias are excruciating, and nausea, vomiting, and abdominal pain become prominent complaints. Aseptic meningitis is the most important manifestation of the second or immune phase of the illness. Suffusion of the bulbar conjunctivae is a useful sign suggesting the diagnosis of leptospirosis. Lymphadenopathy, hepatomegaly, and splenomegaly may occur. Leptospirosis also may pursue a more severe clinical course characterized by renal and hepatic dysfunction and a hemorrhagic diathesis.

Although darkfield examination will reveal leptospires in body fluids, most laboratories do not have the expertise to identify the organisms. The diagnosis is made, rather, by a four-fold rise in indirect hemagglutination antibody titer. Antibiotic treatment shortens the duration of fever and may reduce complications. However, to be effective, antibiotics must be initiated presumptively, before serologic confirmation. Penicillin G 2.4 to 3.6 million units per day or tetracycline 2.0 gm orally per day is effective therapy.

Brucellosis. Brucellosis infects the genitourinary tract of cattle (*Brucella abortus*) and pigs (*B. suis*). Humans are exposed occupationally or by ingestion of contaminated dairy products. Acute disease is characterized by chills, fever, headache, arthralgias, and sometimes lymphadenopathy, hepatomegaly, and splenomegaly. During the associated bacteremia, any organ may be seeded. Epididymo-orchitis is one of the more characteristic findings. With or without antibiotic treatment of the acute infection, brucellosis may relapse or enter a chronic phase. *Brucella* species can be isolated from blood or other normally sterile fluids. However, the laboratory should be alerted to the suspicion of this infection, since the organism requires special conditions for growth. Otherwise, diagnosis must be made serologically. Treatment consists of tetracycline 2 gm orally per day for 21 days and streptomycin 1.0 gm I.M. per day for 14 days. Trimethoprim 480 mg/sulfamethoxazole 2400 mg orally per day is an acceptable alternative regimen.

GRANULOMATOUS INFECTIONS

Tuberculosis. Extrapulmonary and miliary tuberculosis may present as febrile syndromes. In disseminated tuberculosis, initial chest x-rays may be normal and tuberculin skin tests often are nonreactive. Protracted fevers always should suggest this possibility. Liver biopsy and bone marrow biopsy should be performed and have a high yield in miliary disease. Genitourinary and vertebral tuberculosis may present as unexplained fever. However, careful history, urinalysis, intravenous pyelography, and x-ray films of the spine should reveal the site of tissue involvement. Extrapulmonary tuberculosis should be treated with isoniazid 300 mg orally, rifampin 600 mg orally, and ethambutol 15 mg/kg orally per day for nine months. The ethambutol can be discontinued once the organism is shown to be sensitive to isoniazid. Corticosteroids may be a useful adjunctive measure in the patient with severe systemic toxicity. However, they should be tapered as soon as the patient shows symptomatic improvement.

Histoplasmosis. Most individuals living in endemic areas in the Mississippi and Ohio River Valleys will have a subclinical, self-limited febrile illness as a manifestation of acute pulmonary histoplasmosis. Although patients may complain of chest pain or cough, physical examination of the chest usually is unremarkable despite chest x-ray findings of infiltrates and mediastinal and hilar adenopathy. Therefore, in the absence of chest x-rays, the lower respiratory tract component of the illness is easily overlooked. A complement fixation titer of at least 1:32 or a fourfold rise in titer is suggestive of the diagnosis of acute histoplasmosis. Although spontaneous resolution of symptoms is the norm, unusually prolonged illness (more than two to three weeks) may require antifungal treatment with amphotericin B or ketoconazole.

Progressive disseminated histoplasmosis may occur as a consequence of reactivation of latent infection in immunosuppressed individuals or may reflect an uncontained or poorly contained primary infection. The febrile illness in such patients is protracted, and the differential diagnosis is that of "FUO." Oropharyngeal nodules and ulcerative lesions are commonly found in disseminated histoplasmosis. Biopsy of such lesions permits rapid diagnosis. Serologies are less helpful in disseminated histoplasmosis, as they are positive in only one third of cases; cultures and methenamine silver stains of bone marrow biopsy specimens, however, should establish the diagnosis. Disseminated histoplasmosis is treated with amphotericin B 0.5 to 0.6 mg/kg/day intravenously for a total dose of 2 to 3 grams. The role of ketoconazole therapy of this disease requires further evaluation.

Other. Malaria produces febrile paroxysms that in some cases occur every 48 or 72 hours. The diagnosis should be suspected in travellers who

TABLE 85–3. DIFFERENTIAL DIAGNOSIS OF INFECTIOUS AGENTS PRODUCING FEVER AND RASH

Maculopapular Erythematous
  Enterovirus
  Epstein-Barr virus, cytomegalovirus, *Toxoplasma gondii*
  Colorado tick fever virus
  Salmonella typhi
  Leptospires
  Measles virus
  Rubella virus
  Hepatitis B virus
  Treponema pallidum
Vesicular
  Varicella zoster
  Herpes simplex virus
  Coxsackie A
Cutaneous Petechiae
  Neisseria gonorrhoeae
  Neisseria meningitidis
  Rickettsia rickettsii (RMSF)
  R. typhi (murine typhus)
  Viridans streptococci (endocarditis)
Diffuse Erythroderma
  Streptococcus sp. (scarlet fever)
  Staphylococcus aureus (toxic shock syndrome)
Distinctive Rash
  Ecthyma gangrenosum—*Pseudomonas aeruginosa*
  Erythema chronicum migrans—Lyme disease
Mucous Membrane Lesions
  Vesicular pharyngitis—Coxsackie A
  Palatal petechiae—rubella, Epstein-Barr virus, scarlet fever (*Streptococcus* sp.)
  Erythema—toxic shock syndrome (*Staphylococcus aureus*)
  Ulceronodular oral—*Histoplasma capsulatum*
  Koplik's spots—Measles virus

have returned from endemic areas, intravenous drug users, and recipients of blood transfusions. *Plasmodium falciparum* causes a high level of parasitemia and is associated with a high mortality unless recognized and treated promptly. Although *P. vivax* and *P. malariae* may relapse long after primary infection owing to latent extraerythrocytic infection, the course is milder. Demonstration of parasites in blood smears establishes the diagnosis of malaria.

Many, if not most, infectious diseases may present with fever as an early finding, with subclinical or eventual clinical involvement of specific organ systems. Examples include cryptococcosis, coccidioidomycosis, psittacosis, and *Legionella* species and *Mycoplasma pneumoniae* infection. Since pulmonary involvement by these infectious agents tends to produce few signs on physical examination, chest x-rays may reveal more prominent abnormalities than would be suspected clinically.

FEVER AND RASH

Some of the febrile syndromes already discussed may occasionally be associated with a skin rash (Table 85–3). However, this section will consider diseases in which rash is a prominent feature of the presentation.

BACTERIAL DISEASES

Petechial lesions, purpura, and ecthyma gangrenosum are lesions associated with bacteremia (see Chapter 84). Disseminated gonococcemia causes sparse vesiculopustular, hemorrhagic, or necrotic lesions on an erythematous base, typically on the extremities, particularly their dorsal surfaces (see Chapter 94). Meningococcemia is also an important cause of fever and a petechial skin rash that may be sparse.

Bacterial toxins produce characteristic clinical syndromes. Pharyngitis or other infections with an erythrogenic toxin-producing streptococcus may lead to scarlet fever. Diffuse erythema begins on the upper chest and spreads rapidly, although sparing palms and soles. Small red petechial lesions are found on the palate, and the skin has a sandpaper texture owing to occlusion of sweat glands. The tongue at first shows yellowish coating, and then becomes beefy red. The rash of scarlet fever heals with desquamation.

Toxic shock syndrome (TSS) was first recognized as a distinct entity in 1978 and became epidemic in 1980 and 1981, probably because of the marketing of hyperabsorbable tampons. *Staphylococcus aureus* strains producing toxic shock syndrome toxin (TSST-1) cause the syndrome. Most cases have occurred in 15- to 25-year-old females using tampons. Other settings include prolonged use of contraceptive diaphragms and vaginal or caesarean deliveries. TSS in males usually is caused by superficial staphylococcal infections and abscesses. Patients with toxic shock syndrome develop high fever (temperature >40°C), hypotension, severe diarrhea, confusion, and oliguria. Characteristically, diffuse erythroderma is apparent with erythematous mucosal surfaces. Later, intense scaling and desquamation of skin, particularly of the palms and soles, occurs. Diagnosis is based on the clinical findings and requires specific exclusion of Rocky Mountain Spotted fever, meningococcemia, leptospirosis, and measles. Management of the patient consists of restoration of an adequate circulatory blood volume by administration of intravenous fluids, removal of tampons if present, and treatment of the staphylococcal infection with nafcillin 12 gm/day intravenously. Patients must be advised against using tampons in the future, as toxic shock syndrome often recurs within four months of the initial episode.

VIRAL INFECTION (TABLE 85–4)

The rashes associated with viral infections are chiefly important because their appearance may be so typical as to unequivocally establish the cause of the febrile syndrome. Varicella-zoster requires special consideration because of the availability of two effective antiviral drugs, vidarabine and acyclovir. In the normal host, neither chickenpox nor zoster confined within specific dermatomes requires treatment with antiviral agents. Ophthalmic zoster poses an exception, since it is associated with potentially severe side effects including orbital compression syndromes and intracranial extension. The early use of corticosteroids (prednisone 40 mg orally per day for one week, followed by a tapering course for three weeks) decreases the frequency and duration of postherpetic neuralgia and is indicated in patients older than 50 years of age with dermatomal zoster. Both vidarabine and acyclovir have beneficial effects on chickenpox in immunocompromised children and on extradermatomal spread of zoster in immunocompromised adults.

RICKETTSIAL DISEASES

In the United States, three rickettsial diseases are endemic: Rocky Mountain spotted fever (RMSF), Q fever, and murine typhus.

RMSF is a misnomer, as most cases are reported in the southeastern United States. The causative organism, *Rickettsia rickettsii*, is transmitted from dogs (or small wild animals) to ticks to humans. Infection occurs primarily during warmer months, periods of greatest tick activity. About two thirds of patients cite a history of tick exposure. After 2 to 14 days, there is the fulminant onset of severe frontal headache, chills, fever, myalgias, conjunctivitis, and, in one fourth, cough and shortness of breath. At this point, the diagnosis may be particularly obscure. Rash characteristically begins on the third to fifth day of illness as 1- to 4-mm erythematous macules on hands, wrists, feet, and ankles. Palms and soles may be involved. The rash spreads to the trunk and becomes petechial. Intravascular coagulopathy develops in some severely ill patients. Diagnosis and institution of appropriate therapy

TABLE 85–4. FEVER AND RASH IN VIRAL INFECTION

Coxsackie/ECHO virus	*Maculopapular "rubelliform."* 1–3 mm faint pink, begins on face, spreading to chest and extremities. *"Roseoliform."* As fever decreases, 0.5–1.5 cm pink macules appear on face and upper chest. *"Herpetiform."* Vesicular stomatitis with peripheral exanthem (papules and clear vesicles on an erythematous base), including palms and soles (hand, foot, and mouth disease). Herpangina is a vesicular eruption localized to the tonsils and soft palate.	Summertime, no itching or lymphadenopathy. Multiple cases in household or community-wide epidemic. Mostly diseases of children.
Measles	Erythematous, maculopapular rash begins on upper face and spreads down to involve extremities, including palms and soles. Rash becomes confluent in face and neck. Koplik's spots are bluish-grey specks on a red base found on buccal mucosa near second molars. Atypical measles occurs in individuals who received killed vaccine, then are exposed to measles. The rash begins peripherally and is urticarial, vesicular, or hemorrhagic. Pneumonia is frequent.	Incubation period 10 to 14 days. First, severe upper respiratory symptoms, coryza, cough, conjunctivitis. Then, Koplik's spots, then rash.
Rubella	Maculopapular rash beginning on face and moving down. Petechiae on soft palate.	Incubation 12 to 23 days. Adenopathy: posterior auricular, posterior cervical, and suboccipital.
Varicella	Generalized vesicular eruption. Lesions in different stages from erythematous macules to vesicles to crusted. Spread from trunk centrifugally. Zoster—see text.	Incubation 14 to 15 days. Late winter, early spring.
Herpes simplex virus	Oral primary: small vesicles on pharynx, oral mucosa which ulcerate. Painful and tender. Recurrent: vermillion border, one or few lesions. Genital: See Chapter 94.	Incubation 2 to 12 days.
Hepatitis B	Prodrome in one fifth. Erythematous maculopapular rash, urticaria.	Arthralgias, arthritis. Abnormal liver function tests. Hepatitis B antigenemia.

should be based on the clinical findings. The specific complement fixation test will show a rise in titers and allow retrospective confirmation of the diagnosis. Treatment is with chloramphenicol 50 mg/kg orally or parenterally or tetracycline 25 to 50 mg/kg/day orally for seven days.

LYME DISEASE

Lyme disease is a spirochetal infection transmitted by the tick *Ixodes dammini*. Cases occur in the known distribution of the tick (the Northeast, Wisconsin and Minnesota, California and Oregon). Three to 32 days after tick bite, patients develop a febrile illness with headache, stiff neck, myalgias, arthralgias, and erythema chronicum migrans (ECM). ECM begins as a red macule or papule; the surrounding bright red patch expands to a diameter of 15 cm. Partial central clearing often is seen. The centers of lesions may become indurated, vesicular, or necrotic. Several red rings may be found within the outer border. Smaller secondary lesions may appear within several days. Lesions are warm but nontender. Enlargement of regional lymph nodes is common. The skin rash usually fades in about one month. Several weeks after onset of symptoms, neurologic involvement develops in 15 per cent of patients. Most characteristic is meningoencephalitis with cranial nerve involvement and peripheral radiculoneuropathy. CSF at this time shows about 100 lymphocytes/μl. Heart involvement also becomes manifest as atrioventricular block, myopericarditis, or cardiomegaly. Early in the course, arthalgias and myalgias may be quite severe; however, months later, arthritis develops with marked swelling and little pain in one or two large joints, typically the knee. Episodes of arthritis may recur for months or years; in about 10 per cent of patients the arthritis becomes chronic and erosion of cartilage and bone occurs. Diagnosis is suspected on clinical grounds and confirmed by demonstration of IgM antibody to the spirochete which peaks by the third to sixth week. Total serum IgM is increased, as are IgM-containing immune complexes and cryoglobulins. The level of IgM is reflective of disease activity and predictive of neurologic, cardiac, and joint involvement. Synovial fluid contains approximately 25,000 cells/μl, most of them neutrophils. Serum glutamic-oxaloacetic transminase is elevated in most patients.

Treatment with tetracycline 1.0 gm orally per day for 10 days prevents late complications. Meningitis or arthritis should be treated with aqueous penicillin G, 20 million units intravenously per day for 10 days. Repeated courses may be necessary if relapses occur.

TABLE 85–5. INFECTIOUS DISEASES ASSOCIATED WITH GENERALIZED LYMPHADENOPATHY BUT OTHER DOMINANT FEATURES

Viral—measles, rubella, hepatitis B
Bacterial—scarlet fever, brucellosis, leptospirosis, tuberculosis, syphilis, Lyme disease

FEVER AND LYMPHADENOPATHY

Many infectious diseases are associated with some degree of lymphadenopathy (Table 85–5). However, in some, lymphadenopathy is a major manifestation of the disease. These can be further divided according to whether lymphadenopathy is generalized or regional.

GENERALIZED LYMPHADENOPATHY

The mononucleosis syndromes are important causes of fever and generalized lymphadenopathy.

MONONUCLEOSIS SYNDROMES

Epstein-Barr Virus (EBV)

Approximately 90 per cent of American adults have serologic evidence for EBV infection; most infections are subclinical and occur before the age of five years or midway through adolescence.

Clinically manifest infectious mononucleosis usually develops late in adolescence after intimate contact with asymptomatic oropharyngeal shedders of EBV. Patients develop sore throat, fever, and generalized lymphadenopathy and sometimes experience headache and myalgias. About one in 20 patients has a transient rash that may be macular, petechial, or urticarial. Palatal petechiae often are present, as is pharyngitis, which may be exudative. Cervical lymphadenopathy, particularly involving the posterior lymphatic chains, is prominent, although some involvement elsewhere is common. The spleen is minimally enlarged in about 50 per cent of patients. Although rare, autoimmune hemolytic anemia, thrombocytopenia, encephalitis or aseptic meningitis, Guillain-Barré syndrome, hepatitis, or splenic rupture may dominate the clinical presentation. Three fourths of patients present with an absolute lymphocytosis. At least one third of their lymphocytes are atypical in appearance: large, with vacuolated basophilic cytoplasm, rolled edges often deformed by contact with other cells, and lobulated, eccentric nuclei. Immunologic studies indicate that some circulating B cells are infected with EBV and that the cells involved in the lymphocytosis are mainly cytotoxic T cells capable of damaging EBV-containing lymphocytes. Atypical lymphocytes are not restricted to infectious mononucleosis but may be seen in other viral illnesses (Table 85–6).

B-cell infection with EBV is a stimulus to production of polyclonal antibody. Antibodies to foreign red cells (heterophile) are helpful in diagnosis. The finding of sheep red cell agglutinins with differential absorption characteristics at a titer of at least 1:40 is good evidence for infectious mononucleosis. Recently, rapid diagnostic tests, such as the Monospot test, have become available and have replaced the need for heterophile determination in most patients. The Monospot test is sensitive and specific; false positives occur rarely in patients with lymphoma or hepatitis. Some patients with EBV infection will show de-

TABLE 85-6. DIFFERENTIAL DIAGNOSIS OF HETEROPHILE-NEGATIVE MONONUCLEOSIS

Epstein-Barr virus mononucleosis (particularly in
 children)
Cytomegalovirus
Acute toxoplasmosis
Streptococcal pharyngitis
Hepatitis

layed development of heterophile antibodies. Recourse to determination of antibodies to EBV is necessary only in atypical, heterophile-negative cases. The presence of IgM antibody to viral capsid antigen is diagnostic of acute infectious mononucleosis. The appearance of antibody to EBV nuclear antigen also is indicative of EBV infection.

Infectious mononucleosis pursues a surprisingly benign course even in patients with neurologic involvement. The fever resolves after one to two weeks, although residual fatigue may be protracted. Occasional patients have a persistent or recurrent syndrome with fever, headaches, pharyngitis, lymphadenopathy, arthralgias, and serologic evidence for chronic active EBV infection. Patients should be managed symptomatically. Acetaminophen may be useful for sore throat. Antibiotics, particularly ampicillin, should be avoided. The use of ampicillin is associated with skin rash in almost all patients with EBV infection. Corticosteroids are indicated only in the rare individual with serious hematologic involvement (i.e., thrombocytopenia, hemolytic anemia).

Acute bacterial superinfections of the pharynx and peritonsillar abscesses occur and should be considered when the course is unusually septic.

The differential diagnosis of heterophile-negative mononucleosis is shown in Table 85-6.

Cytomegalovirus (CMV)

Serologic surveys indicate that most adults have been infected with CMV. The ages of peak incidence of CMV infection are in the perinatal period (transmission by breast milk) and during the second to fourth decades. CMV shares with the other Herpetoviridae the propensity to reactivate, particularly in immunosuppressed patients.

Two modes of transmission of CMV are particularly important in the development of lymphadenopathy in otherwise healthy adults. CMV can be transmitted sexually. In fact, semen is an excellent source for viral isolation. The frequency of antibody to CMV and active viral excretion are particularly high in male homosexuals. Blood transfusions carry a risk of approximately 3 per cent per unit of blood for transmitting CMV infection. This becomes substantial in the setting of open heart surgery or multiple transfusions for other indications.

Primary infection with CMV causes about 50 per cent of heterophile-negative mononucleosis. The distinction between CMV and EBV may be impossible on clinical grounds alone. However, CMV tends to involve older patients (mean age

29), produce milder disease, and may be typhoidal in its presentation, that is, cause fever with little or no adenopathy. The infrequent but serious forms of neurologic and hematologic involvement that occur in EBV infection also can occur with CMV. Additionally, pneumonitis and hepatitis (which may be granulomatous) may be found. Isolation of CMV from urine or semen and demonstration of conversion of serologies from negative to positive (indirect fluorescent antibody test or complement fixation) are useful in establishing etiology. However, in groups such as male homosexuals in whom asymptomatic excretion of CMV is found frequently, viral isolation alone is inadequate for determining the etiology of lymphadenopathy. CMV mononucleosis is a self-limited disease that does not require or respond to specific therapy.

Acute Acquired Toxoplasmosis

Toxoplasma gondii is acquired by ingesting oocysts contaminating meat and other foods or by exposure to cat feces. In certain geographic areas, such as France, 90 per cent of individuals have serological evidence for *Toxoplasma* infection. In the United States, the figure is closer to 50 per cent by age 50. Ten to 20 per cent of infections in normal adult hosts are symptomatic. Presentation may take the form of a mononucleosis-like syndrome, although maculopapular skin rash, abdominal pain due to mesenteric and retroperitoneal lymphadenopathy, and chorioretinitis also may occur. Striking lymph node enlargement and involvement of unusual chains (occipital, lumbar) often necessitates lymph node biopsy to exclude lymphoma. Histologically, focal distention of sinuses with mononuclear phagocytes, histiocytes blurring the margins of germinal centers, and reactive follicular hyperplasia indicate *Toxoplasma* infection. Acute acquired toxoplasmosis is suggested by conversion of indirect fluorescent antibody test from negative to positive or a four-fold increase in titer. Usually the titer is greater than 1:1000 and is associated with increased specific IgM antibody. Acute acquired toxoplasmosis generally is self-limited and does not require specific therapy. Significant involvement of the eye is an indication for treatment with pyrimethamine plus sulfadiazine.

GRANULOMATOUS DISEASE

Disseminated tuberculosis, histoplasmosis, and sarcoidosis may be associated with generalized lymphadenopathy, although involvement of certain lymph node chains can predominate. Lymph node biopsy shows granulomas or nonspecific hyperplasia.

IDIOPATHIC LYMPHADENOPATHY SYNDROME (ILS)

Patients in groups at risk for AIDS (see Chapter 98) may develop lymph node enlargement in at least two extrainguinal sites, persisting for at least three months, thereby fulfilling the standard diagnostic criteria for ILS. Additional symptoms such as fever, night sweats, fatigue, diarrhea, and weight loss establish the diagnosis of AIDS-related complex (ARC). ILS and ARC are usually caused by HTLV-III infection. Most patients with these syndromes have seroreactivity to HTLV-III, and HTLV-III can be isolated from blood lymphocytes of some. Among male homosexuals, intravenous drug users, and other individuals belonging to groups at risk for AIDS, the presence of generalized lymphadenopathy also could represent Kaposi's sarcoma, cytomegalovirus infection, toxoplasmosis, cryptococcosis, B-cell lymphoma, or syphilis.

All patients in high-risk groups with lymphadenopathy should have a VDRL performed to exclude syphilis. If this is negative and the lymph nodes increase in size over a one- to two-month period of follow-up, a lymph node biopsy should be performed. Lymph node histology in patients with ILS may indicate follicular hyperplasia, follicular involution, or a mixed pattern. Follicular involution is a worrisome finding, as many such patients will progress to AIDS. The findings of seroreactivity to HTLV-III, lymphocytopenia, decreased numbers of T-helper cells, and skin test anergy suggest ILS/ARC but do not establish the diagnosis. Approximately 10–20% of patients with ILS/ARC will go on to develop opportunistic infections.

REGIONAL LYMPHADENOPATHY

Pyogenic Infection. Staphylococcus aureus and group A streptococcal infections produce acute suppurative lymphadenitis. The most frequently affected lymph nodes are submandibular, cervical, inguinal, and axillary, in that order. Involved nodes are large (>3 cm), tender, and firm or fluctuant. Pyoderma, pharyngitis, or periodontal infection may be present and the presumed primary site of infection. Patients are febrile and have a leukocytosis. Fluctuant nodes should be aspirated. Otherwise, antibiotic therapy should be directed at the most common pathogens. Penicillin G therapy is appropriate if pharyngeal or periodontal origin implicates a streptococcal infection. Skin involvement suggests possible staphylococcal infection and is an indication for nafcillin (or dicloxacillin) therapy. The route of administration of drug and dose should be determined by the severity of the infection.

Tuberculosis. Scrofula or tuberculous cervical adenitis presents in a subacute to chronic fashion. Fever, if present, is low-grade. A large mass of matted lymph nodes is palpable in the neck. If *Mycobacterium tuberculosis* is the causative organism, other sites of active infection usually are present. The most common causative agent in children in the United States is *M. scrofulaceum.* Infection with this and other drug-resistant nontuberculous mycobacteria requires surgical excision.

Cat-Scratch Disease. Chronic regional lymphadenopathy following cat exposure or cat scratch should suggest this diagnosis. Histopathological studies indicate a bacterial origin of this syndrome, although the causative agent has not been cultured. About one week after contact with the cat, a local papule or pustule may develop. One week later, regional adenopathy appears. Lymph nodes may be tender (sometimes exquisitely so) or just enlarged (1 to 7 cm). Fever is low-grade if present at all. Lymph node enlargement usually persists for several months. Lymph node biopsy shows necrotic granulomas with giant cells and stellate abscesses surrounded by epithelial cells. The diagnosis must be established on clinical grounds. The course usually is self limited and benign. No form of treatment is known to be effective.

Ulceroglandular Fever. Tularemia is the classic cause of ulceroglandular fever. The syndrome is acquired by contact with tissues or fluids from an infected rabbit or the bite of an infected tick. Patients have chills, fever, an ulcerated skin lesion at the site of inoculation, and painful regional adenopathy. When infection is acquired by contact with rabbits, the skin lesion usually is on the fingers or hand, and lymph node involvement is epitrochlear or axillary. In tick-borne transmission, the ulcer is on the lower extremities, perianal region, or trunk, and the adenopathy is inguinal or femoral. Most cases are diagnosed serologically, as Gram's stained preparations usually are negative and cultivation of the causative organism, *Francisella tularensis,* is hazardous. A four-fold rise in agglutination titer is diagnostic. Patients should be treated presumptively with streptomycin 15–20 mg/kg/day for 7 to 10 days.

Oculoglandular Fever. Conjunctivitis with preauricular lymphadenopathy can occur in tularemia, cat-scratch disease, sporotrichosis, LGV infection, listeriosis, and epidemic keratoconjunctivitis due to adenovirus.

Inguinal Lymphadenopathy. Inguinal lymphadenopathy associated with sexually transmitted diseases (see Chapter 94) is bilateral or unilateral. In primary syphilis, enlarged nodes are discrete, firm, and nontender. Early LGV causes tender lymphadenopathy with later matting of involved nodes, and sometimes fixation to overlying skin, which assumes a purplish hue. The lymphadenopathy of chancroid is very painful and composed of fused lymph nodes. Tender inguinal lymphadenopathy also occurs in genital herpes simplex virus infection.

Plague. Bubonic plague usually presents as fever, headache, and a large mat of inguinal or axillary lymph nodes which goes on to suppurate and drain spontaneously. Plague is an important consideration in the acutely ill patient with possible exposure to fleas and rodents in the western United States. If plague is suspected, blood cultures and aspirates of the buboes should be obtained and tetracycline 30 to 50 mg/kg/day plus streptomycin 30 mg/kg/day therapy instituted. Gram's stained preparations of the aspirate reveal gram-negative rods in two thirds of cases. A fluorescent antibody test allows rapid specific diagnosis and is available through the Centers for Disease Control.

INFECTIONS OF THE NERVOUS SYSTEM

86

Infections of the central nervous system range from fulminating, readily diagnosed septic processes to indolent illnesses requiring exhaustive searches to define their cause. Neurologic outcome and survival depend largely on the extent of CNS damage present before effective treatment begins. Accordingly, it is essential that the physician move quickly to achieve a specific diagnosis and institute appropriate therapy. The initial evaluation, however, must take into account both the urgency of beginning antibiotic treatment in bacterial meningitis and the potential hazard of performing a lumbar puncture in focal neurologic infection or mass lesions.

Patients with CNS infection present with some combination of fever, headache, altered mental status, depressed sensorium, focal neurologic signs, and stiff neck. The history and physical examination, results of lumbar puncture, and neuroradiographic procedures provide the mainstays of diagnosis. The order in which the latter two procedures are performed is critical. A subacute history, evolving over seven days to two months of unilateral headache with focal neurologic signs, implies a mass lesion that may or may not be infectious. A brain-imaging procedure should be performed first; lumbar puncture is potentially dangerous, as it may precipitate cerebral herniation, even in the absence of overt papilledema. By contrast, patients admitted with the fulminant onset of fever, headache, lethargy, confusion, and stiff neck should have an immediate lumbar puncture and institution of antibiotics for presumed bacterial meningitis. If the distinction between focal and diffuse CNS infection is unclear or not adequately evaluable, as in the comatose patient, cultures of blood, throat and nasopharynx should be obtained, antibiotic therapy started, and an emergency scanning procedure performed. If the latter is unavailable, lumbar puncture should be delayed pending evidence that no danger of herniation exists. Inevitably, this approach means that some patients will receive parenteral antibiotics several hours before a lumbar puncture is performed. Fifty per cent of CSF cultures will be negative by 4 to 12 hours after institution of antibiotics; negative CSF cultures are even more likely if the causative organism is a very sensitive pneumococcus. Should the CNS infection actually represent acute bacterial meningitis, however, the characteristics of the CSF still would suggest the diagnosis, since neutrophilic pleocytosis and hypoglycorrhachia (low CSF sugar) usually persist at least 12 to 24 hours after instituting antibiotics. Furthermore, Gram's stained preparation (or counterimmunoelectrophoresis) should indicate the causative organism even after antibiotics have rendered the CSF culture-negative. Blood and nasopharyngeal cultures obtained before therapy also are likely to be positive in view of the high frequency of isolation of causative or-

ganisms from these fluids. This approach, therefore, does not significantly compromise management, although some patients will require broad-spectrum treatment because of absence of positive cultures and the resultant lack of data regarding antibiotic sensitivity tests. This approach to the use of scanning procedures is only germane for adults with community-acquired CNS infection. In children, technically adequate CT scans require heavy sedation; therefore, scanning procedures must be reserved for more stringent indications.

MENINGITIS

Definition. Meningitis is an inflammation of the leptomeninges caused by infectious or noninfectious processes. The most common types of infectious meningitis are bacterial, viral, tuberculous, and fungal. The most common noninfectious causes are subarachnoid hemorrhage, sarcoidosis, and cancer. Infectious meningitis will be considered in three categories: acute bacterial meningitis, aseptic meningitis, and chronic meningitis.

BACTERIAL MENINGITIS

Epidemiology. Three fourths of cases of acute bacterial meningitis occur before the age of 15 years. *Neisseria meningitidis* causes sporadic disease or epidemics in closed populations. Most cases occur in winter and spring and involve children or adults less than 50 years of age. *Haemophilus influenzae* meningitis is even more selectively a disease of childhood, most cases developing by the age of 10 years. Infections are sporadic, although secondary cases may occur in close contacts. In contrast, pneumococcal meningitis is a disease seen in all age groups. Extensive clinical series of adults hospitalized 20 years ago showed a relative frequency of 68 per cent pneumococcal, 18 per cent meningococcal, and 10 per cent *Haemophilus influenzae* meningitis. At University Hospitals of Cleveland in the period 1972 to 1981 the relative frequencies were 40 per cent, 30 per cent, and 20 per cent, in keeping with the general experience that serious *Haemophilus influenzae* infections are increasingly common in adults.

Close contact with a patient with meningococcal or *Haemophilus influenzae* disease is particularly important in the development of secondary cases of meningitis as in the case of *Haemophilus influenzae* Type B and other severe disease manifestations (sepsis, epiglottitis) as well. For example, the risk of meningococcal disease is 500 to 800 times greater in a close contact of a patient with meningococcal meningitis than in a noncontact. Asymptomatic pharyngeal carriers of *Haemophilus* species also can spread infection to their contacts.

TABLE 86–1. MENINGITIS AND MENINGOENCEPHALITIS IN THE IMMUNOCOMPROMISED HOST

ABNORMALITY	INFECTIOUS AGENT
Complement deficiencies (C6-C8)	Neisseria meningitidis
Splenectomy	Haemophilus influenzae Streptococcus pneumoniae Neisseria meningitidis
Sickle cell disease	Streptococcus pneumoniae Haemophilus influenzae
Impaired cellular immunity	Listeria monocytogenes Cryptococcus neoformans Toxoplasma gondii Cytomegalovirus JC virus (progressive multifocal leukoencephalopathy)

Pathogenesis and Pathophysiology. The bacteria that cause most community-acquired meningitis transiently colonize the oropharynx and nasopharynx of healthy individuals. Meningitis may occur in nonimmune hosts following bacteremia from an upper respiratory site (meningococcus or Haemophilus species) or pneumonia and by direct spread from contiguous foci of infection (nasal sinuses, mastoids).

The pathogenesis of acute bacterial meningitis is best understood for meningococcal disease. The carrier state occurs when meningococci adhere to pharyngeal epithelial cells via specialized filamentous structures termed pili. The production of IgA protease by pathogenic Neisseria species favors adherence by inactivating a major host barrier to colonization. Organisms enter and pass through epithelial cells to subepithelial tissues, where they multiply in the nonimmune individual and produce bacteremia. The localization of organisms to the CSF is not well-understood but presumably depends on invasive properties of the capsular polysaccharide which permit penetration of the blood-brain barrier. Immunity is conferred by bactericidal antibody and presumably is acquired by earlier colonization of the pharynx with nonpathogenic meningococci and cross-reacting bacteria. The presence of blocking IgA antibody may increase susceptibility transiently in some individuals. Table 86–1 summarizes host factors conferring a particular risk of bacterial meningitis. Bacterial meningitis remains confined to the leptomeninges and does not spread to adjacent parenchymal tissue. Focal and global neurologic deficits develop because of involvement of blood vessels coursing in the meninges and through the subarachnoid space; in addition, cranial nerves and cerebral tissue can be affected by the attendant inflammation, edema, and scarring as well as by the development of obstructive hydrocephalus.

Gram-negative enteric meningitis occurs mainly in severely debilitated persons or individuals whose meninges have been breached or damaged by head trauma, a neurosurgical procedure, or a parameningeal infection.

Clinical Presentation. Patients with bacterial meningitis present with fever, headache, lethargy, confusion, irritability, and stiff neck. Three syndromes predominate. About 25 per cent of cases begin abruptly with fulminant illness; mortality is high in this setting. More often, meningeal symptoms progress over one to seven days. Finally, meningitis may superimpose itself on one to three weeks of an upper respiratory–type illness; diagnosis is difficult in this group. Occasionally, no more than a single additional neurologic symptom or sign hints at disease more serious than a routine upper respiratory infection. Stiff neck is absent in about one fifth of all patients with meningitis, notably in the young, the old, and the comatose. A petechial or purpuric rash is found in one half of patients with meningococcemia; while not pathognomonic, palpable purpura is very suggestive of Neisseria meningitidis infection. About 20 per cent of patients with acute bacterial meningitis have seizures and a similar fraction focal neurologic findings.

Laboratory Diagnosis. The CSF in acute bacterial meningitis usually contains 1,000 to 10,000 cells/μl, mostly neutrophils (Table 86–2). Glucose content falls below 40 mg/dl and protein rises above 150 mg/dl in most patients. The Gram's stained preparation of CSF is positive in 80 to 88 per cent of cases. However, certain cautionary notes are appropriate. Cell counts can be lower (occasionally zero) early in the course of meningococcal and pneumococcal meningitis. Also, predominantly mononuclear cell pleocytosis may occur in patients who have received antibiotics before the lumbar puncture. A similar mononuclear pleocytosis may be seen in Listeria monocytogenes meningitis, a disease often associated with impaired cellular immunity. For several reasons, Gram's stained preparations of CSF may be negative or misinterpreted when meningitis is caused by Haemophilus influenzae, Neisseria meningitidis, or Listeria monocytogenes; the presence of gram-negative diplococci and coccobacilli

TABLE 86–2. TYPICAL CSF FINDINGS IN CNS INFECTION

	CELLS	PER CENT NEUTROPHILS	GLUCOSE	PROTEIN
Bacterial meningitis	1,000–10,000/μl	>50%	<40 mg/dl	>150 mg/dl
Aseptic meningitis	10–2,000/μl	early 2/3 >50%	normal	<100 mg/dl
Herpes simplex virus encephalitis	0–1,100/μl	<50%	normal	<100 mg/dl
TBC meningitis	100–500/μl	early >50% late <50%	<40 mg/dl	>150 mg/dl

may be difficult to appreciate, particularly when the background consists of amorphous pink material. Also, bacteria tend to be pleomorphic in CSF and may assume atypical forms. In the case of *Listeria*, CSF colony counts are low (10^3/ml). If interpretation of the Gram's stained CSF is not clear-cut, broad-spectrum antibiotics should be instituted while awaiting the results of cultures. If the initial Gram's stained preparation does not contain organisms, examining the stained sediment prepared by concentrating up to 5 ml of CSF with a cytocentrifuge may reveal the causative organism.

Cultures of CSF, blood, fluid expressed from purpuric lesions, and nasopharyngeal swabs have a high yield. The last mentioned is particularly valuable in the patients who have received antibiotic therapy before hospitalization, since most such drugs do not achieve substantial levels in nasopharyngeal secretions.

Recognition of meningitis may be difficult following head trauma or neurosurgery, since the symptoms, signs, and laboratory findings of infection can be difficult to separate from those of trauma. A low CSF glucose usually indicates infection. The causative organism, characteristically an enteric rod, may already have been cultured from an extraneural site, such as a wound or urine. The known antibiotic sensitivities of such isolates may provide a valuable guide to initial treatment of meningitis.

All patients with meningitis should have x-ray films of nasal sinuses and mastoids to exclude a parameningeal focus of infection.

Differential Diagnosis. Classic acute bacterial meningitis resembles few other diseases. Ruptured brain abscess should be considered, particularly if the CSF white blood cell count is unusually high and focal neurologic signs are present. Parameningeal foci of infection usually cause fever, headache, and local signs, but stiff neck occurs only if the meninges are penetrated. In the absence of that catastrophe, a modest pleocytosis may be present. CSF glucose, however, is normal. In patients with bacterial meningitis already given antibiotic treatment, the CSF may be sterile, but neutrophils commonly are present in CSF and the glucose is depressed. Early in the evolution of viral or tuberculous meningitis, the pleocytosis may be predominantly neutrophilic. Serial examinations, however, will show a progressive shift to a mononuclear cell predominance. Acute viral meningoencephalitis may be difficult to distinguish clinically from bacterial meningitis; the evolution of CSF findings and the ultimate clinical course usually decide the matter.

Treatment and Outcome. Bacterial meningitis requires the prompt institution of appropriate antibiotics. If the Gram's stained smear of CSF indicates pneumococcal or meningococcal disease, penicillin G should be administered intravenously in a dose of 25,000 units/kg q2h (up to 24 million units per day). The alternative drug for penicillin-allergic patients is chloramphenicol (25 mg/kg intravenously q6h). Suspected cases of *Haemophilus influenzae* meningitis should be treated with ampicillin 50 mg/kg intravenously q4h plus chloramphenicol. The latter drug can be stopped unless the isolate produces beta-lactamase. In a case of community-acquired meningitis, if the Gram's stained preparation of CSF is negative, but the clinical and laboratory findings suggest bacterial meningitis, penicillin therapy should be started as above and followed by chloramphenicol one hour later. This combination will be effective against beta-lactamase–producing *Haemophilus influenzae*; the delay in starting chloramphenicol offsets possible antagonism with penicillin. Third-generation cephalosporins such as cefotaxime may provide an alternative for the treatment of *Haemophilus influenzae* and Gram's stain–negative meningitis. However, the third-generation agents vary in their antibacterial spectrum and penetration into CSF so that they cannot be used interchangeably. Third-generation cephalosporins are the indicated choice for treating sensitive gram-negative enteric organisms causing meningitis. If the organism is resistant to cephalosporins, the patient should be treated with a combination of intraventricular plus parenteral aminoglycoside and a beta-lactam antibiotic selected on the basis of the sensitivity of the isolate (ticarcillin or piperacillin). The placement of an intraventricular reservoir facilitates treatment of such patients. Regardless of the results of in vitro sensitivity testing, chloramphenicol is not an adequate drug for treatment of gram-negative bacillary meningitis; its use has been associated with unacceptably high mortality rates.

The management of bacterial meningitis extends beyond the patient. Contacts must be protected, as they are at substantial risk of developing meningococcal meningitis or serious *H. influenzae* disease. At the time one first suspects bacterial meningitis, respiratory isolation procedures should be initiated. One should begin antibiotic prophylaxis of contacts when the clinical course or Gram's stained preparation of CSF suggests meningococcal or *H. influenzae* meningitis. Recommended doses for household and other intimate contacts of patients with meningococcal meningitis are rifampin 10 mg/kg (up to 600 mg) twice daily for two days. The goal of prophylaxis of contacts of *H. influenzae*, Type B meningitis is to protect children less than four years of age. Since the organism may be passed from patient to asymptomatic adult to at-risk child, rifampin 20 mg/kg (up to 600 mg) daily for four days should be given to all members of the household and day care center of the index case having contact with children less than four years old. Despite parenteral antibiotic therapy, patients with *N. meningitidis* or *H. influenzae* meningitis may have persistent nasopharyngeal carriage and should receive rifampin treatment before discharge from the hospital.

Although hospital contacts of patients with meningococcal meningitis are at low risk of acquiring the carrier state and disease, occasional secondary cases do occur. Accordingly, personnel with close contact with the patient's respiratory secretions should receive prophylactic antibiot-

TABLE 86–3. SEQUELAE OF BACTERIAL MENINGITIS

	DEAFNESS	MAJOR CNS DEFICITS*
Neisseria meningitidis	11%	1%
Haemophilus influenzae	6%	9%
Streptococcus pneumoniae	31%	18%

*Hydrocephalus (3%), epilepsy (6%), mental retardation (10%), motor defects.

ics. All individuals receiving rifampin prophylaxis should be warned that their urine will turn orange and that oral contraceptives will be inactivated temporarily by the anti-estrogen effects of the drug.

About 30 per cent of patients with bacterial meningitis will die of the infection. Of the survivors, deafness and other serious neurologic sequelae are common (Table 86–3). As noted, the prognosis in individual cases depends largely on the level of consciousness and extent of CNS damage at the time of first treatment. Misdiagnosis (40 per cent of patients) and attendant delays in starting antibiotics are factors in morbidity which the physician must try to offset. Patients with fulminant meningitis ideally should be treated with antibiotics within 30 minutes of reaching medical care. Even after antibiotic therapy and presumed cure, bacterial meningitis may recur. The pattern of recurrence usually suggests a parameningeal infective focus or dural defect (Table 86–4).

Bacterial meningitis can be prevented by vaccinating susceptible individuals. Effective polysaccharide vaccines are available for some strains of N. meningitidis and S. pneumoniae. A vaccine for H. influenzae is undergoing evaluation.

ASEPTIC MENINGITIS

Leptomeningitis associated with negative Gram's stains of CSF and negative cultures for bacteria has been designated aseptic meningitis, a somewhat unfortunate designation implying a benign illness that resolves spontaneously. It is important, however, to assume a high level of vigilance in this group of patients, as they may have a potentially treatable but progressive illness.

Epidemiology. Viral infections are the most

TABLE 86–4. 3 R's OF CNS INFECTION

R	DETERIORATION	POSSIBILITIES
Recrudescence	During Rx, same bacteria	Wrong Rx
Relapse	3–14 days after stopping treatment, same bacteria	Parameningeal focus
Recurrence	Delayed, same or other bacteria	Congenital or acquired dural defects

frequent cause of aseptic meningitis. Of those cases in which a specific causal agent can be established, 97 per cent are due to enteroviruses (particularly Coxsackie B and ECHO), mumps, lymphocytic choriomeningitis virus (LCM), herpes simplex virus, and leptospirosis. Viral meningitis is a disease mainly of children and young adults (70 per cent of patients are less than 20 years of age). Seasonal variation reflects the predominance of enteroviral infection, so that most cases occur in summer or early fall. Mumps occurs in winter and LCM in fall or winter.

Pathogenesis/Pathophysiology. Localization to the meninges occurs during systemic viremia. The basis for the meningotropism of those viruses that cause aseptic meningitis is not understood. Herpes simplex virus, Type 2 may cause meningitis during the course of primary genital herpes.

Clinical Presentation. The syndrome of aseptic meningitis of viral origin begins with the acute onset of headache, fever, and meningismus associated with CSF pleocytosis. The headache usually is described as the worst ever experienced and is exacerbated by sitting, standing, or coughing. In typical cases, the course is benign. The development of changes in sensorium, seizures, or focal neurologic signs shifts the diagnosis to encephalitis or meningoencephalitis. Additional clinical features may suggest a particular infectious agent. Patients with mumps may have or develop parotitis or orchitis and usually give a history of appropriate contact. LCM infection often follows exposure to mice, guinea pigs, or hamsters and causes severe myalgias; an infectious mononucleosis-like illness can ensue with rash and orchitis. Leptospirosis follows exposure to rats or mice or swimming in water contaminated by their urine; aseptic meningitis occurs in the second phase of the illness.

Laboratory Diagnosis. In viral meningitis, the CSF shows a pleocytosis of 10 to 2,000 WBC/μl (5/6<1,000/μl). Two thirds will have mainly neutrophils in the initial CSF specimen. However, serial lumbar punctures will reveal a rapid shift (within six to eight hours) in the CSF differential count toward a mononuclear cell predominance. CSF protein is normal in one third of cases and almost always less than 100 mg/dl. CSF glucose characteristically is normal, although minimal depression occurs in mumps (30 per cent), LCM (60 per cent), and less frequently in ECHO virus and HSV meningitis. Serial lumbar punctures will show a 95 per cent reduction in cell count by two weeks. Stool cultures have the highest yield for viral isolation (40 to 50 per cent); CSF and throat cultures each are positive in about 15 per cent of cases. Serologies also may indicate a specific causative agent.

Differential Diagnosis. Partially treated bacterial meningitis and a parameningeal focus of infection may be particularly difficult to distinguish from aseptic meningitis. Serial lumbar punctures may be helpful in establishing the former and x-ray films of paranasal sinuses and mastoids in the latter.

Treatment and Course. Viral meningitis is benign and self-limited. HSV meningitis associated with primary genital herpes occasionally causes sufficient symptoms to warrant treatment with vidarabine or acyclovir.

CHRONIC MENINGITIS

Although technically "aseptic" meningitis, granulomatous and other infectious and noninfectious diseases can present as a subacute or chronic meningitis. These entities will be described in Chapter 124.

ENCEPHALITIS

Definition. Acute viral and other infectious causes of encephalitis usually produce fever, headache, and stiff neck, and additionally alterations in consciousness, focal neurologic signs, and seizures.

Epidemiology. A large number of viral and nonviral agents can cause encephalitis (Table 86–5). Seasonal occurrence may help to limit the differential diagnosis. Arthropod-borne viruses peak in the summer (California encephalitis and western equine encephalitis in August, St. Louis encephalitis slightly later). The tick-borne infections (Rocky Mountain spotted fever) occur in early summer, enterovirus infections in later summer and fall, and mumps in the winter and spring. Geographic distribution is also helpful. Eastern equine encephalitis is confined to the coastal states. Serologic surveys indicate that many viruses that cause encephalitis most often occur as subclinical infections. It is not clear why a few among infected subjects develop encephalitis.

Herpes simplex virus (HSV) is the most frequent and devastating cause of sporadic, severe focal encephalitis; overall it is implicated in 10 per cent of all cases of encephalitis. There is no age, sex, seasonal, or geographic preference.

Pathogenesis. Viruses reach the CNS by the bloodstream or peripheral nerves. HSV presumably reaches the brain by cell-to-cell spread along recurrent branches of the trigeminal nerve which innervate the meninges of the anterior and middle fossae. Although this would explain the characteristic localization of necrotic lesions to the inferomedial portions of the temporal and frontal lobes, it is not clear why such spread is so rare, one case of HSV encephalitis occurring per million in the population.

Clinical Features. The course of HSV encephalitis will be considered here in detail because of the importance of establishing the diagnosis of this now treatable entity. Patients affected by HSV commonly describe a prodrome of one to seven days of upper respiratory tract symptoms followed by the sudden onset of headache, fever, behavioral abnormalities, delirium, difficulty with speech, and seizures, often focal.

Laboratory Diagnosis. The CSF shows a predominantly lymphocytic pleocytosis. In HSV encephalitis, the cell count is 0 to 1100 WBC/µl (me-

TABLE 86–5. INFECTIOUS AGENTS COMMONLY CAUSING ENCEPHALITIS AND MENINGOENCEPHALITIS

VIRUSES	NONVIRAL
Herpes simplex	Rickettsia rickettsii
Epstein-Barr	Rickettsia typhi
Varicella-zoster	Mycoplasma pneumoniae
Cytomegalovirus	Leptospira species
Mumps	Brucella species
Measles	Mycobacterium tuberculosis
St. Louis	Histoplasma capsulatum
Eastern Equine	Cryptococcus neoformans
Western Equine	Naegleria species
Coxsackie	Acanthamoeba species
ECHO	Toxoplasma gondii
Rabies	Trypanosoma species
	Plasmodium falciparum
	Lyme agent

dian 130). Protein is moderately high (median 80 mg/dl). CSF glucose is reduced in only 5 per cent of individuals within three days of onset but becomes abnormal in additional patients later in the course. In about 5 per cent the CSF is normal. Laboratory findings at onset are of little help, although focal abnormalities may be present in the EEG and develop in technetium brain scans or CT images by the third day in most patients (Fig. 86–1). Clinical diagnosis of HSV is confirmed in about two thirds of patients undergoing brain biopsy, and few patients with other treatable diseases run a similar early course. Some authorities recommend brain biopsy before treatment. Acyclovir offers such high therapeutic benefit (55 per cent success) with such little risk in this highly fatal and neurologically damaging disease that our approach is to biopsy only patients who deteriorate despite antiviral therapy. The main impetus for biopsy is to establish alternate treatable etiologies. A low CSF glucose should increase suspicion that a granulomatous infection is present (tuberculosis, cryptococcosis); earlier recourse to brain biopsy seems appropriate in this setting.

Viral cultures of stool, throat, and buffy coat and brain biopsy specimens may provide a specific diagnosis, but both these and serologic evidence of a rise in antibody titer come too late to guide initial treatment. In the case of HSV encephalitis, serologies are particularly helpful in the 30 per cent of individuals with a primary infection. Also, CSF titers of antibody to HSV, which reflect local production of antibody, may show a diagnostic four-fold rise.

Differential Diagnosis. Acute (demyelinating) encephalomyelitis, acute bacterial endocarditis producing diffuse brain embolization, acute thrombotic thrombocytopenic purpura, cerebral venous thrombosis, vascular disease, and primary and metastatic tumors most often simulate HSV encephalitis.

Treatment and Outcome. The course of viral encephalitis depends on the etiologic agent. Untreated HSV encephalitis has a high mortality (70 per cent), and survival is associated with severe neurologic residua. Acyclovir therapy improves

FIGURE 86—1. *A*, The most common finding on CT scan of patients with HSV encephalitis is a hypodense mass lesion. Streaked contrast enhancement also may be seen (not shown). *B*, In severe cases of HSV encephalitis, involvement may be quite extensive.

survival and lessens morbidity in patients if initiated early, before deterioration to coma. Prognosis is particularly favorable in patients less than 30 years old.

RABIES

Rabies encephalitis is always fatal, requiring one to place major attention on prevention. Currently, zero to six cases of rabies occur each year in the United States, and approximately 20,000 people receive postexposure prophylaxis.

The incubation period for rabies is 20 to 90 days, during which the rabies virus replicates locally and then migrates along nerves to the spinal cord and brain. Rabies begins with fever, headache, fatigue, and pain or paresthesias at the site of inoculation; confusion, seizures, paralysis, and stiff neck follow. Periods of violent agitation are characteristic of rabies encephalitis. Attempts at drinking produce laryngospasm, gagging, and apprehension. Paralysis, coma, and death supervene. When rabies is suspected, protective isolation procedures should be instituted to avoid additional exposure of the hospital staff to saliva

and other infected secretions. Confirmation of the diagnosis is possible by assaying rabies-neutralizing antibody or isolating virus from saliva, CSF, and urine sediment. Immunofluorescent rabies antibody staining of a skin biopsy taken from the posterior neck is a rapid means of establishing the diagnosis.

Deciding on indications for prophylaxis is based on the following principles: (1) The patient must have been exposed. Nonbite exposure is possible if mucous membranes or open wounds are contaminated with animal saliva; exposure to bat urine in heavily contaminated caves has been followed by rabies. (2) Small rodents (rats, mice, chipmunks, squirrels) and rabbits rarely are infected with rabies and never have been associated with human disease. Dogs and cats in New York City and Philadelphia are rabies-free. In other areas, if rabies is present in wild animals, dogs and cats have the potential to transmit rabies. Domestic dogs and cats should be quarantined for 10 days after biting someone; if no signs of illness develop, there is no risk of transmission by their earlier bite. Other animals should be destroyed and their brains examined for rabies virus by direct fluorescent antibody testing. If the biting animal escapes, postexposure prophylaxis is usually indicated. Bat bites require treatment unless the animal is caught. Unusual behavior of animals and truly unprovoked attacks (as opposed to those incurred during handling or feeding) increase the likelihood of rabies.

Currently, postexposure management consists of (1) thorough wound cleansing, (2) human rabies immune globulin 20 IU/kg, one half infiltrated locally in the area of the bite and one half intramuscularly, and (3) human diploid cell rabies vaccine, 1.0 ml intramuscularly five times during a one-month period. Individuals at high risk of exposure to rabies should be vaccinated. Veterinarians, laboratory workers, and those who frequent caves belong in this category.

MYELITIS

Dermatomal varicella-zoster infection is discussed in Chapter 85. In some instances, the infection spreads from the dorsal root sensory ganglia into the spinal cord. If anterior horn cells are affected, paralysis may develop in muscles supplied by the same dermatomal segment involved by the rash. More widespread infection of the spinal cord causes transverse or diffuse myelopathy. Varicella-zoster also can lead to trigeminal or facial nerve palsy (Ramsey-Hunt syndrome, see Chapter 124) or arteritis of the internal carotid artery followed by hemiplegia.

Poliomyelitis was at one time a major public health problem in the United States. Small epidemics still are reported, however, when patients refuse vaccination for religious reasons; occasional sporadic cases result from vaccination. The disease is characterized by symptoms of acute viral meningitis, including headache, fever, and stiff neck, followed in about 10 per cent by paralysis of voluntary muscles supplied by anterior horn cells of either spinal cord or brain stem. Muscle paralysis is asymmetrical and often patchy and may be profound. The spinal fluid contains an increased number of lymphocytes with an elevated protein and a normal glucose concentration. The disorder should not ·be mistaken for Guillain-Barré syndrome (p. 124), which is a nonfebrile,

essentially symmetrical paralytic illness, often accompanied by sensory abnormalities. Both poliomyelitis and Guillain-Barré syndrome produce their most serious symptoms by paralyzing respiratory muscles so as to require respiratory support.

Brain abscess and focal CNS infection are discussed in Chapter 124.

REFERENCES

Bacterial Meningitis

Carpenter RR, and Petersdorf RG: The clinical spectrum of bacterial meningitis. Am J Med 33:262, 1962.
Olsson RA, Kirby JC, and Romansky MJ: Pneumococcal meningitis in the adult. Clinical, therapeutic and prognostic aspects in 43 patients. Ann Intern Med 55:545, 1961.
Spagnuolo PJ, Ellner JJ, Lerner PI, et al: *Hemophilus influenzae* meningitis: The spectrum of disease in adults. Medicine 61:74, 1982.
Swartz MN, and Dodge PR: Bacterial meningitis—a review of selected aspects. N Engl J Med 272:725, 779, 842, 954, 1965.

Aseptic Meningitis

Adair CV, Gauld RL, and Smadel JE: Aseptic meningitis, a disease of diverse etiology: Clinical and etiologic studies on 854 cases. Ann Intern Med 39:675, 1953.
Lepow ML, Carver DH, Wright HT, Woods WA, and Robbins FC: A clinical, laboratory and epidemiologic investigation of aseptic meningitis during the 4-year period 1955–1958. N Engl J Med 266:1181, 1962.
Meyer HM, Johnson RT, Crawford IP, Dascomb HE, and Rogers NG: Central nervous system syndromes of "viral" etiology. Am J Med 29:334, 1960.

Encephalitis

Johnson R: Viral infections of the nervous system. New York, Raven Press, 1982.
Nahmias AJ, Whitley RJ, Visintine AN, et al: HSV encephalitis: Laboratory evaluations and their diagnostic significance. J Infect Dis 145:829–836, 1982.
Whitley RJ, Soonj S-J, Hirsch MS, et al: Herpes simplex encephalitis: Vidarabine therapy and diagnostic problems. N Engl J Med 304:313–318, 1981.
Whitley RJ, Soonj S-J, Linneman C Jr, et al: Herpes simplex encephalitis. Clinical assessment. JAMA 247:317–320, 1982.

INFECTIONS OF THE HEAD AND NECK

87

INFECTIONS OF THE EAR

Otitis externa is an infection of the external auditory canal. The process may begin as a folliculitis or pustule within the canal. Staphylococci, streptococci, and other skin flora are the most

common pathogens. Some cases of otitis externa have been associated with swimming or hot tubs. This infection (swimmer's ear) is usually due to *Pseudomonas aeruginosa*.

Patients with otitis externa complain of ear pain that is often quite severe, and they may also complain of itching. Examination reveals an inflamed external canal; the tympanic membrane may be uninvolved. (Patients with otitis media, in contrast, will not have involvement of the external canal unless the tympanic membrane is perforated.) Otitis externa with cellulitis can be treated with systemic antibiotics such as dicloxacillin or erythromycin and local heat. In the absence of cellulitis, irrigation and administration of topical antibiotics such as neomycin and polymyxin are sufficient. Patients with diabetes mellitus are at risk for an invasive external otitis (malignant otitis) due to *P. aeruginosa*. In malignant otitis externa, pain is a presenting complaint and infection rapidly invades the bones of the skull and frequently results in cranial nerve palsies, invasion of the brain, and death. Treatment must include debridement of as much necrotic tissue as is feasible and at least four to six weeks of treatment with an aminoglycoside plus a pencillin derivative active against *Pseudomonas* (e.g., carbenicillin).

Otitis media is an infection of the middle ear seen primarily among preschool children but occasionally in adults as well. Infection caused by upper respiratory tract pathogens is facilitated by obstruction to drainage through edematous, congested eustachian tubes. *Streptococcus pneumoniae, Haemophilus influenzae,* and *Branhamella catarrhalis* are the most common pathogens, and virus infection may predispose to acute otitis media. Fever, ear pain, diminished hearing, vertigo, or tinnitus may be seen. In young children, however, localizing symptoms may not be appreciated. The tympanic membrane may appear inflamed, but to diagnose otitis media with certainty, either fluid must be seen behind the membrane or diminished mobility of the membrane must be demonstrated by tympanometry or after air insufflation into the external canal.

Treatment with ampicillin, trimethoprim-sulfamethoxazole, or cefaclor is generally effective; addition of decongestants is of no proven value. Complications of otitis media are uncommon but include infection of the mastoid air cells (mastoiditis), bacterial meningitis, brain abscess, or subdural empyema.

INFECTIONS OF THE NOSE AND SINUSES

Rhinitis is a common manifestation of numerous respiratory virus infections. It is characterized by mucopurulent or watery nasal discharge that may be profuse. When due to respiratory virus infection, there may be associated pharyngitis, conjunctival suffusion, and fever. Rhinitis can also be caused by hypersensitivity responses to airborne allergens. Patients with allergic rhinitis often have a transverse skin crease on the bridge of the nose a few millimeters from the tip. The demonstration of eosinophils in a wet preparation of nasal secretions readily distinguishes allergic rhinitis from rhinitis of infectious origin. (Eosinophils can be identified by the presence of large refractile

cytoplasmic granules.) Occasionally, following head trauma or neurosurgery, cerebrospinal fluid (CSF) may leak through the nose. "CSF rhinorrhea" places patients at risk for bacterial meningitis. CSF is readily distinguished from nasal secretions by its low protein and high glucose concentrations.

Sinusitis is an infection of the air-filled paranasal sinuses that may complicate viral upper respiratory infections. Allergic rhinitis and structural abnormalities of the nose that interfere with sinus drainage also predispose to sinusitis. Acute sinusitis is primarily caused by upper respiratory tract bacterial pathogens, *Streptococcus pneumoniae* and *Haemophilus influenzae,* and less often by anaerobes and staphylococci.

Sinusitis may be difficult to distinguish from a viral upper respiratory illness that, in many instances, precedes sinus infection. Patients may complain of headache, "stuffiness," and purulent nasal discharge. Headache may be exacerbated by bending over. There may be tenderness over the involved sinus, and pus may be seen in the turbinates of the nose. Failure of a sinus to light up on transillumination may suggest the diagnosis; sinus radiographs revealing opacification, mucosal thickening, or air-fluid levels establish the diagnosis of sinusitis. Most patients with sinusitis can be treated with a 10-day course of ampicillin, amoxicillin, or trimethoprim-sulfamethoxazole, and nasal decongestants. Patients who appear toxic or otherwise are severely ill should undergo sinus puncture for drainage, Gram's stain, and culture. Sinusitis may be complicated by bacterial meningitis, brain abscess, or subdural empyema. Therefore, patients with sinusitis and neurologic abnormalities must be evaluated carefully for these complications.

INFECTIONS OF THE MOUTH AND PHARYNX

Stomatitis

Stomatitis or inflammation of the mouth can be caused by a wide variety of processes. Patients with stomatitis may complain of diffuse or localized pain in the mouth, difficulty swallowing, and difficulty managing oral secretions. Various nutritional deficiencies can also produce stomatitis and soreness of the mouth (Table 87–1).

Thrush is an infection of the oral mucosa by *Candida* species. Thrush may be seen among infants and also in patients receiving broad-spectrum antibiotics or corticosteroids (systemic or inhaled), among patients with leukopenia (e.g., acute leukemia), and among patients with im-

TABLE 87–1. DEFICIENCY STATES PRODUCING STOMATITIS

Niacin (pellagra)
Vitamin C (scurvy)
Folate
Vitamin B_{12}

pairments in cell-mediated immunity (e.g., AIDS). In its milder form, thrush is manifested by an asymptomatic white, "cheesy" exudate on the buccal mucosa and pharynx, which when scraped leaves a raw, bleeding surface. In more severe cases, there may be pain and also erythema surrounding the exudate. The diagnosis is suggested by the characteristic appearance of the lesions and is confirmed by microscopic examination of a KOH preparation of the exudate, which reveals yeast and the pseudohyphae characteristic of *Candida*. Thrush related to administration of antibiotics and corticosteroids should resolve after the drugs are withdrawn. Otherwise, thrush can be managed with clotrimazole troches. Refractory thrush or *Candida* involving the esophagus should be treated with ketoconazole or intravenous amphotericin B.

Oral Ulcers and Vesicles
(Table 87–2)

Aphthous Stomatitis. Aphthae are discrete shallow ulcers on erythematous bases which may be single or multiple and are usually present on the labial or buccal mucosa. Attacks of aphthous stomatitis may be recurrent and quite debilitating. Symptoms may last for several days to two weeks. The cause of these ulcerations is unknown, and treatment is symptomatic with saline mouth wash or topical anesthetics.

Herpes Simplex Virus Infection. Although most recurrences of oral herpes simplex infections occur on or near the vermillion border of the lips, the primary attack usually involves the mouth and pharynx. Generalized symptoms of fever, headache, and malaise often precede the appearance of oral lesions by as much as 24 to 48 hours. The involved regions are swollen and erythematous. Small vesicles soon appear which rupture, leaving shallow, discrete ulcers that may coalesce. The diagnosis can be made by scraping the base of an ulcer. Wright's or Giemsa stain of this material may reveal the multinucleated giant cells characteristic of herpes simplex infection. Viral cultures are more sensitive but also expensive. Treatment of primary infection with acyclovir will decrease the duration of symptoms but has no effect on the frequency of recurrence.

Vincent's Stomatitis. This is an ulcerative infection of the gingival mucosa due to anaerobic fusobacteria and spirochetes. Breath is often foul, and the ulcerations are covered with a purulent

TABLE 87–2. ORAL VESICLES AND ULCERS

Aphthous stomatitis
Primary herpes simplex infection
Vincent's stomatitis
Syphilis
Behçet's syndrome
Erythema multiforme
Pemphigus
Pemphigoid
Coxsackie A virus (herpangina)
Fungi (histoplasmosis)

exudate. Gram's stain of the exudate reveals the characteristic gram-negative fusobacteria and spirochetes. Treatment with penicillin is curative. Untreated, the infection may extend to the peritonsillar space (quinsy) and even involve vascular structures in the lateral neck (see below).

Syphilis. Syphilis may produce a painless primary chancre in the mouth or a painful mucous patch that is a manifestation of secondary disease. The diagnosis should be considered in the sexually active patient with a large (>1 cm) oral ulceration and should be confirmed serologically, since darkfield examination may be confounded by the presence of nonsyphilitic oral spirochetes.

Herpangina. This is a childhood disease that causes tiny discrete ulcerations of the soft palate and is due to infection with coxsackie A viruses.

Fungal Disease. Occasionally, an oral ulcer or nodule may be a manifestation of disseminated infection due to histoplasmosis. These ulcers are generally mildly or minimally symptomatic and are overshadowed by the constitutional symptoms of disseminated fungal illness.

Systemic Illnesses Causing Ulcerative or Vesicular Lesions of the Mouth. Recurrent aphthous oral ulcerations may be part of Behçet's syndrome. Although isolated oral bullae and ulcerations may be seen in patients with erythema multiforme, pemphigus, and pemphigoid, almost all patients will have an associated skin rash. The "iris" or "target" lesion of erythema multiforme is diagnostic. Otherwise, biopsy will establish the diagnosis. Corticosteroids may be life-saving for pemphigus and are used in the treatment of erythema multiforme majorum (Stevens-Johnson syndrome), although proof of their efficacy is not available.

APPROACH TO THE PATIENT WITH "SORE THROAT"

This section will discuss the clinical approach to patients with sore throat and will also discuss several less common but serious illnesses that can present as a "sore throat." When evaluating a patient with a sore throat, it is first important to distinguish between the relatively common and benign sore throat syndromes (viral or streptococcal pharyngitis) and the less common but more dangerous causes of sore throat. Patients with viral or streptococcal pharyngitis often give a history of exposure to individuals with upper respiratory tract infections. Symptoms of cough, rhinitis, and hoarseness (indicating involvement of the larynx) suggest a viral upper respiratory tract infection, although it is important to remember that hoarseness may also be seen with more serious infections such as epiglottitis.

Examination of the Throat. Two points regarding examination of the throat need emphasis. The first is that complete examination of the oral cavity is important. Not only will a thorough examination give clues as to the etiology of the complaint, but it may also provide early diagnosis of an asymptomatic malignancy at a time when cure is feasible. The second point is that the normal

TABLE 87–3. SEVEN DANGER SIGNS IN PATIENTS WITH "SORE THROAT"

1. Persistence of symptoms longer than one week without improvement
2. Respiratory difficulty, particularly stridor
3. Difficulty handling secretions
4. Difficulty in swallowing
5. Severe pain in the absence of erythema
6. A palpable mass
7. Blood, even in small amounts, in the pharynx or ear

tonsils and mucosal rim of the anterior fauces are generally a deeper red than the rest of the pharynx in healthy subjects. This should not be mistaken for inflammation. Patients with pharyngitis often have a red, inflamed posterior pharynx. The tonsils are often enlarged and red and may be covered with a punctate or diffuse white exudate. Lymph nodes of the anterior neck are often enlarged.

If any of the seven *danger signs* listed in Table 87–3 is present, the clinician must suspect an illness other than viral or streptococcal pharyngitis. Symptoms persisting longer than one week are rarely due to streptococci or viruses and should prompt consideration of other processes (see "Persistent or Penicillin-unresponsive Pharyngitis" below). Respiratory difficulty, particularly stridor, difficulty handling oral secretions, or difficulty swallowing should suggest the possibility of epiglottitis or soft tissue space infection. Severe pain in the absence of erythema of the pharynx may be seen with some of the "extrarespiratory" causes of sore throat, as well as in some cases of epiglottitis or retropharyngeal abscess. A *palpable mass* in the pharynx or neck suggests a soft tissue space infection, and *blood in the ear or pharynx* may be an early indication of a lateral pharyngeal space abscess eroding into the carotid artery.

A good history and careful examination will distinguish between the common and benign causes of a sore throat, and the unusual but often more serious causes.

Pharyngitis

A list of agents that have been associated with pharyngitis is shown on Table 87–4. Almost half

TABLE 87–4. CAUSES OF PHARYNGITIS

Viral
    Respiratory viruses*
    Herpes simplex
    Epstein-Barr virus
    Coxsackie A virus (herpangina)
Mycoplasma pneumoniae
Bacterial
    Group A streptococcus*
    Vincent's fusospirochetes
    Corynebacterium diphtheriae
    Neisseria gonorrheae
Fungal
    Candida species (thrush)

* Most frequent identifiable causes of pharyngitis

are due to respiratory viruses or group A streptococci. Most of the remainder of the cases are without defined etiology. Most cases occur during the winter months. In practice, once a diagnosis of pharyngitis is established clinically, it is most important to distinguish between group A streptococcal infections, which should be treated with penicillin, and viral infections, which should be treated symptomatically (e.g., salicylates, saline gargles). Since clinical criteria do not reliably distinguish streptococcal from nonstreptococcal pharyngitis, all patients with pharyngitis should have a throat swab cultured for streptococci.

Pharyngitis and Respiratory Virus Infections. Many patients with common colds due to rhinovirus or coronavirus or with influenza will have an associated pharyngitis. Other cold symptoms—rhinorrhea, conjunctival suffusion, and mild cough—suggest a cold virus; fevers and myalgias suggest influenza. Symptoms generally resolve in a few days without treatment.

Infectious mononucleosis due to Epstein-Barr virus is often associated with pharyngitis. Patients will often also complain of malaise and fever. On examination, the pharynx may be inflamed and the tonsils hypertrophied and covered by a white exudate. Cervical lymph node enlargement is often prominent and generalized lymph node enlargement and splenomegaly are common. Examination of a peripheral blood smear reveals atypical lymphocytes, and the presence of heterophil antibodies (e.g., Monospot) or a rise in antibodies to EBV viral capsid antigen will confirm the diagnosis.

Streptococcal Pharyngitis. Streptococcal pharyngitis may produce mild or severe symptoms. The pharynx is generally inflamed, and exudative tonsillitis is common but not universal. Fever may be present and cervical lymph nodes may be enlarged and tender. Clinical distinction between streptococcal and nonstreptococcal pharyngitis is inaccurate, and patients with pharyngitis should therefore have a swab of the posterior pharynx cultured on sheep blood agar plates. The growth of group A beta-hemolytic streptococci is an indication for treatment with penicillin (or erythromycin if the patient is penicillin-allergic). Antibiotics may shorten the duration of symptoms due to this infection but are given primarily to decrease the frequency of rheuumatic fever, which on occasion follows bouts of streptococcal pharyngitis.

Diphtheria. Diphtheria is a rare disease in the United States, with only three cases reported to the CDC in 1980. The grey pseudomembrane bleeds when removed and rarely may cause death via airway obstruction. Most morbidity and mortality in diphtheria are related to the elaboration of a toxin with neurologic and cardiac effects. Treatment consists of antitoxin plus erythromycin.

Epiglottitis

Epiglottitis, usually an aggressive disease of young children, occurs in adults as well. Early recognition of this entity is critical, because delay in diagnosis or treatment frequently results in death, which may occur abruptly, within hours after the onset of symptoms. This diagnosis must be considered in any patient with a sore throat and any of the following key symptoms or signs: (1) difficulty in swallowing, (2) copious oral secretions, (3) severe pain in the absence of pharyngeal erythema (the pharynx of patients with epiglottitis may be normal or inflamed), and (4) respiratory difficulty, particularly stridor. Patients with epiglottitis often display a characteristic posture; they will lean forward in order to prevent the swollen epiglottis from completely obstructing the airway and will resist any attempt at placement in the supine position. The diagnosis can be confirmed by lateral x-rays of the neck or by indirect laryngoscopy with visualization of the swollen erythematous epiglottis. This should be performed with the patient in the sitting position to minimize the risk of laryngeal spasm. Furthermore, the physician must be prepared to perform emergency tracheal intubation or tracheostomy should spasm occur. Therapy has two major objectives: protecting the airway and providing appropriate antimicrobial coverage. As the most likely pathogen is *Haemophilus influenzae*, good antibiotic choices would be chloramphenicol, trimethoprim-sulfamethoxazole, or a third-generation cephalosporin. Corticosteroids may relieve some inflammatory edema; however, their role in this disease remains unproven. Patients with respiratory difficulty should have their airway protected by endotracheal intubation or tracheostomy. Patients without respiratory complaints may be monitored continuously in an intensive care setting and intubated at the first sign of respiratory difficulty.

Soft Tissue Space Infections

Quinsy. Quinsy is a unilateral peritonsillar abscess or phlegmon that is an unusual complication of tonsillitis. The patient has pain and difficulty swallowing and often trouble handling oral secretions. Trismus (inability to open the mouth due to muscle spasm) may be present. Examination reveals swelling of the peritonsillar tissues and lateral displacement of the uvula. Digital examination may reveal a mass. When in the phlegmon stage, penicillin therapy may be adequate; abscess requires surgical drainage. Untreated, quinsy may result in glottal edema and respiratory embarrassment or lateral pharyngeal space abscess.

Lateral Pharyngeal Space Abscess. This rare infection is associated with serious morbidity because of its proximity to vascular structures. Extension to the jugular vein may result in thrombophlebitis with septic pulmonary emboli and bacteremia (syndrome of "postanginal sepsis"). Erosion of the carotid artery may also complicate this infection with resultant exsanguination. This is often preceded by small amounts of blood in the ear or pharynx. This infection is generally associated with tenderness and a mass at the angle of the jaw. Prompt surgical intervention may be life-saving.

Retropharyngeal Space Abscess. This complication of tonsillitis is rare in adults, since by adulthood the lymph nodes that give rise to this infection are generally atrophied. Most cases in adults are secondary to trauma (e.g., endoscopic) or extension of a cervical osteomyelitis. The patient often has difficulty swallowing and may complain of dyspnea, particularly when sitting upright. Diagnosis may be suspected by the presence of a posterior pharyngeal mass and confirmed by lateral neck films.

Ludwig's Angina. This cellulitis/phlegmon of the floor of the mouth generally is secondary to an odontogenic infection. The tongue is pushed upward, and there is often firm induration of the submandibular space and neck. Laryngeal edema and respiratory compromise may also occur and necessitate protection of the airway. Penicillin is the antibiotic of choice; some patients may require a broad guillotine incision across the submandibular space to provide decompression and adequate drainage, although incision may be unnecessary if the airway can be protected.

Extrarespiratory Causes of Sore Throat

Several extrarespiratory causes of sore throat should be kept in mind. The older patient who complains of soreness in his throat when he climbs stairs or when he is upset may be suffering from angina pectoris with an unusual radiation. The hypertensive patient who presents with an abrupt onset of a "tearing pain" in his throat may have a dissecting aortic aneurysm. In these patients, swallowing is generally unaffected. Patients with DeQuervain's subacute thyroiditis may present with fever and pain in the neck radiating to the ears. In patients with thyroiditis, the thyroid is generally tender and the sedimentation rate is increased. Patients with vitamin deficiencies may complain of soreness in the mouth and throat (see Table 87–1). Examination may reveal a red "beefy" tongue with flattened papillae, resulting in a smooth appearance.

Persistent or Penicillin-unresponsive Pharyngitis

Most cases of viral or streptococcal pharyngitis are self-limited, and symptoms generally resolve within three to four days. Persistent sore throat should prompt consideration of the following possibilities:

Soft Tissue Abscess or Phlegmon. Rarely, an untreated tonsillitis will extend to the soft tissues of the pharynx, producing one of these potentially life-threatening infections (see above).

Pharyngeal Gonorrhea. Although most cases of pharyngeal gonorrhea are asymptomatic, mild pharyngitis may be seen occasionally. This infection will not respond to doses of penicillin used for pharyngitis; moreover, the gonococcus is relatively resistant to phenoxymethyl penicillin (PenV). The gonococcus will not likely be identified on routine culture medium; isolation generally requires culture of a fresh throat swab on a selective medium such as Thayer-Martin.

Infectious Mononucleosis. One virus that can produce a more protracted exudative pharyngitis is the Epstein-Barr virus, causative agent of infectious mononucleosis. Adenopathy, splenomegaly, generalized malaise, and rash may accompany this illness. Peripheral blood smear usually reveals numerous atypical lymphocytes. The patient should be advised to abstain from contact sports, as traumatic rupture of the enlarged spleen may be fatal.

Acute Lymphoblastic Leukemia. Persistent exudative tonsillitis may be a presentation of acute lymphoblastic leukemia (ALL). Diagnosis can be suspected by examination of the peripheral blood smear; however, some experience may be required to distinguish between the blasts of ALL and the atypical lymphocytes of infectious mononucleosis.

Other Leukopenic States. Stomatitis/pharyngitis may be the presenting complaint of patients with *aplastic anemia* or with *agranulocytosis*. As some of these cases are drug-induced (e.g., propylthiouracil, phenytoin, etc.), a complete medication history on initial presentation may suggest this possibility. Prompt discontinuation of the offending drug may be life-saving.

Although sore throat is a common complaint of patients with relatively benign illness, rarely it is the presenting complaint of a patient with a serious or life-threatening disease. Any of the key signs or symptoms shown in Table 84–3 should alert the clinician to the possibility of an extraordinary process.

REFERENCES

Cherry JD: Acute epiglottitis, laryngitis, and croup. In Remington JS, and Swartz MN (eds): Current Clinical Topics in Infectious Diseases. Vol 2. New York, McGraw-Hill Book Co, 1981.

Evans FO, Sydnar JB, Moore WEC, et al: Sinusitis of the maxillary antrum. N Engl J Med 293:735–739, 1975.

Krause RM: Streptococcal diseases. In Wyngaarden JB, and Smith LH Jr (eds): Cecil Textbook of Medicine. 17th ed. Philadelphia, WB Saunders Co, 1985.

Portions of the section on epiglottitis were reprinted from Lederman MM, Lowder J, and Lerner PI: Bacteremic pneumococcal epiglottitis in adults with malignancy. Am Rev Resp Dis 125:117–118, 1982, with permission.

88 INFECTIONS OF THE LOWER RESPIRATORY TRACT

Pneumonia currently accounts for about 10 per cent of admissions to adult medical services in North America and is one of the leading causes of death during the productive years of life. Although pneumonia ranks sixth among the causes of death in the United States today, it is first among the potentially lethal illnesses that are readily reversible by the alert physician. Every physician must therefore be adept at the *rapid* diagnosis and management of the patient with pneumonia. Viruses, chlamydia, rickettsia, mycoplasma, bacteria, protozoans, and parasites can all produce serious infection of the lower respiratory tract. Careful history and physical examination can provide clues to the likely etiology of infection. The clinical spectra of pneumonias caused by different pathogens overlap considerably, however. Microscopic examination of respiratory secretions provides a rapid and essential step in the differential diagnosis of pneumonia.

PATHOGENESIS OF PNEUMONIA

Microbes can enter the lung to produce infection by hematogenous spread, by inhalation of aerosolized particles, or, most commonly, by aspiration of oropharyngeal secretions. In the latter instance, the organisms colonizing the oropharynx will determine the flora of the aspirated secretions and presumably the nature of the resultant pneumonia. Some organisms like *Streptococcus pneumoniae* may transiently colonize the oropharynx in healthy individuals. Others such as gram-negative bacilli are more prevalent in the upper respiratory tract of debilitated and hospitalized patients. Aspiration of normal oropharyngeal flora may lead to necrotizing pneumonia caused by mixtures of oral anaerobic bacteria.

Inoculum size (the number of bacteria aspirated) may be an important factor in the development of pneumonia. Studies using radioisotopes have demonstrated that up to 45 per cent of healthy men aspirate some oropharyngeal contents during sleep. In most instances, back-up defenses, including cough and mucociliary clearance, are adequate to prevent the development of pneumonia. Individuals with structural disease of the oropharynx or patients with impaired cough reflexes due to drugs, alcohol, or neuromuscular disease are at particular risk for the development of pneumonia due to aspiration. The specialized ciliated cells of the bronchial mucosa are covered by a layer of mucus that traps foreign particles, which are propelled upward by rhythmic beating of the cilia to a point where a cough can expel the particles. Denuding of the respiratory epithelium by infection with the influenza virus may be one mechanism whereby influenza predisposes to bacterial pneumonia.

Infection by *Mycobacterium tuberculosis* is usually acquired through inhalation of aerosolized infected droplet nuclei. A primary infection is established in the parenchyma of the lungs and in the draining lymph nodes which may result in a progressive primary infection, but in most instances it resolves after producing a mild respiratory illness. The organism remains alive, sequestered within host macrophages, and contained by host cell-mediated defenses. Reactivation of infection may never occur or may occur without apparent precipitating events or at times when host cell-mediated immune responses are impaired. Examples of these impairments include starvation, intercurrent viral infections, administration of corticosteroids or cytotoxic drugs, and illnesses associated with immunosuppression such as Hodgkin's disease, hairy cell leukemia, and AIDS.

EPIDEMIOLOGY

Common pathogens of community-acquired and nosocomial pneumonia are shown in Table 88–1. As a general rule, the pneumococcus is an important pathogen in all age groups, and influenza and tuberculosis become more frequent with increasing age. Although *Mycoplasma* occasionally produces pneumonia in the elderly, it is primarily a pathogen of the young. Certain systemic disorders appear to be associated with pneumonias due to particular organisms (Table 88–2). The exposure history may be helpful in suggesting specific causative agents (Table 88–3). Pneumonias associated with bone marrow suppression and malignant disorders are discussed in Chapter 97.

DIAGNOSTIC APPROACH TO THE PATIENT

A critical historical point in the differential diagnosis of pneumonia is the duration of symptoms. Pneumonia due to the pneumococcus, *Mycoplasma*, or virus is usually an acute illness. Symptoms are measured in hours to a few days, although there may occasionally be a longer viral prodrome before bacterial superinfection. In contrast, symptoms of pneumonia lasting 10 days or more are rarely due to the common aerobic pulmonary pathogens and should raise suspicion of mycobacterial, fungal, or anaerobic pneumonia (anaerobes can produce acute or chronic infection) or the presence of an anatomic defect such as an endobronchial mass.

Occupational, exposure, and travel history often provide clues to the etiology of some less common pneumonias (Table 88–3). Although these pneumonias are uncommon, they should be

TABLE 88–1. IMPORTANT PATHOGENS CAUSING PNEUMONIA

Young healthy adult	*Streptococcus pneumoniae, Mycoplasma pneumoniae,* virus
Elderly	*Streptococcus pneumoniae,* influenza, *M. tuberculosis*
Debilitated	*Streptococcus pneumoniae,* influenza, oral flora, *M. tuberculosis,* gram-negative bacilli
Hospitalized	Oral flora, *Staphylococcus aureus,* gram-negative bacilli

TABLE 88–2. SPECIFIC DISORDERS AND ASSOCIATED PNEUMONIAS

Seizures	Aspiration (mixed anaerobes)
Alcoholism	Aspiration, *Streptococcus pneumoniae,* gram-negative bacilli
Diabetes mellitus	Gram-negative bacilli, *M. tuberculosis*
Hemoglobinopathy	*Streptococcus pneumoniae, Mycoplasma pneumoniae*
Chronic lung disease	*Streptococcus pneumoniae, Haemophilus influenza, Pasteurella multocida,* gram-negative bacilli
Chronic renal failure	*Streptococcus pneumoniae, M. tuberculosis*

considered in the appropriate setting because, if improperly treated, some may be fatal.

A history of rhinitis or pharyngitis suggests respiratory virus or *Mycoplasma* pneumonia, although influenza may predispose to bacterial pneumonia. Diarrhea has been associated with Legionnaires' pneumonia in some but not all outbreaks. A persistent hacking, nonproductive cough characterizes some *Mycoplasma* infections; symptoms of grippe—malaise and myalgias— are common in influenza and may also be seen with *Mycoplasma* pneumonia. A true rigor is very suggestive of a bacterial (often pneumococcal) pneumonia. Whereas pleural effusions may be seen in nonbacterial pneumonias, severe pleuritic pain in a patient with pneumonia is suggestive of bacterial infection. Night sweats are seen in chronic pneumonias and suggest tuberculous or fungal disease.

Most patients with pneumonia have fever and tachycardia. Fever without a concomitant rise in pulse rate may be seen in Legionnaires' disease, *Mycoplasma* infections, and other "nonbacterial" pneumonias. Patients with pulmonary tubercu-

TABLE 88–3. EXPOSURES ASSOCIATED WITH PNEUMONIA

Cattle, goats, sheep	Q fever, brucellosis, anthrax
Rabbits	Tularemia
Birds	Psittacosis, histoplasmosis*
Southwestern United States	Coccidioidomycosis
Mississippi and Ohio River valleys	Histoplasmosis
Southeast Asia	Tuberculosis, melioidosis

*Exposure to bird and bat droppings.

losis often maintain high fevers in relative comfort when compared to patients with acute bacterial pneumonia. Respirations may be shallow in the presence of pleurisy. Tachypnea, cyanosis, and the use of accessory muscles for respiration suggest serious illness. Foul breath suggests anaerobic infection. Jaundice may be seen in any bacterial infection and occurs frequently in pneumococcal pneumonias. Mental confusion in a patient with pneumonia should immediately raise the suspicion of meningeal involvement, which occurs most commonly in patients with pneumococcal pneumonia. Any infection may cause confusion in an elderly patient. Nonetheless, patients with pneumonia who are confused must be evaluated by examination of cerebrospinal fluid.

Physical evidence of consolidation—dullness to percussion, bronchial breath sounds, increased fremitus, and whispered pectoriloquy—suggest bacterial pneumonia. Early in the course of pneumonia, however, physical examination may be normal.

RADIOGRAPHIC PATTERNS IN PATIENTS WITH PNEUMONIA

Clinical/radiographic dissociation is seen often in patients with *Mycoplasma pneumoniae* pneumonia. Chest radiographs of patients with *Mycoplasma* infection often suggest a more serious infection than does the appearance of the patient or the physical examination. The converse is true in patients with *Pneumocystis carinii* infection, who may appear quite ill despite normal or nearly normal chest radiographs. This may also be true early in the course of acute bacterial pneumonias, when pleuritic chest pain, cough, purulent sputum, and inspiratory rales may precede specific x-ray findings by many hours. A "negative" x-ray can never "rule out" the possibility of acute bacterial pneumonia when the patient's symptoms and signs point to this diagnosis. A lobar consolidation suggests a bacterial pneumonia; however, patients with chronic lung disease often fail to manifest clinical or radiographic evidence of consolidation during the course of bacterial pneumonia. Interstitial infiltrates suggest a nonbacterial process but may also be seen in early

staphylococcal pneumonia. Enlarged hilar lymph nodes suggest a concomitant lung tumor but may also be seen in primary tuberculous, viral, or fungal pneumonias. Large pleural effusions should suggest streptococcal pneumonia or tuberculosis. Pneumatoceles are seen in patients after respirator-mediated barotrauma but occur frequently in the evolution of staphylococcal pneumonia, particularly among children. The presence of cavitation identifies the pneumonia as necrotizing. This virtually excludes viruses and *Mycoplasma* and makes pneumococcal infection unlikely (Table 88–4).

OTHER LABORATORY FINDINGS

In patients with bacterial pneumonia, the white blood cell count is often (but not reliably) elevated. Among patients with pneumococcal infection, WBC counts of 20,000 to 30,000 per μl or more may be seen. A left shift with immature forms is common. Patients with nonbacterial pneumonias tend to have lower WBC counts. Modest elevations of serum bilirubin (conjugated) may be seen in many bacterial infections but are particularly common in patients with pneumococcal pneumonia.

DIAGNOSIS AND MANAGEMENT OF THE PATIENT WITH PNEUMONIA

When the patient presents with abrupt-onset of shaking chills, followed by cough, pleuritic chest pain, fever, rusty or yellow sputum, and shortness of breath, and the physical examination reveals tachypnea and even minimal signs of alveolar inflammation (e.g., harsh breath sounds at one lung base), the presumptive diagnosis of bacterial pneumonia should be made, sputum should be examined, and appropriate therapy should be begun regardless of radiographic findings. The x-ray abnormalities may lag for several hours after the clinical onset of pneumonia.

EXAMINATION OF RESPIRATORY SECRETIONS

Examination of respiratory secretions is essential for accurate diagnosis and proper treatment of pneumonia. When history and physical examination suggest pneumonia, a specimen of sputum must be Gram-stained and examined immediately. The adequacy of the specimen can be ascertained by (1) the absence of squamous epithelial cells (shown in Fig. 88–1), and (2) the presence of polymorphonuclear leukocytes (10 to 15 per high-power field). The presence of alveolar macrophages (Fig. 88–2) and bronchial epithelial cells (Fig. 88–3) confirms the lower respiratory tract source of the specimen. A specimen with many (more than five per high-power field) squamous epithelial cells is of no value for either cul-

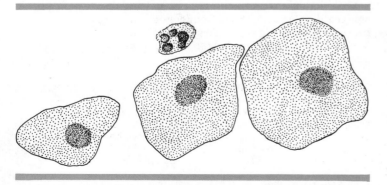

FIGURE 88–1. Three squamous epithelial cells and one polymorphonuclear leukocyte.

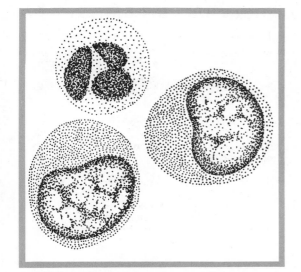

FIGURE 88–2. Two alveolar macrophages and one polymorphonuclear leukocyte.

TABLE 88–4. CAVITARY NECROTIZING PNEUMONIAS

COMMON	RARE	? NEVER
Tuberculosis	Streptococcus pneumoniae	Mycoplasma
Staphylococcus	Legionella	pneumoniae
Gram-negative bacilli	Pneumocystis carinii	Virus
Anaerobes		
Fungi		

ture or Gram's stain, since it is contaminated with upper respiratory tract secretions.

In some cases, the patient cannot produce an adequate sputum sample. Unless the patient appears quite well and by all clinical criteria has a mild viral or *Mycoplasma* pneumonia, a nasotracheal aspiration should be performed. This is done by placing the patient supine, hyperextending the neck, and passing a well-lubricated red rubber suction catheter from the nose to the posterior pharynx. During inspiration, the tube is then passed swiftly past the glottis into the trachea, suction is applied, and secretions are collected in a Lugen's trap. The vigorous coughing stimulated by this procedure often produces an additional excellent expectorated specimen.

If nasotracheal aspiration still fails to provide a good specimen for analysis, transtracheal aspiration should be considered. The sicker the patient and the greater the likelihood of a penicillin-resistant pathogen, the more important it is to get an adequate sample of sputum for examination and culture. With the patient supine and with his

neck hyperextended, local anesthetic is injected over the cricothyroid membrane. A small gauge blade is used to make a tiny nick in the skin. A 14-gauge needle containing a large-bore plastic catheter is then inserted through the incision and directed toward the coccyx with the bevel of the needle facing upward. The catheter is then threaded down the trachea and the needle is withdrawn. With the catheter in place, a 50-cc syringe is used to aspirate tracheal contents. If this is not successful, 2 ml of sterile saline (without preservatives) is injected through the catheter and aspirated. This specimen should be Gram's stained and cultured aerobically and anaerobically. (Note: Expectorated sputum and sputum obtained through nasotracheal aspiration cannot be cultured anaerobically because of universal contamination with oral flora.)

The Gram's stained specimen should be examined using an oil immersion lens. The presence of a predominant organism, particularly if found within white blood cells, suggests that this is the pathogen. In cases of aspiration of mouth flora, there is a mixture of oral streptococci, gram-positive rods, and gram-negative organisms. In some cases, there may be inflammatory cells and no organisms seen on Gram's stain. This finding suggests a number of possibilities, many of which are nonbacterial pneumonias (Table 88–5). Unless the diagnosis of acute bacterial pneumonia is clear, an acid-fast stain or fluorescent auramine-rhodamine stain of sputum for mycobacteria should be performed. If Legionnaires' disease is suspected, immunofluorescence stains for *Legionella* can be performed, although the yield on expectorated sputum is low. The demonstration of elastin fibers in a KOH preparation of sputum (see Figure 82–2) establishes a diagnosis of necrotizing pneumonia (see Table 88–4). Importantly, this test can be positive in the absence of radiographic evidence of cavitation. A tuberculin skin test and control skin tests such as mumps, *Candida*, and *Trichophyton* should be applied in all cases of pneumonia. If the tuberculin is negative but tuberculosis remains a diagnostic possibility, a second strength tuberculin (250 TU) should be placed. In the absence of anergy (no response to control skin tests), a negative 250 TU tuberculin makes reactivation tuberculosis unlikely but does not exclude the diagnosis.

TREATMENT AND OUTCOME

As soon as the organism is identified on Gram's stain, antibiotics must be administered without

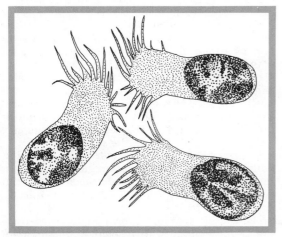

FIGURE 88–3. Three bronchial epithelial cells.

TABLE 88-5. SPUTUM GRAM'S STAIN REVEALING INFLAMMATORY CELLS AND NO ORGANISMS

POSSIBILITIES	CLINICAL SETTING	CONFIRMATION OF DIAGNOSIS	TREATMENT
Prior antibiotic treatment			
Viral pneumonia	Winter months—influenza, may be mild or life-threatening	Serologies, virus culture	Amantadine for influenza
Mycoplasma pneumonia	Hacking, nonproductive cough	Cold agglutinins, serologies	Erythromycin
Legionella	Chronic lung disease—hospital-acquired, summer prevalence	DFA* of sputum or pleural fluid, culture, serologies	Erythromycin
Psittacosis	Exposure to birds, e.g., parrots, turkeys	Culture, serologies	Tetracycline
Q fever	Exposure to cattle, South Africa	Serologies	Tetracycline or chloramphenicol

*Direct immunofluorescence assay

delay. If the pathogen is readily identified, the antibiotic choices are straightforward (see Table 88-6). Patients with *Mycoplasma* and viral pneumonia can generally be treated on an ambulatory basis. An occasional young patient with an uncomplicated pneumococcal pneumonia without underlying disease or other risk factors such as alcohol abuse can also be managed at home, provided that the patient is reliably attended by friends or family and has ready access to a physician or hospital. Otherwise, patients with bacterial pneumonia should be hospitalized.

Supplemental oxygen should be provided if the patient is tachypneic or hypoxemic. Patients at risk for the development of respiratory insufficiency should be monitored in a critical care setting. Patients who are not capable of adequately coughing up respiratory secretions should have frequent clapping and drainage; meticulous attention must be paid to suctioning of oral secretions. Patients with suspected pulmonary tuberculosis should be isolated from other patients until treatment is instituted.

Patients treated for pneumococcal pneumonia should begin to improve within 48 hours after institution of antibiotics; patients with pneumonia caused by gram-negative bacilli, staphylococci, and oral anaerobes may remain ill for longer periods after initiation of treatment. Several possibilities should be considered among patients who fail to improve or who deteriorate while on treatment:

Endobronchial Obstruction. Physical examination may fail to reveal sounds of consolidation, and radiographs may show evidence of lobar collapse. Bronchoscopy can establish the diagnosis.

Undrained Empyema. Radiographs may not always distinguish between fluid and consolidation; ultrasonography and computerized tomography scans can identify the fluid and provide direction for its drainage.

Purulent Pericarditis. This should be suspected in a very ill patient with pneumonia involving a lobe adjacent to the pericardium. Chest pain and electrocardiographic evidence of pericarditis are usually absent. Distended neck veins and pericardial friction rubs are present in a minority of cases. Echocardiogram or chest ultrasonography reveals fluid in the pericardium. If purulent pericarditis is suspected, emergency pericardiocentesis can be life-saving.

Incorrect Diagnosis or Treatment. In cases in which clinical response is poor, the patient's hospital course and admission sputum stains should be reviewed by a clinician with expertise in diagnosis and treatment of pneumonia. Misinterpretation of sputum Gram's stained preparations—either failure to recognize an important pathogen or a treatment decision based upon ex-

TABLE 88-6. INITIAL ANTIBIOTICS FOR TREATMENT OF PNEUMONIA

PATHOGEN	TREATMENT
Streptococcus pneumoniae	Penicillin G, 1.2 million units/day[1]
Mycoplasma pneumoniae	Erythromycin, 500 mg P.O. q.i.d.
Haemophilus influenzae[2]	Trimethoprim-sulfamethoxazole, 80 mg/400 mg q6h, or ampicillin, 1–1.5 gm q4h
Staphylococcus aureus	Nafcillin, 3 gm I.V. q6h
Legionella pneumophila	Erythromycin, 750 mg q6h
Mixed oral flora (anaerobes)	Penicillin, 2–10 million units/day[3]
Gram-negative rods	Aminoglycoside (e.g., gentamicin, 1.7 mg/kg I.V. q8h) plus third-generation cephalosporin, 8–12 gm/day[4]
Tuberculosis	Isoniazid, 300 mg/day, plus either rifampin 600 mg/day or ethambutol 1 gm/day

[1]Erythromycin, 500 mg q6h for penicillin-allergic patients

[2]Beta-lactamase producing *H. influenzae* has caused disease in adults. If patient is very ill, avoid ampicillin and use instead trimethoprim-sulfamethoxazole or chloramphenicol 3 to 4 gm/day.

[3]Clindamycin, 600 mg q6h, if patient is seriously ill or fails to respond to penicillin.

[4]Add penicillin active against *Pseudomonas* (e.g., carbenicillin 30 gm/day) if *Pseudomonas* is a possibility. Antibiotics can be adjusted when sensitivity data are available.

amination of an inadequate specimen—are avoidable pitfalls of medical practice.

Approach to the Patient with Pleural Effusion and Fever

The approach to such patients is quite straightforward: the fluid must be examined. If any organism other than *Streptococcus pneumoniae* is seen on Gram's stain of pleural fluid or grown in culture, chest tube drainage is required. A pleural effusion infected with the pneumococcus can often be treated with simple needle aspiration and antibiotics. Among patients with pneumonia, even fluids that do not reveal organisms on Gram's stain but that have a pH of less than 7.00 and a glucose concentration below 40 mg/dl may require chest tube drainage for satisfactory resolution.

Pleurisy caused by *Mycobacterium tuberculosis* is often an acute illness. In most cases, a pneumonia is not present or readily appreciated. Inflammatory cells—polymorphonuclear leukocytes, mononuclear leukocytes, or both—are present in the pleural fluid. Notably absent are mesothelial cells, whose presence in numbers exceeding 0.5 per cent of the total cell count makes a tuberculous effusion unlikely. Pleural fluid glucose levels are often depressed but may be normal. Mycobacteria are rarely seen on stains of pleural fluid. As many as one third of patients do not have positive tuberculin skin tests. Other possible causes of pleural effusion in this setting include pulmonary infarction (less than half of these cases produce a hemorrhagic exudate), malignancy (most do not have fever), and connective tissue disorders such as SLE and rheumatoid arthritis. If the etiology of the effusion is not apparent, a biopsy of the pleura is required.

PREVENTION

Pneumococcal pneumonia may be preventable by immunizing patients at high risk with polyvalent pneumococcal polysaccharide vaccine. The current polyvalent vaccine is 60 to 80 per cent effective in individuals with normal immune responses. Booster immunizations should not be given because of the possibility of serious reactions. Yearly immunization with influenza vaccine is also recommended for many of these patients; by decreasing the attack rate of influenza, immunization also decreases morbidity and mortality due to bacterial pneumonia (Table 88–7).

Patients without active tuberculosis but with skin test reactivity to tuberculosis are at risk for reactivating their infection. The development of active tuberculosis can be prevented in most instances by treatment for one year with isoniazid 300 mg/day. Indications for prophylaxis are shown in Table 88–8.

TABLE 88–7. PREVENTION OF PNEUMONIA: CANDIDATES FOR PNEUMOCOCCAL AND INFLUENZA VACCINES

	PNEUMOCOCCAL VACCINE (ONE TIME ONLY)	INFLUENZA VACCINE (YEARLY)
Patients ≥ 65 years	Yes	Yes
Chronic lung or heart disease	Yes	Yes
Sickle cell disease	Yes	Consider
Asplenic patients	Yes	No
Hodgkin's disease	Yes	Consider
Multiple myeloma	Yes	Consider
Cirrhosis	Yes	Consider
Chronic alcoholism	Yes	Consider
Chronic renal failure	Yes	Consider
Cerebrospinal fluid leaks	Yes	No
Residents of chronic care facilities	Consider	Yes
Diabetes mellitus	Yes	Yes

TABLE 88–8. INDICATIONS FOR PROPHYLAXIS WITH INH

Documented new skin test conversion to tuberculin over past two years
Tuberculin-positive contacts of patients with active TB
Tuberculin-negative contacts (less than 5 years of age) of patients with active TB[1]
Positive tuberculin skin test of unknown duration
    Patients under 35 years of age
    Patients with radiographic evidence of inactive tuberculosis who have never received an adequate course of antituberculous drugs
Consider INH prophylaxis for patients with positive tuberculin skin tests and:
    gastrectomy
    diabetes mellitus
    prolonged (> one month) administration of corticosteroids or immunosuppressive drugs
    renal transplantation
    silicosis

[1]These children should have repeat skin tests three months after INH is begun. If the repeat test is negative, INH may be discontinued.

REFERENCES

Wolinsky E. Tuberculosis. In Wyngaarden JB, and Smith LH Jr (eds): Cecil Textbook of Medicine. 17th ed. Philadelphia, WB Saunders Co, 1985, pp 1620–1630.

Reynolds HY, Durack DT, Baum SG, and Fraser DW: Pneumonia. In Wyngaarden JB, and Smith LH Jr (eds): Cecil Textbook of Medicine. 17th ed. Philadelphia, WB Saunders Co, 1985, pp 1494–1519.

89 | INFECTIONS OF THE HEART AND VESSELS

INFECTIVE ENDOCARDITIS (IE)

Infective endocarditis ranges from an indolent illness with few systemic manifestations, readily responsive to antibiotic therapy, to a fulminant septicemic disease with malignant destruction of the heart valves and life-threatening systemic embolization. The varied features of endocarditis relate in large measure to the different infecting organisms. Viridans streptococci are the prototype of bacteria that originate in the oral flora, infect previously abnormal heart valves, and may cause minimal symptomatology despite progressive valvular damage. *Staphylococcus aureus*, in contrast, invades previously normal valves and destroys them rapidly.

Epidemiology

The average age of patients with endocarditis has increased in the antibiotic era owing to the greater frequency of underlying degenerative heart disease and nosocomial endocarditis. Rheumatic heart disease remains a predisposing factor in 20 to 30 per cent of patients with IE. About 15 per cent of patients have congenital heart disease. The propensity to develop endocarditis varies with the congenital lesion. For example, infection of a bicuspid aortic valve accounts for one fifth of cases of IE occurring over the age of 60; a secundum atrial septal defect, however, rarely becomes infected. Mitral valve prolapse is the predisposing condition in over one third of cases of endocarditis restricted to the mitral valve. Intravenous drug users have a unique propensity to develop IE of the tricuspid valve, although infection of the mitral or aortic valve also is common.

Pathogenesis

Endocarditis ensues when bacteria entering the blood stream from an oral or other source lodge on heart valves that may already bear platelet-fibrin thrombi. The frequency of bacteremia is quite high after dental extraction (18 to 85 per cent) or periodontal surgery (32 to 88 per cent) but also is significant following everyday activities such as tooth brushing (0 to 26 per cent) and chewing candy (17 to 51 per cent). The production of extracellular dextran by some strains of *Streptococcus* is responsible for their adherence to dental enamel and also is a factor in the pathogenesis of endocarditis; dextran facilitates entrapment of circulating organisms on damaged valves and platelet-fibrin thrombi. Once infection begins, bacteria proliferate freely within the interstices of the enlarging vegetation; in this relatively avascular site they are protected from serum bactericidal factors and leukocytes.

Clinical Features

Most cases of streptococcal endocarditis become manifest clinically within two weeks of initiating events such as dental extraction. Diagnosis usually is delayed an additional four to five weeks or more, however, because of the paucity of symptoms. If the causative organism is slow-growing and produces an indolent syndrome, symptoms may be extremely protracted (six months or longer) before definitive diagnosis. The symptoms and signs of IE relate to systemic infection, emboli (bland or septic), metastatic infective foci, congestive heart failure, or immune complex–associated lesions. The most common complaints in patients with IE are fever, chills, weakness, shortness of breath, drenching night sweats, loss of appetite, and weight loss. Musculoskeletal symptoms develop in nearly one half of patients and may dominate the presentation. Proximal arthralgias are typical and are frequently accompanied by oligoarticular arthritis of the lower extremities. Fever is present in 90 per cent of patients. Fever is often absent in elderly or debilitated patients or in the setting of underlying congestive heart failure, renal dysfunction, or previous antibiotic treatment. Heart murmurs are frequent (85 per cent); changing murmurs (5 to 10 per cent) and new cardiac murmurs (5 per cent) are unusual but highly suggestive of the diagnosis of IE. Congestive heart failure occurs in two thirds of patients. At least one of the peripheral manifestations of endocarditis occurs in one half of patients (Table 89–1). Splenomegaly (25 to 60 per cent) is more likely when symptoms have been prolonged. Clubbing occurs in 10 to 20 per cent of patients.

The clinical syndrome of IE differs in users of intravenous drugs. Tricuspid valve infection is most common. Patients often present with pleuritic chest pain caused by septic pulmonary emboli. Round, cavitating inflitrates may be found on chest x-ray. The infective foci are initially centered in blood vessels; only after they erode into the bronchial system does cough develop, productive of bloody or purulent sputum.

Serious systemic emboli may cause dramatic findings, at times masking the systemic nature of IE. Embolism to the splenic artery leads to left upper quadrant pain, sometimes radiating to the left shoulder; a friction rub; and left pleural effusion. Renal, coronary, and mesenteric arteries are frequent alternative sites of clinically important emboli. CNS embolization is one of the most serious complications of IE, however, since it may produce irreversible and disabling neurologic deficits.

Overall, neurologic manifestations occur in one third of patients with IE. In addition to stroke due to vascular occlusion by an embolus, toxic encephalopathy, which may mimic psychosis, and meningoencephalitis also occur. The consequences of embolization depend on the site of lodging and the bacterial pathogen. Organisms such as viridans streptococci initially produce a

TABLE 89–1. PERIPHERAL MANIFESTATIONS OF INFECTIVE ENDOCARDITIS

PHYSICAL FINDING (frequency)	PATHOGENESIS	MOST COMMON ORGANISMS
Petechiae (20–40%) (red, nonblanching lesions in crops on conjunctivae, buccal mucosa, palate, extremities)	Vasculitis or emboli	Streptococcus, Staphylococcus
Splinter hemorrhages (15%) (linear, red-brown streaks most suggestive of IE when proximal in nailbeds)	Vasculitis or emboli	Staphylococcus, Streptococcus
Osler's nodes (10–25%) (2–5 mm painful nodules on pads of fingers or toes)	Vasculitis	Streptococcus
Janeway lesions (<10%) (macular, red or hemorrhagic, painless patches on palms or soles)	Emboli	Staphylococcus
Roth's spots (<5%) (oval, pale retinal lesions surrounded by hemorrhage)	Vasculitis	Streptococcus

syndrome entirely attributable to the vascular occlusion; however, damage to the blood vessel can result in formation of a mycotic aneurysm that may leak or burst at a later date. S. aureus, in contrast, produces progressive infection extending from the site of embolization; brain abscess and purulent meningitis are common sequelae.

The kidney can be the site of abscess formation, multiple infarcts, or immune complex glomerulonephritis. When renal dysfunction develops during antibiotic therapy, drug toxicity is an additional possibility.

Laboratory Findings

Nonspecific laboratory abnormalities occur in IE and reflect chronic infection. These include anemia, reticulocytopenia, increased erythrocyte sedimentation rate, hypergammaglobulinemia, and circulating immune complexes and rheumatoid factor. Urinalysis frequently shows proteinuria (50 to 65 per cent) and microscopic hematuria (30 to 50 per cent).

The bacteremia of IE is continuous and low-grade. Three sets of blood cultures should be obtained in the first 24 hours of hospitalization. Additional blood cultures are important if the patient has received antibiotic therapy in the preceding one to two weeks and if initial blood cultures are negative at 48 to 72 hours. In most series, 15 to 20 per cent of patients with the clinical diagnosis of IE have negative blood cultures, usually because of previous antibiotic therapy.

Echocardiography is a useful technique for identifying vegetations in endocarditis. The finding of vegetations is helpful diagnostically and also indicates an increased risk of valvular destruction with congestive heart failure, systemic embolization, and death. Echocardiographic findings may be misleading, however, and the finding of vegetations does not constitute an independent indication for cardiac surgery. Furthermore, the absence of vegetations on echocardiogram does not exclude the diagnosis of IE.

Differential Diagnosis

The diagnosis of IE usually is firmly established on the basis of the clinical findings and results of blood cultures. In fact, in streptococcal infection, the speciation of the blood culture isolate may provide circumstantial evidence for or against infection of the heart valves (Table 89–2). The identity of the causative organism may be helpful for other bacteria as well; the ratio of IE to non-IE bacteremias is approximately 1:1 for Staphylococcus aureus, 1:7 for group B streptococci, and 1:200 for Escherichia coli.

The initial presentation of IE can be misleading: the young adult with a stroke, pneumonia, or meningitis, or the elderly patient who is afebrile but confused. The index of suspicion of IE, therefore, must be high and blood cultures should be obtained in these varied settings, particularly if antibiotic usage is contemplated.

Major problems in diagnosis arise if antibiotics have been administered before blood is cultured or if blood cultures are negative. Attempts to culture slow-growing organisms, including those with particular nutritional requirements, should be planned by discussion with a clinical microbiologist. The differential diagnosis of culture-negative endocarditis includes acute rheumatic fever, multiple pulmonary emboli, atrial myxoma, and nonbacterial thrombotic endocarditis. These diagnoses should be considered and excluded, if possible, before beginning therapy for presumed culture-negative IE.

Management and Outcome

The outcome of endocarditis is determined by the extent of valvular destruction, the size and friability of vegetations, and the choice of antibiotics. These, in turn, are influenced by the na-

TABLE 89–2. RELATIVE FREQUENCY OF IE AND NON-IE BACTEREMIAS FOR VARIOUS STREPTOCOCCI*

SPECIES	IE/NON-IE
S. mutans	14:1
S. bovis I	6:1
S. sanguis	3:1
S. faecalis	1:1
S. bovis II	1:2
S. milleri	1:3
Group B streptococci	1:7
Group A streptococci	1:32

* Modified from Parker MT, and Ball LC: Streptococci and aerococci associated with systemic infection in man. J Med Microbiol 9:275, 1976.

TABLE 89–3. SYNDROMES SUGGESTING SPECIFIC BACTERIA CAUSING INFECTIVE ENDOCARDITIS

Indolent Course
   Viridans streptococci
   Streptococcus bovis
   Streptococcus faecalis
   Fastidious gram-negative rods
Aggressive Course
   Staphylococcus aureus
   Streptococcus pneumoniae
   Streptococcus pyogenes
   Neisseria gonorrhoeae
Drug Users
   Staphylococcus aureus
   Pseudomonas aeruginosa
   Streptococcus faecalis
   Candida sp.
   Bacillus sp.
Frequent Major Emboli
   Haemophilus sp.
   Bacteroides sp.
   Candida sp.

ture of the causative organism and delays inherent in diagnosis. The main importance of antibiotics is to halt further valvular damage and to cure the infection. Surgery may be necessary for hemodynamic stabilization, prevention of embolization, or control of drug-resistant infection.

Antibiotics should be selected on the basis of the clinical setting (Table 89–3) and started as soon as blood cultures are obtained if the diagnosis of IE appears highly likely and the course is suggestive of active valvular destruction or systemic embolization. The antibiotics can be adjusted later on the basis of culture and sensitivity data.

Antibiotics

Most viridans streptococci and nonenterococcal group D streptococci, such as S. bovis, are exquisitely sensitive to penicillin. The penicillin concentration inhibiting growth of such organisms is less than 0.1 μg/ml, and they are killed by similar concentrations of penicillin. A variety of antibiotic regimens have been advocated to treat this form of IE and appear to be equally effective. Aqueous penicillin G, 12 million units intravenously per day for four weeks, is curative in almost all patients. In the stable patient at low risk of complications, some or most of the antibiotic course can be administered on an outpatient basis.

Treatment of enterococcal endocarditis and IE caused by other penicillin-resistant streptococci is much less satisfactory because of frequent relapses and high mortality. The recommended regimen is aqueous penicillin G, 20 million units I.V. per day, plus gentamicin or tobramycin, 3 to 5 mg/kg I.V. per day. The lower dose of aminoglycoside is associated with less nephrotoxicity. Tobramycin is the preferred aminoglycoside because of its slightly lower risk of nephrotoxicity unless sensitivity testing reveals greater potency of genta-

micin. The aminoglycoside dose should be adjusted according to measured serum levels and the bactericidal activity of serum. Streptomycin, 0.5 gm I.M. q12h, can be substituted as the aminoglycoside if the organism is sensitive; however, streptomycin is associated with irreversible vestibular and auditory toxicity in some patients.

Although the value of serum bactericidal determinations has not been established vigorously, most experts rely on them as a general guide to the adequacy of antibiotic regimens. A drug regimen is considered adequate for treatment of IE if serum bactericidal activity is present at dilutions of 1:8 or greater. In view of the high frequency of relapses, regimens to treat enterococcal infection should be continued for six weeks. Culture-negative endocarditis should be treated similarly.

Staphylococcus aureus endocarditis should be treated with nafcillin, 12 gm I.V./day. The addition of an aminoglycoside hastens clearance of bacteremia and is indicated in the patient with a fulminant septic presentation and in the initial treatment of left-sided endocarditis. Once sepsis is controlled, the aminoglycoside should be discontinued. Minimal bactericidal concentrations of antibiotic should be determined. If the bactericidal concentration is over 32 times the bacteriostatic concentration, the organism can be considered drug-tolerant. Patients with IE caused by tolerant staphylococci may have a more complicated clinical course. If the organism fulfills the criteria for tolerance, determination of serum bactericidal activity is appropriate; if this proves inadequate (i.e., bactericidal activity <1:8 dilution of serum), addition of a drug (aminoglycoside or rifampin) or substitution of vancomycin for nafcillin should be considered. The duration of antibiotic therapy for staphylococcal endocarditis of the mitral or aortic valve is a minimum of six weeks.

In the patient with streptococcal or staphylococcal IE and history of serious penicillin allergy, vancomycin frequently can be substituted for penicillin. Outcome generally is comparable, although auditory and nephrotoxicity may occur with vancomycin.

Pseudomonas endocarditis is a particular problem in intravenous drug users. Therapy should be initiated with tobramycin, 8 mg/kg/day I.V., and ticarcillin, 250 mg/kg/day I.V. The unusually high doses of aminoglycosides have improved the outcome of medical therapy of Pseudomonas infection of the tricuspid valve with surprisingly few side effects such as nephrotoxicity. Left-sided Pseudomonas aeruginosa infections, however, generally require surgery for cure. Although third-generation cephalosporins may have attractive in vitro efficacy against Pseudomonas species, in vivo development of resistance and clinical failure have limited their usefulness in this setting. Some drug addicts have rapid clearance of aminoglycosides, so it is particularly critical to evaluate pharmacokinetics and adjust dosages as appropriate when these agents are employed.

Fungal endocarditis is refractory to antibiotics

and requires surgery for management. Amphotericin B generally is administered to such patients but is not in itself curative.

Surgery

The indications for early surgery in IE need to be individualized and forged by discussions with the cardiac surgeon. Refractory infection is a clear indication for surgery; as noted, the requirement for surgery is predictable in IE caused by certain organisms. Persistence of bacteremia for longer than 7 to 10 days, despite the administration of appropriate antibiotics, frequently reflects paravalvular extension of infection with development of valve ring abscess or myocardial abscesses. Medical cure is not possible in this setting. A prolonged febrile course is not unusual, however, and is not an independent indication for surgery, particularly when tricuspid endocarditis is complicated by multiple septic pulmonary emboli with necrotizing pneumonia.

Congestive heart failure is the most frequent indication for early cardiac surgery. The extent of valvular dysfunction may be difficult to gauge clinically, particularly in patients with acute aortic regurgitation (AR); in the absence of compensatory ventricular dilatation, classic physical signs associated with AR such as wide pulse pressure may not be present. Echocardiography, fluoroscopy, and cardiac catheterization may be necessary to evaluate the extent of aortic regurgitation in some instances. However, when congestive heart failure develops in the patient with S. aureus IE, aortic valvular destruction usually is extensive, necessitating early surgery. Delaying surgery to prolong the course of antibiotic therapy is never appropriate if the patient is hemodynamically unstable. Prosthetic valve endocarditis seldom occurs following cardiac valve replacement for IE, and its incidence is not influenced by duration of preoperative antibiotics.

Recurrent major systemic embolization is another indication for surgery. If valvular function is preserved, vegetations sometimes can be removed without valve replacement.

PROSTHETIC VALVE ENDOCARDITIS (PVE)

PVE complicates approximately 3 per cent of cardiac valve replacements. Two separable clinical syndromes have been identified. Early PVE occurs within 60 days of surgery and most often is caused by S. epidermidis, gram-negative enteric bacilli, S. aureus, or diphtheroids. The prosthesis may be contaminated at the time of surgery or seeded by bacteremia from extracardiac sites (intravenous cannula, indwelling urinary bladder catheter, wound infection, pneumonia). The combination of vancomycin, 2 gm/day I.V., and tobramycin, 3 to 5 mg/kg/day I.V., plus rifampin, 600 mg/day orally, is indicated to treat S. epidermidis infection. Other infections should be treated with synergistic combinations of anti-

biotics based on in vitro sensitivity testing. Surgery is mandatory in the presence of moderate to severe CHF. The mortality of early PVE is approximately 75 per cent.

Late PVE usually is caused by viridans streptococcal bacteremia from an oral site that seeds a re-endothelialized valve surface. Treatment with aqueous penicillin G, 20 million units I.V. daily, plus tobramycin, 3 to 5 mg/kg/day I.V., is appropriate. Prognosis for cure with antibiotic therapy alone is better in patients infected with penicillin-sensitive streptococci. Moderate to severe CHF is the main indication for surgery. The mortality of late PVE is approximately 40 per cent.

PROPHYLAXIS OF IE

Patients with prosthetic heart valves or mitral or aortic valvular heart disease are at relatively high risk of developing IE. Mitral valve prolapse associated with a systolic murmur is another significant risk factor. Neither the value of antibiotic prophylaxis nor the optimal regimens have been established definitively. Recommended regimens are presented in Table 89–4.

Devices that are associated with high rates of

TABLE 89–4. PROPHYLAXIS OF INFECTIVE ENDOCARDITIS

REGIMEN*	INDICATIONS
Oral	
1. Penicillin V 2.0 gm orally 1 hr before and 1.0 gm 6 hr after procedure	Aortic or mitral valve disease in patients undergoing dental procedure with bleeding gums
2. Erythromycin 1.0 gm orally 1 hr before and 0.5 gm orally 6 hr after procedure	As above for penicillin-allergic patient or when chronic penicillin prophylaxis has been used to prevent rheumatic fever
Parenteral	
1. Ampicillin 2.0 gm I.M. or I.V. plus gentamicin 1.5 mg/kg I.M. or I.V. 30 min before procedure	Patient with prosthetic heart valve undergoing dental, gastrointestinal, or genitourinary procedure. Patient with aortic or mitral valve disease undergoing gastrointestinal surgery or genitourinary instrumentation or surgery
2. Vancomycin 1.0 gm I.V. over a 1-hr period beginning 1 hr before procedure	Penicillin-allergic patient with prosthetic heart valve undergoing dental procedure
3. Vancomycin 1.0 gm I.V. plus gentamicin 1.5 mg/kg I.V. beginning 1 hr before procedure	Penicillin-allergic patient with aortic or mitral valve disease undergoing gastrointestinal surgery or genitourinary instrumentation or surgery. Penicillin-allergic patient with prosthetic valve undergoing gastrointestinal or genitourinary procedure

*These are empiric suggestions. Additional doses of antibiotic may be given if there is risk of prolonged bacteremia.

infection and bacteremia (intravenous cannulas, indwelling urinary bladder catheters) should be avoided in hospitalized patients at risk for IE if at all possible; established local infections should be treated promptly and vigorously.

BACTERIAL ENDARTERITIS AND SUPPURATIVE PHLEBITIS

Bacterial endarteritis usually develops by one of three mechanisms: (1) Arteries, particularly those with intimal abnormalities, may become infected as a consequence of transient bacteremia. (2) During the course of IE, septic emboli to vasa vasorum may lead to mycotic aneurysms. (3) Blood vessels also may be infected by direct extension from contiguous foci and trauma.

A septic presentation is characteristic of endarteritis due to organisms such as S. aureus. Besides sepsis, the major problem caused by endarteritis is hemorrhage. About 3 to 4 per cent of patients with IE develop intracranial mycotic aneurysms. Mycotic aneurysms in IE typically are situated peripherally and in the distribution of the middle cerebral artery. Focal seizures, focal signs, or aseptic meningitis may herald catastrophic rupture of such aneurysms. These premonitory findings, therefore, indicate the need for evaluation with arteriography; neurosurgical intervention should be contemplated if accessible lesions are demonstrated. Other forms of bacterial endarteritis also require combined medical and surgical management; antibiotic selection should be based on the results of in vitro sensitivity testing.

Suppurative thrombophlebitis usually is a complication of the use of intravenous plastic cannulas. Burn patients, especially those with lower extremity catheterization, are at particular risk. Typically, intravenous cannulas have been left in place five days or more. Symptoms may be delayed until several days after removal of the catheter and reflect septicemia, septic pulmonary emboli, or metastatic abscess formation. Local findings at the site of infection are present in only one third of burn patients with this complication. Therefore, surgical exploration is imperative when the diagnosis of suppurative phlebitis first is suspected. Involved segments of vein must be excised. Antibiotics should be selected so as to assure coverage of the most common pathogens, Staphylococcus aureus (nafcillin, 12 gm/day I.V.) and Enterobacteriaceae (gentamicin, 5 mg/kg/day I.V.). When infection of an intravenous cannula is suspected, the catheter should be removed and two-inch segments rolled across a blood agar plate. The growth of more than 15 colonies suggests infection. Intravenous fluids also should be cultured.

Suppurative phlebitis is preventable. Steel "scalp vein" needles are associated with 40-fold less risk of infection than plastic cannulas and should be used preferentially for intravenous therapy. When plastic intravenous cannulas are necessary, they should be inserted aseptically and replaced at least every 48 hours.

PERICARDITIS AND PERIMYOCARDITIS

The major infectious and noninfectious causes of pericarditis are shown in Table 89–5. Ascertaining the precise cause in a patient, when necessary, usually requires pericardial biopsy, although the clinical presentation may narrow the list of possibilities considerably. Pericarditis may occur with no or minimal effusion (pericarditis sicca), or the effusion may dominate the clinical presentation. In patients with pericarditis, the major goals are to assess and reverse hemodynamic compromise, if it exists, and to treat the underlying cause of pericarditis.

Pathogenesis

The pericardium may be involved as part of a generalized enterovirus or other infection. Alternatively, contiguous bacterial infection may extend to involve the pericardial sac; pneumococcal pneumonia leading to purulent pericarditis is one example. Cardiac valve ring abscesses, particularly those caused by virulent organisms such as Staphylococcus aureus, also can extend to the surface of the visceral pericardium and produce pericarditis. Infection may be limited to the pericardium, for example, when a tuberculous node erodes into the pericardial space. Pericarditis also can occur following vaccination or infection, apparently as an allergic or autoimmune process. An aseptic pericarditis sometimes develops two to four weeks following S. aureus or meningococcal septicemia.

Clinical Features

Acute pericarditis often causes severe chest pain that may simulate acute myocardial infarction. The characteristic pain is a sharp, left anterior precordial pain with radiation to the left shoulder, specifically, the left trapezius ridge. It is relieved by sitting up, leaning forward, and breathing out. Fever is common and, in purulent pericarditis, associated with signs of systemic toxicity. Complaints of previous or concurrent upper respiratory infection, nausea, vomiting, cough, myalgias, and arthralgias are infrequent, even in cases attributed to enterovirus infection. Patients with cardiac tamponade may complain of shortness of breath. In tuberculous pericarditis, symptoms are subacute in three fourths of patients. Anorexia, weight loss, and night sweats are prominent complaints, whereas acute chest pain is less frequent.

The presence of pulsus paradoxus is a critical finding, since it suggests cardiac tamponade. Pulsus paradoxus refers to an inspiratory decline in systolic blood pressure of at least 10 mm Hg. Pulsus is assessed with the patient breathing normally; forced respiration increases swings in intrathoracic pressures, leading to faulty determinations. The sphygmomanometer is inflated above systole. During gradual deflation of the cuff, the pressure at which sounds are first transmitted is noted (sounds will be extinguished during inspiration), as well as the pressure at which all sounds are transmitted. The difference is the pulsus paradoxus. The precordium is quiet in the presence of a large pericardial effusion, and heart sounds are distant. The characteristic pericardial rub is scratchy and grating and heard best at the left midsternal border during expiration. It usually is triphasic, reflective of movement of the heart during atrial systole, ventricular systole, and rapid ventricular filling. However, one fourth of patients will have biphasic and one fourth monophasic rubs. Physical examination may reveal a displacement of the left border of cardiac dullness. Subacute to chronic effusive and constrictive pericardial disease can lead to jugular venous distension, hepatomegaly, ascites, and peripheral edema.

Laboratory Findings

The presence of leukocytosis and shift to the left is suggestive of a pyogenic process, but also may be seen in viral pericarditis. The electrocardiographic findings are helpful in the diagnosis of pericarditis, although they do not suggest a specific cause. Characteristically, concave RS-T elevations occur in a diffuse distribution (leads I, II, III, and V_2-V_6) with depression in aV_F or aV_L. The evolution of electrocardiographic abnormalities also is helpful, as the T waves are upright initially and flatten or invert only after RS-T abnormalities subside.

Most cases of acute pericarditis, particularly those occurring as sporadic cases, resolve without the establishment of a specific diagnosis and are classified as idiopathic. Coxsackie B and ECHO viruses cause pericarditis during epidemics. Adenovirus, influenza, mumps, poliovirus, Epstein-Barr virus, *Mycoplasma*, and fungi are less common causes of pericarditis. Viral cultures of pharyngeal and rectal swabs should be obtained, and acute and convalescent serum samples should be assayed for type-specific viral antibodies. Since viral pericarditis usually occurs during epidemics, establishment of the cause of pericarditis based on cultures and serologies is circumstantial. The patient may have had a viral infection, but the pericarditis may have some other cause. Even when pericardial fluid or tissue is obtained, viral cultures usually are negative. Heterophile and *Mycoplasma* complement fixation antibodies should be determined. Intermediate-strength tuberculin skin testing should be performed and usually is positive in patients with tuberculous pericarditis. The diagnosis of tuberculosis requires biopsy of pericardium or demonstration of acid-fast bacilli at some other site (such as sputum).

Pericardiocentesis should be performed through a subxiphoid approach as an emergency procedure for two indications: (1) to relieve pericardial tamponade, and (2) to evaluate the possibility of purulent pericarditis in the toxic-appearing patient (see below). The cytology and culture of the fluid are helpful in establishing a specific etiologic diagnosis in carcinomatous and bacterial pericarditis.

The diagnostic yield is greatest from biopsy of pericardium. Biopsy of pericardium and drainage

TABLE 89–5. FREQUENT CAUSES OF PERICARDITIS

Infectious
  Viral: Coxsackie B, ECHO virus
  Granulomatous: *Mycobacterium tuberculosis, Histoplasma capsulatum*
  Bacterial: *Streptococcus pneumoniae, Staphylococcus aureus, Streptococcus pyogenes, Neisseria meningitidis, Haemophilus influenzae*
Postinfectious
  Neisseria meningitidis, Staphylococcus aureus, rheumatic fever
Collagen-vascular diseases
  Systemic lupus erythematosus
Carcinomatous
Metabolic
  Uremia
  Hypothyroidism
Post–myocardial infarction
Post–cardiac surgery
Idiopathic

of pericardial fluid are indicated in all cases of chronic pericarditis and in the presence of moderate to large pericardial effusions. The subxiphoid approach generally allows biopsy of sufficient tissue for diagnosis and establishment of a small pericardial window that aids in drainage; general anesthesia and the requirement for chest tube placement also are avoided in most patients.

Differential Diagnosis

Many noninfectious diseases cause pericarditis and have clinical manifestations overlapping with those due to living agents (Table 89–5). Differentiation among some of these syndromes may be possible on clinical grounds. Recourse to biopsy of the pericardium sometimes is necessary, however, to exclude tumor and tuberculosis.

Management and Outcome

Initial management of patients with pericarditis requires hospitalization, determination of the presence and hemodynamic significance of pericardial effusions, and consideration of the possibility of purulent pericarditis. Hospitalization is appropriate for all patients, even the young, otherwise healthy individual with apparent viral pericarditis sicca. Both Coxsackie B and ECHO viruses can cause a severe cardiomyopathy with congestive heart failure and arrhythmias. Hospitalization allows observation and prompt initiation of appropriate medications.

If tamponade leads to hypotension, emergency pericardiocentesis should be performed. Delays to obtain echocardiography are not justifiable. With severe tamponade and hypotension, pulsus paradoxus sometimes cannot be demonstrated. The physician must move swiftly to preserve life. If pericardial fluid reaccumulates after drainage, a more definitive procedure such as placement of a pericardial window is appropriate. Pericardial stripping is an extensive operative procedure and rarely is necessary. Patients with idiopathic subacute effusive-constrictive pericarditis or tuberculosis may develop enlarging effusions and progressive tamponade. This often occurs in the hospital and at times requires emergency pericardiocentesis.

Suspicion of purulent pericarditis is another indication for immediate pericardiocentesis. The diagnosis may be missed if fever and hypotension are attributed to sepsis or recognized infection in the lung or elsewhere. Most cases of purulent pericarditis, in fact, are diagnosed at autopsy. Therefore, a high index of suspicion is appropriate in septic-appearing patients. A pericardial rub is present in only about one third of patients with bacterial pericarditis; its absence should not deter one from pericardiocentesis. If purulent pericarditis is confirmed, drainage of the pericardial effusion with a catheter or pericardial window is obligatory. Antibiotics should be selected on the basis of the appearance of Gram's stained sediments of pericardial fluid.

The pain of acute idiopathic pericarditis may respond to indomethacin; otherwise narcotic analgesics sometimes are necessary. If symptoms are protracted (longer than two weeks) corticosteroids should be administered (prednisone, 60 to 80 mg orally per day, in divided doses) and tapered over two to four weeks. The development of congestive cardiomyopathy is another possible indication for corticosteroids.

Tuberculous pericarditis should be treated with isoniazid, 300 mg orally, plus rifampin, 600 mg orally per day. Ethambutol, 15 mg/kg orally per day, is added if isoniazid (INH) resistance occurs with significant frequency in the geographic area where the infection has been acquired (e.g., in Southeast Asia) or INH resistance is suspected because the patient has been treated previously with antituberculous drugs. If the suspicion of tuberculosis is reasonably high, antituberculous drugs should be started pending the results of cultures. A pericardial drainage procedure and corticosteroids (prednisone, 60 to 80 mg orally per day) are important in the management of tuberculosis in

an attempt to avoid chronic constriction of the heart. Tuberculous pericarditis often is a patchy disease, and granulomas may not be found in the pericardial biopsy specimens obtained; therefore, antituberculous drugs should be continued even if histology of the pericardium does not show granulomas or acid-fast bacilli. The duration of treatment with these drugs is determined on the basis of the results of cultures, serial tuberculin skin tests, clinical course, and establishment of alternative diagnoses.

Most patients with pericarditis will have a satisfactory response to medical management with or without a drainage procedure. Chronic constrictive pericarditis usually presents de novo without a clear history of previous acute pericarditis. Idiopathic pericarditis probably is the most common antecedent, although tuberculosis and histoplasmosis account for some cases. Once established, chronic constriction is difficult to diagnose and treat; pericardial stripping has significant morbidity and mortality and frequently unmasks severe congestive cardiomyopathy. Therefore, major attention should be placed on avoidance of chronic constriction by appropriate management of patients with acute and subacute pericardial disease.

REFERENCES

Klacsmann PG, Bulkley BH, and Hutchins GM: The changed spectrum of purulent pericarditis. An 86-year-old autopsy experience in 200 patients. Am J Med 93:666, 1977.
Scheld WM, and Sande MA: Endocarditis and intravascular infection. In Mandell GL, Douglas NG Jr, and Bennett JE (eds): Principles and Practice of Infectious Diseases. New York, John Wiley & Sons, 1985, p 504.
Spodick DH: Differential diagnosis of acute pericarditis. Prog Cardiovasc Dis 14:192, 1971.

90 SKIN AND SOFT-TISSUE INFECTIONS

Normal skin is remarkably resistant to infection. Most common infections of the skin are initiated by breaks in the epithelium. Hematogenous seeding of the skin by pathogens is less frequent.

Some superficial infections, such as folliculitis and furuncles, may be treated with local measures. Other superficial infections (e.g., impetigo

and cellulitis) require systemic antibiotics. Deeper soft-tissue infections such as fasciitis and myonecrosis require surgical debridement. As a general rule, infections of the face and hand should be treated particularly aggressively because of the risks of intracranial spread in the former, and the potential loss of function due to closed-space infection in the latter.

SUPERFICIAL INFECTIONS OF THE SKIN

Circumscribed Infections of the Skin

Vesicles, pustules, nodules, and ulcerations are the lesions in this category (Table 90–1).

Folliculitis is a superficial infection of hair follicles. The lesions are crops of red papules or pustules; careful examination using a hand lens reveals hair in the center of most papules. Staphylococci, yeast and, occasionally, *Pseudomonas* species are the responsible pathogens. Local treatment with cleansing and hot compresses is usually sufficient. The skin lesions of disseminated candidiasis seen in neutropenic patients may resemble folliculitis. In this setting, skin biopsy readily distinguishes these two processes; in disseminated disease, yeast are found within blood vessels and not simply surrounding the hair follicle.

Furuncles and carbuncles are subcutaneous abscesses due to *Staphylococcus aureus*. The lesions are red, tender nodules that may have a surrounding cellulitis and occur most prominently on the face and back of the neck. They often drain spontaneously. Furuncles may be treated with local compresses. The larger carbuncles require incision and drainage if fluctuant. Antistaphylococcal antibiotics should be given if the patient has systemic symptoms such as fever or malaise, if there is accompanying cellulitis, or if the lesions are on the face.

Impetigo is a superficial infection of the skin due to group A streptococci, although occasionally *Staphylococcus aureus* may also be found in the lesions. The disease is seen primarily among children who initially develop a vesicle on the skin surface; this rapidly becomes pustular and breaks down, leaving the characteristic dry golden crust. This infection is highly contagious—usually spread by the child's hands to other sites on the child's body or to other children. Gram's stain reveals gram-positive cocci in chains (streptococci); occasionally, clusters of staphylococci are also seen. The differential diagnosis includes herpes simplex infection and varicella. These viral lesions may become pustular; Gram's stain of an unruptured viral vesicle or pustule should not, however, contain bacteria. Tzanck prep (see below) can establish the diagnosis of herpes simplex or varicella if the differential diagnosis is uncertain. Penicillin is the treatment of choice for impetigo, since staphylococci represent secondary infection and will disappear when the streptococci are eradicated.

Ecthyma gangrenosum (see Fig. 84–2) is a cutaneous manifestion of disseminated gram-negative rod infection, usually due to *Pseudomonas aeruginosa* in neutropenic patients. The initial lesion is a vesicle or papule with an erythematous halo. Although generally small (<2 cm), the initial lesion may exceed 20 cm in diameter. In a short time the vesicle ulcerates, leaving a necrotic ulcer with surrounding erythema or a violaceous

TABLE 90–1. CIRCUMSCRIBED CUTANEOUS INFECTIONS

DESCRIPTION	PREDOMINANT ORGANISM
Folliculitis	*Staphylococcus aureus*
Furuncles, carbuncles	*Staphylococcus aureus*
Impetigo	Group A streptococci
Ecthyma gangrenosum	Gram-negative bacilli (systemic infection)

VESICULAR OR VESICULO-PUSTULAR LESIONS OF THE SKIN

Impetigo
Folliculitis
Herpes simplex virus infection
Varicella-zoster virus infection
Rickettsialpox

ULCERATIVE LESIONS OF THE SKIN

Pressure sores
Stasis ulcerations
Diabetic ulcerations
Mycobacterial infection
Fungal infection
Ecthyma gangrenosum

rim. Gram's stain of an aspirate may reveal gram-negative rods; cultures of the aspirate are generally positive. Biopsy of the lesion shows venous thrombosis, often with bacteria demonstrable within the blood vessels. Since these lesions are manifestations of gram-negative rod bacteremia, treatment should be instituted immediately with an aminoglycoside plus an extended spectrum penicillin (e.g., carbenicillin) and cephalosporin until the results of culture and sensitivity studies are known. (See also Chapter 84.)

Herpes Simplex Virus. Oral infections due to this virus are discussed in Chapter 87, and genital infection in Chapter 94. On occasion, infection with this virus occurs on extraoral or extragenital sites, usually on the hands. This is most often the case in health care workers, but also may result from sexual contact or from autoinoculation. The virus produces a painful erythema, usually at the junction of the nail bed and skin (whitlow). This progresses to a vesiculopustular lesion. At both stages of infection, herpetic whitlow can resemble a bacterial infection—paronychia. When more than one digit is involved, herpes is much more likely. It is important to distinguish between herpetic and bacterial infections, since incision and drainage of a herpetic whitlow is contraindicated. Puncture of the purulent center of a paronychia and Gram's stain of the exudate allow prompt and accurate diagnosis. In the case of herpetic whitlow, bacteria are not present unless the lesion has already drained and become superinfected. In the case of a bacterial paronychia, bacteria are readily seen. Recurrences of herpetic whitlow may be seen but are generally less severe than the primary infection. Treatment with oral acyclovir may shorten the duration of symptoms.

Varicella-zoster Virus (see also Chapter 85). Primary infection with varicella-zoster virus (chickenpox) is thought to occur via the respiratory route but may also occur through contact with infected skin lesions. Viremia results in crops of papules that progress to vesicles, then pustules followed by crusting. The lesions are most prominent on the trunk. This is almost always a disease of childhood. Systemic symptoms may precede development of the characteristic rash by one or two days but are mild except in the case of an immunocompromised patient or primary infection in the adult. In the immunocompromised, chickenpox can produce a fatal systemic illness. In otherwise healthy adults, chickenpox can be a serious illness with life-threatening pneumonia. Clinical diagnosis is based on the characteristic appearance of the rash. Impetigo and folliculitis are readily distinguished clinically or by Gram's stain of the pustule contents. Disseminated herpes simplex virus infection is seen only in the immunocompromised host or in patients with eczema. Only viral culture will distinguish herpes simplex from herpes zoster in these settings. Most patients with rickettsialpox, which is confused with chickenpox rarely, will also have an ulcer or eschar that precedes the generalized rash by three to seven days and represents the bite of the infected mouse mite, which transmits the disease.

Immunocompromised children exposed to varicella should receive prophylaxis with zoster immune globulin. Immunocompromised patients with varicella should be treated with acyclovir.

After primary infection, the varicella-zoster virus persists in a latent state within sensory neurons of the dorsal root ganglia. The infection may reactivate, producing the syndrome of zoster (shingles). Pain in the distribution of the affected nerve root precedes the rash by a few days. Depending upon the dermatome, the pain may mimic pleurisy, myocardial infarction, or gallbladder disease. A clue to the presence of early zoster infection is the presence of dysesthesia—an unpleasant sensation when the involved dermatome is gently stroked by the examiner's hand. The appearance of papules and vesicles in a dermatomal distribution confirms the diagnosis. Herpes zoster infections of certain dermatomes merit special attention. The Ramsay Hunt syndrome can be caused by infection involving the geniculate ganglia and presents with painful eruption of the ear canal and tympanic membrane and an ipsilateral seventh cranial nerve (facial nerve) palsy. Infection involving the second branch of the fifth cranial nerve (trigeminal nerve) often produces lesions of the cornea. This infection should be treated promptly with systemic acyclovir to prevent loss of visual acuity. A clue to possible ophthalmic involvement is the presence of vesicles on the tip of the nose. A rare late complication of infection in this dermatome is a granulomatous angiitis of the intracranial arteries.

In most instances, dermatomal zoster is a disease of the otherwise healthy adult. However, immunocompromised patients are at greater risk for reactivation of this virus. Patients with zoster should receive a careful history and physical evaluation; in the absence of specific suggestive findings, these patients do not require an exhaustive evaluation for a malignancy or immune deficiency.

Cutaneous Mycobacterial and Fungal Diseases. Mycobacteria and fungi can produce cutaneous infection, manifesting generally as papules, nodules, ulcers, crusting lesions, or lesions with a combination of these features. *Mycobacterium marinum*, for example, can produce inflammatory nodules that ascend via lymphatic channels of the arm among individuals who keep or are exposed to fish; similar lesions due to *Sporothrix schenckii* may be seen among gardeners. *Blastomyces dermatitidis* and *Coccidioides immitis* are other fungi that produce skin nodules or ulcerations.

As a general rule, a chronic inflammatory nodule, crusted lesion, or nonhealing ulceration that is not readily attributable to pressure, vascular insufficiency, or venous stasis should be biopsied. Mycobacteria and fungi should be carefully sought, using acid-fast and silver stains and appropriate cultures.

Ulcerative Lesions of the Skin. A common factor in the pathogenesis of many skin ulcers is the presence of vascular insufficiency. Microbial infection of these lesions is secondary but often extends into soft tissue and bone.

Pressure sores occur at weight-bearing sites among individuals incapable of moving. Patients with strokes, quadriplegia, or paraplegia or patients in coma who remain supine will rapidly develop skin necrosis at the sacrum, spine, and heels, since pressures at these weight-bearing sites can exceed local perfusion pressure. Patients kept immobile on their sides will ulcerate over the greater trochanter of the femur. As the skin sloughs, bacteria will colonize the necrotic tissues; abetted by further pressure-induced necrosis, the infection will extend to deeper structures. Infected pressure sores are common causes of fever and occasional causes of bacteremia in debilitated patients. Not infrequently, a necrotic membrane hides a deep infection. The physician should probe the extent of a pressure sore using a sterile glove; potential sites of deeper infection should be probed with a sterile needle. Necrotic material must be debrided and the ulceration may be treated with topical antiseptics and relief of pressure. Systemic antibiotics are indicated when bacteremia, osteomyelitis, or significant cellulitis is present. Anaerobes and gram-negative rods are the most frequent isolates. Skin grafting can be used to repair extensive ulceration in patients who can eventually be mobilized. Prevention of pressure sores by frequent turning and by inspection of pressure sites among immobilized patients is far more effective than treatment.

Stasis Ulceration. Patients with lower extremity edema are at risk for skin breakdown and formation of stasis ulcers. These may become secondarily infected; but unless cellulitis is present, systemic antibiotics are not necessary and treatment is aimed at reducing the edema.

Diabetic Ulcers. Patients with diabetes mellitus

often develop foot ulcers. Peripheral neuropathy may result in distribution of stress to sites on the foot not suited to weight-bearing and may also result in failure to sense foreign objects stepped on or caught within the shoe. The resulting ulceration heals poorly. This may be related to vascular disease, poor metabolic control, or both. Secondary infection with anaerobes and gram-negative bacilli progresses rapidly to involve bone and soft tissue. Prevention of these events requires meticulous foot care, avoidance of walking barefoot, the use of properly fitting shoes, and checking the inside of the shoe before use. Once an ulcer develops, the physician should evaluate the patient promptly. Bed rest and topical antiseptics are always indicated. Systemic antibiotics active against anaerobes and gram-negative bacilli should be employed for all but the most superficial and clean wounds. In most instances, this requires admission to the hospital. Aggressive management is indicated, since, if left untreated or improperly treated, the proximate bones and soft tissues of the entire foot may become involved. Once this occurs, the chances of cure without amputation are low.

More Diffuse Lesions of Skin (Table 90–2)

Erysipelas. Erysipelas is an infection of the superficial layers of the skin; it is almost always caused by group A streptococci. This infection, seen primarily among children and the elderly, most commonly occurs on the face. Erysipelas is a bright red to violaceous raised lesion with sharply demarcated edges. This sharp demarcation distinguishes erysipelas from the deeper tissue infection—cellulitis—the margins of which are not raised and merge more smoothly with uninvolved areas of skin. Fever is generally present, and bacteremia is uncommon; rarely, the pathogen can be isolated by aspiration of the leading edge of the erythema. Penicillin, 2 to 6 million units/day, is curative, but defervescence is gradual.

Cellulitis. Cellulitis is an infection of the deeper layers of the skin. Cellulitis has a particular predilection for the lower extremities, where venous stasis predisposes to infection. Cellulitis predisposes to recurrent infection, perhaps by impairing lymphatic drainage. A breakdown in normal skin barriers almost always precedes this infection. Lacerations, small abscesses, or even tiny fissures between the toes due to minor fungal infection antedate the onset of pain, swelling, and fever. Although shaking chills often occur, bacteremia is infrequently documented. Linear streaks of erythema and tenderness indicate lymphatic spread. Regional lymph node enlargement and tenderness are common. Patches of erythema and tenderness may occur a few centimeters proximal to the near edge of infection; this is probably due to spread through subcutaneous lymphatics. Cellulitis of the calf is often difficult to distinguish from thrombophlebitis. Rupture of a Baker's cyst or inflammatory arthritis may also mimic cellulitis. Pain within the joint on passive motion

TABLE 90–2. DIFFUSE CUTANEOUS AND SUBCUTANEOUS BACTERIAL INFECTIONS

DESCRIPTION	PREDOMINANT ORGANISM
Erysipelas	Group A streptococci
Cellulitis	Group A streptococci, *Staphylococcus aureus*, *Haemophilus influenzae*, *Clostridium perfringens*, other anaerobic organisms, gram-negative bacilli
Fasciitis	Group A streptococci, *Clostridium perfringens*, other anaerobic organisms, Enterobacteriaceae
Myonecrosis	*Clostridium perfringens*, other anaerobic organisms

suggests arthritis, but after Baker's cyst rupture, examination of the joint may be relatively benign. Lymph node enlargement and lymphatic streaking virtually confirm the diagnosis of cellulitis. Most cases of lower extremity cellulitis are due to group A beta-hemolytic streptococci, but on occasion, *Staphylococcus aureus* is responsible. Gram-negative bacilli often cause cellulitis in neutropenic and other immunosuppressed patients. Cellulitis of the face or upper extremities, particularly among children, may be due to *Haemophilus influenzae*. Among patients with diabetes mellitus, streptococci and staphylococci are the predominant pathogens of cellulitis. However, if the cellulitis is associated with an infected ulceration of the skin, there is a good chance that anaerobic bacteria and gram-negative rods are also involved.

As in the case of erysipelas, cultures of blood and clysis cultures of the leading edge of infection rarely yield the pathogen. Almost all patients with cellulitis should be hospitalized and treated with a semisynthetic penicillin active against staphylococci and streptococci, such as nafcillin 6 to 12 gm/day. If *Haemophilus* is suspected, trimethoprim-sulfamethoxazole, moxalactam, or chloramphenicol is an effective agent. Diabetics with foot ulcers complicated by cellulitis should be treated with agents active against anaerobes (e.g., clindamycin) plus agents active against enteric gram-negative rods (e.g., an aminoglycoside). Radiologic studies should be performed on patients with ulcers to determine if osteomyelitis is present (see Chapter 95). Prevention of cellulitis can be achieved by institution of measures aimed at reducing venous stasis and edema. Patients with recurrent cellulitis may benefit from eradication of fungal infection of toes or interdigital regions if present. Repeated attacks of cellulitis may be prevented by monthly one-week courses of an oral antibiotic such as erythromycin.

Soft Tissue Gas

Crepitus on palpation of the skin indicates the presence of gas in the soft tissues. Although this generally reflects anaerobic bacterial metabolism, subcutaneous gas can also be found after respirator-induced barotrauma or after application of hydrogen peroxide to open wounds.

In the setting of soft tissue infection, crepitus suggests the presence of gas-forming anaerobes. Roentgenograms will occasionally demonstrate gas before crepitus is appreciated (Fig. 90–1). The presence of gas requires emergent surgical incision to determine the extent of necrosis and requirements for debridement. Involvement of the muscle establishes the diagnosis of myonecrosis (see below) and mandates extensive debridement. Despite the often extensive crepitus seen in clostridial cellulitis, exploration reveals the muscles to be uninvolved, and proper treatment is limited to debridement of necrotic tissue, open drainage, and antibiotics, usually penicillin G 10 to 20 million units/day and chloramphenicol 4 grams/day. Thus the principles of treatment for anaerobic soft tissue infections are (1) removal of necrotic tissue, (2) drainage, and (3) appropriate antibiotics. These apply to superficial anaerobic infections (clostridial cellulitis), deeper anaerobic infections (anaerobic fasciitis—see below), and deepest infections (anaerobic myonecrosis—see below).

DEEPER INFECTIONS OF THE SKIN AND SOFT TISSUE

Fasciitis is a deep infection of the subcutaneous tissues that generally occurs following trauma, sometimes minor, or surgery. Most cases are caused by beta-hemolytic streptococci with or without staphylococci; some are due to mixtures of anaerobic organisms and gram-negative bacilli. Because fasciitis involves subcutaneous tissues, the skin may appear normal or may have a red or dusky hue. The clue to this diagnosis is the presence of subcutaneous swelling. In some instances, crepitus is present. The patient appears more toxic than one would expect from judging only the superficial appearance of the skin. Radiographs may reveal gas within tissues; its absence does not exclude the diagnosis. Men with diabetes

mellitus, urethral trauma, or obstruction may develop an aggressive fasciitis of the perineum called Fournier's gangrene. Perineal pain and swelling may antedate the characteristic discoloration of the scrotum and perineum. Prompt debridement of all necrotic tissue is critical to cure of these infections. Once the diagnosis is suspected, the patient must be taken to the operating room, where incision and exploration will determine if fasciitis is present. Gram's stain of necrotic material will guide antibiotic choice.

INFECTIONS OF MUSCLE

Pyomyositis. Pyomyositis is a deep infection of muscle usually caused by *Staphylococcus aureus* and occasionally by group A beta-hemolytic streptococci or enteric bacilli. Most cases occur in warm or tropical regions, and most occur among children. Nonpenetrating trauma may antedate the onset of symptoms, suggesting that infection of a minor hematoma during incidental bacteremia may be causative. Patients present with fever and tender swelling of the muscle; the skin is uninvolved or minimally involved. In older patients, myositis may mimic phlebitis. Diagnosis can be readily made, if suspected, by needle aspiration or ultrasonography. Drainage and appropriate antibiotics are usually curative.

Clostridial Myonecrosis (Gas Gangrene). This anaerobic infection generally occurs following a contaminated injury to muscle. Within a day or two of injury, the involved extremity becomes painful and begins to swell. The patient becomes toxic appearing, often delirious. The skin may appear uninvolved at first, but eventually may develop a bronzed-blue discoloration. Crepitus may be present but is not as prominent as in patients with clostridial cellulitis (a more benign lesion). Rarely clostridial myonecrosis occurs spontaneously in the absence of trauma; most of these patients have an underlying malignancy, usually involving the bowel. Regardless of etiology, this illness progresses rapidly, producing extensive necrosis of muscle. Hypotension, hemolytic anemia caused by bacterial lecithinase, and renal failure can complicate this illness. Gram's stain of the thin and watery wound exudate reveals large gram-positive rods and very few inflammatory cells. Emergency surgery with wide debridement is essential if the patient is to survive. Large doses of penicillin (10 to 20 million units/day) may prevent further spread of the bacilli. Hyperbaric oxygen therapy is of uncertain value.

REFERENCES

Finegold DS: The diagnosis and treatment of gangrenous and crepitant cellulitis. In Remington JS, and Swartz MN: Current Clinical Topics in Infectious Diseases. Vol 2. New York, McGraw-Hill Book Co, 1981.
Swartz MN: Cellulitis and superficial infections. In Mandell GL, Douglas RG, and Bennett JE (eds): Principles and Practice of Infectious Diseases. 2nd ed. New York, John Wiley and Sons, 1984.

FIGURE 90–1. Radiograph in a case of clostridial myonecrosis showing gas within tissues. (Courtesy of Dr. J. W. Tomford.)

HEPATIC ABSCESS

Abscesses of the liver are generally due to infection by bacteria or, less commonly in the United States, due to amebae. The diagnosis is often missed, since many patients have only subtle clinical indications of liver disease or none at all.

Pathogenesis

Pyogenic liver abscess is a disease seen predominantly among individuals with other underlying disorders. Structural and neoplastic diseases involving the biliary tract predominate. Obstruction to biliary drainage allows infected bile to produce ascending infection of the liver. Inflammatory diseases of the bowel such as appendicitis and diverticulitis also predispose to hepatic abscess via spread through portal veins. On occasion, penetrating or blunt trauma predisposes to hepatic abscess: tissue injury during incidental portal bacteremia may allow bacterial infection in this setting.

Hepatic abscess complicates fewer than 2 per cent of cases of colitis due to *Entamoeba histolytica*, presumably occurring via portal spread.

Clinical and Laboratory Features

Clinical findings in patients with hepatic abscess are often nonspecific. Most are febrile, but only about half have abdominal pain and tenderness; two thirds have palpable hepatomegaly; less than one in four is jaundiced, although half have elevated serum bilirubin levels. About half of patients with pyogenic liver abscess have positive blood cultures. In patients with liver abscess the alkaline phosphatase is generally elevated and disproportionate to the modest elevation in bilirubin. In contrast, patients with the nonspecific jaundice that occasionally accompanies bacterial infection at other sites generally have elevated bilirubin levels (as much as 5 to 10 mg/dl or more) and only slightly elevated alkaline phosphatase levels.

In liver abscess, chest roentgenogram may reveal an elevated right hemidiaphragm and atelectasis or effusion at the right lung base. The diagnosis is best achieved by contrast-enhanced computerized tomography of the abdomen. Pyogenic abscesses may be single or multiple; amebic abscesses are generally single. Only a minority of patients with amebic liver abscess have concurrent intestinal amebiasis; a positive stool examination for amebae, however, may suggest the diagnosis. Antibody titers against *E. histolytica* are usually positive in patients with amebic liver abscess.

Microbiology

Anaerobes, microaerophilic streptococci, and gram-negative bacilli are the predominant agents of pyogenic liver abscess. Occasionally *Staphylococcus aureus* causes multiple hepatic abscesses during the course of bacteremic seeding of multiple organs. Of the protozoa, only *Entamoeba histolytica* is known to cause amebic abscess.

Differential Diagnosis

In patients with bacteremia and abnormal liver function studies, the jaundice of sepsis may be distinguished from the mild jaundice of liver abscess by a relatively high bilirubin/alkaline phosphatase ratio and clinical indications of a primary extrahepatic source of bacteremia. Patients with cholecystitis and cholangitis are at risk, albeit low, for the development of hepatic abscess. In both cholecystitis and cholangitis the onset of illness is more abrupt than in patients with hepatic abscess. Tenderness among patients with cholecystitis is generally quite localized over the gallbladder. Patients with cholangitis are often very ill and jaundiced.

The Fitz-Hugh-Curtis syndrome or gonococcal perihepatitis may share some clinical manifestations of hepatic abscess and should be suspected in the young sexually active woman with fever and right upper quadrant tenderness. Tumors involving the liver may produce fever and a clinical and radiologic picture mimicking hepatic abscess. This is complicated by the occasional concurrence of malignancy with hepatic abscess.

Diagnosis and Treatment

If pyogenic abscess is suspected, needle aspiration is indicated. Using ultrasound or CT guidance, a percutaneous catheter can be inserted into the abscess cavity for both diagnostic and therapeutic purposes. The pus should be Gram's stained and cultured aerobically and anaerobically. Unless the Gram's stain indicates otherwise, initial therapy for pyogenic liver abscess should include a drug active against anaerobes (clindamycin, chloramphenicol, or metronidazole) plus an aminoglycoside. Antibiotics should be continued for at least four to six weeks. Duration of therapy may be guided by serial CT scans. Surgery is required to relieve biliary tract obstruction and to drain loculated abscesses or abscesses that do not respond to percutaneous drainage and antibiotics. Patients with a pyogenic liver abscess should be evaluated for an intra-abdominal source of infection.

If epidemiologic features strongly suggest an amebic abscess, metronidazole is the drug of choice. Needle aspiration is necessary only to exclude pyogenic infection or if the abscess is large or close to other viscera into which it may rupture. In the case of amebic abscess, the anchovy paste material obtained by needle drainage is not pus but necrotic liver tissue. Large numbers of white cells suggest pyogenic abscess or bacterial superinfection. Trophozoites of *Entamoeba histolytica* are infrequently seen on aspiration of abscesses but may be cultured on certain enriched media.

REFERENCE

Scharschmidt BF: Parasitic, bacterial, fungal, and granulomatous liver disease. In Wyngaarden JB, and Smith LH Jr (eds): Cecil Textbook of Medicine. 17th ed. Philadelphia, WB Saunders Co, 1985, p 827.

ACUTE INFECTIOUS DIARRHEA

Acute diarrheal illnesses caused by bacterial, viral, or protozoal pathogens vary from mild bowel dysfunction to fulminant, life-threatening diseases. Using the best techniques available, a specific causative agent can be identified in 70 to 80 per cent of cases (Table 92–1).

PATHOGENESIS AND PATHOPHYSIOLOGY: GENERAL CONCEPTS

All pathogens that produce diarrhea must be ingested. Normally, the low pH of the stomach, the rapid transit time of the small bowel, and antibody produced by cells in the lamina propria of the small bowel are adequate to keep the jejunum and proximal ileum relatively free of micro-organisms (although not sterile). Furthermore, the ileocecal valve inhibits proximal migration of the huge numbers of bacteria that reside in the large bowel.

Pathogenic micro-organisms are able to pass through the hostile environment of the stomach if (1) they are acid-resistant (e.g., *Shigella*), (2) they are ingested in huge numbers that allow for a few survivors (e.g., *Vibrio cholerae* or *Escherichia coli*), or (3) they are ingested with food and therefore partially protected in the neutralized environment. People with decreased gastric acidity, either natural or surgically induced, are at an increased risk to develop acute diarrheal disease.

Once in the small bowel, the organisms must either colonize (e.g., *V. cholerae, E. coli*) and/or invade (e.g., rotavirus, Norwalk agent) the local mucosa, or pass through into the terminal ileum (*Salmonella*) or colon (*Shigella*) to colonize and invade the mucosa in those sites. The active peristalsis of the small bowel is an effective deterrent to the successful colonization of most organisms. The organisms (e.g., *V. cholerae, E. coli*) that are able to colonize this area have developed special colonization factors such as fimbria (hairlike projections from the cell wall) or lectins (special proteins that attach to specific carbohydrate-binding sites) that allow them to adhere tightly to the mucosal cell surface.

Organisms that do not have special colonization properties pass into the terminal ileum and colon, where they compete with the established flora. The normal fecal flora produces substances that serve to prevent most newly introduced bacterial species from proliferating. (*Bacteroides*, for example, produces fatty acids; certain other enteric bacteria produce specific colicins). The ability of the colonic enteropathogens to invade intestinal mucosa allows these microorganisms (e.g., *Shigella*) to multiply preferentially.

Diarrheas Caused by Enterotoxigenic Pathogens

In the enterotoxin-induced or secretory diarrheas the patient seldom has fever or other major systemic symptoms, and there is little or no inflammatory response. The diarrhea is watery, often voluminous, with a low protein concentration and an electrolyte content that reflects its source. Rapid loss of this diarrheal fluid results in predictable saline depletion, base-deficit acidosis, and potassium deficiency. The amount and rate of fluid loss determine the severity of the illness. Certain of the secretory diarrheas, such as those caused by *V. cholerae* or *E. coli* enterotoxins, can result in massive intestinal fluid losses, exceeding 1 liter per hour in adults.

Characteristically, large numbers of bacteria (10^5 to 10^8) must be ingested with grossly contaminated food or water (although a small inoculum may produce disease in individuals with achlorhydria, whether it be naturally occurring or medically or surgically induced). The enterotoxin-producing bacteria then colonize, but do not invade, the small bowel mucosal cells. After multiplying to large numbers (10^8 to 10^9 organisms per milliliter of fluid), the bacteria produce enterotoxins that bind to mucosal cells, causing hypersecretion of isotonic fluid at a rate that overwhelms the reabsorptive capacity of the colon. The *V. cholerae* enterotoxin rapidly binds to monosialogangliosides of the gut mucosa and causes sustained stimulation of cell-bound adenylate cyclase. This results, via both an increased secretion and decreased absorption of electrolytes, in net secretion of large quantities of isotonic fluid into the gut lumen. The disease runs its course in two to seven days, during which time continued fluid and electrolyte repletion are of critical importance. *E. coli* produces the other two major bacterial enterotoxins. The labile toxin (LT) of *E. coli* is similar in structure and nearly identical in mode of action to cholera enterotoxin. The *E. coli* heat-stable toxin (ST) is much smaller than LT and acts via a different biochemical pathway (stimulation of cellular guanylate cyclase), but also stimulates secretion of isotonic fluid into the gut lumen.

Three conditions provide well-recognized exceptions to the above schema of enterotoxigenic

TABLE 92–1. MAJOR ETIOLOGIC AGENTS IN ACUTE DIARRHEAL ILLNESSES

INVASIVE/DESTRUCTIVE PATHOGENS	NONINVASIVE PATHOGENS	BACTERIAL TOXINS (FOOD POISONING)
Shigella	*Escherichia coli*	*Staphylococcus aureus*
Salmonella	*Vibrio cholerae*	*Clostridium perfringens*
Campylobacter jejuni		
Vibrio parahaemolyticus		*Bacillus cereus*
Yersinia enterocolitica		
Clostridium difficile		
Rotavirus		
Other viruses		
Protozoa		

diarrheas. In each of these exceptions, the culpable enterotoxin exerts its effect by some means other than stimulation of one of the known secretory mechanisms of the small bowel mucosa, and the resulting fluid losses are seldom voluminous.

1. Enterotoxins may be ingested directly in food, as with staphylococcal and *Bacillus cereus* food poisoning. These organisms grow to high concentration in the food rather than the small intestine and often cannot be recovered from the stool. Distinctive features of staphylococcal food poisoning include a short incubation period (two to six hours), high attack rates (up to 75 per cent of population at risk), and prominent vomiting (probably due to direct effect of absorbed toxin on the CNS). *Bacillus cereus* produces two distinct enterotoxins, one of which is similar to the *E. coli* LT, and the other to the staphylococcal enterotoxin; therefore two different clinical syndromes may be produced, one indistinguishable from staphylococcal food poisoning, and the other similar to the diarrhea caused by enterotoxigenic *E. coli*. The former syndrome is usually associated with ingestion of contaminated rice.

2. *Clostridium perfringens*, contracted by eating contaminated meat and poultry, produces an enterotoxin in the small bowel. Like staphylococcal food poisoning, *C. perfringens* has a short incubation period and a high attack rate. However, unlike staphylococcal enterotoxin, *C. perfringens* enterotoxin damages gut mucosa and causes a short-lived diarrhea with a small volume and a high protein content.

3. *Clostridium difficile*, unlike the previously described organisms, colonizes the large bowel. This organism produces enterotoxins that cause severe mucosal damage, yielding colonic lesions that may be indistinguishable from those caused by *Shigella*. *C. difficile* diarrhea is usually associated with antibiotic usage. Diagnosis is reliably made by assaying stool for toxin. Inflammatory cells may be present on methylene blue–stained stool samples.

Diarrheas Caused by Invasive Pathogens

Diarrheas caused by mucosal invasion by micro-organisms are often accompanied by fever and myalgias. Cramping abdominal pain may be prominent, and small amounts of stool are passed at frequent intervals, often associated with tenesmus. These organisms induce a marked inflammatory response, so that the stool contains pus cells, large amounts of protein, and often gross blood. Significant dehydration rarely results from this kind of diarrhea, since the diarrheal fluid volume is small relative to that caused by the secretory enterotoxins, seldom exceeding 750 ml per day in adults. Although certain clinical features are statistically more frequent in invasive diarrheas caused by specific enteropathogens (i.e., more severe myalgias with shigellosis, higher temperature spikes with salmonellosis), epidemiologic characteristics are more helpful than signs or symptoms in determining the etiologic agent in invasive diarrheal illnesses (Table 92–2).

Acute shigellosis occurs when susceptible individuals ingest fecally contaminated water or food. Unlike *Salmonella* infections, which require a large inoculum, shigellosis can occur after ingestion of only 10 to 100 micro-organisms. Largely for this reason, direct person-to-person transmission (e.g., in day-care centers) is more common with shigellosis than with other bacterial enteric infections. The organism multiplies in the small intestine, during which time a watery noninflammatory diarrhea may occur. Later, the organisms invade the colonic epithelium, causing the characteristic bloody stool. Unlike *Salmonella*, *Shigella* rarely causes bacteremia. The disease usually resolves spontaneously after three to six days, but the clinical course can be shortened by antimicrobials (Table 92–2).

Acute salmonellosis usually results from ingestion of contaminated meat, dairy, or poultry products. In the industrialized world, *Salmonella* is often transmitted via commercially prepared dried, processed foodstuffs. Unlike *Shigella*, *Sal-*

TABLE 92–2. EPIDEMIOLOGIC CHARACTERISTICS OF INVASIVE ENTERIC PATHOGENS

MICROORGANISMS	EPIDEMIOLOGIC FEATURE	ANTIBIOTICS
Shigella	Outbreaks in child-care centers or custodial institutions. Person-to-person transmission	Yes
Salmonella	Zoonosis. Survives dessication in processed dairy, poultry, and meat products	No
Campylobacter jejuni	Zoonosis. Worldwide distribution. Transmitted in dairy products	Maybe
Yersinia enterocolitica	Zoonosis. Occasionally transmitted in dairy products	Maybe
Vibrio parahaemolyticus	Coastal salt waters. Transmitted by inadequately cooked shrimp and shellfish	No
Escherichia coli (invasive)	Unusual. Caused by nonenterotoxigenic strains. Reservoir uncertain	No
Clostridium difficile	Almost always follows antimicrobial therapy	Yes
Rotavirus	Outbreaks among children. Worldwide distribution. Unusual and mild in adults	No
Norwalk virus	Microepidemic pattern. No specific age predilection	No
Giardia lamblia	Enzootic, with limited species distribution. Common in travelers to endemic areas (e.g., Rocky Mountain states, Leningrad)	Yes
Entamoeba histolytica	Person-to-person transmission. Very rare in North America and Western Europe	Yes

monella is remarkably resistant to dessication. The nontyphoidal salmonellae, unlike S. typhi, invade primarily the distal ileum. The organism characteristically causes a short-lived (two to three days) illness characterized by fever, nausea, vomiting, and diarrhea. (This is in marked contrast to the three- to four-week febrile illness, usually not associated with diarrhea, that is caused by Salmonella typhi.)

Campylobacter jejuni may be responsible for up to 10 per cent of acute diarrheal illnesses worldwide. This organism may invade both the small intestine, most commonly the terminal ileum, and the colon, which may account for the broad spectrum of symptoms, ranging from an acute shigella-type syndrome to a milder, but more protracted, diarrheal illness. Since the organism is enzootic in domestic animals, epidemiologic features are helpful only in occasional point-source outbreaks.

In addition to Shigella, Salmonella, and Campylobacter, three other organisms—Yersinia enterocolitica, Vibrio parahaemolyticus, and invasive E. coli (distinct from the enterotoxigenic E. coli)—also cause tissue invasion and acute diarrheal illnesses that may be clinically indistinguishable from those caused by the more commonly recognized invasive bacterial enteropathogens (Table 92–2).

Viruses must grow in host cells; by definition, therefore, both the rotavirus and the Norwalk agent produce invasive diarrheal disease. Both these organisms damage the villous epithelial cells, with the degree of injury ranging from modest distortion of epithelial cells to sloughing of villi. Presumably both the rotavirus and the Norwalk agent cause diarrhea by interfering with the absorption of normal intestinal secretions. Affected patients may have low-grade fever and mild to moderate cramping abdominal pain. The stool is usually watery and its contents resemble those of a noninvasive process, with few inflammatory cells, probably because of lack of damage to the colon.

While few protozoa cause acute diarrheal illness, Giardia lamblia is an important pathogen. In North America, Rocky Mountain water sources are frequent origins of microepidemics. As is the case in shigellosis, ingestion of only a few organisms is required to establish infection. The organisms multiply in the small bowel, attach to and occasionally invade the mucosa, but do not cause gross damage to the mucosal cells. Clinical manifestations span the spectrum from an acute, febrile diarrheal illness to chronic diarrhea with associated malabsorption and weight loss. Diagnosis may be made by identification of the organism in either the stool or duodenal mucus or by small bowel biopsy. Entamoeba histolytica may cause intestinal syndromes ranging from mild diarrhea to fulminant amebic colitis with multiple bloody stools, fever, and severe abdominal pain. Although E. histolytica has a worldwide distribution, it is an uncommon cause of diarrhea in the United States.

Although most diarrheagenic pathogens pro-duce either invasive (cytopathic) or enterotoxic (secretory) diarrhea, both processes contribute to the illness in some situations. Certain strains of Shigella, nontyphoidal Salmonella, Y. enterocolitica, and C. jejuni both invade and possess the capacity to produce enterotoxins in vitro. Such enterotoxins may play a contributory role in the acute disease process. The invasive capacity of these organisms is, however, of paramount importance in their ability to produce disease.

GENERAL EPIDEMIOLOGIC CONSIDERATIONS

In developing countries, where sanitation is generally inadequate, young children (up to two years of age) contract multiple episodes of diarrhea (often four to eight per year), a process which engenders intestinal immunity to the majority of enteropathogens in their immediate environment. Most of these diarrheal episodes are mild, but some are life-threatening. In these areas, enterotoxigenic E. coli and rotavirus together cause the large majority of diarrheal illnesses. Shigella infections are far less common during this period.

In the industrialized world, infants and small children have fewer episodes of diarrhea, and the most common etiologic agent is the rotavirus. Most episodes are mild. Enterotoxigenic E. coli and Shigella infections infrequently occur except in a few defined population groups (e.g., individuals in custodial institutions). On the other hand, throughout the world, clinically significant diarrhea in adults is relatively unusual except in specific defined epidemics or common-source outbreaks due to contaminated food or water. The same etiologic agents are largely responsible for the acute diarrheas of both adults and children. This is made apparent by immunologically inexperienced adults from the developed world who visit developing countries. Such tourists have an extremely high incidence of diarrheal disease (traveler's diarrhea), and the organisms responsible are the same ones as those causing most childhood diarrhea in the country visited.

DIAGNOSIS

In managing acute diarrheal illnesses, determining the specific etiologic agent is much less important than promptly repleting lost electrolytes. All pathogens that cause serious diarrheal disease produce similar electrolyte losses. The fluid losses represent the chief cause of serious morbidity and mortality. Determination of the specific cause is less important, since antimicrobial therapy has proven value in only a minority of cases (Table 92–2). Discerning the epidemiology of the illness is often more helpful than laboratory techniques in identifying cases in which antimicrobial therapy is likely to be helpful.

The examination of a methylene blue-stained stool preparation for erythrocytes and pus cells may be helpful in distinguishing between acute diarrheal illnesses caused by invasive and non-invasive pathogens. This is easily accomplished by adding one drop of methylene blue dye to one drop of liquid stool or mucus, allowing the preparation to air dry, and examining under the high dry microscope lens. Few, if any, leukocytes or red cells will be seen in the stools of patients with diarrhea caused by noninvasive organisms (e.g., enterotoxigenic E. coli and V. cholerae). Variable numbers of leukocytes and red cells will be present in diarrheas secondary to invasive bacteria (e.g., Shigella) or cytopathic toxins (C. difficile toxin).

The precise diagnosis of any diarrheal illness lasting longer than four to five days is important, as specific antimicrobial therapy may be helpful, e.g., with giardiasis. Additionally, Crohn's disease or ulcerative colitis may be present.

MANAGEMENT: GENERAL PRINCIPLES OF ELECTROLYTE REPLETION THERAPY

Intravenous Fluids

All acute diarrheal diseases respond to a similar fluid repletion regimen. Voluminous infectious diarrhea in adults consistently produces the same pattern of fecal electrolyte loss. The electrolyte characteristics differ somewhat in diarrhea in young children in that the mean sodium and chloride concentrations are 15 to 20 mEq/L less than in adults. Sodium and chloride concentrations in stool may be even less with diarrheal diseases of viral etiology, in which massive fluid loss seldom occurs.

The fluid losses of massive diarrhea can rapidly be corrected by infusing fluids intravenously that approximate those that have been lost. Lactated Ringer's solution is readily available and provides uniformly good results. With patients who are hypotensive, the intravenous fluids should initially be infused rapidly, at a rate of up to 100 ml/min, until a strong radial pulse is restored. The rate can then be slowed until skin turgor has returned to normal. Subsequent maintenance fluid administration can be guided by the patient's clinical appearance, including his vital signs, the appearance of neck veins, and skin turgor. Clinical evaluation alone provides an adequate guide to fluid replacement in most acute diarrheal illnesses. If intravenous fluids are administered in adequate quantities throughout the diarrheal illness, virtually every patient with diarrhea caused by toxigenic bacteria should be restored to health. Complications (e.g., acute renal failure secondary to hypotension) are exceedingly rare if these principles are followed.

Oral Fluids

In many patients with acute diarrheal illness, fluid repletion can also be achieved via the oral route, using isotonic glucose-containing electrolyte solutions. Oral therapy is based upon the fact that glucose facilitates sodium absorption by the small bowel and that glucose-facilitated sodium absorption remains intact during enterotoxigenic diarrheal illnesses. A uniformly effective solution can be prepared by the addition of 20 gm glucose, 3.5 gm sodium chloride, 2.5 gm sodium bicarbonate, and 1.5 gm potassium chloride to a liter of drinking water (Table 92–3). Such fluids should be administered initially in large quantities, 250 ml every 15 minutes in adults, until clinical observations indicate that fluid balance has been restored. Thereafter, one administers fluids in quantities sufficient to maintain normal balance; if stool output is measured, roughly 1.5 liters of glucose-electrolyte solution should be given orally for each liter of stool. The oral fluid regimen does not decrease the volume of fluid lost via the intestinal tract, but rather provides hydration to counterbalance the toxin-induced fluid secretion.

Since a similar pattern of fluid loss occurs in diarrheal illnesses caused by other intestinal pathogens, patients with fluid depletion caused by invasive microbial agents (e.g., rotavirus, Salmonella) also respond well to oral glucose-electrolyte therapy. Although the pathogenesis of diarrheal disease caused by the rotavirus is quite different from that caused by enterotoxigenic bacteria, patients with rotavirus illness consistently respond well to oral glucose-electrolyte replacement.

Antimicrobial Therapy

Most acute infectious diarrheas do not require antibiotic therapy (Table 92–2). Of the noninvasive bacterial diarrheas, only in cholera do appropriate antibiotics dramatically decrease the volume of diarrhea. Oral tetracycline, 40 mg/kg in four divided doses daily for 48 hours, is the drug of choice.

Of the invasive bacterial diarrheas, short-term antimicrobial treatment significantly decreases the duration and severity of shigellosis. In North America, ampicillin, 40 mg/kg in four divided doses daily for 48 hours, is the drug of choice. Because of the increasing frequency of plasmid-mediated antimicrobial resistance, sensitivity testing is necessary to determine the appropriate antibiotic in many other areas of the world.

Antimicrobial therapy may be helpful in decreasing the duration and severity of enteritis caused by Yersinia and Campylobacter. Oral erythromycin appears to be the drug of choice for Campylobacter jejuni, and trimethoprim-sulfamethoxazole is the preferred treatment for Yer-

TABLE 92–3. ORAL REHYDRATION FLUID

CONSTITUENTS (gm/L)	ELECTROLYTE CONTENT (mmol/L)
NaCl—3.5 gm	Na—90
NaHCO$_3$—2.5 gm	Cl—80
KCl—1.5 gm	K—20
Glucose—20 gm	HCO$_3$—30
	glucose—110

sinia enterocolitica. Antimicrobials are of no known value in *V. parahaemolyticus* infections and are contraindicated in uncomplicated nontyphoidal *Salmonella* enteritis, as they may prolong the fecal shedding of salmonella.

Antimicrobials decrease the duration and severity of giardiasis. In adults, metronidazole, given 750 mg every eight hours for three days, and quinacrine, 300 mg/day for seven days, appear to be equally effective in adults. Acute intestinal amebiasis demands antimicrobial therapy. Metronidazole, 750 mg every eight hours for five days, is the drug of choice in adults.

Antimicrobial Prophylaxis

Prophylactic antimicrobials are effective in preventing traveler's diarrhea, a generally self-limited illness caused most often by enterotoxigenic *E. coli*. Both doxycycline and trimethoprim-sulfamethoxazole (TMP/SMX) are effective. However, because of the rapid response of most patients to early treatment with either TMP/SMX or doxycycline, the advantages of prophylactic drugs are, in most instances, outweighed by their potential risks (adverse reactions).

Symptomatic Therapy

Adjuvant symptomatic therapy is not essential but may provide modest symptomatic relief in acute infectious diarrheas associated with cramping abdominal pain. Bismuth subsalicylate, 0.6 gm every six hours, may ameliorate symptoms of traveler's diarrhea. Agents that decrease intestinal motility (e.g., codeine, diphenoxylate, loperamide) also relieve the cramping abdominal pain associated with many acute diarrheal illnesses, but are potentially hazardous because they may enhance severity of illness in shigellosis, the prototype of invasive bacterial diarrheas.

REFERENCES

Carpenter CCJ: Shigellosis. In Wyngaarden JB, and Smith LH Jr (eds): Cecil Textbook of Medicine. 17th ed. Philadelphia, WB Saunders Co, 1985, pp 1596–1598.

Pierce N: Cholera. In Wyngaarden JB, and Smith LH Jr (eds): Cecil Textbook of Medicine. 17th ed. Philadelphia, WB Saunders Co, 1985, pp 1598–1600.

Sack RB: Human diarrheal disease caused by enterotoxigenic *Escherichia coli.* Annu Rev Microbiol 29:333–353, 1975.

Santosham M, Daum DS, Dillman L, et al: Oral rehydration of infantile diarrhea: A controlled study of well-nourished children hospitalized in the United States and Panama. N Engl J Med 306:1070–1076, 1982.

Stevens DP: Giardiasis: Host-pathogen biology. Rev Infect Dis 4:851–856, 1982.

93 INFECTIONS OF THE URINARY TRACT

The urethra, bladder, kidneys, and prostate are all susceptible to infection. Most urinary tract infections cause local symptoms, yet clinical manifestations do not always pinpoint the site of infection. In addition, the criteria used by different clinical laboratories to define infection of the urinary tract are also variable. This chapter will attempt to simplify the clinical and laboratory approach to diagnosis and treatment of urinary tract infections. Infections associated with indwelling urinary catheters are discussed in Chapter 96.

Urethritis

Urethritis is predominantly an infection of sexually active individuals, usually observed in males. The symptoms are pain and burning of the urethra during urination, and there is generally some discharge at the urethral meatus. Urethritis may be gonococcal in origin. However, nongonococcal urethritis (NGU) is now more frequent in North America. NGU may be due to *Chlamydia trachomatis* or *Ureaplasma urealyticum* and less commonly to *Trichomonas vaginalis* or *Herpesvirus hominis.*

Gram's stain of a sample of urethral discharge should reveal white blood cells and, if the gonococcus is the responsible pathogen, plump gram-negative intraleukocytic diplococci. Culture on selective media that inhibit the growth of most nongonococcal isolates (e.g., Thayer-Martin) confirms the diagnosis of gonococcal infection. The discharge in cases of NGU reveals white blood cells and no or few mixed bacteria on Gram's stain. NGU should be treated with tetracycline, 500 mg q.i.d. for seven days. Gonococcal urethritis should be treated with a single oral dose of amoxicillin, 3.0 gm plus 1 gm probenecid. Since NGU cannot be readily diagnosed in the presence of gonorrhea and the two often coexist, simultaneous treatment for NGU is also advocated for patients receiving treatment for gonococcal urethritis. A VDRL should be obtained and all the patient's recent sexual contacts (beginning with contacts two weeks before the onset of symptoms) should be notified and treated as well, even if initial examination fails to reveal evidence of infection.

Cystitis and Pyelonephritis

Epidemiology. Bacterial infection of the bladder (cystitis) and kidney (pyelonephritis) is more frequent in females, and the incidence of infection increases with age. Factors that predispose to urinary tract infection include instrumentation (e.g., catheterization, cytoscopy), pregnancy, and possibly diabetes mellitus.

Pathogenesis. Although some infections of the kidney may arise as the result of hematogenous dissemination, most urinary tract infections "ascend" via a portal of entry in the urethra. Most pathogens responsible for community-acquired urinary tract infections are part of the subject's normal bowel flora. *Escherichia coli* is the most common isolate and, in the female, colonization of the vaginal and periurethral mucosa may antedate infection of the urinary tract. The longer and protected male urethra may account for the lower incidence of urinary tract infection in men. Motile bacteria may swim "upstream," and reflux of urine from the bladder into the ureters may predispose to the development of kidney infection. Congenital anomalies or obstruction of urine flow at any level also predisposes to infection.

Clinical Features. Pain, discomfort, or burning sensation on urination and frequency of urination are common symptoms of infection of the urinary tract. Back or flank pain or the occurrence of fever suggests that infection is not limited to the bladder (cystitis), but involves the kidney (pyelonephritis) or prostate as well. However, clinical presentation often fails to distinguish between simple cystitis and pyelonephritis. Elderly or debilitated patients with infection of the urinary tract may have no symptoms referable to the urinary tract and may present only with fever, altered mental status, or hypotension.

Laboratory Diagnosis of Urinary Tract Infection. Analysis of a midstream urine sample obtained from patients with infection of the bladder or kidney should reveal white blood cells and may also have red cells and slightly increased amounts of protein. The presence of an increased number (see below) of white cells (pyuria) in a midstream urine sample indicates the likelihood of a urinary tract infection. However, since most laboratories count white blood cells by examining the sediment of a centrifuged urine sample, and since urinary white blood cell count may vary according to the degree of urine concentration, quantitation of pyuria is imprecise. As a general rule, more than 5 to 10 white blood cells per high-power field on a centrifuged specimen of urine is abnormal. Resuspending a sedimented urine should be done gently using a Pasteur pipette; in this way casts are not disrupted; the presence of white blood cell casts in an infected urine sample indicates the presence of pyelonephritis. Bacteria may be seen in sedimented urine and can be readily identified using Gram's stain.

At present, most clinical laboratories will consider bacterial growth of greater than 10^5 colony-forming units/ml as indicative of infection. Recent studies suggest that smaller numbers of bacteria can produce lower urinary tract infections (see below). A hazard in interpreting results of urine culture is that if the sample is allowed to stand at room temperature for a few hours before planting on culture plates, bacteria can multiply. This results in spuriously high bacterial counts. For this reason, urine for culture should not be obtained from a catheter bag. Specimens that are not plated immediately may be refrigerated. Biochemical tests to detect bacteriuria are not reliable. Detection of antibody on the surface of bacteria freshly voided in urine is an indication that the kidney (or occasionally the prostate) is infected.

Treatment and Outcome. Patients with cystitis may be treated with a 7- to 10-day course of antibiotics such as sulfisoxazole, ampicillin, or trimethoprim-sulfamethoxazole. Black men should not be treated with sulfa drugs because of the frequency of glucose-6-phosphate dehydrogenase deficiency in this population. Recent studies suggest that most patients with cystitis will be cured by a single high dose of antibiotic (e.g., 3 gm amoxicillin or 2 gm sulfisoxazole). Culture and sensitivity will confirm the diagnosis and ascertain if the antibiotic is active against the pathogen.

Occasionally, urine culture obtained from a patient with symptoms of urinary tract infection and pyuria will be reported as "no growth" or "insignificant growth." This has been labeled the "urethral syndrome." Low numbers of bacteria (as few as 100/ml urine) may produce such infections of the urinary tract. In other instances, the urethral syndrome may be caused by *Chlamydia* or *Ureaplasma*, which will not grow on routine culture media. Thus, if a patient with the urethral syndrome has responded to antibiotics, the course should be completed; otherwise, if symptoms and pyuria persist, the patient should receive a 7- to 10-day course of tetracycline, which is active against *Chlamydia* and *Ureaplasma*. Other considerations for patients with lower urinary tract symptoms and no or "insignificant" growth on cultures of urine include vaginitis, herpes simplex infection, and gonococcal infection. (*Neisseria gonorrhoeae* will not grow on routine media used for urine culture.) Thus, a pelvic examination and culture for gonoccocci may be indicated in this setting if the patient is sexually active.

The presence of fever suggests that infection involves more than just the bladder. Young, febrile patients with UTI may be treated on an ambulatory basis, provided that (1) they do not appear toxic, (2) they have friends or family at home, (3) they have good provisions for follow-up, and (4) they have no potentially complicating features such as diabetes mellitus, history of renal stones, history of obstructive disease of the urinary tract, or sickle cell disease. Gram's stain of urine in patients hospitalized for pyelonephritis will guide initial therapy. Gram-negative rod infection may be treated initially with an aminoglycoside. The finding of gram-positive cocci in chains suggests that enterococci are the pathogens. This infection should be treated, at least initially, with ampicillin plus an aminoglycoside, since enterococci are resistant to aminoglycosides unless combined with a penicillin. Gram-positive cocci in clusters may be staphylococci. *Staphylococcus saprophyticus* is a likely agent in otherwise healthy women and is sensitive to most antibiotics used in the treatment of UTI. In the older patient, *Staphylococcus aureus* should be considered, and this infection may be treated with a penicillinase-resistant penicillin such as nafcillin. Gram-positive cocci in the urine may represent a case of endocarditis with septic embolization to the kidney.

Therapy may be simplified when reports of antimicrobial susceptibility are available. Repeat urine culture after two days of effective treatment should show sterilization or marked decrease in urinary bacterial count. If the patient fails to demonstrate some clinical improvement after two to three days of treatment or if the patient presents with the clinical picture of sepsis or has been febrile for more than one week, a complicating feature should be suspected. Intra- or perinephric abscess or obstruction due to a stone or an enlarged prostate may underlie this presentation. Plain films of the abdomen may occasionally reveal a radiopaque stone, but ultrasonography is a good first diagnostic procedure in this setting. This will generally detect obstruction and collections of pus and may also detect stones greater than 3 mm in diameter. Obstruction must be relieved and abscesses drained to result in cure.

All patients with UTI should have repeat urine cultures one to two weeks after treatment is completed to check for relapse. If relapse occurs, the patient may have pyelonephritis, prostatitis, or structural disease of the urinary tract. If a six-week course of antibiotics active against the bacterial isolate is not effective in eradicating infection, the possibility of structural abnormalities or prostatic infection should be investigated.

Some patients have frequent episodes of urinary tract infection due to different bacterial isolates. In some instances, these reinfections are related to sexual activity. A single dose of an active antibiotic such as cephalexin just after sexual contact and voiding after sexual contact can decrease reinfection rate in these women. In other cases where no precipitating factor can be found and infections are frequent, prophylaxis with one half a tablet of trimethoprim-sulfamethoxazole nightly has been effective.

On occasion, urine cultures will reveal bacterial growth in the absence of symptoms. If the sample has been obtained properly and repeat culture reveals the same organism, this is termed *asymptomatic bacteriuria*. This is generally observed in elderly or middle-aged individuals and, in the absence of structural disease of the urinary tract or diabetes mellitus, may not require treatment. Asymptomatic bacteriuria occurring during pregnancy should be treated.

The occurrence of pyuria in the absence of bacterial growth on culture of urine ($<10^2$ colonies/ml) may be termed *sterile pyuria*. If this occurs in the patient with lower urinary tract symptoms, chlamydial or gonoccocal infection, vaginitis, or herpes simplex infection should be considered. In the absence of lower urinary tract symptoms, sterile pyuria may be seen among patients with interstitial nephritis of numerous causes, or tuberculosis of the urinary tract. Patients with renal tuberculosis often have nocturia and polyuria. About half of male patients will also have involvement of the genital tract, most commonly the epididymis. Diagnosis can be made by biopsy of genital masses, when present, and by three morning cultures of urine for mycobacteria.

Prostatitis

Although prostatic fluid has antibacterial properties, this gland can become infected, usually by direct invasion through the urethra. Symptoms of urinary tract infection, back or perineal pain and fever, are common. Some patients will experience pain with ejaculation. Rectal examination usually reveals a tender prostate. Patients with acute prostatitis generally have an abnormal urinary sediment and pathogenic bacteria (usually gram-negative rods) in cultures of urine.

Acute prostatitis may be due to the gonococcus but is most often due to gram-negative bacilli. Treatment is directed against the pathogen observed on Gram's stain of urine and is generally effective. Chronic prostatitis should be suspected in men with recurrent urinary tract infection. The urine may be relatively benign in patients with chronic prostatitis. In this instance, comparison of the first part of the urine sample, midstream urine, excretions expressed by massage of the prostate, and postmassage urine should reveal bacterial counts more than 10-fold greater in the prostatic secretions and postmassage urines than in first-void and midstream samples. Treatment of chronic prostatitis is hampered by poor penetration of most antimicrobials into the prostate. Long-term treatment with trimethoprim-sulfamethoxazole has cured approximately one third of patients and prevented symptomatic relapse in another third.

REFERENCES

Andriole VT: Urinary tract infections and pyelonephritis. In Wyngaarden JB, and Smith LH Jr (eds): Cecil Textbook of Medicine. 17th ed. Philadelphia, WB Saunders Co, 1985, pp 619–623.
Komaroff AL: Acute dysuria in women. N Engl J Med 310:368–374, 1984.

SEXUALLY TRANSMITTED INFECTIONS

Changes in sexual attitudes and practices have contributed to a resurgence of all venereal infections. Gonorrhea, for example, has tripled in incidence in the United States since 1963; approximately three million cases now occur each year.

Sexually transmitted diseases can be considered in broad groups according to whether major initial manifestations are (a) genital sores, (b) urethritis, cervicitis, and pelvic inflammatory disease, or (c) vaginitis.

GENITAL SORES

Six infectious agents cause most genital lesions (Table 94–1). The appearance of the lesions, natural history, and laboratory findings allow a clear-cut distinction among the possible causes in most instances. The two most common and significant infections are syphilis and herpes simplex virus infection.

SYPHILIS

Syphilis is of unique importance among the venereal diseases because early lesions will heal without specific therapy; however, serious systemic sequelae pose a major risk to the patient, and transplacental infections to the offspring.

Epidemiology

Primary syphilis occurs mostly in sexually active 15- to 30-year olds. At least one third of new cases are in homosexual males. Approximately 50 per cent of the sexual contacts of a patient with syphilis will become infected. The long incubation period of syphilis becomes a key factor in designing strategies for contact tracing and management. Unless successful follow-up seems certain, contacts of proven cases must be treated with penicillin.

Pathogenesis

Treponema pallidum penetrates intact mucous membranes or abraded skin, reaches the bloodstream via the lymphatics, and disseminates. The incubation period for the primary lesion depends on inoculum size.

Natural History and Clinical Presentation

Primary syphilis is considered in Table 94–1. Secondary syphilis develops six to eight weeks after the chancre. Skin, mucous membranes, and lymph nodes are involved. Skin lesions may be macular, papular, papulosquamous, pustular, follicular, or nodular. Most commonly they are generalized, symmetrical, and of like size and appear as discrete erythematous, macular lesions of the thorax or red-brown hyperpigmented macules on the palms and soles. In moist intertriginous areas, large, pale, flat-topped papules coalesce to form highly infectious plaques or "condylomata"; they are teeming with spirochetes as assessed by darkfield microscopy. Mucous patches are painless, dull erythematous patches or grayish-white erosions. They too are infectious and darkfield-positive. Systemic manifestations of secondary syphilis include malaise, anorexia, weight loss, fever, sore throat, arthralgias, and generalized, nontender, discrete adenopathy. Specific organ involvement also may develop: gastritis (superficial, erosive), nephritis or nephrosis (immune complex–mediated, remits spontaneously or with treatment of syphilis), and asymptomatic meningitis. One fourth of patients have relapses of the mucocutaneous syndrome within four years of onset. Thereafter, infected patients become asymptomatic and noninfectious except via blood transfusions or transplacental spread.

Late syphilis develops after 1 to 10 years in 15 per cent of untreated patients. The skin gumma is a superficial nodule or deep granulomatous lesion that may develop punched-out ulcers. Superficial gummas respond dramatically to therapy. Gummas also may involve bone, liver, and the cardiovascular or central nervous system. Deep-seated gummas may have serious pathophysiological consequences; treatment of the infection often does not reverse organ dysfunction.

Cardiovascular syphilis occurs after 10 years in 10 per cent of patients, most frequently males. Patients develop aortitis with medial necrosis secondary to an obliterative endarteritis of the vasa vasorum. There may be asymptomatic linear calcifications of the ascending aorta or (in decreasing frequency) aortic regurgitation, aortic aneurysms (saccular or fusiform, most commonly thoracic), or obstruction of coronary ostia.

Central nervous system syphilis develops in 8 per cent of untreated patients 5 to 35 years following primary infection and includes meningovascular syphilis, tabes dorsalis, and general paresis (see Chapter 124). Although classified as separate neurologic syndromes, many patients show elements of both general paresis and tabes. Late CNS syphilis also may be asymptomatic despite cerebrospinal fluid abnormalities indicating active inflammation.

Diagnosis and Treatment

The clinical diagnosis of syphilis must be confirmed by darkfield examination and/or serologies. Spirochetes are seen in darkfield preparations of chancres or moist lesions of secondary syphilis. Saprophytic treponemes confuse darkfield diagnosis of oral lesions. Serologic diagnosis is considered in Table 94–2.

The presence of neurosyphilis requires modifying the standard antibiotic treatment of syphilis. For this reason, a lumbar puncture should be performed in all patients with late latent syphilis (at

TABLE 94–1. DIFFERENTIATION OF DISEASES CAUSING GENITAL SORES

DISEASE	PRIMARY LESION	ADENOPATHY	SYSTEMIC FEATURES	DIAGNOSIS/Rx
Syphilis, 25,000 cases U.S./yr caused by *Treponema pallidum*	Incubation 10–90 days (m. 21). Chancre: papule that ulcerates. Painless, border raised, firm, ulcer is indurated, base smooth. Usually single. May be genital or almost anywhere. Persists 3–6 wk, leaving thin atrophic scar.	1 wk after chancre appears. Bilateral or unilateral. Firm, discrete, moveable, no overlying skin changes, painless, nonsuppurative. May persist for months.	Later	Cannot be cultured. Pos. darkfield. VDRL pos. 77%; FTA-ABS, 86% (see Table 94–3).
Herpes genitalis, frequent, due to *Herpes-virus hominis* (II) Primary	Incubation 2–7 days. Multiple painful vesicles on erythematous base. Persist 7–10 days.	Tender, soft adenopathy.	Fever	Tzanck smears pos. Tissue culture isolation, over four-fold rise antibodies to HSV. Rx: acyclovir.
Recurrent	Grouped vesicles on erythematous base, painful. Last 3–21 days.	None	None	Tzanck, tissue culture pos. Titers not helpful.
Chancroid, 1,000 cases U.S./yr caused by *Haemophilus ducreyi*	Incubation 3–5 days. Vesicle or papule to pustule to ulcer. Soft, not indurated. Very painful.	1 wk after primary in 50%. Painful, unilateral (2/3), unilocular, suppurative.	None	Organism in Gram's stains of pus. Can be cultured (75%) but contaminating bacteria inhibit so yields highest in males and from lymph node. Erythromycin 2 gm/day or trimethoprim-sulfamethoxazole 160/800 mg b.i.d. × 10–14 days.
Lymphogranuloma venereum, 600–1,000 cases U.S./yr due to *Chlamydia trachomatis*	Incubation 5–21 days; painless papule, vesicle, ulcer, evanescent (2–3 days), noted in only 10–40%.	5–21-day post primary, 1/3 bilateral, tender, matted iliac/femoral "groove sign," multiple abscesses, coalescent, caseating, suppurative, sinus tracts, thick yellow pus, fistulas, strictures, genital ulcerations.	Fever, arthritis, pericarditis, proctitis, meningoencephalitis, Parinaud's oculoglandular syndrome (keratoconjunctivitis, preauricular adenopathy, edema of eyelids), erythema nodosum.	LGV C.F. pos. 85–90% (1–3 wk); must have high titer (>1:16) as crossreacts with other *Chlamydia*. Also pos. STS, rheumatoid factor, cryoglobulins, high gamma globulins, IgA. Rx tetracycline 2 gm/day × 2–4 wk.
Granuloma inguinale, 50 cases U.S./yr caused by *Calymmatobacterium granulomatis*	Incubation 9–50 days. At least one painless papule that gradually ulcerates. Ulcers are large (1–4 cm), irregular, nontender, with thickened, rolled margins and beefy red, friable, exuberant cobblestone granulation tissue at base. Older portions of ulcer show characteristic depigmented scarring, while advancing edge contains new papules. May be vegetative, always chronic. Occasional "kissing lesions."	No true adenopathy. In 1/5, subcutaneous spread via lymphatics leads to indurated swelling or abscesses of groin— "pseudobuboes."	Metastatic infection of bones, joints, liver.	Scraping or deep curetting at actively extending border— Wright's/Giemsa stain reveals short, plump, bipolar staining "Donovan bodies" in macrophage vacuoles. Rx tetracycline 2 gm/day × 10 days or trimethoprim-sulfamethoxazole.
Condyloma acuminatum, (genital warts). Frequent, due to papillomavirus	Characteristic large, soft, fleshy, cauliflower-like excrescences around vulva, glans, urethral orifice, anus, perineum.	None	None	Chief importance is in distinction from others. Topical podophyllin ± cryosurgery.

least four years after primary syphilis) or syphilis of unknown duration. An elevated CSF white blood cell count, elevated protein, and positive VDRL on diluted samples of CSF establish the diagnosis of neurosyphilis. A patient with persistent positive blood VDRL and a positive CSF VDRL or FTA-ABS should be considered and treated as a case of neurosyphilis. Because the VDRL may be negative in late syphilis, the presence of a positive serum FTA-ABS in a patient with a neurologic syndrome consistent with syphilis is a sufficient indication for treatment. Patients with neurosyphilis may undergo abrupt deterioration following treatment with penicillin; this Jarisch-Herxheimer reaction, due to the release of toxic spirochetal products, can be mitigated by pretreatment with corticosteroids. Lumbar puncture should be repeated at six-month intervals for three years to assure adequacy of treatment as reflected by normalization of CSF and progressive decline in CSF VDRL titer. Retreatment may be necessary if CSF abnormalities persist or recur. Treatment protocols are shown in Table 94–3.

Syphilis serologies must be followed after treatment. Using the recommended treatment schedules, 1 to 5 per cent of patients with early syphilis will develop recurrence (? relapse, ? reinfection). Serologies in adequately treated primary syphilis should be negative by two years after therapy (usually by 6 to 12 months). Seventy-five per cent of patients with secondary syphilis will be seronegative by two years. If the VDRL does not become negative or achieve a low fixed titer in patients with primary, secondary, or early latent syphilis, lumbar puncture should be performed to evaluate the possibility of asymptomatic neurosyphilis, and the patient should be retreated with penicillin. Patients with late or late latent syphilis should show a decline in antibody titer or low fixed titers by two years. Two to 10 per cent of patients with CNS syphilis will relapse following treatment. However, it is rare for asymptomatic patients to develop symptomatic disease after penicillin therapy. Every patient should be seronegative or "serofast" with a low fixed titer before termination of follow-up. If not, therapy should be repeated.

HERPES SIMPLEX VIRUS INFECTION (HSV)

Genital herpes infection has reached epidemic proportions, causing a corresponding increase in public awareness and concern. Genital herpes differs from the other sexually transmitted disease in its tendency for spontaneous recurrence. Its importance stems from the morbidity, both physical and psychic, of the recurrent genital lesions, the danger of transmission of a fulminant, often fatal disease to newborn infants, and the association with cervical carcinoma.

Epidemiology

HSV has a worldwide distribution. Humans are the only known reservoir of infection, which is

TABLE 94–2. SEROLOGIES IN SYPHILIS

	VDRL	FTA-ABS
Technique:	Standard nontreponemal test. Antibody to cardiolipin-lecithin.	Standard treponemal test. Antibody to Nichol's strain *Treponema pallidum* after absorption on nontreponemal spirochetes.
Indications:	Screening and assessing response to therapy. Should be quantified by diluting serum.	Confirmation of specificity of positive VDRL. Remains reactive longer than VDRL. Useful for late syphilis, particularly neurosyphilis.
Per Cent Positive in Syphilis		
Primary	77%	86%
Secondary	98%	100%
Early latent	95%	99%
Late latent and late	73%	96%
False Positives	Weakly reactive is nonspecific (positive treponemal serologies in 30%). Positive VDRL should be repeated and, if positive, FTA-ABS performed. Frequency of false positive determined by incidence of syphilis in the population.	Borderline positive is frequent (80%) in pregnancy. Should be repeated.

spread by direct contact with infected secretions. Of the two types of HSV, HSV-2 is the more frequent cause of genital infection. The major risk of infection is in the 14- to 29-year-old cohort and varies with sexual activity. The prevalence of HSV-2 antibody is 3 per cent in nuns and 70 per cent in prostitutes.

TABLE 94–3. TREATMENT FOR SYPHILIS

CLINICAL CATEGORY	REGIMEN OF CHOICE	HISTORY OF PENICILLIN ALLERGY
Primary Secondary Early latent Healthy contact*	Benzathine penicillin 2.4 MU I.M. once	Tetracycline or erythromycin 2 gm/day × 15 days
Late latent or late	Benzathine penicillin 2.4 MU I.M. q week × 3	No regimen adequately evaluated ? Tetracycline or erythromycin 2 gm/day × 30 days
Neurosyphilis	Aqueous penicillin G 20 MU I.V. q.d. × 10 days	Same as for late latent or late

* Contact of patient with active skin or mucous membrane lesions.

Pathogenesis

After exposure, HSV replicates within epithelial cells and lyses them, producing a thin-walled vesicle. Multinucleated cells are formed with characteristic intranuclear inclusions. Regional lymph nodes become enlarged and tender. HSV also migrates along sensory neurons to sensory ganglia, where it assumes a latent state. Inside the sacral ganglia, HSV DNA can be demonstrated, but the virus does not replicate and is inactive metabolically. Just how viral reactivation occurs is uncertain. The virus, however, appears to migrate back to skin along sensory nerves.

Clinical Presentation

Primary genital lesions develop two to seven days after contact with infected secretions. In males, painful vesicles appear on the glans or penile shaft; in females, on the vulva, perineum, buttocks, cervix, or vagina. A vaginal discharge frequently is present, usually accompanied by inguinal adenopathy, fever, and malaise. Sacroradiculomyelitis or aseptic meningitis can complicate the primary infection. Perianal and anal HSV infections are common, particularly in male homosexuals; tenesmus and rectal discharge often are the main complaints.

The precipitating events associated with genital relapse of HSV infection are poorly understood. In individual cases, stress or menstruation may be implicated. Overall, genital recurrences develop in about 60 per cent of HSV-infected patients. Recurrences are more frequent in males and with HSV-2 infection. Many patients describe a characteristic prodrome of tingling or burning for 18 to 36 hours before the appearance of lesions. Recurrent HSV genital lesions are fewer in number, usually stereotyped in location, often restricted to the external genitalia, and associated with few systemic complaints.

Laboratory Diagnosis

The appearance of the characteristic vesicles is strongly suggestive of HSV infection. However, diagnosis should be confirmed by Tzanck smear, Pap smear, or viral isolation. Serologies for HSV may be useful in the diagnosis of primary infection.

Treatment

Acyclovir shortens the course of primary genital HSV infection. Intravenous or oral administration is recommended for severe cases with fever, systemic symptoms, and extensive local disease. Antiviral agents do not purge the latent stage of virus, however, and cannot prevent recurrent infections. Prophylactic oral acyclovir decreases the frequency of recurrences by 50 to 75 per cent when used over a four- to six-month period; oral acyclovir also hastens recovery from severe recurrent episodes. The role of acyclovir in management of HSV infections needs further evaluation. Cervical shedding of HSV late in pregnancy, near the time of parturition, is an indication for Caesarean section.

URETHRITIS, CERVICITIS, AND PELVIC INFLAMMATORY DISEASE

These syndromes can be considered broadly as gonococcal and nongonococcal in etiology.

GONORRHEA

Gonorrhea is among the most common of venereal diseases. The morbidity of gonococcal infections now exceeds that of syphilis.

Epidemiology

The incidence of gonorrhea reached a plateau in the United States between 1975 and 1980, possibly reflective of a decrease in the size of the at-risk cohort. Reinfection is the norm, and it is not unusual for one patient to have 20 or more discrete infections. Particular risk factors are urban habitat, low socioeconomic status, unmarried status, number of different sexual contacts, and male homosexuality. Fifty per cent of females having intercourse with a male with gonococcal urethritis will develop symptomatic infection. The risk for males is 20 per cent after a single sexual contact with an infected female. Orogenital contact and rectal intercourse also transmit disease. Forty per cent of male contacts of symptomatic women have asymptomatic urethritis. About one quarter of them develop symptomatic infection within seven days; a like number spontaneously become culture-negative within this period. The remaining 50 per cent remain culture-positive and asymptomatic but capable of transmitting infection for periods of up to six months.

Pathogenesis

Neisseria gonorrhoeae is a gram-negative, kidney bean–shaped diplococcus. Specialized projections from the organism, the pili, aid in attachment to mucosal surfaces, contribute to resistance to killing by neutrophils, and constitute an important virulence factor. Production of an IgA protease by the organism is another factor in pathogenicity. In females, several factors alter susceptibility to infection. Group B blood type increases susceptibility, while diverse factors such as vaginal colonization with normal flora, iron and IgA content of vaginal secretions, and progesterone levels may be protective. Spread from the cervix to the upper genital tract is associated with menstruation because changes in the pH and biochemical constituents of cervical mucous lead to increased shedding of gonococci; cervical dilatation, reflux of menses, and binding of the gonococcus to spermatozoa may be additional factors in ascending genital infection and dissemination. Intrauterine contraceptive devices increase the risk of endometrial spread of infection two- to nine-fold (oral contraceptives are associated with a two-fold decrease).

Clinical Presentation

In males, symptomatic urethritis usually develops two to seven days following sexual contact and causes disturbing symptoms of spontaneous purulent discharge and severe dysuria. Prompt treatment usually follows so that more extensive genital involvement is uncommon.

In females, cervicitis is the most frequent manifestation and results in a copious yellow vaginal discharge. Overall, 20 per cent of females with gonococcal cervicitis develop pelvic inflammatory disease (PID), usually beginning at a time close to the onset of menstruation. PID is manifest as endometritis (abnormal menses, midline abdominal pain), salpingitis (bilateral lower abdominal pain and tenderness), or pelvic peritonitis. Salpingitis can cause tubal occlusion and sterility. Gonococcal perihepatitis (Fitz-Hugh-Curtis syndrome) also may complicate pelvic inflammatory disease and present as right upper quadrant pain.

Females also may develop urethritis with dysuria and frequency. One fourth of women complaining of urinary tract symptoms and 60 per cent of those with symptoms but no bacteriuria will have urethral cultures positive for *N. gonorrhoeae*.

Anorectal gonorrhea occurs in homosexual males and heterosexual females. In males, the resultant rectal pain, tenesmus, mucopurulent discharge, and bleeding may represent the only site of infection. Anorectal disease also may be asymptomatic and recognized only by cultures of asymptomatic contacts of patients with gonorrhea. In females, asymptomatic anorectal involvement is a frequent complication of symptomatic genitourinary disease (44 per cent); isolated anorectal infection (4 per cent) as well as acute or chronic proctitis (2 to 5 per cent) are rare. Treatment failures are frequent in anorectal gonorrhea (7 to 35 per cent).

Pharyngeal gonorrhea occurs in homosexual males or heterosexual females following fellatio and less frequently in heterosexual males. Symptoms of pharyngitis occurring in this setting may be due to associated trauma or to gonococcal pharyngitis. Pharyngeal gonorrhea rarely is the sole site of gonococcal infection (5 to 8 per cent). Infection of the pharynx is important, however, as a source of dissemination.

Extragenital dissemination occurs in approximately 1 per cent of males and 3 per cent of females with gonorrhea. The predisposition in females is discussed above. Strains of *N. gonorrhoeae* causing dissemination differ from other gonococci in several respects. They are more penicillin-sensitive, are of the auxotype (require for growth) arginine⁻, hypoxanthine⁻, and uracil⁻, and resist the normal bactericidal activity of antibody and complement. The latter finding may be due to their binding of a naturally occurring blocking antibody. Dissemination of gonococcal infection may take the form of the "arthritis-dermatitis syndrome" with 3 to 20 papular, petechial, pustular, necrotic, or hemorrhagic skin lesions, usually found on the extensor surfaces of the distal extremities (Fig. 94–1). Associated findings are an asymmetric polytenosynovitis, with or without arthritis, which predominantly involves wrists, fingers, knees, and ankles. Joint fluid cul-

FIGURE 94–1. Typical skin lesion of disseminated gonococcal infection.

tures usually are negative in the arthritis-dermatitis syndrome, leading to speculation that circulating immune complexes, demonstrable in most patients, are important in its pathogenesis. Biopsy of skin lesions reveals gonococcal antigens (by immunofluorescent antibody staining) in two thirds of cases. Blood cultures are positive in 50 per cent. Septic arthritis is another manifestation of dissemination; *N. gonorrhoeae* is the most frequent cause of septic arthritis in 16- to 50-year-olds. Sometimes the history indicates an antecedent syndrome suggestive of bacteremia. The joint fluid cultures usually are positive (particularly when the leukocyte count in joint fluid exceeds 80,000/μl), and blood cultures are negative. Gonococcemia rarely may lead to endocarditis, meningitis, myopericarditis, or toxic hepatitis.

Laboratory Diagnosis and Management

Gram's stain of the urethral discharge will determine the cause of urethritis in most males with gonorrhea, typical intracellular diplococci being diagnostic (Fig. 94–2). The finding of only extracellular gram-negative diplococci is equivocal. The absence of gonococci on smear of a urethral discharge from a male virtually excludes the diagnosis. Diagnosis by Gram's staining of cervical exudates is relatively specific but insensitive (<60 per cent). Modified Thayer-Martin medium contains antibiotics that inhibit the growth of other organisms and increases the yield of gonococci from samples likely to be contaminated; it is not necessary for culture of normally sterile fluids such as joint fluid, blood, and cerebrospinal fluid. The addition of 3 per cent trimethoprim to Thayer-Martin medium inhibits fecal *Proteus* and is useful for anorectal cultures. Other important considerations for the isolation of gonococci include the use of synthetic swabs (unsaturated fatty acids in cotton may be inhibitory), the introduction of a very thin swab or loop 2 cm into the male urethra, and the avoidance of vaginal douching (12 hr), urination (2 hr), and vaginal speculum lubricants before culture. In all suspected cases of gonorrhea, the urethra, anus, and pharynx should be cultured. In females, 20 per cent of cases in which initial cultures were negative yield *N. gonorrhoeae* when cultures are repeated. Current recommendations for the treatment of uncompli-

FIGURE 94–2. Gram's stains of urethral discharge showing typical intracellular diplococci associated with neutrophils.

cated gonorrhea are 4.8 million units procaine penicillin intramuscularly or 3.0 gm amoxicillin orally, plus 1.0 gm probenecid. The addition of a course of tetracycline (2 gm/day orally for seven days) is appropriate to treat concurrent chlamydial infection. In fact, tetracycline alone appears to be adequate for treatment of male urethritis. Spectinomycin, 2.0 gm intramuscularly as a single injection, is an effective alternative except in pharyngeal infections. Acute pelvic inflammatory disease should be treated with procaine penicillin followed by tetracycline, 2 gm/day orally for 10 days. Seriously ill females with PID should be hospitalized. If they appear toxic, the initial antibiotic regimens should be broad-spectrum. The combination of gentamicin, ampicillin, clindamycin, and tetracycline should be effective. Surgery may be required, however, to drain a tubo-ovarian or pelvic abscess. Disseminated gonococcal infection should be treated with aqueous penicillin G, 20 million units per day for three to five days, followed by oral ampicillin (2 gm/day) to complete a 10-day course. In the penicillin-allergic patient, tetracycline is an acceptable alternative for the treatment of PID and cefazolin for dissemination. Cephalosporins should not be used, however, if the history suggests an IgE-mediated allergy to penicillin (anaphylactoid reaction, angioedema, urticaria). In such a case, tetracycline or chloramphenicol is indicated. Erythromycin has been associated with treatment failures and should be avoided.

A VDRL should be obtained in all patients with gonorrhea. If negative, no further follow-up is necessary, since procaine penicillin in the dosage used is effective in treating incubating syphilis. This is not true of therapy with alternate drugs; if they are used, the VDRL should be determined serially. Because of both intrinsic and beta-lactamase—mediated penicillin resistance of gonococci, cultures should be repeated after treatment. In males, these should be obtained at 7 to 14 days; in females at 7 to 14 days and again at six weeks. Anal cultures should be part of the routine follow-up of females, since persistent anorectal carriage may be the source of delayed relapse. Postgonococcal urethritis occurs in 30 to 50 per cent of males two to three weeks after penicillin therapy. It usually is caused by *C. trachomatis* or *U. urealyticum*.

NONGONOCOCCAL URETHRITIS, CERVICITIS, AND PID

The diagnosis of nongonococcal urethritis (NGU) requires the exclusion of gonorrhea, since considerable overlap exists in the clinical syndromes.

Epidemiology

At least as many cases of urethritis are nongonococcal as gonococcal. Typically, NGU predominates in higher socioeconomic groups. *Chlamydia trachomatis* causes 30 to 50 per cent of NGU and can be isolated from 0 to 11 per cent of asymptomatic, sexually active males. *C. trachomatis* also can be isolated from 20 per cent of males with gonorrhea and presumably represents a concurrent infection. Some cases of *Chlamydia*-negative NGU are due to *Ureaplasma urealyticum* or *Trichomonas vaginalis*.

Clinical Syndromes

NGU is less contagious than gonococcal disease. The incubation period is 7 to 14 days. Characteristically, patients complain of urethral discharge, itching, and dysuria. Importantly, the discharge is not spontaneous but becomes apparent after stripping the urethra in the morning. The mucopurulent discharge consists of thin, cloudy fluid with purulent specks; these characteristics do not always allow clear distinction from gonococcal disease. *Trichomonas vaginalis* causes a typically scanty discharge.

C. trachomatis also is a common cause of epididymitis in males under 35 years of age and can produce proctitis in homosexual males.

Chlamydial infections are more common than gonococcal infections in females but frequently escape detection. Two thirds of females with mucopurulent cervicitis have chlamydial infection. Similarly, many females with the acute onset of dysuria, frequency, and pyuria, but sterile bladder urine, have *C. trachomatis* infection. *C. trachomatis* is at least as common a cause of salpingitis as is the gonococcus.

TABLE 94–4. ORGANISMS CAUSING THE GAY BOWEL SYNDROME

CAUSATIVE AGENTS	SIGMOIDOSCOPIC FINDINGS			
	PROX. TO 15 CM	DISTAL 15 CM ONLY	ULCERS	ABDOMINAL PAIN
Neisseria gonorrhoeae		+		
Chlamydia trachomatis	+	+	+	
Herpesvirus hominis		+	+	
Treponema pallidum			+	
Shigella species	+			+
Salmonella species				+
Campylobacter species	+			
Entamoeba histolytica	+		+	
Giardia lamblia				+
Cryptosporidium species				+
Strongyloides stercoralis				+

Laboratory Diagnosis

Ordinarily the distinction between gonococcal and nongonococcal infections relies mainly on Gram's stained preparations of exudate and cultures. In a male with urethritis and typical gram-negative diplococci associated with neutrophils, the diagnosis of gonococcal urethritis is clear-cut and culture unnecessary. Coincident NGU cannot be excluded, however. If interpretation of the Gram's stain is not straightforward in males and in all females, culture on Thayer-Martin medium is appropriate. Again, however, the presence of N. gonorrhoeae does not preclude concurrent NGU. Techniques for isolation of chlamydia are more widely available and should become a routine means of evaluating genital infections.

Treatment

The patient and all sexual contacts should be treated with a seven-day course of tetracycline, 2 gm per day orally.

GAY BOWEL SYNDROME

Male homosexuals may present with proctitis/proctocolitis causing anorectal pain, mucoid or bloody discharge, tenesmus, or abdominal pain. Constipation or diarrhea can occur, too. Sigmoidoscopy should be performed with culture and Gram's stain of discharge. Clues to the causative organism are shown in Table 94–4. The diarrheal syndromes are considered in detail in Chapter 92. Ten per cent of patients harbor two or more path-

TABLE 94–5. VAGINITIS

DISEASE	EPIDEMIOLOGY/ PATHOGENESIS	CLINICAL FINDINGS	LABORATORY DIAGNOSIS	TREATMENT
Candidiasis	Yeast are part of normal flora. Overgrowth and disease favored by broad-spectrum antibiotics, high estrogen levels (pregnancy, before menses, oral contraceptives), diabetes mellitus, tight clothing.	Itching, little or no discharge, occasional dysuria. Labia pale or erythematous with satellite lesions. Vaginal discharge thick, adherent with curds. Balanitis in 10% of male contacts.	Vaginal pH = 4.5 (normal), negative whiff test, yeast seen on wet mount in 50%, culture positive.	Miconazole cream or clotrimazole for 7 days.
Trichomonas vaginalis	STD. Incubation 5–28 days. Symptoms begin or exacerbate with menses.	Discharge, soreness, irritation, mild dysuria, dyspareunia. Copious loose discharge, 1/5 yellow/green, 1/3 bubbly.	Elevated pH. Wet mount shows large numbers of WBC, trichomonas. Negative whiff test.	Metronidazole 2 gm as single dose. Treat sexual contacts.
Nonspecific	Synergistic infection, Gardnerella vaginalis and anaerobes.	Vaginal odor, mild discharge, little inflammation. Greyish, thin, homogeneous discharge with small bubbles.	Elevated pH, 10% KOH causes fishy odor (pos. whiff test). Wet prep contains clue cells (vaginal epithelial cells with intracellular coccobacilli), few WBC.	Metronidazole 500 mg b.i.d. × 7 days. Do not treat contacts unless recurrent vaginitis.

ogens. Proctitis also may occur in male homosexuals without a definable pathogen (42 per cent).

VAGINITIS

Table 94–5 considers salient features in the diagnosis and management of patients with vaginitis.

REFERENCES

Holmes KK, Counts GW, and Beaty HW: Disseminated gonococcal infection. Ann Intern Med 74:979–993, 1971.

Jacobs NF, and Kraus SJ: Gonococcal and nongonococcal urethritis in men. Clinical and laboratory distinction. Ann Intern Med 82:7–12, 1975.

Quinn TC, Stamm WE, Goodell SE, et al: The polymicrobial origin of intestinal infections in homosexual men. N Engl J Med 309:576, 1983.

Schacter J: Chlamydial infection. N Engl J Med 298:428–435; 490–498; 540–549, 1978.

Sparling PF: Diagnosis and treatment of syphilis. N Engl J Med 284:642–653, 1971.

Stamm WE, Guinan ME, Johnson C, Starcher T, Holmes KK, and McCormack WM: Effect of treatment regimens for *Neisseria gonorrhoeae* on simultaneous infection with *Chlamydia trachomatis*. N Engl J Med 310:545–549, 1984.

95 INFECTIONS INVOLVING BONES AND JOINTS

ARTHRITIS

In adults, almost all cases of infectious arthritis occur via hematogenous seeding of the joint. Rarely, intra-articular trauma results in septic arthritis. Bacteria, viruses, mycobacteria, and fungi can all produce an arthritis by infection of the joint. Additionally, certain viruses such as hepatitis B virus can produce a polyarthritis via immune complex deposition. Immune mechanisms may also underlie arthritis syndromes seen after diarrhea due to *Salmonella*, *Shigella* and *Yersinia* infections; the majority of individuals with this syndrome share the HLA B27 antigen.

ACUTE ARTHRITIS

Underlying joint disease, particularly rheumatoid arthritis, predisposes to septic arthritis. Many patients with septic arthritis give a history of joint trauma antedating symptoms of infection. Conceivably, disruption of capillaries during an unrecognized and transient bacteremia allows bacteria to spill into hemorrhagic and traumatized synovium or joint fluid, resulting in the initiation of infection.

Microbiology of Acute Infectious Arthritis (Table 95–1)

Staphylococcus aureus is the most common cause of septic arthritis. Patients with underlying joint disease and intravenous drug abusers are at particular risk for infection with this organism. *Pseudomonas aeruginosa* is another important cause of septic arthritis among intravenous drug abusers.

Other gram-negative bacilli are infrequent causes of septic arthritis and are seen primarily among elderly debilitated patients with chronic arthritis. In adults under 30, *Neisseria gonorrhoeae* is the most likely pathogen. Isolates causing disseminated gonococcal infection (DGI) with arthritis are generally resistant to killing by normal serum.

Clinical Presentation

Symptoms of septic arthritis are generally present for only a few days before the patient seeks medical attention. Fever is usual; shaking chills may occur. The knee is the most commonly affected joint and is generally painful and swollen. Fluid can be demonstrated in most infected joints, and there is marked limitation of motion. In some cases, however, particularly among patients with underlying rheumatoid arthritis who are receiving corticosteroids, physical findings indicating infection may be subtle. In these individuals, who are at particular risk for septic ar-

TABLE 95–1. INFECTIOUS ARTHRITIS—ACUTE

	ETIOLOGIC AGENT	CHARACTERISTICS
Bacterial	*Staphylococcus aureus*	Most common overall. Usually monoarticular, large joint involvement.
	Neisseria gonorrhoeae	Most common in young, sexually active adults. Commonly polyarticular in onset. Often associated with skin lesions.
	Pseudomonas aeruginosa	Largely restricted to intravenous drug users. Often involves sternoclavicular joint.
Viral	Hepatitis B, rubella, mumps	Usually polyarticular, with minimal joint effusions, normal peripheral WBC.

thritis, superimposed infection may be difficult to distinguish from a flare-up of underlying disease. Symmetrical symptoms in multiple joints are more indicative of a rheumatoid flare-up. Approximately 10 per cent of cases of septic arthritis, however, involve more than one joint.

Differential Diagnosis of Acute Monoarticular or Oligoarticular Arthritis

Crystal deposition (uric acid—gout, calcium pyrophosphate—pseudogout), rheumatoid arthritis, systemic lupus erythematosus, and degenerative joint disease can also produce an acute monoarticular arthritis. All red, warm, tender joints must be aspirated. The synovial fluid should be cultured anaerobically and aerobically. A Gram's stain should be examined; a wet mount of fluid should be examined using a polarized microscope to look for crystals. Synovial fluid leukocyte counts and chemistries are of limited value in the differential diagnosis of a suspected septic joint. As a general rule, however, synovial fluid WBC counts in excess of $100,000/\mu l$ suggest either infection or crystal-induced disease. Blood cultures should be obtained in all cases of suspected septic arthritis.

Treatment of Acute Infectious Arthritis

The two major modalities for treatment of acute septic arthritis are drainage and antibiotics. During the first needle aspiration of a septic joint, one should remove as much fluid as possible. Initial antibiotic choice should be based upon the clinical presentation and results of Gram's stain. Staphylococcal infection can be treated with penicillinase-resistant penicillin or vancomycin. Gonococcal infections respond to high doses of penicillin (10 to 20 million units/day). Arthritis due to gram-negative rods should be treated with an aminoglycoside plus another drug active against gram-negative bacilli, such as a cephalosporin. In I.V. drug users, the second drug should be active against *Pseudomonas*; therefore, an extended-spectrum penicillin such as carbenicillin is indicated. Arthritis due to *Staphylococcus aureus* or gram-negative bacilli should be treated with antibiotics for four to six weeks. Otherwise, two to three weeks of antibiotics are sufficient to eradicate infection.

Septic joints (with the notable exception of joints infected with the gonococcus) generally reaccumulate fluid after treatment is initiated. These reaccumulations must be removed by repeated needle aspirations as often as necessary. Indications for open surgical drainage of the joint include failure of the synovial fluid white blood cell count to fall after five days of antibiotic treatment and repeated needle aspirations, and presence of loculated fluid within the joint. Septic arthritis of the hip is generally drained surgically because of the difficulty and potential hazard of repeated needle aspirations of this joint. Osteomyelitis is an uncommon complication of untreated or inadequately treated septic arthritis. In instances in which the diagnosis and treatment have been delayed, radiographs of the involved joint should be obtained at the beginning and termination of treatment.

POLYARTICULAR ARTHRITIS

Arthritis involving multiple joints is infrequently attributable to direct microbial invasion. In many instances, a polyarticular arthritis represents an immunologically mediated process. *Acute rheumatic fever*, a delayed immune-mediated response to group A streptococcal infection, may present with a migratory, often asymmetric, arthritis of the knees, ankles, elbows, and wrists. Heart involvement, subcutaneous nodules, or erythema marginatum is present in a minority of cases. Most have serologic evidence of recent streptococcal infection. Antistreptolysin O, anti–DNA-ase, and antihyaluronidase antibodies are usually present. The importance of making this diagnosis lies primarily in the requirement for long-term prophylaxis against streptococcal infection and the clinical response of this process to salicylates.

Viral infections such as *hepatitis B*, *rubella*, and *mumps* may be associated with polyarthritis. These processes are self-limited. Serum sickness, polyarticular gout, sarcoidosis, rheumatoid arthritis, and other connective tissue disorders must be considered in the differential diagnosis. Since 10 per cent of cases of septic arthritis involve more than one joint, all acutely inflamed joints containing fluid should be tapped to exclude bacterial infection.

Disseminated gonococcal infection (DGI) (see Chapter 94) may present with fever, tenosynovitis, or arthritis involving several joints and a characteristic rash. The rash may be petechial but usually consists of a few to a few dozen pustules on an erythematous base. Cultures of the joint fluid are usually negative at this stage, but blood cultures are often positive; Gram's stain of a pustule may reveal the pathogen. High-dose penicillin is curative.

CHRONIC ARTHRITIS (Table 95–2)

Mycobacteria and fungi may produce an indolent, slowly progressive arthritis, usually involving only one joint or contiguous joints such as those of the wrist and hand. Fever may be low-grade. Cultures of joint fluid may be negative. Some patients with tuberculous arthritis have no evidence of active disease in the lungs. As a general rule, patients with inflammatory chronic

TABLE 95–2. INFECTIOUS ARTHRITIS— CHRONIC

Tuberculosis
Nontuberculous mycobacteria
Fungi
Lyme disease (polyarticular)

monoarticular arthritis should have a synovial biopsy for culture and histology. Granulomas indicate the likelihood of fungal or mycobacterial infection. Cultures should confirm the diagnosis. Serologic studies may be helpful when coccidioidomycosis is suspected, as synovial cultures are often negative.

Fungal arthritis is treated with amphotericin B. Mycobacterial arthritis must be treated for 18 months with at least two drugs active against the isolate. Since many mycobacterial isolates causing joint disease are nontuberculous, extensive susceptibility testing may be needed to guide antimicrobial therapy.

A recently discovered spirochete is the pathogen responsible for Lyme disease. Several months to two years after the bite of the ixodid tick and the characteristic rash of erythema chronicum migrans, some patients develop an intermittent arthritis involving one or more joints—usually including the knees. This chronic arthritis may result in joint destruction, but fever is unusual. This diagnosis should be considered in areas endemic for this tick, such as parts of the Northeast, Wisconsin, Minnesota, California, and Oregon. Treatment with high doses of penicillin (20 million units/day) for 10 days will halt the progression of disease in the majority of cases (see Chapter 85).

SEPTIC BURSITIS

Septic bursitis is almost always due to *Staphylococcus aureus* and involves either the olecranon or prepatellar bursa. In most instances, there is a history of antecedent infection or irritation of the skin overlying the bursa. On examination, the skin over the bursa is red and often peeling. The bursa has a doughy consistency and may reveal fluid on careful examination. Needle aspiration and antistaphylococcal antibiotics are generally curative.

OSTEOMYELITIS

Infections of the bone occur either as a result of hematogenous spread or via extension of local infection.

Hematogenous Osteomyelitis (Table 95–3)

This infection occurs most commonly in the long bones or vertebral bodies. The peak age distributions are in childhood and old age. Individuals predisposed to hematogenous osteomyelitis include I.V. drug abusers who are at risk for infections with *Staphylococcus aureus* and *Pseudomonas aeruginosa* and patients with hemoglobinopathy in whom nontyphoidal *Salmonella* and *Staphylococcus aureus* often infect infarcted regions of bone. Like patients with septic arthritis, patients with hematogenous osteomyelitis often give a history of trauma antedating symptoms of infection, suggesting that transient, unrecognized bacteremia might allow initiation of infection in traumatized tissue.

Patients with acute hematogenous osteomyelitis generally present with acute onset of pain, tenderness, and fever; there may also be soft tissue swelling over the affected bone. In the first two weeks of illness, roentgenograms may be negative or show only soft-tissue swelling; technetium scans or gallium scans are almost always positive, but technetium scans may also be positive in the setting of increased vascularity or increased bone formation of any etiology. After two weeks of infection, radiographs generally show some abnormality, and untreated osteomyelitis may produce areas of periosteal elevation or erosion followed by increased bone formation (sclerosis). The erythrocyte sedimentation rate is generally elevated, as is the white blood cell count.

A patient with back pain and fever must be considered to have a serious infection until proven otherwise. Spasm of the paravertebral muscles is common in patients with vertebral osteomyelitis, but nonspecific. Point tenderness over bone suggests the presence of local infection. A good history should be obtained and a careful neurologic examination performed. Abnormalities of bowel or bladder or of strength or sensation in the lower extremities suggest the possibility of spinal cord involvement via spinal epidural abscess with or without osteomyelitis. Spinal epidural abscess is a *surgical emergency*. The challenge is to make the diagnosis before neurologic signs appear. Emergency myelogram will confirm the diagnosis and mandates prompt surgical decompression to avoid disastrous neurologic sequelae.

Although most cases of hematogenous osteomyelitis have an acute presentation, some cases, particularly those involving the vertebral bodies among I.V. drug abusers, may have an indolent course. These patients may have an illness of over one year's duration characterized by pain and low-grade fever. Radiograms are abnormal but may reveal only collapse of a vertebral body. This most often occurs in infections due to *Pseudomonas aeruginosa*, but *Candida* species and *Staphylococcus aureus* may also occasionally present in this manner.

Blood cultures are positive in about half of acute cases of osteomyelitis. Patients with acute osteomyelitis should have a needle biopsy and culture of the involved bone unless blood culture results are known beforehand. Antibiotic treatment should be continued for four to six weeks using agents active against the pathogen.

TABLE 95–3. FACTORS PREDISPOSING TO HEMATOGENOUS OSTEOMYELITIS

SETTING	LIKELY PATHOGENS
Intravenous drug abuse	*Staphylococcus aureus*
	Pseudomonas aeruginosa
Chronic urinary tract infection	Gram-negative bacilli
Sickle cell anemia	*Salmonella* species

OSTEOMYELITIS SECONDARY TO EXTENSION OF LOCAL INFECTION

There are three major settings in which local infection predisposes to osteomyelitis (Table 95–4). The first is after penetrating trauma or surgery where local infection gains access to traumatized bone. In postsurgical infections, staphylococci and gram-negative bacilli predominate. Generally, there is evidence of wound infection with erythema, swelling, increased postoperative tenderness, and drainage. A traumatic incident often associated with osteomyelitis is a bite—either human or animal. Human bites, if deep enough, may result in osteomyelitis due to anaerobic mouth flora. Cat bites notoriously result in the development of osteomyelitis because thin, sharp, long cat's teeth often penetrate the periosteum. *Pasteurella multocida* is a frequent pathogen in this setting. A four- to six-week course of penicillin G, 10 million units/day, is indicated.

The intimate relationship of the teeth and periodontal tissues to the bones of the maxilla and mandible may predispose to osteomyelitis following local infection. Debridement of necrotic tissue and penicillin comprise the treatment of choice, since penicillin-sensitive anaerobes are the usual agents of these infections.

The third setting in which local infection predisposes to osteomyelitis is that of an infected sore or ulcer. Pressure sores of the sacrum or femoral region may erode into contiguous bone and produce an osteomyelitis (see Chapter 90) due to a mixed flora containing anaerobic organisms. Patients with diabetes mellitus often develop ulcerations of their toes and feet, with eventual development of osteomyelitis. Anaerobes, streptococci, staphylococci, and gram-negative bacilli are often involved in these infections (see Chapter 90). Treatment involves debridement (often amputation in the case of diabetics) and antibiotics active against the pathogens involved.

CHRONIC OSTEOMYELITIS

Untreated or inadequately treated osteomyelitis results in avascular necrosis of bone and the formation of islands of nonvascularized and infected bone called sequestra. Patients with chronic osteomyelitis may tolerate their infection reasonably well, with intermittent episodes of disease activity manifested by increased local pain and the development of drainage of infected material through a sinus tract. Some patients have toler-

TABLE 95–4. OSTEOMYELITIS SECONDARY TO CONTIGUOUS SPREAD

SETTING	LIKELY MICRO-ORGANISMS
Surgery, trauma	*Staphylococcus aureus*, aerobic gram-negative bacilli
Cat or dog bites	*Pasteurella multocida*
Human bites	Penicillin-sensitive anaerobes
Periodontal infections	Penicillin-sensitive anaerobes
Cutaneous ulcers	Mixed aerobic and anaerobic organisms

ated chronic osteomyelitis for decades. A normochromic normocytic anemia of chronic disease is common in this setting, and occasionally amyloidosis and rarely osteogenic sarcoma will complicate this disorder.

Staphylococcus aureus is responsible for the great majority of cases of chronic osteomyelitis; the major exception is among patients with sickle cell anemia, in which nontyphoidal salmonellae may cause chronic infection of the long bones.

Cultures of sinus tract drainage do not reliably reflect the pathogens involved in the infection. Diagnosis and cure are best effected by surgical debridement of necrotic material followed by long-term administration of antibiotics active against the organism found in the surgical specimens.

Mycobacteria, especially *Mycobacterium tuberculosis*, can produce a chronic osteomyelitis. The vertebral bodies are the most common site of infection. Hematogenous dissemination and lymphatic spread are the most likely routes of infection. Paravertebral abscess may complicate this infection. Diagnosis is usually confirmed by histologic examination and culture of biopsy material. Long-term (two years) treatment with antituberculous drugs is usually curative.

REFERENCES

Goldenberg DL, and Reed JI: Bacterial arthritis. N Engl J Med 312:764–770, 1985.
Malawista SE: Infectious arthritis. In Wyngaarden JB, and Smith LH Jr (eds): Cecil Textbook of Medicine. 17th ed. Philadelphia, WB Saunders Co, 1985, p 1922.
Waldvogel FA: Osteomyelitis. In Wyngaarden JB, and Smith LH Jr (eds): Cecil Textbook of Medicine. 17th ed. Philadelphia, WB Saunders Co, 1985, p 1566.

NOSOCOMIAL INFECTIONS

A nosocomial or hospital-acquired infection is an infection, not present on admission to the hospital, which first appears 72 hours or more after hospitalization. A patient admitted to a hospital in the United States has an approximately 5 to 6 per cent chance of developing a nosocomial infection. These infections result in significant morbidity and mortality (approximately 1 per cent of these infections are fatal and an additional 4 per cent contribute to death) and greatly increased medical costs (over 1 billion dollars per year).

Numerous factors are associated with a greater risk of acquiring a nosocomial infection. These include factors that are not avoidable by optimal medical practice such as age and severity of underlying illness. Contributing factors that can be minimized by thoughtful patient management include prolonged duration of hospitalization, the inappropriate use of broad-spectrum antibiotics, the use of indwelling catheters, and the failure of health care personnel to wash their hands.

APPROACH TO THE HOSPITALIZED PATIENT WITH SUSPECTED NOSOCOMIAL INFECTION (Table 96–1)

The first clue to the presence of a nosocomial infection is often a rise in temperature. The only sign of infection, particularly in the elderly or demented patient, may be a change in mental status (Table 96–2). Some patients with serious infection will not initially develop fever but will instead become tachypneic or confused for no apparent reason. Analysis of arterial blood gases may reveal at first a respiratory alkalosis, followed by a metabolic acidosis due to increased levels of lactate. Arterial oxygen content may be normal or depressed.

TABLE 96–1. SIGNS OF INFECTION IN THE HOSPITALIZED PATIENT

Fever
Change in mental status
Tachypnea
Hypotension
Leukocytosis

TABLE 96–2. COMMMON CAUSES OF FEVER IN THE HOSPITALIZED PATIENT

Pneumonia
Catheter-related infection
Surgical wound infection
Urinary tract infection
Drugs
Pulmonary emboli
Infected pressure sores

When evaluating a hospitalized patient for a new fever or suspected nosocomial infection, the physician should first assess the stability of the patient. Hypotension, tachypnea, or new obtundation mandate rapid evaluation and treatment. Review the patient's problem list; ascertain if the patient was subjected to a potentially hazardous intervention recently (e.g., genitourinary tract instrumentation or administration of blood products). If the patient can cooperate, elicit a history directed at possible etiologies of the fever. Often the patient will have a specific complaint that helps identify the source of the fever. Examine the skin carefully. Maculopapular rashes often accompany drug fevers; ecthyma gangrenosum can be a sign of gram-negative sepsis (see Chapter 84). Surgical wounds should be examined for the presence of infection. Among debilitated patients, pressure sores located near the sacrum or over the greater trochanters may become infected and produce fever. Abscesses at these sites may be covered by a necrotic membrane so that exploration with a gloved finger or sterile needle may be required to demonstrate a focus of pus. Headache or sinus tenderness may be present in patients with sinusitis—this may be a problem among patients after nasogastric or nasotracheal intubation. Nuchal rigidity may be a sign of nosocomial meningitis, although it may be absent in some cases, and generalized rigidity is often seen in elderly demented patients without CNS infection. Examine the nose and oropharynx and attempt to elicit symptoms of viral upper respiratory tract infections. These do occur in hospitals. A pleural friction rub may indicate a recent pulmonary thromboembolism as a cause of fever; rales or other evidence of consolidation may indicate a nosocomial pneumonia; basilar rales and even egophony and bronchial breath sounds may also be due to atelectasis in debilitated patients. A new S_4 gallop or pericardial friction rub may be the only clinical manifestation of a myocardial infarction. The abdomen may also be a source of fever in the hospitalized patient. The patient with antibiotic-induced colitis generally has fever, diarrhea, and abdominal pain. Patients with indwelling urinary catheters are at particular risk of infection. These patients should have a careful examination of the prostate—looking for abscess or tenderness—and of the urine—looking for white blood cells and bacteria.

The extremities must be examined carefully, particularly the sites of current and old intravenous catheter placements, for evidence of phlebitis. If no other source of fever is found and an intravenous catheter has been in place for 48 hours, it should be replaced and a segment of the catheter should be rolled on an agar plate for culture.

Deep vein thrombophlebitis and pulmonary thromboemboli are life-threatening complications of hospitalization whose only clinical manifestations may be fever. The lower extremities should be examined and measured carefully. An asymmetry in leg or calf circumference, which may not be obvious without a measurement, may be an important clue to an underlying thrombosis. A gouty attack is another potential source of fever in a hospitalized patient. Gout may be precipitated by acute infections.

The patient's medication list should be reviewed for drugs likely to produce fever. In this regard antimicrobial agents (particularly penicillins, sulfa drugs, and cephalosporins) are among the most common causes of drug-induced fevers. A drug fever can occur at any time but usually occurs within the first two weeks of drug administration. A review of the peripheral blood smear can give important clues as to the etiology of the fever. Eosinophilia may suggest drug-reaction; lymphocytosis—a viral process. A left shift and vacuolization within neutrophils suggest a bacterial infection. Unless the etiology of the fever is apparent and bacteremia is unlikely, cultures of blood should be obtained.

NOSOCOMIAL PNEUMONIA

Although some hospital-acquired pneumonias occur as a result of bacteremic spread, the vast majority occur via aspiration of oropharyngeal contents. The oropharynx of the patient admitted to the hospital rapidly becomes colonized with aerobic gram-negative bacilli and often staphylococci. The administration of broad-spectrum antibiotics, severe underlying illness, respiratory intubation, and prolonged duration of hospitalization predispose to colonization.

Sedation, loss of consciousness, and other factors that depress the gag and cough reflexes place the colonized patient at greater risk for aspiration and the development of nosocomial pneumonia. The development of a new pulmonary infiltrate in a hospitalized patient may represent pneumonia, atelectasis, aspiration of gastric contents, drug reaction, or pulmonary infarction. If pneumonia is suspected, prompt definition of the pathogen and appropriate treatment are critical, since nosocomial pneumonia carries a 20 to 50 per cent mortality. If the patient cannot produce good quality sputum, nasotracheal or transtracheal aspiration should be performed (see Chapter 88). Antibiotic therapy is guided by the results of Gram's stain of the sputum or of the tracheal aspirate. Gram-negative rods are the predominant pathogens in this setting; these infections should be treated with an aminoglycoside plus an extended-spectrum penicillin or cephalosporin until results of culture and sensitivity are known. In certain hospitals, nosocomial pneumonia due to *Legionella* species is frequent, and erythromycin should be included in the initial treatment regimen. Patients with nosocomial pneumonia should also receive respiratory therapy consisting of clapping, postural drainage, and promotion of coughing to assist in bringing up secretions. The patient in the intensive care unit with an endotracheal tube in place is at particular risk for nosocomial pneumonia. This patient has an ineffective gag reflex and often a depressed cough as well. He is therefore entirely dependent upon suctioning by the staff to clear secretions from his airways. The airways of these patients become rapidly colonized with bacteria. Epidemics of nosocomial pneumonia have sometimes been associated with contamination of tubing and machinery used for ventilation or respiratory therapy, but more often infection is due to transmission of pathogens on the hands of medical personnel. Patients whose airways are simply colonized but whose lower respiratory tract is not infected should not be treated with antibiotics, despite positive sputum cultures. Premature treatment of colonization results in replacement of the initial colonists by more resistant organisms, whereas delay in treatment of nosocomial pneumonia can result in death due to overwhelming infection. The physician must therefore be able to distinguish accurately between colonization and infection. The development of new fever, leukocytosis, pulmonary infiltrate, and/or deterioration of respiratory status as ascertained by blood gas determinations suggest infection (pneumonia) rather than colonization. The appearance of elastin fibers (see Fig. 82–2) in KOH preps of sputum is a very specific indicator of bacterial infection in this setting. The appearance of these fibers may actually precede the development of infiltrates on chest x-ray. This test will, however, detect only about one half of nosocomial pneumonias in the ICU.

Nosocomial pneumonias are best prevented by (1) avoiding excessive sedation; (2) providing frequent suctioning and respiratory therapy—drainage and clapping—to patients who have difficulty managing secretions; (3) avoiding the injudicious use of broad-spectrum and/or high-dose antibiotic therapy; (4) frequent handwashing by medical and nursing personnel.

INTRAVASCULAR CATHETER–RELATED INFECTIONS

Infections related to intravascular catheters may occur via bacteremic seeding or through infusion of contaminated material, but the vast majority of these infections occur via bacterial invasion at the site of catheter insertion.

Intravenous catheters may produce a sterile phlebitis. Certain drugs such as tetracycline or erythromycin, when administered intravenously, are particularly likely to produce phlebitis. Bacteria migrating through the catheter insertion site may colonize the catheter and then produce a septic phlebitis or bacteremia without evidence of local infection. Factors associated with a greater risk of I.V. catheter–related infection are shown in Table 96–3. *Staphylococcus epidermidis* and *Staphylococcus aureus* are the predominant pathogens in this setting, followed by the enteric gram-negative rods. A peripheral catheter should be changed if bacteremia occurs and no other primary site of infection is found. The catheter

TABLE 96–3. FACTORS ASSOCIATED WITH GREATER RISKS OF INTRAVENOUS CATHETER–RELATED INFECTION

Duration of catheterization > 72 hours
Plastic catheter > steel needle
Lower extremities and groin > upper extremity
Cutdown > percutaneous insertion
Emergency > elective insertion
Breakdown in skin integrity, e.g., burns
Inserted by physician > I.V. therapy teams

should also be removed if fever without an obvious source occurs or if local phlebitis develops. The value of culturing a peripheral catheter tip is uncertain unless semiquantitative techniques are used (i.e., rolling the catheter across an agar plate). During the evaluation of a hospital-acquired fever, an inflamed vein should be examined carefully, and after the catheter is removed the inflamed portion of the vein should be compressed in an attempt to express pus through the catheter entry site. If pus can be expressed or the patient remains febrile or bacteremic while on appropriate antibiotics, the vein should be surgically explored and excised if septic phlebitis is found. Central venous catheters remain in place longer than peripheral catheters and are therefore associated with a greater overall infection rate. This is particularly true if total parenteral nutrition is provided by this route. Patients receiving parenteral nutrition are at particular risk for systemic infection with *Candida* species and gram-negative bacilli as well as with staphylococci. Pus at the catheter insertion site or positive blood cultures without another source are indications for catheter removal. In an attempt to decrease percutaneous spread of bacteria to intravascular sites, most centers are now placing long Silastic catheters into the subclavian vein after subcutaneous tunneling. These catheters may be kept in place for prolonged periods with a lower infection risk. Management of a patient with such a catheter in place who has a fever without an apparent site of infection poses difficult problems. As a general rule, persistent bacteremia while on appropriate antibiotics, bacteremia without another likely primary site, fungemia with *Candida* or related yeasts, or fever without alternative explanation are indications for catheter removal.

TABLE 96–4. FACTORS PREDISPOSING TO NOSOCOMIAL URINARY TRACT INFECTION

Indwelling catheters
Duration of catheterization
Open drainage (versus closed-bag drainage)
Interruption of closed drainage system
Use of broad-spectrum antibiotics (*Candida*)

PRESSURE SORES

See Chapter 90.

NOSOCOMIAL URINARY TRACT INFECTION

Placement of an indwelling catheter into the urethra of a hospitalized patient facilitates access of pathogens to an ordinarily sterile site. Factors that predispose to infection are shown on Table 96–4. The most common pathogens are enteric gram-negative rods; however, among immunocompromised patients and patients receiving broad-spectrum antibiotics, *Candida* species are also important causes of infection. Prophylactic antibiotics, irrigation, urinary acidification, and use of antiseptics are of no value in prevention of infection in this setting. Nosocomial urinary tract infections can be best prevented by instituting the following:

1. Catheterize only when necessary. (Monitoring of intake and output or urinary incontinence is rarely an indication for catheterization.)
2. Remove the catheter as soon as possible.
3. Emphasize handwashing.
4. Use sterile catheters and insert aseptically.
5. Maintain a closed and unobstructed drainage system. (Urine specimens for culture and analysis may be obtained by inserting a 22-gauge needle aseptically through the distal end of the catheter wall.) Do not disconnect the catheter from the drainage bag.
6. Secure the catheter in place.
7. Keep the catheter bag below the level of the bladder.
8. Irrigate the catheter only if obstructed.

Asymptomatic bacterial colonization of the catheterized bladder need not be treated. If the patient has fever or local symptoms, antibiotic treatment is indicated. *Candida* infection will often resolve once broad-spectrum antibiotics are discontinued. If *Candida* infection persists, the catheter may be changed; if infection still persists, twice daily irrigation of the catheter with amphotericin B can eradicate the organism.

The best way to prevent catheter-related infections of the urinary tract is to avoid catheterization unless absolutely necessary.

REFERENCE

Wenzel RP: Prevention and treatment of hospital-acquired infections. In Wyngaarden JB, and Smith LH Jr (eds): Cecil Textbook of Medicine. 17th ed. Philadelphia, WB Saunders Co, 1985, pp 1485–1492.

Immunosuppression is an increasing byproduct of diseases and modern approaches to their treatment. The immunocompromised host suffers from increased susceptibility to opportunistic infection, defined as infection caused by organisms of low virulence that comprise normal mucosal and skin flora or microbial agents usually maintained in a latent state.

Immunocompromise is not an all-or-none phenomenon. The extent of immunosuppression varies with the underlying cause and must exceed a threshold to predispose to opportunistic infections. Importantly, the type of immunosuppression predicts the spectrum of agents likely to cause infections. Accordingly, opportunistic infections can best be considered in categories that reflect the nature of immunocompromise.

DISORDERS OF CELL-MEDIATED IMMUNITY

Cell-mediated immunity is the major host defense against facultative intracellular parasites, as discussed in Chapter 81. The list of diseases and situations that produce impaired cell-mediated immunity is presented in Table 97–1. However, only certain of these result in increased susceptibility to infection with intracellular parasites. Foremost among acquired immunodeficiencies are Hodgkin's disease and other lymphomas, hairy-cell leukemia, and advanced solid tumors; severe malnutrition, as well as treatment with high-dose corticosteroids, cytotoxic drugs, or radiotherapy, can produce a similar predilection to infections. Congenital immunodeficiencies are associated with severe infections early in childhood and will not be considered here. Patients with impaired cell-mediated immunity are susceptible to organisms shown in Table 97–2.

Thus, with depression of cell-mediated immunity, organisms ordinarily constituting the normal flora such as *Candida* species act as virulent opportunistic pathogens capable of causing deep-seated infections. Latent viruses, fungal infections, and tuberculosis reactivate to cause disseminated disease. Often there are few specific signs, symptoms, and laboratory abnormalities to suggest the diagnosis.

The association between defective cell-mediated immunity and disease produced by the infectious agents listed in Table 97–2 is clear-cut. Sometimes, treatment of the underlying disease causing immunodeficiency or progression of this disease tends to produce a more severe and generalized compromised state, which predisposes to infection by other agents. For example, during chemotherapy for lymphoma, bacterial infections predominate. Disease progression also results in local factors favoring bacterial infections such as mucosal breakdown and tumor masses obstruct-

ing bronchi, ureters, or the biliary tract. The result is a marked increase in severe bacterial infection and septicemia late in the course of most diseases associated with impaired cell-mediated immunity.

DISORDERS OF HUMORAL IMMUNITY

The acquired disorders of antibody production associated with increased frequency of infection are common variable immunodeficiency, chronic lymphocytic leukemia, lymphosarcoma, and multiple myeloma. The paraproteinemic states belong in this category because of secondary decreases in levels of functioning antibody. Therapy with cytotoxic drugs may produce a similar immunocompromise.

Infections due to the pneumococcus, *Haemophilus influenzae*, streptococci, and staphylococci predominate early in the course of the humoral immunodeficiency. As the underlying disease itself progresses, infections due to gram-negative bacilli become more frequent. Treatment of the underlying condition with corticosteroids and cytotoxic drugs also causes additional defects in cell-mediated immunity, providing susceptibility to infections with the group of pathogens discussed above (Table 97–2).

In sickle cell anemia, heat-labile opsonic activity is abnormal. Complement depletion by erythrocyte stroma causes impairment of opsonization of pneumococci and *Salmonella* species, leading to frequent infections with these organisms. Im-

TABLE 97–1. CONDITIONS CAUSING IMPAIRED CELL-MEDIATED IMMUNITY

Infectious diseases—measles, chickenpox, typhoid fever, tuberculosis, leprosy, histoplasmosis, acquired immunodeficiency syndrome
Vaccinations—measles, mumps, rubella
Malignancies—Hodgkin's disease, lymphomas, advanced solid tumors
Drugs—corticosteroids, cytotoxic drugs
Miscellaneous—sarcoidosis, uremia, diabetes mellitus, malnutrition, old age

TABLE 97–2. INFECTIONS IN PATIENTS WITH IMPAIRED CELL-MEDIATED IMMUNITY

Viruses—varicella-zoster, herpes simplex, cytomegalovirus
Fungi—Pathogenic: *Histoplasma, Coccidioides*; Saprophytic: *Cryptococcus, Candida, Aspergillus, Zygomycetes*
Bacteria—*Listeria, Nocardia, Mycobacterium tuberculosis, Legionella pneumophila*
Protozoa—*Pneumocystis carinii, Toxoplasma gondii, Cryptosporidium* species
Helminths—*Strongyloides stercoralis*

paired reticuloendothelial system function due to erythrophagocytosis and functional asplenia also may predispose patients with sickle cell disease to serious bacterial infections. The predisposition to infection is age-related; once children with SS disease develop antibodies to pneumococcal capsular polysaccharide, they lose their thousand-fold increased susceptibility to severe pneumococcal infection.

IMPAIRED NEUTROPHIL FUNCTION

Many inherited and acquired diseases impair neutrophil function. The defect may be extrinsic or intrinsic to the neutrophil. Impaired chemotaxis is a significant factor predisposing patients with inherited C3 and C5 deficiencies to frequent bacterial infections. Corticosteroid therapy also interferes with chemotaxis. Whereas circulating neutrophil counts may be normal or increased in patients treated with corticosteroids, these cells are dysfunctional, since they do not localize normally to the site of infection. Defective cell-mediated immunity also contributes to the spectrum of infections promoted by corticosteroids.

Intrinsic defects in neutrophils are rare but provide insights into the microbicidal mechanisms of these cells. Neutrophils from patients with chronic granulomatous disease (CGD) cannot develop an oxidative burst. Catalase-negative organisms produce sufficient hydrogen peroxide to permit their own killing by CGD neutrophils through the myeloperoxidase pathway. Catalase-producing organisms such as staphylococci, Serratia, Nocardia, and Aspergillus scavenge the hydrogen peroxide that they produce; these infectious agents, therefore, cannot be killed by CGD neutrophils and produce serious, deep-seated infections.

The most severe intrinsic neutrophil defects occur in the Chédiak-Higashi syndrome. Patients have giant granules in their leukocytes and defective microtubule assembly. The result is impaired chemotaxis, abnormal phagolysosomal fusion, delayed bacterial killing, and recurrent infections. Diagnosis of this rare syndrome is aided by phenotypic abnormalities: partial albinism, depigmentation of the iris, peripheral neuropathies, and nystagmus.

NEUTROPENIA

As the neutrophil count falls below 500/μl, an exponential increase occurs in the frequency and severity of infections. Most reliable data originate from patients with acute leukemia. However, granulocytopenia of other etiologies produces a comparable risk of infection. In patients with chronic and cyclical neutropenias, the susceptibility to infection varies inversely with the monocyte count; the mononuclear phagocytes provide some of the antibacterial capacity of the missing neutrophils. Following chemotherapy of acute leukemia, neutropenia usually is sustained and associated with damage to mucosal barriers to infection. Patients become susceptible to organisms that are ubiquitous in the environment and ordinarily compose the normal flora (Table 97–3).

DIAGNOSTIC PROBLEMS IN THE COMPROMISED HOST

PULMONARY INFILTRATES

The immunocompromised patient with pulmonary infiltrates presents a particularly vexing diagnostic problem. The pulmonary infiltrates could represent infection, extension of underlying tumor, complication of chemotherapy, or some combination of these. Specific diagnosis is necessary. Unfortunately, noninvasive serodiagnostic tests rarely are helpful in this setting, yet concomitant thrombocytopenia too often increases the risk of lung biopsy.

The clinical setting and radiographic appearance of the pulmonary infiltrate influence the probable yield of lung biopsy and the decision as to whether to proceed. For example, in patients with leukemia, parenchymal infiltrates occurring before or within three days of initiating chemotherapy usually are bacterial, as are focal infiltrates developing later in the course. Major efforts should be directed at obtaining adequate sputum samples for Gram's stain and culture; the evolution of the pneumonitis during antibiotic therapy becomes a useful factor in deciding whether to proceed with lung biopsy.

In contrast, diffuse infiltrates occurring after treatment of leukemia are more suggestive of opportunistic infection. Furthermore, Pneumocystis carinii is the most common cause of diffuse infiltrates due to infectious agents in immunocompromised hosts. In this situation, empirical therapy with trimethoprim-sulfamethoxazole should be initiated. The decision as to whether and when to perform a lung biopsy then can be based on the patient's response.

The indications and timing of lung biopsy, therefore, must be individualized. On the other hand, delay in proceeding with the biopsy, to a point at which the patient is significantly hypoxic, nullifies the chances of affecting the outcome with therapy, even if the biopsy shows a potentially treatable disease.

Once the decision has been made to biopsy, the next question is which procedure to use. Fiberoptic bronchoscopy with transbronchial biopsy has had a good diagnostic yield in some centers, particularly in the evaluation of diffuse pulmo-

TABLE 97–3. INFECTIOUS AGENTS THAT CAUSE INFECTIONS IN NEUTROPENIC PATIENTS

Bacteria—Pseudomonas, Klebsiella, Serratia, Escherichia coli, Staphylococcus aureus
Fungi—Candida, Aspergillus, Zygomycetes
Viruses—cytomegalovirus, Herpesvirus hominis
Protozoa—Pneumocystis carinii

nary lesions. This technique should not be performed in the thrombocytopenic patient. If the local experience favors the transbronchial biopsy, it is imperative that the tissue obtained be processed and examined quickly. Open lung biopsy has an additional yield of 50 to 75 per cent in the patient with a nondiagnostic transbronchial biopsy and should be performed without any further delay if the tempo of progression of the patient's illness mandates an immediate diagnosis. Open lung biopsy generally is safe in thrombocytopenic patients if prophylactic transfusions can achieve an increment in the platelet count and diminish the bleeding time. Recent experience indicates that early treatment of most pulmonary infections in immunocompromised hosts, even aspergillosis (Fig. 97–1), is associated with an initially favorable outcome. The long-term result, however, is totally dependent on the natural history of the underlying leukemia or other condition.

DISSEMINATED MYCOSES

Disseminated mycoses represent another major diagnostic problem in the immunocompromised host. Fungal infections are found post mortem in over one half of patients with leukemia and lymphoma; usually the nature of the infection has not been established ante mortem. Culture of a saprophytic organism such as *Candida* from superficial sites does not establish pathogenicity. Even in patients with widespread infection, however, fungemia is a late and often agonal event.

How, then, can the diagnosis of fungal infection be established early, at a time when the infection is potentially curable? It is important to search for superficial lesions accessible to scraping, aspiration, or biopsy (Fig. 97–2). Dissemination of *Candida tropicalis* frequently causes hyperpigmented macular or pustular skin lesions that show the organism on biopsy. Cryptococcal polysaccharide antigen may be present in serum or CSF of the patient with disseminated cryptococcosis. Serodiagnosis has, in general, been disappointing, although other tests for circulating fungal antigens may soon become available. In the absence of adequate diagnostic procedures, empirical use of antifungal drugs is indicated, with appropriate clinical suspicion of disseminated mycoses, for example, in the neutropenic patient with prolonged fever despite broad-spectrum antibiotic therapy.

FIGURE 97–2. Skin lesion in a 76-year-old woman treated with corticosteroids and cytotoxic drugs for chronic lymphocytic leukemia and presenting with nodular pulmonary infiltrates and lymphocytic meningitis. Fluid expressed from the lesion contained encapsulated yeast seen on India ink preparation and yielded *Cryptococcus neoformans* on culture.

PREVENTION AND TREATMENT OF INFECTIONS IN THE NEUTROPENIC PATIENT

PREVENTION

Acute bacterial infections and septicemia arising from organisms comprising the gut flora occur frequently in granulocytopenic patients and may have fever as their sole manifestation. Prophylactic nonabsorbable antibiotics and protective isolation have failed to prevent such infection in most studies. Recently, trimethoprim-sulfamethoxazole has been given prophylactically and has been shown to decrease the number of infections and bacteremic episodes in some neutropenic patients. Trimethoprim-sulfamethoxazole prophylaxis is not as effective in patients with acute nonlymphocytic leukemia, however, and enthusiasm for its use in other settings has waned because of its bone marrow toxicity and selection of resistant organisms.

Prophylactic granulocyte transfusions decrease the occurrence of bacterial sepsis in patients with acute myelogenous leukemia but are costly, increase the frequency of fatal pneumonitis, and do not affect overall remission rate and duration of survival.

TREATMENT

Empirical antibiotic therapy is indicated in febrile granulocytopenic patients, since two thirds

FIGURE 97–1. Fruiting head of *Aspergillus fumigatus* on lung biopsy. Aspergillosis usually causes an expanding perihilar pulmonary infiltrate. Prompt institution of amphotericin B therapy may lead to a good clinical response.

have an underlying infection. Selection of two drugs such as tobramycin and ticarcillin with activity against *Pseudomonas aeruginosa* is essential. This two-drug regimen also provides adequate initial antibiotic coverage of staphylococcal infections, although clinical experience favors the use of other drugs for their definitive therapy. Despite the early empirical use of antibiotics, the outcome of bacterial infections is poor unless the initial neutrophil count exceeds 500/μl, or the count rises during treatment.

The appropriate duration of antibiotic therapy of febrile neutropenic patients has been questioned recently. Patients who become afebrile during seven days of empiric antibiotics should have the regimen continued for the duration of neutropenia. When antibiotics are stopped earlier, over one third will develop infectious sequelae within the next two days. Empiric addition of amphotericin B therapy is indicated in the neutropenic patient who remains febrile for at least one week despite broad-spectrum antibiotics. Granulocyte transfusions are a useful adjunct to antibiotics in neutropenic patients with gram-negative septicemia.

REFERENCES

Pizzo PA, Robichand KJ, Gill FA, et al: Empiric antibiotic and antifungal therapy for cancer patients with prolonged fever and granulocytopenia. Am J Med 72:101, 1982.

Singer C, Armstrong D, Rosen PP, Walzer PD, and Yu B: Diffuse pulmonary infiltrates in immunosuppressed patients. Prospective study of 80 cases. Am J Med 66:110–120, 1979.

Toledo-Pereyra LH, DeMeester TR, Kinealey K, MacMahon H, Chung A, and Golumb H: The benefits of open lung biopsy in patients with previous non-diagnostic transbronchial lung biopsy. Chest 77:647–650, 1980.

98 THE ACQUIRED IMMUNODEFICIENCY SYNDROME AND RELATED DISORDERS

The acquired immunodeficiency syndrome (AIDS) is defined by the presence of opportunistic infections and unusual neoplasms that have arisen in epidemic proportions among persons with no previously recognized cause of immunodeficiency. The clinical AIDS syndrome probably represents only the most serious expression of a series of related disorders that will be more clearly defined as the etiology and pathogenesis of AIDS become better understood.

EPIDEMIOLOGY

The first cases of AIDS were recognized in 1979 among sexually active homosexual men residing in the cities of New York, Los Angeles, and San Francisco. Since that time, the disease has spread throughout the nation and the world. As of January 1986, over 16,000 cases fulfilling strict diagnostic criteria were reported to the United States Centers for Disease Control. Approximately three fourths of these cases occurred among homosexual or bisexual males (Table 98–1). Intravenous drug abusers comprise the next largest group of AIDS patients. The disease has also been found among Haitian immigrants to the United States and among hemophilic recipients of pooled antihemophilic factor concentrates and recipients of blood transfusions. In many of the latter instances, units of transfused blood have been traced back to "healthy" donors who later developed AIDS themselves. AIDS also has occurred among female sexual contacts of men belonging to groups at risk for AIDS, and among newborn children, offspring of individuals at risk. All these instances make it clear that AIDS is a transmissible disease. The precise mode of sexual transmission of this illness remains uncertain at present, but it appears that receptive anal intercourse may carry a particular risk of disease. The incubation period varies. In transfusion-related cases, where time of exposure can be identified most precisely, the incubation period averages between 12 and 18 months but may be five years or more. There is no evidence that routine nonsexual, nonparenteral contact (e.g., with household members or medical personnel) carries any risk of transmitting the disease.

TABLE 98–1. GROUPS AT RISK FOR AIDS

Homosexual or bisexual men
Intravenous drug abusers
Hemophiliacs
Recipients of blood transfusions
Female sexual contacts of men belonging to groups at risk
Newborn offspring of individuals at risk for AIDS

Recently, a retrovirus belonging to the human T lymphotrophic virus (HTLV) family, named HTLV-III or lymphadenopathy-associated virus (LAV), has been implicated as the probable causative agent of AIDS. Serologic studies among individuals belonging to groups at risk for the disease suggest that only a minority of individuals exposed to the virus now have AIDS. The prognosis for these seropositive individuals is uncertain; most will, in all likelihood, not develop opportunistic infections. The virus is not endemic in the United States and apparently was only recently introduced into this country. Individuals not belonging to groups at risk for AIDS have no serologic evidence of exposure to the virus, and serum samples obtained before 1978 from groups now at risk show no evidence of viral exposure. High rates of seropositivity, however, are present among healthy Central Africans, suggesting that this virus may be endemic in that part of the world.

PATHOPHYSIOLOGY

The retrovirus HTLV-III is trophic for and selectively infects human T lymphocytes of the helper phenotype; in vitro infection of T helper cells results in cytopathic effects and cell lysis. Patients with AIDS almost always have a striking deficiency in the number of T helper lymphocytes. Whether the loss of T helper cells is sufficient to explain the generalized impairment of cell-mediated immunity that characterizes AIDS is not known. Laboratory evidence of immunodeficiency is striking. Anergy—the failure to demonstrate delayed-type hypersensitivity to a battery of recall antigens—is seen in more than 90 per cent of AIDS patients. The ability of T lymphocytes to proliferate in response to various stimuli is generally impaired. The ability of lymphocytes from AIDS patients to kill virus-infected cells and tumor cells in vitro also is generally abnormal, as is the capacity of their T cells to produce the lymphokines interleukin-2 and gamma interferon. B lymphocyte function may be abnormal, since polyclonal hyperglobulinemia is common, and some in vitro tests of B lymphocyte function are also impaired. Clinically, however, the most relevant impairment is the persistent cell-mediated immunodeficiency.

Among clinically well individuals at risk for AIDS, such as homosexual males living in epidemic areas and patients with hemophilia, there is a high frequency of subclinical immunodeficiency. Such persons have in vitro immunologic abnormalities that are similar to, but less severe than those seen among AIDS victims. In these clinically well, susceptible populations, an increase in the frequency of generalized lymph node enlargement has developed concomitant with the AIDS epidemic. Most of these patients with generalized lymph node enlargement show laboratory evidence of immune abnormality; anergy is present in 90 per cent. Furthermore, some patients with lymph node enlargement go on to develop

AIDS. It is likely that in many individuals, subclinical immunodeficiency and generalized lymph node enlargement represent manifestations of exposure to the AIDS agent. It is possible that other agents such as *Toxoplasma*, cytomegalovirus, and Epstein-Barr virus sometimes produce these clinical and laboratory findings. At this time, the contributory role of infection with these agents to the development of clinical immunodeficiency among AIDS patients is unknown.

CLINICAL MANIFESTATIONS

Some patients with AIDS have a prodrome including generalized lymph node enlargement, episodes of fever, night sweats, weight loss, and diarrhea lasting weeks to months before the development of opportunistic infections or neoplasms.

Mucocutaneous Disease

Candida stomatitis (thrush) or herpes zoster are occasionally forerunners of AIDS. The occurrence of esophageal candidiasis, manifesting clinically as pain or difficulty swallowing, fulfills criteria for the diagnosis of AIDS. Thrush often can be suppressed successfully by clotrimazole troches. Esophageal involvement necessitates treatment with ketoconazole or amphotericin B. Chronic perioral or perianal herpes simplex infection, often producing extensive ulcerations, occurs among patients with AIDS. Diagnosis can be established by viral culture or less expensively by Wright's staining of a scraping obtained from the base of an ulcer. Systemic acyclovir is the treatment of choice. *Kaposi's sarcoma*, a malignancy of endothelial cell origin, occasionally occurs as an indolent skin tumor in elderly men of Mediterranean descent. Cytomegalovirus DNA has been found in Kaposi's sarcoma cells. Kaposi's sarcoma in AIDS is histologically identical to Mediterranean Kaposi's sarcoma but follows a more aggressive course, affecting primarily homosexual males, a group known to have a high prevalence of cytomegalovirus infection. The lesions of Kaposi's sarcoma can arise anywhere on the skin or in the mucosa of the mouth or gastrointestinal tract; occasionally they first appear in enlarged lymph nodes. The lesions are vascular, can be raised or flat, pink, brown or blue, and often resemble insect bites, bruises, or nevi. Some have responded favorably to administration of alpha interferon.

Nervous System Diseases

Neurologic manifestations of AIDS are common and often fatal. Patients with cryptococcal meningitis may complain of persistent headache, difficulty concentrating, and lethargy. Prior to the appearance of AIDS, approximately half of cases of cryptococcal meningitis occurred among individuals without underlying immunosuppressive conditions. Thus, the occurrence of cryptococcal meningitis in a previously healthy individual is not necessarily diagnostic of AIDS. AIDS patients with cryptococcal meningitis, however, often have cryptococcal fungemia, an indication of serious immunodeficiency. The infection can be suppressed with amphotericin B, but relapses are the rule. *Toxoplasmosis* of the central nervous system, presenting as single or multiple brain abscesses, is seen in AIDS patients. Serologic tests may not be diagnostic, and brain biopsy may be required to establish the diagnosis. Pyrimethamine and sulfadiazine are the treatments of choice. *Progressive multifocal leukoencephalopathy*, a demyelinating disease due to papovavirus, can produce progressive dementia and long tract signs in AIDS patients. CT scanning may reveal the characteristic low-density lesions of white matter. No known treatment is effective. Dementia is common in patients with AIDS, generally occurring after the onset of opportunistic infection. The etiology of the dementia is uncertain, and histopathologic findings are nonspecific. HTLV-III may directly infect brain cells. Primary lymphoma of the central nervous system also occurs with increased incidence among patients with AIDS. Blindness due to choroidoretinitis often affects patients with advanced AIDS. Some cases have been linked to cytomegalovirus infection; in others, the cause is not clear.

Pulmonary Disease

Pneumocystis carinii pneumonia (PCP) is the most common opportunistic infection complicating AIDS. Affected patients complain of shortness of breath and nonproductive cough. In contrast to the often acute onset of PCP in other immunocompromised patients, AIDS patients with PCP may have pulmonary symptoms for weeks or more before presentation. Arterial hypoxemia is common; chest x-ray generally reveals a mixed, often subtle interstitial and alveolar pattern. Diagnosis is readily made by bronchial lavage or transbronchial biopsy. Treatment with high doses of trimethoprim-sulfamethoxazole is generally effective, but these drugs produce an unusually high frequency of side effects in AIDS patients, including marrow depression, rash, and fever, which limit their effectiveness. Pentamidine is comparably effective and may have fewer side effects. Organisms persist in repeat biopsy specimens and relapse is frequent. Prolonging treatment for three weeks or more may improve results.

Gastrointestinal Disease

The sexual habits of homosexual men predispose to a variety of gastrointestinal pathogens (see Chapter 94). Homosexuals with AIDS often have intermittent or persistent severe watery diarrhea. In some instances, the fluid contains ordinary pathogens; in others, unusual ones can be found such as the protozoan *Cryptosporidium*, *Mycobacterium avium-intracellulare*, or cytomegalovirus (CMV). Often, no cause is identified. Spiramycin (a macrolide antibiotic) may relieve diarrhea in some patients infected with *Cryptosporidium*.

Other Infections

Disseminated CMV infection is common among AIDS patients. The virus can be cultured from the urine of many and has been found in biopsy or postmortem examination of lung, liver, gut, and brain. No effective treatment exists for CMV. *Mycobacterium avium-intracellulare* (MAI) is a saprophytic mycobacterium that, on rare occasion, produces an indolent pneumonia in otherwise healthy individuals. In patients with AIDS, MAI frequently produces disseminated infection. The organism can be cultured from blood but may require several weeks to grow. Acid-fast smears of stool sometimes reveal it. Culture and histologic examination of bone marrow may be more sensitive in the diagnosis of this infection. MAI resists the action of most antibiotics. Combinations of antimycobacterial drugs, including ansamycin (an experimental drug related to rifampin) and clofazamine (a drug used in the treatment of leprosy), can eradicate bacteremia in some patients but almost never provide a cure. MAI bacteremia was distinctly unusual before the AIDS epidemic, even among patients with severe immunodeficiency. By contrast, infections such as listeriosis, aspergillosis, and nocardiosis, common among other groups of patients with impaired cell-mediated immunity, rarely affect patients with AIDS. These observations suggest that "cell-mediated host defenses" are heterogeneous and can be selectively impaired.

DIAGNOSIS AND LABORATORY FINDINGS

At present, one makes a clinical diagnosis of AIDS based upon criteria indicated in Table 98–2. Abnormal distribution of lymphocyte phenotypes, with absolute decreases in T helper cells and relative increases in T suppressor cells, is generally but not invariably present. Anergy to skin test antigens is observed in almost all patients.

Anemia and leukopenia are common. Some patients with AIDS and many belonging to groups at risk have a syndrome resembling immune thrombocytopenic purpura (ITP), probably due to binding of immune complexes to platelets, resulting in their clearance from the circulation by reticuloendothelial cells. Abnormal tests of liver function are common and could be related to infection with cytomegalovirus or *Mycobacterium avium-intracellulare* or to the administration of hepatotoxic drugs for the treatment of opportunistic infections. Serum albumin is often low, and total globulins are often elevated, reflecting a polyclonal increase in immunoglobulins. An unusual acid-labile alpha interferon is often found in the serum of AIDS patients; its significance is unknown. Virtually all AIDS patients have serum antibody against the HTLV-III retrovirus.

APPROACH TO THE PATIENT AT RISK FOR AIDS AND TREATMENT

The long incubation period of AIDS and the absence of definitive predictive tests produce great uncertainty among individuals with AIDS-related syndromes such as generalized lymph node enlargement. Persons with oral thrush, unexplained fevers, weight loss, and night sweats are at high risk for the development of opportunistic infections. Asymptomatic individuals should be informed of means of minimizing their exposures to the causative agent. Homosexuals should be advised to limit the number of sexual partners and to consider avoiding anal intercourse or using a condom. I.V. drug abusers should be told that sharing needles is dangerous. Hemophiliacs should avoid the use of pooled antihemophilic factor concentrates and, in regions where the incidence of AIDS is low, use cryoprecipitates (or in the case of Factor IX deficiency, fresh frozen plasma) prepared locally from the plasma of volunteer donors. Screening of donors for antibody to HTLV-III is an additional safeguard of particular importance in areas of high incidence of AIDS. Recent data suggest that heat treatment of Factor VIII concentrates markedly reduces the infectivity of retroviruses. This may provide a safer treatment method than unheated preparations. There is no evidence that individuals at risk for AIDS who may be harboring the AIDS agent or AIDS patients pose any risk to household members who are not their sexual partners.

Treatment of AIDS is aimed at its specific infectious or neoplastic complications. At present, the disease appears to be uniformly fatal. Although the infection may be controlled, the immunodeficiency persists and patients remain at

risk for more infections. Lymphocyte infusions, bone marrow transplantation, and alpha interferon have not been successful. Ongoing trials are evaluating the effects of interleukin-2 and gamma interferon. The identification of the likely etiologic agent of AIDS and the ability to produce large quantities of viral antigen may allow production of a vaccine for testing in susceptible populations. In vitro assays of viral infection will allow testing of drugs with potential antiviral activity, which may be of value in the treatment of this disease.

TABLE 98–2. CRITERIA FOR THE DIAGNOSIS OF AIDS

An illness suggestive of impaired cell-mediated immunity occurring in an individual without an underlying immunosuppressive disorder, who is not receiving corticosteroids or other immunosuppressive medication. Examples of these illnesses include:

Pneumocystis carinii pneumonia
Esophageal candidiasis
Toxoplasma brain abscess
Mycobacterium avium-intracellulare bacteremia
Cryptococcal fungemia
Disseminated cytomegalovirus infection
Chronic ulcerative herpes simplex infection
Chronic cryptosporidial diarrhea
Kaposi's sarcoma in a patient less than 60 years of age
Primary central nervous system lymphoma

REFERENCES

Fauci AS, Macher AM, Longo DL, et al: Acquired immunodeficiency syndrome: Epidemiologic, clinical, immunologic and therapeutic considerations. Ann Intern Med 100:92–106, 1984.
Gottlieb MS, Groopman JE, Weinstein WM, et al: The acquired immunodeficiency syndrome. Ann Intern Med 99:208–220, 1983.

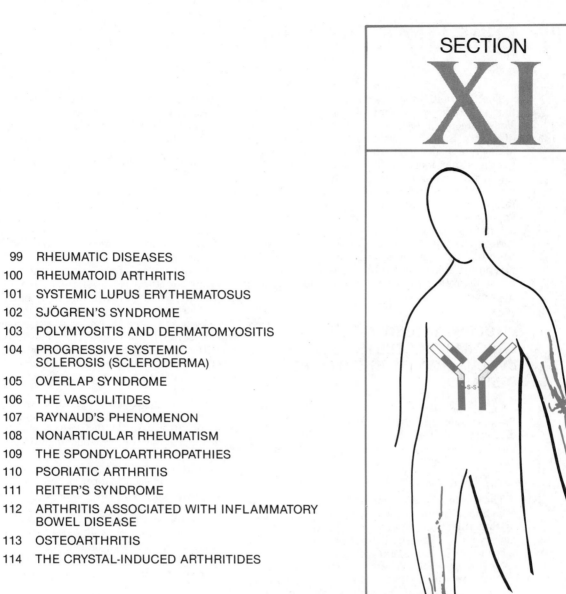

SECTION XI

MUSCULOSKELETAL AND CONNECTIVE TISSUE DISEASES

RHEUMATIC DISEASES

The rheumatic diseases are a group of disorders that affect the supporting or connective tissues. These are often referred to as collagen vascular disorders. Since they encompass a large number of discrete disorders, their clinical manifestations can be either localized or systemic. In practice, the symptoms and signs that attend these disorders tend to be variable and overlapping. A prolonged *latent interval* during which symptoms and signs wax and wane before diagnosis is a characteristic feature of the rheumatic diseases. Also, certain rheumatic diseases exhibit a wide spectrum of symptoms over time. Finally, fluctuating symptoms, that is, episodic exacerbations and remissions, reflect the periodicity of the rheumatic disorders.

UNDERSTANDING LABORATORY TESTS USED IN EVALUATION OF RHEUMATIC DISEASES

Laboratory tests are an important component in the diagnosis and management of the rheumatic diseases. This section will address those laboratory studies of particular interest in the basic evaluation of a rheumatic disease.

The Acute Phase Response

The acute phase response is a complex, time-dependent group of events that is mounted following infection, trauma, or idiopathic inflammatory states. The initial responses have been observed within hours, and the total duration may extend over weeks. There is often fever and an increase in the absolute numbers of circulating polymorphonuclear leukocytes and platelets. Changes in metabolism may include increased rates of synthesis of certain hormones, augmented protein catabolism, and gluconeogenesis. At times, variable immunosuppression is observed, in part due to depressed reticuloendothelial integrity and to altered lymphocyte function.

The concentration of certain plasma proteins derived from the liver increases. The rates of synthesis of the third component of complement and of ceruloplasmin may increase by 50 per cent. The concentration of haptoglobin and fibrinogen can double or quadruple. The concentration of C-reactive protein and serum amyloid A-protein can be augmented several hundred-fold. The measurement of certain acute phase reactants is useful to indicate a systemic inflammatory response and to monitor the response to treatment.

The Erythrocyte Sedimentation Rate (ESR)

In the absence of a laboratory test able to identify a specific etiologic agent, other tests are performed to provide an index of the inflammatory response. The ESR is the most commonly employed test for the presence of a systemic inflammatory response.

Of the methods for measuring the ESR, the Westergren method is the simplest and most reproducible. Some of the factors that contribute to an accelerated rate of sedimentation of red cells in disease are listed in Table 99–1. Of these factors, an elevated fibrinogen correlates most closely with an accelerated sedimentation rate. Similarly, certain factors are known to produce a falsely low sedimentation rate, as summarized in Table 99–1.

In most laboratories, the normal ESR for men is between 0 and 10 mm/hr, and for women between 0 and 20 mm/hr. With increasing age, the range of normal for the ESR becomes wider. Thus, in healthy persons in the seventh decade or older, the ESR may be elevated in the absence of illness.

The clinical indication for the use of the ESR is the suspicion of an inflammatory disorder. Other processes in which the ESR can be elevated include disorders associated with catabolic activity, pregnancy, cancer, and vascular disease. Conversely, the ESR can be unexpectedly normal or only slightly accelerated in certain viral illnesses, including infectious mononucleosis and hepatitis. The ESR should be interpreted as only a crude index of disease activity.

C-Reactive Protein

A second test associated with a systemic inflammatory response is the C-reactive protein (CRP). CRP is produced in the liver in small amounts in all healthy individuals. The normal concentration of plasma CRP is less than 1 mg/dl. Its biological role(s) is unclear; however, the protein behaves as an acute phase reactant, for during tissue injury its concentration in plasma can exceed 1000-fold normal levels. Thus, the CRP is a useful test to establish the presence of a systemic inflammatory process.

In contrast to the ESR, serum CRP concentrations rise rapidly and subsequently fall rapidly. A significant correlation exists between the ESR and CRP levels in chronic, but not acute, inflammatory disorders. Thus, the relative values of the two tests vary with the stage of the rheumatic disorder.

Serum Immunoglobulins

Serum immunoglobulins are composed of four polypeptide chains; the two larger chains are

TABLE 99–1. SOME FACTORS THAT CAN ALTER THE ERYTHROCYTE SEDIMENTATION RATE

ACCELERATION	DECREASE
Rouleaux formation	Increased serum viscosity
Hyperfibrinogenemia	Sickle cell disease
Hyperglobulinemia	Anisocytosis
Lipemia	Hypochromasia
	Interaction of lipase with red cell membrane

termed the heavy chains and the two smaller chains are designated the light chains. Based upon structural differences of the heavy chains, immunoglobulins have been divided into five classes: IgG, IgA, IgM, IgD, and IgE. The heavy chains are termed gamma, alpha, mu, delta, and epsilon, respectively. The two light chains are designated kappa and lambda. Approximately 60 to 65 per cent of all IgG light chains are composed of kappa light chains. The classification and known biological functions of the immunoglobulins are summarized in Table 99-2.

Two techniques are routinely utilized in the clinical laboratory for the characterization and quantitation of serum immunoglobulins. Serum protein electrophoresis separates the serum proteins into characteristic zones; then, scanning of the profile by a densitometer provides a useful technique to identify alterations in the proportions of these proteins. Thus, serum protein electrophoresis is often employed as a screening technique to identify the absence of components, monoclonal immunoglobulin spikes, or beta-gamma bridging. A detailed classification of the alterations of normal serum protein electrophoresis during disease has been developed. In the evaluation of rheumatic diseases, the most common pattern encountered on serum protein electrophoresis is nonspecific, polyclonal increases in IgG, IgM, and/or IgA that occur in response to either acute or chronic inflammation.

Quantitation of the serum immunoglobulins is useful in certain rheumatic diseases. Both systemic lupus erythematosus and rheumatoid arthritis can be associated with partial or complete deficiencies of IgA. Similarly, a seronegative inflammatory arthritis resembling rheumatoid arthritis occasionally complicates hypogammaglobulinemia.

Rheumatoid Factors

Rheumatoid factors are antibodies directed against antigenic determinants on the Fc fragment of IgG. Although IgG and IgM rheumatoid factors are the most common, rheumatoid factors can be of the IgM, IgG, and IgA classes.

The role of rheumatoid factors in homeostasis is not known. Yet the presence of such factors in 5 to 10 per cent of normal persons and their increased incidence during chronic infections suggest that rheumatoid factors operate in concert with other immune mechanisms. Rheumatoid factors are known to activate complement, to convert soluble immune complexes into insoluble complexes, and to enhance phagocytosis, chemotaxis, and kinin generation. The observation that rheumatoid factor exhibits a wide range of functions underscores the concept that these antiglobulins can mediate physiological responses, as well as form antigen-antibody complexes that can contribute to inflammation in rheumatoid arthritis.

Rheumatoid arthritis patients with positive tests for rheumatoid factors (i.e., "seropositive" patients) develop more severe disease, in general, than those individuals without rheumatoid factors, termed "seronegative" patients. Also, IgM rheumatoid factors are associated with more severe and more progressively disabling disease than IgG rheumatoid factors. Thus, the measurement of IgM rheumatoid factors is the most helpful determination.

The presence of a rheumatoid factor is not tantamount to the diagnosis of rheumatoid arthritis. IgM rheumatoid factors are present in approximately 30 per cent of other rheumatic diseases. Moreover, there is a variable incidence of these antiglobulins in the elderly well population, in certain acute and chronic infections, and in hepatic and pulmonary disorders.

TABLE 99-2. CHARACTERIZATION AND BIOLOGICAL FUNCTIONS OF HUMAN IMMUNOGLOBULINS

	IgG	IgA	IgM	IgD	IgE
Heavy chain	gamma	alpha	mu	delta	epsilon
Light chain	K or L*	K or L	K or L	K or L	K or L
Subclasses	gamma 1-4	alpha 1, 2	mu 1, 2	—	—
Molecular weight	150,000	150,000-350,000	900,000	180,000	190,000
Serum concentration (mg/dl)	550-1900	60-330	45-145	2-5	0.01
Plasma half-life (days)	21	6	5	3	2
Placental transfer	yes	no	no	no	no
Activation of classic complement cascade	yes	no	yes	no	no
Biological functions	opsonize agglutinate neutralize bactericide	? opsonize agglutinate neutralize mucosal action	Ag receptor lymphocytes agglutinate neutralize bactericide	Ag receptor B lymphocytes	reaginic

* K = kappa; L = lambda.

Autoantibodies Directed Against Nuclear and Cytoplasmic Antigens

Autoantibodies directed against nuclear and/or cytoplasmic antigens are frequently observed in the sera of individuals with rheumatic diseases. Serological tests to detect autoantibodies are routine in the evaluation and monitoring of treatment.

When the clinical symptoms and signs point to a specific connective tissue disease, an antinuclear antibody (ANA) test may be indicated to delineate the disorder further. The ANA should not be indiscriminately used to "rule out" a connective tissue disorder, because the ANA can be positive in other, unrelated diseases. The ANA is detected by indirect immunofluorescence. Routinely, a thin section of frozen rodent kidney or liver is adhered to a glass slide, test sera serially diluted more than 1:10 are overlayed and incubated, and the excess sera rinsed away. Fluorescein–labeled anti-human immunoglobulin is then overlayered and incubated and the unbound sera washed away. If immunofluorescence is present, the highest dilution giving a visual fluorescent pattern is reported as the titer of ANA. Depending upon the tissue substrate used, a titer of 1:10 or 1:20 is considered significant.

Autoantibodies have been divided into two major groups: those directed against antigenic determinants within the nucleus and those against cytoplasmic antigens. To date, autoantibodies specific for various nuclear antigens have commanded more clinical interest. Anti–native DNA (nDNA) antibodies are routinely used to assess disease activity in SLE and to monitor the progress of therapy. Although the titer of ANA is not a reliable indicator of active disease, the level of circulating anti-nDNA does correlate more closely with disease activity. Furthermore, the occurrence of anti-nDNA, which is present in 60 to 70 per cent of patients with SLE, is almost specific for SLE, although it is occasionally present in low concentrations in other disorders. Although anti–single-strand DNA is present in SLE and may be operative in the pathogenesis of the disease, the antibody is not specific for SLE, since it is also found in other rheumatic and nonrheumatic disorders.

Anti-histone antibodies occur in drug-induced LE, SLE, and rheumatoid arthritis. Of the ANA's present in drug-induced LE, the majority are directed against histones. Moreover, the incidence of these antibodies in drug-induced LE is 95 to 100 per cent. The frequency of anti-histone antibodies in SLE is 30 to 60 per cent and in RA 15 to 20 per cent.

The anti-Sm antibody is directed against an RNase-resistant nonhistone nuclear antigen. Although the antibody is regarded as specific for SLE, it is present in only 30 to 40 per cent of lupus sera.

Anti-nRNP antibody is also directed against a nonhistone nuclear antigen, but, unlike anti-Sm antibody, anti-nRNP is sensitive to RNase and protease digestion. Although found in highest frequency in the overlap syndrome comprising SLE, scleroderma, and polymyositis and in SLE, anti-nRNP can be observed less frequently in rheumatoid arthritis, Sjögren's syndrome, scleroderma, and discoid lupus.

Autoantibodies to SS-A (Ro) and SS-B (La), which exhibit a speckled immunofluorescence pattern, are directed against nuclear antigens. The techniques used to identify these autoantibodies are immunoprecipitation in double diffusion or counterimmunoelectrophoresis. Anti–SS-A is present in nearly 100 per cent of infants with neonatal lupus, in Sjögren's syndrome (60 to 70 per cent), and in SLE (30 to 40 per cent). Anti–SS-B (La) occurs with less frequency in all of these disorders.

Anti–Scl-70 and anti-centromere/kinetochore are antibodies directed against a chromosome-related 70,000-dalton protein and the inner and outer kinetochore plates, respectively. The autoantibodies can be regarded as serological markers for scleroderma and CREST syndrome (calcinosis, Raynaud's, esophageal dysmotility, sclerodactyly, telangiectasia), respectively. The incidence of anti–Scl-70 is only 15 to 20 per cent of scleroderma patients. In contrast, the incidence of anti-centromere/kinetochore is 70 to 90 per cent of patients with CREST.

Anti-nuclear antibodies also occur in adult polymyositis and dermatomyositis. PM-1 occurs in 50 per cent of patients with myositis, and in 87 per cent in overlap syndromes comprising scleroderma and polymyositis. The JO-1 antibody is present in about one third of patients with polymyositis but only 5 per cent of those with dermatomyositis. However, Mi-2 is found in 30 per cent of dermatomyositis patients.

The Classic and Alternative Complement Pathways

The complement cascade contains at least 18 individual serum proteins that interact with and modify the function of the immune system. The cascade is divided into three portions: (1) the classic arm, (2) the alternative or properdin arm, and (3) the terminal attack sequence.

The classic pathway can be activated by immune complexes. Although not all antigen-antibody complexes bind complement equally, larger immune complexes attach to C1q, resulting in the sequential activation of C1r, C1s, C4, C2, and the fragments C3a and C3b.

The alternative or properdin arm of the complement system can be activated by IgA, bacterial polysaccharides and endotoxins, and perhaps IgE. The activated intermediate products factor B, factor D, and properdin (P) finally interact with C3, resulting in the cleavage fragments C3a and C3b.

The terminal attack sequence is activated upon cleavage of C3. This results in the sequential activation of C5, C6, C7, C8, and C9. Adherence to the target of the C5-9 complex results in lysis.

Complement measurements are helpful in gauging the activity of certain rheumatic diseases. The CH50, or total hemolytic complement, depends upon intact and functional classic and terminal pathways, resulting in effective target (red blood cell) lysis. In general, normal CH50 levels imply that there is no enhanced activation of the pathway leading to "consumption" of individual complement components, and that there are normal levels of these components. In contrast, decreased CH50 levels suggest either depletion of complement proteins by an immune-mediated process or an inherited deficiency of an individual protein. In the presence of decreased CH50 levels due to an immune mechanism, low levels of C1q, C4, C2, and C3 are ordinarily observed.

Assessment of the complement system in a patient with a suspected or documented rheumatic disorder is best provided by determining the CH50, C3, and C4 levels. Under certain clinical circumstances, as when monitoring the results of therapy of lupus glomerulonephritis, the clinician may serially follow C4 and C3 levels as well as CH50. Whatever complement levels are measured, it is important to monitor them at regular intervals over time to establish a response to therapy.

In the evaluation of individuals with symptoms of an obscure connective tissue disorder, it is often useful to consider an inherited complement component deficiency disorder. Isolated deficiencies of nearly all components have been recognized. This can be assessed by the CH50, which is usually low or absent. Subsequently, the presence of a heterozygous or homozygous deficiency of an isolated complement protein can be established by family studies.

REFERENCES

Atkinson JP, and Frank MM: Complement. In Parker CW (ed): Clinical Immunology. Philadelphia, WB Saunders Co, 1980, p 219.

Tan EM: Autoantibodies to nuclear antigens: Their immunobiology and medicine. Adv Immunol 33:167, 1982.

RHEUMATOID ARTHRITIS 100

Rheumatoid arthritis (RA) is an inflammatory synovitis of unknown etiology. While the predominant symptoms and signs may involve virtually all synovial joints, RA is often associated with extra-articular involvement of other organ systems. The organs frequently affected include the skin, eye, cardiovascular system, bronchopulmonary system, spleen, and nervous system. Thus, RA is a systemic inflammatory disorder.

IMMUNOPATHOLOGY

The initial event inciting the synovitis is not known. The earliest synovial response to the inciting event is inflammation. In the initial phase, there is hypertrophy of the synovium characterized principally by synoviocyte hyperplasia and increased numbers of blood vessels. Polymorphonuclear leukocytes, B and T lymphocytes, and occasional plasma cells infiltrate the synovium. Upon phagocytosis of immune complexes, polymorphonuclear leukocytes release proinflammatory prostenoids, oxygen radicals, and leukotrienes, which interact synergistically with other mediators to produce vasodilation, edema, heat, and loss of function. Simultaneously, the lining synoviocytes augment the production of synovial fluid, resulting in the accumulation of an effusion. The effusions of RA are characterized by translucent or yellow fluid with a low viscosity; leukocytes, often more than 10,000, with greater than 90 per cent polymorphonuclear cells; a markedly depressed glucose; and normal or low complement levels. Rheumatoid factor is also frequently present.

If untreated, the synovitis of rheumatoid arthritis becomes self-perpetuating and chronic. The synovium becomes thickened and boggy, and the predominantly neutrophilic infiltrate is replaced by macrophages, fibroblasts, lymphocytes (approximately 70 to 75 per cent T lymphocytes), and plasma cells. On pathologic section, the synovium takes on a villous appearance. Inward overgrowth of the hypertrophic synovium across the surface of the articular cartilage results in the formation of pannus. The inflammatory reaction at the cartilage-pannus junction may eventually result in articular cartilage degradation, para-articular osteopenia, and ultimately the characteristic marginal erosions observed on x-ray. The degradation of cartilage leaves large, gaping surface ulcers, and with articulation, the rubbing of bone against bone produces crepitus and pain.

Rheumatoid nodules are granulomatous lesions that occur in approximately 20 per cent of individuals with RA and characteristically form at surface sites of friction, such as the extensor surfaces of the arms and tendon sheaths. Moreover, rheumatoid nodules also form in various organ systems, including the heart, lung, and brain. The origin of rheumatoid nodules is controversial. Pathologic studies indicate that these lesions develop about capillaries. Histopathologically, there is a central area of necrosis, an intermediate layer of palisading histocytes, and a superficial layer comprising lymphocytes and plasma cells. Thus, the rheumatoid nodule could reflect a local response to vasculitis.

CLINICAL MANIFESTATIONS OF RA

RA affects 2 to 3 per cent of the general population. The disease afflicts women in the childbearing years three times more frequently than men. In the older age groups ($\geq$ seventh decade), there is a trend toward more equal involvement of men and women.

RA is an idiopathic, symmetric synovitis affecting similar joints bilaterally. The criteria for the diagnosis of RA are presented in Table 100–1. Occasionally, however, the disease presents as a monoarthritis or asymmetric oligoarthritis. Over time, the arthritis is additive and assumes a symmetric distribution. Very early in its course, the predominant symptoms may be vague: variable aching, polyarthralgias, and fatigability with little, if any, definitive clinical evidence of synovitis. It is during this early phase that alternative diagnoses such as fibrositis and polymyalgia rheumatica are considered. Over months, synovitis insidiously evolves, usually in the feet and hands. A second, commonly observed onset is frank synovitis in an otherwise healthy individual. The synovitis most commonly affects the metatarsophalangeal joints of the feet, and the metacarpophalangeal and proximal interphalangeal joints of the hands, although other joints can be simultaneously involved. A third, but uncommon mode of presentation is that of a rapidly progressive and debilitating polyarticular synovitis, often associated with extra-articular organ system involvement. The fourth and least common onset is

the occurrence of extra-articular disease in the absence of clinical evidence of synovitis. An example of the latter is the histopathologic diagnosis of a rheumatoid nodule prior to the occurrence of synovitis. While these modes of onset may or may not be associated with the early presence of IgM rheumatoid factors, the aggressive form of RA is often characterized by high titers of rheumatoid factor.

The clinical course of RA is highly variable but usually pursues one of three patterns. The most common is a sporadic course punctuated by variable intervals of disease inactivity. The periods of spontaneous remission extend for months to years. This course holds the most favorable prognosis. A second commonly observed pattern is the insidious and relentless progression of synovitis and periodic, debilitating flares. Such flares are accompanied by severe polyarticular pain, flagrant synovitis, joint effusions, marked stiffness, low-grade fevers, and prostration. Because the synovitis involves the joints and tendon sheaths alike, joint subluxations can occur. Pannus formation leads to erosive articular disease and progressive loss of joint function and integrity with eventual fibrosis of tendon sheaths creating joint contractures. The prognosis depends upon the severity and is directly related to treatment intervention. The third, less common clinical course is rapid and aggressive and has been termed "malignant." There is severe polyarticular synovitis, rheumatoid nodules, weight loss, very high titers of rheumatoid factor, and hypocomplementemia. Extra-articular organ involvement of the skin (vasculitis), eyes (scleritis, corneal ulcers), lungs (nodules, interstitial fibrosis), heart (myopericarditis), blood (Felty's syndrome), and nervous system (neuropathy) frequently complicate this aggressive disease (Table 100–2). In the absence of effective treatment, the disease is debilitating and disabling owing to joint contractures, deformities, and the complications of the extra-articular involvement.

The small joints of the hands and feet are the earliest and most common diarthrodial articulations affected. Initially, the synovitis of the proximal interphalangeal (PIP) joints results in fusiform swelling associated with warmth, erythema, pain, and limitation of motion. Independent of PIP involvement, the metacarpophalangeal (MCP) joints develop soft-tissue swelling, squeeze tenderness, and limitation of motion due to synovitis. With the exception of severe RA, the distal interphalangeal (DIP) joints are rarely affected.

Chronic synovitis of joints and tendon sheaths often leads to permanent deformities. Because the metatarsophalangeal (MTP) joints of the feet are commonly affected, subluxations of the heads of the MTP's and foreshortening of the extensor tendons give rise to "hammer toe" or "cock-up" deformities, respectively. A similar process in the hands results in volar subluxation of the MCP joints and ulnar deviation of the fingers. An exaggerated inflammatory response of an extensor tendon can result in a spontaneous, often asymptomatic rupture. Hyperextension of a PIP joint and

TABLE 100–1. CRITERIA FOR RHEUMATOID ARTHRITIS

CRITERIA	CLASSIFICATION
Morning stiffness	Classic rheumatoid arthritis: 7 criteria
Pain on motion or tenderness in at least one joint	Definite rheumatoid arthritis: 5 criteria; joint signs or symptoms continuous for at least six weeks
Swelling (soft tissue or fluid) of at least one joint	
Swelling of at least one other joint	
Symmetric joint swelling, same joint on both sides of body (excluding terminal phalangeal joint)	Probable rheumatoid arthritis: 3 criteria; joint signs or symptoms continuous for at least six weeks
Subcutaneous nodules	Possible rheumatoid arthritis: 2 criteria; joint signs or symptoms continuous for at least three weeks
Roentgenographic changes (at least bony decalcification)	
"Rheumatoid factor" (any method)	
"Poor" mucin precipitate	
Characteristic histologic changes—synovium	
Characteristic histologic changes—nodules	

After Kellgren et al (eds): The Epidemiology of Chronic Rheumatism, Vol 1, 1963. Courtesy of Blackwell Scientific.

flexion of the DIP joint produces a *swan-neck deformity*. The *boutonniere deformity* is a fixed flexion contracture of a PIP joint and extension of a DIP joint.

The radiocarpal, intercarpal, and carpometacarpal joints of the wrists are frequently affected in RA. There is variable tenosynovitis of the dorsa of the wrists, and ultimately, interosseous muscle atrophy and diminished movement due to articular destruction and/or bony ankylosis. Volar synovitis can lead to a compression neuropathy termed carpal tunnel syndrome.

Chronic synovitis of the elbows, shoulders, hips, knees, and/or ankles each creates special secondary disorders. Destruction of the elbow articulations can lead to flexion contractures, loss of supination and pronation, and/or subluxations. When the shoulder is involved, limitation of shoulder mobility, dislocation, and spontaneous tears of the rotator cuff resulting in chronic pain can occur. A result of long-term synovitis of the knee is hypertrophy of the gastrocnemius-semimembranous bursa (Baker's cyst) of the popliteal fossa. Dissection of the cyst distally into the leg and rupture can mimic acute thrombophlebitis.

Involvement of the cervical spine by RA tends to be a late occurrence in more advanced disease. Pain localized to the lateral neck just inferior to the mastoid bone may be the first indication of inflammation of the C1-2 articulation. Chronic inflammation of the supporting ligaments of C1-2 eventually produces laxity, sometimes giving rise to atlantoaxial subluxation. There is posterior displacement of odontoid process, with a consequent increase in the predontoid space of greater than the normal range of 2 to 3 mm. Spinal cord compression can result from anterior dislocation of C1 or by vertical subluxation of the odontoid process of C2 into the foramen magnum.

TREATMENT

RA is an eminently treatable disorder, especially if the medical regimen is initiated early in the course of the disease. The objectives of treatment are (a) pain relief, (b) reduction or suppression of inflammation, (c) avoidance or early recognition of side effects, (d) preservation or restoration of function, and (e) maintenance of life style. The response to therapy can be gauged by the physician's global assessment of the patient's well being and by the criteria listed in Table 100–1.

The conservative therapy of RA requires a multifaceted approach. The importance of an ongoing educational program in RA cannot be overstated. Education should emphasize the benefits of a balanced daily program of rest and exercise. Physical and occupational therapy instruction in the appropriate exercises, along with the judicious application of splinting, can prevent and treat deformities, enhance muscle tone and strength, and preserve or improve function.

The pharmacologic therapy of RA often necessitates a combination of agents. It has been useful to approach therapy logically utilizing a "treat-

TABLE 100–2. EXTRA-ARTICULAR ORGAN SYSTEM INVOLVEMENT IN RHEUMATOID ARTHRITIS

ORGAN SYSTEM	EXTRA-ARTICULAR MANIFESTATIONS
Skin	Cutaneous vasculitis
	Rheumatoid nodules
Eye	Episcleritis
	Scleritis
	Scleromalacia perforans
	Corneal ulcers/perforation
	Uveitis
	Retinitis
	Glaucoma
	Cataract
Lung	Pleuritis
	Diffuse interstitial fibrosis
	Vasculitis
	Rheumatoid nodules
	Caplan's syndrome
	Pulmonary hypertension
Heart and blood vessels	Pericarditis
	Myocarditis
	Coronary arteritis
	Valvular insufficiency
	Conduction defects
	Vasculitis
	Felty's syndrome
Nervous system	Mononeuritis multiplex
	Distal sensory neuropathy

ment pyramid." Treatment is initiated with either aspirin or a nonsteroidal anti-inflammatory agent. The use of aspirin should result in a therapeutic serum salicylate level of 20 to 30 mg/dl. Because of the potential side effects of acetylated salicylates such as gastrointestinal hemorrhage secondary to peptic ulcer or gastritis, or a bleeding diathesis resulting from aspirin-induced inhibition of platelet aggregation, the use of a nonacetylated derivative, choline magnesium salicylate, should be considered. A second group of agents includes the antimalarials and gold salts. Hydroxychloroquine is the most common antimalarial in use in the United States. Although the specific mechanism(s) by which these agents reduce synovitis in RA remains unknown, antimalarials do produce anti-inflammatory activity by stabilizing lysosomal membranes, reducing phagocytic and chemotactic functions of polymorphonuclear leukocytes, and inhibiting prostaglandin formation. If an efficacious response is not obtained within six months, the agent is discontinued. The major toxicity of the antimalarials is their potential to deposit on the cornea, to produce macular pigmentation, or to result in field defects. Although emphasis has been placed upon these potential adverse reactions, the occurrence of visual impairment due to hydroxychloroquine is rare and can be prevented by routine ophthalmologic exams.

Gold salts are the standard disease-modifying therapeutic agents used in RA. Although the precise mode(s) of action in RA is unknown, these agents appear to alter macrophage function and complement metabolism. Two intramuscular forms of the agent are currently available: gold thioglucose and gold sodium thiomalate. The indication for initiating treatment with gold salts remains controversial. In general, the agents are more efficacious when begun early in the course of seropositive disease. In the absence of significant side effects, a total of 1 gm is given and the response to therapy is then assessed. If there is improvement in disease activity (Tables 100–1 and 100–2), therapy is maintained with an increasing time interval between injections. Since there are multiple potential adverse reactions to the gold salts, these agents should be carefully monitored for hematologic and urinary side effects at regular intervals.

Other chemotherapeutic agents are also utilized in the therapy of RA. These include penicillamine, methotrexate, azathioprine, and corticosteroids. Since these agents produce untoward side effects, it is necessary to monitor the blood count, differential, platelet count, and urinalysis twice monthly.

Corticosteroids are routinely used in both the acute and chronic management of RA. Although these agents are clearly beneficial in the therapy of an acute flare, their long-term use is not warranted, since steroids neither cure nor alter the natural course of the disease. In fact, the prolonged use of corticosteroids, even in small or "maintenance" doses, is fraught with numerous unwanted complications, including cataracts, osteopenia, myopathy, and accelerated atherosclerosis. Nevertheless, corticosteroids are indicated in the immediate therapy of rapidly progressive RA complicated by anorexia, weight loss, fever, anemia, leukopenia, vasculitis, pleuropericarditis, Felty's syndrome, and/or hypocomplementemia. Moreover, intra-articular corticosteroids are useful following arthrocentesis to quell the synovitis, reduce pain, and improve function.

REFERENCES

Cohen AJ, Brandt KD, Krey PB: Synovial fluid. In Cohen AS (ed): Laboratory Diagnostic Procedures in the Rheumatic Diseases. 2nd ed. Boston, Little, Brown & Co, 1975.
Greenberg PD, and Zvaifler NJ: Rheumatoid arthritis. In Cohen S, McCluskey R, and Ward P (eds): Mechanisms of Immunopathology. New York, John Wiley & Sons, 1979.
Hurd ER: Extraarticular manifestations of rheumatoid arthritis. Sem Arthritis Rheum 8:151, 1979.

101 SYSTEMIC LUPUS ERYTHEMATOSUS

Systemic lupus erythematosus (SLE) is an acute and chronic inflammatory process of unknown etiology which involves multiple organ systems. This disorder, which afflicts women eight times more frequently than men, predominantly strikes women during their childbearing years. While the general prevalence is approximately 1 in 2100, the disease is observed three times more often in black than white women.

There is a strikingly wide spectrum of disease activity in SLE. When the lesions are confined to the skin, the disorder has been previously termed discoid lupus erythematosus. Although this terminology is still in use, discoid LE is now regarded as a part of the broad spectrum of SLE. In contrast to this benign form of the disease, SLE can be a fulminant, debilitating, and life-threatening disease. Acute proliferative glomerulonephritis can be associated with severe hypertension and the rapid onset of end-stage renal failure, a cause of death. Other common causes of death include hemorrhage secondary to thrombocytopenia, nervous system involvement, and infection. With improved management during the past two decades, the 10-year survival rate is now greater than 85 per cent, and the quality of life has been vastly improved.

IMMUNOPATHOLOGY

Several distinct skin lesions have been observed in SLE. Among these, discoid lesions and vasculitis are commonly observed. In discoid lesions there is a characteristic vacuolar appearance to the dermoepidermal junction where immunoglobulin and complement can be deposited. Using immunofluorescence techniques, a band of granular deposits comprising IgG, IgA, IgM, and/or complement is found. This skin biopsy staining technique, the lupus band test, signifies the deposition of immune complexes in tissue, and the presence of IgG and C3 correlates with active systemic disease, particularly glomerulonephritis.

Vasculitis affects several organ systems in SLE. The presence of inflammation of the capillaries, arterioles, or venules of the skin is called leukocytoclastic vasculitis. Depending upon the age of the lesions, there is either a polymorphonuclear leukocytic or lymphocytic infiltrate of the vessel wall, fibrinoid necrosis, red blood cell extravasation, endothelial cell hypertrophy, interruption of the vessel wall, and deposition of immunoglobulins, complement, and fibrin.

CLINICAL COURSE

Both the clinical presentation and course of SLE are highly variable. Since SLE is a syndrome, not a specific disease entity, the disorder can present as symptoms and signs involving one or more major organ systems. Moreover, SLE can manifest as a single symptom that resolves spontaneously, not to be followed by another symptom for months or years, long after the initial ailment is forgotten. Such an insidious onset is common in SLE. By contrast, SLE can present precipitously de novo as a rapidly progressive, multisystem illness. The ARA Diagnostic and Therapeutic Criteria Committee have published revised criteria for the classification of SLE, which can be used by the clinician as a guide in establishing the diagnosis (Table 101–1).

Nonspecific constitutional symptoms often accompany disease activity in SLE. Skin lesions of SLE are among the commonest signs of the disease, occurring in 85 per cent of individuals. They include alopecia, painless oral ulcers, a discoid rash, photosensitive skin eruptions, and the classic butterfly rash.

Polyarthralgias and polyarthritis are the most common manifestations of SLE, occurring in 95 per cent of patients. A symmetric, nondeforming arthritis affecting the small joints of the hands, wrists, knees, and metatarsophalangeal joints occurs and, during early disease, is often confused with rheumatoid arthritis. The presence of prolonged morning stiffness in one half of patients, rheumatoid nodules (7 per cent), and rheumatoid factors (15 to 20 per cent) in persons with active disease often makes the distinction of SLE from RA difficult, especially in the absence of other distinguishing features of SLE.

Other musculoskeletal disorders also complicate SLE. Myalgias occur in up to one fourth of patients and tend to be unrelated to the degree of disease activity. In contrast to muscle aching, a true inflammation of muscles occasionally is observed in SLE. It is characterized by painless proximal muscle weakness and is clinically similar to idiopathic polymyositis. When SLE coexists with scleroderma and polymyositis, it is termed an overlap syndrome.

Renal disease occurs in approximately one half of patients with SLE. Usually presenting within the first 24 months of disease, the findings on urinalysis include proteinuria, microscopic hematuria, and cylindruria. The presence of red and white cell casts, proteinuria, and hematuria in the urine reflects active glomerulonephritis. The four principal types of glomerulonephritis—(1) minimal change, (2) focal proliferative, (3) diffuse proliferative, and (4) membranous glomerulonephritis—are considered in Chapter 33.

Polyserositis refers to inflammation of the serosal surfaces of the pericardium, thorax, and abdomen and is characterized by pain. Involvement of the pericardium can often be documented by the presence of a pericardial friction rub, echocardiogram, and electrocardiogram findings characteristic of pericarditis. Pericarditis is commonly associated with myocarditis, and this can lead to a transient or persistent tachyarrhythmia and electrocardiographic evidence of myocardial ischemia. Pleurisy and pleural effusion can result from inflammation of the pleura. Pleuritic pain can also be secondary to acute lupus pneumonitis, which occurs in fewer than 5 per cent of SLE patients. Diffuse abdominal pain and ascites reflect inflammation of the abdominal serosa. However, the pain of serositis must be differentiated from other causes of abdominal pain, especially mesenteric arteritis, acute pancreatitis due to pancreatic vasculitis, or occult perforation of a viscus due to corticosteroid therapy.

Hepatosplenomegaly and systemic adenopathy are commonly observed in SLE. Clinically significant liver disease has been regarded as unusual in SLE. However, there is a relationship between the symptoms of SLE and chronic active hepatitis, and this has long been known as "lupoid hepatitis." Although such patients have often not been included in studies of SLE, chronic active hepatitis should be considered in SLE patients with abnormal liver function studies.

The neuropsychiatric manifestations of SLE vary greatly. Psychosis and seizures can start at any time in the course of SLE. Vascular headaches tend to be associated with active disease, although milder forms are seen during periods of remission as well. Other neurologic disorders that may complicate SLE include CVA, chorea, cranial nerve palsies, peripheral neuropathies, transverse myelopathy, and aseptic meningitis. Although the intracranial arteries can exhibit a perivascular cellular infiltrate producing a vasculopathy, cerebral vasculitis is uncommon.

Raynaud's phenomenon of varying severity is observed in about one third of SLE patients. Only a small proportion of patients exhibit fixed Raynaud's phenomenon in warm surroundings or develop digital ulcers.

The relationship between SLE and pregnancy continues to be an important issue. Women with active SLE, especially glomerulonephritis, who become pregnant have an increased frequency of exacerbation of their disease as well as missed abortions, stillbirths, and fetal wastage. In addition, they more often have premature labor and delivery. Children born to mothers with SLE have an increased risk of congenital heart block, and this appears to be associated with the transplacental transfer of anti–SS-A. However, women with SLE in remission can have normal pregnancies and do not appear to have an increased rate

TABLE 101–1. 1982 REVISED CRITERIA FOR CLASSIFICATION OF SYSTEMIC LUPUS ERYTHEMATOSUS*

CRITERION	DEFINITION
1. Malar rash	Fixed erythema, flat or raised, over the malar eminences, tending to spare the nasolabial folds
2. Discoid rash	Erythematous raised patches with adherent keratotic scaling and follicular plugging; atrophic scarring may occur in older lesions
3. Photosensitivity	Skin rash as a result of unusual reaction to sunlight, by patient history or physician observation
4. Oral ulcers	Oral or nasopharyngeal ulceration, usually painless, observed by a physician
5. Arthritis	Nonerosive arthritis involving 2 or more peripheral joints, characterized by tenderness, swelling, or effusion
6. Serositis	a) Pleuritis—convincing history of pleuritic pain or rub heard by a physician or evidence of pleural effusion OR b) Pericarditis—documented by ECG or rub or evidence of pericardial effusion
7. Renal disorder	a) Persistent proteinuria greater than 0.5 gram per day or greater than 3 + if quantitation not performed OR b) Cellular casts—may be red cell, hemoglobin, granular, tubular, or mixed
8. Neurologic disorder	a) Seizures—in the absence of offending drugs or known metabolic derangements; e.g., uremia, ketoacidosis, or electrolyte imbalance OR b) Psychosis—in the absence of offending drugs or known metabolic derangements, e.g., uremia, ketoacidosis, or electrolyte imbalance
9. Hematologic disorder	a) Hemolytic anemia—with reticulocytosis OR b) Leukopenia—less than 4,000/mm³ total on 2 or more occasions OR c) Lymphopenia—less than 1,500/mm³ on 2 or more occasions OR d) Thrombocytopenia—less than 100,000/mm³ in the absence of offending drugs
10. Immunologic disorder	a) Positive LE cell preparation OR b) Anti-DNA: antibody to native DNA in abnormal titer OR c) Anti-Sm: presence of antibody to Sm nuclear antigen OR d) False-positive serologic test for syphilis known to be positive for at least 6 months and confirmed by *Treponema pallidum* immobilization or fluorescent treponemal antibody absorption test
11. Antinuclear antibody	An abnormal titer of antinuclear antibody by immunofluorescence or an equivalent assay at any point in time and in the absence of drugs known to be associated with "drug-induced lupus" syndrome

* The proposed classification is based on 11 criteria. For the purpose of identifying patients in clinical studies, a person shall be said to have systemic lupus erythematosus if any 4 or more of the 11 criteria are present, serially or simultaneously, during any interval of observation. (After Tan EM, Cohen AS, Fries JF, et al: The 1982 revised criteria for the classification of systemic lupus erythematosus. Arthritis Rheum 25:1271, 1982.)

of exacerbation of their disease nor of fetal wastage or stillbirths.

Drug-induced lupus is a disorder in which a pharmacologic agent induces the symptoms and signs of SLE over time. A list of the agents reported to be associated with an SLE-like syndrome is presented in Table 101–2. Although there is convincing evidence that certain drugs induce a lupus syndrome, the data for the remainder are speculative. Review of some cases diagnosed as drug-induced lupus suggests that a number of these patients had premorbid signs of SLE.

Hydralazine and procainamide are the prototype agents associated with a drug-induced lupus syndrome. The incidence of hydralazine-induced lupus in an unselected group of hypertensive patients was approximately 10 per cent and in patients taking procainamide long term 5 to 30 per cent. Hydralazine causes a syndrome characterized by fever, arthritis, erythematous skin rashes, pleurisy, leukopenia, hypergammaglobulinemia, a positive LE cell test, ANA, and a biological false-positive VDRL. Procainamide, considered the most potent inducer of the drug-induced lupus syndrome, is characterized by arthralgias or arthritis, pleuropericarditis (with or without effusions), rashes, pulmonary infiltrates, and ANA. In both types of drug-induced lupus syndrome, neurologic and renal disease are uncommon, and anti-nDNA and anti-Sm antibodies are absent. In general, withdrawal of the offending agents leads to resolution of the symptoms within days to weeks. However, the ANA can persist for months to years.

IMMUNOPATHOGENESIS

The mechanism by which the immune system is regulated by the presence of genetically determined cell surface molecules encoded by the major histocompatibility loci has been an area of intense interest and research. Since the prevalence of SLE in first-degree relatives of SLE probands is approximately 1.5 per cent and the concordance of SLE in monozygotic twins is about 70 per cent, there appears to be a genetic basis for SLE. The relationship between genetically determined complement component deficiencies and SLE also supports this hypothesis. An association clearly exists between SLE and the major histocompatibility complex. There is a significant increase in HLA-A1, B8, DR2, and DR3 antigens.

Both the cellular and humoral effector arms of the immune system are impaired in SLE. Several experimental approaches have identified a defect of suppressor T lymphocyte function during active SLE. Although the suppressor dysfunction improves with disease remission, a residual defect appears to persist even during remission. A disorder of helper T lymphocyte function has also been demonstrated. By contrast, there is exaggerated B cell activity in SLE characterized by the production of antibodies directed against numerous immunogens. One hypothesis to explain the hypergammaglobulinemia resulting from B cell

TABLE 101–2. DRUGS ASSOCIATED WITH A LUPUS-LIKE SYNDROME*

DEFINITE	POSSIBLE	UNLIKELY
Hydralazine	Anticonvulsants	Griseofulvin
Procainamide	Chlorpromazine	Phenylbutazone
Isoniazid	Methyldopa	Oral contraceptives
	Penicillamine	Gold salts
	Quinidine	Sulfonamides
	Propylthiouracil	Penicillin
	Practolol	
	Lithium carbonate	
	Nitrofurantoin	

* After Weinstein A: Drug-induced SLE. Prog Clin Immunol 4:1, 1980.

hyperactivity holds that impaired suppressor cells cannot regulate B cell function, and, in particular, fail to suppress autoantibody production by forbidden B cell clones.

Immune complexes play a central role in the inflammatory response in SLE. Upon deposition or in situ formation, antigen-antibody complexes induce the activation of the classic complement cascade, the release of various vasoactive peptides and anaphylotoxins, the ingress of polymorphonuclear leukocytes, and the aggregation of platelets. This inflammatory response may ultimately result in destruction of the vessel wall, thrombosis, ischemia, and end organ destruction.

TREATMENT

When the diagnosis of SLE is made, it is necessary to make a decision as to whether therapy is indicated. This decision rests largely on the degree of disease activity. The SLE patient who is asymptomatic, has no physical stigmata of active disease, but manifests certain abnormal laboratory studies may present a perplexing problem. Under these circumstances, the decision to treat depends upon the type of abnormal studies. Persistently low complement levels by themselves do not require therapy, whereas hemolytic anemia or thrombocytopenia does. In contrast, falling complement levels, rising titers of anti-nDNA, and a change in the urinary sediment suggesting active renal disease signify activation of the disease and demand a prompt therapeutic decision.

Several different drugs are utilized in the management of SLE. Aspirin and the nonsteroidal anti-inflammatory agents are indicated for the treatment of arthralgias or mild synovitis, pleurisy, headache, myalgia, and low-grade fever. Side effects include a modest rise in hepatic transaminases or deterioration in renal function studies, which are reversible with alteration of dosage.

Hydroxychloroquine, an antimalarial agent, has long been recognized to be effective in the treatment of arthralgias, arthritis, and skin disease in SLE. The major drawbacks to this agent are its slow onset of action (about three months) and potential ocular toxicity.

The use of adrenal corticosteroids in SLE has gained prominence because of their potent anti-inflammatory effect. Although the indications for initiating corticosteroids are imprecise, clinical, serologic, and biochemical evidence for enhanced disease activity constitutes a general guideline. The principal objective of corticosteroid therapy is control of the inflammatory response in order to prevent end organ damage and deterioration. High dose intravenous bolus therapy with methylprednisolone (1 gm/day for three consecutive days) has been efficacious in the therapy of poorly responsive glomerulonephritis.

The decision about when to taper the dosage of corticosteroids depends upon the patient's response to therapy. Improvement or resolution of symptoms and signs, a reduction of the anti-nDNA titer, and an increase of the complement levels toward normal concentrations constitute evidence of lessening disease activity. In general, corticosteroids are tapered slowly to prevent a flare of SLE. At a dosage of approximately 10 to 12.5 mg/day, disease activity may break through. Such an occurrence, far from uncommon, may re-

quire readjustment of the dosage upward, a time interval to re-establish control, and an even slower decrement in dosage. In fact, at a level of 10 mg/day, tapering by 1 mg weekly or more slowly may be necessary.

Lupus nephritis may progress, and there can be continuous deterioration of kidney function despite appropriate corticosteroid therapy. Under these circumstances immunosuppressive agents should be considered. Evidence now indicates that these agents, which principally include azathioprine and cyclophosphamide, when combined with steroids, significantly improve outcome of therapy by preventing further end organ destruction.

REFERENCES

Schur PH: The Clinical Management of Systemic Lupus Erythematosus. New York, Grune and Stratton, 1983.

Tan EM, Cohen AS, Fries JF, et al: The 1982 revised criteria for the classification of systemic lupus erythematosus. Arthritis Rheum 25:1271, 1982.

102 SJÖGREN'S SYNDROME

Sjögren's syndrome is a chronic connective tissue disorder characterized by inflammation of the exocrine glands, particularly the salivary and lacrimal glands. The disease is categorized as (a) the primary form, or (b) the secondary form, which is commonly associated with RA, SLE, or, less commonly, other connective tissue disorders. The combination of xerophthalmia and xerostomia is referred to as the sicca complex. Keratoconjunctivitis sicca refers to loss of integrity of the corneal epithelium due to dessication. The diagnostic criteria for Sjögren's syndrome are summarized in Table 102–1.

CLINICAL FEATURES

Round cell infiltration of the lacrimal and salivary glands produces insidious destruction of glandular tissue, resulting in the sicca complex. There is dryness of the eyes due to decreased and

altered tear production, giving the sensation of grittiness or of the presence of a foreign body. With time, there is variable conjunctival injection, reduced visual acuity, and photosensitivity. Prolonged dessication leads to the development of erosions and sloughing of the corneal epithelium (filamentary keratitis), as demonstrated by rose bengal staining and slit lamp examination. The extent of xerostomia appears to be more variable, even in the presence of striking xerophthalmia. The frequency of dental caries is increased due to diminution of the volume of saliva, which possesses antibacterial factors.

Dryness of other mucosal surfaces as a result of the same inflammatory response is common. In the respiratory tract there may be epistaxis, dysphonia, bronchitis, or pneumonia. Inspissation of secretions in the eustachian tubes leads to obstruction, chronic otitis media, and hearing impairments. Mucosal gland involvement of the gastrointestinal tract produces dysphagia, reduced gastric acid output, constipation, and pancreatic insufficiency. Dyspareunia may occur due to vaginal dryness.

Several prominent extraglandular features can complicate the course of Sjögren's syndrome. Renal tubular acidosis results from infiltrative interstitial nephropathy. Both peripheral and cranial neuropathy have been attributed to vasculitis of the vasa nervorum. Other associated neuro-

TABLE 102–1. DIAGNOSITC CRITERIA OF SJÖGREN'S SYNDROME*

Keratoconjunctivitis sicca
Labial gland biopsy, focus score ≥1
Associated connective tissue or lymphoproliferative disorder

* After Strand V, and Talal N: Advances in the diagnosis and concept of Sjögren's syndrome (autoimmune exocrinopathy). Bull Rheum Dis 30:1046, 1979–80.

TABLE 102–2. DISORDERS ASSOCIATED WITH SJÖGREN'S SYNDROME

Rheumatoid arthritis
Systemic lupus erythematosus
Progressive systemic sclerosis
Overlap syndrome
Polymyositis/dermatomyositis
Graft-versus-host disease
Malignant lymphoma
Chronic Hashimoto's thyroiditis
Chronic active hepatitis
Biliary cirrhosis
Grave's disease
Premature ovarian failure
Celiac disease
Dermatitis herpetiformis
Myasthenia gravis
Pemphigus
Lipodystrophy

muscular disorders include myopathy, polymyositis, and cranial vasculitis. Dyspnea may be the presenting symptom of underlying diffuse interstitial pneumonitis due to lymphocytic infiltration. An obstructive ventilatory defect has been attributed to peribronchial lymphocytic infiltration. Nonthrombocytopenic purpura of the dependent regions is associated with a polyclonal hypergammaglobulinemia. Raynaud's phenomenon occurs in about one fifth of patients. Chronic Hashimoto's thyroiditis is present in a small proportion of patients with Sjögren's syndrome. Also, hepatomegaly, chronic active hepatitis, biliary cirrhosis, and adult celiac disease have been occasionally observed with Sjögren's syndrome. Table 102–2 lists disorders associated with Sjögren's syndrome.

Systemic lymphadenopathy may reflect benign lymphatic hyperplasia, a pseudolymphoma, or frank lymphoma. Although these can occur early in the course of Sjögren's syndrome, death due to lymphoma often ensues after years of illness. Although the histologic type of the lymphoma is variable, the lymphoma is of B cell origin. Other lymphoproliferative disorders observed with Sjögren's syndrome include Waldenström's macroglobulinemia and myeloma. Markers of increased risk of malignancy include persistent parotid swelling, systemic lymphadenopathy, splenomegaly, and a progressive decrement of a previously elevated class of immunoglobulin and/or rheumatoid factor.

DIAGNOSIS

The diagnosis of Sjögren's syndrome is based upon the results of Schirmer's filter paper test, ophthalmologic exam, and minor salivary gland biopsy. Xerophthalmia is confirmed by the wetting of 5 mm or less of filter paper in 5 minutes in an unanesthetized eye. The demonstration of superficial corneal erosions by rose bengal staining and filamentory keratitis by slit lamp examination indicates more advanced keratoconjunctivitis sicca.

Biopsy of the minor salivary glands of the lower lip in Sjögren's syndrome demonstrates lymphocytic infiltration of the acinar glands and progressive destruction of glandular tissue. The extent of inflammation can be quantitatively scored using the "focus score." Each aggregate of 50 or more lymphocytes equals a focus, and the number of foci per 4 sq mm of tissue represents the focus score. A score of greater than 1 is compatible with Sjögren's syndrome.

Sjögren's syndrome appears to exhibit a genetic basis. Immunogenetic studies have identified an excess of the HLA antigens B8, DR3, and MT2 (DRw52). The relationship between these B cell alloantigens and DR3 and Sjögren's syndrome suggests that the development and expression of disease is regulated, in part, by immune response genes.

Autoantibodies are commonly found in both primary and secondary Sjögren's syndrome. Antinuclear antibodies are present in up to 80 per cent of persons. IgM rheumatoid factor is found in 75 to 90 per cent. Antibodies to SS-A occur in 50 to 75 per cent in primary Sjögren's syndrome, in 70 to 85 per cent of SLE with Sjögren's syndrome, and in 30 to 40 per cent of patients with SLE overall. Antibodies to SS-B occur in 50 to 60 per cent of Sjögren's syndrome patients, and in only 10 per cent of SLE patients without Sjögren's syndrome.

THERAPY

The treatment of Sjögren's syndrome is directed at the alleviation of symptoms and complications of xerophthalmia and xerostomia. Xerophthalmia can be treated with artificial tears or with surgical punctal occlusion. Staphylococcal blepharitis should be immediately treated with topical or, if necessary, systemic antibiotics. Xerostomia is managed by maintaining oral hydration and the liberal use of sialogogues. Bronchopulmonary infections require both supportive regimens and antibiotics. Dyspareunia is treatable with commercial water-soluble vaginal lubricants. The use of corticosteroids or immunosuppressive agents is confined to more severe disease of the kidneys or bronchopulmonary tract and systemic vasculitis.

REFERENCES

Strand V, and Talal N: Advances in the diagnosis and concept of Sjögren's syndrome (autoimmune exocrinopathy). Bull Rheum Dis 30:1046, 1979–80.
Talal N: Sjögren's syndrome and connective tissue disease with other immunologic disorders. In McCarty DJ (ed): Arthritis and Allied Conditions. Philadelphia, Lea and Febiger, 1985, p 1037.

103 POLYMYOSITIS AND DERMATOMYOSITIS

Polymyositis (PM) and dermatomyositis (DM) are inflammatory myopathies of striated muscle of unknown etiology. Although the onset of disease can occur in any age group, the clinical course of these disorders in childhood differs from that in adulthood. Women are afflicted twice as often as men. The incidence in the general population has been estimated to be between 1:200,000 and 1:280,000 per year.

CLASSIFICATION

A classification has been devised for PM and DM based upon their association with other diseases (Table 103–1).

CLINICAL COURSE

There is no single presentation or course that typifies either PM or DM. The majority of persons with PM typically manifest proximal muscle weakness. In dermatomyositis, both the skin rash and proximal muscle weakness occur early in the course. The skin rash consists of a scaly, erythematous eruption over the PIP and MCP joints (Gottron's sign), elbows, knees, medial maleoli, face, and elsewhere. Involvement of the upper eyelids, appearing as a dusky lilac suffusion, is termed a heliotrope rash. Both disorders may be punctuated by spontaneous exacerbations and remissions. Moreover, either disorder can present precipitously with rapid loss of muscle strength leading to acute respiratory distress and death.

When these inflammatory myopathies are associated with another connective tissue disorder, it is designated an overlap syndrome. Interestingly, the ratio of females to males affected increases to 9:1. In addition, PM occurs three times more often than DM. The associated disorders include, in descending order of frequency, scleroderma, SLE, and RA. Although relatively uncommon in PM or DM alone, arthralgias, Raynaud's phenomenon, and myalgias are actually more common than proximal muscle weakness in the overlap syndrome.

The occurrence of malignancy with inflammatory myopathy is relatively uncommon (8.5 per cent) but increases with age. When present, about two thirds of malignancies coexist with dermatomyositis. Carcinomas of the breast, lung, ovaries, colon, endometrium, prostate, and stomach are the leading tumors. In 70 per cent the myositis precedes the diagnosis of malignancy by nearly two years. It is currently recommended that a search for malignancy be conducted in persons with PM or DM over age 50 years.

Cardiopulmonary manifestations include nonspecific ST-T wave changes (23 per cent), arrhythmias (6 per cent), altered Q waves (6 per cent), bundle branch block (5 per cent), congestive heart failure (3.3 per cent), heart block (2.2 per cent), and restrictive lung disease (20 per cent).

The leading cause of death in these disorders is metastatic malignant disease followed by sepsis. Other causes include profound muscle weakness and cardiovascular failure.

LABORATORY FINDINGS

The CPK is the most reliable serum enzyme and correlates with the activity of disease. The occurrence of a normal CPK in the presence of active myositis is exceedingly uncommon (< 2 per cent). A normal enzyme level may be accounted for by advanced muscle atrophy and loss of muscle mass. ANA is present in 25 per cent and the rheumatoid factor in up to 40 per cent. The sedimentation rate correlates poorly with disease activity and the clinical course. The triad of EMG findings includes (a) small-amplitude, short-duration polyphasic motor unit potentials; (b) fibrillations, positive sharp waves, and insertional irritability; and (c) bizarre, high-frequency discharges. A normal EMG in the presence of active disease is uncommon (10.7 per cent).

The muscle biopsy is an essential component in confirming the clinical diagnosis of PM or DM. The commonest histopathologic abnormality is degeneration of muscle fibers. Other pathologic findings include an inflammatory infiltrate, centralization of nuclei, regeneration, and interstitial fibrosis.

THERAPY

Treatment of PM or DM includes physical therapy, corticosteroids, and, if indicated, immunosuppressive agents. An intensive course of physical and occupational therapy improves muscle strength and tonus and assists in activities of daily living once muscle inflammation is suppressed.

The initial dosage of corticosteroids depends

TABLE 103–1. CLASSIFICATION OF POLYMYOSITIS AND DERMATOMYOSITIS*

GROUP	DESCRIPTION
1	Primary idiopathic polymyositis
2	Primary idiopathic dermatomyositis
3	Dermatomyositis or polymyositis associated with neoplasia
4	Childhood dermatomyositis or polymyositis associated with vasculitis
5	Polymyositis or dermatomyositis associated with connective tissue disorder (overlap group)

* After Bohan A, Peter J, Bowman R, and Pearson C: A computer-assisted analysis of 153 patients with polymyositis and dermatomyositis. Medicine 56:255, 1977.

upon the severity of disease but often is the equivalent of 60 mg of prednisone. Approximately three quarters of patients normalize the CPK within 57 to 102 days. Muscle strength progressively improves with this regimen. The dosage of corticosteroids is tapered on the basis of clinical and biochemical evidence of resolution of disease activity.

An indication for the addition of immunosuppressive therapy is failure of therapy with corticosteroids alone within a four- to six-week interval. The addition of an immunosuppressive agent often provides a "steroid-sparing effect," allowing the daily corticosteroid dosage to be reduced to lower levels. The agents of choice include methotrexate and azathioprine. It is often necessary to maintain long-term therapy with corticosteroids and/or immunosuppressive agents to control disease activity.

PROGNOSIS

The prognosis of PM and DM has improved substantially with the introduction of corticosteroid and immunosuppressive agents. A recent study demonstrated a survival rate of 87 to 91 per cent with the exception of malignancy associated with myositis (46 per cent) over a 15-year interval.

REFERENCES

Kagen L: Polymyositis/dermatomyositis. In McCarty DJ (ed): Arthritis and Allied Conditions. 10th ed. Philadelphia, Lea and Febiger, 1985, p 971.
Messner RP: Dermatomyositis and polymyositis. In Wyngaarden JB, and Smith LH Jr (eds): Cecil Textbook of Medicine. 17th ed. Philadelphia, WB Saunders Co, 1985, p 1947.

PROGRESSIVE SYSTEMIC SCLEROSIS (SCLERODERMA)

104

Progressive systemic sclerosis (PSS) is characterized by (a) inflammation, (b) fibrosis, and (c) degeneration of the integument. These pathologic alterations are associated with similar changes and prominent vascular lesions in the gastrointestinal tract, synovium, heart, lung, and kidneys. As a result of progression of these lesions, there is thickening (collagenous), tightening and induration (sclerosis) of the skin, and destruction of the normal architecture of visceral organs, culminating in death due to hypertensive renal disease, malabsorption and cachexia, heart failure, or pulmonary disease.

CLINICAL FEATURES

PSS is a disorder of indeterminate etiology which affects women three times more frequently than men. The onset of disease ranges between the third and fifth decades.

Several sequential phases of the disorder occur in the integument over time. The initial phase, characterized by bilateral, painless pitting edema of the hands, forearms, legs and feet, generally extends over a few weeks to several months. The swollen fingers appear tight and demonstrate variable but limited function. During the second phase, the edema is gradually adsorbed, leaving indurated skin. The integument is thickened, tight, and inelastic. This represents the well-known sclerodermatous stage. The third phase is characterized by a taut and shiny appearance. A melanotic hyperpigmentation often develops in a patchy distribution in the affected areas. There is

loss of the skin folds, creases, and hair of the fingers. The face takes on the classic appearance of the Mauskof (mouse-head), in which there are pursed lips, bitemporal muscle atrophy, loss of subcutaneous tissue and muscle of the face and neck, and a taut and shiny skin of the malar region and forehead. Other prominent changes in the skin include calcinosis circumscripta (subcutaneous calcifications) and telangiectasias of the fingers, face, lips, and forearms. Raynaud's phenomenon is present in virtually all persons with PSS. This phenomenon is discussed in a following chapter.

Rheumatic symptoms occur commonly in PSS. Although polyarthralgias are a frequent accompaniment of PSS, active synovitis leading to joint effusions, limitation of range of motion, and severe flexion contractures can present a difficult management problem. Radiographs demonstrate bony resorption of the tufts of the terminal phalanges and subcutaneous calcinosis. Severe, relentless disease often leads to autoamputation of digit(s).

A prominent loss of subcutaneous tissue and muscle bulk steadily progresses over time with consequent weight loss. The myopathy of PSS is the result of an inflammatory myositis indistinguishable from polymyositis and is often referred to as sclerodermatomyositis.

Cardiovascular disorders may complicate the course of PSS. Progressive fibrosis of the myocardium eventually results in the development of a cardiomyopathy. In addition, fibrosis of the conducting pathways can lead to arrhythmias and conduction disturbances. Other disorders include pulmonary arterial hypertension, pericarditis, and pericardial effusions.

Several pulmonary complications of PSS can lead to pulmonary insufficiency and death. Chest radiographs demonstrate a reticular or reticulonodular pattern of interstitial fibrosis. The earliest and most sensitive indicator of pulmonary involvement is a reduced diffusing capacity of carbon monoxide. Progressive diminution of the diffusing capacity with time often predicts gradual progression of the restrictive ventilatory defect.

The gastrointestinal tract is a major target organ in PSS. Esophageal dysfunction may be asymptomatic or be manifested by dysphagia, esophagitis, and/or esophageal reflux. Radiographic visualization by barium contrast and esophageal motility studies often demonstrates disordered or absent motility. There may be marked dilatation of the inferior two thirds of the esophagus and strictures may result from chronic reflux esophagitis, ulceration, and healing by fibrosis. Histopathology of the esophagus reveals loss of smooth muscle and increased collagen deposition in the lamina propria and submucosa. Similar histopathologic alterations elsewhere in the gastrointestinal tract result in reduced motility, causing bacterial overgrowth that leads to malabsorption, weight loss, and inanition. Classic radiographic findings on barium contrast studies include the loop sign (dilatation of the second and third segments of the duodenum due to atony) and widemouth diverticula of the large bowel (due to atrophy of the muscularis).

Progressive involvement of the kidneys, leading to severe hypertension, renal failure, and death, is a common sequence of events in PSS. Often precipitous and unheralded by prior clinical renal disease, the hypertension can result in encephalopathy and rapid, irreversible renal failure associated with markedly elevated renin levels. Histopathology of the kidney demonstrates arteriolar lesions characterized by intimal hyperplasia, fibrinoid necrosis of the arcuate and interlobular vessels, and infarction. Prior to the recent availability of the angiotensin-converting enzyme inhibitor, captopril, the outlook for patients developing scleroderma hypertensive crises was poor.

LABORATORY FINDINGS

Although no laboratory tests are specific for PSS, several abnormalities can be observed. Anemias occur owing to autoimmune hemolytic mechanisms, a microangiopathic process, or chronic disease. Hypertensive renal disease results in proteinuria, cylindruria, and microscopic hematuria.

Antinuclear antibodies exhibiting speckled or nucleolar patterns occur in more than 65 per cent of PSS patients. In particular, autoantibodies directed against the Scl-70 nonhistone nuclear protein occur in 15 to 20 per cent of patients and are regarded as a marker for PSS.

VARIANTS OF PSS

Disorders that manifest certain clinical stigmata of PSS are now well recognized and can be properly termed PSS variants. CREST syndrome refers to calcinosis, Raynaud's phenomenon, esophageal dysfunction, sclerodactyly, and telangiectasia. It is distinguished by cutaneous thickening, confined to the fingers, slow evolution over decades, lack of visceral involvement, and autoantibodies to centromere in 70 to 90 per cent of patients. In contrast to PSS, the early edematous phase characterized by swollen fingers can persist for prolonged intervals in CREST. The calcium deposits may be more diffuse and larger, and the telangiectasia may appear on the face and trunk as well as the extremities. Raynaud's phenomenon is a prominent sign of CREST. Bony erosions leading to dissolution of the tufts or, in more severe cases, the phalanges can complicate the course of CREST. Moreover, the pulmonary hypertension observed in long-standing CREST can be more severe than that of PSS, owing to marked sclerosis of small pulmonary arteries often unassociated with interstitial fibrosis. Although hepatic parenchymal disease is rare in CREST, biliary cirrhosis is found in some women. Cranial neuropathies and sensory neuropathies, especially involving the trigeminal nerve, are more commonly observed in CREST than PSS. When compared with PSS, CREST patients enjoy a relatively benign prognosis.

Linear scleroderma is a localized form of the disease that usually develops during childhood and is characterized by a band of sclerosis of one or more extremities or in the frontoparietal region of the forehead and scalp (scleroderma en coup de sabre). Involvement of the face and scalp can result in ipsilateral hemiatrophy of the face. Linear scleroderma can also co-exist with morphea and may induce an unusual form of hyperostosis (melorheostosis). A nonerosive arthritis of the fingers is occasionally observed. However, visceral involvement does not occur, nor is there a transition to PSS.

Finally, a newly recognized scleroderma-like disorder characterized by induration and inflammation of the fascia has been designated diffuse fasciitis with eosinophilia. The hands, forearms, legs, and feet are predominantly affected; however, over time, the face and trunk can also become involved. During the formative stage of eosinophilic fasciitis, peripheral eosinophilia and a polyclonal hypergammaglobulinemia are often observed. Corticosteroids reduce the symptoms, eliminate the eosinophilia, and reverse the fascial thickening, in striking contrast to their ineffectiveness in PSS.

TREATMENT

Although no therapy is available that can induce remission of the skin and visceral manifestations of PSS, several different measures are available that provide partial relief of symptoms and control end organ damage. The more recent availability of effective antihypertensive agents has resulted in improved control of hypertensive crises and stabilization of renal function. Hypertension should be aggressively and promptly treated. Moreover, there is evidence that control of blood pressure in some patients has resulted in reduction of skin thickening, lending support to the hypothesis that a defective microcirculation plays a role in the pathogenesis of PSS. Because of its inhibition of angiotensin-converting enzyme and the reduction of renin, captopril is the agent of choice in the hypertensive crises due to scleroderma kidney.

The use of corticosteroids in PSS has yielded disappointing results. In general, corticosteroids are reserved for use in controlling the myopathy or signs associated with the overlap syndrome.

REFERENCES

Medsger TA Jr: Systemic sclerosis (scleroderma), eosinophilic fasciitis, and calcinosis. In McCarty DJ (ed): Arthritis and Allied Conditions. 10th ed. Philadelphia, Lea and Febiger, 1985, p 994.
Rodnan G, Myerowitz R, and Justh G: Morphologic changes in the digital arteries of patients with progressive systemic sclerosis (scleroderma) and Raynaud's phenomenon. Medicine 59:393, 1980.

OVERLAP SYNDROME 105

The overlap syndrome, also designated mixed connective tissue disease, refers to the concurrent expression of selected symptoms and signs of polymyositis (PM), SLE, and PSS in a single individual. Although the overlap syndrome has been observed in virtually all age ranges, it occurs most commonly in women during the fourth decade.

CLINICAL FEATURES

Like SLE and RA, the overlap syndrome often develops insidiously over a prolonged period. Therefore, it is not until a group of findings is recognized by the physician that the diagnosis is entertained. The most common features of the syndrome are listed in Table 105–1. In general, any of the features described in SLE, PSS, and polymyositis may be found in such patients.

Clinically significant renal disease is uncommon in the overlap syndrome (Table 105–1). Proteinuria and microscopic hematuria have led to kidney biopsies, which usually demonstrate minimal change disease of the mesangium. Diffuse membranous or membranoproliferative glomerulonephritis similar to that observed in SLE is rare.

LABORATORY FEATURES

Laboratory abnormalities found in SLE, PSS, and polymyositis are variably found in patients with the overlap syndrome. Antinuclear antibodies exhibiting a speckled immunofluorescent pattern directed against nuclear ribonucleoprotein (RNP) are often present. The titers of antibody are characteristically high and persist during periods when disease is quiescent.

TREATMENT

The therapy of the overlap syndrome combines supportive and medical regimens. Considering the wide range of potential stigmata that can occur in each patient, it is apparent that the therapeutic regimen should be tailored to the individual and that it should be flexible should new manifestations develop.

REFERENCE

Sharp GC, and Singsen BH: Mixed connective tissue disease. In McCarty DJ (ed): Arthritis and Allied Conditions. 10th ed. Philadelphia, Lea and Febiger, 1985, p 962.

TABLE 105–1. CLINICAL FEATURES OF OVERLAP SYNDROME*

SIGN	FREQUENCY (%)
Polyarthralgia/polyarthritis	95
Raynaud's phenomenon	85
Esophageal dysmotility	67
Decreased pulmonary diffusing capacity	67
Swollen hands	66
Myositis	63
Lymphadenopathy	39
Skin rash	38
Sclerodermatous change	33
Fever	33
Serositis	27
Splenomegaly	19
Hepatomegaly	15
Neurologic abnormalities	10
Sicca complex	7
Hashimoto's thyroiditis	6
Renal disease, definite or possible	5

* After Sharp GC: Mixed connective tissue disease. Bull Rheum Dis 25:828, 1975.

THE VASCULITIDES

The term vasculitis refers to inflammation of a blood vessel. When the inflammation specifically involves only arterial vessels, it is designated arteritis. Similarly, an inflammatory response of a dermal venule is a venulitis. Often, vasculitis is described as necrotizing when there is obliteration of the vessel by the byproducts of inflammation, resulting in local thrombosis, hemorrhage, and infarction.

CLASSIFICATION OF THE VASCULITIDES

The vasculitides are classified anatomically based upon the predominant size and distribution of the affected vessel. Although the concept of the clinical syndromes developed from the detailed elucidation of the histopathology, the size of the involved vessel does not necessarily dictate the clinical syndrome. For example, medium muscular arteries are involved in polyarteritis nodosa, allergic granulomatosis, and Wegener's granulomatosis. Despite this overlap, the classification of the vasculitides presented in Table 106–1 is clinically useful.

IMMUNOPATHOGENESIS

Although the precise immunopathogenesis of the vasculitides remains incompletely understood, the fundamental event that triggers an inflammatory response of vessels appears to be the deposition or in situ formation of antigen-antibody complexes. In humans, circulating immune complexes of varying size and capability of binding complement have been isolated from individuals with different clinical vasculitic disorders. Moreover, immunofluorescent studies of biopsied tissue have conclusively demonstrated the presence of immunoglobulins and complement in the vessel wall. The finding of the hepatitis B surface antigen and antibody in the serum as well as the hepatitis B surface antigen, immunoglobulin, and complement in the vessel walls of individuals with polyarteritis nodosa suggests that the hepatitis B virion may be directly involved in the pathogenesis of this disorder. Yet, despite the presence of the hepatitis B surface antigen in polyarteritis nodosa and native DNA in systemic lupus erythematosus as two putative antigens, the identification of the antigens comprising the vast array of circulating immune complexes is yet to be elucidated.

HYPERSENSITIVITY ANGIITIS

Hypersensitivity angiitis is the most common form of vasculitis and is usually localized to the integument. It is characterized by infiltration of the dermal arterioles, capillaries, and/or venules with either polymorphonuclear or mononuclear leukocytes. Pathologically, there is infiltration of the vessel wall, leukocytoclasis, red blood cell extravasation, thrombosis of the vessel lumen, and fibrinoid necrosis. Thus, this process is often referred to as a necrotizing leukocytoclastic vasculitis.

The distinctive dermal lesions of hypersensitivity angiitis are purpuric papules and urticaria. Other types of cutaneous lesions associated with this form of vasculitis include infarcts, hemorrhagic or nonhemorrhagic bullae, and superficial erosions. The lesions of cutaneous vasculitis usually appear first on the lower extremities as erythematous macules that evolve into *palpable purpura*. Although the lesions preferentially concentrate in the dependent regions inferior to the knees, a similar process can be observed less often on the upper extremities, particularly on the fingers.

There are no specific laboratory tests that identify cutaneous vasculitis. The ESR can be either normal or elevated. Similarly, the total hemolytic complement can be normal or depressed. Circulating immune complexes can be detected, usually in low concentrations. The hepatitis B surface antigen and antibody are absent. Skin biopsy can confirm the diagnosis of cutaneous vasculitis.

Certain discrete disorders exhibit a cutaneous necrotizing vasculitis. *Henoch-Schönlein purpura*, also referred to as anaphylactoid purpura, is a hypersensitivity vasculitis characterized by fever, abdominal pain, nonthrombocytopenic purpura, arthralgia, and renal disease. The classic triad of purpura, arthritis, and abdominal pain occurs in about 80 per cent of patients. Although the disorder can afflict persons of any age, children and young adults are most commonly affected, the peak age being four to eight years. The disease occurs most often in the spring, and may be preceded by an upper respiratory tract infection. Although the average duration of disease is 6 to 16 weeks, 5 to 10 per cent of persons who recover will relapse with renal disease characterized by glomerulonephritis.

Mural vasculitis of the gastrointestinal tract can result in colicky abdominal pain, intestinal bleeding, obstruction, infarction, intussusception, or perforation. The glomerulonephritis of Henoch-Schönlein purpura is usually self-limited but can progress to fatal renal failure or nephrotic syn-

TABLE 106–1. CLASSIFICATION OF VASCULITIS*

Hypersensitivity angiitis
Allergic granulomatosis
Wegener's granulomatosis
Polyarteritis nodosa
Giant cell (cranial, temporal) arteritis

* After Zeek PM: Periarteritis nodosa: A critical review. Am J Clin Pathol 22:777, 1952.

drome. Immunofluorescence studies have demonstrated the deposition of immunoglobulin and complement in both the kidneys and cutaneous vessels. Serum complement levels are ordinarily normal in Henoch-Schönlein purpura. However, the serum IgA level may be elevated, and IgA is often deposited in the skin and kidney.

A second disorder characterized by hypersensitivity vasculitis is a syndrome of arthralgia, purpura, weakness, and mixed cryoglobulinemia termed *essential mixed cryoglobulinemia*. There are recurrent bouts of palpable purpura of the lower extremities, hepatosplenomegaly, lymphadenopathy, and polyarthralgias. A diffuse proliferative glomerulonephritis may lead to terminal renal failure. The laboratory findings include a moderate anemia, IgM rheumatoid factors, ANA, hypocomplementemia, and cryoglobulins containing IgG and IgM. Certain autoimmune and neoplastic disorders have been associated with this syndrome: lymphoma, renal tubular acidosis, Sjögren's syndrome, rheumatoid arthritis, thyroiditis, and primary biliary cirrhosis.

Hypersensitivity vasculitis, characterized pathologically as either an arteriolitis or venulitis, can also be associated with drug reactions, bacterial infections (i.e., streptococcal), serum sickness, subacute bacterial endocarditis, chronic active hepatitis, ulcerative colitis, Sjögren's syndrome, retroperitoneal fibrosis, and Goodpasture's syndrome.

POLYARTERITIS NODOSA

Polyarteritis nodosa is a vasculitis involving primarily the medium muscular arteries, and to a lesser extent, small muscular arteries. Although the disease principally affects males of middle age, it can occur in any age group of both sexes.

The kidneys are the most commonly involved organ system. Inflammation of the arcuate arteries as well as other medium-size vessels may or may not result in segmental aneurysmal dilatations. A rapidly progressive, necrotizing glomerulonephritis can lead to the sudden onset of severe hypertension, nephrotic syndrome, and renal failure. Spontaneous rupture of aneurysms can result in peritoneal hemorrhage or a perinephric hematoma.

The heart becomes involved during polyarteritis nodosa in approximately 70 per cent of patients. Coronary arteritis can produce angina pectoris or frank myocardial infarction. Pericarditis, often diagnosed post mortem, is another source of retrosternal chest pain.

Polyarteritis nodosa also involves the gastrointestinal tract in about 65 per cent of patients, causing abdominal pain, intestinal bleeding, obstruction, or perforation. Rupture of mesenteric aneurysms can lead to retroperitoneal hemorrhage, hypovolemic shock, and death.

Neurologic involvement contributes significantly to the morbidity of the disease in about 60 per cent of patients. Disorders of the peripheral nervous system are attributable to arteritis of the vasa nervorum and ultimate occlusion. The peripheral neuropathies include mononeuritis multiplex, distal sensorimotor polyneuropathy, cutaneous neuropathy, and extensive mononeuritis. Mononeuritis multiplex is characterized by paresthesias, pain, weakness, and sensory loss of the affected limb due to infarction of several peripheral nerves.

Vasculitis of the central nervous system (CNS) in polyarteritis nodosa is estimated to occur in 20 to 40 per cent of cases. Encephalopathy secondary to severe hypertension and/or primary neuronal dysfunction produces a global cognitive disorder. Vasculitis affecting different anatomical structures of the CNS presents as focal or multifocal defects in function of the brain or spinal cord. Such defects can lead to seizures and hemorrhagic or ischemic strokes.

Polyarteritis nodosa affects the integument in only 5 to 15 per cent of patients. The commonest sign of skin involvement is nodules of the legs or, less commonly, the arms. These nodules, which measure 0.5 to 1.0 cm, pulsate and are painful. Livedo reticularis and peripheral gangrene also occur.

The laboratory findings of polyarteritis nodosa often reflect the presence of a severe systemic inflammation. The erythrocyte sedimentation rate, serum immunoglobulin levels, C-reactive protein, white blood cell count, and platelet count are all frequently elevated. The presence of anemia may be due to blood loss or renal failure. Microscopic hematuria, cylindruria, and proteinuria result from glomerulonephritis. Hypocomplementemia may be present, but the ANA and rheumatoid factor are absent. Thirty per cent exhibit hepatitis B surface antigenemia. The cerebrospinal fluid is normal unless there has been a subarachnoid hemorrhage.

The definitive diagnosis necessitates biopsy of an affected organ, such as the skin, muscle, testis, sural nerve, or kidney. Angiography of the renal, hepatic, and mesenteric arteries is often performed to seek evidence of aneurysmal formation and/or tapering and "cut-offs" of vessels due to vasculitis. However, the absence of aneurysms does not exclude the diagnosis of polyarteritis. If CNS vasculitis is suspected, angiography will also be necessary, since neither the EEG nor CT scan provides sufficient evidence to formulate a diagnosis.

ALLERGIC GRANULOMATOUS VASCULITIS OF CHURG AND STRAUSS

The Churg-Strauss syndrome is characterized by (a) hypereosinophilia, (b) allergic rhinitis and/or asthma, and (c) a systemic vasculitis of the medium and small muscular arteries involving two or more extrapulmonary sites.

Three phases of the disease have been identified. A prodromal period may exist over many years during which the predominant clinical findings are atopic. Allergic rhinitis usually precedes the onset of extrinsic asthma. During the second phase, hypereosinophilia and eosinophilic tissue infiltration occur. The final phase is characterized by the development of a systemic necrotizing vasculitis.

Asthma occurs in all cases of Churg-Strauss syndrome and is therefore regarded as a criterion for the diagnosis. At the onset of vasculitis, asthma may remit or exacerbate. Hypereosinophilia and tissue infiltration with eosinophils is a second criterion of the Churg-Strauss syndrome. Treatment with corticosteroids usually abolishes the eosinophilia.

The vasculitis of Churg-Strauss syndrome involves both the medium and smaller muscular arteries, and, in this way, can be similar to Wegener's granulomatosis and PAN with involvement of cardiac, renal, gastrointestinal, or nervous systems. The onset of vasculitis may be preceded by constitutional symptoms, weight loss, and fever.

The treatment of Churg-Strauss syndrome is similar to that of the other systemic necrotizing vasculitides. The Churg-Strauss vasculitis generally responds readily to high-dose coricosteroids (i.e., prednisone, 60 mg per day). A dramatic drop in the eosinophil count, the white blood cell count, and ESR documents this response. Less often, the disease responds only partially, and it becomes necessary to add cyclophosphamide.

WEGENER'S GRANULOMATOSIS

Wegener's granulomatosis is a systemic necrotizing vasculitis primarily involving the medium and small muscular arteries. It is characterized by (a) granulomatous vasculitis of the upper and lower respiratory tract, and (b) a necrotizing glomerulonephritis.

The disease occurs in equal proportions of males and females. Although the peak incidence is in the fourth and fifth decades with an average age of 40, the range varies between the ages of 15 and 75 years.

The majority of individuals in whom the diagnosis of Wegener's granulomatosis is eventually made present with symptoms of upper respiratory tract disease (Table 106–2). The commonest complaints include nasal ulcers, rhinorrhea, and sinus pain. Sinusitis and otitis media can both occur. Biopsy of sinus mucosa often demonstrates the necrotizing granulomata.

Ocular inflammation also develops in more than half of all patients. The findings include conjunctivitis, episcleritis, scleromalacia, corneal ulcers, and retinal artery thrombosis.

The lungs become involved in the majority of patients. Common symptoms of pulmonary disease include hemoptysis, cough, and pleurisy. Although variable and often nonspecific, the radiographic findings of solitary or multiple infiltrates or nodules and multilocular, irregular cavities re-

TABLE 106–2. FREQUENCY OF ORGAN SYSTEM INVOLVEMENT IN WEGENER'S GRANULOMATOSIS*

ORGAN	PER CENT
Respiratory tract	100
Kidneys	85
Eyes	55
Joints	48
Skin/muscle	40
Ear	36
Heart	17
Nervous system	15

* After Kornblut AD, Wolff S, Defries HO, and Fauci A: Wegener's granulomatosis. Laryngoscope 90:1453, 1980.

flect the presence of a necrotizing granulomatous process in the absence or presence of vasculitis. Biopsy of the lung usually provides documentation of the process.

Kidney disease, which occurs in about 85 per cent of cases, is a later manifestation of Wegener's granulomatosis. The pathologic lesions are a focal or diffuse proliferative glomerulonephritis and interstitial nephritis. The glomerulonephritis often results in an active urinary sediment characterized by proteinuria, hematuria, and cylindruria. If left untreated, a rapidly progressive and terminal renal failure results.

Dermal vasculitic lesions have been observed in more than one third of persons with Wegener's granulomatosis. Both nodular lesions and purpuric papules suggest a granulomatous vasculitis.

Joint pains in the absence of active synovitis are a complaint in about one half of patients. Although synovitis occurs, it is very uncommon.

There is no laboratory test that is specific for the diagnosis of Wegener's granulomatosis. Because of the presence of widespread inflammation, the ESR is elevated and a normochromic, normocytic anemia is often observed. A polyclonal hypergammaglobulinemia is characterized by elevated IgG and IgA levels. Abnormalities of urinalysis, BUN, and creatinine reflect renal disease.

The diagnosis of Wegener's granulomatosis is made on the basis of the clinical signs of upper and lower respiratory tract disease (i.e., sinusitis, rhinitis, otitis, pulmonary nodules or infiltrates) associated with glomerulonephritis and a biopsy demonstrating necrotizing vasculitis with granuloma formation. In addition, other organ systems can be simultaneously involved.

The current therapy for Wegener's granulomatosis utilizes cytotoxic chemotherapy. Cyclophosphamide is the agent of choice and critically ill patients should be treated with intravenous cyclophosphamide until the course of the disease is stabilized and it is deemed advisable to switch to oral therapy.

Although treatment with corticosteroids alone is insufficient to control disease activity and induce remission, these agents are useful in relieving the sequelae of inflammation, particularly that of the eye, skin, and serosa.

POLYMYALGIA RHEUMATICA AND TEMPORAL ARTERITIS

Polymyalgia rheumatica (PMR) is an idiopathic disorder characterized by aching and myalgias of the shoulder and pelvic girdle musculature, neck, and proximal extremities. Usually having its onset in women (2:1) in the sixth decade or older, the yearly incidence is approximately 54 per 100,000 population. Although the onset of the disease usually occurs in persons over the age of 50, occasional cases are reported of documented PMR in younger persons.

Symptoms of aching, stiffness after rest, and myalgias often begin precipitously, although the disease may progress relatively slowly over time. Polyarthralgias or a true synovitis can be present; their presence should not detract from the diagnosis. Other commonly observed constitutional features include fever, weight loss, malaise, and anorexia.

The physical examination reveals tender muscles, but no weakness or atrophy. Synovitis of the knees with or without small effusions can be observed. In contrast, synovitis of the small joints of the hands and feet is rare.

There are no specific laboratory tests to identify PMR. However, the Westergren sedimentation rate is elevated above 35 mm/hr in nearly all patients. A normochromic, normocytic anemia is present in one half of patients. There is no increase in the incidence of rheumatoid factor, ANA, or other autoantibodies. Complement levels are normal or elevated. The muscle enzymes (CPK, aldolase, SGOT) are normal. Neither electromyographic evaluation nor muscle biopsy has provided diagnostic benefit. Synovial fluid analysis usually reveals a noninflammatory or mildly inflammatory picture (WBC = 0–9000/cu mm, predominantly lymphocytes) with normal glucose and complement levels. Synovial biopsy may show a nonspecific, mild synovial hyperplasia.

The differential diagnosis includes infections, neoplasia (i.e., plasma cell dyscrasia), fibromyalgia, and painful myopathies. In 15 to 78 per cent of patients with PMR, temporal arteritis can co-exist. Temporal arteritis can present or be associated with PMR in 41 to 62 per cent of patients.

Temporal arteritis is a granulomatous vasculitis that usually affects individuals over the age of 50. The approximate annual incidence of the disease is 11.7 cases per 100,000 individuals over age 50. The mean age of onset is 65 to 73 years, with a range of 48 to 90 years. Sixty-four per cent of patients with temporal arteritis are women.

The onset of temporal arteritis may be precipitous or insidious. When the disorder co-exists with PMR, proximal extremity aching, stiffness, fatigue, and headache are the presenting symptoms in 20 to 40 per cent of patients. Other constitutional symptoms include recurrent and unexplained fevers, anorexia, weight loss, and malaise. The low-grade fever is often present as an early sign of disease activity in one half of patients.

Neuropsychiatric signs include confusion, depressive reactions, psychosis, and dementia. The synovitis observed with temporal arteritis is a manifestation of PMR.

The symptoms of claudication, headache, visual changes, and scalp tenderness are the result of arteritis. Claudication can occur in muscle groups in which the blood flow is compromised by vasculitis. The most common sites include the muscles of mastication, deglutition, the extremities, and the tongue. Jaw claudication, a symptom in one third to one half of patients, is a consequence of impaired blood flow of the temporal or maxillary arteries.

The visual alterations of temporal arteritis include transient blurring, ptosis, diplopia, and transient, permanent partial, or complete blindness. These symptoms are the result of arteritis affecting the posterior ciliary or ophthalmic vessels or, less commonly, the central retinal artery. Although blindness is usually preceded by other visual changes for weeks or months, it can occur precipitously without warning.

Headache and scalp tenderness, very common symptoms in temporal arteritis, are due to arteritis of the temporal or occipital vessels. Headache may be one of the earliest symptoms of temporal arteritis, since it is reported as an initial complaint in 30 to 45 per cent of patients. The new onset of an ill-defined headache of variable severity in an older person should raise the suspicion of temporal arteritis.

Although several laboratory abnormalities can be observed in temporal arteritis, none is specific for the disorder. Hematologic abnormalities often present are a normochromic, normocytic anemia, leukocytosis of less than 20,000/cu mm, and a thrombocytosis of less than 1,000,000/cu mm. Alterations in plasma proteins result from the response to inflammation and include elevated fibrinogen, α-2-globulin, IgG, total hemolytic complement, C4, and C3. The erythrocyte sedimentation rate is often greater than 60 mm/hr and remains a sine qua non for the diagnosis of temporal arteritis.

When the diagnosis of temporal arteritis is suspected, a biopsy of a clinically involved or symptomatic portion of the temporal artery should be obtained. If the temporal artery appears clinically uninvolved, biopsy of a 5-cm segment should be taken to obtain sufficient tissue to identify the commonly observed "skip" lesions of temporal arteritis. Temporal arteriography has demonstrated low sensitivity, gives frequent false-positive results, and does not appear to enhance the value of the temporal artery biopsy. However, a history of claudication of an extremity and the presence on examination of a bruit implicates large vessel arteritis and should be confirmed by angiography.

The treatment of choice for temporal arteritis is corticosteroids. The usual initial daily dosage is the equivalent of prednisone, 60 mg. If there is a moderate to high likelihood of temporal arteritis, corticosteroid therapy should be instituted immediately, even prior to biopsy, to avert the dreaded potential of blindness. Although prior steroid therapy can alter the histopathologic changes after one week of treatment, the findings are usually discernible, especially if biopsy is performed within one week. The response to therapy is monitored clinically by resolution of symptoms as well as by the ESR. Upon remission and return of the ESR to normal levels, the corticosteroid dosage can be tapered as the ESR is periodically monitored. Whether the corticosteroid therapy can be discontinued in temporal arteritis depends upon the clinical course.

REFERENCES

Cupps T, and Fauci A: The Vasculitides. Philadelphia, WB Saunders Co, 1981.
Fauci A, Haynes B, Katz P, and Wolff S: Wegener's granulomatosis: Prospective clinical and therapeutic experience with 85 patients for 21 years. Ann Intern Med 98:76, 1983.
Lanham J, Elkan K, Pusey C, and Hughes G: Systemic vasculitis with asthma and eosinophilia: A clinical approach to the Churg-Strauss syndrome. Medicine 63:65, 1984.
Travers RO, Allison D, Brettle R, and Hughes G: Polyarteritis nodosa: A clinical and angiographic analysis of 17 cases. Sem Arthritis Rheum 8:184, 1979.

107 RAYNAUD'S PHENOMENON

Raynaud's phenomenon is a disorder characterized by a triphasic color change of the affected anatomical region due to local arterial vasospasm. When unassociated with another disorder, this phenomenon is commonly designated Raynaud's disease.

Raynaud's phenomenon is a relatively common malady, affecting 5 to 10 per cent of the normal population. Approximately 1000 new cases are identified yearly per million adults. When compared with the annual incidence rates of rheumatoid arthritis (750), systemic lupus erythematosus (75), progressive systemic sclerosis (10), and dermatomyositis/polymyositis (10), Raynaud's phenomenon is a relatively common connective tissue disorder. Three out of four affected persons are female, and the median age of onset is 39.5 years.

CLINICAL FEATURES

Raynaud's phenomenon is usually triggered by a stimulus such as exposure to cold or emotional stress. Occasionally, the reaction occurs de novo. Raynaud's phenomenon primarily affects the acral regions, including the hands and feet. Other less commonly involved structures include the ears, nose, nipples, and tongue. The process is classically divided into three phases: initial pallor of the skin resulting from vasoconstriction and subsequent reduced cutaneous blood flow. Following arterial constriction, the second phase of cyanosis results from limited blood flow through the dermal vessels. Upon rewarming, the third stage of hyperemia can be appreciated as the dermal arterial vessels dilate and blood flow returns to baseline. The duration of the reaction is quite variable, from minutes to hours. Indeed, severe Raynaud's phenomenon can exhibit a predominant phase of cyanosis, even in the absence of an ongoing stimulus, and this has been termed "fixed" Raynaud's phenomenon. Thus, neither the duration of each phase nor the extent of dermal changes of each phase need be equivalent. Moreover, pain may or may not accompany an episode of Raynaud's phenomenon.

The severity and frequency of attacks of Raynaud's phenomenon are often dependent on the presence of an associated disorder. In its primary form, Raynaud's disease can be unilateral or bilateral, long-standing, and uncommonly complicated by cutaneous gangrene. However, the occurrence of vasospastic signs well in advance of a connective tissue disorder is common. Thus, more severe vasospastic disease may be premonitory to an insidiously evolving disorder such as scleroderma. Advanced Raynaud's phenomenon can result in gangrene and/or autoamputation of the affected structure.

PATHOPHYSIOLOGY

The precise etiopathogenesis of Raynaud's phenomenon remains unknown. Segmental, often widely distributed local defects of small arterial vessels have been postulated. Histopathology demonstrates variable degrees of intimal thickening with luminal narrowing, endothelial swelling, increased numbers of intracellular cytoplasmic filaments that may be contractile elements, and adventitial fibrosis.

The roles of the various vasoactive mediators in the etiopathogenesis of Raynaud's phenomenon are currently under investigation. Since this disorder is characterized by vasospasm, vasodilation, and thrombosis, prostaglandins may mediate, in part, these exaggerated local responses. Thromboxane A2, synthesized by the endothelium and platelets, promotes vasoconstriction and platelet aggregation. By contrast, prostacyclin, also synthesized by endothelium, produces vasodilation and inhibits platelet aggregation. An inhibitor of thromboxane, dazoxiben, has been shown in clinical trials to produce temporary improvement of the vasospasm. Similarly, prostacyclin has been shown to promote vasodilation, providing temporary resolution of the process.

DISORDERS ASSOCIATED WITH RAYNAUD'S PHENOMENON

The individual presenting for diagnosis of Raynaud's phenomenon should be comprehensively evaluated for a disorder associated with this process.

The initial evaluation must include a comprehensive history and physical exam aimed at identifying remote or recent symptoms and signs of other disorders that can be related to Raynaud's phenomenon. The use of particular drugs or the exposure to certain toxins should be sought. A knowledge of the patient's occupational exposures is critical, since workers in certain trades, such as vinylchloride workers, have an increased incidence of Raynaud's phenomenon. The examination may reveal evidence of an evolving connective tissue disorder or neurovascular compression.

The use of particular laboratory tests in the initial and subsequent evaluation of Raynaud's phenomenon is warranted. A complete blood count, Westergren sedimentation rate, urinalysis, ANA, anti–SS-A and anti–SS-B, serum protein electrophoresis, and cryoglobulins can provide evidence of a connective tissue disorder or paraproteinemia. A chest x-ray and cervical spine films assist in excluding the diagnosis of a thoracic outlet syndrome due to an aberrant first cervical rib, but do not rule out compression due to a hypertrophied scalenus anticus muscle. Arteriography is rarely efficacious in diagnosis or treatment.

Since Raynaud's phenomenon may precede the onset of an associated disorder, the patient with apparent Raynaud's disease should be monitored yearly for an indefinite period. Surveillance of such persons often permits the early recognition and treatment of complicating diseases such as rheumatoid arthritis or monoclonal gammopathy.

THERAPY

The management of Raynaud's phenomenon often requires the use of simple general measures and, on occasion, the addition of medical treatment. The direct exposure both to cold and to extremes of emotional stress should be avoided. Multiple layers of warm clothing, especially gloves, should be recommended. The continued use of tobacco should be discouraged owing to the relationship between thromboangiitis obliterans and Raynaud's phenomenon. The use of beta-adrenergic blocking drugs in the treatment of hypertension should be discontinued owing to their capacity to promote vasoconstriction.

If these measures still fail to control Raynaud's phenomenon, medical therapy should be considered. The application of a quarter inch of a nitroglycerin-containing ointment to the skin prior to cold exposure can reduce or eliminate the vasospasm without producing untoward side effects. More advanced disease may necessitate agents that promote vasodilation. Recent trials have examined the calcium channel blocking agents and captopril, an angiotensin-converting enzyme inhibitor. The calcium channel blocking agents appear to inhibit smooth muscle contraction by regulating the slow calcium channel influx. Although the numbers of patients rigorously studied have been small, preliminary results with nifedipine indicate efficacy.

Another mode of management is sympathectomy. Although previously resorted to in the treatment of this disorder, the results of sympathectomy have been variable and complicated by a high recurrence rate. The efficacy of the newly developed superselective digital sympathectomy awaits further analysis.

REFERENCES

Lafferty K, Roberts V, DeTrafford J, and Cotton L: On the nature of Raynaud's phenomenon. Lancet 2:313, 1983.
Spencer-Green G: Raynaud's phenomenon. Bull Rheum Dis 33:1, 1983.

NONARTICULAR RHEUMATISM 108

Nonarticular rheumatism is the currently preferred designation for a group of disorders that affect the soft or supporting tissues: fascia, tendons, ligaments, bursae, and intervertebral disks. These disorders are very common in the general population and often produce acute and chronic pain syndromes. While certain types of nonarticular rheumatism are readily recognizable and easily treatable, others often remain undiagnosed

for prolonged periods and/or are very difficult to manage effectively. The prototype disorder of nonarticular rheumatism is the myofascial pain syndrome, also referred to as fibromyalgia.

THE FIBROMYALGIA SYNDROME

The fibromyalgia syndrome is a disorder of unknown etiology characterized by chronic and generalized muscular aching, stiffness, joint pains, variable fatigability, paresthesias, poor sleep habits, headaches, anxiety, and irritable bowel syndrome. This disorder occurs in women of child-bearing age (20 to 50 years) six times more frequently than in men. Until recently, the disorder was regarded as psychosomatic in origin; however, carefully conducted clinical studies have further defined and characterized fibromyalgia, and suggested that, although the disorder lacks precise pathologic definition, an organic etiology appears likely.

The person with fibromyalgia describes fatigue upon arising in the morning and prolonged morning stiffness lasting several hours. Some individuals experience both morning and evening stiffness. Certain forms of exercise or manual labor tend to aggravate the muscular soreness and stiffness. There is a sensation of swelling of the joint, especially the small joints of the hands. The nonrheumatic symptoms of headache, sleep disorder, paresthesias, anxiety, and irritable bowel syndrome occur independently. Factors that augment fibromyalgia include changing weather conditions, humid or cold weather, stress, fatigue, overactivity, or sedentary periods. Symptoms tend to be relieved by rest, warm weather, amelioration of stress, hot showers, massage, and, in some persons, stretching exercises.

The physical examination of persons with fibromyalgia unassociated with other disorders (primary fibromyalgia) usually reveals a healthy-appearing adult. The locomotor exam characteristically demonstrates (a) tenderness with palpation of joints with no evidence of synovitis, deformity, or limitation of range of motion; (b) tender zones over distinct muscle groups; (c) tenderness of certain costochondral junctions; and (d) marked cutaneous erythema following palpation of tender zones. Most persons with fibromyalgia exhibit about 12 tender zones.

The laboratory evaluation in fibromyalgia is unrevealing. Tests for the identification of inflammation are negative. Studies examining biopsies of skin, fascia, and muscle demonstrate either nonspecific findings or no pathologic changes.

Similarly, the electromyographic exam may demonstrate some insertional activity but is generally unrevealing.

The management of fibromyalgia should begin with an explanation of the disorder to the patient. It should be emphasized that fibromyalgia characteristically runs a course punctuated by exacerbations and remissions; that it is not strictly a psychosomatic disorder, but that anxiety and stress can exacerbate symptoms; and that the disorder does not produce crippling or disability. Patients should be encouraged to continue gainful employment, but the type of job may have to be changed if it requires manual labor or other activities that are recognized to exacerbate symptoms. The importance of regular periods of rest, vacation, and relaxation, which are known to ameliorate symptoms, should be explained. The participation in a regular program of nonstressful stretching exercises can be tried, since this has proven effective in partially relieving symptoms in a subset of patients.

Medical and psychiatric treatment may be useful in the long-term management of fibromyalgia. Brief psychotherapy is being evaluated for its effectiveness in coping with the disorder. The use of amitriptyline, 10 to 25 mg, in the early evening has been found clinically to improve the sleep disorder and to reduce aching. Other modalities that have been utilized to reduce pain include salicylates and nonsteroidal anti-inflammatory agents. The disorder does not respond to either parenteral ACTH or corticosteroids. Additional adjunctive treatments that have provided relief include transcutaneous electric stimulation (TENS), biofeedback, and acupuncture.

REFERENCES

Smythe H: Nonarticular rheumatism and psychogenic musculoskeletal syndromes. In McCarty DJ (ed): Arthritis and Allied Conditions. 10th Ed. Philadelphia, Lea and Febiger, 1985, p 1083.

Yunus M, Masi A, Calabro J, et al: Primary fibromyalgia (fibrositis): Clinical study of 50 patients with matched normal controls. Sem Arthritis Rheum 11:151, 1981.

109 THE SPONDYLOARTHROPATHIES

The spondyloarthropathies are a group of interrelated disorders that share certain epidemiologic, pathogenetic, clinical, and pathologic features. The entities that compose this group include (a) ankylosing spondylitis, (b) Reiter's syndrome, (c) psoriatic arthritis, (d) arthritis associated with chronic inflammatory disease of the intestine, (e) Whipple's disease, and (f) post infectious "reactive" arthropathies. Ankylosing

spondylitis will be discussed in this chapter and the other disorders in subsequent chapters.

ANKYLOSING SPONDYLITIS

Ankylosing spondylitis (AS) is the prototype of the spondyloarthropathies. It is characterized by *enthesopathy*, the presence of inflammation at the site of ligamentous insertion into bone; sacroiliitis; spondylitis; inflammatory ocular disease; an asymmetric oligoarthritis predominantly of the large joints of the lower limbs; and an association with HLA-B27.

Prevalence

The prevalence of AS in Caucasians is 1 per cent of the general population. Among American blacks, the prevalence of AS is approximately one quarter that of Caucasians. Although the ratio of affected males to females is equal in sacroiliitis, the ratio is 3 : 1 in the presence of spondylitis. The disease usually has its onset in the second and third decades. There is a prominent familial incidence of AS and of other seronegative spondyloarthropathies among first-degree family members of affected persons.

Clinical Features

AS usually presents during young adulthood with vague symptoms of mid- and low-back stiffness and pain. There is often a history of long-standing soreness and stiffness of the back after prolonged rest, which is partially alleviated with mobility and exercise. Radiation of the pain into the buttocks and down the posterior aspect of the leg may occur. The prominent stiffness after rest may prompt the patient to arise from bed at night to walk about.

Thoracic cage pain also occurs in AS. Owing to involvement of the central cartilaginous joints of the anterior thoracic cage, the pain can have a pleuritic quality. In particular, pain from the manubriosternal and sternoclavicular joints is very common.

Enthesopathic pain is also common in AS and is frequently a presenting complaint. The pain is due to dactylitis, Achilles tendinitis, plantar fasciitis, and iliac crest involvement.

Polyarthralgias and/or polyarthritis is another frequent complaint during the course of AS. The proximal synovial joints, including the shoulders, hips and knees, are more often involved than the smaller distal joints. As in RA, there is prolonged early morning stiffness and swelling of joints; however, the synovitis can be asymmetric and only uncommonly results in severe, erosive articular disease.

Acute anterior uveitis occurs in approximately one quarter of patients with AS. There is pain, redness, and photophobia that is usually episodic and may be unilateral or bilateral.

Examination of the patient with early AS can demonstrate reduced spinal mobility, partial or complete loss of the physiologic lumbar lordosis, and increased thoracic and cervical kyphosis. Later findings include restriction of chest wall expansion during deep inspiration (<2.5 cm), the gradual development of a stooped posture, fixation of the spine with head held in flexion, and a shuffling gait. The presence of peripheral joint synovitis is variable.

Pathology

AS is a chronic inflammatory arthritis predominantly affecting the axial skeleton. The target joints are both synovial and nonsynovial. The inflammatory arthritis of the axial skeleton induces an exuberant fibrotic response. Over time, the fibrotic scar calcifies, leading to ossification of ligaments, bony bridging between vertebral bodies (syndesmophytes), and irreversible skeletal immobility.

Radiologic Features

The long-standing pathologic changes produce characteristic radiographic features in AS. Inflammation of the sacroiliac joints leads to gradual destruction of cartilage and subchondral erosions, giving the radiographic appearance of "pseudo-widening." An osteoblastic response of the affected bone then results in sclerosis of the joint margins. Subsequent fusion of the joint results from the ingrowth of osteoid tissue, calcification, and bony bridging of the joint margins. The final radiographic feature is juxta-articular osteopenia.

Osteitis of subchondral vertebral bone and periostitis of the anterior face of the vertebral body can destroy the superior and inferior margins, flattening the normal concave surface and giving the radiographic picture of squaring of the bodies. This finding, most common in thoracic vertebrae, can be the earliest radiographic change of AS.

Healing of the chondritis and osteitis is associated with fibrosis, calcification, new bone formation with replacement of the annulus fibrosus, and development of syndesmophytes that bridge the margins of adjacent vertebral bodies. The gradual ossification of the annulus fibrosus, formation of syndesmophytes, and ossification of the perispinal ligaments eventually immobilize the spine and give the radiographic appearance of the "bamboo" spine.

Laboratory Studies

There is no laboratory test that is specific for AS. Early in the disease process the elevated sedimentation rate reflects the inflammatory process; in the presence of chronic disease, the sedimentation rate may or may not be raised. A mild or moderate rise in the alkaline phosphatase indicates the presence of bony resorption during osteitis.

There is an excellent correlation between AS and the presence of HLA-B27. Approximately 90 per cent of Caucasian patients with AS possess B27, compared with 8 per cent of the general population. In black Americans with AS the incidence of B27 approximates 50 per cent, in contrast to a 4 per cent incidence in the black population at large. Thus, in patients in whom the diagnosis is uncertain, determining the presence of B27 may assist in making the early diagnosis of AS; in contrast, testing for the presence of B27 in persons with clinically evident AS is unnecessary, since it does not alter management.

Treatment

The management of AS is predicated upon a vigorous approach to physical therapy and the judicious use of certain nonsteroidal anti-inflammatory agents. Although nonsteroidal anti-inflammatory drugs do not alter the course of AS, by providing analgesia they promote function. The long-term objective of the exercise regimen is to halt the insidious development of disabling axial immobility and to preserve maximal motion and function. At times, the use of a custom-designed "spondylitic" jacket to maintain maximal upright posture and to relieve distressing paravertebral muscular pain is beneficial.

REFERENCE

Calin A: Ankylosing spondylitis. In Kelley W, Harris E, Ruddy S, and Sledge C (eds): Textbook of Rheumatology. Philadelphia, WB Saunders Co, 1981, p 1017.

110 PSORIATIC ARTHRITIS

Psoriatic arthritis (PsA) is an inflammatory arthritis that occurs in approximately 5 to 7 per cent of patients with psoriasis. Because its prevalence is estimated at one in 1000, the disease is diagnosed far less frequently than rheumatoid arthritis (RA), which has a prevalence of two per 100. Based on clinical, epidemiologic, and immunogenetic findings, PsA is a distinct rheumatic disease and not a variant of RA or other inflammatory spondyloarthritides. Yet patients with PsA often share clinical, radiographic, pathological, and immunogenetic features with Reiter's syndrome and other spondyloarthritides.

Clinical Presentation

The diagnosis of PsA remains a clinical one, dependent on symptoms and findings on examination.

Because PsA is a systemic disorder, patients often describe multiple constitutional complaints. Such symptoms usually include early fatigability, morning stiffness of the affected joints, joint swelling, limitation of range of joint motion, joint pain, and less frequently, myalgias, weight loss, fever, and malaise. The severity and extent of psoriasis and onychodystrophy do not necessarily parallel the activity of the arthritis, however. To be sure, the symptoms of fatigability, morning stiffness, and articular pain and swelling are similar to those found in RA. Thus, the frequent family or personal history of psoriasis or both help provide the initial clue to the diagnosis of PsA.

Because ankylosing spondylitis (including sacroiliitis) occurs in one fifth to one third of individuals with PsA, the symptoms of back pain should be thoroughly investigated. Spondylitis, however, is rarely the presenting feature of PsA. Such complaints as low back pain and stiffness after resting, improvement of soreness and stiffness with exercise, and chest wall pain suggest an inflammatory rather than a structural etiology of the back pain (Table 110–1). Other less common complaints include gradual limitation of range of motion of the low back or neck, or both, alternating radiation of pain into the buttocks, and variable dyspnea with effort.

Three different distributions of synovitis at the onset of disease typify PsA. Patients with PsA classified as group I have an asymmetric oligo- or polyarticular synovitis involving any joint, especially the DIP joints, PIP joints, or both, of the hands and feet. About one half of all individuals with PsA exhibit an asymmetric arthritis at disease onset. Although PsA was classically described as affecting the DIP joints of the hands, in actuality, distal involvement alone occurs in only a small minority of patients. Some patients who initially present with an asymmetric oligo- or polyarticular synovitis develop a symmetrical pattern over time. Other common findings on physical examination include "sausage digits" and onychodystrophy. Sausage digits of the fingers or toes, or both, result from interphalangeal involvement and attendant flexor tendon sheath effusion. Onychodystrophy, a manifestation of psoriasis, occurs in about two thirds of patients with an asymmetric arthritis.

In general, the course of disease in persons with an asymmetric synovitis is less aggressive and disabling than in other forms of PsA. One fourth, however, develop a progressive, destructive arthritis punctuated by recurrent bouts of synovitis.

PsA presents as a symmetric arthritis (group II)

TABLE 110–1. SYMPTOMS AND SIGNS IN PSORIATIC SPONDYLOARTHRITIS*

Symptoms
Back stiffness and pain >3 months
Improved back pain and stiffness with exercise
Thoracic pain
Radiation of pain to buttocks
Dyspnea with effort

Signs
Chest expansion ≤2.5 cm, resulting in restrictive pulmonary defect
Limitation of motion of spine
Inflammatory ocular disease

---

* After Kammer GM: Clinical significance of subgroups in psoriatic arthritis. IM—Int Med for the Specialist 2:40, 1981.

affecting any pairs of joints, including the DIP joints, PIP joints, or both, of the hands and feet, in about 25 per cent of affected individuals. In contrast to individuals with an asymmetric distribution of arthritis, one half may experience an erratic, destructive, deforming, and progressively disabling disease course. The remaining one half of patients, however, experience a variable course characterized by minimal synovitis with few constitutional symptoms to moderate synovitis with a remittent course complicated by occasional flares.

Psoriatic spondyloarthritis (Group III) is the coexistence of either sacroiliitis or ankylosing spondylitis with psoriasis. With the exception of their psoriasis, persons with psoriatic spondyloarthritis have physical stigmata similar to those with idiopathic ankylosing spondylitis or sacroiliitis. Not all persons with spondyloarthritis develop peripheral arthritis.

A major complication of PsA is arthritis mutilans. This is a severe, deforming, and destructive arthritis that has a relentless course and principally affects the small joints of the hands and feet; it occurs with approximately equal frequency in the three groups. Radiographically, it is characterized by osteolysis and bone resorption of the metacarpals, metatarsals, phalanges, and tufts and by ankylosis and osteoporosis. Unfortunately, history or physical examination gives no clues that can predict the eventual occurrence of arthritis mutilans.

Laboratory and Radiographic Findings

No laboratory studies are specific for PsA. Thus, the diagnosis is based on the clinician's observations and often is confirmed by certain radiographic features usually present in PsA. Because of the presence of widespread inflammation, the Westergren erythrocyte sedimentation rate, the C-reactive protein, and other acute phase reactants (i.e., complement) are elevated during disease activity. With remission, these tests often become normal. The occurrence of rheumatoid factors in a patient with otherwise definite PsA should not dissuade the clinician from that diagnosis. Other commonly observed but nonspecific abnormal laboratory findings include the anemia of chronic disease, polyclonal hypergammaglobulinemia, hyperuricemia, low titer ANA, and circulating immune complexes.

The radiographic features of the peripheral joints include soft-tissue swelling, demineralization, loss of cartilage space, erosions, bony ankylosis, subluxation, and subchondral cysts. Several radiographic findings are classically observed in arthritis mutilans. These findings include "whittling," "pencil-in-cup," "la main en lorgnette" (opera-glass hand), and "doigt en lorgnette" (telescope finger). Of particular interest is the usual simultaneous occurrence of osteoporosis, osteolysis, and bony ankylosis.

Immunogenetic Findings

In Caucasian patients with psoriatic spondyloarthritis, the frequency of B27 is about 60 per cent, significantly higher than the incidence of 6 to 8 per cent in the general population. Moreover, the frequency of B27 in all individuals with PsA is about one in three. More recent genetic studies have also shown that the HLA antigens B17, Bw38, Bw39, and DRw4 are significantly increased in persons with PsA. It remains to be demonstrated, however, what the role of these tissue antigens is in the inheritance, susceptibility, and severity of the disease.

Treatment of PsA

Optimal management of acute PsA or a flare of the disease currently combines several modalities: bed rest, a program of physical therapy, orthotics, and drug therapy. The agents used for short-term treatment provide anti-inflammatory action to reduce synovitis and control pain. Such agents include aspirin and nonsteroidal anti-inflammatory drugs.

A minority of patients fail to respond to the conservative regimen outlined above. To control the inflammatory process, corticosteroids are often used either orally or intra-articularly after arthrocentesis. It should be emphasized that low dose corticosteroids may be used short term for the resolution of synovitis failing to respond to the regimen discussed initially.

For long-term management, anti-inflammatory agents alone can be employed in mild, nonerosive PsA. Such agents include aspirin, nonsteroidal anti-inflammatory agents, and/or hydroxychloroquine. In the presence of more severe disease with attendant erosive arthritis, a remittive agent should be used. Several agents, including gold salts, 6-mercaptopurine, and methotrexate, have been successfully employed. Methotrexate has been used extensively in the treatment of both severe psoriasis and PsA. Caution is urged in the use of remittive agents in PsA. The use of these agents may be complicated by dermatoses, bone marrow toxicity, and hepatotoxicity. Care must be taken to follow the clinical course at regular intervals and to obtain appropriate laboratory studies to exclude toxicity.

REFERENCES

Kammer G, Soter N, Gibson D, and Schur P: Psoriatic arthritis: A clinical, immunologic, and HLA study of 100 patients. Sem Arthritis Rheum 9:75, 1979.

Trentham D, Kammer G, McCune J, and David J: Autoimmunity to collagen: A shared feature of psoriatic and rheumatoid arthritis. Arthritis Rheum 24:1363, 1981.

111

REITER'S SYNDROME

Reiter's syndrome is a seronegative spondyloarthritis characterized by (a) urethritis, (b) conjunctivitis, and (c) arthritis. The disease most commonly affects young males (male to female ratio approximates 10–15 : 1) during the third and fourth decades but can rarely be observed in women, adolescents, and elderly persons.

Epidemiology and Immunogenetics

The onset of Reiter's syndrome often occurs following venereal exposure or dysentery. The venereal relationship appears more frequently in the United States and is associated in one third of cases with *Chlamydia trachomatis* urethritis. However, there is no direct evidence to confirm that *Chlamydia* is the etiologic agent of Reiter's syndrome. The postdysenteric form of Reiter's syndrome, which is found more frequently in Africa, Europe, and the Far and Middle East, usually results from a gastrointestinal infection with *Shigella flexneri*. Because the joint fluids of Reiter's syndrome usually yield no bacterial growth, postdysenteric Reiter's syndrome has been regarded as a reactive arthritis.

The observation that Reiter's syndrome can, in some cases, be familial and is associated with sacroiliitis or ankylosing spondylitis led to immunogenetic analysis of the disorder. The genotype HLA-B27 is found by serotyping in 75 per cent of Caucasian and 37 per cent of black patients. Although the precise significance of the B27 allotype remains uncertain, this cellular surface antigen may predispose individuals with certain bacterial infections (i.e., *Shigella, Salmonella, Yersinia enterocolitica*) to the eventual development of a reactive arthritis such as Reiter's syndrome.

Clinical Features

Characteristically, Reiter's syndrome develops one to four weeks following venereal exposure or diarrhea. Urethritis, often the earliest symptom, is characterized by burning and frequency. A concurrent cystitis can be found in both females and males. Since the penile discharge is clear and mucoid, it resembles a postgonorrheal nonspecific urethritis. A notable association with the urethritis is a perimeatal erosion of the glans penis.

A profuse and watery diarrhea can precede the onset of urethritis in Reiter's syndrome. Following an epidemic of *Shigella* dysentery, approximately 2 out of every 1000 affected persons can be expected to develop Reiter's syndrome.

The conjunctivitis of Reiter's syndrome is a mild, noncatarrhal, bilateral inflammation of the bulbar and palpebral conjunctiva. It is characterized by an evanescent irritation with burning usually lasting one to two days, or, less commonly, as long as several weeks. The process is ordinarily self-limiting. In contrast, the development of an acute anterior iridocyclitis, which occurs in less than one third of persons, can be complicated by pain and potential visual loss if not treated.

Mucocutaneous lesions are commonly observed during Reiter's syndrome. Lesions of the oropharynx can be identified on the buccal mucosa, tongue, palate, and pharyngeal mucosa. Such lesions can take the form of *painless* vesicles, elevated erythematous papules, or superficial ulcers. The lesions of the penis, termed *circinate balanitis*, begin as small, painless vesicles that can coalesce to form larger, painless lesions. Once present, balanitis generally resolves within a few weeks but can last several months. The third cutaneous lesion of Reiter's syndrome is keratodermia blennorrhagica. This painless rash, which occurs in 20 per cent of patients and is found most often on the plantar surfaces of the feet, has the appearance of a brown or yellow cone-shaped papule. Coalescence of the papules leads to large desquamating lesions.

The arthritis of Reiter's syndrome often presents precipitously and frequently affects the knees and ankles. The distribution of the arthritis is asymmetrical and can be monarticular or pauciarticular. The synovitis can also involve any other joint, including the small digital articulations and the sacroiliac joints. When involved, the joints become hot, swollen, and painful and can develop effusions.

A particularly notable feature of Reiter's syndrome is the enthesopathy. Although enthesopathic signs are present in other forms of spondyloarthritides, these symptoms are present so often, especially during the early phase of the disorder, as to suggest the diagnosis of Reiter's syndrome. Enthesopathic signs include tendinitis of the extensor hallucis longus; tendinitis at the insertion of the Achilles tendon on the calcaneus; pain on the anterior surface of the patella; periostitis of the digital bones of the feet; and pain over the surfaces of the distal tibias.

The onset of Reiter's syndrome can be abrupt, occurring over several days, or more gradually over several weeks. Patients sustaining the precipitous onset can appear quite toxic and exhibit hectic fevers, weight loss, malaise, and debilitation. The recognition of Reiter's syndrome in a young male presenting in this manner can be difficult in the absence of the complete clinical picture. Yet the presence of urethritis and diarrhea, especially if a history of enthesopathy can be elicited, should suggest the diagnosis of Reiter's syndrome.

The long-term outcome of Reiter's syndrome is variable. Approximately two thirds of patients experience no further acute episodes, while the remaining one third experience recurrent or sustained disease activity. Ankylosing spondylitis complicates the course of Reiter's syndrome in 15 per cent of cases.

Laboratory Findings

There are no laboratory tests that specifically identify Reiter's syndrome. During active disease a normocytic, normochromic anemia, leukocytosis (<30,000/cu mm), and elevation of the ESR are often observed. IgM rheumatoid factors are absent. The urinalysis can show microscopic hematuria and pyuria, but cultures are sterile. Serum and synovial fluid complement levels can be elevated on the basis of an acute phase response but are of no diagnostic significance.

Radiographic Findings

Radiographic changes are notably absent early in the disease course. Later, after the appearance of peripheral synovitis, juxta-articular osteoporosis can be observed about affected joints. Periostitis of the os calcis is common but not diagnostic. The sacroiliitis associated with Reiter's syndrome tends to be asymmetrical, later becoming symmetrical. The ankylosing spondylitis is notable radiographically for nonmarginal syndesmophytes bridging the vertebrae.

Treatment

The management of Reiter's syndrome requires both supportive and preventive measures. In general, the mucocutaneous lesions do not necessitate treatment unless there are ulcerations or extensive spread of the skin lesions. In this situation, the use of a topical corticosteroid preparation is often beneficial. The eyes should be carefully examined by an ophthalmologist and treatment initiated if there is iridocyclitis. Failure to diagnose iridocyclitis or to effectively manage this complication can lead to progressive visual impairment. A regimen of bed rest, physical therapy, and nonsteroidal anti-inflammatory agents is often very effective in the symptomatic management of the arthritis. The use of corticosteroids in the treatment of synovitis is of limited benefit and therefore should be avoided. However, the local injection of corticosteroids and an anesthetic in regions of tendinitis temporarily ameliorates the pain. In the absence of a response of the synovitis to this regimen, low-dose oral methotrexate can be used.

REFERENCES

Sharp J: Reiter's syndrome (reactive arthritis). In McCarty DJ (ed): Arthritis and Allied Conditions. 10th ed. Philadelphia, Lea and Febiger, 1985, p 841.

Wilkens R, Arnett F, Bitter T, et al: Reiter's syndrome. Evaluation of preliminary criteria for definite disease. Bull Rheum Dis 32:31, 1982.

ARTHRITIS ASSOCIATED WITH INFLAMMATORY BOWEL DISEASE

112

Inflammatory bowel disease (IBD) is an idiopathic chronic inflammatory process involving the gastrointestinal tract. It is divided into two groups or disorders, ulcerative colitis and regional enteritis. Both ulcerative colitis and regional enteritis can be associated with an inflammatory arthritis. Two distinct types of arthritis are observed in these disorders: a peripheral arthritis and ankylosing spondylitis.

PERIPHERAL ARTHRITIS AND ULCERATIVE COLITIS

Peripheral synovitis occurs in about 11 per cent of patients with ulcerative colitis. A term that has commonly been applied to this extra-intestinal complication is enteropathic arthritis. Although the arthritis generally complicates pre-existent bowel disease, it may precede the onset of ulcerative colitis by months or years. The process characteristically is a mono- or oligoarticular, asymmetric synovitis affecting the knees or ankles. The onset is sudden, the synovitis is recurrent, and the flares of synovitis are often temporarily related to recurrences of bowel disease. Once present, the synovitis may persist for several months, gradually resolving over time. However, the arthritis uncommonly produces erosive, deforming articular disease. Peripheral synovitis tends to occur in patients with more severe ulcerative colitis, especially when complicated by pyoderma gangrenosa, erythema nodosum, uveitis, pseudopolyposis, or perianal disease.

Unlike AS associated with ulcerative colitis, there is no immunogenetic predisposition to peripheral arthritis in ulcerative colitis. Thus, the frequency of HLA-B27 is no greater in patients with peripheral arthritis and ulcerative colitis than in healthy Caucasian persons.

Management of the peripheral arthritis depends upon effective treatment of the ulcerative colitis. Conservative therapy includes rest, splinting of affected joints, arthrocentesis, and the use of nonsteroidal anti-inflammatory agents. If these drugs cannot be tolerated, corticosteroids, used for a short duration, usually produce resolution of the synovitis. If colectomy is performed, the peripheral synovitis usually resolves.

ANKYLOSING SPONDYLITIS (AS) IN ULCERATIVE COLITIS

AS occurs in approximately 5 per cent of individuals with ulcerative colitis. In contrast, sacroiliitis is observed in about 17 per cent, can be asymptomatic, and can persist without the development of spondylitis. Of interest is the lower male-to-female ratio when spondylitis complicates colitis. However, both sacroiliitis and AS occur predominantly in persons possessing HLA-B27.

The clinical and radiographic findings in sacroiliitis and AS associated with ulcerative colitis are similar to those observed in the idiopathic process. Both can be associated with peripheral arthritis and iridocyclitis. Although peripheral arthritis usually complicates pre-existent colitis, AS more often antedates the onset of ulcerative colitis.

PERIPHERAL ARTHRITIS ASSOCIATED WITH REGIONAL ENTERITIS

Peripheral synovitis complicates about 20 per cent of cases of more extensive regional enteritis. The synovitis, which most frequently involves the knees, ankles, shoulders, and wrists, often accompanies active bowel disease in which iridocyclitis, erythema nodosum, or oral ulcers are observed. The distribution of the arthritis can be mono-, pauci-, or polyarticular. The onset of the arthritis is often abrupt, and, in contrast to AS, the flare of peripheral arthritis tends to occur concomitant with active bowel disease. The peripheral arthritis does not cause erosive, deforming articular disease. Furthermore, its duration is relatively short-lived; the usual flare of synovitis resolves within several months. Examination can show acutely inflamed joint(s) with an effusion but well-maintained range of motion.

Immunogenetic studies have found no relationship between the peripheral arthritis of regional enteritis and HLA-B27.

The management of the peripheral arthritis of regional enteritis is similar to that described for the arthritis complicating ulcerative colitis. Of particular importance is the control of the underlying bowel disease.

ANKYLOSING SPONDYLITIS (AS) IN REGIONAL ENTERITIS

Sacroiliitis and AS occur in about 9.5 and 7 per cent of patients with regional enteritis, respectively. The course of the axial disease is independent of the activity or extent of the bowel disease. Sacroiliitis may or may not develop into AS. In most ways, these disorders resemble the idiopathic forms clinically and radiographically. Moreover, as in idiopathic AS, the majority of persons with regional enteritis and AS exhibit HLA-B27.

The treatment of the sacroiliitis or spondylitis associated with regional enteritis is identical to the idiopathic form. Since the capacity to tolerate the nonsteroidal anti-inflammatory agents in regional enteritis is often problematic, the potential for untoward effects must be monitored. Unlike the peripheral arthritis, surgical bowel resection does not alter the course of the axial disease.

REFERENCE

Ferguson R: Enteropathic arthritis. In McCarty DJ (ed): Arthritis and Allied Conditions. 10th ed. Philadelphia, Lea and Febiger, 1985, p 867.

113 OSTEOARTHRITIS

Osteoarthritis is the most frequently encountered disorder of connective tissue affecting the joints in human beings. Although the disease has been described as a "wear and tear" process leading to the degeneration of articular cartilage in the elderly age range, this characterization is an imprecise oversimplification. Instead, osteoarthritis should be viewed as an insidious, slowly evolving disorder of the articular cartilage occurring over decades, which becomes *symptomatic* during the sixth through ninth decades. More specifically, osteoarthritis is a disease of both articular cartilage and subchondral bone. There is structural disorganization and deterioration of cartilage leading to focal and, later, diffuse erosions of the surface cartilage. The erosions are a result of pitting and fissuring of the cartilage. Contiguous erosions become larger ulcerations, finally resulting in large areas of destroyed cartilage over the articular surface. The progressive loss of cartilage is often associated with proliferation of new bone and cartilage at the joint margins, the result of which is osteochondrophyte spur formation. In general, there is little, if any, primary synovitis associated with the destruction of cartilage and osteophyte formation, and, therefore, osteoarthritis is not regarded as an inflammatory arthritis but as a structural arthritis. The underlying subchondral bone, when directly exposed following cartilage loss, shows drop-out of osteocytes; osteoblastic and osteoclastic activity; and regions of osteolysis adjacent to subarticular osteosclerosis. Thus, osteoarthritis is an insidious, slowly advancing disease resulting in progressive destruction of articular cartilage, osteophyte formation, subchondral bone collapse, and sclerosis, which produces variable clinical disability of an affected joint.

Osteoarthritis is a worldwide disorder found in approximately the same frequency in all geographic regions. Pathologic studies have demonstrated that by age 40 many persons exhibit some asymptomatic degenerative changes in the cartilage of weight-bearing joints. However, by age 75 virtually all persons have developed osteoarthritis in one or more joints. Thus, the prevalence of symptomatic osteoarthritis does increase with age. When all ages are considered, the prevalence of the disease is equal among males and females. However, certain stresses applied repetitively over long periods of time, as occur in certain occupations, appear to predispose to the development of osteoarthritis.

Osteoarthritis is classified as primary (Table 113–1) or secondary. The disorder is considered primary when it occurs in the absence of any identifiable underlying process. In contrast, it is termed secondary when it complicates a previously established pathologic process such as congenital hip dysplasia or slipped femoral epiphysis.

More recently, primary osteoarthritis has been recognized to exist in clinically different forms, or subsets. On the basis of clinical, histopathologic, and radiographic findings, four types have been identified: primary generalized osteoarthritis, erosive osteoarthritis, diffuse idiopathic skeletal hyperostosis, and chondromalacia patellae (Table 113–1).

The most common distribution of joint involvement in osteoarthritis is the distal interphalangeals, proximal interphalangeals, the first carpometacarpals, hips, knees, first metatarsophalangeals, and the cervical and lumbar apophyseal joints. Although most individuals with osteoarthritis have only a few affected joints, primary generalized osteoarthritis often involves the majority of joints listed above sequentially over time. Unlike inflammatory arthritides such as rheumatoid arthritis, there are no systemic signs of early morning stiffness and profound fatigability. Instead, there is a gradual increase in the degree of a deep, poorly localized pain. Pain is worse following use of the affected joint and better with rest. With progression of the disease, every little motion of the affected joint induces pain, and there is often nocturnal pain. The pain is the result of several co-existent factors, including direct pressure upon exposed subchondral bone; trabecular microinfarcts; periosteal elevation; distortion of the joint capsule; and, when present, a secondary inflammatory synovitis.

Examination of the affected joint reveals several notable clinical findings suggestive of osteoar-

TABLE 113–1. CLASSIFICATION OF PRIMARY OSTEOARTHRITIS*

Peripheral joints: first CMC, first MTP, DIP, PIP, hip, knee
Spine: intervertebral and apophyseal joints
Variant subsets
    Erosive inflammatory osteoarthritis
    Generalized osteoarthritis
    Diffuse idiopathic skeletal hyperostosis
    Chondromalacia patellae

* After Moskowitz RW, Howell DS, Goldberg VM, and Mankin HJ (eds): Osteoarthritis: Diagnosis and Management. Philadelphia, WB Saunders Co, 1984, p 3.

thritis. Tenderness upon palpation often affects widely separated areas of the joint. There may be joint enlargement due to proliferative changes in the cartilage and bone with osteophyte formation. Although large effusions are uncommon, the joint, especially the knee, can exhibit a mild synovitis with a small effusion. Palpation of the para-articular structures may demonstrate medial or lateral joint line tenderness and anserine bursitis. Passive range of motion can elicit variable crepitus and limitation of motion. Varus or valgus deformities are observed during the more advanced stages of osteoarthritis of the knees due to cartilage loss and collapse of subchondral bone. Thus, gait disturbances of variable severity can be observed. Similarly, advanced joint disease, with attendant splinting, often results in muscle atrophy, enhancing the characteristic limp.

Specific joints are commonly affected in osteoarthritis. Osteophyte formation and loss of the joint space of the distal interphalangeal joint are termed a Heberden's node, and involvement of the proximal interphalangeal joint is called a Bouchard's node.

There are no specific identifying laboratory features of osteoarthritis. Because there is no substantial inflammatory response, there are no acute phase reactants such as an accelerated sedimentation rate or elevated serum complement levels. The blood count is also within normal limits. Synovial fluid analysis generally shows a clear yellow fluid and a good mucin clot formation. The leukocyte count is usually less than 500 to 750/cu mm, with fewer than 25 per cent granulocytes. The total protein is often less than 3.0 to 3.5 gm/dl. The synovial fluid glucose is more than one half the value of the simultaneous blood sugar, a normal value. Fibrosis and fragments of cartilage embedded in the synovium are often present.

Optimal management of the osteoarthritic joint requires the sequential or simultaneous use of several treatment modalities. These include physical and occupational therapy, drug therapy, and reconstructive surgery. The application of such modalities as exercise, the use of orthoses and adaptive devices, and education in conjunction with a capable therapist will prevent the devastating loss of joint and muscle function which leads to disability. A program of exercises will be more effectively carried out if the patient has sufficient symptomatic relief of pain with appropriate drug therapy. At present, there are no known pharmacologic agents that can reverse or block the natural course of osteoarthritis. Therefore, agents are selected which provide analgesic and/or anti-inflammatory properties. If assessment indicates primarily a mechanical joint dysfunction, but little inflammation, then use of a non-narcotic analgesic agent is sufficient. The presence of more advanced disease with evidence of synovitis as well as pain is an indication for a nonsteroidal anti-inflammatory agent.

Although the majority of patients with osteoarthritis can be successfully managed conservatively, an increasing proportion of individuals is requiring reconstructive joint surgery. In general, three indications for considering a surgical pro-cedure include (a) progressive and irreversible loss of joint function; (b) pain, especially nocturnal pain; and (c) diminishing capacity to carry out activities of daily living independently.

The surgical management of osteoarthritis can be divided into four basic approaches: (a) osteotomy, (b) debridement, (c) arthrodesis, and (d) arthroplasty.

REFERENCES

Howell DS, and Talbott JH: Osteoarthritis symposium. Sem Arthritis Rheum, Vol 11, 1981.
Moskowitz RW, Howell DS, Goldberg VM, and Mankin HJ (eds): Osteoarthritis. Diagnosis and Management. Philadelphia, WB Saunders Co, 1984.

114 THE CRYSTAL-INDUCED ARTHRITIDES

CHONDROCALCINOSIS AND ASSOCIATED DISORDERS

Crystal-induced arthritides include gout, discussed in Chapter 61, and chondrocalcinosis, which will be considered here. Chondrocalcinosis results from the deposition of calcium pyrophosphate dihydrate (CPPD) crystals in cartilage. The disorder is polyarticular, most often idiopathic, but is also associated with aging and certain metabolic disorders (Table 114–1). It affects about 5 per cent of the adult population and is commonly found to resemble clinically gout, rheumatoid arthritis, neurotrophic arthritis, and osteoarthritis.

Pseudogout is an acute inflammatory arthritis that results from the phagocytosis of IgG-coated CPPD crystals by synovial fluid neutrophils and the subsequent release of inflammatory mediators. Pseudogout accounts for approximately one quarter of all cases of CPPD deposition disease and predominantly affects men. Initially monoarticular, the attack soon becomes oligo- or polyar-ticular. Although the acute arthritis can be self-limiting, lasting for one to several days, more severe attacks involving both the peripheral and axial joints can more slowly resolve over several weeks. The precipitating factors are often similar to those inducing an acute gouty arthritis. The large joints of the lower extremities are more likely to be affected as opposed to the small joints in acute gout. The knee joint is involved in over one half of all cases of pseudogout. The diagnosis of pseudogout should not depend upon the radiographic findings alone, since chondrocalcinosis is observed in only 75 per cent of pseudogout. The presence of chondrocalcinosis can be identified radiographically by the characteristic punctate or linear radiodensities in the joint fibrocartilaginous lateral menisci of the knees or hyaline articular cartilage. Other areas frequently exhibiting these findings include the wrists and pelvis.

The diagnosis of pseudogout and its differentiation from other acute inflammatory arthritides make arthrocentesis a necessary procedure in its evaluation. Acute infectious arthritis and gout can clinically resemble pseudogout. Moreover, both monosodium urate and CPPD crystals can coexist within the same joint. CPPD crystals are rhomboid in shape and produce weakly positive birefringence under compensated polarizing microscopy. The crystals can be observed within neutrophils or are free-floating. The synovial fluid exhibits a leukocytosis of 3,000 to 50,000/cu mm with a predominance of neutrophils, has a low viscosity, and shows no difference in its glucose concentration from serum. See Tables 114–2 and 114–3 for joint fluid analysis.

TABLE 114–1. RELATIONSHIP OF CPPD DEPOSITION TO METABOLIC DISORDERS

Hemochromatosis
Hyperparathyroidism
Hypothyroidism
Gout
Hypomagnesemia
Hypophosphatasia
Wilson's disease
Ochronosis

CPPD crystal disease can also exhibit a symmetrical polyarticular distribution and can clinically resemble rheumatoid arthritis in about 5 per cent of cases. Patients having this form of the disease describe prolonged morning stiffness, fatigability, and malaise. The course of the disease is punctuated by mild attacks of many months in duration. Examination reveals polyarticular synovitis and, less often, flexion contractures. Although there can be elevation of the sedimentation rate and IgM rheumatoid factors (10 per cent), radiographs show secondary osteoarthritic changes of affected joints, and the synovial fluid has a normal glucose and complement in the presence of CPPD crystals.

Progressive osteoarthritis complicated by flexion contractures occurs in about one half of all cases of CPPD crystal disease. This form, known as pseudo-osteoarthritis, usually affects women and involves the knees, wrists, MCPs, hips, shoulders, elbows, and ankles. The process can be symmetrical or asymmetrical. Although radiographs may or may not demonstrate the punctate or linear calcifications of the cartilage, CPPD crystals are found in synovial fluid even in radiographically negative joints.

TABLE 114–2. SYNOVIAL FLUID ANALYSIS*

DIAGNOSIS	APPEARANCE	TOTAL WHITE CELL COUNT PER CUBIC MILLIMETER†	POLYMORPHONUCLEAR CELLS	MUCIN CLOT TEST	SYNOVIAL FLUID-BLOOD GLUCOSE DIFFERENCE (MEAN MILLIGRAMS PER DECILITER)	MISCELLANEOUS (CRYSTALS, ORGANISMS)
Normal	Clear, pale yellow	0–200 (200)	<10%	Good	No significant difference‡	—
Group I (noninflammatory effusions)						
Degenerative joint disease; traumatic arthritis	Clear to slightly turbid	50–4000 (600)	<30%	Good	No significant difference	—
Group II (noninfectious, mildly inflammatory)						
Systemic lupus erythematosus; scleroderma	Clear to slightly turbid	0–9000 (3000)	<20%	Good (occasionally fair)	No significant difference	Occasional LE cell; decreased complement
Group III (noninfectious severe inflammatory effusions)						
Gout	Turbid	100–160,000 (21,000)	~70%	Poor	10	Monosodium urate crystals
Pseudogout	Turbid	50–75,000 (14,000)	~70%	Fair-poor	Not enough data	Calcium pyrophosphate dihydrate crystals
Rheumatoid arthritis	Turbid	250–80,000 (19,000)	~70%	Poor	30	Decreased complement
Group IV (infectious inflammatory effusions)						
Acute bacterial	Very turbid	150–250,000 (80,000)	~90%	Poor	90	Culture positive for gram-positive or gram-negative bacteria
Tuberculosis	Turbid	2500–100,000 (20,000)	~60%	Poor	70	Culture positive for M. tuberculosis

* From Cohen AS: Specialized diagnostic procedures in the rheumatic diseases. In Wyngaarden JB, and Smith LH Jr (eds): Cecil Textbook of Medicine. 17th ed. Philadelphia, WB Saunders Co, 1985, p 1907.

† Averages in parentheses.

‡ Less than 10 mg/dl difference.

Asymptomatic persons found inadvertently to have CPPD crystal deposits by radiographs are said to have lanthantic CPPD deposition disease. In contrast, the combination of tabes dorsalis, Charcot knee joint deformities, and CPPD crystal deposits produces a painful, disabled joint. The finding of CPPD crystals in these destructive joint processes is referred to as pseudoneurotrophic.

The management of CPPD deposition disease is similar to that of gout. Clinically symptomatic disease responds to rest, joint protection, and the initiation of a nonsteroidal anti-inflammatory agent. Colchicine has been found to be efficacious in pseudogout as well as gout. Following aspiration of a joint with marked synovitis, the instillation of a corticosteroid preparation may hasten resolution of the inflammatory process. Maintenance therapy, when necessary, consists of a nonsteroidal anti-inflammatory agent and colchicine.

REFERENCE

McCarty DJ: Diagnostic mimicry in arthritis—patterns of joint involvement associated with calcium pyrophosphate dihydrate crystal deposits. Bull Rheum Dis 25:804, 1974—75.

NEUROLOGIC DISEASE

115 EVALUATION OF THE PATIENT

Disorders of the nervous system are not easy to define. In the broadest sense, all symptoms of disease are neurologic, since the ability of the patient to recognize that he is ill requires that (1) sensory pathways carry information from the diseased organ to the brain and (2) the brain interpret that information as a symptom of something wrong. By convention, however, neurologic diseases are defined as those in which there is either a structural or a physiological abnormality in the central or peripheral nervous system. Exceptions exist: most headache is caused by extracranial nonneural dysfunction, but is considered a neurologic disease; the same holds true for much back pain, a condition caused most often by abnormal muscle or joint function.

Disorders of the nervous system place special requirements upon the physician's clinical skills. Symptoms of nervous system disease can be mimicked by those of systemic or psychiatric illness (e.g., somewhat similar headaches may be caused by brain tumor, giant cell arteritis, or involutional depression). The physician must systematically approach patients whose complaints are potentially neurologic and answer four fundamental questions (Table 115–1): (1) *Is a nervous system disorder present* or are the symptoms merely nonspecific signals of a systemic disorder? To answer this question, one must consider whether the symptoms are explicable in terms of what he knows about the physiology of the nervous system. If they are, the disorder affects the nervous system; if not, it is likely that the disorder arises elsewhere. There is an important caveat: the physician should not attribute to the patient's imagination his own failure to understand the mechanisms of the complaints. An easy trap is to diagnose a conversion reaction (hysteria) because one lacks a clear understanding of the pathophysiology of the symptoms. Equal care must be taken not to overreact to physical symptoms that may simply prove a manifestation of psychological stress. (2) *Make an anatomic diagnosis.* If neurologic disease is present, can one identify where in the nervous system it arises? Is it monofocal, multifocal, or diffuse? Are the lesions peripheral or central? If central, does the disease affect structures above or below the foramen magnum, above or below the tentorium, on the right or left side? Is the process static, worsening, or improving? (3) *What is the mechanism of that lesion?* Does the evidence suggest that the disorder is structural, physiological, or psychophysiological? Is the fundamental disorder genetic, developmental, traumatic, environmental, toxic, infectious, immunologic, degenerative, neoplastic, metabolic, or nutritional? (4) *What specific tests can one conduct* to determine or confirm the cause of the disorder and its etiologic agent?

While the physician is considering the nature of the neurologic disorder, he must pay close attention to the patient's psychological state. Few illnesses frighten patients as much as those of the nervous system, with its threat of dementia, paralysis, and loss of control of bodily functions. Kindness, reassurance, and control of symptoms such as pain mark the humane physician's approach to the diagnosis of a patient with neurologic disease. A final requirement is to recognize that the nervous system regenerates poorly and that once neurologic function is lost, it will never be regained. Therefore, an appropriate combination of care and speed are necessary to make the correct diagnosis and institute appropriate treatment. At times, in the presence of severe and potentially irreversible crises, one must attempt to stabilize the nervous system even before beginning the diagnostic exercise.

THE NEUROLOGIC HISTORY

In most respects, the neurologic history is similar to the general medical history. The purpose (to supply diagnostic information that will direct the physical and laboratory examinations and lead to an appropriate diagnosis) and the format (e.g., chief complaint, present illness, past history, social history, review of systems) are the same (Table 115–2). However, the neurologic history usually supplies a greater proportion of the diagnostically relevant information than does a medical history. Many neurologic diseases are not accompanied by abnormal physical or laboratory findings. Even when a neurologic disease is marked by physical signs and/or laboratory abnormalities, the history usually supplies about 80 per cent of the total diagnostic information. Furthermore, because neurologic abnormalities affect such important functions as thinking, moving, and feeling, most important abnormal physical signs have already created symptoms perceived by the patient. (Exceptions occur in demented patients and those with lesions of the dominant parietal lobe, characterized by denial of disability.) Findings on examination not previously recognized by the patient (or his family) are likely to be irrelevant or even misleading. By contrast, recent symptoms, such as mild weakness or alterations of sensation, often mean disease even if too subtle to be detected by the most meticulous neurologic examination. Because neurologic symptoms are so keenly sensed, a careful history often allows the examiner to localize the disease anatomically and to understand its pathophysiology even before he begins the physical examination.

TABLE 115–1. APPROACH TO THE PATIENT WITH NERVOUS SYSTEM SYMPTOMS

1. Does the patient have a nervous system disorder?
2. Where in the nervous system is the disorder?
3. What is the mechanism (pathophysiology)?
4. What is the cause (etiology)?

TABLE 115–2. ELEMENTS OF THE NEUROLOGIC HISTORY

Chief Complaint and Present Illness (be precise)
  Onset sudden or gradual
  Progressive, remitting, improving
  Aggravating and relieving factors
Past History
  Previous neurologic illness
  Previous similar or relevant complaints
Social and Psychological History
  How does illness affect daily life
Review of Systems
  Mood
  Sexual function
  Diet, weight, nutrition
  Drugs and medicinals
  Sleep habits

Taking the neurologic history ordinarily occupies the majority of the time initially spent in evaluating a patient suffering a neurologic disorder. At the completion of the history, the physician should be able either to make a definitive diagnosis or to formulate three or four diagnostic hypotheses that can be tested by physical and laboratory examinations. Because an almost infinite number of potential questions can be asked of a patient with a neurologic disorder, one must develop a strategy to achieve maximal useful information in a reasonable period of time. Specific questions should be tailored to the patient's complaints and to the physician's knowledge of neurologic illness. Certain guidelines aid in taking complete and accurate histories:

Require Precision. Do not accept jargon or diagnoses from the patient. For example, a patient who complains of dizziness may mean vertigo (a vestibular symptom), lightheadedness (potentially caused by cardiovascular disease), syncope, ataxia, diplopia, or psychogenic dissociation—all of which have very different implications. "Sinus headache" is a diagnostic term often given to describe headaches that are rarely caused by sinusitis but are usually migraine or tension headache.

Both Listen and Ask. Elicit the history in the patient's own words and, whenever possible, without interruption. Excessive interruptions can imply that one is hurried or disinterested and may lead patients to exclude vital information. When the patient is allowed to tell his story, important information often emerges about fears and anxieties. However, the physician must ask direct questions to encourage relevance, achieve precision, and place each symptom in its correct context. If the information is not volunteered, ask about the temporal profile of the complaint (was the onset abrupt or gradual?; is it static, progressive, waxing and waning, or improving?), inquire into the intensity and frequency of the symptoms and the events and factors that precipitate or relieve them, and determine how the symptoms affect the patient's daily life and any other symptoms associated with the major complaint. For example, a patient who complains only of severe, disabling headaches may reveal on careful ques-

tioning that the headaches occur in two-to-three-month clusters once or twice a year, characteristically appear three times a day, are always localized in and around the left eye, last no more than 30 to 40 minutes, are the most intense pain ever experienced, frequently awaken him at night, and are precipitated by alcohol intake during the cluster period. Such a precise history allows no other diagnosis than cluster headache.

Form Hypotheses. Do not be a passive recipient of the patient's story. Most patients supply excessive information, much not diagnostically pertinent. One must sift and distill the information in order to retain what is relevant and weed out the irrelevant. Concurrently, one must form anatomic and/or pathophysiological hypotheses about the nature of the symptoms and gradually refine them into etiologic terms as the history develops. For example, in a patient complaining of weakness of the right arm and leg, the hypotheses might include a lesion of the left hemisphere, the brain stem, or the cervical cord. As the history discloses weakness in the face and difficulty with language, the latter two hypotheses can be discarded and the left hemispheral lesion accepted. An additional history of slowly progressive weakness accompanied by headaches and lethargy suggests an intracranial mass, possibly hematoma, tumor, or abscess, and a history of heavy smoking with recent cough could imply a metastatic lung tumor. Hypotheses should favor illnesses that are *probable* (i.e., common diseases are more likely than rare diseases), *serious* (e.g., brain tumors should be excluded before diagnosing tension headache), *treatable* (e.g., combined systems disease and spinal cord meningioma should be ruled out before making a diagnosis of multiple sclerosis), and *novel* (some patients do have rare diseases, and these should not be forgotten in taking the history).

Always Take a Complete History. Even if the diagnosis seems clear from the chief complaint and the present illness, check other aspects of the history to ensure that other physical or psychological disabilities are not playing a role. In particular, inquire about the patient's mood (e.g., is he depressed or suicidal?), his usually daily activities (and whether the illness interferes with them), his sexual function, the nature of psychological and physical support at home, and his own view of his illness and how it affects him.

End by Summarizing. Summarize for the patient the history, asking if the summary is correct and if anything has been missed. Such a summary offers a chance to supply information and to correct misunderstandings. It also tends to reassure patients and allows them to present sensitive or embarrassing material.

Obtain Further History from the Family and Friends. If the history appears incomplete, and particularly if part of the illness involves changes in mental state or consciousness, the family, friends, and colleagues should be asked to corroborate the story and to supply missing elements, giving their views on how the signs and symptoms affect the patient's daily life.

Gear the Neurologic Examination to Hypotheses Generated by the History. It is neither possible nor desirable to perform all elements of the neurologic examination on every patient. Thus, the hypotheses generated during the course of the history determine which of the nonroutine neurologic maneuvers the physician will carry out during his examination. For example, a complaint of intermittent numbness in an upper extremity should lead to tests for thoracic outlet compromise, even though that is not part of the routine neurologic examination. Hypotheses generated during the history also will direct subsequent laboratory testing, even in the presence of a normal neurologic examination. For example, if the history strongly suggests dysfunction of the left cerebral hemisphere (e.g., local seizures), failure to find a hemiparesis on examination does not rule out a brain tumor and a CT scan should be performed. Even if such tests are initially uninformative, a strongly suggestive history requires that the doctor follow the patient closely, repeating the test if necessary.

THE NEUROLOGIC EXAMINATION

All major aspects of the nervous system must be examined systematically (Table 115–3). The *level of arousal* must be noted: is the patient awake and alert, drowsy and lethargic, responsive only when externally stimulated (stuporous), or psychologically unarousable, even to vigorous external stimulation (comatose). The *mental state* can be examined during the history. A person who gives an articulate and comprehensive history with accurate attention to both detail and dating of the complaints almost always has normal cognitive functions. Still, one may occasionally be fooled and it is useful to check (1) orientation, particularly for place and date, (2) short-term memory (the most vulnerable memory function)

TABLE 115–3. ELEMENTS OF THE NEUROLOGIC EXAMINATION

Level of Arousal
Mental Status
  Orientation, mood, language, memory, intellect, thought
Station and Gait
Cranial Nerves
Motor System
  Strength, tone, bulk, adventitious movements
Sensory System
  Pin, temperature, vibration, object identification, proprioception
Reflexes
  Deep tendon
  Plantar
  Anal wink
Autonomic System
  Blood pressure
  Sphincter
Vascular System
  Carotid pulse and bruits; distal arteries

by asking the patient to repeat three unrelated words five minutes after he has heard them, and (3) capacity to abstract, by interpreting proverbs and by recognizing similarities and differences (boy-dwarf, apple-pear). Because anxiety can interfere with cognitive functions, one must be patient and reassuring. Patients usually do not object to cognitive tests if one begins gently by indicating that he is going to test the patient's memory. Those patients who do object usually are hiding cognitive abnormalities.

Observe the patient's *stance and walk.* If possible this should be done with the patient at least partially undressed so that the alignment of the spine can be observed. A patient who can turn briskly, walk on heels and toes, do a deep-knee bend, and tandem walk has no substantial disability of motor or coordinative functions of the lower extremities. In the absence of specific complaints, these functions need not be tested further.

Examine the *cranial nerves;* visual acuity and visual fields should be tested in all patients and the optic fundi scrutinized for abnormalities of the blood vessels, retina, or optic discs. Pupillary activity, ocular movements, corneal reflexes, jaw movement, facial movement, hearing, swallowing, speaking, and breathing should be tested quickly as well. On the other hand, postural tests of labyrinthine function need not be assessed in the absence of a history of dizziness or vertigo.

Abnormalities of *upper extremity* form, strength, and proprioception can easily be assessed by having the patient extend his arms forward in a supinated position and spread his fingers. If, with the eyes closed, neither arm drifts and there are no tremors or adventitious movements of the fingers, and if the patient can accurately touch his index finger in rapid succession to his nose and the examiner's outstretched finger, it is likely that, in the absence of complaints, no neurologic abnormalities affect the upper extremities. If, however, there is a complaint of weakness or sensory loss, one must test individual muscles.

Sensation can further be assessed by testing in succession the ability of the patient to identify objects placed in his hand when his eyes are closed, to perceive position and vibration in the hands and feet (for vibration, the examiner can use his own perception as the norm, recognizing that in older persons vibration perception normally declines slightly), and to recognize the sharp from the dull end of a pin in all four extremities. Any significant sensory loss of the extremities will almost certainly have been described by the sentient patient during the history and demands careful sensory testing of each dermatome and peripheral nerve in the area of complaint. *Deep tendon reflexes* from biceps, triceps, brachioradialis, knees, and ankles are a sufficient screening test. Test the plantar responses, recalling that an equivocal Babinski sign is more likely to be misleading than helpful. *Autonomic activity* and *sphincter functions* are usually examined as part of the general medical examination, but one seeks a history of sphincter disturbance, and careful assessment of sphincter tone, voluntary sphincter contraction, and the anal wink reflex is essential. Always test for postural hypotension when evaluating autonomic impairment or dizziness. The carotid arteries, the aorta, and peripheral pulses should be palpated and auscultated for evidence of vascular disease.

A screening neurologic examination, as outlined above, takes but a few minutes. More time may be required to evaluate areas that the history suggests may be disordered. The physician should be careful not to be misled by equivocal neurologic signs. In office practice the neurologic examination can mislead almost as often as it helps, particularly when subtle sensory or reflex asymmetries are found. Patients, in their anxiety to be helpful, often hyperdiscriminate, so that they interpret mild changes in the pressure of the examining pin as differences in sensation and falsely interpret as vibration the pressure of the unstruck tuning fork. When persons complain of sensory disturbance, it is often wise to let them map its distribution before the examiner attempts to do so.

DIAGNOSTIC TESTS: SCOPE AND LIMITATIONS

New technology has remarkably increased the accuracy of diagnosis and physiological evaluations. However, if used inappropriately, high technology tests needlessly raise the cost of medical care; furthermore, their results threaten to become the goals of care rather than a means to diagnosis. Since the doctor's practice influences this aspect of health care costs, a judicious physician must consider, before ordering, the precise advantages that each positive or negative test can confer on a patient's evaluation and treatment (Table 115–4).

Tissue Analysis

Lumbar Puncture (LP). LP, a safe and simple technique for analyzing cerebrospinal fluid (CSF), indirectly assesses biochemical abnormalities in the extracellular fluid of the central nervous system. Because headache and backache can follow lumbar puncture, the procedure is not routine but is done for a specific indication (Table 115–5). The test is mandatory and usually diagnostic when the leptomeninges or surface of the brain are infiltrated by infectious agents or tumor. The test also establishes the diagnosis (in the presence of a normal CT scan) of pseudotumor cerebri (p. 779) or idiopathic intracranial hypotension (p. 780). The total protein concentration gives nonspecific information about the presence of nervous system disease and assists in the diagnosis of polyneuropathies. Protein electrophoresis may assist in the diagnosis of multiple sclerosis and other inflammatory diseases of the nervous system. No patient should be anticoagulated for a presumed stroke unless an LP (or a CT scan) have

TABLE 115–4. COMMON NEUROLOGIC LABORATORY TESTS: APPROXIMATE 1985 COSTS*

Lumbar Puncture (spinal tap)	$125
Myelogram	$790–$1000
Computerized Tomography (CT)	
Brain	$383 head
Vertebral-paravertebral area	$410 body (spine)
Magnetic Resonance Imaging (MRI)	$800
Brain	
Spinal cord	
Angiography	
Arteriograms	$1,075
Cerebral, spinal	
Digital intravenous angiogram (DIVA)	$639
Vessels of neck	
Cerebral venous sinuses	
Electrodiagnostic Tests	
EEG	$119
EMG and nerve conduction velocity	$334
Neuromuscular transmission	$182
Evoked potentials	
Visual	$178
Auditory	$178
Sensory	$348
Muscle Biopsy	$87 for processing + surgeon's fee

* Cost includes mean laboratory and professional fees at major New York City hospitals.

ruled out intracranial hemorrhage. There are only a few contraindications. In every patient who undergoes LP, sufficient fluid should be obtained and sampled to procure maximal information. The tests in Table 115–5 are those most commonly ordered.

Tissue Biopsy. Diagnostic biopsies of muscle, less often of peripheral nerve or brain, can give information achievable in no other way. Care should be taken to select for biopsy those patients in whom the test is likely to yield information that is not only diagnostic and prognostic but also of therapeutic benefit.

Muscle Biopsy. Muscle biopsy is a simple and safe procedure that can be performed under local anesthesia. It helps distinguish myopathic from neuropathic weakness and often indentifies a particular myopathy. The muscle selected for biopsy should be clinically affected but not so weak and atrophic that the only yield will be fibrous tissue. The biopsy should be done with great care so that the resected muscle is not allowed to contract excessively, which obscures diagnostic information. When appropriate, materials should be obtained for biochemical, histochemical, and ultrastructural analysis as well as routine light microscopy. Myopathy is distinguished from chronic neuropathy by the fact that the latter process leads to grouped areas of atrophy within normal muscle, the groups being of the same histochemical type. By contrast, myopathic changes occur randomly and produce great variation in fiber size. In myopathy the nuceli often migrate from their normal position in the periphery to the center of the muscle fiber. Inflammatory cells suggest the diagnosis of an inflammatory myopathy (e.g., polymyositis—p. 578). Histochemical alterations in the my-

TABLE 115–5. CONSIDERATIONS FOR PERFORMING A LUMBAR PUNCTURE (LP)

Indications for Test

Absolute
 Suspicion of central nervous system infection
 Before anticoagulant therapy for cerebrovascular disease (if no CT)
Relative
 Suspicion of nervous system disease
 Intrathecal therapy for meningeal leukemia or fungal meningitis
 Symptomatic treatment of severe headache from subarachnoid
  hemorrhage or pseudotumor cerebri

Contraindications

Absolute
 Tissue infection in region of puncture site
Relative
 Spinal cord tumor, known or probable brain tumor
 Bleeding tendency (anticoagulant or thrombocytopenia)
 Increased intracranial pressure

Diagnostic Evaluation of Cerebrospinal Fluid

Sediment
 Cell count and differential
 Cytologic examination for neoplastic cells
 Stains for bacteria and fungi
 Culture for organisms
Supernatant Fluid
 Protein concentration
 Protein electrophoresis (gamma globulin, oligoclonal bands)
 Glucose concentration
 Serologic tests for syphilis
 Viral antibodies and cultures
 Spectrophotometric test for bilirubin, oxyhemoglobin, or
  methemoglobin

Complications of Test

Common
 Headache
 Backache
Rare
 Transtentorial or foramen magnum herniation
 Worsening of spinal tumor symptoms
 Spinal epidural hematoma (patients with bleeding tendency)
 Herniated or infected disc
 Reaction to anesthetic agent
 Meningitis (contaminated needle)

opathies may permit a specific etiologic diagnosis of one of the metabolic or congenital muscle disorders.

Peripheral Nerve Biopsy. A peripheral nerve biopsy is indicated to identify a specific cause of peripheral neuropathy; the procedure generally is reserved for certain specialized medical centers. Amyloid infiltrates, sarcoid, leprosy, and vasculitis can often be identified by biopsy of the nerve, although for peripheral neuropathy in general the procedure has a low yield. The nerve commonly biopsied is the sural nerve at the ankle, and this may be done in conjunction with a muscle biopsy of the lower extremity. The tissue can be sampled under local anesthesia and should be processed for electron microscopy as well as light microscopy. Nerve fibers can be teased individually and long segments can be examined for demyelination. Since cutting the sural nerve produces an area of numbness in the foot which in some instances may be painful, some surgeons cut the nerve longitudinally and biopsy only half, decreasing the sensory complications.

Brain Biopsy. Brain biopsies are undertaken to make diagnoses that may affect therapy. With mass lesions the brain may be biopsied either through an open craniotomy or by stereotaxic needle biopsy using the CT scanner. Biopsy material can distinguish inflammatory from neoplastic lesions and can identify the nature of the neoplasm. Many investigators believe that brain biopsy is required for a definitive diagnosis of herpes simplex encephalitis, since errors in the clinical diagnosis are frequent. Others believe that an empirical trial of antiviral agents (pp. 555–556) is indicated before biopsy is undertaken. Several dementing illnesses can be diagnosed by open brain biopsy, including Alzheimer's disease and Creutzfeldt-Jakob disease. However, since at the present time most dementing illnesses are not treatable, such biopsies are rarely justified except in special research centers.

Imaging Techniques (Fig. 115–1)

Computed Tomography. Computed tomography (CT scan) is a computerized x-ray that produces tomographic pictures of slices of the brain (and other portions of the body) a few millimeters thick. Differences in density delineate CSF, gray matter, and white matter. Depending on their density, lesions as small as 5 mm can be seen, and abnormal permeability of the blood-brain barrier can be identified by intravenous injection of iodinated contrast material into a vein (contrast enhancement). The CT scan is the diagnostic test of choice for assessing the presence of structural disease of the brain. It can identify mass lesions and ventricular size, distinguish hemorrhage from infarct, identify most subdural hematomas and brain tumors, and assess the degree of cerebral atrophy. Subarachnoid blood is usually detected, and lesions of the pituitary gland and orbits can be identified readily. The CT scan often does not detect lesions less than 5 mm in diameter or infiltrating brain tumors that do not alter the blood-brain barrier. Very recent infarcts and isodense hematomas also show up poorly.

Magnetic Resonance Imaging (MRI). MRI is rapidly becoming available in many centers and promises to replace CT scanning as the imaging technique of the future. MRI is unaffected by bone and does not require the injection of contrast material. Furthermore, images can be procured in any plane, whereas CT images are limited to horizontal and coronal planes. MRI also has better resolution than CT and frequently reveals lesions, including tumors, arteriovenous anomalies, and areas of demyelination that CT scanning fails to detect. A complete MRI requires 30 to 45 minutes of immobility on the part of the patient. Because of the high magnetic field, the test is contraindicated in patients harboring cardiac pacemakers or metal aneurysm clips. There are no other known risks and no irradiation is involved.

FIGURE 115–1. A comparison of imaging techniques in a patient suffering from radiation necrosis of the temporal lobe. The patient had received a combination of photon and neutron beam radiation therapy to the left palate, nasopharynx, and paranasal sinuses two years before the sudden onset of confusion and aphasia. *A,* Contrast-enhanced CT scan demonstrating a ring-enhanced lesion in the anterior temporal lobe (opposing black and upper white arrow—right side) surrounded by an area of low density (lower white arrow), presumably edema. One cannot determine by inspection whether the ring-enhanced mass is neoplasm, abscess, or radiation damage. The density in the left frontal area (black arrow—left side) is normal bone of the skull base. *B,* A magnetic resonance image (MRI) reveals that the area of abnormality is much larger than indicated by CT scan. The increased signal (black arrow) does not distinguish the primary lesion from surrounding edema. *C,* Positron emission tomograph using a glucose analogue labelled with fluorine-18. The entire left temporal lobe picks up less isotope (arrow), indicating decreased glucose metabolism and suggesting that the lesion, being hypometabolic, is neither tumor nor abscess but necrosis. (Note that CT and MR images are reversed from top-down horizontal views so that the right side of the image shows the left side of brain and vice versa.)

Spinal canal and paravertebral plexus lesions can be detected by CT and MRI. CT is excellent for bony lesions of the spinal canal and, particularly after the injection of intrathecal contrast material, may identify areas of cord compression. Unlike MRI, CT cannot visualize the spinal cord directly and is relatively poor in detecting intrinsic disease of the spinal cord.

Myelography. Suspected abnormalities of the spinal cord should first be assessed by a plain x-ray. Substantial lesions of bone can thus be identified. In order to identify compression of the spinal cord, nerve roots, or cauda equina, myelography is performed by injection of iodinated contrast material, either oil- or water-soluble, into the spinal canal. The contrast material is run up and down the canal and visualized fluoroscopically, and x-rays are taken. The test is particularly valuable for identifying herniated discs; compression of the spinal cord, cauda equina, or nerve roots; and intrinsic or extrinsic tumors and vas-

cular malformation of the spinal cord. MRI will probably replace myelograms in the future.

Angiography. The blood vessels of the brain and spinal cord can be visualized either by injection of contrast material directly into an artery or by the injection of a larger amount of contrast material intravenously and enhancement of the image by computerized subtraction techniques. The latter approach, digital intravenous angiography (DIVA), can be used as an outpatient test in the search for surgically treatable causes of cerebrovascular disease and is the technique of choice for identifying cerebral venous sinuses. Arterial angiography is required for the identification of most small intracranial aneurysms and for definitive outlining of spinal arteriovenous anomalies.

Electrodiagnostic Studies

Electroencephalography (EEG). EEG records the electrical activity of the cerebral cortex (Fig.

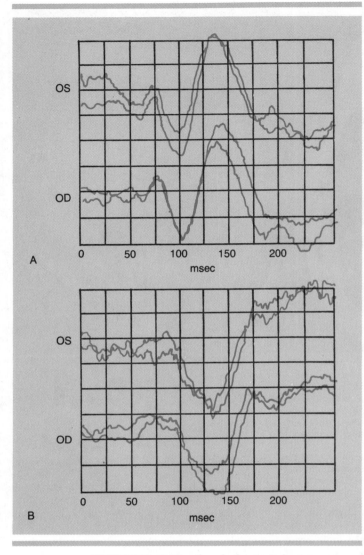

FIGURE 115—2. Visual evoked potentials. *A*, In a normal patient potentials from the two eyes are identical. The large downward deflection (P 100 wave) is seen exactly at 100 msec. *B*, In a patient suffering from multiple sclerosis there are abnormal wave forms from both eyes, with a striking delay of the P 100 wave, indicating abnormal optic nerve transmission.

22–1). Noninvasive and relatively inexpensive, EEG is a sensitive but nonspecific test for abnormal brain activity. It is particularly helpful in the diagnosis of epilepsy, especially if a seizure occurs spontaneously or can be evoked during the recording process. EEG often identifies the presence and type of epilepsy. It also helps differentiate seizures from metabolic encephalopathy, and it aids in distinguishing between organic and psychogenic causes of unresponsiveness. The absence of EEG activity, properly recorded, supports the diagnosis of brain death. A new, still experimental technique, *magnetoencephalography*, records the magnetic field produced by the brain's electrical activity and promises to localize epileptic activity better than does EEG.

Sensory Evoked Potentials. Sensory evoked potentials are averaged EEG responses to a series of visual, auditory, or somatosensory stimuli. The potentials so generated are highly reproducible and provide information on the integrity of the peripheral and central pathway carrying the signal.

Visual Evoked Responses (VER) (Fig. 115–2) are elicited by having the subject fixate on a screen showing a reversing checkered pattern. Electrodes placed over the scalp record a positive potential, the latency of which is related to the conduction velocity in the optic nerve and central visual pathways. The method is highly sensitive for detecting altered conduction of the optic nerve even in asymptomatic patients. It is useful in supporting the early diagnosis of multiple sclerosis.

Brain Stem Auditory Evoked Responses (BAER). BAER detect and often localize abnormalities of the acoustic nerve or brain stem auditory pathways. A click stimulus to the ear generates a series of potentials from the brain stem auditory relay pathway which can be recorded over the scalp at the vertex. Clinically relevant potentials occur from the auditory nerve, superior olive, lateral lemniscus, and inferior colliculus.

Somatosensory Evoked Responses (SER). Stimulation of a peripheral nerve gives rise to potentials that can be recorded over the spine and scalp. The median or peroneal nerves are most often stimulated. The latency of the recorded potential increases progressively from lumbar to cervical spine and brain. The result permits calculation of a conduction velocity thought to reflect transit times in the large sensory fiber pathways of peripheral nerve, nerve plexus, spinal cord, and brain.

Electromyography

Nerve Conduction Studies. Percutaneous electrical stimulation of a peripheral nerve generates an action potential. For motor nerves, electrodes are placed over a muscle to record the evoked muscle action potential. One stimulates the nerve innervating that muscle at various points along its length and determines the conduction velocity from the time required to travel from each site of stimulation to the onset of the evoked muscle response. For sensory nerves, one stimulates cutaneous nerve branches distally and places recording electrodes over the nerve at various proximal sites. The *F-response* provides a measure of conduction in the proximal portions of a motor nerve and ventral root. The *H-reflex* provides the electrical equivalent of the stretch reflex by stimulating sensory fibers of the posterior tibial nerve in the popliteal fossa and recording the efferent evoked action potential from the soleus muscle. These peripheral nerve and muscle electrophysiologic studies assist in determining whether disease involves nerve, muscle, or both and in determining the distribution of the abnormality. They facilitate the differentiation of demyelinating neuropathy from axonal neuropathy, neuropathy from radiculopathy, and primary muscle disease from disease of the motor unit. Demyelinating neuropathies affect mainly large fibers and slow the conduction velocity. When disease

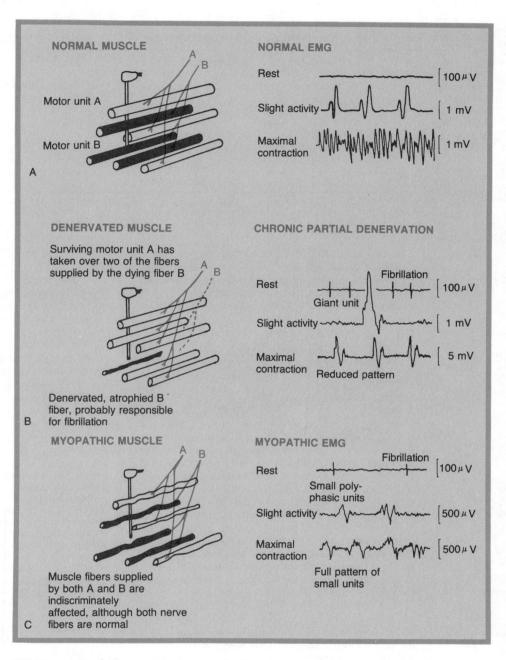

FIGURE 115–3. Electromyogram from normal and abnormal muscle. *A*, The trace shows two normally innervated motor units (left) and the needle electromyogram shows those units at rest, with minimal activity (only one unit is active) and during maximal contraction. When all units are active the normal baseline cannot be seen (complete interference pattern). *B*, Denervated muscle after damage to the motor neuron or peripheral nerve supplying motor unit B. The surviving motor unit has taken over two of the fibers supplied by B; other fibers have become atrophied. The resting tracing shows fibrillation potentials (spontaneous discharge of denervated fibers). Minimal voluntary activity fires a giant motor unit, indicating that there has been sprouting of motor neuron A. With maximal contraction, loss of motor units leads to an incomplete interference pattern. *C*, Myopathic muscle. There is random loss of muscle fibers in all motor units, although the nerve remains normal. Fibrillation potentials are rarely seen unless there is involvement of nerve terminals as well. Minimum voluntary activity fires a small motor unit of short duration. With maximal contraction there is a complete interference pattern of smaller than normal amplitude. (Modified from Patten J: Neurological Differential Diagnosis. New York, Springer-Verlag, 1977.)

TABLE 115–6. DIFFERENTIATION AMONG MYOPATHY, AXONOPATHY, MYELINOPATHY, AND RADICULOPATHY USING ELECTROPHYSIOLOGIC STUDIES

	MYOPATHY	AXONOPATHY	MYELINOPATHY	RADICULOPATHY
Nerve conduction velocity	Normal	Normal	Slow	Normal
F-response	Normal	Normal	Delayed-absent	Delayed-absent
H-reflex*	Normal	Normal	Delayed-absent	Delayed-absent
EMG				
Voluntary contraction	Predominance of small motor units	Predominance of large motor units	Normal	Normal, some large motor units
Spontaneous activity	Fibrillations	Fibrillations, fasciculations	Normal	Fibrillations, fasciculations

* Usually studied with posterior tibial nerve stimulation, recording the soleus contraction, thus providing an index of S1 root function only.

damages axons in addition to myelin, there is a decrease in the number of axons that can be electrically activated, resulting in a diminution in the size of the compound action potential.

Electromyography (EMG). EMG is performed by inserting a needle electrode into a muscle to record the structure's electrical activity (Fig. 115–3). Normal muscle is silent at rest, but denervated or diseased muscle membranes become spontaneously excitable, generating *fibrillation potentials* of small amplitude. When the nerve itself is diseased, entire motor units may become spontaneously active. The resulting *fasciculations* are often visible percutaneously and can be detected by the electrode. Furthermore, when damaged axons cease to innervate muscle fibers, the remaining axons gradually sprout collaterals that reinnervate the denervated fibers; as a result, during voluntary contraction the few remaining muscle units show a decrease in their number and an increase in the size of their electrical potentials. When the patient voluntarily contracts the muscle being examined, action potentials appear and with full voluntary contraction cannot be distinguished one from the other (interference pattern). With neurogenic weakness, the interference pattern is reduced or disappears because of the paucity of voluntary reaction potentials. By contrast, as muscle fibers degenerate in primary disease of muscle, the size of motor units decreases, since each nerve now innervates fewer fibers. During voluntary contraction the number of activated units is normal, but their amplitude is smaller; the interference pattern remains normal. In primary myopathies, the distribution of abnormality helps in characterizing the myopathy itself. Table 115–6 provides guides to the usefulness and pertinent changes in electrophysiologic tests in various neuromuscular disorders. The EMG must be interpreted in light of the clinical findings, since occasional fibrillation potentials may be found in normals and confusingly similar changes sometimes are found in myopathies and neuropathies. Table 115–6 indicates how the above electrical

tests are used to differentiate nerve from muscle disease.

Neuromuscular Transmission Studies. Diseases of the neuromuscular junction (p. 702) are characterized by normal nerve conduction velocity and usually a normal EMG. Repetitive electrical activation of the neuromuscular junction, however, will produce either an abnormal diminution (myasthenia gravis) or an abnormal facilitation (Lambert-Eaton pseudomyasthenia, botulism) of the successively evoked muscle action potential.

REFERENCES

Barrows HS, and Robyn MT: Problem-Based Learning, An Approach to Medical Education. Springer Series on Medical Education, Vol 1. New York, Springer, 1980. *Good chapters in history taking and clinical problem solving.*

Bradbury M, Radda GK, and Allen PS: Nuclear magnetic resonance techniques in medicine. Ann Intern Med 98:514–529, 1983. *A well-written summary of this rapidly advancing field.*

Chiappa KH: Evoked Potentials in Clinical Medicine. New York, Raven Press, 1983. *A good summary supplemented by extensive references.*

Mayo Clinic and Mayo Foundation: Clinical Examinations in Neurology. 5th ed. Philadelphia, WB Saunders Co, 1981. *Provides an excellent detailed consideration of the clinical and laboratory evaluation of the neurological patient according to the technology available in 1980.*

Plum F (ed): Neurologic and behavioral diseases. In Wyngaarden JB, and Smith LH Jr (eds): Cecil Textbook of Medicine. 17th ed. Philadelphia, WB Saunders Co, 1985, pp 1965–2216. *An extensive multiauthored description of diseases of the nervous system.*

Plum F, and Posner JB: Neurology. In Smith LH, and Thier SO (eds): Pathophysiology: The Biological Principles of Disease. 2nd ed. Philadelphia, WB Saunders Co, 1985. *Gives detailed consideration to the physiology and pharmacology of neurological symptoms, signs, and diseases.*

Weisberg LA: Computed tomography in the diagnosis of intracranial disease. Ann Intern Med 91:87–105, 1979. *A recent summary article.*

A. ALTERED STATES OF CONSCIOUSNESS

SUSTAINED LOSS OF CONSCIOUSNESS

Consciousness reflects two functions, the level of arousal and the mental content of the aroused state. Arousal is a vegetative activity, regulated by nuclei lying in the reticular formation of the middle brain stem tegmentum and the basal diencephalon. Mental content comprises the higher brain functions that determine our recognition of the inner and outer world and how we adapt to it. These higher functions are regulated mainly by the primary and association areas of the cerebral cortex together with their immediate subcortical nuclei.

Disorders of Arousal

The critical region for pathological interruption of arousal lies in the tegmental reticular formation, extending from the most rostral third of the pons through the midbrain tegmentum and into the region of the paramedian posterior hypothalamus. Acute bilateral injury or functional depression of this centrally located gray matter reduces or temporarily abolishes arousal and produces, at least temporarily, the facial appearance of sleep. Transient, sleeplike coma also ensues if the eventual reticular target organ, the cerebral cortex, is acutely bilaterally damaged or functionally depressed. In fact, unless one takes other signs into account, the level of reduced arousal does not distinguish clinically between the coma of diffuse cortical damage and the unresponsiveness caused by lesions of the reticular activating system. The anatomy of the lesion, however, does influence the duration of pathological unarousability as well as the pattern of associated signs of motor and neuro-ophthalmologic dysfunction and the mental content of the awake state when arousal returns.

Consciousness describes an awake state accompanied by awareness of self and the environment. Behaviorally, self-awareness must be distinguished from purely reflex responses to noxious or special sensory stimuli such as occur in the vegetative state (see below).

Coma describes an eyes-closed condition of psychological unresponsiveness with no recognizable learned responses to stimuli. Except in a small number of persons with structural damage affecting the posterior hypothalamic area, eyes-closed coma always is transient, lasting days or occasionally weeks before wake-sleep cycles return. No consistent pharmacological system in the brain has been identified in the pathogenesis of coma, although both dopamine agonists and amphetamine congeners sometimes produce partial nonspecific arousal in stuporous persons.

Stupor is a state of psychological unresponsiveness interruptable only by sustained exogenous stimulation.

Obtundation describes reduced arousal with or without an associated impairment in awakened psychological functions. Drowsiness, hypersomnia, and pronounced reduction in alertness fall into this category.

Confusion implies partial disorientation coupled with misperceptions of stimuli, of events, and in the accuracy of memories. Delusions may be present, agitation usually is lacking, and sleep is increased. When prolonged, confusional states pass imperceptibly into dementia.

Delirium classically describes a more agitated and severely disoriented condition than confusion. Affected patients commonly are fearful, boisterous, and hallucinating, most often visually but sometimes for sounds or voices as well. A dream-like state lacking self-recognition is frequent, as is reversal of sleep-wake cycles and, sometimes, prolonged insomnia or excessive daytime sleep.

The vegetative state describes a condition in which the patient regains or retains wake-sleep cycles but provides no evidence of possessing psychological awareness of self or the environment. Persons in the vegetative state may demonstrate inconsistent emotional responses to the environment, and they may withdraw from noxious stimuli or even intermittently follow moving objects with the eyes or head. These responses are mediated subcortically, however, and consistent conditioned responses to psychological stimuli are lost. Vegetative persons do not respond appropriately to verbal command. Neuropathologically, such individuals show extensive bilateral damage to cerebral cortex and/or thalamus but retain an intact lower diencephalon and brain stem. The vegetative state can be transient or permanent, but its presence almost always implies an

TABLE 116–1. CRITERIA FOR DIAGNOSIS OF BRAIN DEATH

1. Nature and duration of coma is known
   a. Known structural disease or irreversible systemic metabolic cause
   b. No chance of drug intoxication or hypothermia; no paralyzing or sedative drugs recently given for treatment
   c. Six-hour observation of no brain function is sufficient in cases of known structural cause when no drug or alcohol is involved in cause or treatment; otherwise, 12 to 24 hours plus a negative drug screen is required
2. Absence of cerebral and brain stem function
   a. No behavioral or reflex response to noxious stimuli above foramen magnum level
   b. Fixed pupils
   c. No oculovestibular responses to 50 ml ice water calorics
   d. Apneic during oxygenation for 10 minutes
   e. Systemic circulation may be intact
   f. Purely spinal reflexes may be retained
3. Supplementary (optional) criteria* (any one acceptable)
   a. EEG isoelectric for 30 minutes at maximal gain
   b. Auditory-evoked responses reflect absent function in vital brain stem structures
   c. No cerebral circulation present on angiographic examination

* May be useful if medicolegal issues are in question or when taking organs for transplantation, especially at six-hour intervals.

TABLE 116–2. COMMON CAUSES OF STUPOR AND COMA

I. Supratentorial lesions
   A. Directly invading or destroying the posterior ventromedial diencephalon
      1. Neoplasms
      2. Infarcts
      3. Encephalitis
   B. Compressing or herniating diencephalon against the upper brain stem
      1. Cerebral hemorrhage
      2. Large cerebral infarction
      3. Subdural hematoma
      4. Epidural hematoma
      5. Brain tumor
      6. Brain abscess (rare)
II. Subtentorial lesions (compressing or destroying the midbrain–upper pontine reticular formation)
   A. Pontine or cerebellar hemorrhage
   B. Infarction
   C. Tumor
   D. Cerebellar abscess
III. Metabolic and diffuse lesions
   A. Anoxia or ischemia
   B. Hypoglycemia
   C. Nutritional deficiency
   D. Hepatic, renal, pulmonary, pancreatic insufficiency
   E. Exogenous poison
   F. Infections
      Meningitis
      Encephalitis
   G. Ionic and electrolyte disorders
   H. Mixed encephalopathies: aging, postoperative state, systemic infection, drugs in various combinations
   I. Multifocal small structural lesions, e.g. metastases, emboli, thrombi, etc.
   J. Concussion and postictal states
IV. Psychogenic unresponsiveness

extremely poor outcome if it lasts for more than two weeks.

The locked-in state describes a sustained condition wherein complete or nearly complete damage to efferent neural pathways prevents the patient from communicating except sometimes by coded, most often vertical, eye movements; consciousness remains but cannot be tested in a satisfactory manner. Either bilateral interruption of the cortical spinal tracts at the midbrain-pontine level or overwhelming motor polyneuropathy can produce the condition. An equivalently helpless and frightening state results when diffusely weak, conscious persons are intubated and passively ventilated. In both instances humane considerateness must comprise a major aspect of care of the patient.

Brain death is a twentieth-century phenomenon. Modern resuscitation techniques make it possible to maintain the vitality of the heart, lungs, and visceral organs for a prolonged period after effective brain function has been irreversibly lost. The circumstance has led to world-wide acceptance of the principle that when the brain is dead the person is dead. In the United States, the presence of brain death has been legally accepted by statute or precedent in many states, and in no instance has it been successfully challenged. Diagnostic criteria as given in Table 116–1 must be followed explicitly, and the determination of brain death should be confirmed by an experienced, qualified consultant.

Types of Coma and Approach to Diagnosis

Only a limited number of disorders can damage the brain so extensively or strategically that they interrupt consciousness (Table 116–2). Those that do fall into three general categories: (1) Supratentorial mass lesions that either (a) directly invade or destroy the posterior ventromedial diencephalon or (b) enlarge sufficiently to compress these medial basal areas or herniate them through the tentorial notch. (2) Subtentorial lesions that bilaterally damage or destroy the midbrain–upper pontine reticular activating system. (3) Metabolic, diffuse, or multifocal abnormalities that cause widespread cerebral hemispheric dysfunction with or without accompanying depression of the brain stem. Now that accurate brain imaging has become widely available to identify mass or destructive lesions, this third group produces the greatest number of problems in the diagnosis and management of altered states of consciousness.

Once consciousness is impaired, an evaluation of motor and neuro-ophthalmologic signs plus an appraisal of the breathing pattern provides the most useful clinical approach to making localizing diagnoses and estimating cause and prognosis. Brain imaging abets clinical localization and, in the case of mass or destructive lesions, often points to specific etiologies. Systematic studies of blood, urine, CSF, and other tissues potentially offer specific answers to the causes of metabolic encephalopathies.

Supratentorial Lesions. Primary lesions of the

posterior basal diencephalon are a well-established but unusual cause of stupor and coma. Acute infarcts resulting from the occlusion of rostrally directed branches from the apex of the basilar artery sometimes produce bilateral thalamic infarction, causing brief loss of arousal followed by permanent amnesia. Neoplasms, particularly primary lymphomas, granulomas such as those of sarcoid, or encephalitis can affect the posterior hypothalamus to cause gradually or acutely progressing hypersomnia, sometimes with patterns of nearly unarousable sleep lasting most of the 24-hour day. The conditions are diagnosed on the basis of other signs of hypothalamic dysfunction plus etiologic information gained from CT or MRI studies. Other than the above uncommon disorders, large supratentorial masses impair consciousness when they expand sufficiently to shift and squeeze the surrounding brain, a process that gradually leads to compression of the diencephalon. If not reversed, this sequence eventually produces the syndrome of central transtentorial herniation.

With supratentorial mass lesions, localizing symptoms and signs such as frontotemporal headache, focal seizures, or contralateral motor sensory abnormalities usually precede or accompany the development of impaired consciousness. Even when diencephalic compression begins to produce diffuse changes in motor reflexes and muscle tonus, brain stem mechanisms, reflected by intact pupillary and eye movements, remain preserved or consist of abnormal conjugate ocular deviation that can be overcome by oculovestibular (caloric) testing.

Central compression-herniation consists of displacement and compression of the diencephalon caudally toward the tentorial notch so that it eventually herniates against the midbrain. As a result, the level of arousal is reduced early, bilateral upper motor neuron signs tend to supplement early focal changes produced by the initial cerebral lesion, and signs of hypothalamic dysfunction, including small, equal pupils, ensue (Table 116–3). *Uncal (lateral) herniation* occurs when a lesion occupying the temporal fossa expands, pushing the uncus over the edge of the ipsilateral tentorium so as to compress the third nerve and midbrain. Reduced consciousness and bilateral motor signs appear relatively late, the earlier harbinger of serious trouble extending beyond the temporal lobe usually being incipient autonomic paralysis of the pupil. In either form of herniation, progressive stupor or coma associated with supratentorial mass or destructive lesions warns of impending upper brain stem compression and implies that unless quick and successful action can be taken irreversible neurologic damage may ensue.

Subtentorial Lesions. Subtentorial lesions causing coma (Table 116–4) almost always can be diagnosed anatomically by clinical signs. The midbrain-pontine reticular activating system (RAS) lies immediately adjacent to the brain stem oculomotor pathways and other cranial nerve nuclei. In its caudal extent, the RAS impinges upon

TABLE 116–3. SIGNS OF CENTRAL AND UNCAL HERNIATION

	CENTRAL	UNCAL
Arousal	Declines early	Declines late
Pupils	Small, equal, reactive	Ipsilateral dilatation
Oculocephalics	Full, conjugate	Unilateral third nerve palsy
Motor	Decerebrate early	Decerebrate late
Breathing	Sighs, yawns, periodic	Central hyperventilation, late

the autonomic respiratory control centers. Accordingly, abnormal pupils, disconjugate eye movements, and, often, motor and breathing difficulties accompany or even can precede the onset of stupor or coma. Such abnormalities almost always are structural, and brain imaging usually distinguishes among infarcts, hemorrhages, and mass lesions.

Metabolic, Diffuse, and Multifocal Disorders Causing Altered Consciousness. These include the conditions listed in Table 116–2, as well as several processes producing multifocal cerebral damage such as acute encephalitis, rapidly evolving multiple cerebral infarctions or metastases, severe brain trauma, and others. More details can be found in the reference material. All these conditions share the principle of functionally depressing or physically damaging so much of the cerebral sensory and association cortex that they globally affect the psychological capacities of the forebrain. Concurrently, by a process of transient caudal inhibition, they reduce or suppress the normal arousal mechanisms of the brain stem and the diencephalon. Several also directly depress certain aspects of brain stem function but almost none paralyze pupillary control. As a group, the disorders produce various aspects of the syndrome known as *acute metabolic encephalopathy.*

SIGNS AND SYMPTOMS. Neurologic signs and symptoms in metabolic encephalopathies characteristically reflect selective functional abnormalities of several different anatomic levels of the brain while sparing other functions that originate at similar levels. The most prominent features are alterations in arousal and mental content. Incipiently affected patients demonstrate reduced attention and can be perplexed, indifferent, distractible, or agitated. Almost always they have problems in maintaining the sustained social in-

TABLE 116–4. SIGNS OF BRAIN STEM DYSFUNCTION ACCOMPANYING SUBTENTORIAL COMA

Always present
  Caloric responses disconjugate or absent
  Pupils abnormal: pinpoint (pons), fixed (midbrain), irregular and/or unequal (pontine-midbrain)
Often present
  Ocular bobbing, irregularly irregular breathing, cranial fifth or seventh nerve paralysis, unilateral cerebellar signs, bilateral motor signs (decerebrate or flaccid)

tercourse necessary to complete a satisfactory history and cooperative physical examination. Disorders of cognition include impaired intermediate recall ("What were this morning's news stories?") and poor abstract and step-wise thinking ("Differentiate between character and reputation," "recite reverse serial sevens," "spell 'world' backwards"). Disorientation, first for time, then place, then person; confabulation; and obtundation and stupor follow in varying degrees and combinations depending on the intensity of the disorder and the rate at which it progresses. Fluctuations in behavior are common; symptoms of confusion or delirium tend to be accentuated by nightfall and unfamiliar surroundings.

Characteristic motor changes include tremor, asterixis, and multifocal myoclonus, as defined on page 703. Tremor tends to be coarse, irregular, rapid at 8 to 10 Hz, and brought out by movement. Asterixis or multifocal myoclonus arising acutely or subacutely and accompanying a recent impairment of consciousness is nearly pathognomonic for metabolic encephalopathy.

Psychomotor activity ranges widely from the extremes of restless, agitated, boisterous, hallucinating tremulous delirium (delirium tremens) to apathetic lethargy bordering on motionless mutism. Seizures, hyperactive stretch reflexes, and even focal signs sometimes can accompany several of the metabolic encephalopathies (e.g., drug withdrawal, global cerebral anoxia, hypoglycemia, hyperosmolar coma, fulminating hepatic encephalopathy). The focal signs, however, usually are transient and always are accompanied by other neurologic changes that reflect diffuse or multifocal brain disease.

The state of neuro-ophthalmologic functions can provide major clues in the metabolic encephalopathies. Pupillary light reflexes always are preserved except following the ingestion of a few drugs possessing anticholinergic properties (e.g., hyoscine, street drugs, or glutethimide, an uncommon sedative), the deliberate or accidental contact with mydriatics, or exposure to severe anoxia-asphyxia. Except for severe overdose of barbiturates or certain other sedatives, spontaneous conjugate eye movements or conjugate oculovestibular reflexes are preserved until the terminal phases of most metabolic comas.

Breathing alterations are common: vigorous hyperpnea (Kussmaul breathing) accompanies the metabolic acidosis of diabetes, uremia, lactacidosis, and organic alcohol ingestion, while less prominent overbreathing characterizes the alkaloses of hepatic disease, septic shock, and early salicylism. Hypoventilation is prominent in CO_2 encephalopathy whether due to pulmonary disease or medullary respiratory depression.

Psychogenic Unresponsiveness

Psychogenic unresponsiveness includes states of catatonic withdrawal in schizophrenia or severe depression as well as hysteria and malingering. All can superficially resemble metabolic coma. Such patients, however, possess a normal general physical and neurologic examination. They may resist answers during attempts to appraise mental status but unless hysterical do not give wrong ones. Those with closed eyes resist passive opening, and when the lids are passively raised they abruptly shut again: neither is a phenomenon of organic coma. Pupils are briskly reactive unless mydriatics have been self-instilled, ice water calorics give normal responses, and the EEG is normal. However, fear, anxiety, or other emotions commonly superimpose prominent psychiatric symptoms on those caused by acute organic disease and must be allowed for when evaluating acutely ill patients.

DIAGNOSIS AND MANAGEMENT

A systematic history and careful general medical examination plus screening blood counts and immediate analyses of blood glucose, electrolytes, and respiratory gases rapidly discriminate among most of the conditions identified in Table 116–2. Where the past history is unknown, certain findings immediately suggest a line of pursuit (Tables 116–5 and 116–6). Once emergency life-support measures are taken, a CT scan of the brain usually quickly settles doubts about the presence or absence of acute space-occupying lesions that may require emergency surgical treatment. Conversely, a negative CT scan provides strong reassurance that lumbar puncture (LP) carries little risk. In any event, LP is best withheld if one suspects an acute intracerebral mass, including cerebral hemorrhage. If meningitis is suspected, however, one must proceed with lumbar puncture immediately; to delay diagnosis and appropriate antimicrobial therapy invites serious complications or death. The EEG helps diagnose only a few

TABLE 116–5. HELPFUL CLUES IN EARLY DIAGNOSIS OF COMA

Fever:	Meningitis, encephalitis, postictal state, acute bacterial endocarditis, scopolamine poisoning
Hypothermia:	Myxedema, hypoglycemia, drug poisoning, brain stem infarct
Signs of trauma:	Cerebral contusion; extradural, subdural or parenchymal hematoma
Severe hypertension:	Cerebral or subarachnoid hemorrhage; hypertensive encephalopathy
Hypotension:	Occult (usually gastrointestinal) bleeding, septic shock, hypovolemia, poor cardiac output, depressant drug poisoning Tachycardia > 180 per min, bradycardia < 40 min: poor cardiac output
Arrhythmias:	Tricyclic overdose, myocardial infarction
Hyperventilation:	Diabetic ketosis; uremia; organic alcohol poisoning; lactic acidosis, hepatic coma; salicylate poisoning
Hypoventilation:	Pulmonary insufficiency, depressant drug or opiate poisoning, low brain stem infarct or hemorrhage
Petechiae:	Meningococcemia; thrombocytopenic and nonthrombocytopenic purpura; bacterial endocarditis
Pink skin:	Carbon monoxide
Stiff neck:	Acute meningitis, subarachnoid hemorrhage

altered states of consciousness, being definitive in examples of partial complex or petit mal status epilepticus and suggestive in certain forms of encephalitis and destructive brain injury.

Most coma of unknown cause that arises outside the hospital results from self-induced drug poisoning, and patients lacking definite alternate diagnoses must be managed for this possibility until proved otherwise. Other puzzling metabolic encephalopathies also are common, especially in the hospital setting where confusional, obtunded, or delirious states can complicate the course of many acute medical or surgical diseases. The laboratory profile given in Table 116–6 plus a search for offending medications in doubtful instances frequently gives the answer. Often, several individual abnormalities contribute to the trouble.

Acutely altered states of consciousness can themselves add to the potential ill effects of the underlying disorder and must be treated while proceeding with the diagnosis and specific treatment of the underlying cause. Table 116–7 outlines the major emergency steps to be taken in almost all of the major conditions producing sustained loss of consciousness.

BRIEF AND EPISODIC LOSS OF CONSCIOUSNESS

These conditions usually must be diagnosed in retrospect from the history given by patients and witnesses. Laboratory studies, unless obtained on the spot, provide only inferential evidence and are potentially most useful in detecting unsuspected causes of asystole in older persons.

Syncope. Syncope describes brief loss of consciousness due to a global reduction in cerebral blood flow. The disorder almost always is due to an abrupt or semiabrupt loss of cardiac output, most frequently secondary to acutely impaired right heart filling (cardiac rhythm maintained) or left heart output failure (asystole or severe arrhythmia) (Table 116–8).

Syncope due to reduced right heart filling usually results from pooling of blood in capacitance veins of the lower extremities or the splanchnic abdominal circulation. Vasodepressor reflex mechanisms are the most frequent cause. Orthostatic hypotension secondary to depleted blood volume, hypotensive drugs, or neurologic disease, as well as mechanical increases in pulmonary resistance such as accompany severe coughing or acute pulmonary infarction, provide less frequent mechanisms. Cardiac tamponade interferes with both right and left heart filling and output.

Vasodepressor syncope (simple fainting) exceeds in frequency all other causes of acute brief unconsciousness combined. Simple fainting tends to be a recurrent problem in some individuals; a few give a family history of the disorder. No associated neurologic or cardiologic abnormality can be found in most cases. Attacks are engendered by emotional crises, acute painful visceral stimuli, hyperventilation, and, in susceptible persons, various combinations of alcohol and

TABLE 116–6. LABORATORY TESTS IN METABOLIC ENCEPHALOPATHY

IMMEDIATE	LATER
Glucose	Liver function tests including arterial ammonia
Na^+	Sedative drug levels
Ca^{++}	Blood and CSF culture
BUN	Full electrolytes, including Mg^{++}
Arterial blood pH, P_{CO_2}, P_{O_2}	Coagulation profile
Lumbar puncture	EEG

TABLE 116–7. EMERGENCY MANAGEMENT OF COMA

1. Assure airway and oxygenation
2. Maintain adequate systemic circulation
3. Give glucose after first obtaining blood for analysis
4. Give thiamine 50 to 100 mg intravenously
5. Stop generalized seizures
6. Restore blood acid-base and osmolar balance but do not change serum sodium by more than 20 mOsm per day
7. Treat infection specifically
8. Treat extreme body temperature (>41 or <35°C)
9. Consider naloxone
10. Control agitation-tremulousness with diazepam

hunger. Many persons experience a brief prodrome of anxiety, giddiness, diaphoresis, and nausea before collapsing, while others drop precipitously as heart rate and blood pressure fall and cardiac output declines. True syncope always occurs in the erect or sitting position, never when supine. Patients are pale and sweaty and sometimes have one or two generalized clonic twitches during a profound faint. Incontinence is unusual, but vomiting, micturition, and diarrhea commonly follow the attack. In young persons with a negative physical examination and characteristic history, physiological or structural disease almost never is present and laboratory studies need not be extensive. Hysteria and drug-alcohol intoxication are the chief resemblers. Table 122–4 (page 765) outlines the differences from minor seizures. Simple fainting can affect persons older than age 50 years, but a first episode in that age group

TABLE 116–8. MAJOR CAUSES OF SYNCOPE

I. **Inadequate cardiac return**
   A. *Vasovagal attacks*
   B. *Orthostatic hypotension*
      Inadequate vasoconstriction; hypovolemia
   C. *Mechanical obstruction*
      Cough; Valsalva maneuver; pulmonary infarct
II. **Primary cardiac output failure**
   A. *Arrhythmia*
      Asystole >10 seconds; tachycardia >180/min; bradycardia <30–40/min; glossopharyngeal or carotid sinus reflex
   B. *Other*
      Cardiac tamponade; aortic stenosis plus exercise; acute myocardial infarction; atrial myxoma
III. **Cerebral causes (all rare)**
      Basilar insufficiency; hyperventilation attacks; plateau waves

deserves careful medical evaluation to rule our serious cardiac disorders. Although less than 10 per cent of all syncope can be attributed to heart disease, when the association does exist, it often implies a poor prognosis. Cerebral transient ischemic attacks rarely simulate syncope. Occasionally, vasodepressor syncope accompanies attacks of severe migraine in adolescents and young adults.

Syncope recovers too quickly to treat except by placing the subject supine and elevating the lower extremities; there are no effective preventive measures except when severe cardiac disorders exist. Avoiding offending foods as well as eliminating bouts of prolonged alcoholic ingestion without food helps when the history incriminates such associations.

Other causes of brief unconsciousness are uncommon. *Hyperventilation attacks* stand closer to the syndrome of panic than to syncope. Affected patients may complain of feeling unreal, floating, or dizzy, but they do not lose contact with the environment. Treatment consists of attempts to provide the sufferer with insight and an emphasis on the benign nature of the condition. Propranolol, up to 40 mg three times daily, may help to reduce the frequency of attacks. The drug is especially useful in warding off stage fright.

Hypoglycemia. Hypoglycemia due to exogenous or, occasionally, endogenous hyperinsulinism can produce brief and episodic alterations of consciousness. Characteristic are episodes of confusion, although hypersomnia, excess fatigability, and, rarely, convulsions can occur. Diagnosis depends on suspicion and the finding of blood sugars lower than 30 to 40 mg/dl during an attack or following fasting.

Drop Spells. Drop spells are poorly understood, uncommon attacks that affect persons of middle age or older, chiefly women. A sudden loss of muscular tone affects the lower extremities, leading to abrupt falls without evidence of loss of consciousness. Basilar artery insufficiency may cause some cases, but the mechanism in most remains unknown. Most cases resist treatment.

FOCAL DISTURBANCES OF HIGHER BRAIN FUNCTION

GENERAL CONSIDERATIONS

The human cerebral cortex contains the final receiving areas for somatic and special sensory information as well as the primary motor cortex that executes all voluntary movement. Lying between, making up 80 per cent or more of the cortical mantle, is the association cortex, which converts sensation into perception and integrates instinctive and acquired memory into symbolic communication and planned, emotionally influenced behavior (Fig. 116–1). Increasing evidence indicates that certain areas of the association cortex preferentially serve relatively specific aspects of higher brain function. Damage to these regions often produces symptoms that betray the anatomy of the injury. This principle especially applies to psychological functions that are strongly lateralized in one hemisphere or the other, such as language and orientation to extracorporeal space.

Injury to a frontal lobe produces contralateral focal paresis or hemiparesis if it impinges upon the motor strip. Lesions located immediately anteriorly encroach on premotor areas to interfere with the integration of contralateral learned movement, while frontopolar abnormalities affect functions involved in the anticipation and planning of future behavior. These last-mentioned influences are subtle and often difficult to detect clinically except in the presence of large or bilateral lesions.

Parietal lobe damage to the post-central gyrus impairs contralateral sensory perception for form,

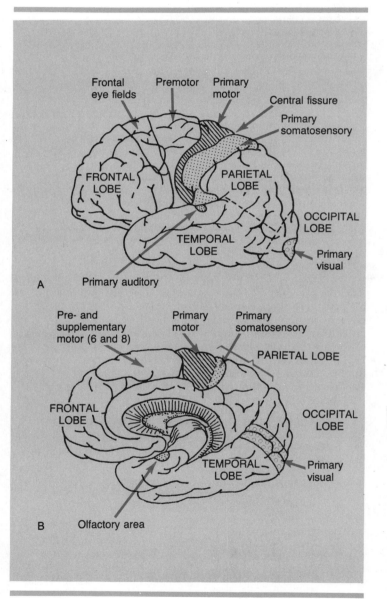

FIGURE 116–1. Major anatomic and functional areas of the cerebral hemispheres. *A*, Lateral surface. *B*, Medial surface.

texture, and shape, producing *astereognosis*. More posteroinferior parietal injury interferes with converging occipital, parietal, and temporal lobe pathways and produces disorders proportional to the size and acuteness of the lesion. Large deficits in this area, especially in the nondominant right hemisphere, can cause spatial neglect, both to the opposite side of the body and to the outside world. Such patients often are confused and inattentive and have difficulty in the ordering of successive spatial acts, as seen in dressing apraxia.

Temporal lobe functions link closely to language, memory, and emotional capacities and are discussed below as well as in the section on complex partial seizures.

LANGUAGE AND APHASIA

Aphasia or dysphasia describes a loss or impairment of language function as a result of damage to the specific language areas of the cerebrum. The condition must be distinguished, respectively, from *dysarthria*, a disturbance in the articulation of speech, from the word salad of schizophrenia, from certain deliria, and from defects in sensory systems that prevent visual or auditory perceptions from reaching the language cortex.

Lesions damaging the posterior superior temporal gyrus of the dominant hemisphere and its adjacent area characteristically destroy the capacity to recognize the sensory symbols of language or to connect words learned with inner thoughts or memories. The classic result is *Wernicke's aphasia*. Affected patients cannot recognize spoken, written, or symbolic instructions except the simplest verbal commands (e.g., "Stop!"). Despite the severe injury to comprehension, expressed words often are chosen correctly. Patient's with Wernicke's aphasia speak nonsense fluently and with a natural rhythm, although neither they nor the examiner can detect understandable syntax or meaning. They cannot repeat phrases given by the examiner. Insight is lost, and prognosis for total recovery is poor. Incomplete or marginal lesions in this area can produce word blocking or fluent aphasia in which comprehension is preserved.

Broca's aphasia is characterized by severe disturbances in the output of either spontaneous or commanded speech and writing. Comprehension is relatively well-preserved, although things spoken usually are understood better than things read. The vulnerable area includes the inferior lateral frontal area of the dominant hemisphere, just anterior to the facial region of the primary motor strip. Largely because of vascular distributions, many patients with Broca's aphasia also have an associated right hemiparesis or hemiplegia, but this is the result of an independent internal capsular lesion.

Conduction aphasia is characterized by a fluent, Wernicke-like aphasia coupled with the ability of the patient to repeat after the examiner phrases and often long sentences. Such an ability implies that Wernicke's and Broca's areas as well as the major connections between them must be relatively intact, so that the responsible lesions must lie near to but not within the primary speech areas.

Global aphasia describes the combined severe loss of all major aspects of language function due to frontotemporal damage in the dominant hemisphere. Affected patients can neither comprehend nor express language except, perhaps, in the form of brief expletives or phrases. Most have a right hemiplegia. Insight is poor, as is prognosis for full recovery.

Mutism, the inability to speak, occurs in several forms. Acutely, it appears in association with vascular lesions of the left frontal lobe involving either part of Broca's area or its conducting pathways. In the absence of hemiplegia, acute mutism characteristically carries a benign prognosis and disappears within a few days to a week or so. Acute mutism also occurs paroxysmally with epileptic attacks involving the left inferior premotor area. More sustained mutism develops as a symptom of bilateral frontal lobe damage. Sustained mutism and behavioral withdrawal also can accompany severe psychiatric disorders recognized by their lack of signs, symptoms, or laboratory findings of structural frontal lobe disease. *Anarthria*, the inability to speak because of abnormal innervation or mechanical disease of the vocal apparatus, differs from mutism in that affected patients make sounds and express their frustration over being unable to speak. Neurogenic causes of anarthria include severe bulbar or pseudobulbar palsy, conditions readily diagnosed by the presence of other signs and symptoms of nuclear or supranuclear paralysis.

The commonest cause of aphasia is vascular damage, either from infarction or from hemorrhage, in the distribution of the middle cerebral artery or, less often, the posterior or anterior cerebral arteries. Other frequent causes are severe head trauma, neoplasms, and other space-occupying lesions. None of these disorders produces very discrete brain injury, and their anatomic variability necessarily leads to an equally inconsistent patterning of the major symptoms of aphasia.

Language function is strongly lateralized in most human brains. In almost all right-handed persons the left hemisphere is heavily dominant for speech. Among the left-handed and strongly ambidextrous, about 70 per cent show a left hemisphere language dominance or predominance. Of the remaining 30 per cent, about half show strong language representation in each hemisphere, while the remainder are right dominant. With many left-handed and ambidextrous persons, damage to the major language area on either side may produce acute symptoms of aphasia, but a higher percentage recover than do right-handed persons with comparable left hemispheric lesions.

Apraxia refers to a disturbance of or an inability to perform learned motor acts despite retention of sufficient sensory and language function to understand the command and the motor capacity to carry it out (praxis). The condition most commonly accompanies deep lesions of the frontal or parietal lobes, often multifocal, such as occur with the degenerative dementias or after multiple strokes.

Agnosia is an uncommon psychological phenomenon characterized by the inability to recognize a complex sensory stimulus despite the preservation of elemental perceptions and the absence of a defect in language. The phenomenon requires either bilateral or extensive impairment of the association cortex for the affected perception. It occurs most often with multiple strokes or as a symptom of one of the degenerative dementias.

MEMORY

Memory and learning are identical processes. Disturbances of memory include defects in past memory, called *retrograde amnesia*, and the inability to form new memories from ongoing events, called *anterograde amnesia*.

Patterns of Memory Failure. Memory can be divided into immediate, intermediate, and remote epochs. *Immediate memory* consists of holding in the mind material just heard or read with no necessary intervening storage process. *Intermediate memory* covers the time span beginning within a few seconds past and extending backward for 24 to 48 hours or more. *Long-term memory* extends beyond that epoch, but this too has its gradations, for many childhood memories tend to be well recalled even as more recent ones begin to fade. Standard I.Q. tests that include definitions of words and functions learned before the age of 14 years often give normal scores in adults who have suffered from diseases that severely damage or destroy recent and anterograde memory.

Memory Mechanisms. Specific structures make important contributions to the anatomy of adult memory. Left hippocampal damage is followed by modest impairments in verbal memory, while right hippocampal damage may produce difficulties in visual spatial memories and the recognition of musical tones. Bilateral damage or surgical removal of the hippocampus in the adult results in profound and usually permanent deficits in intermediate memory affecting especially the verbal-visual-spatial spheres. Proportional defects in anterograde learning accompany the retrograde loss. At the subcortical level, bilateral damage to the dorsal-medial nuclei of the thalamus and, probably, the mammillary bodies, results in a profound multidimensional disturbance of memory. The prominent memory loss that often accompanies Huntington's disease suggests that striatal mechanisms may contribute to the normal memory process.

Cerebral memory mechanisms depend in an incompletely understood way on cholinergic and other autonomic projections that link the subcortical basal forebrain diffusely with the hippocampus and the association cortex of the temporal, parietal, and frontal lobes. Degeneration of these projections is a prominent accompaniment of the dementia of Alzheimer's and certain other dementias.

Clinical Memory Disorders. Many middle-aged and elderly persons report an increasing, relatively isolated difficulty in recalling proper names and recent events of minor importance. This "benign forgetfulness" bears no consistent relationship to the progressive dementias and is best treated with prompt and vigorous reassurance.

The most frequent causes of severe memory loss are the degenerative dementias, severe head trauma, brain anoxia or ischemia, nutritional impairment, encephalitis, and, less frequently, intracranial mass lesions.

Korsakoff's syndrome includes a profound recent memory loss, lack of insight, disorientation to time and place, and confabulation. In Western countries, nutritional Korsakoff's syndrome most frequently affects alcoholics and often accompanies or follows the florid signs and symptoms of acute Wernicke's encephalopathy or delirium tremens. Other causes include global cerebral anoxia-ischemia, status epilepticus, and subarachnoid hemorrhage, all of which can selectively and bilaterally damage vulnerable neurons in the hippocampus and medial diencephalon.

Even modest head trauma temporarily interrupts memory-mediating neural connections. Concussive injuries frequently produce an initially severe degree of retrograde and a lesser degree of anterograde amnesia; in most instances the memory loss almost disappears with time. A less fortunate prognosis accompanies prolonged posttraumatic coma. When this lasts more than two to three weeks, most patients over 25 years old never fully recover from memory impairment.

Permanent or prolonged amnesia occasionally can follow bilateral cerebral infarction, large brain tumors, or surgical operations affecting the hippocampus. Herpes simplex encephalitis has a predilection to produce necrotic-inflammatory lesions in the limbic system lying along the medial surfaces of the temporal lobes and characteristically leaves severe amnesia in its wake.

Transient global ischemia (TGA) is a condition marked by periods lasting from several minutes to as long as 12 hours or so of acute alert confusion. Affected persons can identify themselves but are severely disoriented for time and place. A severe deficit in retrograde memory accompanies the beginning of the attack and gradually disappears as it wears off. Most TGA attacks affect middle-aged or elderly persons and appear to reflect temporary vascular insufficiency affecting the hippocampal memory areas or their immediate neural connections. Affected patients usually remain bright, attentive, and alert and are distressed by their acute confusion. Most attacks neither leave residual limitations nor carry a strong risk of recurrence.

Psychogenic memory impairment can affect either recent or remote recall, usually in clinically recognizable patterns. Preoccupation, forced inattention, or reduced arousal may result in inconsistent responses to testing, with persons accurately recounting some current events but claiming to forget others. In general, organic disturbances in memory are marked by variability in what is remembered, emotionally reinforced material being recalled better than neutral events. With organic memory loss, disorientation is worst for time, less for place and persons, and never for self. In most instances, events of the recent past are unevenly forgotten more than remote memories, and the providing of cues often improves recall. By contrast, psychogenic amnesia tends to be greatest for emotionally important events, may elide from the patient's memory well-defined blocks of past events while leaving intact the recall of preceding or following material, and may affect remote memories equally with recent ones.

Treatment. Patients with acute post-traumatic amnesia show a high rate of spontaneous recovery. Improvement of memory loss from other organic disorders is less predictable except when the amnesia can be traced to an excess use of medication or a temporary systemic disorder such as hepatic, renal, or pulmonary insufficiency. To date, no medications or diets have proved to be clinically useful in the treatment of either the severe fixed amnesias or those that accompany the progressive dementias.

DEMENTIA

GENERAL CONSIDERATIONS

Dementia describes a sustained or permanent decline in several dimensions of intellectual function that interferes seriously with the individual's normal social or economic adjustment.

Static dementia can follow any disease that permanently structurally damages large portions of the association areas of the cerebral hemispheres. Severe head injury, global brain ischemia from cardiac arrest, large intracranial neoplasms or hemorrhages with their surgical removal, or infections such as severe encephalitis or meningitis can injure the brain sufficiently to prevent intelligence from ever returning to a pre-illness level. More frequent are the *progressive dementias* that affect increasing numbers of persons in the United States.

Table 116-9 indicates the most common causes of the progressive dementias and provides rough estimates of their frequencies. The figures emphasize the relatively greater problem of the progressive "primary" dementias, especially of the Alzheimer type.

Early Clinical Manifestations. The diagnosis of dementia implies the deterioration of several aspects of the intellect. Acute, static dementia seldom provides a problem in diagnosis. Most often the diagnostic problem following a sudden brain injury becomes not whether a mental decline has occurred but to what degree and how the patient can restructure his world to his new, possibly permanent limitation.

Early diagnosis in the progressive dementias is often more difficult. Initial symptoms involve deterioration in mood, personality, recent memory, judgment, and the capacity to form abstractions. Families or work associates usually notice a

TABLE 116–9. MAJOR CAUSES OF PROGRESSIVE DEMENTIA

1.	Senile dementia, Alzheimer type	50%
2.	Multi-infarct (arteriosclerotic)	20%
3.	Combination of 1 and 2	
4.	Communicating hydrocephalus	5%
5.	Alcoholic or post-traumatic	5%
6.	Huntington's chorea	5%
7.	Intracranial mass lesions	5%
8.	Uncommon or mixed with above:	10%
	Chronic drug use; Creutzfeldt-Jakob; metabolic (thyroid, liver, nutritional); degenerative (spinocerebellar, amyotrophic lateral sclerosis, parkinsonism, multiple sclerosis, Pick's, Wilson's, epilepsy); static dementia	

change before the patient does, and persons who live by intellectual efforts show their limitations earlier than do those with routine or manual jobs. Some patients become so apathetic as to seem depressed; in others great anxiety or increased irritability disrupts a once pleasant personality. Some persons with early dementia become paranoid or depressed. Loss of recent memory is a universal feature. Appointments are missed, plans forgotten, and stories of recent events become narrated repeatedly with no insight. Eventually orientation fails, first for days, then years, then months, and finally for place. Interest lags. Debts may be accumulated silently, property unwisely sold, accounts lost, and meals cooked twice over or served half-cold. Mental capacities can fluctuate suddenly without apparent relationship to external events. In Alzheimer's disease and some of the other progressive primary dementias, social amenities tend to be retained until late in the course. By contrast, incontinence, soup on the shirt, and a disheveled appearance are more characteristic of the mental deterioration that accompanies frontal lobe disease and intracranial mass lesions.

Diagnosis. The principal questions are: (1) Does a true decline in intellect exist? (2) If so, what is its probable cause?

The clinical examination of all patients with subacute or chronic central nervous system disease should include at least a brief evaluation of mental function. The standard bedside examination measures orientation, language, and memory retention by identifying recent major current events, the spelling of 'world' backwards, and recalling three unrelated words at five minutes. Asking the subject to perform serial sevens backwards tests attention span, while proverbs and definitions (e.g., river from canal) give some idea of abstract capabilities. A standardized approach helps to quantify errors. For further quantitation the Wechsler Adult Intelligence Scale (WAIS) provides useful information but requires the assistance of a trained psychologist. In mild to moderate dementia the verbal score of the WAIS provides an index of learning capacity, while the performance part reflects current mental abilities. A discrepancy of more than 15 points between the two provides a strong indication of acquired brain dysfunction.

The laboratory evaluation of dementia depends on the combined results of the history, general physical and neurologic examination, and preliminary laboratory results. Potentially treatable forms of chronic confusion or potential dementia include acute Wernicke's disease, pellagra, myxedema, hypercalcemia, cyanocobalamin (vitamin B_{12}) deficiency, drugs and toxins, hepatic encephalopathy, Wilson's disease, syphilis, granulomatous meningitis, and hydrocephalus. In the absence of leads from the history or examination, the tests listed in Table 116–10 will detect nearly all of these treatable disorders.

Pseudodementia is a term applied to reversible states in which reduced cognitive functions are caused by chronic drug intoxication or depressive illness. The aging brain is especially susceptible to both conditions. Among drugs, the barbiturates, benzodiazepines, butyrophenones, tricyclic antidepressants, MAO inhibitors, anticholinergics, corticosteroids, and digitalis are most often responsible.

The apathy, semimutism, akinesia, anxiety, and indifference of psychological depression often can be mistaken for dementia (see also Table 116–12). In contrast to demented patients, those with depression complain repeatedly of their poor memory. Patients with depression commonly eat little, often are severely constipated, sleep less than normal, and tend to behave best at night. Errors occur because of indifference or obstinant refusal rather than poor comprehension. Depressed patients may stumble over tests requiring attention, but they rarely forget major recent events or political figures, and when they do cooperate they adequately perform simple tests of language and two- or even three-stage verbal commands. By contrast, patients with incapacitating dementia are disoriented, their nights are more agitated and confused than their days, they have difficulty following commands, attention and recent memory are severely impaired, and they often suffer difficulties in language and specific learned motor functions. Brain imaging procedures show anatomic abnormalities in many of the dementias, and the EEG is slow in most of the dementias but not in depression.

THE MOST FREQUENT DEMENTIAS

Alzheimer's Presenile and Senile Dementia (ASD). The disorder occasionally affects persons younger than 50 years and is uncommon up to age 65. Subsequently, the prevalence increases to affect more than 20 per cent of those who live beyond age 80 years. Pathologically, the condition includes neuronal degeneration in the deeper levels of the cortex as well as in basal forebrain nuclei that project cholinergic fibers to the cortex and other areas of the cerebrum. Noradrenergic and serotonergic projections can be impaired as well. The neuropeptide, somatostatin, is reduced in the cortex. CT scans usually show only moderate cerebral atrophy. Histological examination discloses in the cortex characteristic fibrillary degeneration in neurons, together with amyloid-cored plaques containing cellular debris. Granular vacuoles are seen in some nerve cells; total degeneration affects others. Clinically, the onset usually is insidious, with memory impairment, personality alterations, and affective shallowness giving way to varying rates to severe amnesia, spatial disorientation, and language errors. Social amenities are preserved until late. Focal neurologic abnormalities or convulsions are not a feature. Specific diagnostic laboratory markers are lacking. The duration of ASD varies widely between extremes of 3 to 20 years, with patients declining slowly toward a terminal vegetative state. Death comes from pneumonia or intercurrent illness. Variants have been described in association with parkinsonism and motor neuron disease. There is no effective treatment.

Multi-infarct Dementia. This occurs as a result of successive large and small strokes, most often in association with hypertension or diabetes mellitus, but also with several other disorders capable of causing multiple cerebral arterial occlusions. The usual clinical picture is of successive, cumulative episodes of focal neurologic worsening, resulting in a disheveled condition in which aphasia is common, focal neurologic deficits are the rule, and CT scans show multiple lucencies reflecting past infarctions. Many patients develop pseudobulbar palsy and some, incontinence. Occasionally, successive small strokes in hypertensive patients result in a less episodic decline, but in any event evidence of severe heart and vascular disease is present.

Progressive Hydrocephalic Dementia. This is caused by chronic communicating hydrocephalus resulting from interference with CSF absorption pathways over the surface of the hemispheres. The ultimate cause in some cases is inflammatory or neoplastic meningitis and subarachnoid hemorrhage in others; in many instances the initiating mechanism escapes detection. The condition affects mostly persons older than 55 years and is marked by nonspecific changes in memory and intellect, apathetic fatigability and, usually, the development of a broad-based, moderately spastic ataxic gait, accompanied by extensor plantar responses. Urinary incontinence is common. Diagnosis depends on the clinical findings coupled with CT or MR figures showing abnormal cerebral ventricular dilatation and reduction in vertex sulcal markings coupled with evidence of periventricular edema (Fig. 116–2). Some patients im-

TABLE 116–10. LABORATORY SCREENING TESTS TO IDENTIFY A TREATABLE DEMENTIA

All cases: CBC; full chemistry screen; serum B_{12}; VDRL; serum free T_4 index and TSH. Brain CT or MR image.

If clinical indices suggest: Erythrocyte sedimentation rate, lumbar puncture (cells [including examination of sediment for cytology], protein, glucose, VDRL, culture); EEG

FIGURE 116–2. Communicating hydrocephalus. A 61-year-old woman seven years following uncomplicated removal of carcinoma of the lung developed symptoms of headache and depression of mood in the setting of her husband's catastrophic stroke. Neurologic examination and CT evaluation (A) were unremarkable, although in retrospect the fourth ventricle was slightly dilated. Over the next four months she became increasingly withdrawn, occasionally incontinent, and finally disoriented. She developed a broad-based ataxic gait and CT scan showed (B) absent sulcal markings at the vertex with (C) ventricular dilatation. NMR confirmed the ventricular enlargement (D) and showed periventricular increased signals typical of edema. Spinal fluid contained increased protein, hypoglycorrhachia (glucose 25 mg/dl), and malignant cells. Pressure was 180 mm in the lateral recumbent positions. Her alertness and gait temporarily improved following spinal drainage.

prove following surgical ventricular shunting, but no laboratory test reliably predicts the postoperative outcome.

Other Dementias. *Huntington's disease* is an autosomal, dominantly transmitted disorder producing chorea and dementia, discussed on page 733. *Creutzfeldt-Jakob disease*, a rare, relatively rapidly progressive dementia, affects persons of either sex, mainly between the ages of 40 and 65 years. Intellectual deterioration is accompanied by prominent signs of corticospinal tract dysfunction, myoclonus, and, sometimes, muscle atrophy. In the late stages EEG changes are characteristic. The illness is caused by an infectious particle (slow virus, p. 787) and has been inadvertently transmitted to healthy recipients by corneal transplants and deep brain electrodes taken from unrecognized cases and injections of growth hormone prepared from human pituitary glands taken at autopsy.

REFERENCES

Cummings JL, and Benson DF: Dementia, A Clinical Approach. Boston, Butterworths, 1983. *The most recent comprehensive text on the subject.*

Day SC, Cook ET, Funkenstein H, and Goldman L: Evaluation and outcome of emergency room patients with transient loss of consciousness. *Am J Med* 73:15, 1982. *An analysis of 198 patients gives differential diagnosis, indicates risk groups, and evaluates laboratory tests.*

Kapoor WN, Karpf M, Wieand S, et al: A prospective evaluation and follow-up of patients with syncope. *N Engl J Med* 309:197, 1983. *Among 204 mainly older patients with syncope, 26 per cent had a cardiovas-cular cause. Half of the latter group died within one year, compared to 6 per cent among those of idiopathic origin.*

Katzman R, and Terry RD: The Neurology of Aging. Philadelphia, FA Davis Co, 1983. *The best small monograph on the subject covers most aspects.*

Mesulam M-M (ed): Principles of Behavioral Neurology. Philadelphia, FA Davis Co, 1985. *A comprehensive, up-to-date monograph covering mechanisms and clinical aspects of human cerebral cortical function and disease.*

Plum F, and Posner JB: Alterations of consciousness: The cerebral hemispheres and higher brain function. In Smith LH, and Thier S (eds): Pathophysiology, The Biological Principles of Disease. 2nd ed. Philadelphia, WB Saunders Co, 1985, pp 1137–1167. *Discusses in detail the mechanistic bases of organic disturbances of human behavior.*

Plum F, and Posner JB: The Diagnosis of Stupor and Coma. 3rd revised ed. Philadelphia, FA Davis Co, 1982. *A comprehensive, clinically oriented, thoroughly referenced monograph.*

B.   DISORDERS OF MOOD AND BEHAVIOR

Many patients confront the physician with an abnormality of mood (anxiety, depression, indifference, anger) or behavior (inappropriateness, obsessiveness) that appears to play a major role in their illness. All such moods and behaviors must arise from the brain and therefore ultimately have a neurogenic origin. For pragmatic reasons, however, medicine distinguishes "organic" from "psychogenic" disorders of mood and behavior, the former caused by clearly identifiable structural or metabolic abnormalities of the brain, the latter by more or less identifiable environmental stresses or by endogenous predisposition. The distinction is potentially useful because behavioral symptoms of an organic nature usually require treatment different from those of a psychological nature. There are, however, two major problems with the organic-psychogenic distinction: (1) Often the distinction is clinically difficult. The appearance of psychological depression can be mimicked by frontal lobe brain tumors, and occasional patients with temporal lobe epilepsy develop illnesses indistinguishable from schizophrenia. On the other hand, some patients with conversion reactions develop neurologic signs (i.e., hemiparesis, sensory loss) that closely resemble those of structural brain disease or can even be superimposed on organic signs. (2) The two categories of illness at times overlap so much that the distinction is useless. For example, a patient with structural disease of the brain (e.g., Alzheimer's, post-traumatic) may develop acute anxiety or acute depression because the brain disease has rendered him unable to cope with environmental stresses that he formerly could handle. These psychological abnormalities may be prominent at a time when structural abnormalities are so subtle as to be undetectable by the physician, but sedative drugs used to treat the anxiety may exacerbate the dementia. On the other hand, patients suffering from anxiety or depression related to life stresses may complain only of face, neck, or back pain engendered by muscle tension and postural abnormalities associated with the anxiety (p. 667). A diagnostic work-up may in fact reveal structural disease of the temporomandibular joint, neck, or back which could be responsible for much of the pain. Nevertheless, the physician discovers that only when he appropriately treats the anxiety and depression is he able to ameliorate the somatic symptoms.

Since all mood and behavior *must* be associated with alterations of electrical or biochemical (or both) activity in the brain, it is likely that the future will bring greater knowledge of the physiology of brain function and lead to a clearer understanding of the interface between so-called organic and psychogenic illnesses. In the meantime, however, one must sift out for each patient the relative degrees of psychological as well as physical distress and give due weight to each in devising treatment. This chapter deals with illnesses that are thought to have primarily a psychological origin (organic disorders are described in other chapters) and follows in its classification the Diagnostic and Statistical Manual of Mental

Disorders (American Psychiatric Association, DSM-III) (Table 116–11). This manual provides objective diagnostic criteria for psychiatric disorders which, if rigorously applied, will prevent most diagnostic errors.

SCHIZOPHRENIC DISORDERS

These are a group of symptomatic disorders, possibly of different etiologies, characterized by disturbances of mind and personality, including hallucinations, delusions, and altered behavior toward others. The common thread consists of a disturbance in the form and content of thought. The disorder can be mimicked by structural or physiological-pharmacological disease of the brain, particularly that involving the limbic system, and thus the diagnosis requires that such structural disease be absent. The symptoms of schizophrenia begin before the age of 45, usually during adolescence or early adulthood. Most patients suffer from auditory hallucinations in which they either hear their own thoughts aloud or hear voices commenting on their action, often in a derogatory fashion. At times, several voices discuss the patient, usually in the third person. In addition to the hallucinations, affected patients suffer from delusions, such as, for example, that their actions or thoughts are controlled by outside forces and they are forced to carry out unwanted acts. To the examiner, schizophrenic patients often appear vague, unresponsive, and unemotional, with awkward and slowed thinking and ideas poorly related one to another. The affect is often flat or inappropriate, the patient laughing as he discusses serious problems. In addition, schizophrenic patients may show facial grimaces or tics that at times can resemble chorea or other extrapyramidal disorders. Occasional patients become immobile (catatonia), resembling the apathy and indifference of frontal lobe disturbances.

The cause of the schizophrenic disorders is unknown. Studies of twins have shown a strong genetic basis for the disorder, but no structural or biochemical abnormality of the brain has been identified. Some recent studies employing surveys with CT scans suggest that schizophrenics have atrophic brains, but the finding is far from universal.

The diagnosis rests first on the recognition of the constellation of distinctive symptoms and second on the ruling out of other potential causes for the emotional and personality disorders. Schizophrenic patients, if their cooperation can be assured, are oriented and have no abnormality of cognitive functions; by contrast, careful testing reveals that patients suffering from structural or metabolic disease of the brain manifested by selective symptoms suggesting schizophrenia demonstrate disorientation or other cognitive abnormalities. The clinical problem is that often cooperation cannot be assured in either group. Sometimes it is difficult to distinguish schizophrenia from an affective psychosis (see below).

TABLE 116–11.   PSYCHOGENIC DISORDERS OF MOOD AND BEHAVIOR

1. Schizophrenic disorders
2. Affective disorders
3. Anxiety disorders
4. Somatoform disorders
5. Dissociative disorders
6. Factitious disorders
7. Not attributable to a mental disorder, e.g., malingering

The distinction is important, since the treatment is different and the prognosis is considerably better in the affective psychoses than it is in schizophrenia.

The treatment of schizophrenia requires considerable expertise. Phenothiazine drugs are the mainstay and have been in large measure responsible for allowing most schizophrenic patients to be treated outside mental institutions. However, phenothiazines are difficult to use, in part because of problems with patient compliance. Furthermore, they are fraught with side effects. With the doses required to control the psychotic symptoms, some patients may develop akathisia and/or dystonic reaction or extrapyramidal disorders of the *Parkinson* type. The latter sometimes requires anticholinergic drugs to be added to the phenothiazines. In addition, long-term use of phenothiazines leads in more than 10 per cent of patients to *tardive dyskinesias* in the form of either continuous orolingual facial movements or less commonly dystonic movements of the trunk or extremities. Tardive dyskinesia may persist even when the phenothiazines are discontinued, and it responds poorly to therapy. Thus, one should attempt to control psychotic symptoms with the smallest possible dose of phenothiazines. In addition to drug therapy, it is often useful to try to establish a milieu in which patients can be comfortable and supported without being stressed. The recognition that such therapy is efficacious has led to the founding of halfway houses for chronically ill patients. If appropriate treatment is begun early, one third to one half of patients remit and another 30 per cent are able to live in the community.

AFFECTIVE DISORDERS

This category includes a group of disorders characterized by an excessive disturbance of mood, either elation or depression, the mood abnormality not being due to any other physical or mental disorder. The major affective disorders include recurrent episodes of either manic or depressive behavior, with attacks of either or both kinds repeating on several occasions during a lifetime, but usually clearing after weeks or months even without treatment. The pathogenesis is unknown, although monozygotic twin studies indicate a major genetic component. Unlike the schizophrenic disorders, between episodes most patients appear entirely normal.

Depression. The commonest affective disorder is depression. Depression is a feeling of sadness and misery, usually accompanied by lowered self-esteem and ranging from feelings of inadequacy and incompetence to a full-blown delusion that the patient is evil and responsible for many of the world's ills. The delusions (usually of a bizarre nature) distinguish "psychotic" from situational depressions (i.e., excessive sadness related to a true environmental event). Both groups of patients, however, suffer from physical symptoms as well as depression of mood. Depressed patients often have insomnia, usually falling asleep reasonably promptly but waking early in the morning and being unable to return to sleep. A few are hypersomniac, sleeping 12 to 16 hours a day. There is loss of appetitie, constipation, and frequently weight loss. Severely depressed patients are slow in their responses and appear apathetic and indifferent. They frequently complain of aches, pains, and other somatic symptoms (headache is particularly common) that may be either psychophysiological (p. 668) or delusional. Some patients complain only of the somatic symptoms and deny depression (masked depression). Psychomotor retardation may lead the physician to suspect either that the patient has serious organic disease or that he is suffering from dementia (pseudodementia of depression). However, cognitive functions, if the patient cooperates, are normal.

The diagnosis of depression may be difficult, but it is important. Depression, no matter what its underlying cause, can be treated, but if untreated may lead to prolonged illness, lengthy and unnecessary medical testing, and even suicide. There are several diagnostic problems. The first is to distinguish depression from physical illness. Many patients complaining of somatic symptoms look so ill that the physician searches for a disease such as cancer without considering depression as the primary process. Early morning awakening, loss of appetite, and, particularly, unexplained headache, however, should suggest depression; direct questioning about mood is essential and often rewarding. Patients should be asked if they feel blue or hopeless. If so, patients should be asked gently and supportively if they have considered suicide as an option. An affirmative answer greatly strengthens the diagnosis and increases the gravity. Exploring the nature of the patient's plans for suicide helps determine the level of risk.

The second diagnostic task is to identify depression in the setting of established physical illness or environmental stress. Depression arising in a patient with a chronic illness (e.g., multiple sclerosis or cancer) can too easily be disregarded as merely appropriate to the situation. However, profound depression, even in terminal patients, is not the rule but adds great misery when it occurs. If discovered, the physician should consider it an added illness meriting specific treatment.

The third problem is to distinguish depression from dementia (Table 116–12). Many depressed patients are so inattentive to their environment that they appear to have lost cognitive functions. One particularly important clue is that the pseudodemented depressive patient generally answers a question of cognition with "I don't know," whereas a truly demented patient often will give an answer even though incorrect. Pseudodemented patients also much more frequently ask if they are losing their minds.

Finally, the physician must distinguish structural disease of the brain from psychogenic depression. Patients with large frontal lobe brain tumors, some with hydrocephalus or subdural hematomas and many with myxedema, can give the apathetic appearance of being withdrawn and de-

TABLE 116–12. SOME FEATURES DIFFERENTIATING PSEUDODEMENTIA FROM DEMENTIA

PSEUDODEMENTIA	DEMENTIA
1. Symptoms of short duration suggest pseudodementia	1. Symptoms of long duration suggest dementia
2. Patients frequently complain of cognitive loss	2. Patients rarely complain of cognitive loss
3. Patients' complaints of cognitive dysfunction usually detailed	3. Patients' complaints of cognitive dysfunction usually imprecise
4. Patients usually communicate strong sense of distress	4. Patients often appear unconcerned
5. Memory loss for recent and remote events usually equally severe	5. Memory loss for recent events more severe than for remote ones
6. Memory gaps for specific periods or events common	6. Memory gaps for specific periods unusual*
7. Attention and concentration often well-preserved	7. Attention and concentration usually faulty
8. "Don't know" answers typical	8. "Near miss" answers frequent
9. Patients emphasize disability	9. Patients conceal or ignore disability
10. Patients make little effort to perform even simple tasks	10. Patients struggle to perform tasks
11. Patients highlight failures	11. Patients delight in accomplishments, however trivial
12. Patients do not try to keep up	12. Patients rely on notes, calendars, etc., to keep up
13. Marked variability in performing tasks of similar difficulty	13. Consistently poor performance on tasks of similar difficulty
14. Affective change often pervasive	14. Affect labile and shallow
15. Loss of social skills, often early and prominent	15. Patients often retain social skills
16. On tests of orientation, patients often give "don't know" answers	16. On tests of orientation, patients mistake unusual for usual
17. Behavior often incongruent with severity of cognitive dysfunction	17. Behavior usually compatible with severity of cognitive dysfunction
18. Nocturnal accentuation of dysfunction uncommon	18. Nocturnal accentuation of dysfunction common
19. History of previous psychiatric dysfunction common	19. History of previous psychiatric dysfunction uncommon

* Except when due to delirium, trauma, and seizures.
(Modified from Wells CE, and Duncan GW: Neurology for Psychiatrists. Philadelphia, FA Davis Co, 1977, pp 92–95.)

pressed. Unless accompanied by other neurologic signs, the signs and symptoms of depression may be indistinguishable from those of psychological illness, and some such patients may even respond to antidepressant drugs. Generally, however, one finds other clinical signs of neurologic dysfunction that suggest structural disease of the brain (e.g., with frontal tumors or infarcts, abnormalities of motor function and language, and with hydrocephalus, abnormalities of gait, and sometimes urgency incontinence). In doubtful instances a CT scan provides accurate differentiation.

Depression usually responds to appropriate treatment with antidepressant drugs. This is true not only of "pure" psychogenic depression but also of situational or reactive depression and, to a lesser degree, even that associated with structural disease of the nervous system. The tricyclic antidepressant drugs such as amitriptyline, given in appropriate doses (from 75 to 300 mg/day), often relieve symptoms promptly. These drugs should be started in low doses (e.g., 10 to 20 mg at bedtime) and gradually increased, particularly in elderly patients, to avoid excessive sedation and sometimes hallucinations. If the drug is given as a single dose at night, it promotes sleep, frequently relieving almost immediately one of the most disturbing symptoms of the depressed patient. The full psychologic benefit usually takes two to four weeks. Other antidepressant drugs include monoamine oxidase inhibitors, tetracyclic antidepressants and trazadone, a new drug unrelated to any of the others. Benzodiazepines such as diazepam (Valium) and flurazepam (Dalmane) are *not* useful. Furthermore, if used to treat anxiety or insomnia, they may exacerbate an unrecognized depression. If antidepressant drug therapy fails, electroshock therapy is often efficacious, particularly in patients with psychotic depression. Usually four to eight treatments will terminate an episode.

Mania. Manic symptoms represent the antithesis of depression, producing elation and constant restless activity, transmitting the appearance of alertness and psychic energy. In the earliest stages of mania, patients may in fact become more productive than they had been previously. As the disease progresses, however, they deteriorate. They are easily distracted, show flight of ideas, and become so grandiose and implausible as to be recognized by all around them as "crazy." Such patients have a decreased need for sleep, and with intense mania may go for days without sleep and yet deny fatigue.

The elated mood can suddenly change to anger, and the patient may become violent with little or no provocation. The diagnosis is usually easy because the symptoms are so characteristic and are rarely imitated by other disorders. Occasionally structural disease of the limbic system can mimic mania, and the ingestion of corticosteroid drugs may cause an indistinguishable clinical picture. Sometimes one has difficulty distinguishing a manic episode from schizophrenic illness with agitated behavior, but the extreme self-confidence

TABLE 116–13.   THE PRIMARY ANXIETY DISORDERS

Phobic disorders
  Agoraphobia with panic attacks
  Agoraphobia without panic attacks
  Social phobia
  Simple phobia
Anxiety states
  Panic disorder
  Generalized anxiety disorder
  Obsessive-compulsive disorder
Post-traumatic stress disorder
  Acute
  Chronic or delayed
Atypical anxiety disorder

Modified from Brown JT, Mulrow CD, and Stoudemire CA: The anxiety disorders. Ann Intern Med 100:558–564, 1984.

that accompanies the former usually establishes the diagnosis.

The treatment of mania is difficult, in part because some patients feel so well that they see no need for medicine. Phenothiazines or butyrophenones often control agitated behavior. Lithium is the mainstay. The drug is given in a dose of 900 to 2400 mg/day, with careful monitoring of plasma lithium levels to keep the concentration below 2 mEq/L. Excessive lithium levels lead to confusion, disorientation, tremor, anorexia, and, sometimes, seizures with permanent neurologic damage. Maintenance lithium in patients with a history of manic psychosis often prevents further episodes.

Anxiety Disorders (Table 116–13). Anxiety describes an unpleasant mood of tension and apprehension related to fear but not focused on an object of immediate danger. The symptom is common and frequently is appropriate for a particular life situation or illness and if not excessive or sustained may focus the mind and improve performance. Anxiety is generally accompanied by autonomic symptoms including tachycardia, perspiration, dry mouth, and sometimes hyperventilation. The autonomic symptoms may create a vicious circle in which perception of the autonomic changes, particularly palpitations (tachycardia) and lightheadedness (hyperventilation), increase the anxiety, thus in turn increasing the autonomic symptoms.

The cause of the primary anxiety disorders (those that occur in the absence of identifiable physical or environmental cause) is unknown. Psychoanalytic, behavioral, and metabolic theories each have their champions. There is probably a genetic factor, since anxiety disorders run in families, often associated with alcoholism. At least some evidence supports a physiological underpinning for anxiety attacks in that they can be induced in susceptible subjects by the infusion of lactic acid and appear to occur in a disproportionate number of patients with mitral valve prolapse.

Clinically, anxiety states can be characterized by (1) *phobias*, which can vary from simple phobic fears of particular objects, to agoraphobia, fear of either being alone or being in public places, (2) panic attacks that occur in spontaneous sudden episodes marked by fear, apprehension, and feelings of impending doom without underlying cause (Table 116–14), and (3) a generalized and constant feeling of fear and apprehension.

The diagnosis is usually not difficult. Affected patients complain of attacks of anxiety or panic. Sometimes there are problems in diagnosis: Some patients focus on the physical and autonomic aspects of the panic attacks, complaining of palpitations and dizziness (sometimes misinterpreted as vertigo) rather than the feelings of anxiety. Frequently, having such patients hyperventilate will reproduce their symptoms and distinguish the disorder from a primary cardiac or neurologic abnormality. By contrast, structural disease occasionally may be responsible for attacks of autonomic dysfunction that appear to be panic in origin. Some temporal lobe seizures produce an aura of intense fear or anxiety associated with abnormalities of pulse and respiration, in early stages indistinguishable from panic attacks. In most patients with temporal lobe structural disease, however, the attack culminates in a psychomotor or generalized convulsion, thus establishing the diagnosis. Sudden changes in cardiovascular function, such as arrhythmias or acute hypertension (as from a pheochromocytoma), can mimic panic or anxiety attacks. This is particularly true with pheochromocytomas which release substances that cause the sensation of anxiety.

Behavioral therapy and pharmacologic agents are reported to be efficacious for some panic attacks. Behavioral modification in which the patient is desensitized by exposure to the fear-producing object has been particularly useful in the treatment of phobias. Generalized anxiety disorders and panic attacks respond less well. However, pharmacologic agents are often effective. Useful drugs include beta blockers, monoamine oxidase inhibitors, tricyclic antidepressants, and the anxiolytic agents such as the benzodiazepines. Beta blockers such as propranolol have appeared to be particularly useful in patients with major autonomic symptoms, especially in those suffering from the combination of mitral valve prolapse and panic attacks.

Somatoform Disorders. The essential features of this group of conditions are physical symptoms unexplained by either demonstrable organic findings or known physiological mechanisms, accompanied by evidence of severe psychological conflicts. These disorders differ from factitious disorders or malingering in that the symptom production is believed not to be under conscious control, although this distinction may be difficult to make. Somatoform disorders are often grouped together under the rubric "hysteria," conversion reaction (in which the patient relieves his anxiety by converting psychological to physical symptoms), or Briquet's syndrome.

The pathogenesis of somatoform disorders is not entirely known. Although psychological mechanisms undoubtedly play an important role, a substantial proportion of patients with conversion symptoms suffer a physical, often neurologic, illness as well. The conversion reaction may be either an embellishment of the underlying disorder or a different and more florid sign, both of which serve to call attention to the patient's distress over the physical illness. For example, a patient with weakness of the extensors of the wrist and fingers from a radial nerve palsy may demonstrate paralysis of the entire arm, all but that of the radial nerve distribution being psychogenic in origin.

Somatoform disorders can produce almost any of the symptoms of physical illness. Most conversion reactions produce symptoms that involve the nervous system and consist of sensory loss, paralysis, blindness, hearing loss, speech loss, or seizures. (Many patients with "pseudoseizures" also have true epilepsy.) Abnormalities of consciousness or gait may also be symptoms of a conversion reaction. Even more difficult to diagnose are non-neurologic somatic complaints such as nausea, multiple aches and pains, excessive fatigue, and weakness.

The diagnosis of conversion reactions often is far from easy. When the symptoms are neurologic, the diagnosis must be based on an examination that indicates the findings are inexplicable on a physiological basis. Thus, for example, a patient who complains of complete sensory loss on one side of the body, including absence of vibration and position sense, but who is able to use the arm normally for fine movements with eyes both open and closed, cannot have his symptoms explained by a physiological disease of the nervous system.

TABLE 116–14. DIAGNOSTIC CRITERIA FOR PANIC DISORDER*

I. At least three panic attacks within a three-week period in circumstances other than marked physical exertion or a life-threatening situation. The attacks are not precipitated only by exposure to a circumscribed phobic stimulus.

II. Panic attacks are manifested by discrete periods of apprehension or fear, and at least four of the following symptoms appear during each attack:

  A. Dyspnea
  B. Palpitations
  C. Chest pain or discomfort
  D. Choking or smothering sensations
  E. Dizziness, vertigo, or unsteady feelings
  F. Feelings of unreality
  G. Paresthesias (tingling in hands or feet)
  H. Hot and cold flashes
  I. Sweating
  J. Faintness
  K. Trembling or shaking
  L. Fear of dying, of "going crazy," or of doing something uncontrolled during an attack

III. The disorder is not due to a physical disorder or another mental disorder, such as major depression, somatization disorder, or schizophrenia.

IV. The disorder is not associated with agoraphobia.

* Source: Diagnostic and Statistical Manual III. American Psychiatric Association.

In addition to demonstrating the absence of somatic disease and the nonphysiological nature of the symptoms and signs, every effort should be made to discover a reason for the development of the somatoform disorder at that particular time. For example, the symptoms may have extricated the patient from a difficult environmental situation (secondary gain) or a patient complaining of paralysis may have recently lost a loved one to a stroke. In all instances, however, one must be very careful, even when the evidence suggests conversion symptoms, to be certain that the situation is not caused by an overreaction to or extension of an underlying physical or neurologic illness. At times only careful follow-up will ultimately establish the diagnosis. Perley and Guze state that the physician's diagnosis of hysteria will be correct 90 per cent of the time in patients with a dramatic or complicated medical history beginning before age 35, a total of 25 symptoms in at least 9 of the 10 groups of symptoms indicated in Table 116–15 and no other diagnosis that explains the symptoms.

Conversion reactions are hard to treat. Physical, particularly neurologic, symptoms in their early stages can often be relieved by a matter-of-fact approach in which the physician reassures the patient that he is going to get well but avoids initiating a long discussion of the symptom's pathogenesis. He then demonstrates to the patient his ability to do things that he thought he was unable to do. Firmness and support often restore strength to a hemiplegic hysteric and sight to a blind one. At the same time, psychological support should be given to relieve anxiety and to ameliorate the environmental stresses that produced the symptoms in the first place. Many such patients, however, are intractable to treatment. Even those in whom one eradicates one set of symptoms may return with new and different ones.

DISSOCIATIVE DISORDERS

A dissociative disorder is a sudden, temporary alteration in the normal integration of consciousness or self-identity that is not caused by known structural or physiological disease of the nervous system. Such disturbances can take the form of: (1) *Amnesia*, either for a circumscribed period of time (localized amnesia) or for all of life's events (generalized amnesia). (2) *Fugue states*, episodes in which individuals disappear from home, travel to another place, assume a new identity, and fail to recall their previous identity. Following recovery there is no recollection of the events that took place during the fugue state. (3) *Multiple personalities* (the Three Faces of Eve syndrome), two or more distinct personalities, one of which is dominant at a particular time, controlling the behavior of the individual. (4) *Depersonalization disorders*, in which patients suffer a change in their perception of themselves so that the usual sense of one's reality is temporarily lost or changed ("I

TABLE 116–15. SYMPTOMS OF CONVERSION REACTIONS*

GROUP	SYMPTOMS	GROUP	SYMPTOMS
1	Headaches Sickly most of life	7	Dysmenorrhea Menstrual irregularity, including amenorrhea for at least two months Excessive menstrual bleeding
2	Blindness Paralysis Anesthesia Aphonia Fits or convulsions Unconsciousness Amnesia Deafness Hallucinations Urinary retention Ataxia Other conversion symptoms	8	Sexual indifference Frigidity Dyspareunia Other sexual difficulties Vomiting for all nine months of pregnancy or hospitalized for hyperemesis gravidarum
3	Fatigue Lump in throat Fainting spells Visual blurring Weakness Dysuria	9	Back pain Joint pain Extremity pain Burning pains of sexual organs, mouth, or rectum Other bodily pains
4	Breathing difficulty Palpitation Anxiety attacks Chest pain Dizziness	10	Nervousness Fears Depressed feelings Need to quit working or inability to carry on regular duties because of feeling sick Crying easily Feeling life is hopeless Thinking a good deal about dying Wanting to die Thinking of suicide Suicide attempts
5	Anorexia Weight loss Marked fluctuations in weight Nausea Abdominal bloating Food intolerances Diarrhea Constipation		
6	Abdominal pain Vomiting		

* Modified from Perley MJ, and Guze SB: Hysteria: The stability and usefulness of clinical criteria. N Engl J Med 266:421–426, 1962.

feel as if I am outside my body, watching myself"). There is usually a feeling of unreality ("The world does not seem real").

Depersonalization reactions may be difficult to distinguish from structural or physiological disease of the brain, particularly that arising from temporal lobe and other limbic system disorders (multiple personalities is an exception, almost never being mimicked by neurogenic disease). The differential diagnosis of psychogenic amnesia is discussed on page 660.

A psychogenic fugue state may be confused with temporal lobe or petit mal status epilepticus, in which individuals may also wander long distances with an imperfect knowledge of their environment. During a psychogenic fugue state, the patient is alert, oriented, and purposeful, even when commiting violent acts. On the other hand, patients with prolonged epileptic attacks are usually confused and perplexed and not able to carry out complex acts, merely performing the same automatic activity over and over again and requiring help even to carry out the simplest act. Such patients are rarely violent, although they may strike out if attempts are made to restrain them. Furthermore, in psychogenic fugue states there is usually an identifiable emotional or environmental stress that precipitates the episode. In psychomotor or petit mal status epilepticus, the interictal EEG is often abnormal and other forms of epilepsy including generalized seizures may coexist.

Depersonalization reactions may be described by the patient as dizziness and thus be mistaken for vertigo (p. 698) or may be confused with an aura of temporal lobe epilepsy. A clear description from the patient establishes the difference between depersonalization and vertigo or syncope. The differentiation between a depersonalization reaction and the aura of temporal lobe epilepsy is more difficult. Generally, patients with depersonalization episodes have fewer episodes that last longer and never culminate in automatic activity. Patients with temporal lobe epilepsy are likely to have multiple episodes that are stereotypic and short-lived and often culminate in a psychomotor seizure. The interictal EEG may be abnormal in temporal lobe epilepsy but not in a depersonalization reaction.

In all of the dissociative disorders a meticulous history usually distinguishes neurogenic from psychogenic dissociation. In rare patients, the differentiation from temporal lobe dysfunction may be difficult or impossible. In those rare patients, EEG and CT scan may be indicated. Generally the diagnosis should be made by the examination and the patient treated by psychiatric methods.

FACTITIOUS DISORDERS AND MALINGERING

Factitious disorders are characterized by physical or psychological symptoms under voluntary control of the patient. Factitious disorders are distinguished from malingering because in the former the illness is feigned for no discernible reason, whereas in the latter there is a clear gain to the individual (such as avoiding standing trial, getting out of jail, procuring compensation for an alleged injury). Patients with factitious disorders may feign either psychological (Ganser's syndrome) or physical symptoms (Munchausen's syndrome), with an intensity and self-destructive effect that suggest psychotic thinking. Psychological symptoms include psychosis and/or dementia. Patients may report hallucinations, amnesia, or suicidal ideation. A particularly characteristic symptom of Ganser's syndrome is the tendency to give an approximate but incorrect answer to a question (question: how many legs has a horse? answer: 5; question: what is 8 × 6? answer: 49).

Patients with Munchausen's syndrome may report a symptom (common ones are nausea, dizziness, abdominal pain) or may actually produce abnormal findings. In the days before electronic thermometers, patients caused "fever" by rubbing the thermometer or holding it close to a light bulb. In one series describing patients with fever of unknown cause, over 1 per cent turned out to be factitious. In a particularly malignant form of the syndrome, some patients have been known to take anticoagulant agents to cause bleeding or bruising, to take excessive diuretics to cause potassium loss and muscle weakness, to bleed themselves to cause anemia, or to inject talc into their joints to cause arthritis. Such patients produce these abnormalities in order to be hospitalized and often submit to extensive diagnostic and sometimes surgical procedures. They may travel from hospital to hospital in different parts of the country and many have had 30 or 40 hospitalizations with multiple surgical procedures. Many such patients have a knowledge of medicine from prior work in a hospital. When they are confronted with the correct diagnosis, they usually deny the allegation and sign out of the hospital, only to appear subsequently in another institution with similar complaints. The fixation is often delusional and may be shared by a relative (folie à deux). Even more bizarre are occasional persons who produce symptomatic illness in their children (Munchausen's syndrome by proxy) and submit them to extensive diagnostic and therapeutic work-ups. Reported examples have included the giving of sedative drugs to children to produce episodic coma or the addition of blood or fecal material to urine to cause apparent hematuria or urinary tract infection.

The pathogenesis of Munchausen's syndrome is not known, but the patients, by definition, have underlying major mental illness or personality disorders. The individual's goal is simply to become a patient. Although the diagnosis can be difficult, diagnostic clues usually are available from the beginning to help avoid prolonged work-up. In most such patients, symptoms are vague and out of proportion to the physical findings. There is usually an extensive past history of physical illness and multiple diagnostic and therapeutic procedures. Despite the dreadful background, these patients usually look healthy. Finally, the symptoms and signs are almost always more prominent when medical attention is present. For example, patients writhing in pain from abdominal distress cease to do so once the nurse leaves the room.

The diagnosis is usually made readily once considered. A surreptitious search of the patient's room may disclose the drugs or instruments that lie behind the abnormal laboratory values, or skin lesions may be located only at sites where the medical actor can reach to scratch.

Munchausen's syndrome appears to be relatively intractable to treatment, since patients usually refuse psychiatric assistance. Therapeutic endeavors should be directed toward identifying the illness and attempting to prevent repetitive entry to hospitals. A few victims can be sustained by close contact with a knowledgeable physician.

Malingering is the voluntary production of false or grossly exaggerated physical or psychological symptoms in the pursuit of a goal that is better recognized by understanding the individual's circumstances than unraveling his or her psychology. Examples abound in the military (where physical symptoms can be used to avoid or limit onerous duty), in the last year before retirement from a variety of jobs (particularly persons in uniform, to whom additional compensation is given for physical illness), in patients who have suffered an injury such as an automobile accident (where lawsuits are pending), and in patients who are trying to evade criminal prosecution or to obtain drugs from a physician.

The diagnosis of malingering can be made with certainty only if the patient confesses that he is "faking." Otherwise, even when the physician can determine that the physical sign is not physiological, it may be difficult to distinguish malingering from factitious disorders, conversion reactions, or psychophysiological musculoskeletal syndromes. The diagnosis depends solely on the judgment as to whether the symptom production is in pursuit of a goal that is recognizable and understandable under the circumstances. When the situation is unclear, the patient must be given the benefit of the doubt.

REFERENCES

Benson DF, and Blumer D: Psychiatric Aspects of Neurological Disease, Vol II. New York, Grune & Stratton, 1982. *A description of abnormalities of mood and behavior related to structural disease of the nervous system. There are good chapters on pseudodementia and psychiatric manifestations of epilepsy.*

Brown JT, Mulrow CD, and Stoudemire GA: The anxiety disorders. Ann Intern Med 100:558–564, 1984. *A well-stated review of the pathophysiology, diagnosis, and treatment of the anxiety disorders based on the DSM classification.*

Greist JH, Jefferson JW, and Spitzer RL: Treatment of Mental Disorders. New York, Oxford University Press, 1982. *This excellent monograph uses the DSM-III classification, with an emphasis on the approach to treatment.*

McHugh PR, and Slavney PR: The Perspectives of Psychiatry. Baltimore, Johns Hopkins University Press, 1983. *The authors discuss the concept of disease as it arises in psychiatric thinking and address the methodological problems of psychiatry as a medical discipline.*

Weintraub MI: Hysterical Conversion Reactions. A Clinical Guide to Diagnosis and Treatment. New York, SP Medical & Scientific Books, 1983. *A guide to clinical findings, examination, diagnosis, and treatment of conversion reactions presenting as neurologic disease.*

Williams JBW (ed): Diagnostic and Statistical Manual of Mental Disorders. 3rd ed. Washington, DC, American Psychiatric Association, 1981. *The newest classification of psychological disorders, with good brief descriptions of clinical symptomatology and differential diagnosis.*

C.   DRUG AND ALCOHOL ABUSE

Almost any drug as well as many household substances, including some common plants, can produce toxic changes if taken in large amounts. Most abused drugs, however, as well as those ingested for suicidal purposes, exert their primary effects on the brain.

THERAPEUTIC DRUG OVERDOSE

This condition is frequent, especially among the elderly whose susceptibility is enhanced by poor memories for what they have taken and the development of weakened neurologic and metabolic reserves to handle the pharmacological load. The chief offenders include (1) digitalis glycosides; (2) sedatives, anxiolytics, antidepressants, and antipsychotics, which can blunt and confuse an otherwise sane and well-adjusted mind and sometimes produce an agitated semidelirium as well; recovery following withdrawal can be symptomatically difficult and sometimes requires several weeks; (3) miscellaneous therapeutic agents including salicylates, corticosteroids, levodopa, theophylline, amantadine, cimetidine, and many others that can cause confusion and hallucinations in "standard" therapeutic doses, especially in patients over age 70.

RECREATIONAL STREET DRUG ABUSE

Almost all drugs that affect higher brain function possess in varying combinations and severity the addiction-promoting potentials of *psychological dependence* leading to craving, *tolerance-habituation* leading to the ingestion of increasing amounts of drugs to achieve a constant effect, and *physical dependence* leading to neurogenic *withdrawal phenomena* unless the drug is taken continuously. Individual susceptibility to these changes varies widely and is influenced by both environmental and inherited qualities.

Marijuana

This widely used, predominantly inhaled agent depends primarily on metabolites of delta-9-tetrahydro cannabis for its pharmacological action. Autonomic effects include conjunctival congestion, tachycardia, flushing, orthostatic hypotension, dry mouth, and, sometimes, vomiting. Psychic reactions depend considerably on the user and on the setting in which the drug is inhaled. Users report perceptual enhancement, euphoria, a sense of timelessness, infectious joviality, and drowsiness. Coordination and reaction time are impaired. Mild tolerance and physical dependence usually develop, but most persons suffer only moderately adverse effects. Physiological effects include respiratory tract irritation, tachycardia, decreased sperm formation, and, possibly, reduced fertility. Enduring psychic changes are uncertain. Acutely, depression, panic, paranoia, and toxic psychosis have been reported. Some chronic heavy users show an apathetic inability to undertake goal-directed efforts, but whether the traits precede or follow cannabis use is uncertain.

CNS Depressants

The drugs most frequently abused under this heading include benzodiazepines (diazepam [Valium], chlordiazepoxide [Librium], short-acting barbiturates (pentobarbital [Nembutal], secobarbital [Seconal], amylbarbital [Amytal]), and other sedatives, especially methaqualone (Quaalude), glutethimide (Doriden), and methyprylon (Noludar). The agents are mostly ingested orally and are widely used to counteract insomnia and anxiety. Most self-medicators develop only mild habituation, but severe addiction can develop among secret sedative users, much as it does among secret alcoholics. Street use of all the drugs occurs, usually combined with marijuana, alcohol, or cocaine.

Withdrawal symptoms commonly follow the removal of any of these drugs after heavy usage, usually beginning two to six days after cessation. Symptoms consist of heightened insomnia, anxiety, and apprehension, together with tremulousness and mild autonomic changes. Withdrawal from chronic heavy barbiturate use is most distressing and causes symptoms and signs similar to those of the alcohol abstinence syndrome (p. 675). Treatment is similar to that of alcohol withdrawal syndromes. Addiction to these drugs often is abetted by the physician's overprescribing. Benzodiazepines are best given to patients in limited amounts to curb severe anxiety or insomnia. They should not be prescribed chronically. Barbiturates probably should not be prescribed at all except for the treatment of epilepsy. Since all CNS depressant drugs tend to intensify pre-existing feelings of psychological depression, their use is contraindicated for treating such symptoms.

Cocaine

This powerfully addicting agent is predominantly insufflated but also can be taken by mouth,

vein, or mucous membrane absorption. Its use has increasingly and rapidly spread among adolescents and young adults of both the affluent and impoverished sections of society. Mortality is climbing apace. Physiological effects include local anesthesia, fever, tachycardia, hypertension, pupillary dilatation, peripheral vasoconstriction, tachypnea, and anorexia. Psychologically, users report feelings of increased energy, alertness, and self-confident psychic power, often coupled with irritability and some anxiety. The last-mentioned symptoms often lead to combining cocaine use with sedatives. Reportedly, intravenous use or the smoking of a "free base" alkaline extract induces an intense, euphoric "rush" followed by a craving to repeat the experience. Complications include social dissolution associated with craving, ulceration of the nasal septum, intracranial stroke-causing angiitis, occasionally convulsions and, with high doses, coma and death. Amphetamine abuse can cause many of the same experiences and complications. Treatment of cocaine abuse consists of withdrawal in a protective, supportive environment plus the giving of benzodiazepines or phenothiazines as necessary to control severe agitation. Psychological dependence is strong, leading to repetitive or continuous use, with a "crash" of debilitated disorganization and deep sleep at the end. Postwithdrawal craving reportedly is intense and protracted, leading to frequent recidivism even after weeks or months of abstinence.

Opiates

Heroin, morphine, methadone, and meperidine are the chief offenders, in that order. Two principal medical problems arise with their usage: accidental or intentional overdose and the development of complications resulting from idiosyncratic reactions, infections, and immunologic abnormalities. Efforts by amateur chemists to produce psychedelic congeners have sometimes generated molecular variants with disastrous results, as exemplified by a recent mini-epidemic of chemically induced severe parkinsonism.

Acute overdose with opiates produces stupor or coma, pupillary miosis, and slow, irregular hypoventilation. Body temperature and blood pressure fall, seizures can occur, and some patients develop acute pulmonary edema. Treatment of acute overdose consists of immediately giving naloxone, a powerful opiate antagonist, intravenously or, if no veins can be found, intramuscularly. If no immediate response occurs, the injection should be repeated immediately. Since the effects of naloxone wear off within two to three hours and the depressant effects of the opiates can last much longer, the antagonist should be repeated at two- to three-hour intervals until all evidence of a response disappears. Stuporous or hypoventilating patients who do not respond immediately should be treated according to the general program for care of the patient in coma (p. 656).

Chronic opiate addicts can develop severe withdrawal symptoms consisting of yawning, anxiety, restlessness, rhinorrhea, lacrimation, and influenzal symptoms within minutes after receiving naloxone. In an emergency, the symptoms can be somewhat relieved by clonidine or ameliorated by small doses of narcotics. The use of naloxone should be confined to overdose situations and not employed in a nonemergency setting either as a diagnostic measure or to induce withdrawal.

Complications of illicit narcotic use include arrhythmias, pulmonary edema, and convulsions due to adulterants. Opiate users have a high incidence of bacteriological infections of skin, veins, blood, heart, and lung. Many develop viral hepatitis and AIDS (p. 604). Serious neurologic complications consist of neuropathy, myelopathy, optic neuritis, and a myriad of infections, including tetanus and brain abscess.

Tricyclic Antidepressants

These agents possess potentially serious cardiovascular effects, oral doses of more than 2 gm often being lethal. Since behavioral changes can take some hours to develop and blood levels may not be easily available, patients reporting recent self-destructive ingestion should have an immediate ECG: a widened QRS to greater than 100 milliseconds indicates serious toxicity and a need for intensive supervision and cardiac monitoring. A more common presentation consists of a state of stupor or coma, combined with anticholinergic signs reminiscent of atropine poisoning and the presence of cardiac arrhythmias on the ECG. Treatment in alert patients consists of ipecac-induced vomiting or in stuporous ones of gastric lavage followed by activated charcoal instillation. Convulsions and arrhythmias are treated by appropriate standard measures, including ventricular pacing in the event of serious arrhythmia. Physostigmine given intravenously sometimes produces transient awakening but is inadvisable for treatment, since its action is brief and it risks producing arrhythmias and seizures. Most tricyclics have half-lives of many days, so that monitoring and intensive treatment can be required for as long as a week in severe cases.

Salicylate Poisoning

Salicylate intoxication in adults occurs as accidental overdose in elderly persons taking the drug to relieve pain and with intentional overdose, largely by adolescents and young adults. Salicylates in high doses uncouple oxidative phosphorylation and aspirin itself adds acid radicals. The resulting acid-base disturbance is almost diagnostic: tissue glycolysis produces intracellular lactacidosis, which produces an acid urine and stimulates the brain stem respiratory centers. The result is a mixed respiratory alkalosis—metabolic acidosis with a low $Paco_2$ and low serum bicarbonate. Early symptoms include tinnitus, deafness, disequilibrium, drowsiness, and a moderate delirium. With blood levels greater than 60 mg/dl, stupor, coma, and potentially fatal convulsions can ensue. Treatment of

acute overdose consists of gastric lavage and the giving of bicarbonate solutions in an attempt to achieve alkaline diuresis.

Phencyclidine (PCP)

PCP is currently the most widely abused of the psychedelic-hallucinogenic group of drugs that, in street use, include, among numerous others, LSD, amphetamines, and scopolamine. Users describe various sensations, most prevalent of which is a state of altered perception in which dreams and heightened reality become indistinguishable. Excess inhalation or ingestion of PCP can induce ataxia, confusion, aggressive violence, prolonged psychotic states, coma, or convulsions. Treatment is symptomatic, but the bad trip may be shortened by acidifying the urine with ammonium chloride and applying continuous gastric suction to accelerate excretion of the drug.

Nonethyl Alcohols

Most poisoning from these agents occurs by alcoholics or drug abusers unaware of the toxic nature of the substance. Methanol, isopropyl alcohol, and ethylene glycol all produce potentially fatal metabolic acidosis through their metabolic products. Paraldehyde acidosis may have a similar mechanism. The hepatic enzyme alcohol dehydrogenase acts on all three substrates to produce acid products. Since the enzyme preferentially metabolizes ethanol, the first, potentially life-saving step is to slow metabolism of the poison by administering ethyl alcohol by mouth or vein in intoxicating amounts. Severe poisoning requires that ethanol blood levels of 100 to 150 mg/dl be maintained for at least 48 to 72 hours while stabilizing blood acid-base levels with the bicarbonate buffer. Ethylene glycol may cause subsequent renal damage from oxalate and hippurate crystalluria.

ALCOHOL AND ITS COMPLICATIONS

Ethyl alcohol is the oldest and still most widely taken addicting psychotropic drug. Used by nearly half of all Americans and abused by 1 in 20, the agent creates a huge medical and sociological problem. Alcohol generates a direct and associated death rate that lags behind only vascular disease and cancer and a total work-loss and life-year loss rate that probably exceeds all other illnesses.

Pharmacology

Ethanol is usually ingested as a fraction of some vehicle of distinctive taste such as beer (5 per cent), wine (12 per cent), or various stronger agents containing 20 to 50 per cent alcohol (40 to 100 proof). Ethanol enters the blood within minutes from the stomach and intestine and, being lipid-soluble, quickly penetrates all aqueous body compartments, including the brain and alveolar air. Ethanol is excreted by physical diffusion

TABLE 116–16. BLOOD-ALCOHOL LEVELS AND SYMPTOMS

LEVEL (mg/dl)	SPORADIC DRINKERS	CHRONIC DRINKERS
50 (party level)	Congenial euphoria	No observable effect
75	Gregarious or garrulous	Often no effect
100	Incoordinated. Legally intoxicated	Minimal signs
125–150	Unrestrained behavior Episodic dyscontrol	Pleasurable euphoria or beginning incoordination
200–250	Alertness lost → lethargic	Effort required to maintain emotional and motor control
300–350	Stupor to coma	Drowsy and slow
>500	Some will die	Coma

through the lungs and detoxified by hepatic dehydrogenase at a rate that approximates 8 ml/hour, clearing about 15 mg/dl/hour from blood.

Blood levels of alcohol correlate directly with clinical signs and symptoms, chronic alcoholics showing great tolerance compared to novice drinkers (Table 116–16). Acutely, in less than near-fatal amounts, aside from producing vasodilatation and gastric irritation, alcohol exerts almost all its ill effects on the central nervous system. The molecular action is unknown, but alcohol acts entirely as a depressant, although not simultaneously on all CNS structures. Thus the earlier euphoriant-excitatory stage reflects a removal of higher inhibitory effects from limbic impulses, while larger doses increasingly depress first forebrain and then brain stem functions, including those regulating pain sensation and arousal. Death from acute intoxication usually results from central respiratory depression followed by circulatory failure.

Clinical Features

Acute Intoxication. The behavioral effects of acute intoxication vary with the user, ranging among social drinkers from pleasant conviviality to angry argumentativeness. A small number of younger male drinkers develop pathologically severe, aggressive, violent behavior ("dyscontrol") when intoxicated for which they later claim no memory. The syndrome has potentially dangerous consequences and calls for total abstinence and immediate psychiatric referral. *Alcoholic blackouts,* periods of amnesia lasting for several hours or more during or at the end of a heavy drinking bout, are a sign of serious intoxication bordering on anesthesia. When recurrent, they signify impending or already existing alcoholic addiction.

Treatment of acute alcoholic attacks depends upon the degree of intoxication and the associated blood levels. Mild drunkenness requires no treatment. More severe intoxication producing heavy drowsiness or stupor deserves attention, especially if one does not know whether or not additional drugs have been ingested. The level of CNS depression can increase rapidly as alcohol is absorbed, and stuporous drunks need close attention to potential autonomic depression. Alcoholic

deep stupor or coma requires hospital monitoring until symptoms subside. Patients with associated severe trauma or fever need especially close supervision, as masked neurologic injury, blood loss, or infection can intensify alcohol's depressant effects.

Withdrawal Syndromes. Headache, giddiness, difficulty in concentrating, nausea, and mild tremulousness characterize the well-known hangover. Classic but unproved remedies or preventatives include forcing nonalcoholic fluids while still intoxicated, avoiding agents such as red wines or brandies known to contain idiosyncratically toxic agents, and taking antacids. The ingestion of another alcoholic drink aborts most of the symptoms but represents an early step toward the development of chronic alcoholism.

The serious withdrawal states of chronic alcoholism consist of prominent tremulousness, rum fits, and delirium tremens (DTs). All appear after years of problem drinking and are usually precipitated by a continuous alcoholic ingestion lasting many days or weeks. With an increasing degree of severity, each withdrawal syndrome reflects central hyperexcitation as the inhibitory drug effect declines or disappears.

Tremulousness, insomnia, and agitation, although much more common, symptomatically blend into delirium tremens and are discussed in that section. *Withdrawal convulsions* consist of single or short runs of generalized seizures, usually with no focal features. Their necessary stimulus consists of no more than a falling blood alcohol level and, in contrast to the more delayed appearance of DTs, they can occur during the course of a prolonged spree within hours of the last drink. About one third are followed by the DTs if abstinence continues. Treatment is symptomatic, using diazepam to stop the seizures and dampen the often associated tremulousness. Interictal laboratory tests, including CT scans and EEGs, show no specific abnormality, although if focal seizures occur a CT scan should be obtained to rule out a localized brain lesion such as subdural hematoma. Prophylactic anticonvulsants confer no protection.

Delirium tremens represents the most serious and sometimes fatal withdrawal complication of alcohol, usually appearing only after a decade or more of fairly continuous, heavy drinking. The course is worsened when complicated by systemic infection, hepatic insufficiency, or head trauma. A somewhat similar although less florid condition affects patients withdrawing from chronic heavy barbiturate use, and the treatment described below applies to both that syndrome and alcholic DTs. Either alcoholic or *barbiturate withdrawal* DTs can arise unexpectedly in patients abruptly withdrawn from these drugs because of admission to hospital for other conditions such as trauma, emergency surgery, etc.

In contrast to less severe tremulousness or rum fits, DTs most often follow complete or nearly complete alcohol or drug withdrawal by three to five days, producing severe tremulousness, disorientation, visual hallucinations, and agitation. Signs of beta-adrenergic autonomic hyperactivity are prominent, including fear, sweating, tachycardia, hypertension, tachypnea, and incontinence. Many patients are malnourished and display associated signs of hepatic insufficiency, gastritis, dehydration, infection, polyneuropathy, myopathy, or Wernicke's syndrome (see below). Treatment consists of sedation with a drug cross-tolerant for alcohol, the benzodiazepine diazepam being most useful (Table 116–17). Huge amounts of diazepam may be required: authorities report as much as 15 to 215 mg being necessary to control agitation initially, with as much as 1200 mg given intravenously during the first 60 hours in order to maintain a calm state. In controlled trials, paraldehyde, the agent traditionally used to treat DTs, has been less effective.

Acute alcoholic hallucinosis is less common than the DTs but arises in a similar setting. The disorder is characterized by days or weeks of auditory hallucinations accompanied by comparatively less agitation or mental confusion. Although the auditory hallucinations, which are sometimes paranoid, can resemble an acute schizophrenic reaction, the history of chronic heavy drinking followed by withdrawal indicates the diagnosis.

Chronic Alcoholism. This condition is widespread and requires the physician's constant vigilance to detect it sufficiently early to modify its course. Psychological dependence, closet drinking, increasing social lapses, more than an occasional mild hangover or, among spouses, an increasing number of nights out with the boys (or girls) are danger signals. Blackouts, absenteeism, drunken driving, occupational downgrading, or any medical complications including poorly explained, repeated physical injury imply serious trouble.

Even to get a potential alcoholic to consider that he or she has a psychological-medical problem commonly is a thankless and unsuccessful task. To accomplish sustained and effective treatment usually requires experienced psychotherapy plus the patient's participation in a vigorous reinforcement group, such as Alcoholics Anonymous. Several industries and large universities recently have established such groups, reportedly with success running as high as 70 per cent or higher when persons can be persuaded that their jobs are on the line and that the employer is genuinely interested. Recovery or improvement rate is less once severe social disruption begins. Disulfiram (Antabuse) is a drug that produces conditioned avoidance to alcohol by introducing a violently adverse reaction to its ingestion. Antabuse is reserved for treating the severe alcoholic and is best supervised by experts in its use.

Complications of Alcohol

Drunkenness contributes to a large fraction of death and severe injury from traffic accidents, trauma, murder, suicide, and the inadvertent overdose of other drugs. Chronic complications as

TABLE 116–17. TREATMENT OF SEVERE TREMULOUSNESS OR DELIRIUM TREMENS

1. Attempt control by reassurance and observation.

2. Treat systemic problems promptly.

3. Treat uncontrollable agitation: Control with diazepam 10 mg I.V. given slowly followed by 5–10 mg I.V. slowly every 5 minutes to induce calmness. Once calm, maintain with diazepam 5–10 mg I.V. every 1-4 hours.

4. Continuously supply and balance electrolytes and vitamins, especially thiamine.

TABLE 116–18. MAJOR NON-NEUROLOGIC COMPLICATIONS OF ALCOHOLISM

Heart
  Cardiomyopathy
  Arrhythmia
  Hyperlipidemia

Gastrointestinal
  Gastritis
  Hepatitis-cirrhosis
  Pancreatitis
  Head, neck, and esophageal cancer
  Malabsorption

Blood
  Iron or folate deficiency
  Anemia
  Thrombocytopenia
  Prothrombin deficiency

Endocrine
  Male sexual impairment
  Increased fetal risk

Immune System
  Increased susceptibility to infection and impaired healing

Electrolyte Disturbances
  Hypocalcemia
  Hypomagnesemia
  Hypophosphatemia
  Acute water intoxication
  Alcoholic hyperosmolality
  Alcoholic ketosis

indicated in Table 116–18 can affect many body organs. Some of these may be due to a direct, but tenuously established, toxic effect. Nutritional deprivation, however, causes the majority. Alcohol contains 7 calories per gram, but most of its vehicles include negligible amounts of vitamins, trace metals, or other nutrients, including protein. Alcoholics, supplying their immediate energy needs by carbohydrates, can wear the mask of nutritional good health for years while their brains, nerves, livers, and hearts structurally degenerate in a pattern which, sooner or later, allows no turning back.

TOXIC AND DEFICIENCY NEUROLOGIC DISORDERS RELATED TO ALCOHOLISM AND OTHER NUTRITIONALLY DEPRIVED STATES (Table 116– 19)

In addition to chronic alcoholism, severe nutritional insufficiencies can accompany a number of debilitating, energy-consuming illnesses, including metastatic cancer, disseminated infection, thyrotoxicosis, advanced connective tissue disease, impaired intestinal absorption, and chronic behavioral disorders. Nutritional lack with these illnesses only occasionally is confined to a single vitamin or nutrient fraction, although thiamine lack is perhaps most prevalent. Signs that suggest nutritional insufficiency include apathetic listlessness, darkening of the skin, a sore red tongue, fissuring at the corners of the mouth, burning feet, progressive unexplained weight loss, and unexplained anemia. These problems are discussed at greater length in the *Cecil Textbook of Medicine*. This chapter focuses on the most common neurologic disorders, all of which are associated more with alcoholism than any other single cause.

Chronic severe alcoholics suffer an increased incidence of middle-life onset *optic neuropathy*, with reduced visual acuity, central or paracentral scotomas, and normal optic fundi. Dietary and vitamin therapies sometimes improve the condition. Advanced problem drinkers as young as the fourth decade also develop detectable *cerebral atrophy* as measured by CT scanning and score poorly on psychometric tests designed to detect early dementia. Abstinence sometimes can reverse the severity of these changes.

Alcoholic-Nutritional Peripheral Neuropathy. This disorder can develop in special populations as a pure thiamine deficiency (dry beri-beri), but in the United States it usually occurs only with advanced, mixed deprivation and usually improves only with total nutritional replacement and weight gain. The disorder produces axonal degeneration affecting predominantly the small pain- and temperature-mediating fibers in the distal lower extremities. Since the larger, touch-carrying peripheral fibers determine sensory nerve conduction velocities, that function can remain normal in the early stages of the neuropathy. Distal motor loss occurs relatively early. Spontaneous, often burning, pain is a feature of advanced

neuropathy, as are associated autonomic changes. Deep tendon reflexes disappear in a distal-to-proximal pattern. Recovery, often incomplete, requires months or years of renourishment.

Alcoholic myopathy is confined to chronic, severe alcoholics and can be acute or chronic. The acute form consists of sudden transient rhabdomyolysis, often following a cluster of rum fits or, possibly, other trauma. It includes muscle pain, tenderness, cramping, weakness, and an elevated serum creatine kinase. Severe cases can develop myoglobinuria with associated renal complications. Chronic myopathy, a less blatant and distinctive disorder, consists of diffuse proximal muscle wasting and weakness disproportional to any existing neuritic impairment. It improves gradually with nutritional replacement.

Wernicke-Korsakoff Disease. This condition reflects the acute and chronic nervous system effects of severe, sustained thiamine depletion in the face of a continued caloric intake. Thiamine deprivation produces a similar disorder in experimental animals, in which it can be shown that either repeated episodes or prolonging thiamine deprivation after symptoms begin leads to increasing neuronal damage. The pathological substrate consists of axonal demyelination, neuronal loss, glial proliferation, endothelial thickening, and petechial pericapillary hemorrhages affecting the gray matter of selected areas of the brain stem reticular formation, the diencephalon, and the cerebral cortex. In the brain stem, the oculomotor nuclei, the vestibular nuclei, the medullary autonomic nuclei, and the midbrain periaqueductal gray suffer the greatest damage. At higher levels the mammillary bodies, the mediodorsal thalamic nuclei, and scattered cortical regions including the hippocampus show the worst changes.

The clinical manifestations of Wernicke's disease parallel the major neuropathological alterations. Acutely such patients are confused, often drowsy or semistuporous, ataxic, and dysarthric. Partial or complete external ophthalmoplegia and nystagmus are cardinal features. Further examination often discloses tachycardia, orthostatic hypotension, hypothermia, and a diffuse analgesia. The pupils seldom are affected, but almost any motor cranial nerve can be partially paralyzed. Most patients have at least mild signs of peripheral neuropathy, but these are not requisite to diagnosis. Treatment consists of giving thiamine 50 mg parenterally, upon suspicion of the diagnosis, followed by replenishment of blood volume and electrolytes. Glucose administration should not precede thiamine treatment, as it can precipitate acute worsening. Evidence of severe anemia, hepatic insufficiency, or infection should be corrected and the patient watched closely for evidence of impending seizures or DTs. General good nourishment and efforts to halt the destructive slide of chronic alcoholism necessarily follow.

Differential diagnosis of Wernicke's disease is readily made on clinical grounds, provided one has enough history to suspect thiamine defi-

TABLE 116–19. MAJOR NEUROLOGIC COMPLICATIONS OF SEVERE ALCOHOLISM

Amblyopia and optic atrophy
Progressive cerebral degeneration and dementia
Peripheral neuropathy
Myopathy
Wernicke-Korsakoff disease
Parenchymatous cerebellar degeneration
Cerebral leukodystrophy (Marchiafava-Bignami disease)

ciency. The cause can lie in chronic alcoholism or any other circumstance of prolonged vitamin-free caloric intake, such as occurs with unsupplemented glucose infusions or, rarely, in extreme food faddism or the exclusive ingestion of polished rice. The eye signs provide a critical clue: only acute idiopathic polyneuropathy, myasthenia gravis, botulism, and intoxication with phenytoin are likely to cause a similarly acute symmetric or asymmetric bilateral external ophthalmoplegia. Of these, only Wernicke's disease and, rarely, phenytoin intoxication produce mental changes. Furthermore, the response to thiamine injection is usually diagnostic: the ophthalmoplegia usually begins to improve within a matter of hours to a day or so, a response produced with no other disorder.

Korsakoff's amnestic syndrome usually emerges as the acute confusional delirium of Wernicke's disease subsides. Affected patients show a remarkable and relatively isolated loss of recent memory. This, coupled with a placid lack of insight, often leads to absurd conversations or answers to questions (confabulation). Arousal, language functions, and remote memories are spared. Korsakoff's arises only after either several preceding attacks of Wernicke's encephalopathy or an unusually severe one. Treatment is as for Wernicke's, with about half the patients treated for the first time improving to the point of regaining independence.

Acute Cerebellar Degeneration. This arises most often in male alcoholics as a complication of an acute superimposed severe alcoholic spree rather than following the prolonged drinking periods that usually precede the Wernicke-Korsakoff syndrome. The disease is caused by an unknown mechanism of neuronal degeneration in the anterior and superior cerebellar vermis, leading to a gradually or suddenly appearing broad-based, stiff-legged ataxia unaccompanied by incoordination in the upper extremities or nystagmus. Many patients have an associated nutritional peripheral neuropathy whose treatment sometimes improves their functional difficulties.

Central Pontine Myelinolysis. This reflects a problem in the treatment of the severe alcoholic or nutritionally deprived patient. The disorder consists of the development of a symmetrical zone of demyelination affecting the basis pontis of the brain stem, leading to lethargy or stupor, a quiet confused delirium, and more or less severe quadriparesis. Both in patients and in its experimental reproduction in animals, the condition follows a too rapid (> 15 to 20 mEq per day) correction of hyponatremia. In most instances the lesion becomes visible by CT scan within a week or so after onset. Given proper subsequent systemic therapy and a nonfatal underlying disease, many or most patients treated symptomatically recover in a matter of weeks.

REFERENCES

Dreisbach RH: Handbook of Poisoning. 10th ed. Los Altos, CA, Lange Medical Publishers, 1980. *Succinct and handy, an excellent guide to emergencies.*

Kissin B: Alcohol abuse and alcohol-related illness. In Wyngaarden JB, and Smith LH Jr (eds): Cecil Textbook of Medicine. 17th ed. Philadelphia, WB Saunders Co, 1985, pp 50–54. *A clear, brief outline description of the problems.*

Millman RB: Drug abuse and dependence. In Wyngaarden JB, and Smith LH Jr (eds): Cecil Textbook of Medicine. 17th ed. Philadelphia, WB Saunders Co, 1985, pp 2015–2024. *Gives considerably greater detail on a larger number of drugs than can be covered in this chapter.*

Sellers EM, and Kalant H: Alcohol intoxication and withdrawal. N Engl J Med 294:757, 1976. *Despite the publication date, remains an unusually lucid and informative brief review.*

Tartar RE, and van Thiel DH (eds): Alcohol and the Brain. New York, Plenum Publishing Corp, 1984. *A multiauthored volume that discusses many aspects of the problem.*

Thompson WL, Johnson AD, Maddrey WL, et al: Diazepam and paraldehyde for treatment of severe delirium tremens. Ann Intern Med 82:175–180, 1975. *A model controlled clinical trial demonstrates the superiority of the benzodiazepine and outlines an effective program for management.*

Victor M, Adams RD, and Collins GH: The Wernicke-Korsakoff Syndrome. Philadelphia, FA Davis Co, 1971. *A classic clinical-neuropathologic study illuminating the ravages of nutritional disease and identifying possible structures involved in the amnesic syndrome.*

Vinken PJ, and Bruyn GW: Metabolic and Deficiency Diseases of the Nervous System. Handbook of Neurology, Vol 28. Amsterdam, North Holland Publishing Co, 1976. *Provides comprehensive reviews of the individual problems.*

117 DISORDERS OF AUTONOMIC FUNCTION

A. SLEEP DISORDERS

GENERAL CONSIDERATIONS

Sleep, a biological function regulated by brain stem autonomic mechanisms, normally varies widely from person to person. Some healthy persons require as little as four to five hours of sleep per day, while others seem unable to function with less than nine or ten. Moderate exercise reduces the latent period required to fall asleep and generally increases the depth and somewhat the length as well. Anxiety, preoccupation, depression, drugs such as caffeine, and conditions such as fever, pain, and cardiopulmonary disease all contribute to subjective difficulties in sleeping. Distressing insomnia or hyposomnia can have several aspects. Some insomniacs complain of an increased latent period before sleep occurs, while others report middle-of-the-night or early-morning awakenings. Such experiences may cause subjective distress but usually produce little or no physiological harm. Scientific observations of reported spontaneous hyposomnia indicate that in almost all instances the period of sleep usually lasts longer than the subject believes; what is recalled is the awakenings. Forced severe insomnia, however, whether induced by anxiety, pain, disease, or work requirements, does appear to reduce mental efficiency.

Insomnia of recent origin is best handled by reassurance with attention directed toward correcting underlying medical or psychological problems and, if necessary, the giving of widely spaced medications. Such cautious approaches may fail to please all patients, but the realities are that most chronic insomnia is extremely difficult to treat effectively because tolerance develops to all sedatives. That of recent origin, due to intercurrent illness, acute physical or emotional pain, jet lag, and the like, is best treated in otherwise healthy persons with the short-acting benzodiazepine, triazolam, at bedtime. Elderly patients or those with fever or systemic illness are better treated with milder agents such as chloral hydrate or flurazepam. Tricyclic antidepressants with the entire dose taken in the late evening are helpful in managing the insomnia of depression. Alcohol is a poor choice of sedative; although it shortens the sleep latency interval, it tends to shorten the duration of sleep and to produce unpleasant hangovers. Tolerance often results in the patient's resorting to increasing ingestion to achieve effect.

HYPERSOMNIAS

Increasing hypersomnia of recent origin can be a symptom of overwhelming fatigue or psychological depression but in all instances deserves consideration as possibly reflecting potentially serious neurologic disease. Chronic or recurrent hypersomnia is a symptom most often of narcolepsy or of one of the sleep apnea syndromes described on page 173.

Narcolepsy is a chronic disorder of unknown cause characterized by recurrent uncontrollable drowsiness, usually starting in the late teens or early 20's and associated with one or more of the following experiences: (1) *sleep attacks*, sudden episodes of rapid eye movement (REM)–sleep interrupting wakefulness; (2) *cataplexy*, abrupt muscular hypotonia precipitated by surprise or emotion; (3) *hypnagogic hallucinations*, intense dreamlike experiences occurring during the penumbra between sleep and wakefulness; (4) *sleep paralysis*, the sense during the moments of awakening from sleep that one cannot move. All these features may be experienced to some degree by normals, but in narcolepsy the symptoms intensify to the point of disrupting social and vocational occupations or even producing situations of great danger such as drowsy driving. Narcolepsy appears to be inherited as an autosomal dominant trait but with variable expression. Its cause is unknown, although a defect in central neurotransmission has been postulated. In intractable cases, treatment with monoamine oxidase inhibitors or amphetamines brings at least some relief.

The *Klein-Levin syndrome* is a rare disease of adolescent boys and young men marked by episodic periods of hypersomnia and hyperphagia that can last for days to weeks at a time. No favorable treatment has been established, although anecdotal reports indicate that clonazepam sometimes halts attacks. The condition usually subsides in adulthood.

SLEEP DISTURBANCES

Enuresis (bedwetting), night terrors, nightmares, sleep walking, and sleep talking all are disorders that occur in otherwise normal persons, more often during childhood than adult life. Efforts to establish consistent psychiatric correlations have been unsuccessful. Although tension and anxiety may accentuate the conditions, they are probably not the cause. Imipramine, 25 to 50 mg at bedtime, is beneficial in some cases of enuresis, while several of the other disorders improve with the taking of short-acting benzodiazepines at bedtime. Most of the conditions subside when the person reaches late adolescence or full adulthood.

REFERENCE

Hobson JA: Sleep and its disorders. In Wyngaarden JB, and Smith LH Jr (eds): Cecil Textbook of Medicine. 17th ed. Philadelphia, WB Saunders Co, 1985, pp 1986–1991. *A succinct yet informatively comprehensive discussion of the topic.*

B.   DISORDERS OF AUTONOMIC REGULATION

The autonomic nervous system contains three major components. One operates principally via the hypothalamus and links the brain to the pituitary gland and thence to the peripherally located endocrine organs. Its functions and disorders are discussed in this text with the endocrine system. The second component diffusely projects cholinergic, noradrenergic, and serotonergic pathways that travel rostrally from, respectively, ventral basal forebrain nuclei, the locus ceruleus of the pontine tegmentum, and the raphe nuclei of the midbrain and pons. These ascending projections appear to modulate the activities of higher levels of brain function, but their functions currently are little understood and will not be discussed further at this time. The third, classically known system consists of the descending autonomic sympathetic and parasympathetic pathways that connect the hypothalamus and other brain stem centers to the viscera so as to help regulate internal homeostasis. This section briefly describes this last-mentioned system and describes some of the more common examples of impaired autonomic regulation.

HYPOTHALAMUS (HT)

Direct damage to the HT can impair normal arousal mechanisms, interfere with trophic regulation of the pituitary gland, blunt normal learning memory and emotion, and disrupt the mechanisms that regulate normal water balance, heat regulation, and caloric appetite.

Disorders of Water Balance. Disease of the HT can produce three principal disorders of water balance: (1) Hypoplasia of or direct damage to the supraoptic or paraventricular nuclei or their major connections to the posterior pituitary gland leads to antidiuretic hormone (ADH) deficiency and the disorder *diabetes insipidus* (p. 196). (2) Neurogenic imbalance or biologically erroneous signals from peripheral receptors or their CNS connections can lead to *inappropriately increased ADH* secretion, producing excessive hemodilution and hyponatremia (p. 195). (3) HT-engendered failure of thirst coupled with reduced ADH secretion causes the rare condition of *essential hypernatremia*, in which appetite for water (thirst) is lacking despite pathologically elevated serum sodium levels.

Disturbances of Temperature Regulation. Sustained relative *hypothermia* or *poikilothermia*, with body temperatures varying with the environment and falling below 35°C, follows destructive lesions of the posterior hypothalamus or adjacent midbrain and can also accompany several metabolic comas as well as depressant drug poisoning. In addition, deficiencies in appropriate autonomic responses to both dehydration and ambient cooling frequently affect alcoholics and elderly persons, increasing their susceptibility to exposure and intensifying fluid loss and hypothermia. Recently, several small epidemics of exposure-induced hypothermia have been reported among residents of insufficiently heated nursing homes.

Special low recording thermometers usually are required to quantify the diagnosis of severe hypothermia, although stupor or coma, a reduction in amplitude of vital signs, and the patient's coldness to touch are qualitatively obvious. When core temperature lies between 31° and 35°C, treatment consists of gradual rewarming by blankets in an ambiently warm room. Heating blankets set at 38°C, tub immersions at 40° to 42°C, or warmed peritoneal dialysis can be employed with persons with colder core temperatures. Fluids and auxiliary treatment are guided by specific cardiac or infectious complications.

Paroxysmal hypothermia is an uncommon disorder, probably a form of diencephalic epilepsy, in which body temperature episodically drops to 32°C or less, associated with reduced alertness, mental slowness or confusion, and, usually, cardiorespiratory irregularities. Some affected patients respond to antiepileptic therapy.

Hyperthermia appears in several forms, including an uncommon neurogenic variety as well as heat exhaustion, heat stroke, and malignant hyperthermia. *Neurogenic hyperthermia* occurs as an acute phenomenon in association with acute head injury, surgical trauma, hemorrhages into the hypothalamic region, or encephalitis affecting this area. Fever can rise to potentially fatal levels of 42°C or higher. If standard antipyretic measures fail, small doses of opiates sometimes ameliorate the elevated temperature. Subacute or chronic fever never results from primary noninflammatory central nervous system disease.

Heat exhaustion and heat stroke result from a combination of varying degrees of high environmental temperature, increased body heat generation, and decreased bodily adaptive functions. Muscular heat cramps are common following exhausting exercise in hot weather. They respond quickly to fluid and salt ingestion. More extensive heat exhaustion and heat stroke represent potentially more serious problems. *Heat exhaustion* results from a gradual net water or salt and water loss. Its least serious form consists of muscle cramps progressing to eventual impairment of cardiovascular mechanisms. These anomalies produce feelings of giddiness, dizziness, syncope, and, in a more protracted and severe stage, fever and delirium. The presence of sweating continues until the late stages. Treatment consists of cool spongings or tubs plus salt and water replacement in generous amounts.

Heat stroke, a potentially fatal disorder, characteristically affects its victims during the first severe heat wave of the new season or upon the sudden movement of vigorously active young men from a cool to a hot climate, such as occurs with active troops during war. As is true with heat exhaustion, risk factors include a lack of acclimatization, old age and infirmity, and use of excess alcohol or anticholinergic or antipsychotic drugs. The disorder results when high ambient temperatures and humidity prevent adequate heat loss. Tissue damage ensues when core temperatures rise above 43°C. Clinical signs include hyperpyrexia greater than 41°C; hot, dry skin; and increasing prostration, confusion, stupor and, finally, coma accompanied by signs of brain stem dysfunction. Associated abnormalities can include tachycardia, ST and T wave abnormalities on the EKG, hypotension, consumption coagulopathy, signs of dehydration, and both potassium and sodium depletion as well as hepatic damage. Treatment is aimed at bringing core temperature below 39°C in an ice tub bath and meeting systemic problems, including high-output heart failure, as they arise. Mortality and the development of permanent neurologic disability relate directly to the duration of hyperthermia and whether or not pressor agents are required to support the circulation.

Malignant hyperthermia is a rare disorder that occurs in two drug-related settings, one with anesthetics, the other with neuroleptics. The anesthesia-related disorder most often is associated with an inherited defect in muscle that leads to excessive calcium release from sarcoplasm during anesthetic induction. Immediately following the preoperative giving of succinylcholine followed by an inhalation anesthetic, diffuse, severe skeletal muscle contraction takes place, producing generalized rigidity, increased heat production, and potentially fatal fevers of 39 to 42°C or greater. Treatment consists of quick interruption of anesthesia and surgery, with vigorous measures taken to counteract fever and lactacidosis. Blood relatives should be pretested by anesthesiologists for potential susceptibility before receiving general anesthesia. The *malignant neuroleptic syndrome*, a less frequent idiosyncratic response, follows a similar clinical pattern, with hyperthermia, muscle rigidity, autonomic instability, and reduced consciousness following upon the administration of one or more of the phenothiazine, thioxanthine, or butyrophenone classes of drugs. The pathogenesis in this disorder is less clearly known, but the approach to treatment is similar, consisting of neuroleptic withdrawal plus symptomatic attention to hyperthermia and serum lactacidosis. Dantrolene and, sometimes, procainamide have been reported to counter the muscle rigidity in some but not all examples of both hyperthermic syndromes.

Caloric Control. The ventromedial hypothalamus contains the setpoint mechanisms regulating *caloric intake* and *body weight*. Trauma, neoplasms, or granulomas affecting the region can release ravenous appetites and great weight gain until a new higher setpoint is reached. No satisfactory evidence implicates hypothalamic derangements as a primary cause of anorexia nervosa, emaciation, or simple obesity in adults.

AUTONOMIC SYMPATHETIC AND PARASYMPATHETIC PATHWAYS

Generalized systemic autonomic insufficiency can occur on either a central or a peripheral basis. Diffuse, moderate sympathetic-parasympathetic dysfunction accompanies occasional cases of parkinsonism and several of the late-life cerebellar degenerations. *Shy-Drager disease* is an uncommon midlife, idiopathic system degeneration in which central autonomic systems degenerate accompanied by variable abnormalities in extrapyramidal and, occasionally, other motor systems. Cardinal symptoms and signs include male impotence, anhidrosis, orthostatic hypotension, absent autonomic cardiovascular reflexes, impaired pupillary control, gastrointestinal hypomotility, urinary retention or incontinence, hoarseness, and signs of parkinsonism. Late in the disease the capacitance veins of the abdomen and lower extremities completely lose their constrictor reflexes. Refractory bradycardia develops, and symptoms of lightheadedness or syncope with low blood pressure can occur when assuming the erect or even the sitting position. Treatment is symptomatic and consists of counteracting the hypotension with elastic stockings, increasing fluid intake, and giving mineralocorticoids to assist in blood volume expansion.

Autonomic abnormalities including severe hypotension can accompany a number of peripheral neuropathies, especially those of diabetic neuropathy, syphilitic tabes dorsalis, and inherited amyloid disease. Moderate autonomic dysfunction consisting of tachycardia, impaired volume reflexes, and mild orthostatic insufficiency also accompanies most examples of acute inflammatory neuropathy. A few patients with inflammatory neuropathy have been observed to suffer major defects in peripheral sympathetic and parasympathetic control due to a predominant or selective involvement of these fibers.

Neurogenic Bladder Dysfunction. Micturition represents a parasympathetically regulated reflex act, normally subordinated to higher cerebral control. The afferent and efferent components of the reflex travel between the bladder and the lower sacral spinal cord, and the cord contains all the necessary components for completion of the reflex. Centrally, several levels of the spinal cord and brain stem enhance the reflex and facilitate complete bladder emptying. The cerebrum acts primarily to inhibit the micturition reflex, thereby normally governing its appropriate time and place of action.

Cerebral disorders disinhibit the micturition reflex threshold. Medial frontal lobe lesions often are associated with urgency incontinence (brief warning, full emptying), while diffuse cerebral disorders causing dementia lead to the incontinence of indifference. Subcortical and incomplete spinal disorders causing spasticity lower the micturition reflex threshold and cause urinary urgency, usually with small volumes and complete emptying. (Urinary tract infections produce similar symptoms.) Spinal transection at first inhibits reflex micturition due to spinal shock, then facilitates it as reflex hyperactivity returns in the distal spinal stump. Lacking influences from higher centers, spinal reflex micturition seldom completely empties the bladder unless specific rehabilitation retraining is carried out.

Peripheral bladder denervation occurs with lesions of the sacral cord, cauda equina, or afferent or efferent nerves. Reflex micturition is lost, and the bladder dilates until the intravesicle pressure overcomes urethral resistance to produce overflow incontinence. Within weeks to months multifocal autonomous contractions involve the bladder wall, reflecting parasympathetic denervation hypersensitivity. Urine is ejected as either a semicontinuous dribble or in repeated small, ineffective volumes. The bladder increasingly distends and generally requires recurrent catheterization to avoid chronic infections.

The treatment of neurogenic bladder difficulties varies with its cause. Antispasticity drugs or parasympathetic blocking agents such as oxybutynin chloride sometimes reduce the urgency of cerebral or spinal disorders. Urinary retention and impaired reflex control usually require at least temporary catheterization, best done intermittently to minimize infection. Chronic correction usually requires expert assistance for success.

Male sexual dysfunction has several potential causes, as listed in Table 117–1. Psychogenic

TABLE 117–1. COMMON ORGANIC CAUSES OF MALE SEXUAL FAILURE

Drugs:	Alcohol; anxiolytics and sedatives; antidepressants; sympathetic-parasympathetic blockers; several others
Endocrine:	Primary or secondary hypogonadism; diabetes, myxedema
Chronic Illness:	Disseminated malignancy, cirrhosis, uremia
Neurogenic:	Temporal lobe disorders; intramedullary spinal diseases; disease of the cauda equina or pelvic autonomic nerves
Urologic:	Extensive local surgery; Peyronie's disease
Vascular:	Severe aortic atherosclerosis

problems cause a substantial fraction of cases, especially among men younger than age 50 years. Neurologic abnormalities account for as many as 15 to 20 per cent, especially among older persons. Organic symptoms are limited to loss of libido, failure to sustain an effective erection (impotence), and failure to attain normal ejaculation-emission. The absence of nocturnal penile tumescence is more characteristic of organic than psychogenic causes. Temporal lobe–limbic system damage carries a high association with reduced male libido, while lesions affecting descending or peripheral parasympathetic fibers commonly interfere with the capacity to gain and maintain an erection. If serum testosterone is abnormally low and the neurologic defect partial, hormonal therapy sometimes helps. Some paraplegics can be taught relatively normal reflex erection and ejaculation. Most persons, however, with severely or completely impaired spinal or peripheral parasympathetic pathways will require prosthetic assistance if they are to satisfy a partner in sexual intercourse.

REFERENCES

Bennett AH (ed): Management of Male Impotence. Baltimore, Williams & Wilkins Co, 1982. *A useful, multiauthored monograph covering the organic aspects of the problem.*

Hart GR, Anderson RJ, Crumpler CP, et al: Epidemic classical heat stroke: Clinical characteristics and course of 28 patients. Medicine 61:189, 1982. *A recent study describing clinical aspects of the syndrome and delineating effective approaches to treatment.*

Nelson TE, and Flewellen EH. The malignant hyperthermia syndrome. N Engl J Med 309:416, 1983. *A recent, succinct, informative review of the anesthetic variety.*

Plum F: Autonomic disorders and their management. In Wyngaarden JB, and Smith LH Jr (eds): Cecil Textbook of Medicine. 17th ed. Philadelphia, WB Saunders Co, 1985, pp 2025–2031. *Provides more extensive description and references to material contained in this chapter.*

Plum F, and Van Uitert R: Nonendocrine diseases and disorders of the hypothalamus. Res Publ Assoc Res Nerv Ment Dis 55:415, 1977. *A comprehensive review of the entitled subject, extensively referenced.*

Williams ME, and Pannill FC: Urinary incontinence in the elderly. Physiology, pathophysiology, diagnosis and treatment. Ann Intern Med 97:895, 1982. *A highly practical guide to a common and difficult problem.*

118 DISORDERS OF SENSORY FUNCTION

A. PAIN AND PAINFUL SYNDROMES

GENERAL CONSIDERATIONS

Pain is the most common symptom for which patients seek medical assistance, and chronic pain is among the most vexing problems that physicians face. Pain has two aspects: the first is an emotionally neutral perception of a stimulus which is usually sufficiently strong to produce tissue damage; the second is an affective response to the perception of that stimulus. Pain implies damage to the organism, either physical or psychological, and chronic pain if untreated will itself damage the organism.

DIAGNOSIS OF PAINFUL DISORDERS

Pain is either acute or chronic; over six months duration is usually considered chronic. Several clinical features differentiate acute from chronic pain. Patients suffering from *severe* acute pain usually give a clear description of its location, character, and timing. Signs of autonomic nervous system hyperactivity with tachycardia, hypertension, diaphoresis, mydriasis, and pallor are often present. Acute pain usually responds well to analgesic agents, and psychological factors often play only a minor role in pathogenesis. By contrast, patients suffering from chronic pain describe less precisely the localization, character, and timing of the pain, and, because the autonomic nervous system adapts, signs of autonomic hyperactivity disappear. Furthermore, chronic pain usually responds less well to analgesic agents, and psychological colorings are usually more pertinent than in acute pain. All of these factors may lead the physician to believe that the patient exaggerates his complaints. Since there are no reliable objective tests to assess chronic pain, the physician is advised to accept his patient's report, taking into consideration his age, cultural background, environment, and other psychological background known to alter reaction to pain.

Chronic pain can be divided into three somewhat overlapping categories in decreasing order of frequency: (1) *Psychophysiological disorders.* Structural disease, such as a herniated disc or torn ligaments, may once have been present, but whether structural disease was ever present or not, psychological factors have engendered chronic physiological alterations, such as muscle spasm, which produce pain long after the underlying deficit has healed. Such patients tend to re-spond poorly to analgesic drugs, but often respond well to combination therapy directed at the end-organ (i.e., injection of trigger points in muscles) and at disturbing psychological factors. (2) Chronic pain associated with *structural disease,* such as occurs with rheumatoid arthritis, metastatic cancer, or sickle cell anemia, may be characterized by prolonged episodes of pain alternating with pain-free intervals or by unremitting pain waxing and waning in severity. Psychological factors may play an important role in exacerbating or relieving pain, but treatment of the pain by analgesics or correcting the underlying disease is usually more helpful. (3) *Somatic delusions.* Pain caused by neither structural nor physiological disorders occurs in patients with profound psychiatric disturbances such as psychotic depression or schizophrenia. The history of the pain is so vague and bizarre and its distribution so unanatomical as to suggest the diagnosis. These patients respond *only* to psychiatric therapy. History, examinations, laboratory studies, and management must be pursued with these principles in mind.

Referred pain is perceived at a site remote from the source of the noxious disturbance. It is usually cutaneous and evoked by disease of deep structures innervated by the same dermatome. Referred pain may be associated with cutaneous hyperalgesia and even relieved by procaine injection into the area of referral. When pain is referred to the same dermatome or myotome that includes the diseased structure [e.g., pain down the medial aspect of the arm (T1-T2) produced by myocardial infarction or angina pectoris or diaphragmatic irritation causing shoulder pain (C4)], it is often helpful in diagnosis. However, pain is sometimes referred at a great distance from the primary site to segments not similarly innervated, in which case the mechanism is perplexing (e.g., anginal pain referred to the jaw, gallbladder pain felt in the chest or shoulder). Various theories have been suggested to account for referred pain. Such theories as division of the same nerve into deep (visceral) and superficial branches, release of chemical mediators in the nervous system, and convergence of cutaneous and visceral nerves into common synaptic pools at the spinal cord all might explain the dermatomal referral of pain but fail to explain pain at remote sites.

HEADACHE AND OTHER HEAD PAIN

Headache is one of man's most common afflictions. The frequency of disabling headache is

FIGURE 118—1. Some pain-sensitive structures of the intracranial cavity. The figure shows the superior aspect of the brain with the calvarium removed. The dura and meningeal arteries are shown on the left, the cerebral and tributary veins on the right. The open circles indicate the points of stimulation without pain. Closed circles indicate the point of stimulation causing pain. Painful sites include (1) the margins of the superior sagittal sinus, (2) the meningeal artery, and (3) the tributary veins of the superior sagittal sinus. (From Dalessio DJ: Wolff's Headache and Other Head Pain. 4th ed. New York, Oxford University Press, 1980.)

explained in part by the rich nerve supply to the head (including efferent nerve fibers from trigeminal, glossopharyngeal, vagus, and upper three cervical nerves) and in part by the psychological implications of head pain, causing anxiety about even modest headache, whereas a pain of equal severity elsewhere in the body might be ignored. Head pain can result from distortion, stretching, inflammation, or destruction of pain-sensitive nerve endings as a result of either intra- or extracranial disease in the distribution of any of the aforementioned nerves (Fig. 118–1). Most head pain, however, arises from extracerebral structures and carries a benign prognosis. Table 118–1 classifies the common causes.

Because headache is so common and so rarely due to structural disease, excessive application of expensive and highly technical laboratory procedures to its diagnosis and management substantially increases unnecessary medical costs. Nevertheless, in some instances a timely CT scan or lumbar puncture can give lifesaving information about an otherwise undiagnosable problem. The following principles may help to manage the individual patient:

1. Patients with chronic classic or common migraine or with chronic tension headache rarely require more than a careful history and examination. Even when the unilateral prodromes and headache of long-standing, classic migraine consistently affect the same side, the incidence of associated intracranial lesions remains so low that CT scan is unnecessary and angiography unjustified.

2. Headaches that are of recent origin or progression deserve investigation by CT scan. This principle especially applies to headaches that have a consistently focal distribution, follow trauma, or begin after the age of 30 years.

3. The EEG is almost never useful in the diagnosis of headache. Skull x-rays are useful in diagnosing headache only (a) when searching for abnormalities involving the base of the brain such as sellar or suprasellar lesions or (b) immediately following head trauma. CT scans have superior discriminating capacities and, when available, make x-rays unnecessary.

4. Diagnostic lumbar puncture should be performed with any acute headache that (a) is accompanied by fever or (b) is explosive or the most severe headache ever suffered (a history typical of acute subarachnoid hemorrhage). Lumbar puncture should, if possible, be deferred until after CT scanning with other forms of acute headache, especially if stiff neck but no fever is

TABLE 118—1.   COMMON CAUSES OF HEADACHE

Vascular headache
  Migraine headache
    Classic, common, complicated, variant
  Cluster headache
  Miscellaneous vascular headaches
    Hangover, toxins and drugs, occlusive vascular disease
Muscle contraction (tension) headache
  Tension headache, depressive equivalent
  Conversion reaction, cervical osteoarthritis
Traction/inflammation headache
  Cranial arteritis, increased or decreased intracranial pressure, subarachnoid hemorrhage, meningitis, space-occupying lesions, extracranial structural lesions
Cranial neuralgias
  Trigeminal, glossopharyngeal

present. (This combination may indicate partial herniation of cerebellar tonsils into the foramen magnum secondary to an intracranial mass lesion.)

5. Radioisotopic brain scanning almost never adds useful information and is expensively superfluous.

Migraine and Other Vascular Headaches

The term vascular headache applies to a group of clinical syndromes of unknown etiology in which the final step in pathogenesis of the pain appears to be dilatation of one or more branches of the carotid artery, leading to stimulation of nerve endings supplying that artery. A typical vascular headache is unilateral, throbbing in quality, and recurs over months or years. Individual headaches are frequently precipitated by identifiable environmental or psychological factors. During a vascular headache, the involved arteries may be tender to touch, and compression of the carotid artery may temporarily relieve the pain, only to have it return with increased severity when compression is released. So-called common migraine may affect as many as 25 per cent of the population. Other vascular headache syndromes are less common, but each has distinctive clinical findings. Most acute vascular headaches last only several hours and are best treated by rest in a quiet, dark room accompanied by a mild analgesic agent such as aspirin, if the patient is not too nauseated to take it. Occasionally more potent analgesics such as codeine or Demerol may be required, but such drugs should generally be avoided, in part because they add to the nausea frequently accompanying vascular headaches and in part because of their potential for abuse. Patients with prolonged or severe migraines usually respond to vasoconstrictive agents such as ergotamine given orally, rectally, or subcutaneously. If the headaches recur frequently (twice a week or more), prophylactic agents such as beta-adrenergic blockers (e.g., propranolol), methysergide, calcium channel blockers, or sometimes tricyclic antidepressants (e.g., amitriptyline) may provide effective prophylaxis.

Common migraine is characterized by recurrent headaches, often severe, frequently beginning unilaterally, and usually associated with malaise, nausea and/or vomiting, and photophobia. The disorder often begins in childhood, affects women more often than men, and runs in families. Identifiable factors that often precipitate individual headaches are holidays and weekends, menstrual periods, foods (especially chocolate, nuts, and aged cheese), alcohol (especially red wine), environmental stimuli (such as bright sunlight, too much sleep, and undue emotional stress or resentment). Medical conditions and their treatment may also precipitate attacks. Vasodilators such as nitroglycerin and antihypertensives, serotonin releasers such as reserpine, as well as estrogens and oral contraceptives have all been reported to cause migraine attacks in susceptible individuals. Important historical points that help distinguish migraine from the equally common tension headaches (see below) include their unilaterality, their association with nausea or vomiting, the tendency of migraine to awaken one from sleep, a positive family history, and a favorable response to ergot preparations.

Classic migraine is distinguished by well-defined symptoms of brief (up to 30 minutes) neurologic dysfunction that precede or less often accompany headache. Neurologic symptoms are usually visual, most often consisting of bright flashing lights (scintillation or fortification scotomata) beginning in the center of a homonymous visual half-field and radiating over 10 to 30 minutes outward toward the periphery. Other possible neurologic disturbances include unilateral paresthesias of the hand and perioral area, aphasia, hemiparesis, and hemisensory defects. An uncommon variant named *basilar artery migraine* occurs predominantly in children and adolescents and is characterized by vertigo, ataxia, and diplopia, along with hemiparesis or hemisensory changes and, rarely, confusion, stupor, or even coma. In rare instances neurologic signs may persist for hours or days, throughout and even beyond the headache (complicated migraine).

The diagnosis of classic migraine is made entirely by history. When neurologic disability is severe or prolonged, CT scan or angiography may be required to rule out structural lesions of the brain or its vasculature.

Migraine variants include *ophthalmoplegic migraine*, in which an ocular motor palsy develops during the course of a severe migraine attack.

Cluster headaches are short-lived attacks of extremely severe, unilateral head pain that occur in clusters, often occurring several times daily and lasting several weeks, only to disappear for months or years before recurring. Their pathogenesis is unknown, although they are believed to be vascular headache related to migraine. The diagnosis is established by the characteristic history. The disorder affects men much more than women and usually starts between the third and sixth decades. Clusters characteristically occur in the spring and fall, and last three to eight weeks. Each attack, which lasts 30 minutes to 2 hours, is characterized by the rapid onset of a knifelike pain in the nostril or behind the eye which spreads to involve the forehead. During the attack, the ipsilateral nostril waters and the eye may tear. About 20 per cent of cases develop a homolateral Horner's syndrome. The headache disappears as abruptly as it came, usually leaving no residua. Unlike migraine, patients with cluster headaches neither feel systemically ill nor suffer nausea, vomiting, or exhaustion when the headache ceases. During a cluster epoch but not otherwise, alcohol invariably induces an attack. The individual cluster headache is so brief there is insufficient time for pharmacologic agents to be absorbed. Inhalation of pure oxygen often aborts the headache. Since the headaches frequently recur at known times, the ingestion of ergotamine tartrate prophylactically an hour or two before the expected headache may abort the headache. The serotonin inhibitor methysergide also is often successful in preventing headaches.

Hangover headache is part of a larger syndrome, usually including premature awakening from an overindulging night and often accompanied by a fine tremor of the extremities and mild gastric distress or nausea, mental dulling, and mild incoordination. The pathogenesis is related to alcohol withdrawal, dehydration, and the toxic effect of various congeners found with different intoxicants.

Nitrites can induce pulsating headache and, occasionally, facial flushing, most often after the ingestion of processed foods ("hot dog" headache). *Monosodium glutamate* has been blamed for the "Chinese restaurant syndrome," characterized by postprandial headache, tight sensations about the face and head, and less often giddiness and diarrhea.

True hypertensive headaches occur only in patients with severe, episodic hypertension, such as occurs with pheochromocytoma or reflex sympathetic hyperactivity such as is induced from an isolated distal spinal cord in paraplegics.

Muscle Contraction (Tension) Headache

Muscle contraction or tension headaches are characterized by a steady, nonpulsatile, unilateral or bilateral aching pain, usually beginning in the occipital region but often involving frontal or temporal regions as well. Tension headaches often recur daily, usually in early afternoon or evening, with a dull occipital or frontal pain that, vicelike, may grip the entire head in a constricting band. Unique among headaches, the pain may be constantly present for days, weeks, or months, and often is associated with tenderness in the posterior cervical, temporalis, or masseter muscles. Patients rarely complain of nausea, vomiting, or malaise, but modest dizziness, blurring of vision, and sometimes tinnitus are frequent symptoms. Tension headaches are more frequent in women, in individuals who are tense and anxious, and in those whose work or posture requires sustained contraction of posterior cervical, frontal, or temporal muscles. There is much overlap between the symptoms of common migraine and tension headaches, and many patients suffer from both.

Tension headache variants include muscle contraction and psychological tension as part of their pathogenesis. The so-called temporomandibular joint syndrome belongs to this group and includes unilateral or bilateral head pain, usually in the temporal region and in the jaw, often radiating into the ear. Tenderness affects the masseter and temporalis muscles and may be exacerbated by chewing. Accompanying symptoms often include limitation of full movement at the temporomandibular joint when opening the jaw, bruxism, and malocclusion. The disorder occasionally responds to dental manipulation, particularly use of a mouth guard that prevents bruxism.

For most patients analgesics and antianxiety manipulation effectively treat muscle contraction head pain. *Post-traumatic headaches* are dull, generalized, aching head pains that follow head injury. The disorder can blend into *depressive headache*, a chronic generalized headache, usually vaguely described, sometimes associated with giddiness and unsteadiness, that occurs as a frequent and sometimes predominant manifestation of depression. The headache may have muscle contraction and tension as its pathogenesis or may be a *somatic delusion* in a severely depressed patient. The treatment of choice is an antidepressant drug.

Atypical facial pain or atypical facial neuralgia is a term used to describe a syndrome characterized by steady aching face pain, usually unilateral, localized to the lower part of the orbit, maxillary area, and sometimes the jaw. The pain begins without a known precipitating episode and may last for hours or indefinitely. It may spread to involve the head or neck, and the muscles of the jaw and neck often become tender. Sometimes autonomic symptoms including sweating, flushing, rhinorrhea, and pallor are present. The disorder almost exclusively affects tense, anxious, and often chronically depressed women, often in early middle age. The importance of diagnosis lies in minimizing expensive laboratory tests and avoiding addicting drugs or mutilating surgical or dental procedures.

Traction/Inflammation Headache

Cranial arteritis (giant cell arteritis), a vasculitis of unknown cause, often restricted to cranial vessels, is an important cause of headache in the elderly. The illness almost always appears after age 60, usually after 70, with unilateral or bilateral temporal, occipital, or fronto-occipital head pain of variable intensity, often coupled with tenderness of the painful areas. Many patients have pain in the jaw muscles, making chewing uncomfortable. Nodules are occasionally palpable on affected vessels, especially the superficial temporal artery. The great risk is occlusion of retinal arteries with blindness. The erythrocyte sedimentation rate is usually markedly elevated. Definitive steroid treatment should be started promptly, but since migraine-vascular headaches and depressive headaches also can have their onset in the elderly, a confirmed diagnosis by arterial biopsy is essential.

Acute and subacute meningitis cause gradually developing headache resulting from inflammation of pain-sensitive structures surrounding the brain. The headache is usually generalized, throbbing, and very severe. It may be rapid or gradual in onset, and by the time it is fully developed is associated with nuchal rigidity. The diagnosis is established by lumbar puncture. In *subarachnoid hemorrhage*, the initial sudden headache is caused by an abrupt alteration of intracranial pressure. This immediate pain is succeeded by a chronic persistent headache, often accompanied by gradually increasing nuchal rigidity that results from a chemical meningitis caused by the blood.

Intracranial hypotension, usually from loss of spinal fluid from lumbar puncture or a dural tear, decreases the buoyancy of the brain so that the organ descends when the upright position is assumed, exerting traction on structures at its apex and compression on structures at its base. (In rare instances, the small bridging veins that enter the sagittal sinus may rupture and cause subdural hematomas.) *Intracranial hypertension* causes headaches when vascular and neural structures over the apex or at the base of the brain are compressed by tumor or edematous brain.

Extracranial Structural Lesions

Nasal and Sinus Headache. Most true sinus headache results from acute inflammation of the paranasal sinuses, which produces pain localized over the involved sinus and is associated with the stigmata of acute infection, including fever, swelling, and tenderness over the sinus and engorgement of the turbinates, ostia, nasofrontal ducts, and superior nasal spaces. Most patients diagnosed by a physician or self-diagnosed as having sinus headaches are in fact suffering from either vascular or muscle contraction headache. Sinus x-rays and a physical examination are diagnostic.

Dental Pain. Noxious stimuli in a tooth usually evoke local toothache, but severe dental pain can be extremely difficult to localize because pain may spread to other teeth or distant tissues, which exhibit surface hyperalgesia, tenderness, and vasomotor reactions, such as tender eyeballs, reddening of the conjunctivae, and tenderness of the auricular and temporal tissues. Secondary muscle contraction produces other sites of tenderness and pain behind the ears, behind the lower border of the mastoid process, and in the muscles of the occiput, neck, and shoulders. Patiently tapping each tooth for tenderness, using a blunt object or rod, often gives a localizing clue.

Aural Pain. Pain in the vicinity of the ear can be caused by disease of the teeth, tonsils, larynx and nasopharynx, temporomandibular joint, or cervical spine and its soft tissues. Pain in the ear can be associated with vascular headaches, atypical facial pain, and herpes zoster of the fifth and seventh cranial nerves as well as, rarely, the glossopharyngeal nerve. True glossopharyngeal neuralgia causes severe pain radiating from the tonsil into the ear. Primary ear disease is relatively infrequent—but important—as a source of headache, because it almost always indicates inflammation or destructive disease.

Eye Pain and Headache. Errors of refraction (hypermetropia, astigmatism, anomalies of accommodation), ocular muscle imbalance (strabismus), glaucoma, and iritis are universally described as causing headache. For most, the headache is mild in degree and usually starts around and over the eyes and subsequently radiates to the occiput and back of the head. The pain of glaucoma or iritis begins in the eye, can

become severe, and then later extends to include a periorbital distribution.

Pituitary Pain. Headache caused by pituitary tumors is the result of compression and distortion of pain-sensitive structures at the base of the skull, particularly the diaphragma sella. Pain is generally referred to the frontal or temporal regions bilaterally and may on occasion be referred to the vertex or occipital regions. *Acute headache* occurring with known pituitary lesions (*pituitary apoplexy*) usually results from infarction or hemorrhage into the tumor. Sudden expansion of the tumor may compromise the overlying optic chiasm, leading to visual loss, or invade the laterally lying cavernous sinus, producing ocular palsies. Pituitary apoplexy should be treated surgically by emergency drainage of the hemorrhagic or infarcted material.

Cranial Neuralgias

The term cranial neuralgias refers to several distinctive, extremely severe, paroxysmal head pains that appear to result from sudden episodic, intrinsic, and excessive discharges from the involved nerve. The best known is trigeminal neuralgia. Similar but much rarer disorders than trigeminal or glossopharyngeal neuralgia have been reported to involve the greater occipital nerve and the nervus intermedius portion of the facial nerve. The clinical features and treatment of these rare disorders are similar to those of trigeminal neuralgia.

Trigeminal Neuralgia. Trigeminal neuralgia is characterized by sudden, lightning-like paroxysms of pain in the distribution of one or more divisions of the trigeminal nerve. Most trigeminal neuralgia is probably caused by compression of the trigeminal nerve by tortuous arteries of the posterior fossa. Occasionally the syndrome can result from a gasserian ganglion tumor, multiple sclerosis, or a brain stem infarct.

The history is diagnostic. The pain occurs as brief, lightning-like stabs, frequently precipitated by touching a trigger zone around the lips or the buccal cavity. At times, talking, eating, or brushing the teeth serves as a trigger. The pains rarely last longer than seconds, and each burst is followed by a refractory period of several seconds to a minute in which no further pain can be precipitated. The pains, however, often occur in clusters so that affected patients may report that each pain lasts for hours. The pain is limited to the distribution of the trigeminal nerve, usually involving the second and third division or both. Spontaneous remissions are common. Exacerbations tend to occur in the spring and fall. Between paroxysms of pain, the patient is asymptomatic. The pain rarely occurs at night. Ordinarily, the neurologic examination is entirely normal. Sensory changes in the distribution of the trigeminal nerve should prompt a careful search for structural disease such as tumor.

Carbamazepine is the initial treatment of choice for the treatment of trigeminal neuralgia; phenytoin and baclofen are also sometimes effective. The drugs are not analgesics and are effective only for specific kinds of pain such as trigeminal neuralgia, glossopharyngeal neuralgia, and the lightning pains of tabes dorsalis. If medical treatment fails, surgery, either radiofrequency lesions of the gasserian ganglion (to block sensory conduction) or posterior fossa craniotomy (to relieve the trigeminal nerve of compression by vascular structures), is indicated.

Glossopharyngeal Neuralgia. Glossopharyngeal neuralgia is characterized by pain similar to that of trigeminal neuralgia but in the distribution of the glossopharyngeal and vagus nerves. The trigger zone usually lies in the tonsil or posterior pharynx, and the pain spreads toward the angle of the jaw and the ear. Occasionally patients suffer cardiac slowing or brief arrest (syncope) during attacks of pain as a result of the intense afferent discharge over the glossopharyngeal nerve. Carbamazepine is often effective, but, if drugs fail, glossopharyngeal nerve roots are sectioned in the posterior fossa. Symptomatic glossopharyngeal neuralgia is occasionally the presenting complaint in a patient with a tonsillar tumor, and careful examination of the pharynx and tonsillar fossa for mass lesions must be carried out.

NECK AND BACK PAIN

Neck and/or back pain is one of man's most common afflictions. About 80 per cent of individuals suffer significant low back pain at least once during their life. Pain in the neck or back may arise from one or more of several pain-sensitive structures (Fig. 118–2), including the periosteum of the vertebral body (explaining why compression fractures of the spine are at least initially painful), posterior longitudinal ligament (one source of pain from herniated disc), the nerve roots exiting the intervertebral foramina (the source of dermatomal pain from nerve root compression by herniated discs), the facet joints (a common cause of acute back pain after unaccustomed bending), the sacroiliac joints, and the paravertebral muscles. Table 118–2 lists some

TABLE 118–2. COMMON CAUSES OF NECK AND/OR BACK PAIN

Trauma
  Muscle strain or spasm
  Subluxed facet joints
  Compression fractures (osteoporosis)
Degenerative disorders
  Herniated disc
  Spondylosis
    Spinal stenosis
  Osteoarthritis
Neoplasm
  Extradural (usually malignant)
  Intradural extramedullary (usually benign)
  Intramedullary (either benign or malignant)
Inflammation
  Arthritis
  Osteomyelitis of vertebral body
  Disc infection

common causes of neck or back pain. Most acute neck or back pain is probably caused by muscle strain and spasm due to unaccustomed exercise or stretching, is transient, and is not life-threatening. The pain is probably similar pathophysiologically to muscle contraction headache (see also myofascial pain, below). Patients suffering from such pain usually recover within a few weeks no matter what the treatment, but a few suffer chronic disability. Most chronic neck or back pain is usually associated with vertebral arthritis and/or intervertebral disc disease, the former causing pain by compression of small nerve twigs supplying the facet joints and the periosteum of the vertebral bodies, the latter causing pain by compression of the nerve root. More rarely, tumors and inflammatory or degenerative arthritic lesions of the spine may be responsible.

In patients with acute neck or back pain, particularly when the precipitating cause (such as unaccustomed exercise) cannot be identified, heat and rest suffice without further diagnostic workup. In patients with persistent or recurrent pain, meticulous diagnostic evaluation and vigorous therapy often prevent or reverse serious or potentially lethal neurologic damage.

The diagnostic evaluation begins with a history. Most benign back or neck pain is of acute or subacute onset and frequently follows by minutes to hours some unaccustomed physical activity, particularly lifting or bending. Other patients awaken feeling stiff and sore the morning after unusual exercise. Sometimes low back pain begins acutely, frequently on arising in the morning, without any obvious precipitating event. Most neck pain begins as a stiff neck, often on awakening in the morning, without a previous history of unusual activity. Many patients' neck or back pains occur episodically over many years. Most benign neck or back pain is dull or aching in quality, exacerbated by movement, and relieved by rest. The majority of patients are comfortable when recumbent and immobile or at least are able to find one position that relieves the pain. Pain that is present when the patient is immobile and that cannot be relieved by postural manipulation should lead the physician to search for a serious disorder. Likewise, pain that radiates in a clear dermatomal distribution is probably a result of nerve root compression, especially if there are paresthesias or loss of sensation. Radiating pain in a nondermatomal distribution often accompanies neck and back muscle spasms; it usually does not portend serious neurogenic disease.

A careful physical and neurologic examination may reveal an obvious cause for the pain. Systemic disease such as cancer, urinary tract infection, pelvic disease, or abdominal aneurysm may be a cause of back pain because a lesion impinges on the vertebral body or paravertebral structures. Evidence for neurologic disease such as weakness, sensory loss, or reflex abnormalities suggest spinal cord or nerve root dysfunction. Such evidence of neurologic disability requires a careful laboratory examination, including plain radiographs, CT scan of vertebral and paravertebral

PLL (+)
LF (−)

VB (−)

FA (+)
NR (+)
IVD (−)

FC (+)

ALL (+)
M (+)

ALL (+)
IVD (−)
NR (+)
VB (−)
PLL (+)

AC (+)
FA (+)
LF (−)

M (+)

ISL (+)

FIGURE 118–2. Pain-sensitive tissue in and around the spine. Those tissues labeled with a plus are pain-sensitive because they contain sensory nerve endings that communicate pain when stimulated. The tissues labeled with a minus are devoid of sensory nerve endings. Paravertebral muscles, not shown in this schematic, are also pain-sensitive. (From Cailliet R: Neck and Arm Pain. 2nd ed. Philadelphia, FA Davis Co, 1981.)

Tissue sites of pain production.

PLL = Posterior longitudinal ligament	IVD = Intervertebral disk
LF = Ligamentum flavum	FC = Facet capsule
VB = Vertebral body	ALL = Anterior longitudinal ligament
FA = Facet articulation	M = Muscle
NR = Nerve root	ISL = Interspinous ligament

structures, and, if clinically indicated, myelography. Specific findings resulting from intervertebral disc disease are found on p. 717 and those from spinal tumor and congenital anomalies on p. 725.

In the absence of a clear abnormality on physical examination, conservative treatment of back pain with immobility, heat, analgesics, and sometimes physical therapy will ameliorate symptoms in a short period of time without the necessity of substantial laboratory evaluation. Even in the absence of neurologic signs, however, if pain persists after conservative treatment, x-ray and laboratory evaluation become mandatory.

MYOFASCIAL PAIN

A major part of head, back, and neck pain arises from skeletal muscle, particularly from the paravertebral muscles. Unaccustomed exercise causes soreness and tenderness in the involved muscles but is rarely a source of patient complaint. Prolonged tonic contraction of skeletal muscles, however, has a pathogenesis that originates in psychological tension, resentment, and anxiety and may produce pain whose cause is not immediately apparent to the patient. Examples are tension headache arising from chronic contraction of muscles at the base of the skull, anterior chest pain from contraction of the pectoralis majors, posterior thoracic or lumbar pain from paraspinous muscle contraction, and abdominal pain from rectus muscle contraction. The pain is initially localized over the area of muscle contraction but may spread widely in a distribution characteristic for the muscles involved. The affected muscles are usually tender to palpation, and one often finds a particularly tender area somewhere in the muscle, called a trigger zone, which, when palpated, reproduces the distribution of the spontaneous pain. The pathophysiology of myofascial pain is poorly understood. Some observers have reported microscopic changes at trigger points (so-called fibrous nodules), suggesting that a tonic contraction may lead to structural changes in the muscle. Others have

suggested that release of noxious substances such as lactic acid, potassium, or kinins from chronically contracting muscles might be reponsible for the pain and tenderness associated with this syndrome. The treatment of myofascial pain is often difficult and frustrating. In some patients mild analgesic drugs (aspirin), heat, and massage will yield temporary or long-term relief. In other patients, massage or even injection of trigger points with local anesthetics will give relief. Biofeedback with the patient trying consciously to relax contracted muscles recorded by surface EMG has been reported to be useful. For most patients, a combination of the above physical methods with investigation and treatment of the underlying psychological disorder is necessary if long-term relief is to be achieved.

B. THE SPECIAL SENSORY SYSTEM

SMELL AND TASTE

Smell. Most acquired disturbances of smell result from transient or sustained diseases of the nasal mucous membranes that dry out or deaden the receptor area. Such disorders seldom are complete and commonly respond to local treatment. More severe and often permanent anosmia results from, respectively, basal skull fractures avulsing the olfactory nerves, frontal fossa brain tumors affecting the central pathways, and, much less often, herpes zoster, vitamin B_{12} deficiency, and multiple sclerosis. Sudden idiopathic anosmia usually associated with loss of taste has been reported, probably a result of a local neurotropic viral infection. No satisfactory treatment has been found for such neurogenic anosmias. Affected patients must be warned explicitly to avoid gas heating and to install smoke alarms to compensate for the life-threatening hazards of the defect. *Parosmia* is a distortion of olfactory perception (normal odors perceived as a foul smell) that may occur without prior anosmia or during the recovery phase from anosmia. The cause most often lies in paranasal infections or, sometimes, in psychiatric illness. Hallucinations of smell, usually of a foul quality, occur with epileptogenic lesions affecting the region of the amygdala and are termed uncinate fits.

Taste. Much of what is perceived as taste derives indirectly from olfaction, which should be checked in any patient complaining of taste loss (ageusia or reduction hypogeusia). Disorders that directly cause taste abnormalities include Bell's palsy, an acute, unilateral loss of facial nerve function that usually reduces taste perception on the involved side. Trigeminal dysfunction with somatosensory loss on the tongue usually does not affect taste. Epileptic discharges occasionally cause gustatory hallucinations. Psychologically

depressed or paranoid patients often complain of a foul taste, but taste perception is usually normal. Aging, hepatitis, cancer, and several drugs reduce or distort taste. Unilateral taste loss should prompt a search for facial nerve disease; bilateral taste loss demands investigation of local tongue disease, followed by a systematic review of medications, and, if still necessary, an inquiry into systemic illness. Treatment depends on cause; zinc therapy is not helpful.

VISION AND OCULAR MOVEMENT

VISION

Introduction and Definitions

The visual sensory system is our most important window on the outside world. A knowledge of the anatomy of visual pathways (which can be found in standard textbooks of neurology) is important, because lesions of the visual sensory system can usually be discretely localized by history and visual field examination (Fig. 118–3). In brief, if visual loss can be corrected to 20/40 or better by refraction or by use of a pinhole (the pinhole test done at the bedside requires the patient to look through a small card with a pinhole in it held over his eye and then to read an eye chart), the disorder is caused by abnormalities of the lens or other structures anterior to the retina and is not neurologic. Partial or complete visual loss in one eye, sparing the other, implies damage to the retina or optic nerve anterior to the chiasm, whereas a visual field abnormality affecting both eyes originates at the chiasm or posterior; the more congruent the visual field, the more posterior. *Scotomas* are areas of relative or complete visual loss. *Central scotomas* severely decrease vision be-nasal temporal

Lt Rt

8 (subtotal)

FIGURE 118–3. Visual fields that accompany damage to the visual pathways. (From Plum F: Neuro-ophthalmology. In Wyngaarden JB, and Smith LH Jr (eds): Cecil Textbook of Medicine. 17th ed. Philadelphia, WB Saunders Co, 1985, pp 2032–2037.)

Visual fields that accompany damage to the visual pathways. 1. Optic nerve: Unilateral amaurosis. 2. Lateral optic chiasm: Grossly incongruous, incomplete (contralateral) homonymous hemianopia. 3. Central optic chiasm: Bitemporal hemianopia. 4. Optic tract: Incongruous, incomplete homonymous hemianopia. 5. Temporal (Meyer's) loop of optic radiation: Congruous partial or complete (contralateral) homonymous superior quadrantanopia. 6. Parietal (superior) projection of the optic radiation: Congruous partial or complete homonymous inferior quadrantanopia. 7. Complete parieto-occipital interruption of optic radiation. Complete congruous homonymous hemianopia with psychophysical shift of foveal point often sparing central vision, giving "macular sparing." 8. Incomplete damage to visual cortex: Congruous homonymous scotomas, usually encroaching at least acutely on central vision.

cause the macular fibers are damaged, whereas scotomas away from the macula may hardly be noticed by the patient. Visual field abnormalities impairing half or nearly half of the field are termed hemianoptic. A *homonymous hemianopia* implies a postchiasmal lesion, a *bitemporal hemianopia* a chiasmal lesion, and an *altitudinal hemianopia*, whether unilateral or bilateral, implies vascular damage to retinal structures. Smaller defects involving only a quarter of the visual field are called *quadrantanopsia*. Homonymous *superior quadrantanopsia* implies temporal lobe damage, whereas homonymous *inferior quadrantanopsia* implies parietal lobe damage. *Scintillating scotomas* refer to hallucinations of flashing lights. Such abnormalities imply an ab-

normal discharge of the visual system anywhere along its course. The disorder is common in migraine and also in seizures originating from the occipital lobe.

Diseases Causing Visual Impairment

Corneal, lenticular, or vitreous diseases large enough to produce visual symptoms can usually be detected by funduscopic inspection. Glaucoma with high intraocular pressure causes either slow or rapid visual loss associated with ring or annular scotomas and a deeply cupped optic disc. Visual loss may be preceded by halos seen around illuminated lights and pain in the affected eye. Diagnosis can be made only by tonometry. Retinal detachment gives rise to unilateral distortion of visual images that may be mistaken for monocular scintillating scotomas. Detachment can be usually identified by irregularities seen in the retina on funduscopic examination.

Unilateral Visual Loss. Serious visual loss from optic nerve lesions affects either one eye or both eyes asymmetrically, leading to nonhomonymous visual defects; the pupillary light reflex is diminished to the same degree as is vision. Most acute or subacute optic nerve disease is due to demyelinating (optic neuritis), vascular (e.g., giant cell arteritis), or neoplastic lesions. If the disorder is at the nerve head, it produces papillitis, but if more posteriorly the same disease process can cause a central scotoma or even blindness with no visible change in the optic nerve. *Demyelinating optic neuritis* is usually unilateral. It may be a symptom of multiple sclerosis, but many patients with optic neuritis recover and do not develop other neurologic dysfunction. Demyelinating lesions of the optic nerve appear to have a particular predilection for the myelinated fibers that supply the macula, thus leading to central scotomas. Visual acuity is severely impaired, but the peripheral vision may remain intact. *Ischemic optic neuropathy* may be a symptom of *giant cell arteritis* (p. 685) or may occur in late middle age, usually in hypertensive individuals as an isolated vascular phenomenon. Blinded patients with giant cell arteritis are usually elderly and suffer from headache, malaise, fever, and an elevated sedimentation rate. Emergency treatment with corticosteroids may prevent blindness in the other eye. In patients with ischemic optic neuropathy, the second eye also tends to become involved, but there is no treatment to prevent it. *Tumors* usually produce slowly progressive visual loss rather than acute or subacute loss, and their diagnosis can be made by either funduscopic examination, CT scan, or both. Acute and *transient monocular blindness* is usually a result of embolization of the central retinal artery or one of its branches. The emboli may originate from an atherosclerotic plaque in the carotid or ophthalmic artery or from material on cardiac valves. The disorder has been reported to complicate rheumatic heart disease and mitral valve prolapse.

Bilateral Visual Loss. Bilateral retinal or optic nerve disease occurs with hereditodegenerative conditions, vascular diseases such as diabetes, idiopathic (senile) macular degeneration, or diseases such as retinitis pigmentosa. These disorders can be diagnosed by funduscopic or sometimes slit lamp examination. Acute *transient bilateral blindness* (bilateral visual obscuration) is usually a symptom of increased intracranial pressure; it is almost always associated with severe papilledema and can occur with either brain tumors or pseudotumor cerebri (p. 779).

Acute or subacute bilateral optic neuritis may be demyelinating but usually is not due to multiple sclerosis, being more likely toxic-nutritional or an inherited optic atrophy. Most chiasmal lesions in the adult result from tumors compressing that structure; the commonest are pituitary adenomas, but also include craniopharyngiomas, meningiomas, and large aneurysms of the carotid artery. In small children, optic gliomas are a major cause of chiasmal visual loss. Lesions of the optic tract producing incongruous homonymous field defects are usually caused by infarcts or less commonly tumors. Disorders posterior to the optic tract produce congruent field defects that usually involve macular fibers. When the lesion is occipital, sparing the occipital pole (which often has a bilateral supply from both the middle and the posterior cerebral artery), macular fibers may be spared. The phenomenon cannot be detected at bedside but can be detected by careful visual field testing. Most postchiasmal visual loss is caused by vascular disease or tumor.

Bilateral damage to the visual radiation or occipital cortex produces *cortical blindness.* Such blindness is characterized by a normal funduscopic examination, normal pupillary light reflexes, and often unawareness on the part of the patient that he is, in fact, blind. Most transient cortical blindness is a symptom of basilar artery insufficiency, hypertensive encephalopathy, or more rarely of migraine. The disorder may also occur in the postictal state after a generalized seizure. The reason for the vulnerability of the cerebral cortex to these diffuse cerebral disorders is not clear. Cortical blindness, because of the preservation of pupillary reflexes, may at first be confused with a conversion reaction (hysteria). If there is any question, however, visual evoked responses will establish the diagnosis.

Any complaint of visual loss, particularly unilateral and transient, is an emergency. Lesions that involve one eye can often soon involve the second, and transient or incomplete lesions can become permanent or complete. Many disorders of the visual system are caused by vascular disease, inflammation, or tumors and are thus potentially treatable. Accordingly, a rapid and meticulous examination is necessary first to localize the site of the lesion by funduscopic and visual field examination, and then to identify its pathogenesis (that is done usually by a CT scan or angiography). These steps may lead to appropriate treatment that preserves vision. Examples of sight-saving procedures include reduction of pressure in acute glaucoma, the early use of corticosteroids for the treatment of cranial arteritis, anticoagulation for crescendo carotid or basilar insufficiency, and prompt surgical decompression for the treatment of tumors.

PUPILS

The size of the pupil is determined by the balance between discharges of the sympathetic and parasympathetic (oculomotor nerve) fibers (Fig. 118–4). The pupillary light reaction is determined on the afferent side by visual sensory fibers originating in the retina and traveling through the optic nerve, chiasm, and tract to the midbrain and on the efferent side by parasympathetic fibers that arise in the oculomotor nucleus of the midbrain (Table 118–3).

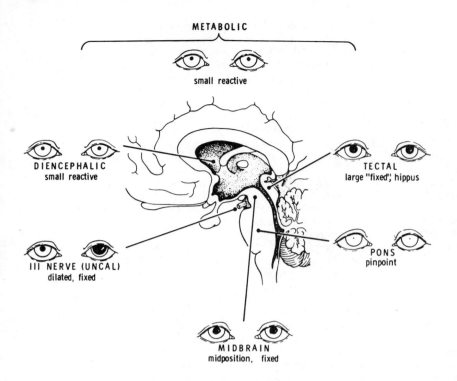

METABOLIC

small reactive

DIENCEPHALIC
small reactive

TECTAL
large "fixed"; hippus

III NERVE (UNCAL)
dilated, fixed

PONS
pinpoint

MIDBRAIN
midposition, fixed

FIGURE 118–4. Responses in comatose patients. The schematic shows pupillary responses resulting from damage to various areas of the central pupillary pathways. In patients with metabolic encephalopathy, pupils are small and reactive, as are pupils resulting from diencephalic damage such as occurs with early herniation. Lesions of the upper brain stem usually produce unilaterally or bilaterally large or mid-position fixed pupils, whereas pontine lesions result in pinpoint pupils. (From Plum F, and Posner JB: Diagnosis of Stupor and Coma. 3rd ed. Philadelphia, FA Davis Co, 1980.)

When *sympathetic fibers* are damaged, the pupil narrows (the light reaction is still normal) and the palpebral fissure becomes smaller as the upper lid descends and the lower lid elevates (Horner's syndrome). The eye, however, does not close as it does with oculomotor nerve lesions. Sweat fibers may be involved as well, leading to anhidrosis on the entire half of the body if the damage is central, on the ipsilateral face and neck if the damage is between the spinal cord and the superior cervical ganglion, or on the medial side of the forehead only if the damage is above the superior cervical ganglion.

Horner's syndrome may be caused by vascular damage to the hypothalamus or brain stem but then is associated with other neurologic signs that point to the disorder. An isolated Horner's syn-

drome may be the first sign of a lung cancer of the superior sulcus or may occur with tumors or other diseases involving the carotid artery. In some instances the cause of the disorder is not found. Horner's syndrome is valuable as a localizing diagnostic sign but in and of itself does not require treatment in that it impairs neither vision nor ocular motor function.

Parasympathetic disorders occur unilaterally with any lesion of the oculomotor nerve, particularly those that compress the nerve, such as tumors or aneurysms. Cerebral herniation leads to pupillary dilatation if it affects the third nerve or to bilaterally midpositioned and fixed pupils if it affects the midbrain.

The pupils are not always equal in size. Essential anisocoria (lifelong difference in the sizes of the pupils with a normal light reaction) occurs in about 15 per cent of normal people. Tonic (Adie's) pupil is a somewhat larger than normal pupil that constricts little or not at all to light and shrinks slowly on accommodation. It constricts more than normal when dilute pilocarpine is instilled, suggesting that the pupil is parasympathetically denervated (denervation hypersensitivity). The disorder may be unilateral or bilateral and when symptomatic is characterized by a long delay in focusing when the patient attempts to move from far to near vision. There may be pain or a dazzling sensation when affected patients exit from a dark to a light room. In some persons the disorder is associated with deep tendon reflex absence (Adie's syndrome), but neither the pupillary nor the reflex disorder causes serious disability.

Argyll Robertson pupils are small (1 to 2 mm), unequal, irregular, and fixed to light. They constrict briskly on accommodation. Their principal cause is neurosyphilis, although partial Argyll

TABLE 118–3. COMMON CAUSES OF PUPILLARY ABNORMALITIES

SIZE		REACTION TO LIGHT
SMALL PUPILS	LARGE PUPILS	
Argyll Robertson pupil	Holmes-Adie pupil	Nonreactive
Pontine hemorrhage	Post-traumatic iridoplegia	
Opiates	Mydriatic drops	
Pilocarpine drops	Glutethimide overdose	
	Cerebral death	
	Atropine poisoning	
	Amphetamine overdose	
Old age	Childhood	Reactive
Horner's syndrome	Anxiety	
	Physiological anisocoria	

Modified from Patten J: Neurological Differential Diagnosis. New York, Springer-Verlag, 1983.

Robertson pupils occur with diabetes and certain of the autonomic neuropathies. Unexplained unilaterally or bilaterally dilated pupils with visual blurring can result from accidental or intentional instillation of mydriatics such as scopolamine or atropine. Such an abnormality is characterized by failure of the pupil to constrict promptly with 1 per cent pilocarpine.

Damage to visual fibers (the afferent arc of the pupillary light reflex) leads to the "paradoxical pupillary response," in which the direct reaction to light is impaired (because the afferent information is not carried to the oculomotor nerve), but the consensual reaction is normal (since the afferent information reaches both oculomotor nerves). The response is best seen when a bright light is rapidly moved from a normal to a visually impaired eye; the consensually constricted pupil in the impaired eye then dilates.

OCULAR MOVEMENT

Definitions

Abnormal disjunctive eye movements can result from disturbances at several levels of the neuraxis. These include abnormalities in the action of individual muscles (ocular myopathies), the myoneural junction (myasthenia gravis), the oculomotor nerve, the three paired nuclei in the brain stem, or the internuclear medial longitudinal fasciculus that yokes the eyes in parallel movement. The term *strabismus* describes an involuntary deviation of the eyes from normal physiological position. Nonparalytic strabismus is due to an intrinsic imbalance of the ocular muscle tone and is usually congenital. Paralytic strabismus results from defects in ocular muscle innervation and thus implies a neuromuscular disorder. A congenital strabismus may be compensated during life only to become manifest with aging, fatigue, or systemic disease. With strabismus, the patient often suppresses vision in one eye in order to prevent diplopia. If this occurs in early infancy, the suppressed eye will develop permanent reduction of vision (amblyopia exanopsia). This does not occur if strabismus develops later in life.

Defects in ocular movement resulting from faulty action of the eye muscles or their peripheral innervation (such as the third, fourth, and sixth cranial nerves) are called ocular paralyses. Abnormalities of conjugate gaze are called gaze paralyses and result from disease of central structures.

Ocular Paralyses

The *abducens* (sixth cranial) nerve subserves the lateral rectus muscle. Selective involvement of the abducens nerve anywhere along its pathway, in or outside the brain stem, leads to isolated weakness of abduction of the affected eye. If the nucleus itself is involved, there is also a gaze paresis to the ipsilateral side as a result of damage to supranuclear structures in the same area. The *trochlear* (fourth cranial) nerve subserves the superior oblique muscle, which intorts the eye and

TABLE 118-4. A. MAJOR CAUSES OF ACUTE (<48 HOURS) OPHTHALMOPLEGIA

CONDITION	DIAGNOSTIC FEATURES
Bilateral	
Botulism	Contaminated food, high altitude cooking, pupils involved
Myasthenia gravis	Fluctuating degree of paralysis; responds to edrophonium chloride I.V.
Wernicke's encephalopathy	Nutritional deficiency; responds to thiamine I.V.
Guillain-Barré	Antecedent respiratory infection; elevated CSF protein
Brain stem stroke	Other brain stem signs
Unilateral	
Carotid-posterior communicating aneurysm	Third cranial nerve, pupil involved
Diabetic-idiopathic	Third or sixth cranial nerve, pupil spared
Myasthenia gravis	As above
Brain stem stroke	As above

B. CAUSES OF OCULAR NERVE PARALYSIS*

CAUSE	Oculomotor (3rd nerve)	Trochlear (4th nerve)	Abducens (6th nerve)	Multiple
Undetermined	67(23.1%)	62(36.0%)	124(29.6%)	10(8.4%)
Head trauma	47(16.2%)	55(32.0%)	70(16.7%)	25(21.0%)
Neoplasm	34(11.7%)	7(4.1%)	61(14.6%)	41(34.5%)
Vascular	60(20.7%)	32(18.6%)	74(17.7%)	6(5.0%)
Aneurysm**	40(13.8%)	3(1.7%)	15(3.6%)	13(10.9%)
Other	42(14.5%)	3(1.7%)	15(3.6%)	13(10.9%)
Total	290(100%)	172(100%)	419(100%)	119(100%)

* Based on 1000 patients (Rush JA, Younge BR: Paralysis of cranial nerves III, IV, and VI. Arch Ophthalmol 99:76–79, 1981.
** Includes diabetes mellitus, hypertension, atherosclerosis.

moves it down when it is medially deviated. All other muscles, including the pupilloconstrictor and the levator of the upper lid, are controlled by the *oculomotor* (third cranial) nerve. Abnormalities of the cranial nerves in the brain stem are almost always associated with other neurologic signs and are usually caused by vascular disturbances, tumors, or demyelinating disease. The peripheral nerves may be involved individually or together by lesions anywhere from their site of exit in the brain stem to their site of entry to the muscle. The nerves are most widely separated in the posterior fossa and run closest to each other in the cavernous sinus and superior orbital fissure. Accordingly, compressive lesions in the cavernous sinus usually cause multiple unilateral ocular palsies, whereas those in the posterior fossa may cause single (sometimes bilateral) nerve dysfunction. Intrinsic lesions of the third nerve (e.g., diabetic vasculopathy) often spare the pupil, whereas compressive lesions (tumors and aneurysms) involve the pupil early. Table 118-4 lists the major causes of acute ophthalmoplegia and also the causes of ocular nerve paralysis, either acute or chronic.

Conjugate Paralysis

Conjugate movement of the eyes is regulated by supranuclear pathways that descend from the forebrain to reach the medial longitudinal fasciculus in the brain stem. Unilateral hemispheral disease resulting from hemorrhage, infarct, or tumor acutely paralyzes conjugate gaze to the contralateral side and often causes deviation of the eyes to the ipsilateral side. Sometimes, particularly in deep-lying hemispheral hemorrhages involving the thalamus, the eyes deviate in the opposite direction. The eye deviation can usually be overcome by vestibular stimulation (p. 697) and is generally transient. Lesions of brain stem pathways cause more permanent conjugate paralysis to the ipsilateral side, with slight eye deviation to the contralateral side. This abnormality usually cannot be overcome by vestibular stimulation.

Lesions of the medial longitudinal fasciculus (MLF), which connects the third and sixth nerves in the brain stem, lead to *internuclear ophthalmoplegia*, in which the eyes at rest may either be parallel or show a mild skew deviation but move disjunctively on lateral gaze. (Skew deviation results from any of a number of lesions involving the brain stem and has little localizing value.) A characteristic of internuclear ophthalmoplegia is that during lateral gaze toward the side of the MLF lesion, the ipsilateral eye abducts and shows nystagmus (see below), whereas the contralateral adducting eye partially or completely fails to move nasally because of the failure of ascending impulses to reach the opposite third nerve nucleus. Internuclear ophthalmoplegia may be caused by an infarct from small vessel disease (e.g., systemic lupus erythematosus) or by demyelinating disease. Bilateral internuclear ophthalmoplegia is almost always a result of multiple sclerosis.

HEARING

Symptoms of Auditory Dysfunction

Only two symptoms result from disease of the auditory system: The first is hearing impairment, sometimes associated with a distortion as well as a decrease in the intensity of sound, and the second is tinnitus, a sound heard in the ear or head not arising from the external environment. Hearing loss is termed conductive (external and middle ear), sensorineural (cochlea and auditory nerve), or central (brain stem and cerebral hemispheres). Most is conductive or sensorineural.

Conductive hearing loss is characterized by equal loss of hearing at all frequencies and by well-preserved speech discrimination once the threshold for hearing is exceeded. The ear often feels full, as if "blocked," with acquired conductive difficulties. Bone conduction exceeds air conduction and, if unilateral, the Weber test (tuning fork in the center of the head) is referred to the deaf ear. With *sensorineural hearing loss*, one typically hears better for low- than for high-frequency tones, and it may be difficult to hear speech that is mixed with background noise; small increases

in the intensity of sound may cause discomfort (recruitment). Air conduction exceeds bone conduction and the Weber test refers to the hearing ear. With hearing loss resulting from cochlear disease (usually due to selective destruction of hair cells), diplacusis and recruitment are common (p. 695). *Central hearing loss* is uncommon and usually characterized by loss of speech more than of pure tone perception. Substantial central hearing loss requires bilateral lesions of such areas as inferior colliculus, medial geniculate bodies, or temporal lobe. When the primary receiving areas (Heschl's gyrus) are destroyed, hearing is diminished or absent even for pure tone. If association areas in the superior temporal gyrus are damaged, a patient may hear the sounds but be unable to comprehend their meaning.

Causes of Hearing Loss

Conductive hearing loss arises from abnormalities of the external or middle ear and can raise hearing threshold no more than 60 dB, since bone conduction is intact. Obstruction in the external auditory meatus (the most common cause of conductive hearing loss) impairs air transmission to the tympanum. This benign condition is most often caused by *impacted cerumen*, but it occasionally results from canal infection or similar causes. A *fluid-filled middle ear*, a result of middle ear infection (otitis media), reduces movement of the ossicles against the oval window. *Otosclerosis* is a process in which the annular ligament that attaches the stapes to the oval window overgrows and calcifies. Chronic tinnitus sometimes marks the early stages of this process, which reduces ossicular transmission via the window to the cochlear basement membrane.

Sensorineural hearing loss from genetically determined deafness, usually from hair cell aplasia or deterioration, may be present at birth or develop in adulthood. The diagnosis of *hereditary deafness* rests on the finding of a positive family history. In many instances the inheritance is transmitted through a recessive gene or a dominant gene with low penetrance, making it difficult to determine the genetic pattern. *Intrauterine factors* resulting in congenital hearing loss include infection (especially rubella); toxic, metabolic, and endocrine disorders; and anoxia associated with Rh incompatibility and difficult deliveries.

Acute unilateral deafness usually has a cochlear basis. Bacterial or viral infections of the labyrinth, head trauma with fracture or hemorrhage into the cochlea, or vascular occlusion of a terminal branch of the anterior inferior cerebellar artery all can damage the cochlea and its hair cells. An acute, idiopathic, often reversible, unilateral hearing loss strikes young adults and is presumed to reflect either a viral infection or a vascular disorder of the cochlea. Sudden unilateral hearing loss, often associated with vertigo and tinnitus, can result from a perilymphatic fistula. Such fistulae may be congenital, follow stapes surgery, or result from severe or mild trauma to the inner ear.

Drugs fairly often cause sudden bilateral hearing impairment. Salicylates, furosemide, and ethacrynic acid can cause intense tinnitus and transient deafness when taken in high doses. Aminoglycoside antibiotics can destroy cochlear hair cells in direct relation to the height of their serum concentrations, thereby causing permanent hearing loss. Some anticancer chemotherapeutic agents, particularly cisplatin, cause severe ototoxicity by a similar mechanism. Subacute, relapsing cochlear deafness occurs with *Meniere's syndrome*, a condition associated with fluctuating hearing loss and tinnitus, recurrent episodes of abrupt and often severe vertigo, and a sensation of fullness or pressure in the ear. Recurrent endolymphatic hypertension (hydrops) is believed to cause the episodes. Pathologically, the endolymphatic sac is dilated and contains atrophic hair cells. The resulting deafness is subtle and reversible in the early stages but subsequently becomes permanent. What hearing remains is characterized by *diplacusis* (a different pitch heard in the affected ear) and loudness recruitment (quiet sounds are not heard but loud sounds are heard as loud as or louder than in the good ear). The disorder is usually unilateral. When bilateral (< 20 per cent of cases), it begins in one ear before the other.

Gradually progressive hearing loss with age (*presbycusis*) reflects deterioration in the cochlear receptor system with degeneration of the hair cells, especially at the base. As a result, higher tones are lost early, a change similar to that which follows the recurrent trauma of noise-induced hearing loss from exposure to loud military or industrial noises or loud blaring modern music. Unilateral hearing loss that arises and progresses insidiously is characteristic of a benign neoplasm of the cerebellopontine angle (e.g., acoustic neurinoma); a high-resolution CT scan usually establishes that diagnosis.

Central hearing loss can be unilateral only if it results from damage to the pontine cochlear nuclei on one side of the brain stem, such as occurs with occlusion of the anterior-inferior cerebellar artery, a plaque of multiple sclerosis or, rarely, invasion or compression of the dorsal lateral pons by a neoplasm or hematoma. Bilateral degeneration of the cochlear nuclei accompanies some of the rare, recessively inherited disorders of childhood.

Because of the extensive cross-innervation of the supranuclear auditory pathways, clinically important unilateral hearing loss never results from neurologic disease arising rostral to the cochlear nucleus. Bilateral hearing loss can be an important early sign of tumors in the pineal region, presumably from compression of the inferior colliculi. Most affected patients also have other signs of brain stem tectal dysfunction, including loss of upward gaze. Bilateral infarctions of the transverse gyrus of the temporal lobe may also cause central deafness; such damage usually is accompanied by aphasia due to involvement of the nearby Wernicke's area in the dominant hemisphere.

Tinnitus

Tinnitus is the term applied generally to extraneous noises heard in one or both ears. Tinnitus is either *objective*, i.e., the patient hears a real sound, one that can usually be heard by the examiner with a stethoscope, or *subjective*, i.e., the sound arises from an abnormal discharge of the auditory system and cannot be heard by the observer. Most objective tinnitus has a benign cause such as noise from temporomandibular joints, opening of eustachian tubes, or repetitive contraction of the stapedius muscle. Sometimes in a quiet room individuals can hear the pulsatile flow in the carotid artery or a continuous fluctuating hum of normal venous outflow through the jugular bulb. The latter can easily be obliterated by gentle compression of the jugular vein. Pathologic objective tinnitus occurs when patients hear turbulent flow in arteriovenous anomalies or tumors (e.g., glomus jugulare tumor). Objective tinnitus may also be an early sign of increased intracranial pressure. Such tinnitus, which can be obliterated by pressure over the jugular vein, probably arises from turbulent flow of compressed venous structures at the base of the brain. The symptom is also relieved transiently by decreasing the intracranial pressure, e.g., by lumbar puncture.

Subjective tinnitus can arise from anywhere in the auditory system. A faint, moderately high-pitched metallic ring can be observed by almost everyone if they concentrate their attention on auditory events in a quiet room. Sustained, louder tinnitus accompanied by audiometric evidence of deafness occurs in association with either conductive or sensorineural disease. The phenomenon can be a manifestation of salicylate, quinine, or quinidine toxicity. Tinnitus observed with otosclerosis tends to have a roaring or hissing quality, while that associated with Meniere's syndrome often produces sounds that vary widely in intensity with time and quality, sometimes including roarings or clangings. Tinnitus with other cochlear or auditory nerve lesions tends to be higher-pitched and ringing in quality. Clanging or tonally fluctuating tinnitus or formed auditory hallucinations can be manifestations of temporal lobe seizures.

DIZZINESS AND VERTIGO

Symptoms of Vestibular Dysfunction

The vestibular system, consisting of the bilateral semicircular canals and otolithic apparatus of the inner ear as well as their central connections, is a finely tuned discharging system. Any imbalance in input-output between the paired vestibular end organs or their primary receiving areas in the vestibular nuclei not caused by a true movement of the head or body produces a mismatch between vestibular stimulation and that going to other sense organs (especially the eyes and proprioceptive organs) and leads to an illusory sensation of movement in space called vertigo. Vertigo is the only direct symptom of a vestibular abnormality, but because the vestibular system influences other neural systems, vertigo may be accompanied by autonomic symptoms (nausea, vomiting, diaphoresis), motor symptoms (ataxia, past pointing, falling), or ocular symptoms (oscillopsia—a visual sensation that the environment is moving). The clinical sign of a vestibular abnormality is *nystagmus*, a rhythmic to-and-fro movement of the eyes. Patients suffering from vertigo and nystagmus have an abnormality, either physiological or pathological, of the labyrinthine-vestibular system. However, many patients cannot distinguish vertigo from other forms of dizziness, and nystagmus can originate from forces other than the vestibular system. Also, neither symptoms nor signs may be present at the time the physician examines the patient. The paragraphs below first classify dizziness and nystagmus and then describe an approach to complaints of dizziness, followed by a discussion of the causes of physiological and pathological vertigo.

Dizziness is a nonspecific term that patients apply to symptoms that may include vertigo (the illusory sensation of movement), lightheadedness (a sensation of floating or of impending syncope caused by anxiety or, more seriously, by global cerebral ischemia or anoxia), ataxia (unsteadiness on one's feet), diplopia, or even a psychological dissociative feeling. Even the most sophisticated person may have difficulty distinguishing mild vertigo from lightheadedness, and many patients are unable to describe their symptoms clearly enough to allow the physician to easily distinguish among the above symptoms.

Nystagmus reflects an imbalance in the complex neural network that involves the visual pathways, the labyrinthine proprioceptive influences from neck muscles, the vestibular and cerebellar nuclei, the reticular formation of the pontine brain stem, and the oculomotor nuclei. It can be of two types: jerk nystagmus consists of a slow phase away from the visual object followed by a quick saccade back toward the target. The quick eye movement describes the direction of jerk nystagmus. *Pendular nystagmus* describes nystagmus usually slow and coarse and equal in rate in both directions. It is usually congenital in origin or develops after birth as a result of severe visual impairment but can occasionally be a symptom of cerebellum or brain stem disease.

Purely horizontal fine nystagmus at the extremes of gaze is a common finding without pathologic significance. It is more common with fatigue or poor lighting. When bidirectional gaze-evoked nystagmus is prominent or involves vertical as well as horizontal movements to an equal degree, excessive sedative or anticonvulsant drug ingestion is most often the cause.

Several unusual forms of nystagmus have neurologic localizing qualities: *Dissociated nystagmus*, i.e., unequal in the two eyes, implies a brain stem lesion. *See-saw nystagmus* involves the eyes reciprocally rising and falling, then reversing their reciprocal directions. The phenomenon accompanies parasellar tumors or, less often, upper brain stem damage. *Convergence or retractory nystagmus* accompanies mesencephalic lesions. *Periodic alternating nystagmus* consists of a horizontal jerk nystagmus that changes its direction periodically. A typical sequence would be spontaneous jerk nystagmus 90 seconds to the left, followed by a 10-second inert pause, followed by jerk nystagmus 90 seconds to the right, with the sequence then repeating itself. The finding has been associated with a variety of posterior fossa abnormalities, especially those involving the region of the craniocervical junction. *Downbeat nystagmus* produces downward jerks with the eyes in the primary gaze position; it often reflects a craniocervical abnormality such as the Arnold-Chiari malformation but can occur with parenchymal lesions such as multiple sclerosis. Some subjects have the capacity to induce *voluntary nystagmus*, which is extremely rapid, occurs in short bursts of 10 to 15 seconds or so, is present on the extremes of gaze, and may be unequal in the two eyes.

Other abnormalities of conjugate eye movements include *ocular bobbing*, consisting of fast conjugate downward eye jerks followed by a slow return to the primary gaze position. The phenomenon accompanies severe displacement or destruction of the pons or, much less often, metabolic CNS depression. *Ocular myoclonus* consists of continuous, rhythmic, pendular oscillations, most often vertical, with a rate of two to five beats per second. Often it accompanies palatal myoclonus and has a similar pathogenesis. *Ocular flutter* consists of brief, intermittent, horizontal oscillations arising from the primary gaze position. It blends into *opsoclonus*, a pattern of rapid, chaotic, conjugate, repetitive saccadic eye movements ("dancing eyes"). Both of these disorders usually reflect cerebellar dysfunction but can emerge as a remote effect of systemic neoplasm, especially neuroblastoma in children. *Ocular dysmetria* consists of saccadic overshoots or undershoots of conjugate eye movement during rapid following of a visual object. The phenomenon reflects cerebellar dysfunction.

Evaluation of the Dizzy Patient

In most patients dizziness is episodic, so that there are neither symptoms nor signs when the physician examines the patient. The physician's first task is to distinguish vertigo from the other symptoms and then, if the patient is suffering from vertigo, to assign a cause (Table 118–5).

Perform a standard physical and neurologic examination. Pay special attention to heart and blood pressure (orthostatic hypotension or cardiac arrhythmias) to evaluate suspected syncope. Look for cerebellar or peripheral nerve dysfunction that may cause ataxia. Visual and oculomotor system abnormalities cause visual vertigo. Nystagmus and past pointing appraise vestibular dysfunction. Try to have the patient simulate the symptoms by provocative tests. *Hyperventilation*

TABLE 118–5. DIFFERENTIAL DIAGNOSIS OF DIZZINESS

Vertigo
  Physiological
  Pathological
Lightheadedness or syncope (see Table 116–8)
Ataxia
  Cerebellar dysfunction
  Proprioception loss
Diplopia and other visual abnormalities
  Anxiety
  Hyperventilation
  Dissociative episodes
  Partial complex seizures (NA)

lowers the Pco_2 and decreases cerebral blood flow, causing a "lightheaded" sensation. Ask the patient to *hyperventilate* maximally for 3 minutes. If the procedure exactly mimics the patient's symptoms, it suggests that anxiety and hyperventilation may be playing an important role. In addition, during the course of hyperventilation the patient may suffer dry mouth, chest tightness, and paresthesias which he may then recognize are part of his spontaneous attacks, thus helping in the diagnosis. *Tandem walking* (heel to toe) with eyes opened or closed intensifies ataxia and simulates the sensation of dysequilibrium. The *Barany rotation maneuver* (rotating the patient about a vertical axis 10 times over 20 seconds), caloric tests (see below), and positional tests (see below) simulate the symptoms of vestibular vertigo.

Examine the patient carefully for nystagmus (p. 696). The patient should fix upon a light successively requiring horizontal and vertical gaze in both the erect and supine positions. Sustained nystagmus suggests pathology of the vestibular system, and vertical nystagmus suggests that it is central rather than peripheral. Nystagmus and vertigo can sometimes be precipitated by rapid movements of the head (*Nylen-Barany test*). The examiner tilts the seated patient so that the head is hanging 45 degrees below horizontal, with first one ear and then the other dependent. He observes for nystagmus and vertigo. In some patients rapid head turning (once from center to side or vice versa or from supine to erect) suffices to bring out positional nystagmus and vertigo. A latency of 15 seconds or so characteristically separates the abrupt head movement from the appearance of the nystagmus.

The laboratory evaluation depends on the clinical findings and can include routine blood studies and chemistries, 24-hour cardiac monitoring, and electroencephalography. Bedside *caloric tests* (Fig. 118–5) will induce vertigo. With the patient lying supine and the head elevated approximately 30 degrees, water either 7 degrees above or below body temperature is douched against the tympanic membrane. In the normal situation, cold water produces nystagmus away from the side of stimulation (because of inhibition of the horizontal semicircular canal) and warm water nystagmus to the side of stimulation (because of stimulation of the semicircular canal). An astute patient suffering from labyrinthine vertigo can often tell which stimulation reproduces the symptoms, thus assisting in the localization of the lesion. Absence of the caloric response on one side suggests labyrinthine failure on that side. Because most peripheral nystagmus is partially inhibited by the visual fixation of the open eyes, accurate quantitative evaluation requires electrical recording of the eye movement with the eyes closed. *Electronystagmography* can be performed in the resting position, with the head rotated into various positions to provoke nystagmus, and before, during, and after caloric stimulation. Electronystagmography is often helpful in identifying the pathology of the vestibular system and localizing it when identified.

The above examinations should identify whether or not a complaint of dizziness reflects vertigo, implying a vestibular lesion. If the symptoms are vestibular, one must decide whether the abnormality is physiological or pathological and its exact cause.

OCULAR REFLEXES

FIGURE 118–5. Ocular reflexes. In the awake, supine patient: Cold water produces nystagmus with the quick component away from the stimulated ear; warm water produces nystagmus with the quick component toward the stimulated ear; bilateral cold water produces upward nystagmus; and bilateral warm water, downward nystagmus. The same responses occur in the patient with simulated coma. In the comatose patient with an intact brain stem, cold water produces tonic deviation of the eyes toward the side of the stimulus; responses to the other stimuli are pictured. With brain stem dysfunction, disconjugate eye movements appear on stimulation or the stimulus produces no response at all. The oculocephalic response is as pictured in the bottom four drawings in the comatose patient with an intact brain stem. Awake patients often have no oculocephalic responses. (From Posner JB: Clinical evaluation of the unconscious patient. Clin Neurosurg 22:281–301, 1975.)

Causes of Vertigo

Physiological vertigo occurs when there is a mismatch among the vestibular, visual, and somatosensory systems induced by an external stimulus. Common examples of physiological vertigo include motion sickness, height vertigo (the sensation that occurs when one looks down from a great height), and visual vertigo (the sensation sometimes felt when one views a motion picture of a roller coaster or other violent movement). In almost all instances, the diagnosis is clear from the history. One exception may be head extension vertigo, a sensation of vertigo or postural imbalance induced with the head maximally extended while standing; the sensation abruptly stops when the head is flexed to a neutral position. The symptoms may mistakenly be attributed to vertebral artery insufficiency. Head extension vertigo does not occur when the head is extended in the lying position and appears rarely when sitting. If physiological vertigo becomes a clinical problem, it is best treated by supplying sensory cues that help to match the various sensory systems. Thus, motion sickness, which is often exacerbated by sitting in a closed space or reading, giving the visual system the miscue that the environment is stationary, may be relieved by looking out at the environment and watching it move. Height vertigo caused by a mismatch between sensation of normal body sway and lack of its visual detection can often be relieved by the patient either sitting or visually fixing a nearby stationary object.

Pathological vertigo usually arises from an abnormality of the vestibular system but less commonly can be produced by visual or somatic sensory disorders. Vestibular vertigo can be caused by disease of either the peripheral or central vestibular apparatus (Table 118–6). In general, peripheral vertigo is more intense, more likely to be associated with hearing loss and tinnitus, and often leads to nausea and vomiting. Nystagmus associated with peripheral vertigo is frequently inhibited by visual fixation. Central vertigo is generally less severe, more sustained, and often associated with other signs of central nervous system disease. The nystagmus of central vertigo is not inhibited by visual fixation and frequently is disproportionately prominent to the degree of vertigo.

Benign positional vertigo is an extremely common disorder of middle and old age which accounts for the symptoms of at least 25 per cent of such patients with this complaint. Typically, the patient first experiences severe whirling vertigo when turning over or first lying down in bed at night. Less commonly, the patient may experience similar symptoms when he sits from a lying position or when he turns suddenly while standing or walking. Usually the symptoms are greatest when the patient lies on his side with the affected ear undermost. The vertigo is delayed for several seconds following the motion, sudden in onset, very severe, and may be accompanied by nausea or vomiting. The patient usually reports that the vertigo ceases when he moves out of the position that causes it, but in fact if he remains in that position, it rarely lasts more than a minute. The pathophysiology of the disorder is not established. Some investigators have postulated that debris from otoliths may enter the posterior canal to artificially stimulate it in the dependent position. The diagnosis is made by the characteristic history and the reproduction of the attack by the Nylen-Barany maneuver. The illness usually runs a course of several weeks and then resolves, but may recur several times over many years. If the patient has the classic history and physical findings, no further evaluation is necessary. If the history or findings are atypical, the condition must be distinguished from other causes of vertigo and nystagmus, such as tumor or infarct of the posterior fossa. Typical benign positional vertigo is very rarely associated with such conditions. The treatment for most patients is simple reassurance. Since the vertigo can be fatigued, many patients find that repetitively reproducing the sudden head movement each day gives them prolonged relief.

Peripheral Vestibulopathy. This disorder, also called acute labyrinthitis or vestibular neuronitis, may occur as a single bout or may recur repeatedly over months or years. The vertigo is acute, severe, and often associated with nausea and vomiting. Attacks sometimes follow a respiratory infection. The vertigo may be so severe that the patient is unable to sit or stand without vomiting and ataxia. He prefers to lie absolutely still in bed with the involved ear uppermost. Nystagmus is invariably present, usually horizontal or rotatory, and directed away from the involved labyrinth. The severe symptoms usually improve substantially within 48 to 72 hours, allowing the patient to be up and about. However, many patients report that for weeks or months following the episode sudden movements of the head produce mild vertigo or nausea. Although the disorder is called *acute labyrinthitis*, suggesting a viral infection of the labyrinth, EMG evoked potential studies suggest that in many patients there are accompanying eighth nerve or brain stem abnormalities, leading some to refer to the disorder as *vestibular neuronitis*. Labyrinthine fistulae have been reported to produce episodic vertigo. Fistula testing by a skilled otolaryngologist should establish that diagnosis. There has been a recent suggestion that some vertigo results from compression of the vestibular nerve by blood vessels of the posterior fossa in a manner analogous to trigeminal neuralgia (p. 686). *Other peripheral causes of vertigo* include Meniere's syndrome (p. 695) and the taking of vestibulotoxic drugs, most of which are also ototoxic (p. 694). Vertigo may be an additional symptom in patients suffering from *sudden hearing loss*. The pathogenesis of the disorder is unknown but may be vascular in some, viral infections in others. Bacterial infection of the labyrinth or occasionally otitis media causes vertigo. Degenerative and genetic abnormalities of the labyrinthine system can cause vertigo. *Cervical vertigo* is the term given to the feelings of dysequilibrium associated with head movement described by some patients with cervical osteoarthritis or spondylosis. The disorder probably is caused by unbalanced input from cervical muscles to the vestibular apparatus. Acute neck strain may be occasionally associated with vertigo. Local anesthetics injected into one side of the neck can produce vertigo and ataxia by a similar lack of balanced input. There is no nystagmus in these disorders.

CENTRAL VERTIGO

Central causes of vertigo, less common than peripheral causes, are usually characterized by less severe vertigo than that resulting from peripheral lesions, no hearing loss or tinnitus, and concomitant neurologic signs of brain stem or cerebellar dysfunction. Central vertigo is usually accompanied by neurologic signs or symptoms of brain stem or cerebellar dysfunction, strongly suggesting the site from which the vertigo arises.

Cerebrovascular Disease. If ischemia, infarction, or hemorrhage affects the brain stem or cerebellum, vertigo accompanied by nausea and vomiting is a relatively common symptom. Occipital headache as well as nystagmus and other neurologic signs suggesting brain stem or cerebellar dysfunction usually accompany vertigo. Rarely, vertigo (nonpositional) is the sole symptom of *transient ischemic attacks* of the brain stem, but most patients suffering such attacks will, if carefully questioned, report headache, diplopia, facial or body numbness, and ataxia as well.

Cerebellopontine Angle Tumors. Most tumors growing in the cerebellopontine angle (e.g., acoustic neuroma, meningioma) grow slowly, allowing the vestibular system to accommodate, and thus they usually produce vague sensations of dysequilibrium rather than acute vertigo. Frequently such neoplasms produce complaints of tinnitus, hearing loss, and a sensation that the person is being pulled or pushed when he walks. Occasionally episodic vertigo or positional vertigo will herald the presence of a cerebellopontine angle tumor. Virtually all affected patients will have retrocochlear hearing loss and decreased or absent caloric responses on the involved side. Careful CT scans through the temporal bone and posterior fossa usually reveal the tumor. The MRI may be an even more sensitive test.

Demyelinating Disease. Acute vertigo may be the first symptom of *multiple sclerosis*, although only a small percentage of young patients with acute vertigo eventually develop multiple sclerosis. Vertigo may also be a symptom of *parainfectious encephalomyelitis* or, rarely, *parainfectious cranial polyneuritis* of the Guillain-Barré type. In this instance, the accompanying neurologic signs establish the diagnosis.

Cranial Neuropathy. A variety of acute or subacute illnesses affecting the eighth cranial nerve can produce vertigo as an early or sole symptom, the most common being *herpes zoster*. The Ramsay-Hunt syndrome (*geniculate ganglion herpes*) is characterized by vertigo and hearing loss, variably associated with facial paralysis and some-

TABLE 118–6. CAUSES OF VESTIBULAR VERTIGO

PERIPHERAL CAUSES	CENTRAL CAUSES
Peripheral vestibulopathy*	Brain stem ischemia
Labyrinthitis and/or vestibular neuronitis	Cerebellopontine angle tumors
Acute and recurrent peripheral vestibulopathy	Demyelinating disease
"Benign" positional vertigo*	Cranial neuropathy
Meniere's syndrome*	Seizure disorders (rare)
Vestibulotoxic drugs	Heredofamilial disorders
Focal labyrinthine–third cranial nerve disease	Spinocerebellar degeneration
Trauma	Friedreich's ataxia
Cancer	Olivopontocerebellar atrophy, etc.
Infection	Other central causes
Otosclerosis	Brain stem tumors
Perilymph fistula	Cerebellar degenerations
	Paraneoplastic syndromes

* Common causes of acute severe vertigo.

times pain in the ear. The typical lesions of herpes zoster, which may follow the appearance of neurologic signs, are found in the external auditory canal and sometimes over the palate. Whether herpes zoster is ever responsible for vertigo in the absence of the full-blown syndrome is not certain. *Granulomatous meningitis* or *leptomeningeal metastases* and cerebral or systemic *vasculitis* may involve the eighth nerve, producing vertigo as an early symptom. In these disorders, cerebrospinal fluid analysis usually suggests the diagnosis.

Seizure Disorders. Patients suffering from temporal lobe epilepsy occasionally suffer vertigo as the aura. Vertigo in the absence of other neurologic signs or symptoms, however, is never caused by epilepsy or other diseases of the cerebral hemispheres.

Other Central Causes. Many structural lesions of the brain stem or cerebellum, particularly if rapid in onset, may cause vertigo. In a few instances, vertigo may initiate the symptoms of *paraneoplastic brain stem or cerebellar degeneration*. As with *brain stem tumors*, *cerebellar degenerative diseases* and other structural disease of the brain stem and posterior fossa, there are usually other neurologic symptoms, almost always including signs of brain stem or cerebellar dysfunction in addition to the vertigo and nystagmus.

Treatment

The best treatment of symptomatic vertigo is to cure the underlying disease. In many instances, however, that is not possible and one must resort to symptomatic treatment only. In acute vertigo, such as occurs with labyrinthitis, most patients will insist on being at bedrest. Vestibulosedative drugs such as meclizine or diazepam may be helpful. Prochlorperazine suppositories can be used to circumvent vomiting. Vestibulosuppressive drugs such as meclizine also sometimes help more chronic vertiginous disorders. Scopolamine, 0.4 to 0.8 mg, together with methylphenidate, 5 mg orally, may give relief of vertigo, particularly motion sickness. Recently, transdermal scopolamine paste-on units placed behind the ear have been reported to be effective in preventing motion sickness for up to 72 hours. These, like all scopolamine products, may produce anticholinergic side effects. If head or neck movement precipitates vertigo, a cervical collar sometimes relieves the symptoms.

REFERENCES

Baloh WR: Dizziness, Hearing Loss and Tinnitus: The Essentials of Neurotology. Philadelphia, FA Davis Co, 1984. *A new monograph with sections on anatomy and physiology, clinical examination, and treatment.*

Cailliet R: Low Back Pain Syndrome. 3rd ed. Philadelphia, FA Davis Co, 1981. *A well-written monograph with schematic drawings illustrating the anatomy, physiology, causes, and treatment of low back pain.*

Cailliet R: Neck and Arm Pain. 2nd ed. Philadelphia, FA Davis Co, 1981. *This short monograph describes the clinical anatomy and physiology of the cervical spine and the causes of pain originating from disorders of that area.*

Diamond S, and Dalessio DJ: The Practicing Physician's Approach to Headache. 3rd ed. Baltimore, Williams & Wilkins, 1982. *This short, up-to-date monograph describes the practical approach to the management of headache. The book is beautifully illustrated.*

Glaser JS: Neuro-ophthalmology. Hagerstown, MD, Harper & Row, 1977. *An excellent one-volume didactic introductory text.*

Schiffman SS: Taste and smell in disease. N Engl J Med 308:1275, 1983. *A two-part, well-referenced review of an often neglected medical problem.*

Wall PD, and Melzack R (eds): Textbook of Pain. New York, Churchill Livingstone, 1984. *A comprehensive monograph on all aspects of pain.*

Zee DS, and Leigh RJ: Disorders of Ocular Movement. Philadelphia, FA Davis Co, 1983. *An up-to-date monograph that gives the clinical and physiological details of modern investigations on ocular control.*

119 MOTOR AND MOTOR-SENSORY DISORDERS

INTRODUCTION AND DEFINITION

Muscles move the world, directed in their action by the brain and its efferent motor pathways. Dysfunction anywhere along the line, including muscle, myoneural junction, efferent motor nerve plexus or nerve roots, afferent proprioceptive systems, craniospinal motor neuron pool, descending corticospinal systems, basal ganglia, or cerebellum can interfere with the normal strength, coordination, and automatic postural controls that are required to complete the voluntary motor act.

At the level of the craniospinal segments, motor control is strongly influenced by proprioceptively governed stretch reflexes that simultaneously inform both the segmental motor pool and higher centers about the speed and position of the muscles and the direction of their movement. Ultimately, the spinal neuron pool integrates much of the final pattern of movement by coordinating segmental reflex activity with descending supraspinal influences and playing out the result via the complex functions expressed by the anterior horn cells, known as the *lower motor neurons*.

At the supraspinal level, the corticospinal system includes the premotor and primary motor cortex of the cerebrum as well as the red and vestibular nuclei of the brain stem and the reticular formation of the brain stem and spinal cord. Col-

lectively, these cortical and subcortical areas transmit *parallel* motor signals that descend to converge upon the segmental craniospinal interneurons and lower motor neurons (Fig. 119–1). In varying degrees, depending upon the individual case and the anatomical distribution of the lesion, their dysfunction results in the syndromes of the *upper motor neuron* as described in a subsequent paragraph.

In contrast to the parallel descending upper motor neuron systems, both the basal ganglia and the cerebellum normally exert their major controls on voluntary movement *in series* with the cerebral cortex (Fig. 119–1); i.e., they project their signals to the latter structure before it sends its final commands caudally to the segmental neuron pools. During the initiation of voluntary movement, signals from the frontal and parietal lobes flash to the basal ganglia and cerebellum and back again to the cortex a few milliseconds before the motor cortex transmits its final message spinalwards. The process guarantees normal postural supports and the coordination of movement. Furthermore, the arrangement means that both basal ganglia and cerebellar hemispheric (neocerebellar) diseases express their symptoms through the descending upper motor neuron systems rather than by directly influencing the spinal motor neuron pool. This feature helps to explain why signs of basal ganglia and cerebellar abnormality tend to disappear during sleep or if a corticospinal hemiplegia develops.

Signs and symptoms of upper motor neuron disease can accompany a variety of structural and metabolic disorders affecting the cerebrum and its connections and are mainly discussed in this text in association with those causative conditions. By contrast, motor syndromes of basal ganglia or cerebellar dysfunction frequently occur in isolation, reflecting diseases that selectively or predominantly affect one or the other of these structures and their specific connections. Before discussing these diseases, it may be useful to define briefly the nature and mechanism of major symptoms and signs of motor dysfunction.

FIGURE 119–1. The principal supranuclear influences on motor control, greatly simplified. The cerebral cortex signals both the basal ganglia and the cerebellum before initiating movement. The latter two structures, in turn, predominantly feed signals forward via the thalamus to the cortex which guarantee the programming of postural activity that makes possible the subsequent skilled movement and automatic acts. The brain stem reticular formation and other major motor nuclei receive corticospinal and cerebellar projections and, in turn, send additional descending fibers that join the corticospinal pathway to make up the upper motor neuron system.

A.   MOTOR SYMPTOMS AND SIGNS

Asthenia consists of an inner sense of subacute or chronic lassitude conveying feelings of undue weakness or motor fatigue before any activity is initiated. The symptom can arise acutely or subacutely during the course of a number of acquired illnesses, including viral infection, hepatitis, myocardial infarction, and endocrine disorders. Several neurologic diseases, including multiple sclerosis, parkinsonism, and acute polyneuritis, produce symptoms of asthenia. Most chronic asthenia unassociated with objective evidence of somatic disease has a psychogenic basis.

Fatigue refers to an abnormal rate or degree of exhaustion following brief or sustained voluntary activity. The symptom tends to be more specific in its associations than asthenia and accompanies many of the same systemic and neurologic disorders, as well as post-traumatic syndromes and chronic sedative drug abuse. Local fatigability most often reflects a regional disorder or deconditioning of the nerves or muscles; when accompanied by detectable, exercise-induced, local reductions in muscle strength, the symptom is characteristic of myasthenia gravis.

Weakness refers to an impaired capacity to carry out a voluntary motor act due to a loss of muscular power. The term paresis is synonymous. *Paralysis* designates a more complete loss of motor function. Most weakness or paralysis results from disease or dysfunction of the central or peripheral nervous system or the muscles. Muscle guarding and immobility that surround injured or inflamed areas of the trunk or extremities sometimes can produce pseudoparalysis when motion accentuates the pain. Hysterical weakness is described below.

Patterns of Weakness

Most persons promptly recognize a recently developing or rapidly progressing muscle motor loss but tend to ignore insidiously developing, painless weakness until it produces substantial functional disability. Families or physicians may sometimes detect such gradually evolving limitations before the patient does.

Upper motor neuron lesions arising at the cerebral level typically produce focal weakness predominating in the hand and arm, the lower face, or the foot and leg, in that order of frequency. A hemiparesis (face, arm, and leg) can originate from the cerebrum, as can face-hand-arm weakness. Face-leg weakness, sparing the arm, implies two anatomically distinct lesions, whereas arm-leg weakness sparing the face can originate anywhere along the corticospinal pathway between the internal capsule and the upper cervical cord. Upper

TABLE 119–1. CLINICAL SIGNS OF UPPER AND LOWER MOTOR NEURON LESIONS

	UPPER	LOWER
Paralysis	Mostly distal, distributed in major body part	Proximal or distal, distributed by nerve root or anterior horn cell anatomy
Atrophy	Minimal, late, disuse	Prominent, early, trophic
Fasciculations	Absent	Often present
Spasticity	Present	Absent
Deep tendon reflexes	Increased	Decreased or absent
Babinski reflex	Present	Absent

motor neuron weakness typically affects skilled movement, with paresis being more marked distally than proximally in the limbs (Table 119–1). Various components of spasticity emerge, including increased muscular resistance to passive stretch with lengthening and shortening reactions, increased deep tendon reflexes, abnormal postural responses to stimulation, including decorticate, decerebrate, and spinal flexor responses, and the classic Babinski sign. Upper motor neuron lesions seldom severely paralyze the face and never completely so. As a result the brow and orbicularis oculi, like other midline muscle groups, are relatively spared. Atrophy of the limbs, if it occurs at all, is mild and due to disuse. The EMG shows no abnormality.

Among *basal ganglia diseases*, asthenia is prominent in parkinsonism and chorea. Some patients in the early stages of parkinsonism complain of a hemiparetic weakness that can misleadingly suggest corticospinal tract dysfunction. Most persons with Parkinson's disease, however, suffer only mild to moderate weakness but report disproportionately prominent difficulty in initiating and continuing movements, "as if starting through molasses." Their limbs show rigidity rather than spasticity, their deep tendon reflexes are at most only moderately increased, and they lack Babinski signs or the other pathological reflex spasticity.

Cerebellar diseases, especially those of the hemisphere and dentate nuclei, also can engender the sense of asthenia and weakness in ipsilateral limbs. Ataxia and incoordination, however, are more prominent. Muscle resistance to passive stretch is, if anything, reduced rather than increased. Deep tendon reflexes may be moderately hyperactive, and impaired cerebellar regulation of the stretch reflex can cause pendularity. Pathological reflexes or muscle atrophy is lacking.

Disease of the lower motor neuron, including the anterior horn cells, the motor nerve root, or the motor nerve, causes a classic syndrome (Table 119–1). Weakness is regionally distributed according to areas of denervation, so that a major clue to anatomical diagnosis lies in distinguishing among the respective paralytic patterns produced by damage to spinal cord, ventral motor root, plexus, or peripheral nerve. Characteristic sensory defects will be added at many of these locations. With severe denervation-weakness, muscle atrophy begins within days. Motor resistance is subnormal, deep tendon reflexes diminish or disappear, and with proximally originating denervation, fasciculations may, in time, become visible through the skin. Electrical signs of denervation, including first fibrillation and then fasciculation, follow within three to four weeks of the time of injury.

Nerve-muscle junctional disease is of two kinds. The more frequent, myasthenia gravis (MG), consists of an autoimmune blockage of the acetylcholine receptor in the muscle. The other, the Eaton-Lambert myasthenic syndrome (ELMS), involves immunological impairment of the release of neurotransmitter from the nerve terminals. Weakness in MG affects most often the oculomotor, bulbar, and proximal limb muscles, which rapidly fatigue with quick successive action. Weakness in ELMS, by contrast, affects mainly the distal limbs, is maximal with first effort, and lessens with repeated tries. Atrophy occurs in neither disorder except when severe chronic MG induces muscle disuse. Muscle tonus is normal, deep tendon reflexes are usually preserved or reduced, and sensation is unaffected. EMG changes are diagnostic.

Myopathies, diseases intrinsic to muscle, produce insidiously beginning weakness that symmetrically affects anatomical groups characteristic of the particular variant of degenerative (dystrophy), metabolic (e.g., thyrotoxic), or inflammatory diseases (myositis). Weakness occasionally remains constant (congenital myopathy) but usually progresses either slowly (dystrophy), rapidly (metabolic or inflammatory myopathy), or episodically (periodic paralysis). Resistance to passive stretch is normal, but the muscles may be tender (myositis), show myotonia (congenital myotonia, myotonic dystrophy), be abnormally soft (thyrotoxicosis), look abnormally large (pseudohypertrophy), or feel unduly firm (connective tissue infiltration). Deep tendon reflexes are preserved until late except in hypokalemic myopathy. Serum enzymes often are abnormal in muscular dystrophy and EMG's in many instances are characteristic. Sensation remains intact.

Major Abnormal Movements

Myotonia comprises a prolonged (seconds) involuntary contraction of a group of adjacent muscle fibers following a self-limited, voluntary effort or an abrupt local percussion as with a reflex hammer. An abnormal postsynaptic muscle membrane producing self-repetitive depolarizations and muscle after discharges causes the sustained fiber shortening.

Muscle fibrillation describes continuously recurrent, spontaneous contractions of single muscle fibers due usually to denervation but sometimes to dystrophic degeneration of single fiber membranes. In either event, the phenomenon reflects membrane and contractile hypersensitivity to circulating or locally diffusing acetylcholine (ACh). *Fasciculations* represent spontaneous, synchronous, recurrent depolarization-contraction of the fibers of a single motor unit or of a group of partially denervated motor units that have been reinnervated by sprouting from adjacent, still conducting motor axons. The pathogenesis reflects denervation hypersensitivity to ACh of the damaged motor axon. Fasciculation of larger motor units and grouped motor units is visible through the skin. Fibrillations and fasciculations produce characteristic EMG changes (p. 650).

Tremor exists in three major forms. *Essential tremor* or *benign familial tremor* is an accentuation of a physiological, 8- to 12-Hz rhythmic oscillation that can affect the distal arms, the head, or, less often, the vocal apparatus. Coarse in its pattern but absent at complete rest, the tremor begins with the maintenance of posture and is accentuated by voluntary movement, sometimes to an incapacitating degree. The abnormality depends on cerebellar mechanisms as well as basal ganglia dysfunction and can be blocked by lesions placed in the ventrolateral nucleus of the thalamus. Essential tremor varies widely in intensity and can appear at any age but becomes more common and prominent in elderly life (*senile tremor*). Accompanied by neither rigidity, akinesia, nor ataxia, its predisposition is transmitted as an autosomal dominant trait. Alcohol in small amounts and, less often, anxiolytic agents suppress the movement. The beta-blocker propranolol reduces the intensity of the tremor in about 25 per cent of affected persons.

Resting or parkinsonian tremor, a 4- to 7-Hz oscillation, reflects the alternating contractions of agonist-antagonist muscles, most often of the distal extremities, especially the hand ("pill rolling"). Less frequently the lower facial muscles, the tongue, or the lower extremities are involved. The tremor worsens with anxiety or fatigue and tends to quiet down or briefly disappear with relaxation or periods of intense manual concentration. As with all abnormal movements of basal ganglia origin, parkinsonian tremor disappears during sleep. Its genesis is believed to reflect excess cholinergic activity in the striatum, leading to an abnormally high GABA output from the putamen to the pallidum. The tremor can be abolished by lesions of the thalamic ventrolateral nucleus and is improved by antiparkinsonian drugs, as discussed below.

Intention (cerebellar) tremor can take three patterns. One relates to damage of the vermis and anterior lobe and results in an oscillating, rhythmic ataxia of the trunk and lower limbs during attempts to walk (titubation). A second, associated with lesions of the afferent spinocerebellar input, produces a more irregular high-steppage tremorous ataxia of the lower extremities, which can blend into titubation. The third, resulting from damage to the dentate outflow pathway of the superior peduncle, produces the classic manual intention tremor, consisting of an irregular, coarse 3- to 6-Hz distal oscillation that increases in amplitude and irregularity as the voluntarily moving hand approaches its object. In all instances, cerebellar tremor reflects a disruption in the balance between afferent impulses that directly stimulate the roof nuclei as they reach the cerebellum and the immediately following inhibitory loop that normally feeds back on these nuclei from the Purkinje cells. Cerebellar intention tremor so far has resisted efforts at pharmacological control.

Asterixis is an irregular, flap-like tremor, distributed more distally than proximally, that involves the extremities, less often the tongue, with a frequency varying from less than 1 to as high as 3 Hz. It is most often observed to accompany the metabolic encephalopathies and usually is accompanied by an accentuated physiological tremor. Its mechanism reflects a brief loss of muscle contraction in muscles controlling extension of the involved member, followed by a rapid myoclonus-like recovery.

Chorea describes involuntary, nonrhythmic, irregularly distributed, coarse, quick twitching movements affecting the face, tongue, and proximal and distal extremities. Slower athetoid twistings sometimes intersperse themselves concurrently. Mild cases may resemble little more than anxiety-provoked fidgets, while the appearance of severe examples blends into generalized dystonia. Efforts at sustained muscular contraction accentuate the disorder, which possesses features of both basal ganglia and cerebellar dysfunction. Pharmacologically, the phenomenon most closely resembles the effects of central dopamine hyperactivity. *Ballism* consists of irregular, abrupt, repetitive, wide-amplitude flinging movements of the limbs initiated predominantly by proximal girdle muscles. Less prominent distal choreiform movements often accompany the condition, which involves body parts opposite to an infarcted or, rarely, otherwise damaged subthalamic nucleus. Usually unilateral in distribution (hemiballismus), the condition is ameliorated by haloperidol or reserpine. Ordinarily it subsides spontaneously within a few weeks after onset.

Dystonia can accompany several basal ganglia disorders and is the major sign of a primary movement disorder of late childhood, adolescent, or adult life, as discussed more extensively in a later section (see Table 119–15). The abnormality is characterized by bizarre twisting or turning motions, most but not all of which affect more distal body parts. The distinctive feature of the movements is that they involve the simultaneous tonic co-contraction of agonist and antagonist muscle groups. The duration of brief dystonia usually lasts for a second or more, a rate somewhat faster than in *athetosis*, the slow, dystonically related, proximally distributed twisting observed most commonly in children who have suffered perinatal or infantile basal ganglia–thalamic damage. Most dystonic movements also tend to recur in longer spasms, sometimes lasting minutes to hours at a time. Dystonia can be generalized or restricted, inherited or acquired. It arises as a specific problem as an accompaniment to several basal ganglia diseases, including Huntington's chorea and Wilson's disease. The pathophysiology and pharmacological basis of the abnormal movements are poorly understood. Several phenothiazine disorders, however, can induce acute dystonia as an idiosyncratic response in susceptible hosts. Structural lesions involving the basal ganglia–thalamic motor pathways sometimes cause a contralateral hemidystonia. The anticholinergic, antihistamine drug diphenhydramine hydrochloride blocks drug-induced dystonia but not the naturally occurring form.

Tics are sudden, quick, irregular, stereotyped movements of variable complexity that repetitively involve similar but not identical groups of muscles. They can come on at any age, most often in adolescence or young adulthood, and most frequently involve the face, eyes, or mouth, seldom the extremities. Some in mild form represent psychologically generated habit patterns. More severe examples, often combined with bizarre barkings or the shouting of scatological and other obscenities, comprise *Gilles de la Tourette's syndrome.*

Myoclonus describes sudden, abrupt contractions of single muscles or restricted groups of muscles, most frequently affecting the limbs, less often the trunk. The phenomenon has many causes and can arise from abnormally excitable gray matter at any level of the nervous system. Single generalized myoclonic jerks occur normally as startle responses or when drifing off to sleep. Such discharges in the cerebrum usually produce distal myoclonus, while myoclonus generated in the lower brain stem or spinal gray matter usually has a proximal distribution that affects the pectoral girdle, trunk, or pelvic girdle. Myoclonic jerks accompany several forms of epilepsy (see page 763). They also occur in a multifocal pattern in association with several metabolic encephalopathies, especially those associated with uremia or penicillin intoxication, and they can follow severe cerebral anoxia or slow virus infection (Creutzfeldt-Jakob disease).

Palatal myoclonus relates more to a form of continuous tremor than to true myoclonus. The condition consists of rhythmic, regular, 2- to 3-Hz contractions of the soft palate, and less commonly, the adjacent pharynx. It arises in association with infarction or degeneration of the pathway that links together the dentate, red nucleus, and inferior olive. Unlike tremor of basal ganglia or cerebellar origin, palatal myoclonus persists during sleep. The serotonin precursor 5-hydroxytryptamine sometimes ameliorates the contractions, which have been attributed to denervation hypersensitivity of olivary neurons.

Hemifacial spasm can affect the motor distribution of either facial nerve, producing rapidly recurring, painless, nonstereotyped fragmentary twitching of any of the facial muscles. The condition persists into sleep and has been attributed to ephaptic cross-conduction of fibers within the nerve secondary to damage caused by its long-standing intracranial compression from an overlying branch of the basilar artery. Surgical decompression sometimes relieves the condition, which is disfiguring but neither painful nor dangerous.

B. DISEASES OF MUSCLE AND MYONEURAL JUNCTION

APPROACH TO THE PATIENT

As in most neurologic disorders, the first approach to diagnosis is the careful and detailed history. (1) Try to establish that the patient is complaining of weakness rather than asthenia by eliciting a description of specific former muscular activities that are more difficult or impossible to carry out. If such activities can be detailed, it is likely that the patient does, in fact, have muscle weakness. (2) Attempt to determine the distribution of the muscle weakness. Patients who have difficulty lifting objects onto high shelves, combing their hair, getting out of low chairs or off the toilet seat but who can grip objects normally and walk on their heels and toes, suffer from predominantly proximal weakness, suggesting myopathic rather than neuropathic illness. On the contrary, patients who drop heavy objects from their hands, cannot press an aerosol can, have trouble opening car doors or turning the ignition key, and those who note that they trip when they walk, particularly in trying to get up over curbs (because of foot drop), have predominantly distal weakness, suggesting neuropathic illness. Nerve functions can be assessed historically as well. Diplopia is common in myasthenia gravis, botulism, and neurogenic disorders, but even with substantial extraocular paralysis, diplopia is not common in ocular myopathy, since paralysis is slow and symmetrical. Difficulty whistling or puckering suggests facioscapulohumeral and muscular dystrophy; dysphagia and dysarthria are more common in polymyositis and myasthenia than in the other myopathic processes. (3) Try to determine the temporal pattern of the weakness. Weakness that progresses slowly for months to years is characteristic of the muscular dystrophies and metabolic myopathies. A more rapid onset of weakness suggests polymyositis, disorders of the neuromuscular junction, and peripheral neuropathies. Weakness of most myopathic and neuropathic processes is constant and unremitting, whereas the major disease of the neuromuscular junction, myasthenia gravis, is remitting and characterized by fatigability with improvement after rest. Periodic paralysis, as the name implies, is characterized by normal muscle function interspersed with attacks of severe paralysis. (4) Ask the patient about unusual muscle contractions. A history of myotonia, even though that disorder is not now present, strongly suggests the diagnosis of myotonic dystrophy. Patients frequently recognize the presence of fasciculations. Repetitive spontaneous cramping and cramping in response to muscle movement suggest neurogenic disease, whereas bilateral and severe cramps always precipitated by exercise (contractures) suggest a metabolic myopathy.

Physical examination is also helpful. Marked atrophy of muscles, with fasciculations and reflex hypoactivity, indicates involvement of the lower motor neuron, whereas pseudohypertrophy, particularly in the calves, strongly suggests Duchenne's dystrophy. The distribution of muscle weakness elicited by history can be confirmed by examination. Characteristic facial configurations mark myotonic dystrophy (temporal and masseter hollowing, long face; sternocleidomastoid weakness giving a swan neck appearance), facioscapulohumeral muscular dystrophy (see page 706), and myasthenia gravis (the appearance of a snarl when the patient attempts to smile). Duchenne's dystrophy and most of the metabolic myopathies are not associated with facial weakness.

The laboratory examination contributes. Elevation of serum muscle enzymes (particularly creatine kinase) suggests myopathy, with high levels being found in Duchenne's dystrophy and sometimes in acute polymyositis. However, creatine kinase levels can be modestly elevated in neurogenic atrophy. Elevation of erythrocyte sedimentation rate and creatinine kinase suggests an inflammatory myopathy such as polymyositis. Thyroid function studies are particularly helpful with periodic paralysis and in some proximal metabolic muscle weaknesses. Acetylcholine receptor antibodies in the serum are diagnostic of myasthenia gravis. Electrical tests (see Table 115–6) help distinguish myopathy from neuropathy. Muscle biopsy with careful attention to enzyme histochemistry as well as the anatomical structure of the muscle may distinguish among the various metabolic myopathies as well as define a lipid and glycogen storage disease.

MYOPATHIES

Muscle, the largest organ in the body, can be affected by several diseases of the muscle itself or by secondary effects of systemic diseases. Fur-

TABLE 119–2. MYOPATHIES

Muscular dystrophy (see Table 119–3)
Myotonias (see Table 119–4)
Inflammatory myopathies
  Infections (e.g., toxoplasmosis, trichinosis, viral)
  Immune processes (polymyositis, sarcoidosis, polymyalgia rheumatica)
Endocrine myopathies
  Hyperthyroidism and hypothyroidism
  Hyperparathyroidism
  Hyperadrenalism
  Hyperpituitarism
Periodic paralysis (see Table 119–5)
Biochemical disorders
  Glycogen storage diseases
  Lipid storage and mitocondrial myopathies
Congenital muscle disorders
Drugs and toxins (see Table 119–6)

thermore, since weakness is so easily recognized by the patient, the myopathy leads to early consultation with the physician even when the primary disease is elsewhere. Table 119–2 classifies the myopathies. Emphasis in this text is on disorders that are common or that have characteristic clinical findings.

MUSCULAR DYSTROPHIES

Muscular dystrophies are inherited myopathies characterized by progressive weakness, usually beginning early in life. The genetics are well-established for most of the dystrophies, but the biochemical defect is unknown and there is neither biochemical nor histological evidence for abnormal products in the muscle such as is found in many of the metabolic myopathies. Table 119–3 classifies the muscular dystrophies.

Duchenne's dystrophy is an X-linked recessive disorder of boys (rarely girls) characterized by painless weakness that is maximal in the pelvic girdle and thighs, less prominent about the shoulders, and least prominent in the distal extremities. The disorder reveals itself with abnormal and increasing clumsiness when the child begins to walk (beyond 18 months). Affected boys run awkwardly and rise from the floor by placing hands on knees and using the hands to walk up the thighs (Gower's sign). With time the calf muscles appear abnormally enlarged (pseudohypertrophy). Gradually the weakness becomes more severe, and adolescents are usually wheelchair-bound. Even with scrupulous care, death occurs in early adulthood, usually from pneumonia. The diagnosis can be made early in life before symptoms appear by an elevated serum creatine kinase. The mutation rate is high, and in about two thirds of individuals, no other family member is affected. The disorder must be distinguished from two similar dystrophies: *Becker's dystrophy* is similarly X-linked but has its onset later in childhood or adolescence and has a slower or more variable tempo (some patients functioning well into adult life). *Emory-Dreyfus dystrophy* also begins later and is more benign than Duchenne's

TABLE 119–3. CLASSIFICATION OF HUMAN MUSCULAR DYSTROPHIES

	DUCHENNE DYSTROPHY	FACIO-SCAPULO-HUMERAL DYSTROPHY	LIMB-GIRDLE DYSTROPHY	MYOTONIC DYSTROPHY
Genetic pattern	X-linked, recessive	Autosomal, dominant	Autosomal, recessive	Autosomal, dominant
Age at onset	Before age 5	Adolescence	Adolescence	Early or late
First symptoms	Pelvic	Shoulders	Pelvic	Distal; hands or feet
Pseudohypertrophy	+	0	0	0
Predominant weakness, early	Proximal	Proximal	Proximal	Distal
Progression	Relatively rapid; incapacitated in adolescence	Slow	Variable	Slow
Facial weakness	0	+	0	Occasional
Ocular, oropharyngeal weakness	0	0	0	Occasional
Myotonia	0	0	0	+
Cardiomyopathy	0 or late	0	0	Arrhythmia, conduction block
Associated disorders	None (?mental retardation)	None	None	Cataracts; testicular atrophy and baldness in men
Serum enzymes	Very high	Slight or no increase	Slight or no increase	Slight or no increase
Prevalence (per million population)	38	5	20	25
Incidence (per million births)	251	5	47	–
Mutation rate	9×10^{-5}	5×10^{-7}	3×10^{-5}	10×10^{-6}

From Rowland LP: Diseases of muscle and neuromuscular junction: Inherited diseases. In Wyngaarden JB, and Smith LH Jr (eds): Cecil Textbook of Medicine. 17th ed. Philadelphia, WB Saunders Co, 1985, pp 2201–2209.

dystrophy; pseudohypertrophy is lacking and serum enzymes are normal or only slightly increased. This form is also characterized by cardiac arrhythmias that can lead to sudden death.

Limb-girdle dystrophy, an autosomal recessive with a high mutation rate, affects muscles of the pelvic and shoulder girdle, usually begins late in childhood or adolescence, affects girls as often as boys, and progresses at extremely variable rates. Pseudohypertrophy is not common. Muscle biopsy and electromyography may be necessary to distinguish this disorder from a similar-appearing, also proximal neurogenic disorder—the Kugelberg-Welander syndrome (page 724).

Facioscapulohumeral dystrophy is characterized by prominent weakness in the perioral muscles of the face and eventually weakness of eye closure. Latissimus dorsi degeneration leads to scapular winging, and the sternal head of the pectoral muscle is affected more than the clavicular. The shoulder and pelvic girdle muscles are affected as well. Weakness of the trunk muscles may cause severe scoliosis. The disorder is transmitted as an autosomal dominant trait with variable but usually extremely slow progression.

Ocular muscular dystrophy is a slowly progressive disorder characterized by ptosis and progressive external ocular paralysis. The pupils are spared, and both eyes are usually affected symmetrically, so that diplopia is not common. Other muscles of the head, neck, and limbs may be affected, but this varies from family to family. Because each oculomotor nerve fiber supplies only

a few muscle fibers, it is exceedingly difficult to distinguish neuropathies from myopathies by either EMG or histological examination of the eye muscles. As a result, the clinical distinction between ocular myopathies and neuropathies rests on findings in other skeletal muscles. In some disorders producing ocular myopathy, the skeletal muscles of the neck or limbs contain abnormally large mitochondria in increased numbers, producing a characteristic "ragged red fiber" appearance on trichrome stains.

Distal myopathy, unlike most muscular dystrophies, affects distal leg and hand muscles first. It is rare and can only be identified by characteristic signs of myopathy on electromyography and muscle biopsy. *Scapuloperoneal dystrophy*, with its distal weakness in the legs, resembles neurogenic peroneal atrophy, but there is no sensory loss and proximal weakness often affects the shoulder girdle. The disorder is transmitted as an autosomal dominant with relatively slow progression.

Treatment

There is no treatment for any of the muscular dystrophies. Physical therapy along with splints and braces may keep many patients walking who would otherwise be confined to a wheelchair. Carriers of Duchenne's dystrophy can sometimes be identified by increased creatinine kinase serum levels, but the fetus at risk cannot reliably be identified in utero. Genetic counseling is valuable in preventing the disease.

MYOTONIAS

Table 119–4 classifies those muscle diseases associated with myotonia. Myotonia results from an abnormality of the muscle membrane leading to delayed relaxation. The diagnosis is easily made clinically by asking a patient to grip one's fingers and then quickly let go. There is also a characteristic electromyogram with repetitive action potentials that may wax or wane over many seconds when the needle is inserted or after the patient attempts to relax from a voluntary contraction. The most common myotonic abnormality is *myotonic dystrophy*, an autosomal dominant disorder characterized by progressive, primarily distal muscle weakness, myotonia, cranial muscle weakness, and endocrine abnormalities. The disorder may begin early in life or be delayed into adulthood. Affected persons have facial weakness with ptosis, difficulty puckering the lips, and dysarthria. In addition, wasting involves the temporalis and masseter muscles, which, when combined with the ptosis, gives the face a characteristic appearance. Selective weakness and wasting affects the sternocleidomastoid muscles, giving the neck a long and thin appearance (swan neck).

Extremity muscles are affected distally. The myotonia occurs primarily in the hands and usually is the first symptom. It becomes less severe as weakness develops and may not be easy to identify clinically in the late stages. In addition to the muscle symptoms, almost all patients eventually develop cataracts, and males experience early frontal baldness and testicular atrophy. Conduction defects in the heart may lead to cardiac arrhythmias, and cardiac myopathy may cause congestive heart failure. The disease runs a long course and does not generally cause disability until well into adulthood. The clinical and electromyographic features are characteristic. *Myotonia congenita* is rarer and occurs in both autosomal dominant and recessive forms. The disease begins early in life and is characterized by diffuse myotonia, which makes the patient stiff when he begins to exercise but loosens as activity continues. Affected persons move clumsily and have a stiff and wooden appearance. Cold generally makes their symptoms worse. The disorder is annoying more than disabling. Drugs such as phenytoin and quinine, which affect neuromuscular transmission, may relieve the symptoms. *Paramyotonia congenita* is a rare disorder of autosomal dominant inheritance that differs only slightly from myotonia congenita. Facial muscles

and muscles of the forearm and hand are predominantly involved; the myotonia shows extreme sensitivity to cold, and indeed may be present only when the patient is exposed to cold. Similar myotonias sometimes occur in hyperkalemic paralysis, and paramyotonia may simply be a manifestation of the more common periodic paralysis. In addition to the congenital disorders, myotonia can be acquired after exposure to a number of toxins, including cholesterol antagonists and the herbicide 2-4D.

INFLAMMATORY MYOPATHIES

Inflammatory myopathies are a group of disorders characterized by the invasion of macrophages and lymphocytes in the muscle or its perivascular space. The commonest is polymyositis.

Dermatomyositis and Polymyositis. These conditions are characterized by the subacute onset of weakness of proximal muscles, affecting the shoulder girdle, pelvic girdle, and neck and sometimes causing profound weakness of truncal and distal extremity muscles as well. The disorder occasionally affects laryngeal and respiratory muscles. There may be myalgias and muscle tenderness. Involved muscles often show spontaneous insertional activity and fibrillation on EMG. Five categories have been recognized: adult polymyositis, dermatomyositis, myositis associated with malignancy, childhood polymyositis, and overlap syndrome, i.e., myositis associated with other connective tissue diseases. The muscle disorder is similar in all forms. In dermatomyositis, there is also an erythematous rash on forehead, neck, shoulders, trunk, and arms, with a lilac or heliotrope component on the upper eyelids and in the malar area of the face. The rash may be associated with edema and reddened, elevated, scaly patches over the extensor surface of hands, elbows, and knees. The nail folds may show periungual telangiectasia, dilated and distorted nail fold capillary loops, and, in some patients, shiny and atrophic finger pads. The *overlap symdrome* is associated with Raynaud's syndrome or, more rarely, can involve the whole spectrum of dermatologic changes in connective tissue disease. About 10 per cent of patients with polymyositis, particularly those with dermatomyositis, suffer from an occult *malignancy*. Malignancies are rare in the childhood form.

The diagnosis of polymyositis should be strongly suspected in any patient with the subacute onset of substantial proximal muscle weakness of upper and lower extremities. Elevation of muscle enzymes in the serum, elevated erythrocyte sedimentation rate, the EMG changes listed above, and an inflammatory infiltrate on muscle biopsy establish the diagnosis. A compulsive search for an occult malignancy is usually unwarranted, although routine chest films, breast examination, and stool guaiac examination are good medical practice. Corticosteroid hormones are often effective in the treatment of polymyositis, but high doses (up to 100 mg prednisone a day) may be required for several weeks or months.

TABLE 119–4. MYOTONIA

Myotonic muscular dystrophy
Myotonia congenita
  Autosomal dominant
  Autosomal recessive
Paramyotonia congenita
Hyperkalemic periodic paralysis
Chondrodystrophic myotonia
Acquired myotonia

Polymyalgia Rheumatica. Polymyalgia rheumatica is a disorder of the elderly, found more commonly in women than in men, and characterized by the acute or subacute onset of pain and stiffness in the neck, back, shoulders, upper arms, and thighs without accompanying weakness. The disorder is associated with an elevated erythrocyte sedimentation rate and responds dramatically to small doses of corticosteroids. In some patients, polymyalgia is part of the giant cell arteritis syndrome, and that disorder should be suspected, particularly if headache or other systemic symptoms are present. Both diseases respond well to corticosteroids.

Myositis Ossificans. Myositis ossificans is a rare disorder with dramatic consequences. Symptoms usually begin in early childhood, with transient and localized swelling of the neck and back. There is progressive rigidity of neck, back, and limbs. Calcification can be identified in the muscles on x-ray. Early in the disease, muscle biopsy reveals necrosis and inflammation. The disorder is believed to be inherited because digital abnormalities, including microdactyly and syndactyly, are present in other members of the family. The disorder can easily be distinguished from the ectopic calcification seen in a variety of other conditions, including the late stages of polymyositis, vitamin D intoxication, and abnormalities of parathyroid function.

Metabolic diseases that affect muscles may involve that organ alone, or the myopathy may be part of a wider, more generalized disorder. Most of the disorders cause nonspecific weakness or cramping, the specific diagnosis being made only by histological and biochemical studies of the involved muscles. A few clinical syndromes are relatively specific, suggesting the diagnosis on history alone.

ENDOCRINE MYOPATHIES

Disorders of thyroid, parathyroid, adrenal, and pituitary can cause profound changes in muscle function. Mild proximal weakness accompanies most cases of florid *hyperthyroidism*, but sometimes myopathy may be the predominant symptom without obvious clinical evidence of either hypermetabolism or ocular changes of Graves' disease. Rarely, muscle twitches accompany the weakness, so-called fasciculating myopathy of thyrotoxicosis. The shoulder girdle is sometimes weaker than hip muscles, and creatine kinase levels in the serum may be normal. Weakness always responds to the treatment of the hyperthyroidism. In young Asian males, hypokalemic periodic paralysis may complicate hyperthyroidism (p. 709). Hyperthyroidism also can precipitate exacerbations of myasthenia gravis.

In *hypothyroidism*, like thyrotoxicosis, the weakness is proximal. Owing to increased muscle viscosity, the deep tendon reflexes relax slowly in a characteristic fashion, and affected patients can experience difficulty in relaxing muscles. The phenomenon lacks the characteristic EMG changes of myotonia. Percussion myoedema of the muscles (a mounding of the percussed muscle associated with the electrical silence of a focal contracture) is also characteristic of hypothyroid myopathy. Muscle enzyme levels in the serum can rise high enough to suggest polymyositis. Hypothyroid myopathy can occur in the absence of other stigmata of hypothyroidism, and the diagnosis must be suspected from the muscle findings and confirmed by appropriate laboratory tests. In children, the hypothyroid state may be associated with muscle hypertrophy. Exacerbations of myasthenia gravis are also occasionally associated with hypothyroidism.

Hypoparathyroidism with its resulting hypocalcemia can cause tetany, usually without associated myopathy. A few reports also suggest that hypoparathyroidism may be associated with anterior horn cell disease, with amyotrophic lateral sclerosis–like weakness affecting both bulbar and axial muscles. *Hyperparathyroidism* commonly produces weakness, and proximal muscle wasting, with the hips more involved than the shoulders, may be the presenting complaint. Myalgias often accompany the myopathies of hyperparathyroidism, potentially causing the endocrine disorder to be mistaken for polymyositis. Usually, however, other signs of hyperparathyroidism, including renal stones, encephalopathy, and peptic ulceration, accompany the weakness and represent a clue to its pathogenesis. A proximal myopathy is also part of the clinical picture of *hyperpituitarism*, but in this disorder acromegalic features overshadow the muscle weakness. *Hyperadrenocorticalism*, whether spontaneous or induced by the ingestion of adrenocorticosteroids as part of therapy for another disorder, also causes proximal weakness and mild muscle wasting involving hips more than shoulders. Muscle enzymes usually remain normal. This so-called *steroid myopathy* complicates the course of almost every patient treated for more than a few weeks with pharmacological doses of corticosteroids and can even occur after a long period of doses that are considered close to replacement. Patients receiving every-other-day steroid therapy seem to have less myopathy. *Adrenal insufficiency* (Addison's disease) causes weakness only when the serum potassium rises to above 7 to 9 mEq/L.

DRUG, NUTRITIONAL, AND TOXIC MYOPATHIES

With the exception of corticosteroids, only a few drugs cause myopathy. These include vincristine, chloroquine, bretylium, emetine, ipecac, carbenoxolone, guanethidine, episilon-aminocaproic acid, penicillamine, and clofibrate. Thiazide diuretics, the repeated use of laxatives, or the ingestion of other drugs that cause potassium loss may lead to chronic hypokalemia and a proximal myopathy that may be acute at onset, with elevated serum enzymes and even necrosis on muscle biopsy. For severe weakness to occur, the serum potassium concentration must fall below 2 mEq/L.

Nutritional deprivation of vitamin E or selenium ingestion causes a myopathy in animals, but these are not clinical problems in humans. However, chronic alcoholism can lead to severe proximal muscle weakness.

PERIODIC PARALYSES

Periodic paralyses are disorders characterized by recurrent attacks of flaccid weakness, often associated with an abnormally high or low serum potassium concentration, although rarely is the potassium level sufficiently abnormal to produce weakness in an otherwise normal individual (Table 119–5). Many of the cases are familial, usually inherited in a pattern consistent with an autosomal dominant trait. Periodic paralysis has two major forms: hypokalemic and hyperkalemic. The former is characterized by sudden attacks of flaccid weakness, usually beginning in late childhood or adolescence and frequently occurring at night after a large carbohydrate meal. The attacks may totally paralyze the extremities and trunk, sparing the respiratory, bulbar, and cranial muscles, and may last a day or more before spontaneously resolving. During the course of the attack, the serum potassium is usually low (e.g., 2.5 to 3 mEq/L), and the patient may respond to oral or intravenous potassium. Repeated attacks can lead to permanent weakness. Muscle biopsy shows vacuoles within muscle fibers. The hyperkalemic variety generally begins in early childhood with attacks that occur more frequently than the hypokalemic variety, are usually milder, and generally last only minutes to hours rather than days. Typically, the hyperkalemic attack begins while the patient is resting after vigorous exercise. Hyperkalemic attacks may begin with paresthesias in the extremities, but no sensory changes are found on examination. Lid lag and Chvostek's sign may be present along with prominent myalgias. During attacks, the serum potassium usually rises to between 5 and 7 mEq/L, and some patients develop myotonia, often limited to percussion myotonia of the tongue. Although the serum potassium levels and the clinical symptoms separate typical examples of the hypo- and hyperkalemic disorders, the conditions overlap, and many patients suffer periodic paralyses without alteration of the serum potassium.

The diagnosis of periodic paralysis is made by the typical history and confirmed by finding an abnormal serum potassium level during an acute attack. If an acute attack is not observed, one may be precipitated (in the hypokalemic form by glucose and insulin or in the hyperkalemic form by potassium), but this should be done only in a hospital setting where one is prepared to deal with complications. Thyroid function should be assessed in all patients suffering hypokalemic periodic paralysis; diuretic ingestion should be suspected if the serum potassium is below 2.5 mEq/L.

TABLE 119–5. PERIODIC PARALYSIS

Primary
  Hypokalemic
  Hyperkalemic (including those with cardiac arrhythmias)
  Normokalemic
Secondary
  Hypokalemic
    Thyrotoxic
    Potassium-losing states
      Urinary potassium wastage
        Hyperaldosteronism
        Licorice intoxication
        Various renal diseases
        Thiazide diuretics
      Gastrointestinal potassium wastage
  Hyperkalemic
  Renal failure
  Adrenal failure
  Drug-induced: triamterene, spironolactone
  Self-induced: geophagia
  Iatrogenic: potassium supplements

OTHER MYOPATHIES

Several rare congenital or inherited biochemical defects cause muscle weakness, which is usually life-long. Among these are congenital myopathies, glycogen storage diseases, lipid storage diseases, and mitochondrial myopathies.

Congenital myopathies are a group of disorders characterized by mild weakness that generally persists unchanged throughout life. The cause is not known: a few are familial and many are sporadic. The disorders are present at birth, and their chief importance lies in distinguishing them from the more severe progressive muscular dystrophies and neonatal anterior horn cell disorders. A number of glycogen storage diseases cause muscle symptoms. *McArdle's disease*, type 5 glycogen storage disease, results from an absence of muscle phosphorylase, so that patients are unable to break down glycogen during anaerobic exercise. They are usually asymptomatic until early adolescence or early adulthood when they develop painful muscle cramps (actually contractures) after exercise. Myoglobinuria and renal failure may ensue, and patients may eventually become weak. A similar deficit results from phosphofructokinase deficiency. The diagnosis of both is established by the failure of venous lactate to rise during ischemic exercise. Biochemical study of biopsied muscle will define the exact enzyme deficiency. *Lipid storage* and *mitochondrial myopathies* usually become symptomatic in childhood and can be responsible for neurologic symptoms in addition to muscle weakness. The references provide sources that discuss these myopathies more extensively.

MISCELLANEOUS DISORDERS OF MUSCLE

Myoglobinuria results when major injuries to muscles lead to rhabdomyolysis and release of myoglobin into the serum and urine, giving the urine a brown-rust color. Myoglobinuria either can occur as a hereditary disease or can complicate a variety of sporadic muscle injuries. Crush injury, such as occurs in accidents, is a common cause, as is pressure injury to muscles, resulting from a patient's lying immobile after poisoning from sedatives or carbon monoxide. Prolonged unconsciousness in the snow likewise can lead to myoglobinuria, as can arterial occlusion by tourniquet or embolism. Snake bites and binge alcohol ingestion also can cause myoglobinuria, as can malignant hyperthermia. Even normal people may develop some degree of myoglobinuria after vigorous exercise. Strenuous exercise among army recruits, during ritual hazing, or in marathon runners leads to myoglobinuria in a small percentage of individuals. In addition to the discoloration of the urine, the clinical syndrome is characterized by muscle aches and swelling as well as some weakness. Symptoms may persist for several days, even though the pigment in the urine rarely lasts more than four hours. The muscles most affected are those most vigorously exercised or crushed, but cranial musculature and respiratory muscles are almost never affected. The major potential problem is kidney injury due to myoglobin plugging the renal tubules. The disorder should be considered as a possible cause of acute renal failure of uncertain etiology. Myoglobin can be identified spectrophotometrically in the urine.

Cramps are a sudden, painful, abrupt shortening of muscles. Motor units during cramps fire at about 300 per second, much faster than the most vigorous voluntary contraction. The high rate of discharge probably causes the palpable muscle tautness and pain. The pain may be relieved by stretching the affected muscle or by massage. Central mechanisms may also be involved, since certain conditions are associated with a propensity to cramps: denervation (especially amyotrophic lateral sclerosis), pregnancy, and electrolyte disorders (especially water intoxication and hyponatremia). Cramps attributed to hypo-osmolarity are seen in some patients treated by maintenance hemodialysis. They respond to treatment with hypertonic solutions of glucose or sodium.

Cramps occur commonly in otherwise normal individuals, and some people with or without a family history of cramps are more susceptible than others for unknown reasons. Cramps that occur only at night can sometimes be prevented by quinine sulfate, 0.3 gm orally at bedtime. Others occur frequently during the day, occasionally so often that the individual is effectively crippled. Phenytoin, 0.3 to 0.6 gm daily, may be helpful in these patients, but some are resistant to this as well as to other drugs that may be tried, including diazepam, carbamazepine, and diphenhydramine. Patients with benign fasciculations (lacking weakness, wasting, or other signs of motor neuron disease) seem especially prone to have frequent cramps.

Tetany is a special form of cramp, identified by its predilection for flexor muscles of the hand and fingers, its association with laryngospasm, and its relationship to hypocalcemia. Tetany can be painful. It differs from other cramps electromyographically because of a characteristic rhythmic grouping of discharging potentials. Hyperventilation-induced tetany is likely to be overlooked as a cause of cramps or laryngospasm.

Myokymia has been used to describe a variety of apparently different disorders characterized by cramps in association with continuous spontaneous twitching of muscle. The EMG of some cases shows prolonged trains of spontaneous potentials, whereas in others grouping of potentials is found. Some of these patients have difficulty in relaxing grip, a phenomenon called neuromyotonia, since, unlike myotonia, the muscular activity is abolished by neuromuscular blocking agents, indicating a neural rather than a muscular origin. Hyperhidrosis is prominent in some patients and is secondary to the increased muscular activity.

In patients with severe myokymia, continuous shortening of muscle leads to abnormal postures and abnormally increased resistance to passive movement. Such abnormalities are often due to central neurologic disorders. There are other patients who suffer fluctuating rigidity of axial and limb muscles and continuous electromyographic activity despite authentic attempts to relax. This syndrome has been called the *stiff man syndrome* (or Isaac's syndrome, quantal squander, armadillo disease, neuromyotonia, and continuous muscle fiber activity). Ordinary cramps may be superimposed upon the persistent stiffness. Phenytoin, carbamazepine or diazepam in therapeutic doses may bring dramatic relief. The cause is unknown.

DISORDERS OF NEUROMUSCULAR JUNCTION

These conditions are caused either by a deficient release of acetylcholine at the neuromuscular junction because of presynaptic disease, by block of action of acetylcholine at the neuromuscular junction, as occurs in poisoning with curare-like drugs (such blocks can be either depolarizing or nonpolarizing), or by abnormalities of the postsynaptic junction such as occurs in myasthenia gravis. Like the myopathies, neuromuscular junction disorders are characterized by weakness and often by fatigability of muscle, so that repetitive use of the muscle often leads to increased weakness. In some, but not all, of the diseases, cranial and respiratory musculatures are peculiarly susceptible. Drugs may cause or exacerbate pre-existing neuromuscular junction disorders (Table 119–6). They are particularly likely to cause postoperative respiratory depression.

Myasthenia gravis is an autoimmune disease caused by circulating antibodies that damage acetylcholine receptors lying within the postsynaptic muscle membrane. The disorder may occur in isolation or be associated with other autoimmune disorders, such as systemic lupus erythematosus

TABLE 119–6. DRUG-INDUCED NEUROMUSCULAR BLOCKADE

CLINICAL PRES-ENTATION	ANTIBIOTICS	CARDIOVASCU-LAR DRUGS	ANTIRHEUMATIC DRUGS	PSYCHOTROPIC DRUGS	ANTICONVUL-SANTS	HORMONAL AGENTS	OTHER DRUGS
Postoperative respiratory depression	Clindamycin Colistin Kanamycin Lincomycin Neomycin Streptomycin Tobramycin	Lidocaine Quinidine Trimethaphan	Chloroquine	Lithium Phenelzine Promazine			Aprotinin Cholinesterase inhibitors Oxytocin
Aggravation or unmasking of myasthenia gravis	Colistin Kanamycin Streptomycin Tetracyclines	Procainamide Propranolol Quinidine	Chloroquine(?)	Chlorpromazine Lithium	Phenytoin	ACTH Corticosteroids Thyroid hormones	Acetylcholinesterase inhibitors Methoxyflurane
Drug-induced myasthenic syndrome	Colistin Gentamicin Kanamycin Neomycin Polymyxin B Streptomycin	Oxprenolol Practolol Trimethaphan	D-Penicillamine		Phenytoin Trimethadione	Oral contraceptives(?)	Tetanus antitoxin

From Argov Z, and Mastaglia FL: Medical intelligence: Drug therapy. N Engl J Med 301:8, 1979.

and hyperthyroidism. The disorder is usually associated with an abnormality of the thymus gland, either hypertrophic germinal centers or a thymoma. It is accompanied by accumulation of lymphocytes in muscle and other organs, an increased frequency of nonspecific antibodies against nuclear antigens, and the presence of an antithyroid antibody. That a circulating substance plays a major role in production of the weakness is proved by two facts: (1) Transplacental passage of a substance occurs, so that infants born to myasthenic women suffer transient myasthenia-type bulbar weakness. Symptoms subside as the antibody supplied to the infant by the mother disappears, usually within a week to a month. (2) Plasmapheresis brings at least a transient relief of symptoms to patients with the disease.

Myasthenia gravis may begin any time in life, including in the newborn, but there are two major peaks of onset, one in young adulthood, when the incidence is about three times more common in women than men, and another in older persons, with men and women about equally affected. There are occasional familial cases, but most are sporadic.

Clinically, the disease is characterized by weakness and fatigability. Weakness usually begins in the extraocular muscles, with ptosis and diplopia. The symptoms may be localized to the ocular muscles or be generalized, mild or severe (Table 119–7). Symptoms tend to become more prominent toward the end of the day, following fatiguing activity, or with continuous use of extraocular muscles, such as in driving or reading. Closing the eyes or relaxing the muscles for a few minutes makes the symptoms disappear. Other bulbar muscles may also be affected, with difficulty in swallowing, chewing, or speaking, becoming more noticeable after sustained activity of the involved muscles or when the patient is otherwise fatigued. If limb muscles are involved, weakness is more often proximal than distal. Respiratory weakness alone or in combination with swallowing paralysis is the most feared compli-

cation of myasthenia gravis. Because all symptoms of the disorder may be exacerbated by fatigue or infection, a patient who is otherwise not severely affected may develop sudden acute respiratory failure during a respiratory infection.

The disorder is suggested by the history, and the diagnosis can usually be confirmed on physical examination, by observing weakness that develops in extraocular or other muscles as repetitive activity continues. The physician asks the patient to look fixedly at an object on the ceiling. After 30 or 40 seconds, the lids begin to droop and the eyes may diverge. Similarly, repetitive contraction of arm muscles may cause weakness of those muscles or may cause ptosis. In a symptomatic patient, an intravenous injection of edrophonium hydrochloride, an anticholinesterase agent, leads to rapid amelioration of clinical symptoms and improved or normal muscle function for a few minutes, until the effects of the drug wear off. When positive, in a fully symptomatic patient, the results are so dramatic that they establish the diagnosis. False-positive tests can result from increased muscular effort by the patient during the test and can sometimes be identified by a similar positive response to a placebo. Occasionally, when the muscles are very weak, they may be refractory to edrophonium, giving rise to a false-negative test. Additional confirmatory evidence is provided by electromyographic re-

TABLE 119–7. CLASSIFICATION OF MYASTHENIA GRAVIS

I.	Ocular myasthenia
IIA.	Mild generalized myasthenia with slow progression; no crisis; drug-responsive
IIB.	Moderate generalized myasthenia; severe skeletal and bulbar involvement, but no crisis; drug response less satisfactory
III.	Acute fulminating myasthenia; rapid progression of severe symptoms with respiratory crisis and poor drug response; high incidence of thymoma; high mortality
IV.	Late severe myasthenia; same as III, but takes two years to progress from Classes I or II; crisis; high mortality

sponse to nerve stimulation. With repetitive stimulation of the nerve, there is a rapid decline in the muscle action potential, the electrical counterpart of muscle fatigability. More recently, single fiber electromyography, which measures the interval between discharges of different fibers within the same motor unit, reveals excessive variation called jitter, believed to be strongly suggestive of myasthenia gravis. Patients with myasthenia gravis harbor in their serum antibodies against the acetylcholine receptor. Such antibodies can be identified in at least half the patients with ocular myasthenia and in over 80 per cent of patients with generalized myasthenia. There are virtually no false-positive tests, although patients in remission from myasthenia may continue to have elevated levels of antibodies.

In a typical patient the diagnosis is not difficult to make once considered. However, the disorder must be distinguished from neurasthenia, a subjective feeling of weakness and fatigability caused by psychological disorders, as well as from other myopathies and neuropathies. Careful attention to the effects of pharmacological agents and studies of the electrical activity of muscle will almost always establish the diagnosis.

The treatment of myasthenia has three components: (1) One can increase the effectiveness of acetylcholine released at the myoneural junction by preventing its breakdown. The anticholinesterase drugs neostigmine and pyridostigmine rapidly ameliorate most myasthenic symptoms. Drugs are given in sufficient doses and with sufficient frequency to keep muscle function as close to normal as possible. An average dose of pyridostigmine is 60 to 120 mg every four to five hours. Dosage is begun low and gradually adjusted upward to achieve maximal function. Unfortunately, excessive treatment itself can cause weakness because cholinesterase inhibitors may produce a depolarizing block at the neuromuscular junction. In addition, the augmented release of acetylcholine may cause distressing abdominal cramping. Because the autonomic acetylcholine receptors are muscarinic, they can be blocked by atropine-like agents (e.g., probanthine) without an effect on the nicotinic neuromuscular receptors. (2) The second approach is to remove the circulating antibody that produces the symptoms. Plasmapheresis has proved to be a safe and beneficial treatment for most patients with myasthenia. Patients who are severely weak may improve within minutes of completion of plasmapheresis and may be free of symptoms for days to weeks. In some patients who are refractory to other treatments, plasmapheresis given once a week to once every two weeks allows the patient to maintain relatively normal function. (3) The third approach is to suppress production of the antibody. That the thymus gland has had a causal role in myasthenia gravis has been known for a long time. Thymectomy is a well-established treatment that improves about 85 per cent of patients. All patients with generalized myasthenia should be considered for thymectomy, although that option may not be chosen in severely ill elderly patients. Another method of suppressing production of the antibody is to use immunosuppressive drugs, either steroids or azathioprine. Corticosteroids in high doses often produce an exacerbation of myasthenia symptoms (rarely even culminating in respiratory paralysis), but after a few days or a week the patients begin to improve. Many patients with myasthenia can be well-controlled on doses (20 to 50 mg) of prednisone every other day. Steroids, in addition to their effect in suppressing acetylcholine receptor antibody concentration, also have direct effects on neuromuscular transmission. Azathioprine is the other drug currently used to suppress antibody formation. Most investigators believe that in doses of 150 to 200 mg per day it can be helpful in the treatment of myasthenia.

Patients with myasthenia are prone to develop sudden worsening of symptoms, particularly associated with respiratory infections. These patients are best treated in intensive care units with respiratory support and without the use of anticholinesterase drugs. Plasmapheresis may be useful in hastening resolution of the myasthenic crisis.

The *Lambert-Eaton or myasthenic syndrome* is an uncommon disorder of neuromuscular transmission that is electrically, in many respects, the opposite of myasthenia gravis. Repetitive stimulation of the nerve leads to a facilitation of the muscle action potential rather than a diminution. In about two thirds of instances, the myasthenic syndrome is a paraneoplastic phenomenon associated with oat cell carcinoma of the lung; in the remaining the disorder occurs without an underlying illness. Patients complain of proximal weakness of limb muscles, particularly in the lower extremities, and increased fatigability. They also complain of paresthesias in the thighs, a dry mouth and, in males, impotence. Cranial nerve muscles are almost never involved. Examination reveals proximal weakness that may increase as the patient attempts to sustain a contraction (the clinical counterpart of the electrical facilitation) and hypoactive or absent deep tendon reflexes, particularly at the knees and ankles. The diagnosis is confirmed by the electrical response. The presence of the Lambert-Eaton syndrome should prompt a careful search for oat cell carcinoma of the lung, since the neuromuscular symptoms occasionally precede other evidence of the cancer by months to years. Some investigators report that injection of serum from patients with myasthenic syndrome into animals produces disorders of neuromuscular transmission. As in myasthenia gravis, plasmapheresis often relieves the symptoms.

Botulism is caused by the exotoxin of *Clostridium botulinum* and occurs following the ingestion of contaminated, improperly canned food. The toxin interferes with adequate release of acetylcholine at the neuromuscular junction. Symptoms usually begin within a few days of ingestion with blurring of vision, diplopia, and difficulty in swallowing and chewing. Gastrointestinal symptoms may precede the neurologic symptoms, and the weakness spreads rapidly to cause paralysis of cranial and respiratory muscles and lesser paralysis of arms and legs. Autonomic fibers, particularly the pupilloconstrictor fibers, are affected early in the disorder, and there is loss of visual accommodation. If electrical neuromuscular transmission studies are performed early, the findings may resemble the myasthenic syndrome. The disease may produce death from respiratory paralysis unless artificial respiration is started promptly. The history, its usually more rapid onset and progression, and normal spinal fluid protein distinguish botulism from the ophthalmoplegic form of the Guillain-Barré syndrome, which it can resemble closely. If the patient's physiological functions, particularly respiration, are supported, there is usually full recovery.

Tick paralysis is a disorder caused by a tick neurotoxin that blocks transmission at the neuromuscular junction. Most cases of tick paralysis occur in children, particularly girls, in whom the tick embeds in the skin near the hairline and goes unnoticed. After five or six days of embedding, paresthesias and progressive weakness develop which may progress to flaccid paralysis of cranial and respiratory muscles and the extremities, resembling botulism or the Guillain-Barré syndrome. Spinal fluid protein is normal and the paralysis subsides promptly following removal of the embedded tick.

Aminoglycoside antibiotics, including neomycin, streptomycin, colistin, and kanamycin, can interfere with neuromuscular transmission. The most common manifestation is postoperative apnea without other evidence of paralysis in patients who have received the antibiotics, particularly in those who have renal failure, leading to high antimicrobial drug levels. Some patients may have a flaccid quadriplegia that responds to administration of calcium and quinidine.

C. PERIPHERAL NERVES, MOTOR NEURON, SPINAL, AND NEUROCUTANEOUS SYNDROMES

PERIPHERAL NERVES

General Considerations

Diseases of the peripheral nervous system may affect one (or more) of three structures: (1) the cell body (neuronopathy), (2) the axon (axonopathy), or (3) the Schwann cells and/or their metabolic product, the myelin sheath (demyelinating neuropathy). Any of these processes may be focal, leading to mononeuropathy (involvement of a single nerve) or multiple mononeuropathy (involvement of several different single nerves), or diffuse, causing polyneuropathy (a diffuse, predominantly symmetrical, and often distal involvement of the nerves of the extremities) (Table 119–8). The distal nature of most polyneuropathies reflects the fact that the longest nerves are the most metabolically active. Although each of the anatomical and pathological disorders listed in Table 119–8 can have distinctive clinical symptoms, there is considerable overlap. Furthermore, individual etiologic agents, such as diabetes or cancer, may cause more than one type of neuropathy. Accordingly, in the pages that follow, the peripheral neuropathies are discussed first pathophysiologically and then etiologically.

In *demyelinating neuropathy* (Fig. 119–2) segments of myelin degenerate to a greater or lesser extent, usually due to immunological or infectious causes. Clinically, demyelinating neuropathy is characterized by failure of large myelinated fibers, leading to decreased light touch, position, and vibration sensation, as well as to weakness and reduction or absence of deep tendon reflexes. A relative sparing of lightly myelinated or unmyelinated fibers partially preserves temperature and pain sensation, although these modalities become involved if the disorder is severe. The onset of demyelinating neuropathy may be rapid, and with Schwann cell proliferation and remyelination, recovery may be equally rapid. Because the myelin sheath can be involved anywhere throughout its peripheral course, the disease, although usually symmetrical, sometimes affects both proximal and distal fibers to a similar degree.

TABLE 119–8. ANATOMICAL AND PATHOLOGICAL CLASSIFICATION OF PERIPHERAL NEUROPATHIES*

LESION	CLINICAL EXAMPLE
Focal	
Mononeuropathy	Median nerve compression (carpal tunnel syndrome)
Multiple mononeuropathies	Periarteritis nodosa
Diffuse (Polyneuropathies)	
Axonopathies	
Distal	Diabetes
Central	Clioquinol poisoning
Myelinopathy	Guillain-Barré syndrome
Neuronopathies	
Sensory	Paraneoplastic sensory neuronopathy
Motor	Amyotrophic lateral sclerosis
Autonomic	Shy-Drager syndrome

* Modified from Schaumburg HH, Spencer PS, and Thomas PK: Disorders of Peripheral Nerve. Philadelphia, FA Davis Co, 1983.

A

PRIMARY MYELINOPATHY (e.g., inflammatory)

Normal

Attack by
Inflammatory Cells

Segmental Demyelination

Remyelinated Fibers

B

TOXIC DISTAL AXONOPATHY

Normal

Early

Late

Recovering

Astrocyte
Proliferation

Axon
Regeneration

CNS

PNS

Cranial nerves are often involved, as well as peripheral nerves. The spinal fluid protein is elevated in diffuse demyelinating neuropathies because of damage to spinal roots. Electrical studies of demyelinated nerves reveal that conduction velocity is slowed, often to 20 or 25 per cent of normal values, and the amplitude of the action potential is small because it is dispersed over a longer duration.

Axonal neuropathy is characterized by degeneration of the distal ends of long axons, with secondary loss and degeneration of the myelin sheath. The disorder usually causes an equal loss of all sensory modalities, although in some instances small axons carrying pain and temperature suffer a loss disproportionate to larger axons. The first symptoms are usually sensory, with paresthesias or sensory loss of the tips of the fingers

FIGURE 119–2. Pathological processes damaging the peripheral nervous system (PNS). *A,* A diagram of the cardinal pathological features of inflammatory PNS myelinopathy. Axons are spared, as in CNS demyelinating illness. Following the attack the remaining Schwann cells divide. The denuded segments of axons are remyelinated, leaving them with short internodes. *B,* The cardinal pathological features of a toxic distal axonopathy. The jagged lines (lightning bolts) indicate that the toxin is acting at multiple sites along motor and sensory axons in the PNS and CNS. Axon degeneration has moved proximally (dying-back) by the late stage. Recovery in the CNS is impeded by astroglial proliferation. *C,* The cardinal features of a rapidly evolving toxic sensory neuronopathy. The jagged lines (lightning bolts) indicate that the toxin is directed at neurons in the dorsal root ganglion (DRG). Degeneration of these cells is accompanied by a fragmentation and phagocytosis of their peripheral central processes. Schwann cells remain. There is no axonal regeneration. (From Schaumburg HH, Spencer PS, and Thomas PK: Disorders of peripheral nerves. Philadelphia, FA Davis Co, 1983.)

and toes. Only later, as the sensory loss spreads more proximally, does motor involvement occur in a typical "stocking and glove" distribution. Unlike demyelinating neuropathy, recovery is usually slow because of the slow rate of regeneration of the damaged axons. Spinal roots usually are not involved and the CSF protein remains normal. Electrically, axonal neuropathies are characterized by normal or only slightly (10 to 15 per cent) slowed conduction velocity and by small sensory action potentials.

A recently described *central axonopathy* caused by several toxic substances may underly some human degenerative diseases. This disorder is characterized by selective vulnerability of that portion of the sensory axon that lies between the dorsal root ganglion and the spinal cord, sparing the peripheral axon. There is a dying back of the axon in the posterior column, proceeding from distal to proximal, with secondary loss of the surrounding myelin sheath and gliosis of the posterior column. Central motor pathways may also be affected, with degeneration of distal portions of the corticospinal tract. The sensory loss usually begins subacutely with paresthesias and loss of large fiber function. Unlike peripheral axonopathies, the deep tendon reflexes are usually hyperactive, and because of corticospinal tract damage, a spastic paraparesis may accompany the disorder.

Neuronopathies can also affect either sensory or motor nerves, or both. Neuronopathies cause either acute or gradual onset of sensory and/or motor loss with little or no recovery.

FOCAL NEUROPATHY

The etiologic agents that cause focal neuropathy usually differ from those causing polyneuropathy, although some diseases, such as diabetes and hypothyroidism, can cause either mononeuropathy or polyneuropathy. Most focal neuropathies result from vascular disease, compression, or trauma. Clinically, the mononeuropathies are characterized by sensory and/or motor loss (usually both) in the anatomical distribution of all or part of a nerve root, nerve plexus, or peripheral nerve. One can determine the site of the injury clinically by observing the anatomical distribution of dysfunction (e.g., an injury to the radial nerve at the humerus causes weakness of the brachioradialis muscle and extensors of the wrist and fingers, but spares the triceps muscle because radial nerve fibers in the triceps depart from the nerve more proximally in the upper arm).

TRAUMA AND COMPRESSION

Most mononeuritides are caused by trauma and result either from compression, transection, or stretching of nerve, or from chronic entrapment by various anatomical structures. Mild injury to a nerve may leave the nerve structurally intact but cause a conduction block first by ischemia and subsequently by demyelination. Acute ischemic lesions recover rapidly when pressure is released; demyelinating lesions may recover more slowly. A more severe injury interrupts the axons but leaves the connective tissue sheaths intact. Such lesions are common in closed crush injuries. Depending on the degree of damage, recovery may be partial or complete, but it proceeds slowly. The most severe injury is transection of both axons and connective tissue sheaths, such as occurs with severe stretch injuries or penetrating wounds. Because of the interruption of the sheath, recovery does not occur unless the nerve is surgically repaired, and even then the prognosis is poor.

Acute Trauma

Any portion of the peripheral nervous system can be damaged by trauma. In wartime, penetrating wounds of peripheral nerves and nerve plexuses are major causes of disability. In peacetime, traumatic peripheral nerve lesions usually result from closed crush or traction injuries. The brachial plexus is a major site of stretch injuries, commonly resulting from motorcycle accidents and compression injury when the arm is hyperabducted, as under anesthesia. The former injuries are usually permanent, the latter transient. Other acute compression injuries that sometimes follow general anesthesia for surgery or are self-induced by alcohol or sedatives include radial nerve palsy from compression of the nerve in the radial groove of the humerus (Saturday night palsy), peroneal nerve palsy from compression between the surface and the head of the fibula (crossed-leg palsies), ulnar palsy (often from compression by an I.V. board in the ulnar groove at the elbow), and sciatic palsies from buttocks compression or ill-placed injections.

Chronic Compression Neuropathies

In order to reach their peripheral targets, many nerves must pass through narrow channels where they can become chronically compressed in fibro-osseous tunnels, angulated and stretched over arthritic joints or bony structures, or recurrently compressed by repeated trauma. Table 119–9 lists the major compression neuropathies. The most common are discussed below.

Carpal Tunnel Syndrome. The median nerve is compressed at the wrist as it passes deep to the flexor retinaculum. The usual symptoms include numbness, tingling, and burning sensations in one or both hands and the fingers supplied by the

TABLE 119–9. COMMON SITES OF NERVE ENTRAPMENT

Median nerve
  Carpal tunnel—wrist
  Pronator muscle—elbow
Ulnar nerve
  Elbow
  Wrist
Radial nerve—humeral groove
Brachial plexus—thoracic outlet
Sciatic nerve—buttocks (sciatic notch)
Peroneal nerve—behind knee
Lateral femoral cutaneous nerve—inguinal ligament
Cervical and lumbar root—intervertebral canal

median nerve, including the thumb, index, middle, and half of the ring finger. Some patients complain that all fingers become numb, but if tested this is usually found not to be the case. Pain and paresthesias are most prominent at night and often interrupt sleep. The pain is prominent at the wrist but may radiate to the forearm or at times to the shoulder. Both pain and paresthesias are relieved by shaking the hands. In some patients, symptoms may persist for years without objective signs of median nerve damage. In others, sensory loss may appear over the tips of the fingers and/or weakness can develop in the thumb muscles in association with atrophy of the lateral aspect of the thenar eminence.

The carpal tunnel syndrome occurs mostly in middle-aged and obese women. It may affect those who use the wrists and hands occupationally, as in gardening, house painting, meat wrapping, or typing. Other predisposing causes include pregnancy, myxedema, acromegaly, rheumatoid arthritis, and primary amyloidosis.

The diagnosis is based on clinical symptoms, the finding of Tinel's sign (paresthesias in the finger with a light tap over the nerve at the wrist), and the demonstration of a conduction block at the wrist by motor nerve velocity studies. The most effective treatment is section of the transverse carpal ligament, decompressing the nerve.

Ulnar Palsy. The ulnar nerve may be injured at the elbow, especially in persons with a shallow ulnar groove and those who rest on their elbows excessively. Injury may also occur years after a "malunited" supracondylar fracture of the humerus with bony overgrowth (*tardive ulnar palsy*). Contrary to the findings in the carpal tunnel syndrome, muscle weakness and atrophy characteristically predominate over sensory symptoms and signs. Patients notice atrophy of the first dorsal interosseous muscle and difficulty performing fine manipulations of the fingers. There may be numbness of the small finger, the contiguous half of the ring finger, and the ulnar border of the hand.

Lateral Cutaneous Nerve of the Thigh. *Meralgia paresthetica* is an entrapment neuropathy resulting from compression of this nerve as it passes under the inguinal ligament. Obese persons wearing tight belts and those with pendulous abdomens are especially prone to develop numbness or burning sensations over the lateral thigh. Sometimes prolonged standing or walking provokes the symptoms. Weight reduction may help, and in many cases the condition subsides spontaneously.

Cervical Rib and Thoracic Outlet Syndrome. The brachial plexus as it passes through the thoracic outlet can be compressed by a cervical rib or by normal bone, muscles, and fibrous tissue. The compression usually occurs when the arm is abducted and may involve the subclavian artery as well as the plexus. Symptoms include paresthesias of ulnar fingers and rarely weakness and wasting of the small hand muscles. The sensory abnormalities usually respond to avoiding the abducted position, but surgical removal of the first rib and fibrous band may occasionally be necessary if weakness persists.

Chronic Compression
Radiculopathies and Myelopathies

Herniated Intervertebral Disc. The disc material herniates into the vertebral canal, generally lateral to the posterior longitudinal ligament, thereby compressing spinal roots as they enter the intervertebral foramen. Occasionally, the disc herniates more centrally, compressing either the spinal cord in the cervical or thoracic area or the cauda equina in the lumbar area. The specific signs and symptoms of herniated discs depend in part on whether the predominant compression is spinal cord or nerve root, and in part on the level at which the neural structures are compressed. The most common sites of herniation are in the lumbar area, between L4 and L5 or L5 and S1, with the ensuing compression being upon the L5 and S1 roots. (Because of the anatomy, a laterally herniated disc between L4 and L5 compresses the L5 root, and a disc between L5 and S1, the S1 root.) L3-L4 herniations are less common. In the cervical area, the common herniations occur between C5 and C6 (C6 root) and most often, between C6 and C7 (C7 root). Less frequently, herniations appear between C3 and C4, C4 and C5, and C7 and T1. Thoracic disc herniations are rare, but when they occur they usually compress the spinal cord as well as the emerging root because of the narrowness of the thoracic vertebral canal. Although clinical localization in the diagnosis of disc disease is usually quite accurate, an extruded disc fragment at times may be large enough to affect several roots, or may migrate from the disc space in which it herniated, causing signs at a distance from the original herniation.

The most common symptom of herniated disc is pain. Local pain is felt as a dull aching in the neck or back, with an associated stiffness of those structures, frequently occurring episodically in response to minor trauma (or no discernible trauma at all) months or years prior to the development of radicular pain. The exact pathogenesis of the local back pain in disc disease is not known, but some believe that it results from compression of the sinuvertebral nerve, a recurrent branch of the nerve root that supplies the dura mater. Radicular pain may occasionally be the first sign of disc disease but is far more likely to follow repetitive bouts of local pain. Radicular pain is perceived as sharp and well-localized and may radiate from the back along the entire distribution of the involved root or affect only a portion of the root. Both local and radicular pain have the characteristics of being exacerbated by activity and relieved by rest.

With cervical disc herniation, most patients hold their necks stiffly and resist passive movement. Lateral bending, either to or away from the side of the herniated disc, frequently exacerbates both the local and the radicular pain. The patient may be more comfortable with his neck slightly flexed but is usually comfortable only when recumbent. Patients with lumbar disc disease are most comfortable lying, most uncomfortable sitting, and a little less uncomfortable standing. The back is held stiffly, reducing or erasing the normal lumbar lordotic curve, and pain is usually exacerbated by extension of the back. Slow forward bending sometimes relieves the pain. Muscle spasm is prominent with both cervical and lumbar disc disease. Raising the intraspinal pressure, as by coughing, sneezing, or straining, increases the pain sharply. Directly stretching the compressed root also aggravates the pain. In the upper extremities, extending the arm and laterally flexing the neck away from the extended arm often reproduces radicular pain. In the lower extremities, raising the extended leg with the patient in the recumbent position frequently reproduces the pain of an L5 or S1 radiculopathy and, if the pain is felt on the opposite side as well (crossed straight leg raising), the sign is very suggestive of herniated disc disease. Symptoms of L4 radiculopathy often can be reproduced by extending the hip or fully flexing the knee (stretching the femoral nerve) when the patient is lying in the prone position. Often tenderness is present along the entire distribution of the nerve(s) supplied by the compressed root, as well as in muscles supplied by the root. In patients with cervical disc disease, palpation or light percussion of the brachial plexus and the supraclavicular fossa or axilla often causes pain. In patients with lumbar disc disease, palpation over the femoral nerve (L4) in the groin or over the sciatic nerve (L5-S1) in the calf, thigh, or buttocks can cause severe pain. Occasionally tenderness in the calf (the posterior tibial nerve) can be so striking as to suggest that the patient is suffering from thrombophlebitis rather than disc herniation. Other neurologic signs that commonly accompany disc disease include paresthesias and sensory loss in the distribution of the involved root and motor weakness in the myotome supplied by that root. The most important sign is a locally diminished or absent deep tendon reflex, giving objective evidence of neurologic disease.

If an intervertebral disc herniates medially, rather than laterally, it may spare the root and involve the spinal cord or cauda equina directly. The lesion then mimics a spinal tumor (see p. 725) except that with disc disease there may be little or no pain. The diagnosis of herniated disc is deduced from the characteristic clinical symptoms and findings. Both CT and MRI are effective in identifying most disc disease (Fig. 119–3). Myelography may be performed before surgical extirpation to localize the site of disc herniation and to determine whether other disc lesions or tumors are present as well, but in many cases the CT scan alone suffices.

No consensus exists about the preferred management of herniated discs. Most physicians believe that the first step is bed rest. Some investigators have reported that adrenocorticosteroids, either taken orally or injected into the epidural space, may hasten resolution of pain and other symptoms. A short course of oral steroids is safe, but there is no unequivocal evidence that it is efficacious. Steroids injected into the epidural or subarachnoid space, particularly those in depot form, may produce severe inflammatory reactions and are inadvisable. Surgery is indicated when (1) bed rest fails, and the patient is incapacitated by severe, intractable pain; (2) a centrally placed lumbar disc compresses the cauda equina, producing urinary dysfunction; or (3) there is motor weakness caused by compression of the spinal cord. Some believe that motor weakness caused by root compression is also an indication for immediate surgery. The best operation removes the

FIGURE 119–3. Cervical disc herniation causing myelopathy. MR image from a middle-aged patient with a one-year history of numbness in the right arm and progressive spastic weakness of both legs. There was no pain. Although magnetic resonance does not image bone, the bone marrow in the vertebral bodies is clearly visible (closed arrow). The herniated disc impinging on the cervical cord between C5 and C6 can be easily seen (open arrow).

involved disc, leaving intact as much bone as possible. Fusion of the lumbar spine is rarely necessary. Lumbar disc operations are done posteriorly via a laminotomy. Cervical disc operations may be done either posteriorly to decompress the cord or anteriorly to remove the disc without disturbing posterior bony elements. The surgical approach for myelopathy should probably be anterior if the disc is in the cervical area and lateral if the disc is in the thoracic area.

A relatively new technique of disc dissolution by the injection of the enzyme chymopapain directly into a lumbar disc space has received enthusiastic support from some centers. The technique is still being subjected to clinical trials, and what role, if any, it will play in the therapeutic armamentarium remains uncertain.

Spondylosis. Spondylosis is a term applied to chronic degenerative disease of intervertebral discs associated with reactive changes in the adjacent vertebral bodies. Spondylotic changes in the neck and low back increase with increasing age and are almost invariably present in the elderly. Most spondylosis causes no symptoms, except when the reaction tissue compresses a nerve root or the spinal cord. When this occurs, the signs and symptoms resemble those of herniated disc disease, but the onset is less abrupt and the treatment often more difficult. In both the cervical and lumbar areas, spondylosis is more likely to produce spinal cord or cauda equina symptoms if the sagittal diameter of the spinal canal is further impinged upon by osteophytes. The signs and symptoms of *cervical spondylosis* result from compression either of the spinal cord or its emerging roots and are thus similar to those of a herniated disc. Most patients suffer either radiculopathy or myelopathy (see p. 725) but not both. Pain is common in patients with spondylotic radiculopathy but usually less acute and severe than with herniated discs, and muscle spasm may be absent. However, the vertebral degenerative changes in the neck often lead to limitation of movement in all directions. The classic picture of cervical spondylotic *myelopathy* is one of little or no pain but slowly developing weakness, atrophy, and fasciculations in the upper extremities, particularly the small muscles of the hand, or an insidiously developing spastic paraparesis with decreased proprioception in the legs. At first the findings may suggest a diagnosis of amyotrophic lateral sclerosis (see p. 723). However, in cervical spondylosis there are sensory changes, particularly vibration loss in the lower extremities, and in amyotrophic lateral sclerosis there are fasciculations arising in areas different from motor roots compressed at the cervical level (e.g., the tongue). The differential diagnosis also includes other compressive lesions of root and spinal cord, (Fig. 119–4).

Plain x-rays of the cervical spine confirm the presence of cervical spondylosis, but many patients without symptoms have similar x-ray findings. Evidence that spondylosis is symptomatic is found by measuring the sagittal diameter of the cervical canal. When the diameter is less than 10

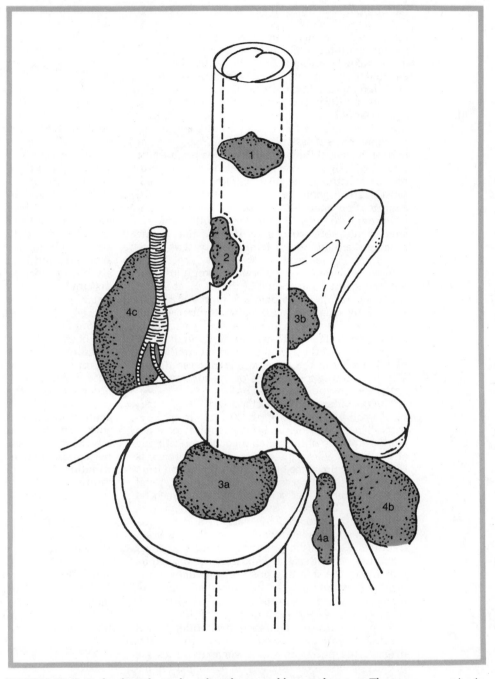

FIGURE 119–4. Pathophysiology of myelopathy caused by neoplasms. *1*, The tumor may arise in or metastasize hematogenously to the substance of the spinal cord (intramedullary). *2*, The tumor may be extraparenchymal but intradural. *3*, The tumor may be extradural, either extending from the vertebral body (*3a*) or from a spinous process (*3b*), and cause symptoms by compressing the spinal cord. *4*, The tumor may originate in or spread to the paravertebral space and produce its symptoms either by (*4a*) invading nerve roots, (*4b*) invading the epidural or subdural space through the intravertebral foramen, or (*4c*) compressing radicular arteries to cause spinal cord ischemia.

mm, cord compression is almost a certainty. If the diameter is over 13 mm, it is unlikely that cord compression is occurring, but a soft disc or tumor not seen on the x-ray may be impinging on the cord. A CT scan sometimes helps to delineate ac-curately the size of the cervical canal. Myelog-raphy determines the size of the lesion and the degree of obstruction, but MRI may be as accurate and decrease the need for myelography.

The natural history of cervical myelopathy and

radiculopathy is not well established. It is known that many patients experience long periods of pain relief and remission or stabilization of neurologic symptoms. Such spontaneous improvement makes it difficult to evaluate the effect of a particular treatment. Many physicians prefer, once having established the diagnosis, to begin conservative treatment with a period of bed rest accompanied by cervical traction and stabilization of the neck with a soft collar. If these approaches are successful, they should be continued. However, if the patient develops progressive neurologic signs, especially weakness and atrophy or spasticity, surgical therapy is indicated. Most neurosurgeons believe that if the spinal cord compression occurs at one or two segments, anterior removal of the disc material with spinal fusion is the preferred course. If more than a few segments are involved, laminectomy with foraminotomy is preferred.

In some patients with cervical spondylosis (or with congenital narrowing of the cervical spinal canal, or both), neurologic symptoms are exacerbated by exercise, with pain, numbness, and weakness appearing when a particular extremity is exercised. The pathogenesis is thought to be compression of the spinal cord so severe that the blood supply to the area cannot increase during activity, leading to ischemia of the cord and root structures (pseudoclaudication).

The considerations described above under cervical spondylosis also apply to *lumbar spondylosis*. The symptoms of lumbar spondylosis are similar to those of herniated disc, often occurring at multiple levels. One outstanding difference is the frequent presence of pseudoclaudication from cauda equina compression in patients with spinal stenosis from either spondylosis or congenital narrowing. Typically, symptoms and signs are evoked or accentuated by walking and include pain, paresthesias, and weakness in the lower extremities. All of the symptoms may disappear when the patient ceases walking, even though he remains in the standing position. At times, however, the symptoms may be exacerbated by prolonged standing and relieved only by sitting or lying down. Pseudoclaudication of the cauda equina may be distinguished from intermittent vascular claudication in several ways. In vascular disease, the pulses in the lower extremities are usually absent or become absent as the patient begins to exercise. With vascular disease, the symptoms are usually reproducible and stereotypic; i.e., the patient can predict the exact distance he can walk at a given speed before symptoms develop. Symptoms of cauda equina pseudoclaudication are less stereotypic, so that on some days patients can walk much longer distances than on others. The reason for this variability is not known. In patients with pseudoclaudication, the neurologic examination may be normal when the patient is at rest, but abnormal signs, particularly absence of deep tendon reflexes, may appear as the patient exercises. In patients with pseudoclaudication the lumbar canal is narrowed on either lateral x-ray or CT scan, and there is a sub-stantial block to the passage of myelographic dye. With severe lumbar stenosis, conservative treatment usually fails and decompressive laminectomy is the treatment of choice.

Immune Focal Neuropathies

A few acute focal neuropathies are believed to have an immune cause. The most common is *acute brachial neuritis*, characterized by the acute onset of severe pain, usually in the distribution of the axillary nerve (over the lateral shoulder) but at times extending into the entire arm. It generally subsides after a few days to a week. Usually coincident with the subsidence of the pain, weakness of the proximal arm becomes apparent. The serratus anterior is the most commonly paralyzed muscle, but other muscles of the shoulder girdle, including the deltoid and muscles of the upper arm, may be paralyzed as well. Rarely, most of the arm and even the ipsilateral diaphragm are paralyzed. Sensory loss is usually restricted to the distribution of the axillary nerve. Weakness may last weeks to months and be accompanied by severe atrophy of the shoulder girdle. Total recovery occurs in most patients within several months to two or three years. The disorder has been reported to follow upper respiratory infection or an immunization, but often there is no antecedent illness. Considerably less common is a similar disorder affecting the *lumbosacral plexus*, causing pain and weakness of a lower extremity. As with acute brachial neuritis, although the pain may be severe and the weakness profound, recovery usually occurs. Differential diagnosis from acute disc herniation is made readily by identifying the distribution, which involves incomplete changes in multiple nerve roots rather than complete changes in a single root.

Infectious Focal Neuropathies

Infection rarely affects the peripheral nervous system directly, although cranial nerves and nerves of the cauda equina may be damaged by acute bacterial meningitis, subacute meningitis (e.g., tuberculosis), or less commonly chronic meningitis (e.g., fungal meningitis). The only common infection of the peripheral nervous system is *herpes zoster*.

Vascular Neuropathies

Several diseases that affect small or medium-sized vessels may lead to ischemia or infarction of isolated peripheral nerves. The most common disorder is a mononeuropathy or multiple mononeuropathies that accompany periarteritis nodosa. Less commonly, rheumatoid arthritis, systemic lupus erythematosus, hypersensitivity angiitis, Sjögren's syndrome, or Wegener's granulomatosis may cause a similar peripheral neuropathy. Vascular neuropathies are characterized by the acute onset of motor and sensory loss in the distribution of one or more single peripheral nerves. With the passage of time, other nerves become involved. Depending on the intensity of the vasculitis, the neurologic deficit may resolve after weeks or months, only to affect another nerve at a distant place. Severe cases can involve so many nerves that the condition resembles a polyneuropathy rather than a mononeuritis multiplex. Usually a careful history will distinguish the focal onset of the latter.

POLYNEUROPATHY

Inflammatory/Immune Polyneuropathies

Several acute and chronic polyneuropathies are associated with inflammatory infiltrates in the peripheral nerves and roots. The mechanism of neurologic dysfunction is usually demyelination, believed usually to have an immune basis. Most of these disorders are rare, the exception being the common Guillain-Barré syndrome (GBS or acute postinfectious polyneuropathy). An acute disorder, GBS has a peak incidence in middle age but can affect all ages and races and both sexes. The disorder is characterized by a rapidly progressive, predominantly motor neuropathy that may paralyze all voluntary muscles, including those supplied by the cranial nerves and those controlling respiration. Sensory changes are usually milder than motor abnormalities and may include no more than tingling paresthesias in the hands and feet. Rarely, sensory loss may be profound and be more significant than motor weakness. Pain is common, as is some degree of autonomic dysfunction. Many patients suffer from hypertension or cardiac arrhythmias, the latter being the usual cause of death in the 5 per cent of patients who die. Bilateral facial paralysis is also common and helps distinguish the GBS from other polyneuropathies.

Characteristically, a previously healthy person who has suffered a mild respiratory infection in the past two or three weeks (other predisposing factors include swine flu vaccine, surgical procedures, and Hodgkin's disease) notes the painless onset of mild weakness in the lower extremities, often accompanied by tingling paresthesias in toes and fingers. Although the patient is aware of weakness, particularly when walking or climbing stairs, the examiner at this early stage may be unable to discern any abnormality save for diminished deep tendon reflexes. Over a matter of a few days, the weakness becomes more profound and often ascends from the lower extremities to the upper extremities and finally to the face (Landry's ascending paralysis). Deep tendon reflexes disappear, and the patient may complain of proprioceptive loss in arms and legs. It may become difficult for him to swallow and breathe. Examination now reveals symmetrical motor weakness of both proximal and distal muscles of all extremities. The spinal fluid protein concentration, which is normal during the first several days, rises often above 100 mg/dl, usually without an accompanying pleocytosis. In most instances the weakness progresses for several days to a couple of weeks and then stabilizes. After a period of stability, recovery begins and in 85 per cent of patients it is complete over several weeks to months.

Some patients require respiratory support and careful monitoring of cardiovascular function during the acute stages. Thus hospitalization is necessary until recovery is well under way. In a small minority of patients, neural function recovers only partially or not at all, and a few patients with persistently high spinal fluid proteins develop headaches and papilledema as a late complication of the illness. The pathogenesis of the latter is believed to be the plugging of arachnoid villi by the persistently elevated protein.

There is an unusual variant of GBS characterized by ataxia, oculomotor paralysis, and reflex absence. Other less common neuropathies that are probably GBS variants include a *chronic inflammatory neuropathy*, which may be progressive or relapsing and, unlike classic GBS, responds favorably to corticosteroid therapy, and acute neuropathies that predominantly involve either sensory or autonomic fibers. Recent evidence suggests that improvement in Guillain-Barré syndrome can be hastened by plasmapheresis, particularly when applied early in the course to rapidly advancing cases.

Other immune polyneuropathies not related to the Guillain-Barré syndrome are those associated with multiple myeloma, particularly of the osteoblastic variety, and benign monoclonal gammopathies. The neuropathy in these instances slowly progresses and has a sensorimotor distribution with no distinct systemic signs other than the alterations of serum proteins. The pathogenesis is thought to be immune in that the gamma globulin produced in excess by the primary disorder deposits on the nerves to react with a myelin-associated glycoprotein and cause demyelination. In the case of multiple myeloma, treatment of the primary disease sometimes leads to amelioration of the neuropathy.

Metabolic Neuropathies

Several metabolic diseases are associated with polyneuropathy. Diabetic neuropathy can take several forms (Table 119–10). The commonest is a distal, primarily sensory disorder that affects as many as 40 per cent of individuals who have had diabetes for more than 25 years. A few patients develop the neuropathy before clinical diabetes mellitus is discovered. One form affects *large fibers* and causes paresthesias in the feet, absence of ankle jerks, and diminished sensation. When severe this variant can cause paresthesias and weakness in the hands as well, although it rarely

---

TABLE 119–10. DIABETIC NEUROPATHIES

Symmetrical polyneuropathy
  Rapidly reversible
  Distal, primarily sensory—small fibers predominant
  Distal, primary motor—large fibers predominant or mixed
  Autonomic
Mononeuropathy and multiple mononeuropathy
  Cranial nerve lesions (especially oculomotor nerve)
  Focal peripheral nerve lesions
  Proximal lower extremity neuropathy (diabetic amyotrophy)

becomes extensive enough to be disabling. Another disorder involves primarily *small fibers*. Affected patients may complain of dull aching or burning pain in the feet, particularly at night. There is usually diminished touch and pin sensation in the lower extremities, but ankle jerks, proprioception, and motor function may be preserved. An *autonomic* form of diabetic neuropathy is characterized by paralysis of gastric emptying, constipation and/or episodic nocturnal diarrhea, orthostatic hypotension and other impaired cardiovascular reflexes, and urinary bladder paralysis. The most common autonomic manifestation is male impotence, which may affect as many as 50 per cent of diabetics and often provides the presenting symptom of the disorder. Autonomic symptoms may become severe enough to be disabling through either gastrointestinal or cardiovascular failure. *Pseudotabetic diabetic neuropathy* is rare. The clinical findings are severe impairment of cutaneous and deep sensation, leading to ulceration of the feet and the formation of Charcot joints, and proprioception so severely involved that patients have difficulty walking in the dark. Deep tendon reflexes are absent in the legs. There may be postural hypotension and Argyll Robertson pupils (p. 692).

In addition to the symmetrical polyneuropathies, which probably have a metabolic basis, diabetics also suffer from *mononeuropathy*, probably on a vascular basis. Unlike the polyneuropathies, most of which appear late in the course of established diabetes, mononeuropathies often occur in mild diabetics in whom the clinical diagnosis of diabetes is not suspected until neurologic symptoms develop. Among the common mononeuropathies are oculomotor palsies, the most frequent of which is third nerve paralysis, which begins abruptly and is associated with retro-orbital and forehead headache (see Table 118–4). All of the striated muscles supplied by the oculomotor nerve may be paralyzed. Pupillary function is usually spared, distinguishing the condition from compressive neuropathies of the oculomotor nerve such as caused by carotid aneurysms. The nerve usually recovers function spontaneously in several weeks. Other isolated lesions in individual nerves that have been reported in diabetes include the ulnar, radial, sciatic, and peroneal nerves, as well as the thoracic and abdominal nerve roots. As with the oculomotor palsy, the onset is abrupt and painful, and there is often complete recovery. *Diabetic amyotrophy* is a syndrome occurring in middle-aged mild diabetics and characterized by painful asymmetrical weakness of the thigh muscles with loss of knee jerks. Patients have characteristically suffered severe weight loss in the weeks preceding the onset of the diabetic amyotrophy. The weight loss suggests cachexia from cancer and the asymmetrical weakness of the lower extremities infiltration by tumor of the lumbosacral plexus. However, a glucose tolerance test will reveal diabetes, and with diet and diabetic control such patients usually recover.

TABLE 119–11. METABOLIC DISEASES OF PERIPHERAL NERVES

Endocrine
  Diabetes (polyneuropathy)
  Hypothyroidism
  Acromegaly (usually entrapment neuropathies)
Nutritional
  Vitamin deficiency
    Thiamine (beri-beri; Wernicke's disease)
    Pyridoxine (isoniazid toxicity)
    Vitamin B_{12} (pernicious anemia, gastrectomy)
  Multiple factors (alcohol)
  Malnutrition
Renal (uremia)
Hepatic
  Porphyria
  Chronic liver failure

Other Metabolic Neuropathies. Subacute or chronic sensorimotor neuropathies are associated with a variety of metabolic and nutritional disorders, as indicated in Table 119–11. The disorders have few individually characteristic signs, and the diagnosis is usually suggested by diagnosing the systemic disease; e.g., most patients with the peripheral neuropathy of acute intermittent porphyria have mental changes and/or abdominal pain preceding the onset of the neuropathy. Likewise the characteristic slow reflexes of hypothyroidism are usually present in addition to the sensorimotor polyneuropathy. In any patient suffering from a chronic progressive sensorimotor polyneuropathy, a careful search for metabolic disorders is essential to establish the diagnosis.

Toxic Neuropathies

Table 119–12 lists some of the toxins associated with polyneuropathies. In general, polyneuropathies produced by toxins are sensorimotor, although a few, such as acrylamide and pyridoxine toxicity, produce predominantly sensory changes. In every instance of obscure polyneuropathy, a careful occupational history and search for intoxicants, either knowingly or unknowingly ingested, is warranted.

Hereditary Neuropathies

Hereditary neuropathies are slowly progressive inherited disorders in which the pathogenesis is not clearly defined. Hereditary disorders may produce sensorimotor neuropathies, relatively pure sensory neuronopathies, or autonomic neuropathies (Table 119–13). In addition to the obvious hereditary disorders of peripheral nerves and sensory and autonomic neurons, several motor neuropathies have a genetic basis and others are of unknown cause. These are considered in the next section on motor neuron diseases.

MOTOR NEURON DISEASES

The term motor neuron disease refers to a group of chronic neurologic disorders affecting the anterior horn cells of the spinal cord and lower brain stem plus, in many instances, involving large motor neurons of the cerebral cortex that give rise to the corticospinal tract. Sensory changes or cerebellar dysfunction is absent. Some apply the term amyotrophic lateral sclerosis to all of the motor neuron diseases of unknown cause beginning in adulthood. Others use the term motor neuron disease to apply to the general condition and subclassify the variations (Table 119–14). If both upper and lower motor neuron abnormalities are found, the disorder is called *amyotrophic lateral sclerosis* (ALS). *Progressive bulbar palsy* causes relatively rapidly advancing upper and lower motor neuron involvement of the muscles of the jaw, pharynx, and tongue. When there are no signs of upper motor neuron disease and only slowly progressive muscle wasting and weakness, the disorder is termed *progressive muscular atrophy* (PMA).

Amyotrophic Lateral Sclerosis

Amyotrophic lateral sclerosis (ALS) affects first bulbar muscles, one or both of the extremities on one side of the body, the lower or upper extremities symmetrically, or all four limbs simultaneously. The disorder's incidence increases with advancing age and progresses over two to seven years until death. The bulbar form has the shortest course, PMA the longest (often more than 10 years), and ALS intermediate. The disease usually is sporadic, but familial groupings have occurred, indicating either a genetic predisposition or common exposure to an unknown causative agent. Familial cases tend to affect younger persons and to progress more rapidly than do sporadic ones. Despite extensive searches to establish ALS as an autoimmune or slow virus disease, no firm leads exist, and the cause of the motor neuron degeneration remains unknown.

The typical patient develops progressive weakness affecting distal more than proximal structures, especially the small muscles of the hand. The disease may develop quite asymmetrically. There is prominent and early atrophy and fasciculations. The patients may have muscle cramps but rarely sensory symptoms. The deep tendon reflexes are usually preserved, at least in the upper extremities, in the early phase of the disease. Signs of upper motor neuron involvement may develop at any time but almost always appear by the time muscle involvement has lasted a year. These include spasticity, particularly in the lower extremities, with associated hyperreflexia, clonus, and extensor plantar responses on one or both sides. Characteristically, the superficial abdominal reflexes and the cremasteric reflexes as well as the bladder and bowel functions remain normal. Generalized fasciculations and muscle atrophy in most instances involve the lower extremities later than the upper. ALS spares the extraocular muscles but in the late stages can interfere with supranuclear oculomotor control. Some patients show signs of emotional lability. Intellectual functions deteriorate in approximately 5

TABLE 119–12. CAUSES OF TOXIC NEUROPATHIES

PHARMACEUTICAL AGENTS	OTHER AGENTS
Chloramphenicol	Acrylamide (truncal ataxia)
Dapsone*	Arsenic (sensory, brown skin, Mees' lines)
Disulfiram	
Dichloracetate	Buckthorn toxin
Ethionamide	Carbon disulfide
Gold	Cyanide
Glutethimide	Dimethylaminopropionitrile (urinary complaints)
Hydralazine	
Isoniazid†	Dichlorophenoxyacetic acid
Lithium	Biologic toxin in diphtheritic neuropathy (pharyngeal neuropathy)
Metronidazole-misonidazole	
Nitrofurantoin*	
Nitrous oxide	Ethylene oxide
Platinum (cis-platinum)†	n-Hexane
Pyridoxine†	Lead (wrist drop, abdominal colic)
Sodium cyanate	Lucel-7 (cataracts)
Thalidomide†	Methyl bromide
Vincristine	Organophosphates (cholinergic symptoms, delayed onset of neuropathy)
	Thallium (pain, alopecia, Mees' lines)
	Trichlorethylene (facial numbness)

* Predominantly motor.
† Predominantly sensory.
Modified from Schaumburg HH: Toxic Neuropathy. In Wyngaarden JB, and Smith LH Jr (eds): Cecil Textbook of Medicine. 17th ed. Philadelphia, WB Saunders Co, 1985, p 2195.

per cent. The cerebrospinal fluid is normal. EMG testing is helpful (see Table 115–6). The motor nerve conduction velocities remain normal even in the presence of severe atrophy, a finding that separates this disorder from the peripheral motor neuropathies, in which conduction velocities are reduced.

In its classic form, ALS, with painless weakness and atrophy of the hands, fasciculations in the entire upper extremities, and spasticity and reflex hyperactivity of the legs with extensor plantar responses, may be mistaken for a cervical spinal cord tumor or other myelopathy. However, in ALS the lack of sensory changes, the frequent presence of fasciculations in the tongue, and EMG findings of denervation in the lower extremities almost always establish the diagnosis. In only a few instances is myelography necessary to rule out a cer-

TABLE 119–13. SOME HEREDITARY NEUROPATHIES

Lipid Disorders
Metachromatic leukodystrophy (sulfatide metabolism)
Krabbe's disease (ceramide galactoside metabolism)
Lipoprotein deficiency
    Bassen-Kornzweig (beta-lipoprotein deficiencies)
    Tangier disease (high density lipoprotein)
Refsum's disease (phytanic acid metabolism)
Fabry's disease (alpha-galactosidase deficiency)
Unknown Cause (hereditary sensorimotor neuropathy)
    Type I—Hypertrophic form of Charcot-Marie-Tooth peroneal muscular atrophy
    Type II—Neuronal form of Charcot-Marie-Tooth peroneal muscular atrophy
    Type III—Dejerine-Sottas hypertrophic neuropathy

TABLE 119–14. MOTOR NEURON DISEASES

Motor neuron disease (amyotrophic lateral sclerosis) includes:
Progressive muscular atrophy
Progressive bulbar palsy
Amyotrophic lateral sclerosis
   Sporadic forms
   Familial forms
   Western Pacific (Guam and Japan)
Spinal muscular atrophies
   Werdnig-Hoffman disease
   Wohlfart-Kugelberg-Welander disease
   Proximal
   Distal
   Scapuloperoneal form
   Facioscapulohumeral form
   Juvenile progressive bulbar palsy
Motor neuron disease associated with other disease of the central nervous system
   Mental disorder
   Extrapyramidal disorders
   Spinal disease including the hereditary spinocerebellar ataxias
Miscellaneous diseases
   Infections
   Metabolic, including hypoglycemia
   Toxicity—heavy metals, organophosphorus compounds
   Ischemic myelopathy, including radiation damage
   Trauma, including electrical injury
   Paraneoplastic

vical cord lesion. Likewise, in its typical form, PMA with its widespread weakness and atrophy affecting primarily distal muscles and both proximal and distal fasciculations, is only rarely confused with peripheral neuropathy or muscle disease. The characteristic neurogenic EMG and the lack of creatine kinase elevation rule out muscle disease. Most peripheral nerve disorders cause sensory impairment and rarely cause fasciculations; they are also associated with slowing of electrical conduction velocity, a finding not found in PMA. Progressive bulbar palsy must be distinguished from myasthenia gravis and myopathies, in particular polymyositis. Upper motor neuron signs such as a hyperactive jaw jerk and emotional lability and spastic speech establish the diagnosis of motor neuron disease. Marked atrophy and fasciculations of the tongue likewise establish that diagnosis. If these findings are absent, an edrophonium test (see p. 711) and EMG of bulbar muscles may be necessary to make the distinction. Early in its course, if motor neuron disease affects only a few contiguous muscles, it must be distinguished from nerve root or plexus disease. The finding of widespread electromyographic abnormalities, when clinical findings are localized, usually establishes the diagnosis of motor neuron disease.

Werdnig-Hoffman Disease

Werdnig-Hoffman disease is a progressive impairment of the motor system occurring in infancy and early childhood. The lower motor neuron is exclusively involved, leading to paralysis of muscles innervated by motor cranial nuclei and anterior horn cells of the spinal cord. Infants and young children may present with this syndrome at birth or in the first few months of life with diffuse flaccidity, muscular atrophy, muscle fasciculations, and reduced to absent myotatic reflexes with associated respiratory and swallowing difficulties. There may be prominent lingual fasciculations and atrophy, and the cerebrospinal fluid is normal. Electromyography shows denervation with normal peripheral nerve conduction velocities. The disorder is an autosomal recessive trait. The cause is not known.

Wohlfart-Kugelberg-Welander Disease

Wohlfart-Kugelberg-Welander disease is an autosomal recessive disorder in which symptoms begin during late childhood, adolescence, or early adulthood and include progressive *proximal* muscle atrophy, weakness, and fasciculations. It is slowly progressive and is usually compatible with a lifespan into the third or fourth decade. Typical examples have been described in families in which other children have Werdnig-Hoffman disease. Thus, varying penetrance of a single genetic mutation inherited in an autosomal recessive manner may produce either an aggressive form of early childhood motor neuron disease (Werdnig-Hoffman disease) or a more benign form of motor neuron disease in later childhood and early adulthood (Wohlfart-Kugelberg-Welander disease). The onset in the first and second decade of life of proximal weakness and atrophy with fasciculations but a very slow progression without evidence of upper motor neuron involvement separates this disorder from amyotrophic lateral sclerosis. Both Wohlfart-Kugelberg-Welander disease and polymyositis may present with progressive proximal weakness and atrophy. If fasciculations are not prominent, electromyography (denervation with the insertional irritability of polymyositis) and muscle biopsy (see p. 647) establish the diagnosis. These tests distinguish the neurogenic disease from acquired or inherited myopathies. The cause of the disorder is unknown, and specific therapy is not available.

Other Anterior Horn Cell Diseases

Monomyeleic amyotrophy is a rare disorder in which lower motor neurons supplying one extremity (usually an arm) are affected. The disease usually begins in the second or third decade and progresses over a period of two to four years and then stops. The patient is left with a variable degree of weakness in the involved extremity, but the disease does not generalize and is usually not disabling. *Poliomyelitis* (see also p. 557) is an acute inflammatory disease of the anterior horn cell which was a major cause of paralysis in the United States before the development of an effective polio vaccine. A similar but much less severe weakness can occasionally be caused by other neurotropic viruses. *Subacute motor neuronopathy*, a remote effect of Hodgkin's disease, is a rare cause of slowly progressive muscle weakness and wasting. The disorder is thought to be caused by a neurotropic virus.

DISORDERS OF THE SPINAL CORD

The spinal cord may be affected by any of the numerous disorders that damage nervous system tissue. Some of these conditions represent only a portion of wide involvement of the nervous system (e.g., spinocerebellar degenerations), whereas others are unique to the spinal cord (spinal neoplasms or arteriovenous malformations).

NEOPLASMS OF THE SPINAL CORD

Neoplastic growths that cause nerve root or spinal cord disorders can begin in the paravertebral, extradural, intradural, or intramedullary compartments. Most neoplasms that cause spinal cord compression are extradural and metastatic. Most extradural neoplasms originate in the vertebral body and compress spinal roots or cord without invading them. Most intradural neoplasms also cause symptoms by compressing spinal roots or cord without invading, but unlike extradural neoplasms, the majority are benign and slow growing. Intramedullary neoplasms cause symptoms by both invading and compressing spinal structures; the tumors may be either benign or malignant.

Paravertebral Tumors. Neoplastic lesions that begin in or metastasize to the paravertebral space often cause serious and perplexing neurologic problems. The tumor may extend longitudinally within the paravertebral space, progressively compressing nerve roots as it grows. At times, the tumor may grow through an intervertebral foramen and compress not only the nerve root but also the spinal cord. Rarely, spinal cord symptoms may be caused by ischemia from compression of radicular arteries that supply the spinal cord. If the tumor lies lateral to the immediate paravertebral space, it may compress the brachial, lumbar, or sacral plexus, causing symptoms similar to root compression but with a different pattern of sensory and motor loss. The symptoms of extravertebral tumors begin insidiously with severe, unrelenting pain, often with a burning quality. The pain is localized just lateral to the spine and radiates, bandlike, in the distribution of the involved dermatome(s). If the lesion involves abdominal or thoracic roots, objective motor and sensory changes often are minimal, but autonomic changes may be prominent or the only neurologic sign. *Hyperhidrosis* occurring in a band coinciding with the site of the pain strongly suggests the diagnosis. When the tumor involves cervical or lumbar roots, the pain may be soon followed by numbness in the fingertips or toes, with accompanying weakness and reflex diminution, depending on the roots involved. Autonomic changes, including anhidrosis or hyperhidrosis, can affect the arm or leg, while Horner's syndrome and/or diaphragmatic paralysis often accompany cervical or upper thoracic paravertebral tumors. The diagnosis of paravertebral tumors is best established by CT or MRI at the level suggested by the clinical findings. The CT scan also can determine whether the lesion has grown through the intervertebral foramen or has eroded vertebral bodies. Myelography may be performed to assess the extent of intravertebral tumors.

The differential diagnosis of paravertebral tumor includes a variety of other disorders that can cause paravertebral pain with or without compression of nerve roots. *Psychophysiological* muscle tension syndromes often cause paravertebral low back or neck pain. In some instances, there may be radiation of the pain, but usually in a nondermatomal distribution. On examination, there is often marked tenderness of muscle, which sometimes can be relieved by injecting the trigger point with saline solution or a local anesthetic. Temporary improvement of pain after such injection does not imply that structural disease is absent, since trigger points can equally well be a reaction to spinal or nerve root disease. In muscle tension syndrome, however, autonomic, sensory, or motor changes are not present. Disease of the kidneys and other viscera lying in the retroperitoneal space may cause pain similar to that of paravertebral tumors, but the pain usually does not radiate and is not associated with autonomic, motor, or sensory changes. Percussion of the involved viscera reproduces the pain that is described as a dull ache rather than a neurogenic burning pain. Entrapment neuropathies occasionally mimic the symptoms of paravertebral tumor. Chronic *post-thoracotomy pain* probably results from entrapment of nerve roots at the time of operation, perhaps with neuroma formation. The pain characteristically appears shortly after surgery and may be unremitting for many years. Motor, sensory, or autonomic changes are rare. Such pain sometimes can be relieved by paravertebral anesthetic blocks.

The management of paravertebral masses depends on the diagnosis. In patients known to have cancer, particularly lymphomas or carcinomas of the breast or lung, the tumor can be assumed to be metastatic and should be treated with radiation therapy and, if available, chemotherapy. If the patient has no known primary lesion, resection may be attempted, both to establish a diagnosis and to decompress the nerve roots. Once biopsy establishes diagnosis, further therapy such as radiation or chemotherapy can be chosen.

Extradural Tumors. Extradural neoplasms can compress spinal roots and cord in one of two ways. Either they arise in vertebrae surrounding the spinal cord and grow into the epidural space, or they arise in the paravertebral space and grow through the intervertebral foramen so as to compress the cord without involving either vertebral or paravertebral structures. Most extradural neoplasms are metastatic from carcinomas of the breast, lung, prostate, or kidney or from malignant melanoma. Some extradural neoplasms arise de novo in the vertebral bodies (e.g., chordoma, osteogenic sarcoma, myeloma, chondrosarcoma). A minority of extradural neoplasms are benign (e.g., chordoma, osteoma, osteoid osteoma, angioma). Pain, the first symptom, may precede other symptoms of spinal cord compression by weeks or months, depending on the rate of growth of the tumor. Rarely, extradural neoplasms may be painless, with the first symptoms being those of spinal cord dysfunction. The first spinal cord symptoms other than pain usually consist of corticospinal tract dysfunction with weakness, spasticity, and hyperreflexia, followed by paresthesias and loss of vibration and position sense. Unless the lesion compresses the conus medullaris or the cauda equina, bladder and bowel dysfunctions are late signs. As with other causes of spinal cord compression, extradural neoplasms cause symptoms first distally and later proximally. Thus, even thoracic and cervical neoplasms generally cause weakness and numbness in the legs before trunk and upper extremity muscles are involved. The diagnosis of extradural spinal cord compression must be suspected by the history of pain followed by signs and symptoms of spinal cord dysfunction and confirmed by radiographic study. In about 85 per cent of patients suffering from extradural spinal cord compression, plain radiographs reveal bone lesions at the site of compression. In the few remaining patients x-ray tomography, radionuclide bone scan, or CT scan may demonstrate a bone lesion. The diagnosis of extradural spinal cord compression and its localization require myelography. A myelogram not only establishes the site of cord compression but also determines that the compression is extradural rather than intradural or intramedullary. The differential diagnosis of extradural neoplasms includes inflammatory disease of bone and epidural abscess (e.g., vertebral tuberculosis, bacterial osteomyelitis), acute or subacute epidural hematomas, herniated intervertebral discs, spondylosis, and, very rarely, extreme extramedullary hematopoiesis (in patients with severe and chronic anemias) or epidural lipomatosis (in patients on chronic steroid therapy). Often a definitive diagnosis can be made only by biopsy of the lesion, either during the course of decompressive laminectomy or by percutaneous needle biopsy of the involved vertebral body.

The treatment of extradural neoplasms depends on the cause. Most neoplasms that cause extradural spinal cord compression are malignant and progress rapidly. Once spinal cord symptoms begin, paraplegia may develop in a matter of days. Complete paraplegia is usually irreversible, whereas patients with only moderate spinal cord dysfunction often recover. Thus, the early diagnosis and vigorous emergency treatment of extradural spinal cord compression is mandatory. The treatment includes corticosteroids (dexamethasone 16 to 100 mg daily) to decrease spinal cord edema. In patients not known to be suffering from a primary cancer, metastatic disease is the most common cause of extradural spinal cord compression, but in these instances a definitive diagnosis must be made by biopsy. Such patients should begin corticosteroid therapy followed by surgery with removal of as much tumor as possible for both diagnostic and therapeutic purposes. When a primary cancer already has been diagnosed treatment consists of radiation therapy and chemotherapeutic agents (if an effective agent is available). In patients in whom radiation therapy and chemotherapy are ineffective, resection of the vertebral body involved by tumor may delay the development of paraplegia. Benign extradural tumors require surgery and usually can be completely removed.

Intradural Extramedullary Tumors. Most intradural tumors are benign. Meningiomas and neurofibromas are the two most common types. Teratomas, arachnoid cysts, and lipomas are less common causes. Meningiomas occur especially in middle-aged and elderly women, predominantly in the thoracic spinal cord. Another common site is the foramen magnum. Meningiomas grow slowly. Pain is the first symptom in most patients, but in about 25 per cent the growth is painless, the first symptoms being those indicating gradually developing spinal cord compression. Because meningiomas most often are located on the posterior aspect of the cord, paresthesias and sensory changes beginning distally in the lower extremities are a frequent early symptom and are often mistaken for peripheral neuropathy. As the disease progresses, however, the development of corticospinal tract signs indicates the spinal origin of the symptoms. Even when spinal cord signs and symptoms are obvious, the occasional lack of pain may lead one to suspect a degenerative or demyelinating disease such as multiple sclerosis rather than a neoplasm. In patients with meningiomas, the lumbar puncture reveals an elevated CSF protein content well above that found in degenerative or demyelinating diseases. CT, MRI, or myelography usually establishes the diagnosis of a tumor. The treatment of spinal cord compression from meningiomas is surgical removal. Because the tumor grows so slowly and the cord has an opportunity to adapt to compression, even patients with severe neurologic disability often recover fully.

The second most common cause of intradural spinal cord compression is neurofibroma. Because these tumors usually arise from the dorsal root, radicular pain is often the first symptom, preceding signs of spinal cord compression by months or years. When spinal cord compression develops, it progresses slowly. Some patients with spinal neurofibromas suffer from neurofibromatosis (see p. 730). That diagnosis may be suspected either by a positive family history or by the cutaneous stigmata of the disorder. As neurofibromas grow through the intervertebral foramen, they enlarge it, a finding appreciated by an appropriately positioned radiograph. The CSF protein is almost always elevated. The diagnosis is established by myelography. Surgical extirpation of the lesion usually leads to recovery.

Occasionally metastatic tumors involving the leptomeninges produce intradural extramedullary mass lesions. Pain is almost always a prominent early symptom, and spinal cord compression develops more rapidly than it does with the more benign intradural tumors. In addition, malignant cells are usually found on cerebrospinal fluid examination. The glucose concentration may be low and the protein concentration elevated. The treatment of intradural malignant neoplasms is by radiation and chemotherapy, since complete surgical extirpation is almost always impossible.

Intramedullary Tumors. The most common intramedullary spinal tumors are astrocytomas (usually benign) and ependymomas. Other tumors that occasionally cause intramedullary spinal lesions are hemangioblastomas, lipomas, and metastases (Fig. 119–5). Pain is an early symptom of most intramedullary tumors, and signs of spinal cord dysfunction progress rapidly or slowly, depending on the growth characteristics of the tumor. Intramedullary tumors are often associated with syringomelia, the syrinx sometimes lying at a distance from the primary tumor and producing its own symptoms of spinal dysfunction (p. 729). The so-called classic signs of intramedullary spinal cord lesions (dissociated sensory loss, sacral sparing, and early onset of bladder and bowel dysfunction) are not reliable enough clinically to distinguish intramedullary from extramedullary lesions; currently that diagnosis must be established by myelography, although MR imaging probably will provide definitive diagnosis in the future. In some patients with long-standing benign intramedullary lesions, plain radiographs of the spine may show widening of the spinal canal and erosion of the pedicles. Myelography reveals an enlarged spinal cord, sometimes with complete block to the passage of myelographic contrast material. If a syrinx is suspected, a CT scan six hours after myelography performed with water-soluble contrast material usually reveals contrast material in the syrinx. The differential diagnosis of intramedullary tumors includes intramedullary abscesses and syringomyelia without tumor. A definitive diagnosis is established by biopsy. Successful surgical removal of intramedullary tumors is possible, particularly with ependymomas and hemangioblastomas but sometimes with gliomas as well. A highly skilled and experienced surgeon, however, is necessary for tumors to be removed without producing increased neurologic symptoms. If the tumor cannot be totally excised, postoperative radiation may delay recurrence.

Ependymomas have a predilection to involve the lower end of the spinal cord and the filum terminale. An unusual symptom sometimes produced by such tumors is *hydrocephalus.* Affected patients may present with headache, papilledema, and enlarged cerebral ventricles without signs of cauda equina dysfunction or with only minor signs such as mild sacral sensory loss or an absent ankle jerk. The pathogenesis of the hydrocephalus is believed to be the plugging of arachnoid granulations by protein exuded from the tumor into the spinal fluid. The diagnosis is suspected in a patient with papilledema and hydrocephalus accompanied by a high CSF protein; myelography establishes the diagnosis.

FIGURE 119–5. An intramedullary metastasis. A man with oat cell carcinoma of lung, in remission, complained of progressive weakness of the lower extremities and loss of bladder, bowel, and sexual function. A metrizamide myelogram revealed an area of enlargement at the conus medullaris (arrow), indicating a hematogenous metastasis to the spinal cord.

INFLAMMATORY DISEASES OF THE SPINAL CANAL (see Chapter 124)

Vascular Disorders of the Spinal Canal

Extradural, intradural, and intramedullary vascular disorders all can cause spinal cord compression. The most common and serious extradural vascular disease is *spinal epidural hematoma.*

Hemorrhage into the spinal epidural space may occur spontaneously or be associated with trauma, a bleeding diathesis, or a vascular malformation. The condition occurs particularly among patients being treated with anticoagulants. It may occasionally follow lumbar puncture, particularly in patients with bleeding abnormalities or receiving anticoagulants. The hemorrhage usually arises from the epidural venous plexus and tends to collect over the dorsum of the spinal cord, covering several segments. The clinical picture is characterized by the sudden or rapid onset of severe localized back pain and spinal cord dysfunction, often leading to complete paraplegia in several hours. If the patient has a known bleeding disorder, the clinical diagnosis is easily established. In patients without known bleeding or clotting disorders, the differential diagnosis includes acute epidural abscess and acute transverse myelopathy. Although occasional patients recover spontaneously from paraparesis related to epidural spinal cord compression, most require emergency surgical evacuation to save spinal cord function. The more rapidly the paralysis develops and the longer the delay in decompression, the less likely is recovery.

Spinal arteriovenous malformations (Fig. 119–6) may cause symptoms by hemorrhage, compression, or ischemia. Spinal subarachnoid hemorrhage is characterized by the sudden onset of back pain, often with a radicular component, with or without the development of signs of spinal cord compression. A lumbar puncture reveals evidence of subarachnoid hemorrhage with red cells, xanthochromic spinal fluid, and usually an elevated protein concentration. In the absence of spinal cord signs, the differential diagnosis includes spontaneous intracranial subarachnoid hemorrhage. The diagnosis of spinal subarachnoid hemorrhage often can be suspected clinically because symptoms begin with back pain rather than with headache as in intracranial hemorrhage.

Vascular malformations within the substance of the spinal cord may give rise to intramedullary hemorrhage (hematomyelia) as well as subarachnoid hemorrhage. The sudden development of partial or complete transverse myelopathy is the most common onset. If there is bleeding into the subarachnoid space, pain in the neck and back and other signs of meningeal irritation occur.

Spinal arteriovenous malformations may also gradually compress the spinal cord or give rise to hemodynamic changes that result in spinal ischemia. In such cases, patients present with slowly progressive, sometimes episodically worsening symptoms of spinal cord dysfunction. Transient exacerbation of symptoms may occur in association with menstrual periods or pregnancy.

Complete or partial recovery of function can follow episodes of spinal cord ischemia or even small hemorrhages. The unchanging localization of the attacks and the prominence of pain help differentiate symptoms caused by arteriovenous malformations from other recurrent neurologic disorders such as multiple sclerosis. Rarely, a bruit may be heard by auscultation of the spine or back over the site of the malformation. Myelography often reveals vascular shadows suggesting the presence of arteriovenous malformation. Angiography with regional catheterization of radicular vessels is necessary to establish the diagnosis and as a preliminary step to surgical treatment. Advances in microsurgery have increased considerably the chances for satisfactory removal or obliteration of spinal vascular malformations. Embolization of the malformation or ligation of feeding arteries has been performed when the lesion cannot be removed surgically.

INHERITED AND DEVELOPMENTAL STRUCTURAL DISORDERS

Congenital anomalies of the spine are common and are often encountered on radiographs of patients suffering from neck or low back pain. Some congenital anomalies such as spina bifida occulta are so common as to be considered variants of normal and are probably never responsible in and of themselves for low back pain. Other congenital anomalies that are usually asymptomatic but are potential causes of neck or back pain include *façet tropism* (misalignment of the facets on the two sides of the corresponding vertebral body; several authorities believe that this increases rotational stress on the facet joints and may cause back pain); *transitional vertebrae* (e.g., sacralization of a lumbar vertebra or lumbarization of a sacral vertebra) altering spinal mechanics, resulting in instability and stress, and sometimes producing back pain; and *spondylolisthesis* (forward slipping of one vertebral body onto another, caused by a defect between the articular facets). A third group of congenital anomalies of the spine consists of those that are likely to cause not only neck or back pain but also neurologic disability. These include basilar impression, which is often associated with Arnold-Chiari malformation (see next section). Severe spinal scoliosis or kyphosis, congenital

FIGURE 119–6. Spinal arteriovenous malformation. A metrizamide myelogram demonstrates a tangle of abnormal vessels (arrows) on the surface of the cord.

stenosis of the lumbar or cervical spinal canal, anterior and lateral spinal meningoceles and diastematomyelia are other causes of back pain and neurologic disability. *Diastematomyelia* is a bony abnormality that divides the spinal canal, leading to duplication of the spinal cord. It is usually associated with spina bifida. Sometimes the bony septum can be identified on plain x-ray. Patients who become symptomatic in adulthood almost always have some cutaneous abnormality, especially hypertrichosis over the sacral area. The disorder may be associated with other congenital abnormalities of the central nervous system as well.

Abnormalities of the Craniocervical Junction

Basilar impression consists of invagination of the odontoid process into the foramen magnum. Occasionally the condition arises from occipital bone softening due to Paget's disease, fibrous dysplasia, or cancer. Much more often basilar impression occurs as a congenital defect, often associated with anomalies of the foramen magnum, the Arnold-Chiari malformation, or syringomyelia. Symptoms of congenital basilar impression often first appear in the third or fourth decade of life and reflect the presence of either vertebral artery compression-ischemia or direct medullopontine compression-displacement. Occipital headache, vertigo, nystagmus, dysarthria, dysphagia, ataxia, abnormalities of central respiratory control, and long tract signs begin insidiously and progress gradually. Many patients develop a secondary obstructive hydrocephalus. Diagnosis is suggested by the clinical findings plus an abnormally short neck on inspection. Confirmation comes from roentgenographic or imaging evidence of protrusion of the odontoid process above the foramen magnum.

The *Arnold-Chiari malformation* type II consists of developmental displacement of the cerebellar tonsils through the foramen magnum, associated with elongation of the medulla and lower end of the fourth ventricle into the cervical canal. Symptoms can resemble those described for basilar impression, can be entirely due to obstructive hydrocephalus, or can reflect a progressive cerebellar ataxia. In any event, signs of spinal long tract dysfunction gradually become added to the above. CT or, especially, MR images disclose the characteristic morphologic abnormality (Fig. 119–7). Treatment of either basilar impression or the Arnold-Chiari malformation causing progressive neurologic deficits consists of surgical decompression or, when appropriate, ventricular shunting to relieve hydrocephalus.

Syringomyelia refers to a cavity within the central spinal cord, arising most often at the cervical level. The lesions often extend into the medulla (syringobulbia) or can penetrate caudally into the thoracic and lumbosacral regions.

Pathologically, the syringomyelic cavity usually is associated anatomically with the central spinal canal; some communicate directly with the floor of the fourth ventricle. As life advances, the

FIGURE 119–7. Midsagittal MR image of Chiari malformation (small black arrows) and syringomyelia (three white-black arrows) in a 33-year-old man. Note the cerebellar tonsils extending below the posterior rim of the foramen magnum (dark structure immediately above the black arrow). The syrinx extends from the medulla well into the thoracic cord.

syrinx progressively replaces the centrally located gray matter of the posterior and anterior horns of the spinal cord and also interrupts the decussating spinothalamic pain-carrying fibers in the anterior commissure. Often, syringomyelia is associated with other congenital malformations, including the Arnold-Chiari malformation (Fig. 119–7), fusion of the cervical vertebrae, or malformations at the lumbosacral region, including spina bifida and associated meningomyelocele.

Clinical manifestations of syringomyelia most often begin in the second or third decade, frequently affecting the hands or upper trunk with a typically dissociated impairment of pain and temperature sensation coupled with preservation of the senses of touch, vibration, and joint position. Progressive muscular atrophy usually develops in the involved segments, especially in the upper extremities, and commonly leads to kyphoscoliosis. The analgesia results in painless ulcers, burns, and traumatic arthropathy. As a rule, areflexia marks the upper extremities, while upper motor neuron signs eventually develop in the legs, accompanied in those members by reduced vibratory and position sensations. In most affected patients the disease process progresses slowly but relentlessly.

In patients with syringobulbia, dissociated impairment of pain and temperature develops over the face, along with nystagmus, pharyngeal and vocal cord paralysis, and lingual atrophy.

Clinical diagnosis is usually not difficult once

considered. Leprosy, other rare and acquired peripheral neuropathies, and intramedullary destructive or neoplastic lesions of the spinal cord and brain stem are the only insidiously developing conditions that cause widespread dissociated loss of pain and temperature sensation. Leprosy can be dismissed if the subject has not been raised in an endemic area, and neither it nor other peripheral neuropathies produce signs of spinal cord dysfunction. The important consideration is whether or not an associated spinal neoplasm exists. MR imaging definitively outlines most syrinxes and neoplasms if present. If unavailable, metrizamide myelography followed by delayed CT scan usually defines the lesion. Treatment generally is unsatisfactory unless a tumor is found and can be removed. Surgical drainage has been claimed to halt the disease process in some patients. Some surgeons believe that plugging the opening of a syrinx into the fourth ventricle improves the prognosis but scant evidence supports the suggestion.

NEUROCUTANEOUS SYNDROMES

Neurofibromatosis, sometimes called Von Recklinghausen's disease, is a common disorder inherited as an autosomal dominant trait and characterized by the occurrence of pigmented skin lesions (café au lait spots), multiple tumors of spinal or cranial nerves (neurofibromas composed of proliferating fibroblasts or neurilemmal sheath cells), skin tumors, and the frequent occurrence of intracranial meningiomas. There is an increased association with pheochromocytomas, cystic lung disease, renal vascular lesions causing hypertension, fibrous dysplasia of bone, and medullary thyroid carcinoma, as well as other tumors of endocrine glands. The tumors can overlap in the region of the brachial or sacral plexus to produce large plexiform neuromas that can evolve into malignant sarcomas. Intracranial astrocytomas and glioblastomas occur with a greater than normal frequency. Stenosis of the aqueduct with noncommunicating hydrocephalus is sometimes observed.

Replacement of normal bone with fibroblasts and fibrocytes in some patients results in bone overgrowth with occlusion of cranial foramina, rarefaction, and cyst formation. Congenital osteoagenesis in various bones, as well as bone cysts, pseudoarthroses of the tibia, local extremity gigantism, and scoliosis can be encountered. Ectopic islands of gray matter and focal gliosis in the cerebrum may be the basis for an increased incidence of mental retardation.

The presence of multiple cutaneous neurofibromas accompanied by macular café au lait spots represent the clinical hallmarks. The pigmented skin lesions occur most commonly over the trunk and in the axilla. If greater than 1.5 cm in diameter and more than six in number, they indicate the presence of the disease. Nerve involvement can be solitary or multiple and diffuse. Multiple cranial nerves can be affected, resulting in facial weakness, numbness, deafness, and optic nerve atrophy. Local confluent tumors with associated fibrosis result in elephantiasis neuromatosa, as well as gross asymmetrical hypertrophy of body parts. Neurofibromas arising from nerve roots can invade the intervertebral foramina to compress the spinal cord or brain stem. Bilateral cerebellar pontine angle tumors are almost always neurofibromatous in origin.

Neurofibromatosis is diagnosed readily by the occurrence of the characteristic neurofibromas and pigmented skin lesions. The tumors vary considerably in size; most are smooth, soft, and multilobulated; and most can be palpated along the course of a peripheral nerve. Biopsy gives the definitive answer.

Hypertensive patients must be evaluated for the possibility of renal artery stenosis as well as for pheochromocytoma. Cranial nerve palsies and hydrocephalus signal the presence of an intracranial neoplasm and the need for imaging studies.

Tuberous sclerosis is a neurocutaneous disorder inherited as an autosomal dominant trait. Its triad of findings, all present by late childhood, include facial nevi (adenoma sebaceum), epilepsy, and mental retardation. The importance of the disorder for adult medicine is that subtle cases occasionally produce problems in the differential diagnosis of early or late adolescent epilepsy, while funduscopic examination can disclose nodules or phakomas of the retina that look neoplastic but in fact are stable and similar in structure to the adenoma sebaceum. Some patients develop intracranial or optic gliomas. Rhabdomyomas of the heart as well as renal tumors and neoplasms of the endocrine organs are sometimes observed.

Sturge-Weber disease produces a port wine–colored capillary hemangioma on the face accompanied by a similar vascular malformation of the underlying meninges and cerebral cortex. The cause is unknown. Diagnosis is made by observing the disfiguring stain involving the sensory dermatomal distribution of the first, second, or third portions of the trigeminal nerve. General or focal motor seizures may occur with or without associated mental retardation and require antiepileptic medication. The disfiguring stain deserves cosmetic repair if possible.

Hippel-Lindau disease is inherited in a simple autosomal dominant pattern producing hemangioblastomas of the cerebellar hemispheres with associated angiomas of the retina and cystic changes in the kidney and pancreas. The condition can produce cerebellar neoplasms, cerebellar hemorrhage, brain stem vascular malformations, or hemangioma of the retina. An association with pheochromocytomas and polycythemia has been noted.

D. DISEASES OF THE BASAL GANGLIA

GENERAL CONSIDERATIONS

The basal ganglia, a group of symmetrically placed large deep cerebral nuclei, include the caudate nucleus and putamen (together known as the striatum), the globus pallidus or pallidum, the subthalamic nucleus, and the substantia nigra of the midbrain (Fig. 119–8). The functions of the basal ganglia are best deduced from their diseases. The ganglia especially influence the control of trunk and proximal appendicular movement by feeding information forward to the frontal cortex before that region sends its final signals to the craniospinal motor neurons via the corticospinal tract. Interruption of the corticospinal pathway ameliorates or interrupts signs of basal ganglia dysfunction. The basal ganglia exert a major influence on the planning of movement and in establishing the postural platform upon which corticospinal influences erect skilled distal activity. An earlier view that the ganglia projected directly to the spinal level led to their designation as the extrapyramidal motor system. Although a more accurate term would be prepyramidal, the older designation has persisted.

The basal ganglia contain a distinct neurotransmitter anatomy. Corticostriatal and thalamostriatal afferents are both excitatory in their action, probably employing glutamine as a transmitter (Fig. 119–8). The well-known nigrostriatal input employs dopamine. Dopaminergic synapses probably exist on all neuronal types within the striatum, although the functionally most important receptors appear to lie on the axon terminals of incoming corticostriate fibers. The striatum also contains many cholinergic interneurons believed functionally to oppose the dopaminergic input. This latter action may help explain why anticholinergic drugs often improve the symptoms of parkinsonism. The major outputs of the basal ganglia to all of their known projection areas predominantly employ the inhibitory transmitter GABA. A number of neuropeptides have been identified in the nuclei, but their functional significance remains unknown.

PARKINSONISM

Parkinsonism is a syndrome consisting, in variable combinations, of slowness of movement (bradykinesia), increased muscle tonus (rigidity), tremor, and impaired automatic postural responses to position or movement. The movement disorder results primarily from a defect in the dopaminergic pathway that connects the substantia nigra to the striatum. In idiopathic or postencephalitic parkinsonism, the deficiency results from degeneration of the pigmented dopamine-secreting neurons in the substantia nigra, while most drug-induced parkinsonism reflects a block-

ing of dopamine receptors in striatal neurons. The rare disease *striatonigral degeneration* clinically somewhat resembles idiopathic parkinsonism but results from degeneration of both nigral transmitter and striatal receptor cells. As a consequence, therapy with dopamine or its congeners brings little relief. Parkinsonian symptoms to a greater or lesser degree accompany several other conditions that structurally damage the nigrostriatal pathway, including advanced vascular diseases, neoplasms, and certain degenerative disorders, such as progressive supranuclear palsy, the Shy-Drager form of generalized idiopathic autonomic insufficiency, and some of the progressive cerebellar degenerations. In most of these conditions treatment with dopamine agonists confers only small benefits.

Parkinson's Disease

This idiopathic disorder of adults has its highest incidence in males over 40 years. The cause is unknown. Although epidemiologic studies have traced some cohorts to long-preceding influenzal epidemics, most patients relate neither a history of past infections, an exposure to toxins, nor a family predisposition. The early motor deficits can be traced to incipient degeneration of nigral dopamine-transmitting cells. Later, refractory motor, autonomic, and mental abnormalities develop in many cases, implying degeneration of

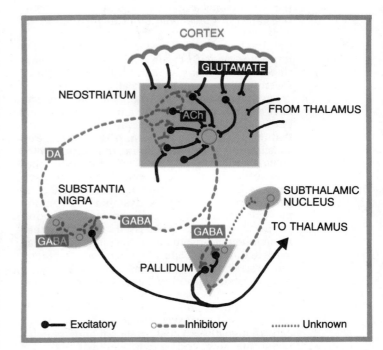

FIGURE 119–8. Simplified diagram of the principal connections and known transmitters of the basal ganglia. ACh = Acetylcholine; GABA = gamma amino butyric acid; DA = dopamine.

striatal receptor mechanisms plus, sometimes, degeneration of the locus ceruleus and the basal nucleus of Meynert.

Symptoms and Signs. Symptoms most often begin and gradually progress with either weakness or tremor. Patients describe motor slowness, stiffness, or easy fatigability in a single limb or hemiparetic distribution. The typical 4- to 7-Hz resting tremor affects approximately 70 per cent but may not present at all in some patients, especially those affected by prominent rigidity. As time passes the voice drops in amplitude and becomes monotonous, and the handwriting diminishes in size.

Patients with parkinsonism often have a diagnostically typical appearance. The body stoops stiffly forward, bent at the knees, hips, and neck, with arms held close to the sides and flexed at the elbows. The outstretched, often trembling hands are extended at the wrist and thumb and flexed at the metacarpophalangeal joints (pill rolling posture). Patients with parkinsonism take small, shuffling steps and turn stiffly, slowly, and unsteadily. Those with advanced cases tend to accelerate their steps (festination) or suffer retropulsion. The face becomes masklike and unblinking, often greasy and sometimes scaly with seborrheic dermatitis. Deep tendon reflexes can be of average, slightly increased, or decreased amplitude. Myerson's sign, the failure of the blink reflex to adapt to repeated gentle percussions of the brow, is present. Other abnormal motor reflexes are absent early, but Babinski signs sometimes emerge late, reflecting the development of corticospinal tract dysfunction. The limbs of most patients display a nonspastic, steadily increasing resistance to movement, often interrupted by an 8-Hz tremor, conferring the classic "cogwheel" rigidity. Behavioral disorders are common. Many if not most patients become depressed in the early stages, and as many as half develop dementia by seven or more years after onset.

Postencephalitic parkinsonism was particularly a problem in the 1930's and 1940's following the worldwide epidemic of lethargic encephalitis that occurred during the years 1918 to 1926. Persons involved with that illness, in addition to the above-mentioned classic signs and symptoms, also suffered a variety of acute behavioral disorders, as well as autonomic abnormalities, oculogyric crises, and various dystonias, choreiform movements, and tics. The illness tended to affect younger persons but progressed less rapidly than idiopathic parkinsonism. In the latter disease, an average duration of 5 to 10 years usually separates the first symptoms from an advanced stage of drug-resistant disability and, often, mental decline.

Drug-induced parkinsonism can follow the taking of several antipsychotic agents given chronically in high doses. Chief present offenders are the phenothiazines and butyrophenones, both of which pharmacologically block dopamine receptors in the striatum and may interfere with the dopamine output of nigral cells as well. Various toxic syndromes can occur with these agents, including a diffuse motor restlessness; acute dystonic reactions that dissipate with anticholinergic, antihistamine, or diazepam therapy; and oculogyric crises, which reflect an oculomotor dystonia, and parkinsonism. The last-mentioned can be clinically typical in all respects except that it fails to subside with levodopa. The late complication of tardive dyskinesia is discussed below.

Treatment. The treatment of Parkinson's disease consists of general measures and specific drugs. These increasingly disabled and fearful patients need considerable emotional support and vigorous encouragement to continue as much physical activity as possible. Every dimension of personal life may require assistance in the later stages.

Drug therapy includes three mainstays that usually are given in some combination. *Amantadine HCl*, 100 mg two to three times daily, usually is tried first in all patients. The agent possesses low toxicity, helps almost two thirds of patients, and sometimes can be used alone in early cases. If no effect or mental dulling is noted by one week, the drug is discontinued. Controversy surrounds the question of whether *levodopa* is the drug of second choice. The agent usually is given combined with a peripheral dopa decarboxylase inhibitor so as to minimize systemic toxicity and provide more drug for CNS absorption. Some authorities believe that levodopa should be given early, since at that time it restores many patients to an asymptomatic state. Others have the impression that levodopa treatment may accelerate the course of parkinsonism and that if it is started later in the course it delays the onset of undesirable side effects. Currently available information fails to resolve these differences. *Anticholinergic drugs* can be used alone in an effort to control the symptoms in some cases of early Parkinson's disease. Most often, however, they serve in low doses as a useful adjunct to levodopa therapy. The anticholinergics often benefit tremor, while levodopa predominantly ameliorates rigidity and some of the postural abnormalities. Several dopamine agonist drugs have been employed in an effort to improve the function of advanced cases. In general, their benefits are modest at best and usually best administered by specialists.

Given in high or prolonged dosages, both levodopa and the anticholinergic drugs exert toxic side effects that potentially limit their benefits. These problems arise especially in the elderly and during the advanced stages of Parkinson's disease. Such patients often walk a tightrope between incapacitating toxic dyskinesias and severe immobility imposed by insufficient neurotransmitter. More extensive discussion of these management problems can be found in the references.

Many patients become depressed during the course of Parkinson's disease, some suicidally so. Tricyclic or other antidepressant medications often ameliorate these symptoms.

Progressive Supranuclear Palsy

This is an uncommon disorder of middle-aged or older persons marked by insidiously developing and progressive degenerative changes in the basal ganglia, basal nuclei, and cerebellum. Clinical features include a Parkinson-like rigidity and a loss of postural reflexes combined with considerable rigidity of the body and a postural dystonia of the head. Masked facies are absent and a progressive external ophthalmoplegia is diagnostically distinctive. The latter consists first of paralysis of voluntary conjugate up and down gaze and later of lateral gaze. Full-range tonic abnormal oculocephalic reflex responses emerge concurrently and are easily elicited by bedside examination. A moderate dementia usually accompanies the motor changes. Dopamine agonist drugs bring symptomatic improvement to some patients.

Huntington's Disease

Huntington's disease, sometimes called Huntington's chorea, is an uncommon inherited disorder transmitted as an autosomal dominant trait with complete penetrance. Recent research has succeeded in bracketing the Huntington gene, giving promise that specific genetic identification soon will follow. Such a step should make it possible to identify those at risk for trials of therapy and appropriate genetic counseling.

Huntington's disease affects striatal neurons, especially the small GABA-transmitting cells and scattered nerve cells in the frontal lobe cortex, claustrum, subthalamus, and cerebellar Purkinje and dentate neurons. Gliosis is prominent. Neurochemically, GABA, acetylcholine, and angiotensin II decline in the striatum, with less severe reductions affecting substance P, cholecystokinin, and enkephalin. Somatostatin-containing neurons are selectively preserved.

The principal clinical changes include dyskinesia, altered behavior, and dementia. The age of onset averages 40 years, with most cases beginning between ages 30 and 50. Motor symptoms in the early stage often include dystonic posturing and rigidity, but these changes give way to prominent choreiform activity in most affected adults. Signs of corticospinal tract dysfunction or sensory changes are lacking. Eccentricity, inappropriateness, a loss of social amenities, excess irritability, and sexual hyperactivity can mark the early stages. Occasionally a schizophreniform illness precedes the motor abnormality by several years. Depression is common and suicide frequently occurs, since the progressing dementia often fails to blunt insight.

Diagnosis comes from recognizing the characteristic progressive generalized choreiform activity accompanied by behavioral or personality changes, especially in a person with a tell-tale family history. Spontaneous mutations are uncommon, but some affected persons inevitably will lack knowledge of their true antecedents. CT or MR scans in fully developed cases show cerebral atrophy, especially of the caudate and putamen, to a degree that is almost specific to the disease. Symptomatic treatment is aimed at minimizing the distressing movements, reserpine or baclofen being the most useful agents. Psychological symptoms may require major antipsychotic drugs for their control. Genetic counseling remains based on statistical probabilities. The principal disorders to be considered in differential diagnosis are as follows: *Gilles de la Tourette's syndrome* (p. 704) occasionally is transmitted in an autosomal dominant pattern, but such patients show motor tics rather than chorea and lack the behavioral-mental changes. *Senile chorea* is a rare disorder beginning in persons older than 60 years. The abnormal movements usually are less prominent than in Huntington's, and there is no comparable degree of dementia. *Hemiballismus* is a disorder of older persons described on page 703. Adult chorea also can develop in association with lupus erythematosus or thyrotoxicosis. In both these instances, the chorea has an abrupt onset and gradually disappears without the associated mental changes of Huntington's disease.

Sydenham's Chorea

This now uncommon, self-limited disorder usually lasts two to six months and is related to rheumatic fever. It occurs most often in children under the age of 15 years but can sometimes affect pregnant women. In contrast to the flowing, more forceful movements in Huntington's disease, which commonly impair walking and standing to the point of causing falls, choreiform activity in Sydenham's chorea more often takes a fidgety, fragmented form, sometimes difficult to separate from habit tics. The children are clumsy and often dysarthric and walk unsteadily. An inability to sustain tonic movement, such as steadily protruding the tongue or sustaining an uninterrupted grasp of the examiner's fingers, is common to all the choreas.

Treatment is symptomatic. Recurrent attacks occur in as many as one third of affected children.

Paroxysmal Choreoathetosis

Paroxysmal choreoathetosis describes a group of conditions in which seizure-like paroxysms of choreodystonic movements recur intermittently in a setting of full consciousness. Most cases are familial in origin. One variety tends to be movement-induced and responds to anticonvulsant drugs. Another type, not sensitive to antiepileptic therapy, is precipitated by alcohol, tea, coffee, excitement, or fatigue.

THE DYSTONIAS

Dystonia can appear either as part of a primary basal ganglia disease or as a secondary symptom to a number of other conditions affecting those structures (Table 119–15). The chronic dystonias include a group of uncommon disorders of inherited or sporadic origin. The specific cause and pathophysiology are unknown for any of these conditions, and no neuropathological changes have been found consistently in the brain. An imbalance of neurotransmitter function in the basal ganglia has been postulated, but specific neurochemical candidates remain elusive, inasmuch as

TABLE 119–15. THE MAJOR DYSTONIAS

PRIMARY DYSTONIA

CONDITIONS	INHERITANCE	AGE OF ONSET
Generalized dystonia	Autosomal recessive Autosomal dominant Sporadic	Childhood Adolescence or adulthood
Focal dystonia Foot-leg or hand-arm	Inherited or sporadic	Mostly adulthood, occasionally late
Blepharospasm	Sporadic	Late adulthood
Facial mandibular (Meige's syndrome)	Sporadic	Late adulthood
Spasmodic dysphonia	Sporadic	Adulthood
Spasmodic torticollis	Mostly sporadic, occasionally autosomal recessive	Middle adulthood
Occupational dystonia Writer's cramp Musician's cramp	Sporadic	Early-middle adulthood

SECONDARY DYSTONIA

CHRONIC	ACUTE
Wilson's disease	Head trauma
Huntington's disease	Phenothiazines
Postencephalitic	Butyrophenones
Severe cerebral anoxia-ischemia	Levodopa
Manganese poisoning	

both dopamine excess and presumed dopamine receptor blockade can induce acute transient dystonic movement.

Severe generalized dystonia, sometimes called *dystonia musculorum deformans*, begins predominantly in young children and adolescents, most often spreading from an equinovarus posturing in the foot or tonically flexed hand to involve the neck, face, and trunk in nearly continuous, recurrent, intense, involuntary, asymmetrical contractions. The movements, which characteristically lead into prolonged spasms, eventually produce bizarre contortions with severe musculotendinous contractures. Ensuing bone deformities can produce scoliosis, chest deformities, and a foreshortening of natural height. Lesser degrees of the illness can arise during adulthood and tend to produce restricted impairments of the lower or upper extremities.

Spasmodic torticollis is the most common of the focal dystonias. It affects predominantly the muscles of the neck and shoulders, which bilaterally and simultaneously contract to produce recurrent unilateral head turning or head extension. Elevations of the shoulder and, often, platysmal contractions may accompany the movements of the head and neck. In mild cases the movement can be restrained by the subject's placing gentle antagonistic pressure against the chin. More severe examples can spread to produce spastic dysphonia and hand-arm dystonia. Discussion of other forms of focal dystonia can be found in the references.

Treatment of the dystonias is largely unsatisfactory. High doses of the anticholinergic drug trihexyphenidyl brings a measure of relief to some patients. The use of carbamazepine or diazepam occasionally has been reported favorably in others. Stereotaxic surgical attacks in the thalamus benefit some children with severe generalized dystonia but carry a high risk of complications and are desperation measures. Recently, investigators have reported success with judiciously repeated fractional injection of botulinum toxin into the periocular muscles of patients with incapacitating blepharospasm.

DYSKINESIA

Tardive dyskinesias consist of abnormal, semirhythmic involuntary movements affecting the mouth (lingual-oral-buccal), trunk, or extremities following the taking and, often, withdrawal of antidopaminergic antipsychotic drugs. Once it appears the condition almost always remains permanently. A few cases are known to have succeeded upon no more than a few days of phenothiazine medication, and weeks, months, or even years sometimes can separate the time when the drugs were taken and the movements emerge. The facial movements most often consist of chewing, tongue darting, and grimacing. Other forms include repeated flexion and extension of the trunk, piano playing–like successive contraction of the fingers and toes, and repetitive steppings of the feet while standing erect. Supersensitivity of the dopamine receptors of the basal ganglia is believed to be the cause. Reserpine or, in the presence of continued psychosis, a higher dose of antidopaminergic antipsychotics sometimes bring partial relief. Tardive dyskinesia is a disfiguring, seriously disturbing, and frequent complication. The potential for producing it should discourage the use of phenothiazine drugs for any but serious medical-psychiatric problems. *Meige's syndrome*, a dystonia involving the jaw and lower face, somewhat resembles tardive dyskinesia but with slower, more twisting movements. There is no necessary history of antipsychotic medication. Baclofen or valproate has been reported to improve selective cases.

WILSON'S DISEASE
(Hepatolenticular Degeneration)

The biochemical changes of this disorder, which results from an inborn error of copper metabolism, are discussed on page 429. Since prominent neurologic changes often precipitate medical attention, they are briefly described here.

In the brain with Wilson's disease, copper is deposited in the pericapillary areas and astrocytes of the basal ganglia and frontal lobe, leading eventually to atrophy of those structures with cystic changes in the putamen. Copper deposits in the cornea produce the pathognomonic Kaiser-

Fleischer ring. Seen best with a slit lamp but often visible to the naked eye, the ring appears as a green-brown, 1- to 2-mm wide, peripheral zone of iridescent pigmentation located a millimeter or so from the outer corneal limbus. The neurologic disease begins usually between ages 11 and 25, occasionally as late as 40 years. Early symptoms and signs consist of an intellectual decline, coupled with a tight, slightly retracted upper lip. Later a characteristic rotating and flapping ("wing beat-ing") tremor appears in outstretched arms. Muscular rigidity, intention tremor, and dystonic posturing often ensue. Diagnosis is suspected on clinical grounds and strengthened by finding abnormal liver function tests, absent or decreased serum ceruloplasmin, and increased urinary copper excretion. If doubt exists, liver biopsy showing elevated copper is definitive. Treatment aimed at reducing body copper stores often induces improvement.

E. THE MAJOR CEREBELLAR ATAXIAS

SIGNS AND MECHANISMS OF CEREBELLAR DYSFUNCTION

Disorders of the cerebellum or its principal connections produce characteristic symptoms and signs, including *asthenia* or easy fatigability; *ataxia* of gait; *dysmetria*, an inability to control the range of movement, producing under- or overshoot; *dysdiadokokinesia*, the impairment of rapidly alternating movements; *decomposition of movement*, the inability to synergize motion around two or more joints; *postural* (*sustention*) or *intention tremor*; *dysarthria* and, possibly, nystagmus with the fast component toward the side of the cerebellar lesion.

Ataxias linked to the cerebellum and its major afferent and efferent connections fall into three major groups (Table 119–16). These include (1) diseases affecting predominantly the afferent spinocerebellar and associated spinal pathways; (2) diseases or disorders involving the cerebellum proper and its immediate outflow tracts; and (3) diseases in which cerebellar involvement comprises only part of a wide degeneration of central nervous system structures. Clinically, the three categories overlap but can be roughly distinguished by their symptoms and signs. Specific etiologic diagnosis then can be reached by laboratory tests or a process of exclusion.

Spinocerebellar disease produces a wide-based, lurching sensory ataxia due to involvement of ascending proprioceptors and spinocerebellar pathways. At their worst, patients stagger from side to side with highstepping, irregularly placed feet that often pound the floor heavily. Large afferent fibers carrying position and vibratory sense disappear from the lower extremities, leading to rombergism and an accompanying loss of deep tendon reflexes. Involvement of descending corticospinal pathways results in pathological reflexes, while direct cerebellar involvement can add additional signs of neurologic impairment affecting ocular control and upper extremity coordination.

TABLE 119–16. PRINCIPAL DISEASES OF THE CEREBELLUM AND ITS CONNECTIONS

I. **Primarily spinocerebellar**
  A. Inherited spinocerebellar ataxias (childhood or adolescent onset, chronic course, few positive sensory symptoms)
    1. Molecular genetic defect uncertain: Friedreich's ataxia and its variants; Roussy-Levy
    2. Genetic defect known: phytanic acid α-oxidase deficiency (Refsum); abetalipoproteinemia (Bassen-Kornzweig); arylsulfate and other deficiencies*
  B. Acquired spinal sensory ataxia (acute, subacute, or insidious onset): polyneuropathy; sensory polyradiculopathy (tabes dorsalis); vitamin B_{12} deficiency; spinal cord damage (multiple sclerosis, neoplasm, etc.)

II. **Primarily cerebellar**
  A. Inherited degenerative (course progressive): restricted olivopontocerebellar atrophy (young to mid-adulthood); ataxia-telangiectasia (childhood onset)
  B. Developmental abnormalities (onset of signs varies, progressive): basilar impression; Arnold-Chiari malformation
  C. Nutritional-immunological (mostly adult onset, acute or subacute course)
    1. Acute, parainfectious cerebellar ataxia of children
    2. Alcoholic-nutritional cerebellar degeneration
    3. Paraneoplastic cerebellar-brain stem degeneration
  D. Structural cerebellar lesions (acute or subacute course): trauma, neoplasms, hemorrhage, anoxia-ischemia, etc.
  E. Intoxication (acute or subacute or chronic): alcohol; sedatives; anxiolytics; phenytoin; anticancer agents

III. **Cerebellar-plus disorders**
  A. Inherited-degenerative system degeneration (middle adult onset, gradual progression)
    1. Olivopontocerebellar atrophy plus, variably, spasticity, parkinsonism, sensory changes, optic atrophy, retinitis pigmentosa, ophthalmoplegia, dementia
    2. Shy-Drager syndrome
    3. Generalized mitochondrial dysfunction with ataxia, ophthalmoplegia, myopathy
  B. Acquired disseminated disorders affecting cerebellar and other systems (Disseminated cancer, abscess, etc.)

* See also Table 490–1 by Rosenberg RN: Spinocerebellar Degenerations. In Wyngaarden JB, and Smith LH Jr (eds): Cecil Textbook of Medicine. 17th ed. Philadelphia, WB Saunders Co, 1985, p 2081.

Within the cerebellum itself, damage or degeneration of the posterior midline *floccular nodular area* rarely is selective. When it is, it produces a narrow-based ataxia with a tendency to fall backwards plus lateral gaze and sometimes downbeat nystagmus. Dysfunction of the more anterior midline *vermis and anterior lobe* is more common, especially with deep midline cerebellar tumors and with alcohol-nutritional or paraneoplastic degeneration in adults. A broad-based, stiff-legged ataxia develops, often accompanied in severe cases by an oscillating, rhythmic sustention tremor of the trunk and lower extremities (titubation). Deep tendon reflexes tend to be accentuated, but nystagmus is uncommon unless the disease concurrently affects the vestibular nuclei.

Lateral hemispheric lesions characteristically produce subtle signs consisting of mild ipsilateral incoordination and perhaps hypotonia. If they expand to compress the brain stem or directly involve the cerebellar roof nuclei and their outflow pathways, they cause in the upper extremities the classic signs of cerebellar incoordination as described in the first paragraph of this section. Lesions that expand the cerebellum so that they compress or extend into the adjacent brain stem add to the above syndromes symptoms and signs of headache, nausea, vomiting, cranial nerve abnormalities, or long tract dysfunction.

PRIMARY CEREBELLAR DEGENERATIONS

This category includes a heterogeneous group of largely genetically caused *system degenerations* in which neuroaxonal death variously affects afferent pathways to the cerebellum, the cerebellum itself, and, often, trans-synaptically connected central nervous system structures. Although one can identify more or less distinct syndromes of spinocerebellar and primary cerebellar degeneration, considerable neuropathologic overlaps occur between the different diseases, as do phenotypic variations in single kindreds. Both these considerations suggest molecular linkages among these disorders and several other degenerative central nervous system diseases. These related conditions include peroneal muscular atrophy, other degenerative neuropathies, hereditary spastic paraplegia, motor neuron disease, atypical forms of parkinsonism, and the Shy-Drager form of progressive autonomic insufficiency (page 680). Fortunately, most of the CNS system degenerations are uncommon, but in only a few is the specific cause known. The following section describes the most frequent types; the references contain more extensive discussions as well as descriptions of the rarer entities.

Friedreich's Ataxia

Friedreich's ataxia represents the prototypical spinocerebellar degeneration. The disease can be transmitted in autosomal dominant and autosomal recessive forms, but sporadic cases are common. Neuronal loss involves the dorsal root ganglia and the spinal cells of origin of the spinocerebellar tracts, with degeneration beginning caudally and progressing rostrally. Axonal loss and demyelination affect the spinal nerves, the dorsal column, and the spinocerebellar tracts as well as the descending corticospinal tract. Some cases show cell loss in the cerebellum and occasionally in brain stem nuclei.

The molecular etiology of the spinocerebellar generations can vary from patient to patient despite considerable similarity in clinical presentations. Although the specific cause remains unknown in most instances, somewhat similar clinical disorders have been observed among small groups of patients showing abnormalities in several tissue enzymes as listed in section IA-2 of Table 119–16.

Friedreich's ataxia typically begins insidiously, usually before age 10 years, and progresses steadily to produce ataxia by the second decade. Most patients become unable to walk unassisted during their third decade. Position and vibratory sense are lost initially in the lower extremities, and this plus the corticospinal defect leads to an increasing sensorimotor staggering ataxia. Concurrently, one finds atrophic, hypotonic lower limbs with areflexia and extensor plantar responses. By the time of their late teens or twenties, most patients develop dysarthria and many have nystagmus. Orthopedic changes include a characteristic pes cavus deformity (which can affect some family members as the sole mark of the abnormal trait) as well as a mild to moderate scoliosis and, sometimes, a high arched palate. Low intelligence affects some victims from the start, while a few appear to decline mentally as the disorder progresses. Associated, less common, individual neurologic abnormalities consist of optic atrophy, retinal degeneration, deafness, and anterior horn cell degeneration. Cardiac enlargement is common, and most patients show conduction defects on the ECG. Some develop heart failure; few survive beyond 40 years. Diagnosis usually is apparent from the patient's appearance and physical findings. Among laboratory tests, none is specific except in the already identified deficiency syndromes, most of which clinically appear sufficiently distinctive to prompt appropriate biochemical study. Visual evoked potentials are abnormally slow in most cases of either spinocerebellar or primary cerebellar ataxia, while somatic evoked potentials tend to be particularly slowed in Friedreich's ataxia but not in olivopontocerebellar atrophy. The spinal fluid is normal.

Roussy-Levy ataxia closely resembles Friedreich's except that the condition runs a much slower course, often with little progression into adulthood. Position and vibration sensations are spared, and extensor plantar responses fail to develop. Other family members may show evidence of the more common peroneal muscular atrophy or hereditary spastic paraplegia.

The Olivopontocerebellar Degenerations (OPCD)

This category includes a group of uncommon degenerative disorders of middle to late adult life characterized by progressive symptoms and signs of cerebellar dysfunction. Considerable clinical and pathological variation separates individual cases, some showing almost pure cerebellar abnormalities, while others have changes reflecting dysfunction of spinal cord, cerebellar outflow pathways, basal ganglia, autonomic nervous system, optic nerves, and even cerebral cortex. The illnesses occur in both sporadic and hereditary patterns.

Pathologically, the most frequent denominator to the OPCD group includes degeneration of the inferior olive and pontine cerebellar relay nuclei, with degeneration and demyelination of their climbing axons into the cerebellum. Trans-synaptic death occurs in the target cells of the cerebellar cortex. Less consistent abnormalities affect neurons and their axons in the more remote neurologic structures mentioned above. Degeneration of the basal ganglia and central autonomic neurons usually is prominent in the Shy-Drager variant.

OPCD can affect either sex, most often between the ages of 40 and 60 years. Progression is relatively rapid, and most patients become totally dependent within six years of onset. Initial symptoms and signs include a relatively wide-based ataxia accompanied by incoordination of the upper extremities and dysarthria. Dysmetria usually remains worse in the lower than in upper extremities. The limbs become hypotonic, and deep tendon reflexes are preserved except when an associated spinal degeneration occurs. Most patients develop nystagmus. Among those with basal ganglia involvement, parkinsonian signs emerge during the moderately advanced stages of the illness. Babinski signs and other manifestations of corticospinal tract dysfunction occur late if at all. Some patients develop palatal myoclonus. A functional dementia accompanies the late stages of approximately one third of cases.

No specific test is diagnostic of OPCD. Brain stem auditory evoked potentials are abnormal in a majority. Differential diagnosis requires ruling out the conditions listed in sections II and III of Table 119–16. CT or MR imaging usually discloses cerebellar and pontine atrophy and rules out other structural lesions. Nutritional disease and possible drug intoxication can be identified by the history. Paraneoplastic syndromes are discussed on page 776.

The cause being unknown, only symptomatic treatment can be offered.

Ataxia-Telangiectasia

This disorder affects spinal cord, cerebellum, and basal ganglia functions. The illness begins in early childhood, inherited as an autosomal recessive trait. Progressive ataxia of gait, incoordinated upper extremities, facial and appendicular choreoathetosis, and opsoclonus are characteristic. Most patients become wheelchair-bound and begin to show mental retardation by the second decade. Prominent telangiectases stud the conjunctivae, the ears, the nose, and the cheek areas. The disease includes thymic hypoplasia with a severe deficiency of IgA. Patients suffer a high incidence of endocrine abnormalities, respiratory infections, chromosomal aberrations, and neoplasms; most die before completing their second decade.

REFERENCES

Aminoff MJ: Spinal Angiomas. Oxford, Blackwell Scientific Publications, 1976. *A comprehensive text on spinal and vascular anomalies.*

Austin GM (ed): The Spinal Cord. 3rd ed. New York, Igaku-Shoin, 1983. *The third edition of a comprehensive multiauthored monograph describing the clinical findings and management of many disorders of the spinal cord, including lumbar and cervical discs.*

Barnett HJM: Syringomyelia. London, WB Saunders Co, 1974. *The standard reference on the problem.*

Dyck PJ, Thomas PK, and Lambert EH: Peripheral Neuropathy. Philadelphia, WB Saunders Co, 1984. *Two-volume authoritative reference on all peripheral nerve diseases.*

Fahn S: The extrapyramidal disorders. In Wyngaarden JB, and Smith LH Jr (eds): Cecil Textbook of Medicine. 17th ed. Philadelphia, WB Saunders Co, pp 2068–2079. *A well-written and informative chapter.*

Gilman S, Bloedel JR, and Lechtenberg R: Disorders of the Cerebellum. Philadelphia, FA Davis Co, 1981. *A thorough, informative reference source.*

Plum F, and Posner JB: Neurology. In Smith LH, and Thier SO (eds): Pathophysiology. The Biological Principles of Disease. 2nd ed. Philadelphia, WB Saunders Co, 1985. *A thorough chapter on normal and abnormal physiology of motor control and motor diseases; supplements the clinical articles of the Cecil Textbook of Medicine.*

Rosenberg RN: Inherited, congenital, and idiopathic degenerative diseases of the nervous system. In Wyngaarden JB, and Smith LH Jr (eds): Cecil Textbook of Medicine. 17th ed. Philadelphia, WB Saunders Co, 1985, pp 2079–2086. *Provides details about genetic abnormalities, where known, in cerebellar and other disorders.*

Schaumburg HH, Spencer PS, and Thomas PK: Disorders of Peripheral Nerve. Philadelphia, FA Davis Co, 1983. *Short, clearly written monograph providing an excellent introduction to peripheral nerves and their disorders.*

Walton J: Disorders of Voluntary Muscle. 4th ed. Edinburgh, Churchill Livingstone, 1981. *An excellent reference on all disorders of muscle, whether originating in nerves or muscles.*

Cerebrovascular diseases include disorders of the arterial or venous circulatory systems or their contents that produce or threaten to produce injury to the central nervous system. The general term *stroke* describes the functional neurologic injury. The cause of stroke can be either *anoxic-ischemic*, the result of vasogenic failure to supply sufficient oxygen and substrate to the tissue, or *hemorrhagic*, the result of abnormal leakage of blood into or around central nervous system structures. *Arteriovenous malformations* of the brain or spinal cord can produce neurologic abnormalities by bleeding, by producing ischemic damage, or by acting as space-occupying lesions.

Anatomy and Pathophysiology of the Cerebral Circulation

Anatomy. The cerebral arterial circulation derives from four major extracerebral (neck) arteries,

the paired internal carotids, and vertebrals (Fig. 120–1). Acute, complete occlusion of these extracranial arteries can result at any age from atherosclerosis, embolization, inflammation, intrinsic arterial disease, or trauma. Age and the effectiveness of the anastomotic pattern of the large arteries at the base of the brain determine whether ischemic brain damage ensues.

The circle of Willis provides in most persons a potentially effective intracranial anastomotic pathway to compensate for sudden focal reductions in blood flow at the base of the brain. Unfortunately, however, the circle sometimes loses some of its effectiveness because of congenital asymmetry of the vertebral arteries or narrowing or absence of its anterior or posterior communicating segments. Beyond the circle, the major intracranial arterial beds anastomose through tiny interconnecting pial arterioles, most of which are

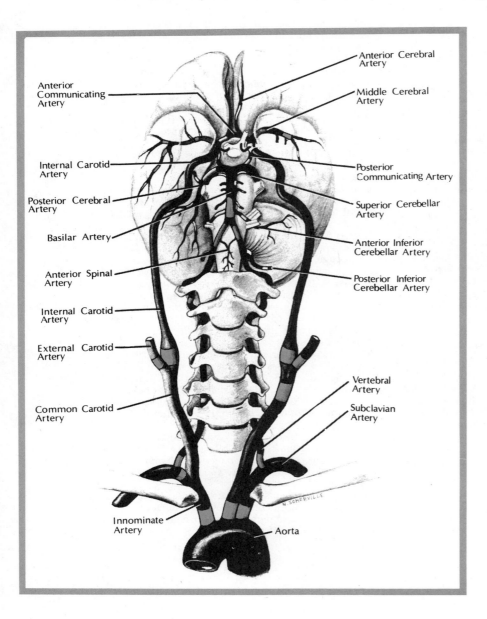

FIGURE 120–1. The major arteries supplying the brain. The light bands around the arteries indicate the most frequent sites of severe atherosclerosis. The two most common sites to cause symptoms are the region of the carotid sinus and the intracranial portion of the carotid artery. (From Barnett HJM: Cerebral ischemia and infarction. In Wyngaarden JB, and Smith LH Jr (eds): Cecil Textbook of Medicine. 17th ed. Philadelphia, WB Saunders Co, 1985, pp 2090–2103.)

too small to compensate for major arterial occlusions. Figures 120–2 to 120–6 diagram the large parent intracranial arteries and their major branches.

Physiology. Cerebral arteries contain less muscle, no elastic tissue, and less adventitia compared to systemic arteries. The reduced musculature especially affects the junctions where major branches diverge from the large arteries at the base of the brain, creating vulnerable points from which most intracranial aneurysms arise. The absence of elastic tissue as an antigen may explain the invulnerability of the intracranial arteries to the common late-life immunologic-inflammatory vascular disease, cranial arteritis (page 685).

The *blood-brain barrier* insulates the brain and its extracellular fluid, including the cerebrospinal fluid (CSF), from many of the chemical perturbations that can affect the systemic circulation, including circulating drugs, immunogenic antigens, and electrolyte changes. The anatomical barrier lies in the intracranial endothelium, where tight intercellular junctions weld the entire inner surface into a continuous membranous sheet. As a result, only nonpolar materials that either have a small molecular size, are lipid soluble, or are transported across the membrane by specific carrier systems or pumps penetrate the endothelium with any rapidity. Transient breaches of the barrier occur under a variety of circumstances and appear to have little ill effect on the brain. Sustained, partial barrier alteration occurs in areas of cerebral neoplasms and inflammation and contributes to the formation of edema associated with such conditions. Severe damage to barrier transport mechanisms is a factor contributing to brain tissue infarction during ischemia.

Autoregulation describes an intrinsic two-

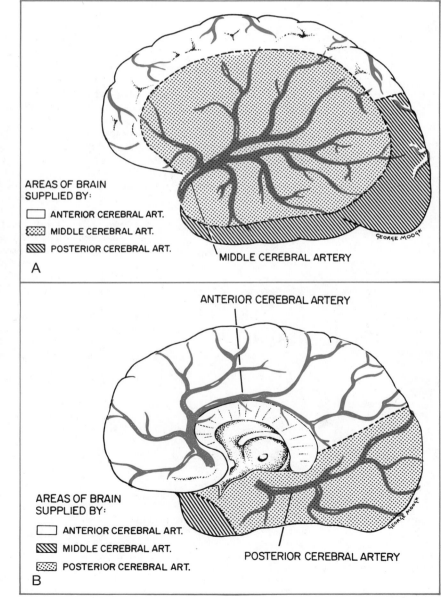

FIGURE 120–2. *A,* The lateral surface of the cerebral hemisphere and the course of the middle cerebral artery. The middle cerebral artery has been elevated from the Sylvian fissure to illustrate its course. *B,* The medial surface of the cerebral hemisphere, showing the course of the anterior and posterior cerebral arteries and the areas of brain supplied by them. (From Barnett HJM: Cerebrovascular diseases: Introduction. In Wyngaarden JB, and Smith LH Jr (eds): Cecil Textbook of Medicine. 17th ed. Philadelphia, WB Saunders Co, 1985, pp. 2086–2090.)

AREAS OF BRAIN SUPPLIED BY:
ANTERIOR CEREBRAL ART.
MIDDLE CEREBRAL ART.
POSTERIOR CEREBRAL ART.

MIDDLE CEREBRAL ARTERY

A

ANTERIOR CEREBRAL ARTERY

AREAS OF BRAIN SUPPLIED BY:
ANTERIOR CEREBRAL ART.
MIDDLE CEREBRAL ART.
POSTERIOR CEREBRAL ART.

POSTERIOR CEREBRAL ARTERY

B

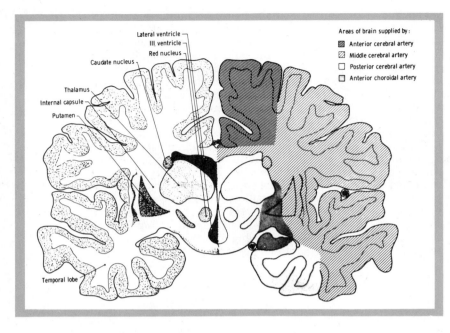

FIGURE 120–3. The vascular supply to the cerebral hemispheres, in coronal section. (From McDowell FH: Cerebral ischemia and infarction. In Beeson PB, McDermott W, and Wyngaarden JB (eds): Cecil Textbook of Medicine. 15th ed. Philadelphia, WB Saunders Co, 1979, pp 778–794.)

dimensional property of the brain's resistance arterioles that helps to guarantee the metabolic requirements of the tissue. The arterioles automatically and locally dilate or constrict in response to increases or decreases in local brain functional activity. The arterioles also normally adjust their diameter in response to changes in systemic blood pressure, dilating when the pressure falls and constricting when it rises. Although the two responses are independently regulated,

they synergize in order to meet constantly the brain's metabolic need. The normal limits of cerebral autoregulation to pressure extend between approximately 60 and 160 mm Hg of systemic mean pressure. Impaired autoregulation to pressure changes can contribute to brain injury in several circumstances, especially with disorders that cause an increased intracranial pressure (ICP). At such times widespread abnormal vasodilatation allows the ICP to rise, sometimes to alarming levels that can approach the arterial blood pressure. Impaired arterial autoregulation also can accompany severe hypertension (mean BP greater than 160 torr), in which case intense elevations of systemic blood pressure cause focal breakthroughs of the resistance vessels to produce vascular and brain tissue injury.

Epidemiology and Risk Factors

Stroke is worldwide in its distribution, affecting especially persons aged 55 years and older. Although the incidence of stroke has declined somewhat in recent years, only heart disease and cancer exceed it as a cause of death and disability in developed countries.

Stroke has several specific causes, listed in Table 120–1. In addition, a number of systemic conditions and social habits predispose to stroke, and early attention to these abnormalities may delay or prevent appearance of the disorder. *Hypertension* both adversely affects the heart and induces progressive narrowing of the cerebral arterioles; it creates the greatest risk factor. The increasingly widespread successful treatment of hypertension probably deserves the greatest credit for the decline in stroke incidence. Population studies show an especially strong association among dietary salt intake, hypertension, and cerebral hemorrhage. Both the length and degree of *smoking* correlate with an increased incidence of stroke as well as of myocardial infarction. *Myo-*

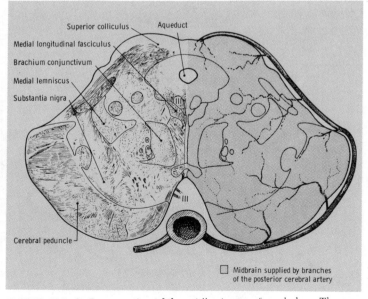

FIGURE 120–4. Cross section of the midbrain seen from below. The medial regions are supplied by short branches from the apex of the basilar artery and the posterior cerebral artery. The posterior cerebral artery supplies the lateral and dorsal areas as it passes around the midbrain. (From McDowell FH: Cerebral ischemia and infarction. In Beeson PB, McDermott W, and Wyngaarden JB (eds): Cecil Textbook of Medicine. 15th ed. Philadelphia, WB Saunders Co, 1979, pp 778–794.)

cardial infarction, atrial fibrillation, and congestive heart failure all predispose to stroke, as does
diabetes mellitus and familial hypercholesterolemia. Possibly predisposing factors include obesity, lack of vigorous exercise, the absence of high
density lipoproteins in the serum, and blood hematocrit levels between 48 and 55 per cent. Hematocrit levels above 55 per cent or white blood
counts greater than 500,000 per cu mm predispose. Alcoholic excess increases stroke risk, with
several studies reporting an increase of severe
strokes immediately following single bouts of
heavy intoxication. Combined progesterone/estro-
gen oral contraceptives increase the risk of stroke
among women of child-bearing age to about three
times the normal rate.

ISCHEMIC STROKE

Etiology and Mechanisms

Focal ischemic stroke is caused by either embolic or thrombotic occlusion of a major artery in
the neck or head. Global ischemic stroke results
in total failure of blood supply, e.g., following cardiac arrest or, rarely, from severe impairments of
the oxygen supply alone to the brain.

Vascular Factors. These can be either primarily
thrombotic or embolic, as listed in Table 120–2.
In either case, the critical event is reduction of
blood flow to the brain.

Hematogenous Factors. These include severe
anoxemia or anemia, abnormalities producing
spontaneous endovascular thrombosis, and
marked increases in blood viscosity. Anoxemia or
anemia by themselves are uncommon causes of
ischemic stroke inasmuch as arterial oxygen supplies must be reduced to about 40 per cent of normal before cerebral insufficiency develops; this
level of anoxemia is likely to produce cardiac as
well as cerebral difficulties. Accordingly, in the
absence of an accompanying low systemic blood
pressure or of anatomical abnormalities in the cer-
vicocranial circulation, isolated hemoglobin levels greater than 7 to 8 gm/dl or Pao_2 values greater
than 40 to 45 mm Hg seldom can be incriminated
as primary causes of stroke. Because of blood flow
adjustments, even lower hemoglobin values may
cause no symptoms in chronically anemic persons. When combined with hypoxemia, electrolyte, or biochemical abnormalities, however, anemia becomes an important cofactor in producing
a metabolic encephalopathy.

Among the coagulopathies causing stroke,
physiological platelet aggregation deserves specific attention. Vascular changes producing partial or complete ischemia in brain stimulate an
immediate increase in platelet aggregation in the
abnormally irrigated areas. Similarly, ulcerated
arteriosclerotic plaques attract fibrin-platelet ag-
gregations to their surface as part of the healing
process. The ensuing detritus provides a potential
source for the extension of a thrombosis or the
formation of artery-to-artery emboli.

Blood Flow and Tissue Factors. The brain and
spinal cord possess the highest basal rate of me-

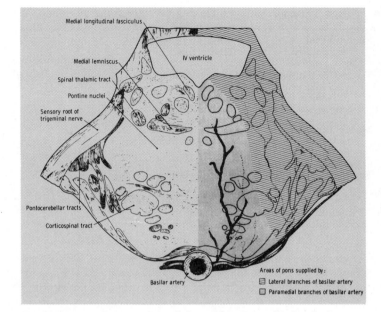

FIGURE 120–5. Cross section of the midpons. At this level, the more
dorsal structures are supplied by the long circumferential branch, the
anterior inferior cerebellar artery. (From McDowell FH: Cerebral ischemia and infarction. In Beeson PB, McDermott W, and Wyngaarden
JB (eds): Cecil Textbook of Medicine. 15th ed. Philadelphia, WB Saunders Co, 1979, pp 778–794.)

tabolism of any large organ in the body, consum-
ing approximately 20 per cent of the body's resting oxygen requirement. The brain contains
practically no reserves of oxygen and only tiny
stores of glucose, its normal substrate. As a result,
any severe reduction of blood supply threatens to

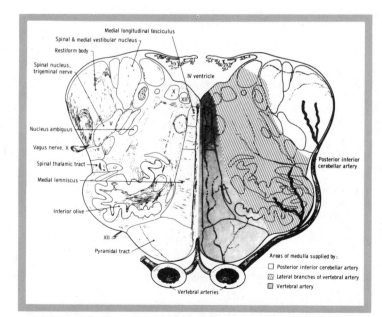

FIGURE 120–6. Cross section of the medulla oblongata seen from above
at the level of the hypoglossal nuclei. (From McDowell FH: Cerebral
ischemia and infarction. In Beeson PB, McDermott W, and Wyngaarden
JB (eds): Cecil Textbook of Medicine. 15th ed. Philadelphia, WB Saunders Co, 1979, pp 778–794.)

TABLE 120-1. CAUSES OF ACUTE CEREBRAL ISCHEMIA

Mainly Focal
Arterial disease, thrombotic or embolic
Cardiac emboli
Functional arterial spasm or constriction
    a. Migraine
    b. Subarachnoid hemorrhage
Intracranial sinus or venous thrombosis

Mainly Global
Absolute or functional (ventricular fibrillation) asystole >8 sec in duration
Severe decline in cardiac output
    Shock; bradycardia <30-40 per minute; cardiac tamponade; severe heart failure
Three- or four-vessel stenosis of cervical arteries plus TIA
Profound anemia, HCT usually <20
Profound hypoxemia: PaO_2 <35-40 mm Hg
Carbon monoxide poisoning
Prolonged status epilepticus
Disseminated intravascular coagulation
Fat embolization

TABLE 120-2. VASCULAR FACTORS CONTRIBUTING TO STROKE

Mural Abnormalities
A. Extracranial-intracranial atherosclerosis
    1. Thrombotic narrowing or occlusion of cervical vessels
    2. Ulcerated aortocervical plaques generating platelet-fibrin or cholesterol emboli
    3. Thrombotic occlusion of intracranial vessels
B. Inflammatory-immunological vascular occlusions
    1. Extracranial only—cranial arteritis
    2. Extracranial and intracranial
        a. Generalized polyarteritis
        b. Septic emboli (bacterial endocarditis)
    3. Intracranial only
        a. Accompanying bacterial or granulomatous arteritis
        b. Amphetamine—cocaine-like drugs
        c. Idiopathic
C. Invasion or compression of arterial or venous vascular walls by trauma, neoplasms, etc.

Embolic disorders
A. Artery to artery: platelet or cholesterol emboli from aortocervical atherosclerotic plaques
B. Cardiogenic
    1. Mural (post–myocardial infarction)
    2. Atrial
    3. Valvular
        a. Septic (endocarditis)
        b. Nonseptic (rheumatic, atherosclerotic, mitral prolapse, marantic)
    4. Neoplastic—arterial myxoma, etc.

TABLE 120-3. FINDINGS SUGGESTING CARDIAC ORIGIN FOR FOCAL STROKE

Persons <45 years of age with no risk factors (mitral prolapse)
Known heart disease: Rheumatic aortic or mitral valve; atrial fibrillation; recent anterior wall infarction; murmur plus unexplained fever (SBE); chronic cardiomyopathy; mitral annular calcification
Multiple cerebral arteries involved
Emboli in other organs
Hemorrhagic infarct

become rapidly lethal. The blood supply to the brain normally averages about 55 ml per 100 gm of tissue per minute. In the absence of anemia (Hb < 12 gm) or hypoxemia (PaO_2 < 65 mm Hg), cerebral autoregulation and increased tissue oxygen extraction can support normal or nearly normal cerebral functions in the face of blood flow reductions down to about 40 per cent of normal. Below this threshold physiological dysfunction appears and only a small additional decline is required to produce membrane failure and death of brain cells. Partial or complete vascular occlusion (focal ischemia) and profound hypotension (global ischemia) represent the commonest causes of such catastrophes, with anemia, hypoxemia, or hypercoagulability often accentuating the effects of reduced blood flow.

The time required to produce permanent anoxic ischemic brain damage is uncertain. Syncope occurs in humans after approximately 8 seconds of asystole. Clinical and experimental evidence, however, suggests that brain tissue sometimes can recover from severe partial ischemia lasting as long as an hour or more.

Heart disease is the single most important associated factor causing clinical stroke (Table 120-3). Most focal stroke comes from emboli, and an estimated 40 per cent of all emboli to the brain emanate from the cardiac chambers. Cardiac arrhythmias account for most instances of syncope or global cerebral ischemia among older persons. Furthermore, heart disease is linked closely to cerebrovascular disease so that among patients with acute stroke the statistical risk of future myocardial infarction is as great as or greater than the risk of a repeated cerebral event. Mitral valve prolapse, which can cause valvular or subvalvular thrombi, occurs six times more frequently than normal among persons below age 45 with acute stroke. Similarly, a greatly increased incidence of focal stroke is associated with atrial fibrillation of whatever cause. Anterior wall myocardial infarction (MI) produces a high incidence of left ventricular thrombi; if not treated prophylactically with anticoagulants, as many as 40 per cent of such patients suffer stroke during convalescence from the MI. Bacterial endocarditis, prosthetic heart valves, nonbacterial (marantic) endocarditis, indwelling pacemakers, mitral or aortic calcific disease, and atrial myxomas all represent additional potential sources of cardiogenic emboli.

Neuropathology of Ischemic Brain Damage.
Cerebral infarction is a pathological process that damages or destroys all tissue elements, including neurons, glial cells, and blood vessels. Within a matter of hours after onset, water leaks into the tissue, increasing the mass by edema. Tissue lactacidosis added to the oxygen lack may be a factor in producing extensive damage. Infarction characteristically follows prolonged anoxia-ischemia such as occurs with vascular occlusion and can be focal or multifocal in nature depending on the pattern of affected vessels. Large infarcts involve the vascular territory of the major intracranial arteries. Small infarcts, 5 to 8 mm or so in diameter,

sometimes called *lacunes*, result from occlusion of arteriolar branches. Lacunes may arise anywhere in the brain but are especially frequent in the deeper circulatory beds of the middle cerebral and basilar arteries.

Hemorrhagic infarcts are marked by scattered areas of escaped red cells in the ischemic tissue, occurring most often at the periphery of an infarcted area. The mechanism is thought to represent reperfusion of an artery in which transient embolization damages the endothelium, allowing diapedetic bleeding to occur.

Selective neuronal necrosis consists of damage confined to nerve cells, sparing glial and vascular elements. The process shows a predilection for selectively vulnerable neurons located in the hippocampus, the deeper level of the cerebral cortex (laminar necrosis), and the cerebellar Purkinje cells. The process characteristically follows brief periods of acute cardiac arrest, prolonged status epilepticus, and profound hypoglycemia. Severe hippocampal damage represents the most frequent cause of memory loss following cardiac arrest, while Purkinje cell damage is a major factor in causing the distressing condition of postanoxic myoclonus.

Postanoxic demyelination of the brain is an unusual condition wherein prolonged exposure to severe, incomplete hypoxemia, usually associated with severe systemic hypotension, damages oligodendroglial cells and leads to diffuse damage to hemispheric white matter. The process largely spares the cerebral neurons. The demyelination produces signs and symptoms similar to those of a severe metabolic encephalopathy and often develops only after a delay of a few days to as much as three weeks following anoxic exposure. Although potentially acutely fatal, most patients recover at least partially. Many, however, suffer residual movement disorders from small, associated infarcts affecting the basal ganglia.

Clinical Definitions of Stroke

Transient ischemic attacks (TIA's) are periods of focal, acute neurologic insufficiency lasting from a few minutes to as much as an hour or so, followed by complete functional recovery. Emboli that lodge in the retinal or small cerebral arteries and then rapidly dissolve represent the main cause. Composed of fibrin, platelets, or, rarely, cholesterol, most such emboli arise from the heart, proximal aorta, or great vessels of the neck. Less frequent sources include fragments of cardiac valvular vegetations or hematogenous abnormalities within the affected vessels. Some workers postulate that greater than 85 per cent narrowing of the common or internal carotid artery in the neck can cause transient ischemia on a hemodynamic basis. Individual TIA's can involve the territorial distribution of either an internal carotid–middle cerebral artery system or the vertebral-basilar system with characteristic symptoms as described below.

Completed stroke refers to a sustained ischemic event sufficient to produce neuronal necrosis or infarction in at least part of the territory of the affected artery. The ensuing neurologic defect can last days, weeks, or permanently; even after maximal recovery, at least minimal neurologic difficulties often remain. The clinical severity of completed strokes depends upon the size of the affected arterial bed, the relative balance between lethal and critical flow reduction to the tissue, and the functional neuroanatomy of the lesion. Completed *minor strokes* involving only distal branches of the middle cerebral or basilar artery, for example, produce much less neurologic damage than do *major strokes* that involve the main middle cerebral or basilar trunk and its associated drainage area. A clinically important point is that minor strokes causing fractional neurologic impairment sometimes warn of impending thrombosis of the larger parent artery. In the early hours following onset of neurologic damage, minor completed strokes may be difficult or impossible to distinguish from reversible ischemic neurologic deficits or even the beginning of a stroke in evolution, as described below.

Between the extremes of TIA's and completed stroke lie two less common conditions. Briefly lasting, completed ischemic events, sometimes called *reversible ischemic neurologic defects* (RIND's), produce neurologic abnormalities similar to acute completed stroke, but the deficit subsides within 24 to 36 hours, leaving few or no detectable neurologic residua. Although less severe in their initial clinical damage than most completed strokes, the favorable outcome of RIND's usually cannot be predicted until rapid recovery begins. RIND's and other minor strokes differ only in that the latter leave more long-lasting neurologic residua. *Stroke in evolution* refers to a condition wherein ischemic neurologic deficits begin in a focal or restricted distribution but thereafter for a period of hours or more spread to affect ever-enlarging contiguous zones within the territory of a middle cerebral or basilar artery. About 15 per cent of patients with acute stroke deteriorate measurably within 24 hours after admission to hospital, making this an important time period for attempted therapy. A small number can evolve for longer periods, rarely lasting up to a week or more after onset. Diagnosis must be reviewed carefully in such instances to rule out other disorders. The pathogenesis of most evolving strokes probably consists of extension of thrombus from an initial clot along the affected artery. Some, especially in the vertebral basilar system, may reflect hemodynamic instability with insufficiency spreading into the penumbral margin of critical but not lethal ischemic zones at the edge of the initially hypoperfused area. Evolving stroke must be differentiated from the less specific neurologic worsening that results from cerebral edema with large, completed strokes (see below).

Major Stroke Syndromes

Ischemia of the Internal Carotid Artery (Anterior Circulation) System. More symptomatic emboli affect the anterior cerebral circulatory vascular bed than any other in the body. This is because of the extent of its supply to the sensorimotor zones of the hemispheres and also because so many emboli from the heart find their first escape up the large common carotid arteries.

Internal carotid artery (ICA) TIA's occur about half the time in association with arteriographically evident stenosis-ulceration or severe stenosis (> 75 per cent) in the ipsilateral common or internal carotid artery, usually at its bifurcation. Thrombi that arise from either the heart or the proximal aorta cause most of the rest. A few carotid TIA's may be caused by hematogenous abnormalities producing small, spontaneous endovascular clots.

Anterior circulation TIA's almost entirely affect either the retinal or middle cerebral artery (MCA) circulations, with the two involved concurrently about 10 per cent of the time. Isolated ophthalmic artery TIA's have the least serious prognosis, often appearing with no accompanying evidence of associated carotid or cardiovascular disease. Symptoms consist of a rapidly developing (10 seconds or so), unilateral graying out of vision of the eye, commonly spreading from the periphery to the center of the field and followed either by total amaurosis or a sense of seeing only shadows through a thick gray mist. Appropriately called *amaurosis fugax,* the episodes usually last for seconds, rarely for more than a few minutes. Retinal examination during the attack may disclose severe narrowing of both arteries and veins, sometimes with segmentation of venous blood. Occasionally one can observe fragments of white or yellow emboli slowly radiating outward through the arteries as the attack clears, usually leaving no residua. Yellow, refractile, residual retinal arterial spots represent cholesterol crystals. Their presence implies cholesterol in an upstream arterial plaque and a greater potential risk for future irreversible embolic ischemia.

Symptoms of TIA's affecting the MCA distribution depend upon the anatomy of the ischemic field. Peripheral cerebral branch occlusions characteristically cause transient, restricted hand-arm or face-hand-arm paresis with or without accompanying somesthetic sensory loss. Occlusions distal to the lenticulostriate artery take-off can cause transient aphasia, while those lodging proximal to or within the lenticulostriate arteries produce transient motor hemiparesis with or without associated language defects. Neither altered consciousness nor confusion ordinarily accompanies ICA-MCA TIA's, most of which last less than 10 to 20 minutes. Seizures are rare.

ICA Occlusion. *Acute* occlusion of the previously fully patent vessel can occur at any age due to immunologic-inflammatory disease, trauma, arterial dissection, massive embolism, or surgical ligation performed in an effort to halt traumatic bleeding or entrap an intracranial aneurysm. Resulting neurologic effects depend upon the patient's age and the anastomotic anatomy of the circle of Willis. In persons under 50 years, acute closure often can be tolerated asymptomatically.

Beyond that age increasing numbers suffer small or large infarcts in MCA distribution, even when cerebral arteriography shows an apparently adequate collateral arterial supply. Most ICA occlusions develop at the site of a previously severe stenosis, either at the carotid bifurcation or, less frequently, in the intracranial siphon.

The neurologic effects of either severe stenosis or total ICA occlusion depend on the rate at which closure occurs, whether or not ulcerated plaques stud the surface of the endothelial lesion, and the degree of intracranial anastomotic compensation. Stenoses that narrow the ICA orifice by less than 85 per cent usually cause little or no reduction in blood flow across the lesion. The stenosing plaques often contain ulcers, however, which can provide a source of TIA-causing emboli. Plaques containing calcification are especially dangerous. Complete occlusions vary widely in their resulting symptoms. Autopsy and arteriographic studies suggest that among ICA occlusions as many as half or more that evolve gradually cause neither remembered symptoms nor structural brain damage. Neurologic injury with the remainder ranges from small, deep focal infarctions to massive strokes that involve the entire distribution of the ipsilateral middle and, sometimes, anterior cerebral arteries.

TIA's or small completed strokes precede symptoms of major acute stroke due to ICA occlusion in as many as 20 per cent of cases, usually reflecting progressive stenosis or plaque formation. If a major hemispheric lesion does occur, neurologic symptoms and signs affecting the MCA distribution characteristically develop rapidly, with their intensity depending on the size of the subsequent brain lesion. Ipsilateral or bitemporal headache may accompany the onset of occlusion. Whether or not language disorders, sensory impairments, confusional states, or altered levels of consciousness develop depends on the distribution and size of the infarct as well as on the associated cerebral tissue reactions. Focal motor or generalized seizures accompany the acute stage of about 5 per cent of large ICA-MCA distribution infarcts.

External palpation of the neck is an unreliable sign in diagnosis of ICA occlusion, since internal and external carotid arteries cannot reliably be distinguished from one another. A total absence of cervical arterial pulsations in the region of the angle of the jaw or over the facial arteries suggests the uncommon event of common carotid or combined internal-external carotid artery occlusion. Bruits heard predominantly or entirely over the carotid bifurcation area below the angle of the jaw suggest an underlying stenosis of either the ICA or ECA or both. Generally, the harsher the bruit the more likely that it reflects severe stenosis, especially if accompanied by a palpable thrill. However, *only bruits that disappear as auscultation moves down the neck from the angle of the jaw toward the clavicle can be regarded confidently as emanating from the carotid bifurcation.*

Middle Cerebral Artery (MCA) Occlusion. Embolism represents the most frequent cause of MCA occlusion. Other mechanisms include extension of clot from an occluded internal carotid artery, intrinsic atherosclerosis, and endovascular thrombosis. The onset of symptoms and signs usually is rapid, taking seconds or minutes to evolve, and commonly silent, producing a lack of function but few positive neurologic symptoms. Affected patients, if asleep at onset, may notice no difficulty until they attempt to arise after awakening. Those who are awake may suddenly find without warning that they cannot speak or use an extremity in some common motor act. The immediate neurologic deficit, as with carotid occlusion or ICA-MCA TIA's, depends upon where along the MCA the occlusion rests. Major MCA strokes in either hemisphere tend to produce contralateral hemiplegia. Those affecting the dominant hemisphere tend to cause aphasia, while those lying in the nondominant right hemisphere tend to produce confusional states, spatial disorientation, and various degrees of sensory and emotional neglect. Psychological unresponsiveness with unilateral cerebral stroke is limited to patients in whom acute, large, dominant-hemisphere lesions produce global aphasia and patients who develop severe secondary brain edema and transtentorial compression-herniation.

ANTERIOR CEREBRAL ARTERY (ACA) OCCLUSION. The anterior cerebral artery has two major parts: (a) the basal portion extending from the ICA to join the anterior communicating artery and (b) the interhemispheric portion supplying the ipsilateral medial frontal lobe as far posteriorly as the sensorimotor foot area. Occlusion of the interhemispheric branch produces an acute focal sensorimotor defect in the contralateral foot and distal leg. Bilateral ACA occlusion distal to the anterior communicating artery causes a moderate spastic paraparesis, urinary incontinence, and behavioral and mental changes consistent with dysfunction of the association cortex of the frontal lobes. Proximal ACA occlusion may cause no neurologic deficits so long as a stout and patent anterior communicating artery carries blood from the opposite carotid supply. Lacking such collateral, ischemia may affect deep frontal lobe nuclei to cause in the dominant hemisphere Broca's or anterior conduction aphasia. TIA's rarely affect the ACA distribution; recurrent paresthesias or weakness involving a single foot-leg is more consistent with cerebral seizures or, occasionally, recurrent ischemia in the vertebral-basilar system.

Ischemia of the Vertebral-Basilar (Posterior Circulation) System. The basilar artery (BA) and two intracranial vertebral arteries (VA) are supplied rostrally by the posterior communicating arteries and caudally from the cervical vertebral arteries, which originate from the subclavians. Variation in the patency of these sources has several possible effects. With both ends of the double supply open, narrowing or even occlusion of a vertebral or even the basilar artery sometimes can occur without causing symptoms. Emboli are less frequent in the posterior than the anterior circu-

TABLE 120–4. COMMONEST SYMPTOMS OF VERTEBRAL BASILAR TIA'S

PARAMEDIAN ARTERIES	CIRCUMFERENTIAL ARTERIES
Transient global amnesia	Nonpositional vertigo
Diplopia	Unilateral face or body
Episodic, paroxysmal	paresthesias
drowsiness	Episodic hemianopia or
Paraparesis or tetraparesis	scintillations
Ataxia	Unilateral posterior headache
Dysarthria	

lation, whereas primary atherosclerotic occlusion affects the BA and VA's more frequently than the carotid systems.

Vertebral-basilar TIA's (VB TIA's) have potentially rich and variable patterns that can produce different symptoms and signs depending upon the anatomical distribution of ischemia. They often result in neurologic changes that vary from attack to attack in the same person (Table 120–4). This variability contrasts with carotid TIA's in which recurrent episodes in the same patient tend to remain stereotyped.

Occlusion of VA or BA and their main branches produces any of a number of somewhat complex syndromes depending on the rostral-caudal brain level of the arterial stoppage, the point of occlusion along the length of the vessel, and whether or not the involvement includes the paramedian vessels, circumferential arteries, or both.

Posterior cerebral artery (PCA) occlusions most often originate at the basilar take-off. More distal occlusions also can result, sometimes from emboli but also from inflammatory arteritis or compression during transtentorial herniation. Neurologic effects depend on the site of PCA closure. Distal obstructions result in homonymous quadrantic or hemianopias, while more proximal stoppage produces infarction of the sensory thalamus and sometimes the lateral midbrain as well.

BA occlusion at the apex has several possible outcomes depending upon whether the obstruction includes the posterior cerebral arteries, the arteries supplying the overlying diencephalon, the vessels feeding the midbrain, or some combination thereof. Loss or reduction of consciousness at the onset is common, often associated with a variety of pupillary, gaze, and oculomotor paralyses. If the cerebral peduncles are affected, decorticate or decerebrate motor posturing and paralysis ensue. During convalescence one finds varying combinations of dementia, memory loss, visual field defects, gaze palsy, and sensory or motor impairments, which individually or together reflect the extent of the eventual damage to the occipital lobe, the diencephalon, and the midbrain. More caudally placed occlusions of the BA, if they selectively affect paramedian vessels, impair consciousness and produce dysconjugate eye movements, unequal pupils, and bilateral signs of upper motor neuron dysfunction. Bizarre irregularities in breathing patterns commonly emerge. Obstruction of individual superior, anterior, and posterior cerebellar arteries characteristically produces contralateral sensory impairment on the body combined with variable lower motor neuron and sensory changes involving ipsilateral cranial nerves 5 through 12. Ipsilateral cerebellar ataxia and some degree of contralateral upper motor neuron deficit affecting at least the lower extremity often are associated.

Complete basilar occlusion affecting both paramedian and circumferential vessels usually produces incomplete ischemic transection of the brain stem. Affected patients usually are in a coma and show pinpoint, irregular, or unequal pupils, bilateral conjugate gaze paralysis, or internuclear ophthalmoplegia and tetraplegia. Mercifully, few survive more than a few days.

Unilateral VA occlusion produces clinical changes indistinguishable from blockage of a posterior inferior cerebellar artery. Postmortem studies suggest that about half such stoppages cause no symptoms. Among the remainder, signs of mild ipsilateral cerebellar dysfunction are accompanied by ipsilateral lower motor neuron paralysis of cranial nerves 9, 10, and 12, coupled with pain and temperature loss contralaterally on the body and ipsilaterally on the face. Ipsilateral miosis usually is present. Hiccup is common.

Acute cerebellar infarction can occur more or less independently of other neurologic difficulties when occlusion strikes any of the three main cerebellar arteries, principally the inferior branch. A grave syndrome ensues if enough ischemic edema affects the organ so that it swells to distort the brain stem and obstruct the normal CSF outflow. Initial symptoms include ipsilateral occipital headache and mild signs of cerebellar dysfunction followed by increasing occipital head pain, often vomiting, and the development of ipsilateral cranial nerve defects, including oculomotor changes. Progression, if it occurs, usually develops within 12 to 36 hours and is marked by more severe bilateral headache, drowsiness or stupor, and the appearance of bilateral upper motor neuron signs in the extremities. CT scans will show an enlarged, hypodense cerebellar hemisphere with obstruction of the fourth ventricle together with dilatation of the third and lateral ventricles. Urgent treatment, consisting of lateral ventricular drainage or occipital decompression, sometimes is required to prevent further damage or death.

Spinal Stroke. Ischemic infarction due to arterial occlusion rarely affects the spinal cord. More common is spinal infarction associated with prolonged hypotension (shock) or compression by intraspinal mass lesions. Arterial lesions, when they occur, almost always involve the anterior spinal artery, atherosclerotic obstruction striking most often at the level of the cervical radicular artery or one or two segments below. Inflammatory and immune arteritides are as frequent as or more frequent than atherosclerotic obstructions, especially in younger persons, and tend to occur at the T4 level. In both instances, neurologic damage develops acutely or rapidly, usually reaching a maximum within 24 hours of onset, and involves primarily the anterior one third of the cord. Lower motor neuron abnormalities sometimes can be detected at the level of the lesion combined with bilateral impairment of pain and temperature sensations beginning one or two dermatomes below. Injury to corticospinal pathways results in upper motor neuron dysfunction caudal to the level of occlusion. Dysfunction of bowel, bladder, and male sexual activities usually accompanies these abnormalities.

Cerebral Venous Thrombosis. Obstruction to the cerebral venous sinuses or their main tributaries has several potential causes (Table 120–5). Most spontaneous examples appear either during the postpartum period, as an idiopathic phenomenon related to little understood "physiological" hypercoagulability, or as a complication of disease-related coagulopathy, especially that associated with cancer or infection. The clinical findings are discussed on page (784).

Hypertensive Encephalopathy (HE). HE represents a serious complication of severe hypertension, now made uncommon by the widespread use of effective antihypertensive drugs. The abnormal cerebral state accompanies an acute rise in blood pressure in excess of previous levels, precipitated most often by acute or chronic renal disease, eclampsia, or the abrupt withdrawal of previously taken antihypertensive drugs. Foods high in tyramine content can precipitate HE in patients taking monoamine oxidase inhibiting drugs for psychiatric illness. Recurrent crises sometimes reflect the presence of an underlying pheochromocytoma and can occur rarely for unexplained reasons in individuals with otherwise only moderate chronic hypertension.

The pathogenesis of HE relates to the effect of the high systemic intravascular pressure on the brain's arterioles. The elevated tension exceeds the upper limits of normal cerebral autoregulation, so that a combination of multifocal arteriolar vasodilatation and vasoconstriction occurs, producing diffusely distributed small zones of microhemorrhages and ischemia.

Florid multifocal and usually transient clinical changes characterize HE and include headache, nausea, vomiting, and visual loss, sometimes with cortical blindness. Focal or generalized seizures, confusional states, stupor, or coma marks the course of severe attacks. Focal, often evanescent monoplegia or hemiplegia may be present. The retinal arterioles usually show abnormal hypertensive changes and sometimes are barely visible

TABLE 120–5. MAJOR CAUSES OF CEREBRAL VENOUS AND SINUS THROMBOSIS IN APPROXIMATELY DECLINING ORDER OF FREQUENCY

Late pregnancy and postpartum state
Contraceptive medication
Coagulant factors associated with malignancy, disseminated intravascular coagulation, thrombotic purpura
Idiopathic
Severe dehydration or intrinsic hyperviscosity
Septic extension from face, sinus, mastoid

because of spasm. Hemorrhages and papilledema can occur, but nowadays are no longer the rule. The BUN is less than 100 mg/dl and often normal. CSF values are usually elevated for pressure (above 180 mm Hg), protein (above 60 mg/dl), and cells (both RBC and WBC). CT is not diagnostic except to rule out an intracranial mass lesion or hemorrhage as the cause of illness.

Differential diagnosis of HE includes acute uremia (BUN > 100 mg/dl), encephalitis (fever, no severe hypertension, usually slower course), cerebral venous sinus thrombosis, and acute lead encephalopathy. Less common causes of acute multifocal encephalopathy must be considered, including disseminated intravascular coagulation and acute bacterial endocarditis.

HE requires urgent treatment using intravenously regulated sodium nitroprusside to lower blood pressure promptly to levels within the upper range of autoregulation (mean 130 ± 10 mm Hg). Later, within 12 hours or so, systemic pressures can be brought further down more gradually so as to allow arterioles to adapt to the reduced pressure and thereby reduce the risk of inducing focal cerebral hypoperfusion. Convulsions can be controlled acutely using diazepam, 10 to 20 mg intravenously. Long-term control of the underlying hypertension must be pursued vigorously.

Diagnosis and Differential Diagnosis in Ischemic Stroke

The major diagnostic questions are several: Has an ischemic event occurred? If so, is it transient, progressive, or completed? If completed, is it minor or major? Finally, what is its cause and what immediately and subsequently must be done?

Clinical understanding plus judiciously chosen confirmatory laboratory tests give accurate diagnosis in nearly all instances. Age, mode of onset, the presence or absence of known risk factors or previous vascular events, and whether or not the neurologic deficit fits a known vascular distribution provide the chief clues. The first minutes or hours of observation tell whether a stroke is a TIA, is progressing, or, for the time being, has completed its ravages. The general history and physical examination often disclose the presence or absence of stroke-causing systemic diseases (Table 120–1), especially those of the heart or great vessels. These steps, combined with routine laboratory studies (urinalysis, CBC and smear, standard chemical and electrolyte screening, ECG, chest x-ray) provide accurate diagnosis in perhaps 90 per cent of instances. To these measures should be added a CT head scan performed with and without contrast agent for any first completed or progressive stroke, since about 4 per cent of patients diagnosed on clinical grounds as having a stroke turn out to have other disorders such as a neoplasm or hematoma. CT is also indicated to verify possible strokes with unusual anatomic patterns. CT or, if unavailable, lumbar puncture should be done before initiating anticoagulant therapy, since some cerebral hemorrhages have a stroke-like onset. Even fairly large areas of brain infarction, however, may not produce CT changes of either necrosis, edema, or contrast enhancement until 24 to 48 hours after onset. Small strokes may never disfigure the scan.

Ischemic stroke affects persons less than age 50 rarely, and those less than 70 uncommonly, except in association with specific risk factors or identifiable toxic or systemic causes. Patients lacking such apparent antecedents deserve especially careful appraisal.

Differentiation among TIA's, progressive stroke, minor completed stroke, and severe completed stroke is implicit in their presentations. TIA's must be differentiated from seizures, usually not a difficult matter, since TIA's rarely cause positive motor signs, are less long-lasting, and produce no postictal effects. Nevertheless, with stereotyped recurrent hemispheric attacks a CT scan is desirable to rule out a structural cause. Glaucoma or other local diseases of the eye, cranial arteritis, and migraine represent alternate potential causes of unilateral visual loss. Basilar migraine, an illness most common in young persons and carrying a strong family predisposition, can produce symptoms suggesting VB TIA's; age, family history, and a longer duration all are distinctive. Benign positional vertigo differs from basilar TIA's by its strict link to positional stimuli and its lack of associated symptoms of brain stem dysfunction. Similar considerations rule out the nonspecific dizzy feelings experienced by many elderly persons. Cardiac arrhythmias rarely cause symptoms resembling TIA's, just as TIA's rarely cause syncope (page 657). Subdural hematomas or large intracranial aneurysms sometimes produce attacks indistinguishable from carotid TIA's and perhaps having a similar pathogenesis. Such episodes are rare, however, without associated specific symptoms of the primary disorder. Minor or major progressive or completed stroke must be distinguished from deep cerebral hemorrhage. Usually, the latter produces more headache, a faster evolution, a higher incidence of seizures, and prominent autonomic changes. Brain tumors can resemble stroke in occasional instances when they internally bleed and suddenly enlarge. Afebrile brain abscesses or granulomas can provide a similar problem. CT scan differentiates in all three instances. Postictal paralysis can give the appearance of stroke, but the history is distinctive. When the seizure is unobserved, age and rapid recovery usually serve to differentiate. Cervical-cerebral angiography has little usefulness in evaluating acute stroke. Its place in managing aftercare is described below.

Etiologic diagnosis in stroke is important for guiding both acute and chronic management. All patients deserve careful evaluation of the cardiovascular system, with one basing the extent of the investigation upon preliminary findings and known risk factors. Echocardiography and wall motion studies can identify potential sources of emboli in patients with mitral prolapse, valvular stenosis, or anterior wall infarctions and will detect the rare unsuspected atrial myxoma. EEG's and other clinical neurophysiological studies seldom provide useful information. Noninvasive investigations, such as ultrasonic or Doppler flow studies, applied to the carotid systems become more useful in planning convalescent than acute management. Generally speaking, the more restricted and reversible the inital neurologic injury, the more assiduously one searches for specific causes for which treatment might reduce the risk of future brain damage.

Management of Acute Stroke

Once ischemic neurologic damage has occurred, no currently available treatment favorably influences the outcome of the brain injury. Management consists of providing good general medical and nursing care, reducing hypertension or hyperviscosity if present, and taking steps to prevent acute or future worsening of the neurologic deficit. Acutely, one attempts to halt progressing stroke, prevent acutely recurring cerebral emboli, and stabilize with the least possible deficit patients with fluctuating neurologic changes. In 24 hours or so after onset, the problem of ischemic brain edema may require therapeutic attention.

The Use and Choice of Anticoagulants. The use of these drugs in acute stroke is a somewhat controversial subject. The treatment can cause dangerous bleeding of about 1 to 2 per cent per year in experienced hands. Anticoagulation is contraindicated in the presence of uremia, any bleeding diathesis, and diastolic blood pressure greater than 100 mm Hg. In other circumstances, the choice and use of anticoagulants are guided by theoretical considerations plus a limited number of incompletely controlled studies and the experience of the therapist. We describe here the approach at the New York Hospital.

Heparin therapy, unless specifically contraindicated, is initiated at the time of admission to hospital in patients describing repetitive, closely spaced TIA's, in those with progression of weakness during the hours before hospitalization, in those observed to have increasing neurologic deficits during the first 12 to 18 hours following admission, and in patients demonstrating fluctuating signs and symptoms of vertebral, basilar, or carotid ischemia. A CT scan is obtained first to rule out hemorrhage. If lumbar puncture has been performed, heparin thereafter is delayed for at least two hours to minimize potential spinal epidural bleeding. Heparin is also given to patients with minor or restricted completed strokes of less than 8 to 12 hours' duration as well as to patients suffering a first stroke accompanied by conditions such as atrial fibrillation that produce a high risk of future embolism.

Heparin therapy is stopped usually within three to five days in patients who turn out to have no neurologic progression or instability, in those who complete a severe stroke with massive cerebral, brain stem, or cerebellar infarction, and in patients with partial defects that clear quickly

(RIND). Heparin is replaced gradually by coumerol derivatives in patients whose evolving stroke halted when they received the drug as well as in those with a high risk of future embolization. Anticoagulation is stopped in most patients except those with atrial fibrillation (AF) after two to three months and continued out of hospital only when adequate supervision can be guaranteed. Chronic anticoagulation is reserved for patients with chronic AF, valvular protheses, and a limited number of other specific thrombogenic disorders.

Platelet Antiaggregant Therapy. Several large trials have suggested that aspirin given to persons previously susceptible to TIA's or coronary artery disease reduces the risk of recurrent cerebral TIA's as well of both cerebral and cardiac thromboembolism. Two other agents, dipyridamole and sulfinpyrazone, also possess theoretically beneficial effects against platelet aggregation. Aspirin exerts long-lasting effects on the arachidonate cascade so as to inhibit platelet aggregation and is given in single daily doses ranging from 80 mg to as much as 1.5 gm. Empirical confirmation of the ideal dose awaits clinical trial. Dipyridamole and sulfinpyrazone possess shorter durations of action than salicylates and are given in divided doses, three to four times daily.

When not specifically contraindicated, platelet antiaggregants are currently used by most authorities to treat all patients experiencing infrequent carotid or vertebral basilar TIA's, for chronic treatment of patients who have had a completed stroke, and for patients considered at high risk for stroke.

Ischemic Cerebral Edema. Some degree of edema surrounds all cerebral infarcts. The necrosis of cells and vascular endothelium releases osmols into the extracellular space while the associated death of astrocytes prevents their normal osmotic pumping action. The combined factors draw water into the extracellular space, sometimes in dangerous proportions. Ischemic edema generally becomes detectable within 12 to 24 hours following infarction and continues to increase for as long as 48 hours thereafter.

Cerebral edema produces hypodense areas by CT scanning surrounding a region of recent infarction. Such changes usually cannot be detected until at least 48 hours after the ictus and by themselves neither produce symptoms nor require treatment. Large, edematous hemispheric infarcts, however, can lead to transtentorial herniation, while similar enlargement in the cerebellum may compress the brain stem or obstruct CSF outflow pathways. Either can be fatal.

Systemic metabolic derangements and pulmonary or urinary infections appear to intensify the edematous process. Treatment consists of correcting or treating these complications and, if herniation threatens, giving intravenously a dehydrating agent such as mannitol in an effort to shrink the brain. Passive hyperventilation will briefly reduce the intracranial pressure by inducing one to two hours of arterial vasoconstriction. Diuretic drugs produce minimal benefit except as they treat systemic fluid overload. The induction of anesthetic coma has no therapeutic value and greatly complicates care. Corticosteroid drugs are contraindicated: they do not benefit necrotic edema and may induce hyperglycemia, which risks worsening of the stroke.

Convalescent Management. Patients whose neurologic disability improves incompletely within two to three weeks will benefit from an organized rehabilitation program. Most improvement can be expected by 8 to 12 weeks, making prolonged rehabilitation measures unjustified. The additional value of speech therapy is uncertain.

Preventive Measures. Even after a first stroke, epidemiologic studies indicate that treatment of hypertension and cessation of smoking reduce the risk of recurrence. Weight loss for the obese and at least some exercise for everyone may be beneficial. Otherwise, careful medical supervision plus daily platelet antiaggregants form the mainstay of most medical treatment.

Arteriography and Vascular Surgery in Stroke Prevention

Arteriography carries a risk of 1 to 2 per cent of serious complications in the stroke age group but is indicated (1) when diagnosis is in doubt, (2) to seek the source of an arteriovenous malformation or an unexplained subarachnoid or lobar cerebral hemorrhage, and (3) to search for potentially surgically treatable stenoses or ulcerations in the carotid arterial system.

Operative repair of internal carotid artery stenosis in the neck has become widely practiced in recent years as a presumed preventive measure against strokes in the ipsilateral cerebral hemisphere. Controversy surrounds both the indications for such procedures and their results, the only existing controlled study on the subject showing no benefit from surgery. Those data may be outdated by modern approaches, although most other analyses also suffer limitations of case selection and other factors. The approach taken by the Stroke Research Center at The New York Hospital–Cornell Medical Center follows.

Treatment of TIA's and Partial or Minor Strokes. A substantial fraction of patients with these disorders have lesions of the carotid arteries. If the ipsilateral internal carotid artery in the neck contains an ulcerated plaque or a greater than 80 per cent stenosis, carotid endarterectomy is recommended so long as no contraindications exist as discussed below. The presence of surface calcium in the ulcer strengthens the recommendation. Patients with exclusively basilar TIA's or partial strokes are not subjected to arteriography or considered for surgery, since no evidence suggests that benefits would follow.

Carotid Bruits and Neurologically Asymptomatic Internal Carotid Lesions. Several studies indicate that careful physical examination discloses a carotid bruit unassociated with cerebrovascular symptoms in about 5 per cent of the population over age 50 years. Only about half of such patients show appreciable internal carotid artery narrowing by arteriography. Present evidence indicates that in asymptomatic patients whose arteriograms show neither ulcerated plaques nor a greater than 80 per cent stenosis of the internal carotid artery the morbidity-mortality risk of arteriography plus surgery is as high or higher than the risk of naturally occurring stroke. Accordingly, the ideal approach to patients with asymptomatic cervical bruits is to obtain noninvasive Doppler or sonographic flow studies of the carotid arteries. If these studies disclose severe ulcerations or tight narrowing, arteriography can then be carried out to determine whether or not a lesion exists that is appropriate for surgical treatment.

Contraindications for Carotid Surgery. These consist of circumstances in which either surgical treatment has no shown measurable benefit or potential complications exceed possible benefits. They include complete internal carotid artery occlusions; acutely evolving strokes; totally asymptomatic carotid narrowing in patients destined for coronary bypass or other major surgery; the presence of an already massive cerebral infarct involving the ICA-MCA vascular field; plaques or narrowing in the intracranial portion of the carotid artery, and unstable general medical conditions such as recent myocardial infarction, congestive heart failure, uncontrolled hypertension, or severe systemic metabolic problems. Such factors double or triple the surgical risk.

Some surgeons have attempted other vascular operations such as bypassing a superficial temporal artery to a distal branch of the middle cerebral artery in efforts to prevent future stroke. Controlled studies indicate that such operations offer no therapeutic value.

Prognosis in Stroke

About one fourth of patients with acute completed stroke will die during hospitalization. Advanced age, severe brain stem dysfunction, coma, and severe associated heart disease all worsen the prognosis. Among survivors about 40 per cent make a good functional recovery, with the degree and rate depending on the initial severity, the degree of improvement within the first two weeks, age, and how much language or cognitive difficulty persists. Few patients with pronounced Wernicke aphasia or functional dementia regain full independence. Motor flaccidity or dense hemisensory defects persisting past the first weeks similarly reduce the chances for future independence.

Prognosis for patients with TIA's depends on the presence or absence of associated risk factors, especially cardiac. A variety of studies indicate a combined risk of about 12 per cent per year for either stroke, myocardial infarction, or death (from either) following the onset of these minor cerebrovascular events. The annual risk of such consequences climbs to about 20 per cent among patients with major strokes.

CEREBRAL HEMORRHAGE

Spontaneous (nontraumatic) cerebral hemorrhage may occur primarily into the substance of the brain (intracerebral or parenchymal) or over its surface (subarachnoid). With rare exceptions, all arise from one of three causes: (1) progressive damage and finally rupture into the parenchyma of a brain-penetrating artery due to hypertension, atherosclerosis, or intrinsic arterial degeneration, (2) "spontaneous" rupture of a penetrating artery associated with either excess circulating anticoagulant or an intrinsic defect in coagulation, (3) rupture of a congenital or acquired arterial anomaly into the subarachnoid space (berry and mycotic aneurysm) or the parenchyma (arteriovenous malformation). Other uncommon mechanisms include hemorrhage into brain tumors, bleeding from inflammatory vasculopathies such as periarteritis nodosa or that associated with amphetamine usage, and bleeding from degenerative amyloid (congophilic) angiopathy in the elderly. Hemorrhagic infarction with arterial or venous obstruction has been discussed in a previous section. Cerebral hemorrhage totals about 15 per cent of all clinically detectable strokes but assumes greater importance because of the serious consequences that often result.

Hypertensive Atherosclerotic (H-A) Cerebral Hemorrhage. Roughly 90 per cent of spontaneous parenchymal cerebral hemorrhages fall into this category; the remainder emanate mainly from vascular malformations and blood dyscrasias, with a small number arising from amyloid (congophilic) degeneration of the arteries. Approximately two thirds affect patients with hypertension, with the incidence of bleeding generally paralleling the intensity and duration of that disorder. With or without hypertension, rupture reflects an area of weakening brought about by a combination of mural wear and tear eventually leading to bleeding from penetrating arterioles of approximately 100 to 150 μm in diameter. The results of CT scanning indicate that spontaneous bleeding can affect almost any part of the brain. Bleeding into the deep cerebral regions of the internal capsule, basal ganglia, and thalamus, as well as into the central pons and the deep nuclear regions of the cerebellum represents the most frequently devastating forms (Fig. 120–7). Most hemorrhages affecting more peripheral or polar regions of the hemisphere either produce few symptoms or cause changes that resemble ischemic stroke. The regions of the lower diencephalon, midbrain, medulla, and spinal cord are unusual sites for H-A bleeding to occur.

In contrast to ischemic stroke, which commonly occurs during sleep, most H-A cerebral hemorrhage begins during wakefulness, often associated with exertion. Sudden severe headache, "the worst in my life," announces the onset, followed within minutes to hours by neurologic signs whose nature and severity reflect the site and extent of the bleeding. Characteristically, systemic examination discloses hypertension, sometimes to a temporarily severe degree, and, commonly, cardiac enlargement as well as hypertensive changes in the retinal arteries.

Basal Ganglia–Internal Capsular Hemorrhage. The onset headache commonly arises ipsilateral to the bleed and is followed shortly by a progressive contralateral hemiparesis, often accompanied by the eyes deviating toward the side of the lesion owing to damage to the frontal eye fields. Convulsions are common and can take either a generalized grand mal pattern or be focal and involve the body contralateral to the bleeding. In the latter case, the eyes often deviate away from the lesion during the seizure. Rupture into the lateral ventricle is frequent and precipitates autonomic symptoms of shivering, nausea, and vomiting. Large hemorrhages greater than 2.5 to 3 cm in diameter frequently produce first coma, leading to signs of transtentorial herniation-compression, followed by severe disability or death. Smaller bleeding causes proportionately less neurologic damage, and ultimate improvement may be considerable.

Thalamic Hemorrhage. While serious, these often are less large or devastating than the above. Contralateral sensory loss, hemianopia, and hemiparesis or hemiplegia are characteristic. Compression of the tectum-midbrain commonly induces drowsiness, which proceeds to coma only in rapidly fatal cases. Gaze palsies are common and include defects in upward gaze. Eyes cast down and laterally at rest provide an almost pathognomonic sign of bleeding in this area. Midbrain compression may transiently cause pupillary inequality or fixation.

Pontine Hemorrhage. The onset usually is cataclysmic with sudden headache followed within seconds to minutes by coma accompanied by stertorous or irregularly irregular breathing, pinpoint pupils, bilateral conjugate gaze paralysis or ocular bobbing, tetraparesis and, often, decerebrate or decorticate rigidity. Most patients die, and those who survive usually are left quadriplegic and totally dependent.

Cerebellar Hemorrhage. Unilateral occipital headache often announces the onset followed by ipsilateral incoordination-ataxia of the extremities, slurred speech, and sometimes nausea and vomiting. Disequilibrium, ipsilateral facial weakness, and diplopia with ipsilateral conjugate gaze paralysis often follow within a matter of hours and may reflect either dissection of the hematoma into the lateral pons or only compression of that structure. The development of a reduced level of consciousness or of signs of upper motor neuron dysfunction in the extremities suggests the possibility of brain stem compression, either because of direct enlargement of the hematoma or secondary to acute obstruction of the fourth ventricle, producing hydrocephalus.

Diagnosis

Only acute ischemic stroke represents a frequent source of potential diagnostic uncertainty, although hemorrhage into brain tumors may be

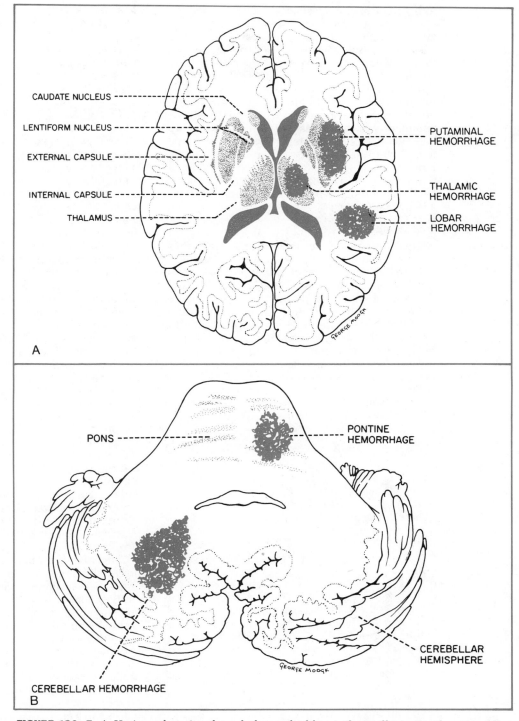

FIGURE 120–7. *A,* Horizontal section through the cerebral hemispheres illustrating the sites of thalamic, putaminal, and lobar hemorrhages. *B,* Horizontal section through pons and adjacent cerebellum showing common hemorrhage sites. In specific instances, hemorrhages can be either smaller or larger than diagrammed. (From Barnett HJM: Intracranial hemorrhage. In Wyngaarden JB, and Smith LH Jr (eds): Cecil Textbook of Medicine. 17th ed. Philadelphia, WB Saunders Co, pp 2103–2111.)

indistinguishable. Headache, severe hypertension, acute prostration, nausea and vomiting, convulsions, autonomic signs, and loss of consciousness are all more characteristic of hemorrhage than ischemia. If blood reaches the subarachnoid space or if downward or upward herniation threatens, the neck will be stiff. The CT scan is diagnostic, leaving only the cause of bleeding in doubt. Patients who are not hypertensive, who are young, or who have less than devastating neurologic deficits deserve arteriography to seek a potentially treatable vascular anomaly. Lumbar puncture can precipitate fatal intracranial herniation and should be avoided unless no CT scan is available and acute bacterial meningitis seems a strong possibility.

Treatment

Treatment consists of lowering the blood pressure deliberately as described under hypertensive encephalopathy and applying supportive measures. Where clinical signs and CT exams suggest that a cerebellar hemorrhage is compressing the brain stem or causing acute hydrocephalus, lateral ventricular decompression may be life-saving. Occasionally, posterior fossa decompression may become necessary. Efforts to drain acute cerebral hemorrhages surgically usually lead to a neurologic outcome worse than otherwise would be the case.

Patients in coma from cerebral hemorrhage seldom survive, and those with extensive brain stem

damage usually remain neurologically devastated. Considerable neurologic recovery, however, often follows even moderately large hemorrhages in the cerebral or cerebellar hemispheres, presumably because the blood dissects between much of the tissue rather than destroying it.

INTRACRANIAL ANEURYSMS

Intracranial aneurysms occur in three characteristic forms: fusiform, mycotic, and congenital "berry" aneurysms.

Fusiform aneurysms represent ectatic dilatations of the basilar or intracranial carotid artery which take a sausage-like or irregular bulbous shape, sometimes reaching a size of 5 to 10 cm in diameter. Usually they produce no symptoms, but sometimes their large size compresses adjacent tissues or cranial nerves to cause local neurologic dysfunction. Large basilar artery aneurysms characteristically cause multiple bilateral asymmetrical cranial nerve dysfunction extending anywhere from the third to the tenth nerve, while those of the carotid artery can cause symptoms reflecting their parapituitary position. In either location, branch occlusion of vessels arising within or adjacent to the aneurysm can occur. Such ectatic aneurysms seldom rupture, and they are rarely amenable to successful surgical therapy.

Mycotic aneurysms result in the course of bacterial endocarditis when septic emboli lodge in a peripherally located cerebral vessel, producing endothelial ischemia at the embolic site. Infecting bacteria subsequently invade the arterial wall, and the resulting weakening invites aneurysmal blowout. Mycotic aneurysms often are multiple and recognized by their peripheral location on the cerebral arterial tree. Some resolve with antibiotic treatment, but those that remain after systemic infection is brought under control should be surgically treated.

Congenital berry aneurysms arise at bifurcation points along the circle of Willis at the base of the brain in the anterior circulation, forming especially at the junctions between the anterior cerebral and anterior communicating arteries; and between the middle cerebral and either the posterior communicating or carotid arteries (Fig. 120–8). Less frequently, similar aneurysms balloon out at one of the several major tributary points along the basilar-vertebral axis. Berry aneurysms vary considerably in size from a few millimeters to 1, 2, or more centimeters in diameter. Those larger than 1.5 to 2 cm in diameter are commonly termed "giant" and carry a particular risk of rupture.

The pathogenesis of berry aneurysms is thought to reflect a congenital defect in elastic tissue and muscle at arterial branch points along the base of the brain which allow aneurysmal formation and eventual rupture secondary to accumulated wear and tear. Similar aneurysms also occur in association with brain tumors; here the mechanism is unknown. Congenital aneurysms are more common in persons with long-standing hypertension,

Internal carotid artery

Anterior communicating artery

Anterior cerebral artery

Middle cerebral artery

Posterior communicating artery

Posterior cerebral artery

Superior cerebellar artery

Paramedian arteries

Circumferential artery

Anterior inferior cerebellar artery

Basilar artery

Vertebral artery

Posterior inferior cerebellar artery

Anterior spinal artery

FIGURE 120–8. The more common sites of berry aneurysm. The diagrammatic size of the aneurysm at the various sites is directly proportional to its frequency at that locus. (From McDowell FH: Intracranial hemorrhage. In Beeson PB, McDermott W, and Wyngaarden JB (eds): Cecil Textbook of Medicine. 15th ed. Philadelphia, WB Saunders Co, 1979, pp 794–801.)

especially those with coarctation of the aorta and polycystic kidney disease. Some persons have multiple intracranial aneurysms. A low but definite family incidence has been reported.

Most intracranial aneurysms are detected only when they rupture, an event that can occur at any age but is most common between the ages of 40 and 65. Most rupture takes place during the waking hours, many examples occurring in association with hypertension-inducing physical activity.

Clinical Manifestations of Aneurysmal Rupture and Subarachnoid Hemorrhage (SAH)

These can be divided into five phases: onset, the first week of acute symptoms, the risk of secondary ischemic infarction, the development of communicating hydrocephalus, and the indications for and outcome of surgery.

The usual first symptom is sudden excruciating headache, sometimes followed by brief syncope or a seizure, the latter symptoms being attributed either to an induced cardiac arrhythmia or to the brief concussion that accompanies the sudden rise in intracranial pressure. Subsequent effects depend on the locus and extent of the bleeding. Small warning leaks sometimes occur, causing a uniquely severe headache that then subsides over the following few days. Larger bleeds confined to the subarachnoid space produce more severe and sustained head pain, followed in 12 to 24 hours by signs of meningeal inflammation as red blood cells lyse and release irritating bile pigments into the CSF. Severe bleeds can immediately produce coma, sometimes caused by a high intracranial pressure, but more often because bleeding dissects into the brain or ruptures into the ventricular system. Persistent coma implies transtentorial herniation and a bad prognosis.

Stiff neck at onset implies a large hemorrhage, perhaps with descent of the cerebellar tonsils. Subhyaloid retinal hemorrhages can appear within minutes of the onset of the subarachnoid bleeding. If either focal neurologic signs or a reduced state of consciousness develops immediately, it implies that blood has dissected into the brain, worsening the prognosis. After the first day, the development of new focal motor or neurologic abnormalities reflects either an episode of rebleeding or a secondary cerebral infarction caused by arterial vasospasm induced by the subarachnoid blood.

After the first few hours of bleeding a variety of systemic and secondary changes complicate the picture. The autonomic storm that accompanies the initial headache releases systemic catecholamines, which produce diffuse myocardial micronecrosis and infarction-like ECG abnormalities. Acutely, systemic hyperglycemia, leukocytosis, and fever have a similar pathogenesis. Subsequently, fever, leukocytosis, and delirium can last a week or more due to the continuing hemorrhagic chemical meningitis. Most severely ill patients with acute SAH secrete inappropriately high lev-

els of antidiuretic hormone. Late symptoms of lethargy, continued delirium, stupor, or diffuse mild upper motor neuron abnormalities may reflect the development of communicating hydrocephalus.

Diagnosis

The first principle is thoroughly to respect the development of sudden severe headache in a previously well adult. Discrimination may be difficult in persons of known hypochondriacal disposition, but when in serious doubt, even if neurologic findings are absent, it is wise to obtain lumbar puncture, taking care to identify intrinsic bleeding by centrifuging bloody fluid and looking for a discolored supernatant.

For more obviously acutely ill patients with typical symptoms, CT scan is the laboratory procedure of first choice. SAH's large enough to threaten transtentorial herniation will show blood by CT evaluation; if none is visualized, lumbar puncture can then be done to seek infection or other potential causes of sudden acute headache. CT scans also will show whether or not large clots exist in the subarachnoid space or brain (they increase the risk of arterial spasm) and provide a baseline for future comparison in the event of subsequent unexplained worsenings. Contrast CT scans performed with contemporary instruments often will outline aneurysms of greater that 5 mm in diameter as well as arteriovenous abnormalities that may have caused the hemorrhage.

Arteriography is indispensable for identifying the presence and location of aneurysms and, where more than one is found, for estimating which has bled. For patients in a hospital staffed with surgeons appropriately skilled for aneurysm work, radiographs should be obtained on suitable surgical candidates as soon as possible after admission. In poor-risk patients or when it is anticipated that surgery will be done elsewhere, no value is gained by adding the hazards of arteriography to the already precarious state. The latter patients should be transferred as early as possible to a tertiary care center.

Prognosis and Management

Prognosis is poor in acute SAH owing to ruptured aneurysm. Careful population studies indicate that of all such patients, two thirds die within one month (many without reaching hospital), with about one fourth of the survivors being severely disabled. The first two weeks after onset carry the greatest risk of rebleeding, amounting to about 30 per cent. Among patients whose aneurysms cannot be treated successfully, rebleeding with a two thirds risk of mortality continues at about 3 per cent per year.

The above considerations imply that as soon as acute SAH is recognized patients should be placed in the hands of an experienced neurologic-neurosurgical team for definitive management. Initially, patients are placed at bed rest, kept quiet with mild benzodiazepine sedatives, and given analgesics short of opiates for pain. Stool softeners or enemas are important for preventing straining. Gentle movement in bed and turning should be emphasized to prevent the complications of immobility. Blood pressure should be controlled at nearly normal levels, but blood volume should be maintained by adequate fluids using 3 per cent saline solutions if necessary to correct hyponatremia.

Most centers do four-vessel cerebral angiography within 24 hours of onset. Definitive treatment consists of surgical isolation and clipping of the leaking aneurysm. Such procedures are technically difficult and carry a high perioperative risk of inducing even more brain damage. Currently, surgical opinion differs as to whether operation is better done immediately, risking more frequent complications, or after 10 to 14 days when the risk of spasm and associated infarction declines but the greatest chance of rebleeding already has passed. Surgery should be deferred or avoided in patients who are neurologically unstable, in those with major neurologic deficits, and in those who are stuporous or comatose. Similarly, most authorities avoid immediate surgery for patients whose arteriograms show arterial vasospasm. Continued obtundation not explained by focal damage and associated with CT evidence of progressive hydrocephalus sometimes can be relieved by ventricular shunting. It is not established whether or not operative treatment initiated more than 30 days following initial bleeding confers any advantage over the natural history of the disease.

ARTERIOVENOUS MALFORMATIONS (AVM's)

In addition to congenital aneurysms, four types of vascular malformations can affect the brain. These include: (1) Capillary telangiectases, seldom a cause of clinical abnormalities. (2) Venous angiomas. One form comprises the Sturge-Weber syndrome; larger ones may rupture or, in the spinal cord, produce tissue compression. (3) Small vessel *cavernous angiomas*, which sometimes provide an occult source of intracerebral hemorrhage. (4) AVM's consisting of snakelike vascular tangles in which arteries connect directly with veins. AVM's can affect any part of the brain or spinal cord. They range in diameter from a few millimeters to structures that occupy most of a cerebral lobe. Most form at the junction points of two or more major intracranial arteries such as in

the deep frontoparietal area where anterior, middle, and posterior circulations converge. The rule is for AVM's gradually to increase in size, which best explains why they most often produce their symptoms in persons over age 30 years.

AVM's can cause three kinds of neurologic disability. As many as half leak intermittently, producing various-sized parenchymal or subarachnoid hemorrhages, usually smaller and less dangerous than results from either hypertensive hemorrhage or ruptured berry aneurysm. Of the remaining, some cause focal epileptic seizures, while others, in the process of their slow enlargement, generate progressive neurologic deficits. A small percentage of AVM's are associated with unilateral headaches resembling classic migraines; among all migraine, however, this is a rare cause.

Definitive treatment of AVM's is technically difficult because many of them reside in neurologically indispensable areas of brain. Moderate-sized AVM's discovered incidentally by CT scan or arteriography and causing no symptoms are best left alone. Although symptomatic lesions lying in the poles of the frontal or occipital lobes often can be amputated safely, larger AVM's usually have many arterial sources and may be difficult or impossible to remove without producing severe postoperative deficits. The risk of neurologic damage or fatal bleeding in intracranial AVM's is relatively low and cases should be judged individually by experienced neurologic centers. Appropriate nonsurgical treatment is necessary to treat seizures and other neurologic deficits.

REFERENCES

Barnett HJM: Cerebrovascular diseases. In Wyngaarden JB, and Smith LH Jr (eds): Cecil Textbook of Medicine. 17th ed. Philadelphia, WB Saunders Co, 1985, pp 2086–2111. *A well-balanced, referenced, and thorough treatment of the subject.*

Barnett HJM, Plum F, and Walton JM: Carotid endarterectomy—an expression of concern. Stroke 15:941, 1984. *The editorial introduces an issue which contains articles pro and con on this debated subject.*

Kassel NF, and Drake CG: Review of the management of saccular aneurysms. Neurol Clin 1:73, 1983. *A comprehensive, up-to-date review of this vexingly difficult clinical problem.*

Ross RW (ed): Vascular Diseases of the Central Nervous System. 2nd ed. New York, Churchill Livingstone, Inc, 1983. *A well-written, multiauthored, detailed monograph.*

TRAUMA TO THE HEAD AND SPINE

Serious craniofacial and spinal injuries create a major source of death and disability in the United States. The annual incidence exceeds 100,000 cases, of whom almost half die, with many of the survivors suffering chronic intellectual or motor-sensory limitations. Furthermore, most of the victims are in the younger, most productive decades of their lives. Emergency and early general medical care influence both mortality and morbidity, making an understanding of these disorders important to almost every physician.

HEAD INJURY

Pathophysiology of the Injury

Severe head trauma threatens life and future well-being in direct proportion to the degree that it injures the brain. Open, focal brain injuries caused by crush or penetrating objects affect specific regions, usually of the cerebrum. Some high-velocity penetrating missiles also send out shock waves that can injure more remote areas of the hemispheres and brain stem, but focal injuries otherwise produce problems requiring largely acute surgical treatment. Closed head injury is a more frequent form of trauma that affects the brain diffusely. The consequences often include systemic problems and depend, respectively, upon the intensity of impact, the direction of the resulting movement of the cranium, and whether or not complications arise. Certain operatives beyond the immediate cerebral trauma also affect outcome. The excessive ingestion of alcohol and/or drugs predisposes to carelessness and sedation. The effect increases the incidence of head trauma and worsens its subsequent severity and associated complications. The presence or absence of serious systemic effects of trauma similarly influences acute and postacute management and outcome.

Damage to the brain in closed head injury comes from sudden acceleration-deceleration forces received at the time of impact. These cannot be judged from external appearances; indeed, many severe brain injuries are accompanied by few external signs of trauma. Conversely, skull fracture per se carries few serious implications unless there are accompanying neurologic signs of underlying brain damage. At the moment of maximal change in velocity, e.g., when a forceful blow suddenly strikes the head or when the forward accelerating head strikes an automobile dashboard after impact, the inertial movement of the gelatinous brain briefly lags behind the onset or offset of the skull's motion. As a result, the brain undergoes a sagittal, lateral, or rotatory shift within the cranium, damaging structures both under the point of injury and 180 degrees away

on the opposite surface of the hemispheres (contra coup) (Fig. 121–1). Strong ensuing implosive-explosive forces affect the tissue, potentially resulting in capillary or neuronal damage. Concurrently, shearing forces threaten to disrupt white matter pathways and produce additional neuronal injury. The distribution and severity of these reactions determine the subsequent clinical course.

Types and Complications of Diffuse Head Injury

The severity of brain trauma usually is judged acutely by whether or not consciousness has been lost and beyond that by the presence or absence of associated neurologic abnormalities, especially those that relate to neuro-ophthalmologic function, motor activities, and breathing patterns. Later on, severity can be judged in retrospect by the duration of coma and how long anterograde or retrograde amnesia lasts. These latter indices, however, have little application in the acute situation.

Cranial injuries in which persons report feeling only dazed or syncopal and have normal neuro-

FIGURE 121–1. MR image showing cerebral edema-contusion at point of impact (two large arrows) and 180 degrees opposite (one large arrow) in a 22-year-old woman. An extradural hematoma had been removed at the impact site six days earlier. Small arrows indicate additional contusions. The patient recovered completely.

logic findings and no localized headache usually need neither hospitalization nor laboratory testing so long as the patient can be depended upon to maintain close medical contact to guard against severe complications. If doubt exists, one is wise to obtain a CT scan to rule out incipient extradural or parenchymal hematoma. When CT is available, skull x-rays usually can be dispensed with in head injury.

Concussion describes brief loss of consciousness with no immediate or delayed residua detectable by radiographic or clinical study. The boxer's knockout, which derives from an abrupt sagittally delivered force, epitomizes the abnormality. One observes immediate, evanescent autonomic paralysis: consciousness disappears, the pupils dilate and fix, breathing stops, the heart slows, and muscles become flaccid. In concussed experimental animals petechial hemorrhages and scattered neuronal loss appear in the lower brain stem. Clinical recovery begins within seconds to minutes and completes itself within hours except for the frequent persistence of psychosensory symptoms such as giddiness, anxiety, and apprehension, which remain for days or longer. Brain imaging studies, if obtained, show no abnormality, and no treatment is indicated other than reassurance.

Intermediate diffuse injuries extend the level of unconsciousness to as much as an hour or so and are followed by the slower recovery of orientation and behavior, sometimes leaving permanent residua. Associated drunkeness can make appraisal more difficult, but in the earliest stages safe evaluation requires that one attribute detectable neurologic changes directly to the trauma. Patients with moderate brain injuries often remain lethargic for a day to a week or more and many go through an agitated stage. Temporarily, they may be partially disoriented, and many transiently will show mild or moderate focal neurologic abnormalities such as extensor plantar responses or unilateral weakness. Signs of brain stem damage are lacking, but the CSF may be bloody, reflecting cerebral contusions or lacerations. CT or, especially, MRI scans show scattered petechiae or contusions (Fig. 121–1), with small hematomas sometimes lying opposite to the side of original impact (contra coup injury). Even with severe injury, however, imaging studies can be normal. Patients affected with intermediate level injuries require hospitalization to guard against complications and to control possibly agitated behavior. More active treatment seldom is necessary unless complications arise as discussed below. Most patients younger than about age 40 years recover completely within days to weeks. Loss of consciousness for as little as 24 to 36 hours in persons older than that age often is followed by permanent functional limitations, especially in psychological and intellectual spheres.

Severe diffuse injury is judged by the patient's response rather than the nature of the trauma. Serious neurologic damage usually is apparent from the start, although exceptions exist. Ilustrating the

latter, after seemingly mild to moderate head trauma, children and adolescents occasionally develop massive and sometimes fatal brain edema coming on within minutes to an hour or so following the injury. Similarly, persons of all ages can develop within several hours or more delayed complications including severe brain edema, ischemic infarction, or parenchymal, subdural, or extradural hemorrhages. Such individuals who "talk and die" comprise as many as 20 per cent of the fatalities in some series of head trauma.

With the above exceptions, most patients suffering from severe brain trauma become deeply unconscious from the onset; many almost immediately develop decerebrate or decorticate posturing responses to noxious stimuli. Signs of associated trauma are common, and at least partial respiratory obstruction due to aspiration of vomitus or oral secretions is almost the rule. Evidence of brain stem damage indicated by bilateral pupillary fixation or impaired oculovestibular responses signifies especially severe injury and a poor prognosis, with fewer than 15 per cent making a satisfactory recovery. Almost half of all patients with such severe trauma will show intracranial hemorrhages by CT scan; it is debatable whether or not early operative removal improves ultimate functional outcome in such instances.

Management of Acute Head Trauma and Its Complications

Emergency Management. Whether at the accident scene or hospital emergency room, proper immediate steps may save both lives and brains. Patients who are awake and do not appear to be seriously injured must be kept quiet and watched until it is certain that no occult damage silently leads to delayed deterioration. At the accident, the more seriously injured should be placed flat and supine, taking care to avoid flexing or twisting a potentially fractured spine or neck. Pulmonary ventilation should be evaluated and guaranteed immediately, and evident systemic hemorrhage should be stopped. The victim must be transported as promptly as possible and, if not in shock, to the most effective rather than merely the nearest emergency facility. Opiates are contraindicated. One must evaluate emergency personnel respectfully: some trained paramedics are more skilled in managing this stage than are untrained or partially trained physicians. In the emergency room, unresponsive persons should be intubated and 30 to 100 per cent oxygen started with or without assisted ventilation depending on circumstances (see Table 116–7). A large-gauge intravenous needle should be placed to draw necessary blood and to treat hemorrhage or shock if either occurs. Dehydration is not an advantage, but specific attention should be directed to preventing the development of hyponatremia or excess hyperglycemia. Seizures, if present, should be treated urgently with diazepam and a full phenytoin dose given intravenously (see Table 122–8). This is the time to complete the emergency neurologic and systemic examinations and to obtain, if possible, brain images and any radiographs. Decisions as to the priority of treating systemic vs. intracranial lesions and whether or not to evacuate intracranial masses are best left to those experienced in trauma care.

Hospital Management. Patients with severe head trauma should be treated in an intensive care setting with appropriate facilities for monitoring vital functions. The level of consciousness, neuroophthamologic status, and motor responses should be monitored at 30- to 60-minute intervals in potentially unstable cases so that complications can be met quickly. Arterial blood gases and electrolytes need close attention. Most brain-injured patients either aspirate gastric contents or suffer neurogenic pulmonary edema, so antimicrobial agents are prescribed after obtaining appropriate cultures. Corticosteroid drugs are contraindicated: they counteract immunity and may worsen traumatic tissue damage. Unless specific complications need attention, the medical care of head injuries focuses on maintaining good physiological balance and allowing the patient's brain and systemic tissues spontaneously to recover their full potentials.

Certain general problems recurrently arise in caring for patients with intermediate or severe head injury. Ventilatory difficulties require constant attention to the upper airway, any associated thoracic trauma, pulmonary edema-pneumonitis, and infection. Renal or bladder trauma often accompanies head injuries, and urinary retention or incontinence is almost universal. Patients with altered consciousness should be placed on indwelling catheterization during the early stages, with the urine cultured at 48-hour intervals. The fluid intake should be balanced against output, and if renal failure is absent, urinary volume should reach at least 1500 ml a day to minimize infection and calculi. Serum electrolytes should be monitored concurrently. Effective bowel emptying may require enemas.

Pain is common as patients recover consciousness, and if severe may require codeine to supplement milder analgesics. Opiates should not be given to spontaneously breathing patients because of the risks of inducing hypoventilation and associated increases in intracranial pressure. Mild agitation is best controlled with diazepam, severe boisterousness with haloperidol. In alcoholics or those addicted to sedative drugs, delirium tremens or withdrawal seizures should be anticipated and countered with benzodiazepines at the first sign of motor tremulousness (p 674).

Management of Complications. Cerebral edema accompanies almost all severe head injuries, causing an increase in brain mass that interferes with the cerebral circulation and threatens to cause central or lateral transtentorial herniation (see Table 116–3). *Traumatic hematomas* can arise acutely in either the subdural, extradural, or parenchymal regions, creating additional space-occupying lesions and producing further blood-induced irritation to the tissue. Such hemorrhages most often signify their presence with signs of in-

creasing neurologic disability that begin at a time when improvement might otherwise be expected. Some centers routinely measure the intracranial pressure in an effort to detect and guide the treatment of these complications. With or without such steps, CT or MR imaging can be invaluable in detecting either intracranial shifts or hypodensities that indicate the development of edema and the presence and size of hematomas. Lacking these imaging devices, arteriography may be desirable. In the presence of known or suspected edema, giving a 20 per cent solution of mannitol intravenously, plus applying passive hyperventilation to reduce cerebral blood volume, can serve as an emergency measure to lower intracranial pressure if surgery is decided upon. Few patients who require such acute surgical treatment make a fully satisfactory social-vocational recovery.

Where imaging is not available, skull x-rays must be done. Fractures by themselves indicate no more than the fact that a fairly severe injury has occurred. Fractures do, however, have several potential complications that may demand attention. Bony breaks across the middle meningeal artery groove in the temporal bone can lacerate the artery, leading to delayed middle temporal fossa *extradural hematomas.* Typically, such clots enlarge progressively to produce signs of neurologic worsening from 12 hours to three days following the initial injury. Unilateral headache followed by restlessness, agitation, or greater obtundation ensues. Unless the hematoma is treated, such changes may lead eventually to uncal and lateral tentorial herniation. *Basal skull fractures* can open channels from the subarachnoid space into the paranasal sinuses or either middle ear. CSF rhinorrhea or secondary meningitis are risks; some neurosurgeons treat such CSF leaks with prophylactic antibiotics until the rhinorrhea stops spontaneously or they repair it surgically. *Depressed skull fractures* displace pieces of skull to a level below the surrounding bone surface. Such lesions confer an increased risk of post-traumatic epilepsy and are best treated by surgical elevation.

Acute bacterial *infections* can follow open skull or spine injuries that either infect the subdural space or penetrate more deeply into the tissue to cause meningitis or brain abscess. Diagnosis is suspected from the nature of the injury and is discussed, along with treatment, in Chapter 124.

Cranial nerve paralyses are common following cranial facial trauma, especially when it affects the ocular structures and the innervation of the face. Anosmia is a frequent result for which there is no treatment. The management of more serious injuries often requires surgical facial reconstruction.

Carotid-cavernous fistulas result from basal skull fractures that lacerate the artery within the cavernous sinus. The condition also may occur spontaneously or in association with intracavernous aneurysms or connective tissue diseases. Chemosis, a painful semi-immobilized eye, and pulsating exophthalmos develop ipsilaterally to the fistula and occasionally contralaterally as well. Vision can decline in either eye associated with secondary glaucoma and stretching of the optic nerve. Treatment, often difficult, consists of surgical ligation or efforts to patch the leak by injecting artificial emboli.

Post–Head Injury Problems

Postconcussion syndrome is a common disorder that characteristically follows mild to moderate, often subconcussional head injuries as well as other forms of potentially severe, psychologically threatening trauma. Headache, giddy sensations, irritability, difficulty in concentration, and vague apprehension comprise major symptoms. Physical and laboratory signs of significant neurologic or systemic dysfunction usually are lacking, and the condition gradually passes with time, medication having no specific effect. No cause is known, although the nature of the symptoms suggests reversible brain stem dysfunction. Compensation or psychological issues appear not to influence the incidence of the disorder; whether they prolong the period of disability is uncertain.

Incomplete recovery in the intellectual and motor sphere affects many patients with severe head injury, including nearly all adults who remain in coma for more than one week's duration. Comprehensive rehabilitation efforts in specialized centers offer such patients the best hope for social and vocational re-entry and should be pursued as soon as acute medical recovery permits.

Post-traumatic epilepsy, mainly associated with generalized tonic-clonic attacks, ranges in incidence from a maximum of 50 per cent after penetrating brain injuries down to about 5 per cent following unconsciousness-producing closed head injury. Most authorities treat both groups of patients prophylactically with full phenytoin therapy for periods up to two years following severe injury. If no seizures occur, treatment is gradually discontinued. If patients do have seizures, antiepileptic medication is strengthened or treatment is lengthened according to the frequency and intensity of the attacks.

Delayed post-traumatic encephalopathy, an unusual syndrome affecting principally children or young adults, begins 15 minutes to two hours or more following usually minor head injuries. The young person becomes obtunded or stuporous, often with nausea or vomiting. Despite these potentially alarming early symptoms, most patients recover uneventfully, but focal neurologic deficits including cortical blindness sometimes can last for several hours or, very rarely, permanently. The cause is not known. Similarly unexplained are rare instances of parenchymal cerebral hemorrhage that can arise from hours to a matter of a week or more following relatively mild cerebral trauma, insufficient initially to cause residual neurologic signs or symptoms.

Chronic subdural hematoma is a late complication of head injuries that are usually mild and sometimes so trivial as to have been forgotten. The interval between injury and symptoms usually varies from weeks to months. Older age, alcoholism, and anticoagulation are important predisposing factors, although many patients give no history of relevant risk factors or even injury. A sustained, new headache and mental dullness are the most common symptoms, often blending into hypersomnia and confusion with or without hemiparesis. The symptoms often fluctuate, presumably because of small rebleedings or the development of abnormal intracranial pressure waves, transient pressure elevations associated with impaired cerebral arterial autoregulation. Diagnosis is best made by brain imaging, which in symptomatic cases usually shows brain shift or, with bilateral hematomas, smaller than normal ventricles and few sulci at the vertex. One must interpret films cautiously, since at certain stages within a matter of a few weeks after injury, the hematoma itself becomes isodense with the surrounding brain and may not be outlined by CT scan (Fig. 121–2). This problem does not arise with MRI scanning. Small or moderate hematomas can be treated by observation with or without the concurrent giving of steroid drugs. Larger clots, particularly those causing abnormal neurologic signs or symptoms, are best treated surgically.

Dementia pugilistica, the "punch drunk" syndrome, affects former boxers. Most reported instances have been in men older than age 55 years, although psychological tests show a high incidence of intellectual deterioration even under age 40. The old fighters develop progressive motor slowness, clumsiness, dysarthria, ataxia, memory loss, and incontinence. Development of the syndrome relates directly to the number of former fights, with the subsequent incidence being about 20 per cent among those who box for six to nine years or more. CT scans show cerebral atrophy and ventricular dilatation. Postmortem findings include neurofibrillary tangles in the brain along with neuronal loss, especially in the cerebellum and temporal lobes. Some subjects improve after ventricular shunt procedures.

SPINAL CORD INJURY

Severe spinal cord injury is relatively uncommon but often devastating and prolonged in its consequences, since most cases affect persons younger than 30 years of age. The intraspinal contents can be concussed, contused, lacerated, macerated, or sheared, depending upon the nature of the initiating injury. Road traffic accidents, domestic falls, and diving accidents are frequent causes. The spinal levels most susceptible to trauma lie at the upper and lower ends of the cervical canal and at the thoracolumbar junction, regions of maximal mobility. Any level, however, can be affected by injuries that strike the spinal column directly or penetrate into the spinal canal.

The principal mechanisms of spinal injury are dislocation with or without fracture at the atlas-axis junction, fracture-dislocations with or with-

FIGURE 121–2. An isodense subdural hematoma invisible on CT scan (*A* and *B*) is readily disclosed by a concurrently obtained MR image (*C* and *D*). The patient, a 61-year-old man with a history of partial complex seizures and a single generalized convulsion one year earlier, had suffered from headache, loss of mental acuity, fatigue, and dysequilibrium for four months. He was unable to tandem walk, but examination otherwise was unremarkable. He recovered completely following drainage of the hematoma.

out bony fragmentation at other spinal levels, and penetrating missile or stab wounds that either concuss the cord and its roots or injure it directly. Less frequent causes are severe hyperflexion or hyperextension injuries that damage the cervical cord in persons who suffer from an abnormally narrow spinal canal (stenosis) due either to congenital factors or age-related progressive spondylosis.

Patterns of Spinal Cord Injury and Their Resulting Disabilities

Complete vs. partial cord injury can usually be discerned almost immediately following injury. With complete injury, neurologic findings are those of functional cord transection. Motor function, with the occasional exception of priapism, disappears altogether distal to the level of damage accompanied by diffuse pananesthesia in the same distribution. Initially, flaccidity and hypoactive deep tendon reflexes reflect profound distal inhibition (spinal shock); extensor plantar responses ordinarily do not appear for several days. Bladder and bowel functions are lost, and prognosis for neurologic recovery is poor no matter what treatment is applied.

Partial spinal injury is more common with cervical than thoracic cord trauma and can take several forms, as described in subsequent paragraphs. Any voluntary movement or sensory perception distal to the injury and discernible at the time of accident means that the injured cord or roots possess a capacity for recovery that only time will define. Treatment must be guided accordingly.

Concussion most often follows high-velocity missile wounds that pass close to the spinal canal but fail directly to damage the cord structurally. Distal neurologic loss never is complete, and recovery occurs within hours to days, occasionally leaving episodic residual paresthesias in the lower extremities secondary to dorsal column scarring (Lhermitte's sign).

Central cord damage due to trauma affects primarily the lower cervical segments, usually with patchy hemorrhage centered along or adjacent to the region of the central canal (hematomyelia). Severe external blows or local fractures without serious canal displacement is the usual cause. The upper extremities become more paralyzed and insensate than the lower, sensory changes affect pain and temperature more than touch, especially at and immediately below the cervical level, and bladder paralysis is common.

Cervical hyperextension injury typically produces mild or inconsequential paraparesis affecting legs more than arms, coupled with painful paresthesias in the arms and hyposensitivity to position and vibratory testing below the lesion. *Hyperflexion injury*, on the other hand, may simulate anterior spinal artery occlusion, producing tetraparesis or tetraplegia accompanied by bilateral pain and temperature impairment below the lesion, often associated with acute urinary retention. Both hyperextension (posterior cord) and hyperflexion (anterior cord) injuries can vary widely in severity and many undergo considerable functional recovery. Mixed or unilateral injuries produce variants of the *Brown-Sequard syndrome* of hemicord damage.

Intraspinal damage at or distal to the first lumbar level injures the *conus medullaris* or *cauda equina*, resulting in various mixtures of flaccid paralysis, distal mixed sensory loss, and autonomic-sexual paralysis affecting the pelvic girdle and lower extremities.

Emergency treatment at the scene of the accident consists of measures that avoid flexing or twisting the spinal column and placing the patient on a hard, flat surface for examination and transportation. Patients with cervical injury commonly require immediate ventilatory assistance, if necessary by mouth-to-mouth breathing. Transport to an experienced center should be arranged immediately, with special attention in patients with cervical injuries being given to immobilizing the neck and counteracting hypoventilation and/or hypotension. In the absence of neurologic damage, patients with cervical fractures or fracture-dislocations should be placed in head traction and managed conservatively pending expert consultation. For patients with partial cervical cord injury and evidence of compression by x-ray or imaging studies, immediate surgical decompression sometimes is beneficial. For most severe cord injuries, however, including all examples of functional transection, open surgical treatment confers little benefit and only adds another trauma. Overall, acute and postacute management for quadriplegics or paraplegics requires elaborate attention to pulmonary, cutaneous, autonomic, musculoskeletal and psychosocial problems, employing techniques that are best carried out in specialized rehabilitation units.

REFERENCES

Becker DP: Injury to the head and spine. In Wyngaarden JB, and Smith LH Jr (eds): Cecil Textbook of Medicine. 17th ed. Philadelphia, WB Saunders Co, 1985, pp 2170–2177. *A lucid, more lengthy presentation of the problem.*

Guttman L: Spinal Cord Injuries. Comprehensive Management and Research. 2nd ed. Oxford, Blackwell Scientific Publications, 1976. *A thorough and well-presented exposition of the varied medical problems and results of these challenging and often tragic problems.*

Jennett WB, and Teasdale G: Management of Head Injuries. Philadelphia, FA Davis Co, 1981. *A clearly written, highly informative, comprehensive monograph on the subject.*

122 EPILEPSY

Definitions

An *epileptic seizure* is an episode of pathological, hyperactive, hypersynchronous brain electrochemical activity, expressed as abnormal motor, sensory, or psychological behavior. All seizures are not epilepsy. Nonrecurrent or only briefly recurrent epileptiform attacks of several kinds can result from a variety of causes such as electroconvulsive therapy, profound syncope, the ingestion or withdrawal of certain drugs or toxins, or any of several kinds of infections of the brain.

The term *epilepsy* refers to a condition of chronically recurrent seizures in which the attacks themselves become a target for specific therapy. Etiologically, seizure disorders fall into two general groups. Those whose cause remains largely or entirely unknown are called *primary* or *idiopathic epilepsy*. Most primary epilepsy reflects an inherited predisposition, the exact genetic mechanism being unknown. The second group consists of cases in which a known structural or metabolic disease of the brain generates *secondary* or *symptomatic epilepsy*.

Incidence and General Etiology

Seizures can begin at any time of life. Neonatal seizures represent a special problem, linked to brain injuries or insufficiency in that age group, and are not directly related to later epileptic disorders. In children under age two, perinatal injury, metabolic disorders, and congenital malformations represent the most frequent causes. Genetic factors act most strongly in older children and adolescents. After the age of 20 years, head trauma, intracranial space-occupying lesions, drug or alcohol withdrawal, and scarring from cerebrovascular disease become important mechanisms. Encephalitis or meningitis can initiate chronic epilepsy at any age.

Population studies in several developed countries worldwide indicate that among older children and adults about one in 200 (0.5 per cent) suffers from recurrent seizures. Third world areas fare worse, the higher rates being caused by infections, poor nutrition, and an increased incidence of severe head trauma.

Pathophysiology

Focal seizures most often originate in association with specific, anatomically restricted lesions of gray matter such as scars, tumors, arteriovenous malformations, or focal areas of inflammation. (An exception to this rule of structural abnormality sometimes occurs in children with a benign and self-limited form of focal motor seizure called rolandic epilepsy.) *Generalized seizures*, by contrast, represent the effects of either a diffuse hyperexcitable propensity of brain cells or the presence of a deep, cryptic epileptogenic abnormality involving centrally located subcortical activating mechanisms. Overlap occurs between focal and generalized seizures in that focally originating ictal discharges can become generalized in their expression when they anatomically project back into the diencephalic reticulum. In this instance, the remote focus quickly transmits its hyperactive hypersynchrony to a central electrophysiological pacemaker, which in turn fires forward to capture both sides of the forebrain and produce a generalized attack. Epileptic discharges arise preferentially in certain anatomical areas of the cerebrum, including the frontal lobes, the medial temporal lobes (limbic system), the diencephalic reticular formation, and, to a lesser degree, the occipital lobe.

Genetic factors influence susceptibility to both generalized and focal epilepsy. Intrinsic generalized epilepsies, such as petit mal absences and febrile convulsions, usually reflect the expression of an autosomal dominant trait with variable penetration. Patients with chronic focal seizures originating in the temporal lobe also show an above-normal incidence of seizure disorders of all kinds in their blood relatives, implying hereditary factors in that disorder as well.

The specific brain mechanisms that cause seizure discharges to start, spread, or stop are poorly understood. Abnormalities that have been suggested include (1) intrinsic neuronal membrane changes that could lead to an abnormality in ionic conductance; (2) abnormal neurotransmitter synthesis leading to deficiencies of inhibitory or excesses in excitatory neurotransmitters; and (3) deficiencies in genetically regulated intracellular enzymes that normally affect the capacity of the neurons or glial cells to pump ions and repolarize.

Clinical Seizure Patterns (Table 122–1)

Epileptic attacks commonly evolve in their symptoms. Individual episodes can last from a few seconds to several minutes in duration, with the pattern of the symptoms reflecting the anatomy and physiology of the underlying cerebral involvement. Seizures and their effects can be divided into several stages: the *aura* or first self-experienced symptom usually reflects the anatomic focus where the seizure begins. *The attack* itself follows and subsequently gives way to the *postictal period*, during which headache, drowsiness, or focal neurologic abnormalities can remain, often for minutes and sometimes for hours or even days.

Partial seizures consist of attacks of focal neurologic dysfunction. The attacks are described as *simple* if only one restricted form of behavior is expressed (equivalent to the aura) and self-aware consciousness remains throughout. They are called *complex* if the pattern of neurologic symptoms and signs changes during the attack (e.g., a hallucination of smell gives way to visceral automatisms or complex motor acts) or if consciousness is lost as the attack evolves. With any seizure the initiating signs and symptoms offer the best localizing evidence for the area of the brain that contains the epileptogenic lesion.

Partial motor seizures arise from epileptogenic foci in the primary motor or the premotor, sup-

---

TABLE 122–1. CLASSIFICATION OF EPILEPTIC SEIZURE PATTERNS

I. **Partial seizures** originate from a focal lesion in brain, usually structural, and may occur either with a single symptom (simple) or symptoms that change in type as well as degree (complex).
    A. Motor (includes monomyoclonic)
    B. Sensory
    C. Psychological
    D. Partial complex. Seizures with changing patterns, usually of limbic-temporal lobe origin.

II. **Generalized seizures**
    A. *Nonconvulsive* (all but some myoclonic attacks cause at least momentary loss of consciousness)
        Absence (petit mal)
        Atypical absence
        Atonic
        Myoclonic
    B. *Convulsive*
        Tonic-clonic (grand mal)
        Tonic only
        Clonic only

III. **Atypical or unclassified seizures.** Consciousness usually remains intact.
    A. Paroxysmal tonic spasms
    B. Spinal myoclonus

plementary motor, or prefrontal areas of either frontal lobe. Lateral prefrontal, supplementary motor, and premotor foci all cause adversive seizures, with only moderate differences distinguishing the respective movement patterns. The frontal lobe possesses many anatomic transcortical and thalamic interconnections. As a result, frontal seizure discharges can either spread to produce progressively larger amounts of contralateral motor activity or fire directly into the diencephalon to precipitate generalized convulsions. With lesions lying far anterior in the frontal lobes, consciousness may be lost concurrently with or even slightly before any focal movements begin. Most patients with seizures arising from supplementary or premotor areas, however, retain awareness for at least the beginning of the attack. Motor components in partial motor seizures can begin and remain as simple aversion of the head and eyes away from the side of the focus, can include extension or raising the contralateral arm and turning of the trunk, and occasionally include crude vocalizations or, in the dominant hemisphere, speech arrest. Head turning alone is not a reliable lateralizing sign.

Primary motor (rolandic) seizures produce the classic jacksonian epileptic attack. Rhythmic, clonic twitching begins in the contralateral thumb or corner of the mouth and slowly spreads to produce adjacent movements, most often from thumb to hand to arm to face, but sometimes jumping in the reverse direction. Spread to a generalized convulsion is common. Many jacksonian seizures are followed by transient or sustained postictal (Todd's) paralysis of the limb affected by the seizure.

Partial sensory seizures produce the classic epileptic aura: a sensory presentiment or fragment that represents the ictal beginning and advertises its origin. Most common are epigastric rising sensations that emanate from discharges affecting the insular cortex, followed in frequency by somatosensory tingling or numbness (postcentral gyrus), simple visual phenomena (mostly occipital), vertigo (superior temporal gyrus), or vague cephalic or generalized body sensations (no localizing value). Lesions in and around the temporal uncus cause foul smelling, olfactory hallucinations that often blend into other temporal lobe symptoms.

Partial complex seizures of temporal lobe–limbic cortex origin represent the most frequent form of chronic epilepsy, amounting to about 40 per cent of total cases. About half begin before age 25 years, and most are associated with discernible structural lesions in the temporal limbic area. Frequent causes are developmental anomalies, residua of early life brain infection or severe febrile convulsions, head trauma, neoplasms, and in later life stroke or focal atrophy. Most partial complex seizures begin along the medial portion of the temporal lobe or the adjacent inferior frontal limbic area and spread posteriorly along the temporal lobe limbic cortex. They often project transcallosally to the opposite medial temporal area. Secondary generalization into deep diencephalic structures to produce chronic convulsions can occur but is less common than complex automatisms. In either event, consciousness and memory are severely dulled or lost during the evolution of the attack.

The aura of partial complex seizures (Table 122–2) commonly reflects their anatomic origin and sometimes comprises the entire episode. More often, it spreads into stereotyped automatic movements that can take several forms, alone or in combination (Table 122–3). Partial complex seizures usually last 1 to 2 minutes, seldom as much as 5, and are followed by the patient's slow reorientation, with headache and drowsiness. The interictal EEG of affected patients shows temporal lobe spikes or slow foci in about 80 per cent, provided that records during sleep are obtained. The frequency of abnormalities increases during or after an attack, but even then deep limbic discharges may go undetected by skull surface electrodes.

Many patients suffering from partial complex seizures display abnormal interictal behavior, including excessive ruminative obsessiveness, religiosity, circumstantiality, hypersensitivity, and self-absorption, as well as hypergraphia.

Differential diagnosis of partial complex seizures includes mainly petit mal absences and psychiatric fugue states. Absence attacks are abrupt

TABLE 122–2. FREQUENT SYMPTOMS OF LIMBIC-TEMPORAL LOBE SEIZURES

SYMPTOM	LOCUS OF ORIGIN
Foul odor, "uncinate fit"	Temporal uncus-amygdaloid area
Micropsia or macropsia	Middle-inferior temporal gyrus
Déjà vu (intense familiarity)	Parahippocampal-hippocampal area
Jamais vu (environmental unfamiliarity)	
Fragments of voices, phrases, songs	Auditory association cortex
Lip smacking, abdominal pain, borborygmi, epigastric rising, cardiac arrhythmia	Insular, temporal-polar limbic cortex
Dreamy feelings, fear, pleasure, anger	Parahippocampal and septal areas

TABLE 122–3. COMMON ICTAL MANIFESTATIONS OF LIMBIC SEIZURES

Autonomic:	Flushing, pallor, tachypnea, nausea, eructation-borborygmi, sweating, cardiac arrhythmia
Cognitive:	Intense déjà vu (familiarity), jamais vu (spatial amnesia), forced thinking, dreamlike states, depersonalization
Affective:	Laughing, fear, rage, depression, elation
Sensory:	Olfactory hallucinations; macropsia, micropsia, familiar voice fragments, visualized objects or scenes, emotional experiences (dreamy states)
Motor:	Staring with lip smacking, chewing, semipurposeful rubbing; confused, bizarre behavior; walking or, occasionally, running; postictal confusion or drowsiness

in onset and offset, last only a few seconds, usually are unaccompanied by subjective self-awareness, do not produce auras or automatisms, and are associated with a diagnostic EEG abnormality. Psychiatric fugues can be more difficult to distinguish, especially when patients with psychomotor attacks have normal EEG's. Psychiatric states, however, include a past history of sustained psychiatric or behavioral aberration, they last longer than seizures, they lack the characteristic evolution from aura to attack to a drowsy and confused postictal state, and they often have a self-rewarding relationship to life situations that is lacking in true epilepsy. Partial complex seizures rarely, if ever, offer a satisfactory explanation for committing crime or carrying out other apparently deliberate departures from the social norm.

GENERALIZED EPILEPSIES

SECONDARY GENERALIZATION

Many partial seizures, especially those that begin in the frontal lobe, but also some that begin in the temporal lobe or other areas, can evolve rapidly into generalized convulsions before the epileptic discharge burns itself out. Occasionally, as noted above with deep frontal lesions, the generalized seizure explodes before any focal behavioral sign has time to appear. In such instances meticulous EEG study, brain imaging, or identifying restricted postictal weakness may be needed to discover the focus and the lesion causing it.

PRIMARY GENERALIZED EPILEPSIES

These can take several forms depending upon the patient's age at onset and the extent and nature of any associated structural or metabolic disease of the brain. Since the clinical features are what most attract the physician's attention and serve as the principal focus for treatment, this chapter divides the generalized epilepsies according to whether or not they produce major convulsions.

Nonconvulsive Generalized Epilepsy

Absence Seizures (Petit Mal). Absence seizures begin in childhood, usually between the ages of 2 and 12 years, and in most instances cease by age 20. They represent the classic example of primary epilepsy: no structural or known generalized metabolic disease exists in the brains of these youngsters. Genetic studies, however, show an approximately 40 per cent incidence of EEG abnormalities among first-degree relatives. Intelligence is not impaired, and other neurologic abnormalities are absent.

Simple absence attacks are brief, lasting no more than one to two seconds, and are characterized by a blank stare, often accompanied by mild 3- to 4-Hz blinking of the eyelids. Unprepared observers commonly note no abnormality, and the child remains unaware of the event. In severely affected children, dozens to 100 or more such ep-

isodes can occur in a single day. More protracted, *complex absence attacks* can last for 15 to 30 seconds, rarely as long as a minute. Such spells are readily detected: the child's head droops, the lids and sometimes the arms jerk rythmically but mildly, and there may be brief motor automatisms and even enuresis.

Both the clinical pattern and the EEG in classic absence epilepsy run true to form. The EEG contains repeated bursts and runs of symmetrical 3.5-Hz activity. Furthermore, both the electrical abnormality and the seizures commonly can be brought on by voluntary hyperventilation for 60 to 180 seconds. Atypical seizures or an EEG that is asymmetrical or contains faster or slower frequencies make one consider an alternate diagnosis of one of the less benign generalized childhood epilepsies.

About half the children with petit mal seizures develop generalized tonic-clonic convulsions before the age of 20. Absence or petit mal status epilepticus is described in a later section.

Myoclonus, a brief, unexpected, and uncontrollable jerk of the entire body or a focal portion of the trunk or one of the extremities, is a common, normal phenomenon e.g., during pre-sleep drowsiness. Diffuse or multifocal myoclonus, however, is abnormal, and occurs in several degenerative toxic and infectious neurologic disorders as well as in several of the severe childhood epilepsies. A more benign form of restricted myoclonus, discussed below, affects the upper extremities and is closely related to generalized primary epilepsy. Partial myoclonus, with distally or proximally located repetitive focal twitchings, can be associated with several disorders of the cerebrum or spinal cord (see Partial Focal Motor Status Epilepticus in a later section).

Bilateral epileptic myoclonus is an uncommon condition consisting of bilateral repetitive myoclonic jerks affecting girls more than boys, and often beginning at the menarche. The symmetrical jerks especially involve the shoulders and arms. Often, the EEG contains bifrontal 3.5- to 4-Hz sharp and slow activity similar to that found in absence seizures. The disorder pathogenetically and genetically lies close to petit mal and carries a similar risk of future tonic-clonic seizures. It responds to similar medication, especially sodium valproate. A more serious form of symmetrical or multifocal massive myoclonus epilepsy affects children with inherited degenerative diseases (Unverricht-Lundborg disease; ceroid lipofuscinosis). Multifocal myoclonus also frequently accompanies progressive encephalitis in either children (subacute sclerosing panencephalitis) or adults (Creutzfeldt-Jakob disease). A variety of other metabolic and degenerative disorders of the brain can produce multifocal or intention myoclonus, including hepatic encephalopathy, uremia, penicillin intoxication, postanoxic encephalopathy, the Ramsay-Hunt form of cerebellar degeneration, and several dementias, including Alzheimer's disease, Hungtington's chorea, and occasionally Wilson's disease.

Atonic-akinetic seizures often accompany severe myoclonic epilepsy in young children between the ages of one and six years. Head dropping attacks, falls, staring spells, prolonged episodes of minor motor seizures, generalized tonic-clonic convulsions, and mental retardation can occur. Treatment is difficult and often incompletely successful.

Infantile spasms consist of brief, frequently repeated massive flexor spasms of the head and extremities. About half the cases are associated with a cerebral degenerative or metabolic disorder, with the remainder being of unknown cause. About 9 out of 10 affected children become mentally retarded, some severely so.

Generalized Convulsive Epilepsy

Generalized convulsive epilepsy can take two forms, tonic-clonic and tonic.

Tonic-clonic (grand mal) seizures can begin at any age. Most produce loss of consciousness at onset, although a fraction of patients report a brief rising epigastric sensation as the attack begins. Prodromal warnings (not auras) sometimes precede the attacks by several hours and can include a change in mood, a sense of apprehension, insomnia, or loss of appetite. Episodes of repetitive myoclonus may anticipate a convulsion. As the convulsion begins, many patients cry out unconsciously. They stiffen tonically in extension, usually with muscles contracted so tightly that breathing is arrested. Deep cyanosis occurs before relaxation and a first post-tonic breath ensues. Such vigorously tonic phases seldom last as much as a minute but may be repeated several times over. Gradually, hyperextension gives way to a minute or so of rapid successive clonic jerks of the neck, trunk, and extremities. Finally, flaccid relaxation ensues, accompanied by stertorous breathing, pallor, and heavy salivation. Hypertension, tachycardia, and heavy perspiration accompany the motor changes. The pupils may be briefly fixed and moderately dilated during the tonic convulsions. Absent oculocephalic reflexes, hyperactive deep tendon reflexes, and extensor plantar responses can outlast the seizure for several minutes but usually disappear along with the reappearance of arousal two to three minutes after the relaxation phase begins. Many patients bite their tongues or lose sphincter control. In addition, the tonic contractions may exert sufficient force to compress dorsal or upper lumbar vertebrae. Other serious injuries are relatively uncommon, but susceptible patients must be warned about tub bathing, since drowning is a hazard, as is suffocation against the bedclothes if a convulsion takes place during sleep. Meticulous search should be given to any focal manifestations in the evolution of the attack or in the postictal period. Either finding suggests a localized structural rather than a generalized cause for the seizure. Fatigue, muscle weakness and soreness, generalized headache, and drowsiness follow grand mal attacks. Sometimes confusion can last for several hours. Most patients sleep postictally and awaken several hours later with only muscle soreness reminding them that a convulsion has occurred. Severe residua can follow multiple successive convulsions or status epilepticus, as discussed below.

During the convulsive movement of generalized seizures EEG recordings disclose rapidly repeating spike discharges followed by sharp-slow activity as clonic contractions supervene. Postictally the record becomes abnormally slow, sometimes for several hours. The interictal EEG can contain spike-slow complexes, bursts of abnormally slow activity, or mixtures of spike and slow activity in bursts or short, 10- to 20-second runs. About 20 per cent are normal. When abnormalities do occur, they appear symmetrically over the scalp.

Unusual Seizures and Other Conditions Responding to Antiepileptic Medication

Reflex epilepsy can affect sensitive persons in response to a variety of sensory stimuli. Photogenic seizures can be triggered by stroboscopic lights, driving past a stand of trees that filters the sun, or even waving the hand in front of eyes fixed upon bright illumination. The ensuing generalized seizure can take the form of myoclonus, an absence attack, or a tonic-clonic convulsion. Closely related are seizures elicited by looking at certain geometric patterns or, rarely, by reading. Polarized glasses may reduce the stimulus intensity of photosensitive attacks; valproic acid is the most effective anticonvulsant. Other rarer forms of responses to sensory stimuli consist of unduly violent, repetitive startle responses to noise and partial complex seizures triggered by particular musical themes.

Familial paroxysmal choreoathetosis is an uncommon disorder, inherited as an autosomal dominant or recessive trait and characterized by paroxysms of choreiform, dystonic, and athetoid body torsions occurring during full consciousness. Stress or sudden movement can precipitate the episodes. The anticonvulsants phenytoin or carbamazepine relieve most cases.

Recurrent torsion spasms consist of episodic dystonic spasms affecting the face, trunk, and extremities in patients with multiple sclerosis. Sometimes attacks include ataxia and dysarthria rather than dystonia. Body movement or startling stimuli can precipitate the attacks, which do not interfere with consciousness. The EEG remains normal, but phenytoin or carbamazepine treatment prevents the episodes, which presumably are caused by plaques involving the lower brain stem reticular formation.

Anticonvulsants also can favorably affect other conditions, including myokymia (page 710) and *lightning pains*—episodic, severe, flashlike pains affecting the extremities, associated most often with neurosyphilis or diabetic neuropathy. Trigeminal neuralgia, a condition in which lightning pains affect one or more divisions of the fifth cranial nerve, is described on page 686.

DIAGNOSIS

Given evidence that a seizure, automatism, or other brief episode of altered brain function has occurred, the major questions are whether it is epileptic and, if so, of what type and cause. Since the physician rarely can observe the attack itself, most of the evidence derives from the history and supplementary, mostly inferential evidence.

The patient's description of his experience plus, if available, a witness's accurate observation of an attack usually provides the most diagnostically rewarding information. The setting of the attack immediately suggests acute causes such as drug withdrawal, CNS infection, trauma, stroke, etc., while a history of past similar seizures implies a more chronically sustained, intrinsically epileptic, disorder. Any partial (focal) feature observed either as an aura or during or following the seizure suggests a structural brain lesion and demands appropriate investigation and, possibly, specific treatment. Similarly, the pattern of an attack as well as the patient's age immediately limits the possible types and causes of the reported episode (Table 122–4).

The physical and neurologic examinations are useful chiefly for identifying evidence of either systemic illness or acute or chronic structural neurologic disease. Having susceptible patients hyperventilate during the examination often will induce diagnostically typical absence attacks and sometimes precipitates partial complex seizures. Laboratory studies should include lumbar puncture in children with seizures of acute onset as well as in any adolescent or adult suspected of developing meningitis or encephalitis. Single seizures seldom affect the CSF fluid content, but major motor status epilepticus can raise the protein concentration and generate up to 100 white cells per cu mm. Any person in whom either the history, findings, or EEG suggest a focal abnormality, as well as all persons whose seizures begin after childhood, deserve a CT scan with contrast enhancement. The older the patient, the higher the yield from CT even when other studies suggest no focus.

The electroencephalogram is particularly helpful in diagnosis. The normal EEG contains fairly rhythmic, bilaterally symmetrical potentials that range in frequency from 1 to 50 Hz, with amplitudes ranging from about 20 to 200 mV. The typical EEG frequencies recorded in healthy adults are 8.5 to 13 Hz, called alpha; 13 to 30 Hz, called beta; 4 to 7 Hz, called theta; and 0.5 to 4 Hz, called delta (Fig. 122–1). Wakeful persons at rest typically show a dominant alpha rhythm, which accelerates into less rhythmic, faster frequencies during concentrated attention and after ingesting certain drugs. Frequencies of 8 Hz and slower occur normally during drowsiness or sleep; such slowing during wakefulness commonly reflects an abnormality of brain function. Regionally localized bursts of slowing, sharp waves, or spikelike waves characteristically reflect focal disturbances in brain function, while paroxysmal and symmetrical slow, sharp, or sharp-slow activity is typ-

TABLE 122–4. MAJOR CLINICAL FEATURES OF POSTINFANTILE EPILEPSY

AGE	MAJOR CAUSE	TYPES OF SEIZURES
Children < 14 years	Idiopathic epilepsy	Generalized (grand mal) Febrile convulsions Petit mal absence Partial complex attacks (?)
	Genetic and developmental defects: birth trauma; inherited biochemical disorders; acute CNS infection-inflammation; post-traumatic or post-infectious	Generalized grand mal Partial motor, sensory or psychological attacks, simple or complex Disseminated myoclonus
	Brain tumors (uncommon)	Partial or generalized
Adults 14–25 + years	Idiopathic epilepsy	Generalized (grand mal) convulsions Partial complex seizures
	Acute CNS infection-inflammation; traumatic—post-traumatic; drug intoxication or withdrawal; brain tumor or arteriovenous malformation	Generalized or partial seizures
Adults > 25 years	Brain tumor; CNS infection-inflammation; traumatic—post-traumatic; withdrawal; acute or post-stroke	Generalized or partial seizures

ical of primary epilepsy (Fig. 122–2). As many as 20 per cent of patients with clinically typical epilepsy can have normal records, however, while the EEG of 2 to 5 per cent of persons who never have a seizure can contain epileptic-like sharp waves or sharp-slow activity. Most laboratories

FIGURE 122–1. Normal EEG rhythms. (From Solomon GE, Kutt H, and Plum F: Clinical Management of Seizures. 2nd ed. Philadelphia, WB Saunders Co, 1983, p 48.)

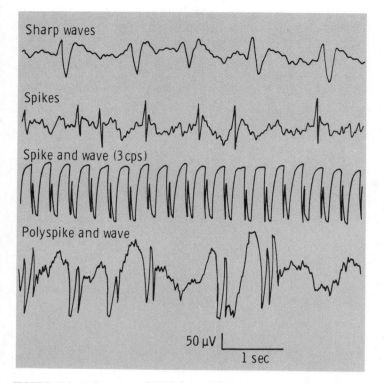

FIGURE 122–2. Paroxysmal EEG abnormalities found in epilepsy. (From Solomon GE, Kutt H, and Plum F: Clinical Management of Seizures. 2nd ed. Philadelphia, WB Saunders Co, 1983, p 52.)

routinely employ hyperventilation and stroboscopic stimulation as EEG activating measures. Special electrode placements, sleep studies, and telemetry are diagnostic tools utilized by specialists.

Chief to be considered in the differential diagnosis of epilepsy are syncope at all ages, pseudoseizures and other factitious attacks among adolescents and younger adults, and cerebral transient ischemic attacks in older patients.

Syncope (p. 657) provides the biggest problem, since one seldom can observe the attack and retrospective histories incline towards ambiguity. Furthermore, the disorder often recurs and, if severe, sometimes is punctuated at the maximum of hypotension by a brief, tonic seizure. As Table 122–5 indicates, however, syncope always occurs when sitting or standing except when associated with episodic cardic arrest. Furthermore, attacks of syncope last a shorter time than seizures, produce characteristic changes in the patient's appearance and motor behavior, cause no postictal confusion or headache, and often are linked to emotional or visceral stimulation. Persons with syncope characteristically lack EEG abnormalities, and neither anticonvulsants nor other medications reliably induce improvement.

Factitious seizures or *pseudoseizures* provide a diagnostic challenge, since they sometimes occur in persons who suffer from organic epilepsy as well. Hysterical seizures most often take place in emotionally stressful settings or to achieve secondary gain. Certain features suggest pseudoseizures: rapidly rolling the head or body from side to side, an alternating thrashing of the extremities or pelvic thrusting. Few hysterics soil or injure themselves during attacks, while many epileptics do. Nevertheless, hysterics or malingerers can be good actors and produce attacks that fool even experienced observers. A dependable but expensive way to differentiate organic from hysterical major motor seizures is to obtain a serum prolactin level immediately postictally: true convulsions but not hysterical attacks elevate the value. In most instances, observing the pattern of the attack coupled with obtaining a normal postictal EEG and employing diagnostic common sense yields the answer.

Episodic fugue states or attacks of behavioral dyscontrol sometimes become confused with partial complex seizures (p. 762). Most such behavioral-psychogenic episodes little resemble the stereotyped automatisms of temporal lobe epilepsy. As with major convulsion-like attacks, a strongly abnormal EEG inclines one toward a diagnosis of epilepsy. In difficult cases, telemetric monitoring of behavior concurrently with EEG recording can assist diagnosis.

Cerebral TIA's (p. 743) only rarely produce symptoms resembling epilepsy, since their principal effects consist of ischemic hypofunction rather than epileptic hyperfunction. Occasionally, however, aphasic speech arrest can occur with TIA's, and a few patients develop contralateral or generalized trembling of the extremities which may resemble epileptic phenomena. The recent development of symptoms, the vascular distribution of the changes, the lack of an epileptogenic lesion by clinical evaluation or brain imaging, and the presence of other signs of systemic or carotid vascular disease almost always lead to the correct diagnosis.

Several other kinds of episodic events may

TABLE 122–5. MAJOR DISTINCTIONS OF SYNCOPE FROM SEIZURES

SIGN	SYNCOPE	SEIZURES
Prodromes	Usually nausea, "swimming" sensation, faintness, sometimes none	Aura or epigastric rise. Often none
Onset	Sitting or erect	Any position
Self-awareness	Always present	Sometimes absent (petit mal absences)
Motor activity	Usually none, occasionally brief clonic. Rare convulsions with cardiac arrests	Focal, tonic, clonic, sustained
Duration	Seconds	0.5 to 2 minutes
Cardiovascular	Pulse slow, weak	Pulse fast, strong
Appearance	Deathly pale, sweating	Flushed, salivating
Postictal	Oriented, sweaty, nauseated, sometimes vomiting, diarrhea	Confused, headache, drowsy
EEG	Normal	Abnormal

briefly suggest seizures but can be dismissed by obtaining a careful history or description of the attack. These include breath-holding attacks in young children; migraine, which in children sometimes causes ataxia, vomiting, visual hallucinations or delirium, and stupor; narcolepsy-cataplexy; hyperventilation spells; and drop attacks in older adults. Nonepileptic causes of recurrent seizures include hypocalcemia, which can occur spontaneously in children and following parathyroidectomy in adults, hypoglycemia at any age, and recurrent alcohol or depressant drug withdrawal in adults.

MANAGEMENT

The management of continuing epilepsy consists of efforts to halt the seizures completely while helping the patient to adjust to a disease that brings fear to most and shame to many.

Control of Seizures

About 60 per cent of patients with chronic epilepsy can have their seizures completely suppressed by medication, and another 15 to 20 per cent can be improved substantially. Many of the uncontrollable patients suffer from a serious underlying disease of the brain, while others for psychological reasons fails to comply with therapeutic instructions. Certain principles guide optimal prescribing of antiepileptic drugs and enhance the likelihood of their success.

1. Many single seizures do not recur, so one does not treat chronically patients who have had only one attack unless a defined cause can be found that is likely to generate recurrences. Special social or vocational circumstances may circumvent this rule. This principle of avoiding chronic treatment for only a single event also applies to uncomplicated febrile convulsions (see below).
2. Diagnose accurately the probable type of epilepsy and give the single preferred medication in full recommended therapeutic doses.
3. If a single drug does not control the seizures, even at toxic levels, try another. Similarly, if the first anticonvulsant causes serious side effects, withdraw it but rapidly initiate the next most effective agent. If efforts at single drug therapy fail, most patients are best referred to a specialized center for consultation, since combined therapy is undesirable. In any event, adjust medications gradually so as to accomplish the maximum of seizure control with a minimum of side effects.
4. Never stop anticonvulsant medication for generalized seizures abruptly. Status epilepticus may result.

Choice of Anticonvulsants. Table 122–6 lists in order of preference the effective anticonvulsants for the various types of chronic epilepsy. Table 122–7 summarizes some of the major pharmacological properties of these agents. They all possess potentially toxic effects and, as with any

TABLE 122–6. CHOICE OF DRUGS IN EPILEPSY

Generalized Tonic-Clonic Seizures
  Phenytoin
  Phenobarbital
  Carbamazepine
  Primidone
Absence Seizures
  Ethosuximide
  Valproate
  Trimethadione
  Clonazepam
Partial Epilepsies
  Carbamazepine
  Phenytoin
  Primidone
  Clonazepam
  Valproate (adjunctive)
Myoclonic Epilepsies
  Infantile spasms
    ACTH or corticosteroids
      clonazepam
      valproate
  Others:
    valproate
    clonazepam

potent medication, physicians should read package inserts before prescribing. Notwithstanding these precautions, one must never forget that recurrent seizures constitute a physically dangerous, emotionally devastating, and intelligence-threatening risk. By comparison, the incidence of potential complications of antiepileptic therapy is trivial.

Use of Drug Levels in Management. The determination of blood levels can be a valuable adjunct to treatment. "Therapeutic" blood levels, however, reflect only empirically established values at which most patients acquire seizure control without toxic side effects. Many patients become well-controlled (or occasionally toxic) below the therapeutic level, while others show no ill effects despite blood values above this point. In all instances the clinical response, not the blood level, defines the goal of the treatment.

Drug level determinations are especially useful within two to three weeks after beginning therapy so as to determine the patient's compliance and his metabolic response to the medication, and to compare the pharmacologic and clinical effects. They also can be helpful when drug dosage is changed, since some individuals quickly saturate their detoxification mechanisms when one increases an antiepileptic drug or drop their levels rapidly to subtherapeutic ranges when the dose is reduced. Blood levels should be rechecked when patients are placed on an additional anticonvulsant or another drug that may influence hepatic enzyme systems.

An occasional blood level determination obtained during the course of chronic, effective therapy helps to reinforce to the patient the need for continued compliance. Most patients with controlled seizure disorders need blood levels checked no more than annually.

TABLE 122–7. PHARMACOLOGIC ASPECTS OF MAJOR ANTIEPILEPTIC DRUGS

	CARBA-MAZEPINE (TEGRETOL)	CLON-AZEPAM (CLONIDINE)	ETHO-SUXIMIDE (ZARONTIN)	PHENO-BARBITAL (LUMINAL)	PHENYTOIN (DILANTIN)	PRIMIDONE (MYSOLINE)	TRIMETH-ADIONE (TRIDIONE)	VALPROATE (DEPAKENE)
Plasma half-life	12–24 h	15–40 h	30–60 h	72–120 h	15–30 h	5–12 h	12–18 h	6–18 h
Active metabolite 10,11-epoxide	6–16 h	0	0	0	0	phenobarbital: 72–120 h; phenyl-ethylma-lonamide: 15–30 h	dimetha-dione: 7–10 days	?
Time to peak blood level (oral dose)	4–18 h	1–4 h	1–4 h	4–12 h	4–8 h	2–4 h	1–2 h	1–2 h
Effective/toxic blood level (ml)	6/12 µg	20/80 µg	50/100 µg	20/40 µg	10/20 µg	5/15 µg (+ pheno-barb.)	600/1200 µg	50/100 µg
Must monitor	CBC, LFT		CBC				CBC, LFT, renal	platelets, CBC, LFT
Adult dose	200–400 mg t.i.d.	2.5–5.0 mg b.i.d. or t.i.d.	250 mg t.i.d.	90–200 mg/day	300–400 mg/day	250 mg t.i.d.–5 × day	300 mg 3–5 × day	250 mg 3–5 × day

STATUS EPILEPTICUS

The rapid succession of seizures so that one begins before the symptoms or after effects of the previous attack have passed is termed *status epilepticus*. Attacks that follow in close succession but with brief periods of reawakening between are designated *serial seizures*. Each condition can occur with either partial or generalized epilepsy. Status epilepticus is of a special concern because in several of its forms the successive or continuous epileptic activity can damage the brain per-

manently. Without actually knowing that several seizures have occurred in rapid succession, however, the diagnosis cannot be made. Accordingly, if an accurate witness is unavailable, one must be sure that epileptic attacks are still continuing before initiating the treatment outlined in Table 122–8.

Partial motor status, an uncommon condition sometimes known as *partial continuous epilepsy*, occurs in several forms and can last for hours, days, or even as long as a year or more. The seizure frequency can range from as little as one every three seconds to as many as several per second. The motor attacks can consist of as little as a highly focal, myoclonic, repetitively localized twitch to jerks that involve most of the limb or even half the body, not always affecting precisely the same muscles. In general, cerebral lesions cause distally distributed partial motor seizures, while brain stem or spinal lesions tend to cause proximal myoclonic activity. Large hemorrhagic or ischemic strokes cause about half the cases, while neoplasms, encephalitic processes, or trauma produce the rest. In some instances, particularly with chronic partial continuous seizures, the cause never becomes clear despite extensive searching. Whatever the cause the seizures often resist treatment. Phenytoin, carbamazepine, diazepam, and clonazepam all have been tried but often with only limited success.

Partial complex status produces a sustained state of confusion or delirium in which stereotyped motor and autonomic automatisms are associated with dull, slow, blunted behavior, often combined with semimuteness or total disorientation. Some attacks may take a schizophreniform or stuporous pattern, while others are marked by

TABLE 122–8. TREATMENT OF ADULT STATUS EPILEPTICUS OR SERIAL SEIZURES

I. Convulsive tonic-clonic or complex partial status
   1. Assure the airway, give O₂, check blood pressure and pulse. Establish a venous line and draw blood for glucose, calcium, hyper- or hypo-osmolar indicants. If indicated, measure pH, Pao₂, Paco₂.
   2. Start infusion and give 50 ml of 50% glucose.
   3. Infuse diazepam intravenously 5 mg/min until seizures stop or to total 20 mg. Also start phenytoin 50 mg/min to total 18 mg/kg.
   4. If convulsions persist, give *either* (1) phenobarbital 100 mg/min or as loading dose to 20 mg/kg, *or* (2) 100 mg diazepam in 500 ml dextrose 5% run in at 40 ml/hr. Monitor ventilation closely.
   5. If convulsions persist, start anesthesia with halothane and neuromuscular blockade. If latter not immediately available, give lidocaine 50–100 mg intravenously.
II. Serial tonic-clonic or partial motor status
   Steps 3 and 4 above but not to induce coma.
III. Petit mal status
   Diazepam as in step 3 followed by oral ethosuximide, valproic acid, or both

bizarre, detached activity. Patients may resist assistance in their fugue-like state, which can last for hours and sometimes days. The EEG usually shows continuous slow and spike activity predominating over one or both temporal areas, commonly in an asymmetrical distribution. Occasionally, surface recordings can be normal, but abnormal activity can be detected on nasopharyngeal leads or from electrodes placed deep in limbic system structures of the brain. Treatment should be initiated promptly, as prolonged seizures can permanently impair memory and intellect.

Absence status (petit mal status) occurs in two forms. The more common is an extension of complex absence seizures discussed earlier in which semiconfused automatic behavior occurs accompanied by closely fused or continuous runs of 3- to 4-Hz spike and wave on the EEG. The condition occurs in patients with known petit mal and usually is confined to adolescents or occasionally young adults. Most episodes last less than 30 minutes. Somewhat similar in behavior are attacks of prolonged (days to months) automatisms associated with confusion and sometimes gradual interictal mental deterioration. These are more likely to occur in older persons, often with no history of epilepsy. Most such attacks can be halted with diazepam given intravenously. Some, however, strongly resist antiepileptic therapy.

Major generalized motor status epilepticus with tonic-clonic convulsions creates a medical emergency, since continuation of the convulsions beyond an hour or so commonly produces residual brain damage. The commonest cause is abrupt withdrawal of anticonvulsant medications from a known epileptic. Almost as frequent are withdrawals of alcohol or drugs in a habitual user, cerebral infection, trauma, hemorrhage, or neoplasms. Treatment of the convulsions and the protection of the brain are of immediate concern and should take the form outlined in Table 122–8 and 116–7. Diagnostic steps to identify and treat the cause must be undertaken as soon as possible after the emergency situation has been brought under control.

SPECIAL MANAGEMENT PROBLEMS

Febrile Convulsions. Convulsions caused by fever occur mainly in neurologically otherwise healthy children between the ages of six months and five years who recurrently develop single generalized seizures when affected by an acute, fever-producing illness. Factors that increase the chance of having a future chronic epileptic disorder include age less than one year at onset, convulsions lasting longer than 15 minutes or coming in clusters, any pre- or postictal sign of neurologic abnormality, or a family history of epilepsy. Ten per cent of children with two or more of these risks go on to have chronic epilepsy, while recurrent nonfebrile seizures affect less than 2 per cent of the remainder. Present practice is to do everything possible to limit the course of the single convulsion but to place only children who have high risk factors on medication, usually phenobarbital.

Menstruation, Genetic Counseling, and Pregnancy. A number of women with epilepsy suffer an increase in seizures during the days immediately preceding and following the onset of menses. Acetazolamide, 250–500 mg daily, taken prophylactically or a modest increase in medication during the susceptible days often counteracts the problem.

Persons with seizure disorders inevitably will ask about the hereditary risks to the fetus. Best available evidence suggests that 4 to 10 per cent of the offspring of patients with generalized primary epilepsy will suffer one or more seizures during their lifetime. This compares to an incidence of approximately 1.5 per cent of the general population. Rates in the partial epilepsies are less clearly different from the norm.

Chronic anticonvulsant medication often requires adjustment during pregnancy. The blood volume increases and drug pharmacokinetics change. Blood level monitoring during the latter half of pregnancy can be useful in managing the difficult-to-control woman. During pregnancy it is advisable to give vitamins and supplements, including folic acid and calcium. Vitamin K, 5 mg twice weekly, should be given orally during the final six weeks, with a parenteral supplement administered to the mother and infant at the time of delivery. Breast feeding is not contraindicated in women taking antiepileptics.

Teratogenic Effects. The overall incidence of important birth defects in children of mothers or fathers taking antiepileptic medication is two to three times higher than in the general population. Trimethadione has been especially incriminated, and experimental studies suggest that the taking of valproate during pregnancy also is inadvisable. Phenytoin carries a demonstrated risk, but the exact rate is unknown. Data on phenobarbital or carbamazepine are too few to allow firm recommendations.

Psychosocial Management. The presence of incompletely controlled epilepsy and the frequent association between seizures and other neurologic limitations create large problems in emotional adjustment. In addition, some patients with partial complex seizures may possess aberrant personality traits that intensify their potential social isolation. Outbreaks of frustration are common, and depression and suicide are more frequent among patients with epilepsy than in the general population. A reduced libido and hyposexuality have been noted in males with partial complex seizures. These limitations notwithstanding, in the absence of associated brain damage most persons with epilepsy score in the normal range on standard intelligence tests. One can cite examples of persons with epilepsy who have performed in an outstanding manner in every level of professional, governmental, artistic, and business life.

Patients with seizure disorders are helped most by bringing the attacks under control, but reassurance, empathy, and optimistic social guidance by the physician aid immeasurably. Once seizures are under control, affected persons should be encouraged to live a normal life using mainly common sense as their guide. Sports carrying a high risk of injury are best avoided unless seizures have been completely controlled for well over a year; high diving, deep water or underwater swimming, high alpine climbing, boxing, and head contact football are ill-advised. Most states grant automobile driver's licenses to patients with epilepsy provided that no seizures have occurred for at least a year. Educational and vocational opportunities depend on whether or not seizures are controlled and upon the person's innate capabilities. Life and health insurance policies are available under special circumstances. The Epilepsy Foundation of America can assist patients with these and other social considerations.

Discontinuation of Medication. One considers stopping antiepileptic medication either (1) because seizures continue and patients believe the drugs are ineffective or (2) because seizures have been completely controlled for a long time. The first condition is uncommon and must be approached cautiously because of the dangers of precipitating status epilepticus. The latter decision can be considered between patient and doctor when absence seizures have been fully suppressed for two or three years and other types of seizures for three to five years. Patient's value systems, economic and social factors, and knowledge of risks all should contribute to the decision. Between 20 and 50 per cent of those who do discontinue treatment will undergo recurrent seizures, which may be more difficult to control than the original attacks. Particularly likely to relapse are persons whose initial seizures lasted longer than six months, were difficult to control, or were associated with any evidence of a focal defect or other neurologic abnormality. A moderate or severely abnormal EEG is an additional sign favoring recurrence if treatment stops. In general, we advise most adult epileptics not to stop anticonvulsant medication no matter how long they have been well-controlled. For most, the cost of relapse is just too high.

REFERENCES

Delgado-Escueta AV, Ferrendelli JA, and Prince DA (eds): Basic mechanisms of the epilepsies. Ann Neurol 16 (Suppl):1–158, 1984. *A workshop proceedings that gives the best available summary of recent scientific advances on the problem.*

Delgado-Escueta AV, Treiman DM, and Walsh GO: The treatable epilepsies. N Engl J Med 308:1508, 1983. *A succinct, lucid account.*

Engel J Jr, Troupin AS, Crandall PH, et al: Recent developments in the diagnosis and therapy of epilepsy. Ann Intern Med 97:584, 1982. *A well-balanced discussion of management and some aspects of diagnosis.*

Laidlaw J, and Richens A: A Textbook of Epilepsy. 2nd ed. Edinburgh, Churchill Livingstone, 1982. *The best comprehensive book in the field, written by an international roster of authoritative contributors.*

Solomon GE, Kutt H, and Plum F: Clinical Management of Seizures. Philadelphia, WB Saunders Co, 1983. *A pocket-sized monograph, didactically describing practical aspects of the problem, well-tabulated and referenced.*

123 INTRACRANIAL NEOPLASMS, CNS COMPLICATIONS OF CANCER, AND STATES OF ALTERED INTRACRANIAL PRESSURE

INTRACRANIAL NEOPLASMS

INTRODUCTION AND DEFINITIONS

Intracranial tumors can arise from any structure within the intracranial cavity. Most begin in the brain, but the pituitary, the pineal region, cranial nerves, and leptomeninges are also sites of neoplastic degeneration. Furthermore, any of these structures may be the site of metastatic spread from tumors that arise outside the nervous system. Intracranial tumors are not rare; they are the second most common cancer in children, and in adults malignant brain tumors are more common than Hodgkin's disease. Recent studies indicate an incidence of 14.1 primary intracranial and spinal tumors per 100,000 population per year in the United States, or about 35,000 new patients. Of these, 12,000 are malignant brain tumors. The incidence of metastatic intracranial tumor is less well-established but at least equals that of primary neoplasms.

Intracranial tumors can be classified both by site of origin and by histologic type (Table 123–1). Most arise from neuroectodermal elements (the precursor of both neurons and glia) of the brain. The commonly encountered brain tumor of adults is glial in origin, a benign or malignant astrocytoma (glioblastoma multiforme). The terms *benign* and *malignant* applied to brain tumors reflect histologic criteria that in turn reflect local growth rate rather than propensity to metastasize. Even highly malignant primary brain tumors rarely metastasize, although they may spread locally from the parenchyma to seed the leptomeninges and spinal cord. Many "benign" brain tumors recur despite treatment and eventually lead to the demise of the patient. Others may undergo "malignant degeneration" and alter their biologic potentiality.

CLASSIFICATION

Neuroectodermal Tumors. The commonest neuroectodermal tumor is the *astrocytoma*. Astrocytomas can arise anywhere in the brain or spinal cord and infiltrate surrounding normal structures. Tumor cells can often be found several centimeters distant from the main bulk of the tumor. Furthermore, in some instances, astrocytomas may have a multicentric origin or, more rarely, infiltrate the entire neuraxis (gliomatosis cerebri). Some, particularly cerebellar astrocytomas of childhood, may become quiescent for decades after only partial resection. About half of astrocytomas are relatively benign. The others consist of rapidly growing tumors that include the anaplastic astrocytoma and, most malignant of all, the glioblastoma multiforme. In adults, benign astrocytomas have a prognosis of four to seven years, anaplastic astrocytomas one and a half to two and a half years, and glioblastoma usually a year or less. *Oligodendrogliomas* may be either benign or malignant. In general, oligodendrogliomas usually grow more slowly than astrocytomas and tend to calcify. Glial tumors are often mixed, so that elements of oligodendroglioma may be found within a tumor that is primarily astrocytic in origin, and areas of benign astrocytoma may be found within a malignant glioblastoma. Because of the heterogeneity of such tumors, small biopsies may give misleading diagnostic and prognostic information. *Ependymomas* also can be either benign or malignant. Common sites of ependymal growth include the fourth ventricle in children and the spinal cord in children and adults. Malignant ependymomas of the fourth ventricle tend to spread to involve the leptomeninges. *Medulloblastomas* arise from a primitive neuroectodermal cell, usually in the cerebellum, and likewise may seed throughout the CSF. They are predominantly tumors of childhood and are highly malignant, but 50 per cent of children treated by surgery and radiation therapy now survive more than five years. In children, astrocytomas represent half of all cerebellar tumors,

TABLE 123–1. CLASSIFICATION OF BRAIN TUMORS

I. Tumors of Neuroepithelial Tissue
   A. Astrocytic Tumors
      1. Astrocytoma
      2. Anaplastic (malignant) astrocytoma
   B. Oligodendroglial Tumors
      1. Oligodendroglioma
      2. Anaplastic (malignant) oligodendroglioma
   C. Ependymal and Choroid Plexus Tumors
      1. Ependymoma
      2. Anaplastic (malignant) ependymoma
      3. Choroid plexus papilloma
      4. Anaplastic (malignant) choroid plexus papilloma
   D. Pineal Cell Tumors
      1. Pineocytoma
      2. Pineoblastoma
   E. Neuronal Tumors
      1. Gangliocytoma
      2. Ganglioglioma
   F. Poorly Differentiated and Embryonal Tumors
      1. Glioblastoma
      2. Medulloblastoma
      3. Primitive neuroectodermal tumors
II. Tumors of Nerve Sheath Cells
   A. Neurilemmoma (schwannoma, neurinoma)
   B. Anaplastic (malignant) Neurilemmoma
   C. Neurofibroma
   D. Anaplastic (malignant) Neurofibroma
III. Tumors of Meningeal Tissues
   A. Meningioma
   B. Meningeal Sarcoma
IV. Germ Cell Tumors
   A. Germinoma
   B. Embryonal Carcinoma
   C. Choriocarcinoma
   D. Teratoma
V. Tumors of the Anterior Pituitary
   A. Pituitary Adenoma
   B. Pituitary Adenocarcinoma

Modified from World Health Organization: International Histologic Classification of Tumors, No. 21, Geneva, Switzerland, 1979. Used with permission.

medulloblastomas and ependymomas making up the rest.

Mesodermal Tumors. The most common mesodermal tumor is *meningioma*. Meningiomas are usually benign and arise in certain favored sites: along the dorsal surface of the brain, the base of the skull, the falx cerebri, the sphenoid ridge, or within the lateral ventricles. Although these tumors are benign, they often reach large size before they are discovered and may be difficult to remove. Furthermore, they may recur even after apparently complete surgical extirpation. The most common cranial nerve tumor is the *acoustic schwannoma* (neurilemmoma, neuroma). Early discovery of such tumors has been possible in recent years because of the development of refined auditory tests and computed tomographic (CT) scans, thereby enabling these tumors to be removed frequently via a translabyrinthine approach. *Pituitary adenomas* may begin as intrasellar masses and extend into extrasellar locations, causing visual loss. *Microadenomas*, asymptomatic except for their hormone secretion, can now be identified by high-resolution CT scan of the pituitary. *Craniopharyngiomas* are developmental tumors derived from Rathke's pouch and may be intrasellar or suprasellar in location; they are frequently calcified and often cystic. *Pineal region tumors* occur primarily in children. They rarely truly originate from the pineal gland but are commonly germinomas, often curable by radiation therapy. The benign *colloid cyst* usually grows in the anterior third ventricle. Vascular tumors include *arteriovenous malformations*, which are not truly neoplastic, and the *hemangioblastomas*, which are. The latter tumors, when located in the brain stem or cerebellum, may be part of the von Hippel-Lindau syndrome that includes hemangioblastomas elsewhere in the body. Congenital tumors include the *craniopharyngiomas*, *chordomas* (which arise at the base of the brain or the lumbosacral area from the primitive notochord), *dermoids*, and *teratomas*. Granulomas and parasitic cysts come from tuberculomas, cryptococcosis (toruloma), sarcoidosis, and cysticercosis.

Metastatic Tumors. These can spread to any part of the intracranial cavity and tend to exhibit growth characteristics similar to their parent neoplasm. There is some clinical and a great deal of experimental evidence, however, to suggest that the same tumor may grow somewhat more slowly in the brain than in the primary organ of origin. Metastatic tumors, unlike primary tumors, tend to be well-circumscribed rather than infiltrative and are easier to remove in toto than are primary neoplasms.

SYMPTOMS AND SIGNS

Because they arise within the closed box of the skull, intracranial tumors tend to cause symptoms and signs while still relatively small. Symptoms may be caused because (1) the tumor invades and replaces normal tissue (Fig. 123–1). This probably accounts for only a minority of symptoms in brain tumors and is particularly characteristic of low-grade infiltrating gliomas. (2) The tumor growth compresses normal tissues. As intracranial tumors grow, they compress surrounding tissues and cause shift of normal brain structures. Blood vessels are compressed as well, leading to ischemia of the surrounding tissue. (3) New vessels formed in the growing brain tumor do not possess a blood-brain barrier (that anatomical-physiological structure that excludes proteins, ionized substances, and many water-soluble chemotherapeutic agents from the normal central nervous system). The blood-brain barrier also breaks down in compressed tissue surrounding a brain tumor. As a result, edema forms both within and around the tumor, which adds to the mass in the brain. Furthermore, because the brain has no lymphatics, removal of edema is slow. That edema produces many of the symptoms of intracranial tumors is attested to by the dramatic response that most brain tumor symptoms show to corticosteroids. These drugs, which decrease brain edema (exact mechanism unknown), substantially ameliorate symptoms for most patients with brain tumors without having a biologically significant effect on the growth of the tumor. (4) Large or small strategically located tumors (third ventricular and fourth ventricular tumors, leptomeningeal tumors) obstruct spinal fluid pathways, leading to hydrocephalus. The resulting inability of normally formed spinal fluid to escape from the ventricular system or the subarachnoid space further

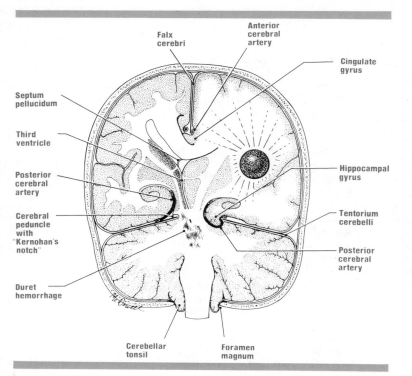

FIGURE 123–1. Schematic representation of the pathophysiology of clinical symptoms caused by a brain tumor. A mass lesion (black sphere) and surrounding edema (dashed lines) enlarge the hemisphere, obliterating normal sulci and shifting normal structures caudally and across the midline. The tumor and surrounding edema destroy and displace normal tissue in the hemisphere, producing contralateral neurologic signs (e.g., weakness and sensory loss). Obliteration of subarachnoid spaces by the mass lesion raises intracranial pressure, producing generalized signs (e.g., headache and papilledema). Shifts of normal brain cause symptoms at a distance and may lead to cerebral herniation (see Chapter 116). (From Cairncross JG, and Posner JB. In Yarbro JW, and Bornstein RS (eds): Oncologic Emergencies. New York, Grune and Stratton, 1981.)

Falx
cerebri

Anterior
cerebral
artery

Cingulate
gyrus

Septum
pellucidum

Third
ventricle

Posterior
cerebral
artery

Cerebral
peduncle
with
"Kernohan's
notch"

Duret
hemorrhage

Hippocampal
gyrus

Tentorium
cerebelli

Posterior
cerebral
artery

Cerebellar
tonsil

Foramen
magnum

adds unwanted mass and raises intracranial pressure.

The mass of a brain tumor plus the attendant edema and hydrocephalus all may lead to herniation of normal cerebral structures under the falx cerebri, through the tentorium or foramen magnum (p. 655).

The symptoms and signs caused by brain tumors depend on the location of the tumor and its histopathology (rapidity of growth). Sudden changes in tumor size resulting from hemorrhage, necrosis, or sudden obstruction of spinal fluid pathways can cause additional symptoms. Symptoms and signs may be divided into three major categories: (1) *generalized*, largely due to increased intracranial pressure, (2) *focal*, a result of ischemia and/or compression of normal brain at the site of the tumor, and (3) *false localizing*, a result of shifts of cerebral structures, causing neurologic abnormalities at a distance from the tumor.

Generalized Symptoms and Signs

The most common symptom of increased intracranial pressure is *headache*. Headache results from compression or distortion of pain-sensitive dural and vascular structures surrounding the brain; the brain itself is insensitive to pain. The head pain may be felt at the site of the tumor but more commonly is diffuse. In its early stages, the typical brain tumor headache is mild, tends to occur early in the morning when the patient first awakens, and disappears as the patient assumes an upright posture and breathes more deeply, thus lowering intracranial pressure. As the tumor enlarges, headaches become more constant and severe and are often exacerbated by coughing, bending, or sudden movement of the head. Later, headaches may awaken the patient at night. Headaches (p. 683) are a common symptom, rarely caused by brain tumors, but their onset in a patient not previously prone to headache or a recent change in headache pattern should alert the physician to the possibility of increased intracranial pressure. *Papilledema* occurs in about one fourth of patients with an intracranial neoplasm, probably as a result of obstruction of CSF pathways. Papilledema is much more common in children and young adults than it is in the elderly. *Vomiting*, with or without preceding nausea, is a common symptom of intracranial hypertension in children but much less so in adults. Vomiting usually occurs early in the morning before breakfast. It is often, but not always, accompanied by headache. Vomiting is more common in posterior fossa tumors but can occur with any tumor that raises intracranial pressure. *Mental changes* are also common. Patients first become irritable and then later quiet and apathetic. They retire to bed early and arise later (unless the early morning is accompanied by headache) and nap during the day. They are forgetful, seem preoccupied, and often appear psychologically depressed. Psychiatric consultation is frequently procured before the diagnosis of brain tumor is suspected. In patients with mass lesions and intracranial pressure, *plateau waves* are a common phenomenon. Plateau waves are rises in intracranial pressure that last between 5 and 20 minutes. They are caused by failure of normal cerebral vascular autoregulation so that an abrupt increase in cerebral blood volume occurs, causing the intracranial pressure to rise. Such pressure waves can increase an already high intracranial pressure by as much as 60 to 100 mm Hg. The wave may be asymptomatic, but more commonly is accompanied by neurologic symptoms including headache, visual obscurations, altered consciousness, and sometimes weakness of the extremities. These episodic changes in neurologic function usually last only a few minutes and may be precipitated by a sudden rise from a lying position, by alterations in intracranial pressure associated with coughing, sneezing, or straining, or even by tracheal suctioning.

Focal Symptoms and Signs

The location of a brain tumor determines not only whether the tumor is more likely to produce generalized or focal signs but also the type of focal signs it will produce. Tumors arising in relatively silent areas of the brain (such as the frontal pole) may grow to large size, raise intracranial pressure, and cause severe signs of generalized brain dysfunction before focal signs are evident. Similarly, tumors arising in the ventricular system, particularly at the outflow of the third and fourth ventricles, also produce generalized signs before focal signs become evident. On the other hand, tumors arising in primary rather than association cortex are more likely at their outset to produce focal symptoms and signs: Tumors of the visual system, whether optic nerve, optic chiasm, or occipital cortex, cause visual loss or visual field deficits before generalized signs develop. Tumors of the sensorimotor cortex cause weakness and sensory change. In addition, because certain areas of the frontal lobe, temporal lobe, and sensorimotor cortex have a relatively low threshold for epileptic discharge, seizures are often an early symptom. If the tumor is in the sensorimotor cortex, the seizures take a focal sensory or motor pattern. Tumors arising in more silent areas can cause unrecognized focal epileptogenic discharges, which generalize to produce a grand mal seizure. Seizures, when they appear, are most often the presenting symptom of meningiomas, where compression of the underlying cortex produces an epileptogenic focus, or of low-grade infiltrating frontal lobe gliomas.

Frontal lobe tumors often grow to a huge size before producing symptoms. Focal symptoms of frontal lobe tumors include personality change, either irritability and facetiousness or depression and apathy (or a combination of both), abnormalities of gait, and sometimes urinary frequency. Frontal lobe gliomas are often bilateral, arising in the corpus callosum and infiltrating the white matter of both frontal lobes. Posterior frontal lobe tumors involving the motor cortex lead to monoparesis or hemiparesis, and if in the dominant hemisphere to Broca's aphasia.

Parietal lobe lesions cause cortical sensory abnormalities in the contralateral half of the body. If the tumor grows to involve the thalamus, all sensory modalities including pin sensation are impaired contralaterally. Large parietal lesions often give rise to apraxia and, if in the nondominant hemisphere, to anosognosia (the failure to recognize the presence of a neurologic deficit). Difficulty with visual-spatial orientation, including inability to dress oneself, is characteristic of nondominant parietal lobe lesions.

Temporal lobe tumors often produce seizures as their first symptom. Hallucinations of smell or hearing as well as déjà vu phenomena are typical focal symptoms of temporal lobe tumors, often followed by a psychomotor or generalized seizure. Superior quadrantanopsia is common in temporal lobe seizures. If the tumor is on the dominant side, patients develop Wernicke's aphasia.

Occipital lobe tumors cause contralateral visual field defects and often contralateral visual seizures.

Brain stem tumors are marked by the combination of upper and lower neuron signs (e.g., in brain stem gliomas, a common problem in children, symptoms such as facial diplegia and ocular palsies appear with or without involvement of sensory and motor long tracts).

Cerebellar tumors are particularly common in children and produce early signs of increased intracranial pressure by compressing the fourth ventricle. Focal signs include ataxia of gait in midline tumors such as medulloblastoma or ataxia of ipsilateral extremities with laterally placed tumors such as cerebellar astrocytomas.

Cranial nerve tumors include trigeminal and acoustic schwannomas or meningiomas. Fifth nerve tumors are characterized by pain and sensory loss in the face, the pain sometimes resembling that of trigeminal neuralgia. Eighth nerve tumors are characterized by slowly progressive hearing loss with or without loss of balance. Both can be treated surgically.

A number of different tumors growing in the *pituitary fossa* and/or the *suprasellar cistern* lead to a combination of neurologic and endocrinologic abnormalities. The most common sellar tumor is the pituitary adenoma, a benign growth that often secretes excessive amounts of the hormone made by its parent cell. The tumors often remain very small, the only symptoms produced being those of hypersecretion of prolactin (amenorrhea-galactorrhea syndrome in women), growth hormone (acromegaly), or adrenocorticotropic hormone (Cushing's disease). Other adenomas, however, can grow to a large size, compressing and destroying the normal pituitary gland and leading to hypopituitarism and diabetes insipidus. As such tumors grow superiorly, they compress the diaphragma sella, a pain-sensitive structure, and cause headache. Immediately above the diaphragma sella is the optic chiasm, compression of which leads to bitemporal hemianopsia.

If the tumor grows laterally, it encounters the oculomotor nerves in the cavernous sinus, producing ocular palsies. Some pituitary tumors outgrow their blood supply. In this instance, patients suffer sudden hemorrhage or a necrosis into the tumor, producing the syndrome of *pituitary apoplexy*: a previously asymptomatic patient presents to the physician with acute headache, visual changes (bitemporal hemianopsia or blindness), and sometimes oculomotor palsies. The patient is often febrile, with a stiff neck from spillage of blood and necrotic tissue into the subarachnoid space. A CT scan usually reveals a pituitary mass, often hemorrhagic. Emergency treatment with hormonal replacement and, often, decompression usually leads to a good outcome. Tumors arising in the *parasellar area* may cause visual loss simultaneous with or even before pituitary failure. The first sign of pituitary failure in these instances is usually diabetes insipidus; in children, failure of sexual development and obesity are common problems, probably resulting from compression of the hypothalamus. Craniopharyngiomas, optic gliomas, meningiomas, and sometimes large carotid aneurysms cause masses in this area, as do germinomas (ectopic pinealoma).

Most tumors arising in the *pineal area* are germinomas, teratomas, or other embryonal growths. These tumors are common in children, boys more than girls. They produce their symptoms by compression of the sylvian aqueduct, leading to hydrocephalus. Compression of fibers in the upper brain stem leads to loss of upward gaze and sometimes pupillary fixation, early signs of pineal region compression. Occasionally compression of the inferior colliculus causes deafness. A definitive diagnosis of pineal region tumor is important, since the germinomas are usually curable with radiation therapy, whereas most of the others are not. *Leptomeningeal* tumors usually result from spread of a primary brain or systemic tumor to the leptomeninges; primary lymphomas or melanomas of the leptomeninges are rare. Metastatic leptomeningeal invasion, however, is common from lymphomas, leukemias, or solid tumors such as carcinomas of the breast or lung and malignant melanoma. Primary tumors of the nervous system that commonly seed the meninges include medulloblastomas, malignant ependymomas of the fourth ventricle, and germinomas. Symptoms of leptomeningeal involvement may occur before the primary tumor has declared itself. The first symptoms are often those of increased intracranial pressure from hydrocephalus (see Fig. 116–2). Additional symptoms include seizures from invasion of the cortex, cranial nerve palsies from infiltration of nerves passing through the subarachnoid space, and spinal root dysfunction, often involving the lower extremities and the bladder as a result of infiltration of the cauda equina. The diagnosis is suspected by the presence of diffuse or multifocal signs of central nervous system dysfunction and usually can be established by the identification of malignant cells in the spinal fluid.

False Localizing Symptoms and Signs

Growing tumors mold the surrounding normal brain and displace adjacent and remote structures from their normal positions. When these structures are shifted, they may be compressed by nearby dura, by bone at the base of the skull, or by the bony foramina through which the cranial nerves pass. Compression of normal structures at a distance from the growing tumor leads to focal neurologic signs that may incorrectly localize the tumor. These false localizing signs usually occur with slow-growing tumors arising in relatively silent areas. Examples of well-recognized false localizing signs include diplopia from abducens nerve palsy as a result of displacement compression of the sixth nerve at the base of the brain, hemianopsia caused by tentorial herniation that compresses the posterior cerebral artery and produces ischemia to the occipital lobe, and tinnitus, vertigo, or hearing loss from compression of the eighth nerves as they pass through the internal auditory canal. False localizing signs rarely produce a diagnostic problem nowadays because of the availability of new imaging techniques. False localizing signs can also occur with pseudotumor cerebri or intracranial hypotension, where their recognition is particularly important if one is to avoid unnecessarily exhaustive laboratory evaluation or inappropriate surgery.

DIAGNOSTIC TESTS

In any patient clinically suspected of harboring an intracranial neoplasm, a CT scan is the first test to be ordered. The procedure should be performed both before and after the injection of iodinated contrast material, and special attention should be given to the region that the clinician suspects is involved. For example, if a pituitary or suprasellar tumor is suspected, the radiologist should take 1-mm sections in both horizontal and coronal planes. Similar fine sections may reveal small posterior fossa or orbital tumors that are missed by routine CT scanning. Meningeal tumors can often be suspected by the development of hydrocephalus and the appearance of contrast enhancement in the subarachnoid space. Radionuclide brain scan, skull x-ray, and electroencephalography add nothing to the diagnosis. If a leptomeningeal tumor is suspected, lumbar puncture should be performed to look for the characteristic changes of pleocytosis, malignant cells in the spinal fluid, elevated protein and hypoglycorrhachia (low glucose content). At times, myelography will identify small tumors on the nerve roots. If an intracranial neoplasm is still suspected on clinical grounds and the CT is nondiagnostic, magnetic resonance imaging (MRI) often can identify an infiltrating tumor (usually a low-grade glioma) when the CT scan is normal (Fig. 123–2). The test also may help to distinguish arteriovenous anomalies of the brain from brain neoplasms.

Imaging techniques reveal the presence but not the exact nature of a lesion. Thus, neither CT nor

FIGURE 123–2. MRI of an 18-year-old man with progressive cranial nerve symptoms suggesting a brain stem tumor. The CT scan was normal. Sagittal magnetic resonance image reveals a mass (arrow) in the pons.

MRI can definitively distinguish between the histological types of tumors, nor can they reliably differentiate between neoplasms and other tumors such as abscesses or granulomas. Angiography is useful primarily to assist the surgeon in defining the proximity of the tumor to nearby arteries and veins. Thus, if a lesion is present and cannot clearly be identified on clinical grounds, biopsy is necessary before treatment is undertaken. When the lesion is accessible, surgical excision will not only establish the diagnosis but also provides the first step in the treatment of the patient. If the lesion is not accessible, CT-directed stereotactic needle biopsy often can establish the diagnosis definitively.

TREATMENT

The treatment of intracranial neoplasms varies, depending on the nature of the neoplasm, its location, and the general status of the patient. Certain general principles apply: When there is a single lesion and it is surgically accessible, it should be removed to whatever degree possible. Although some patients undergoing surgery of intracranial neoplasms suffer increased neurologic dysfunction, the majority improve after compression of brain structures is relieved. The advantages of surgery are that it cures some patients (pituitary adenoma, most meningiomas, cerebellar astrocytomas), that it ameliorates symptoms in the majority of patients, and that the debulking of a large malignant lesion allows time for other slower-acting therapeutic modalities to be effective. It also definitively establishes the diagnosis.

Most intracranial neoplasms cannot be cured surgically (Fig. 123–3). For them the second line of treatment is radiation therapy (RT). RT is delivered either to the local site of the tumor (some recurrent meningiomas) or by a combination of whole-brain and local radiation (most malignant

FIGURE 123–3. Results of treatment of glioblastoma multiforme. A 32-year-old man presented in the fall of 1982 with headaches, seizures, and papilledema. A large contrast enhancing bifrontal mass was partially extirpated and then treated with radiation therapy and chemotherapy. *A,* The mass prior to therapy. *B,* The mass shortly postoperatively, indicating that there had been a major but incomplete resection. A residual tumor is indicated by the arrows. *C,* CT scan 2.5 years later. The site of surgical extirpation is indicated by the lucent area. There is no evidence of contrast enhancement, suggesting that the residual tumor has been eradicated. The patient is asymptomatic.

gliomas) or to the entire neuraxis (medulloblastomas, malignant ependymomas). RT improves both survival and the quality of life in most patients with highly malignant tumors. It probably also favorably affects the course of more benign tumors such as astrocytomas and recurrent meningiomas.

Chemotherapy, when added to RT, appears to enhance both survival and quality of life in patients with malignant astrocytomas, but its role in other intracranial neoplasms is not yet well-established.

SPINAL NEOPLASMS

Spinal tumors originate from the same cell types as do intracranial tumors, and the same principles of diagnosis and treatment apply to them as to intracranial tumors. They are discussed in detail on pages 725–727.

PARANEOPLASTIC SYNDROMES

When patients with systemic cancer (i.e., cancer that arises outside the central nervous system) develop nervous system dysfunction, metastasis is usually the cause. However, cancer also exerts deleterious effects on the nervous system in the absence of direct metastatic involvement (paraneoplastic syndrome). Recognition of these nonmetastatic neurologic complications can prevent inappropriate and perhaps harmful therapy directed at a nonexistent metastasis. Since at times the nervous system symptoms precede the discovery of the cancer, they can also lead the physician to the diagnosis of an otherwise occult neoplasm. An almost bewildering variety of neurologic disorders have been ascribed to effects of systemic cancer (Table 123–2). Most patients with nervous system dysfunction not caused by metastases are eventually found to be suffering from systemic infections, from vascular or metabolic disorders that affect the nervous system secondarily, or from unwanted side effects of cancer therapy. This section discusses two types of nervous system damage related to cancer and not described elsewhere in this book: "remote effects" and radiation injury.

REMOTE EFFECTS

Remote effects of cancer on the nervous system is a term used to describe nervous system dysfunction of unknown cause occurring exclusively or at higher frequency in patients with cancer.

Remote effects are not common, probably affecting less than 1 per cent of patients with cancer. Their cause is unknown. Circulating antibodies against the target nervous system organ can be found in some patients suffering from remote effects. In a few instances, injection of the antibody or extracts of tumor into experimental animals has reproduced portions of the clinical syndrome, suggesting an autoimmune mechanism, with the antigen originating in the tumor. Not all patients harbor such antibodies, and other suggestions for etiology have included viral infections, toxins secreted by the tumor, and nutritional deprivation.

A few neurologic syndromes are highly characteristic of remote effects. These include subacute cerebellar degeneration, subacute sensory

TABLE 123–2. NONMETASTATIC EFFECTS OF CANCER ON THE NERVOUS SYSTEM

I. "Remote effects"
 A. Brain and cranial nerves
  1. Dementia
  2. Bulbar encephalitis
  3. Subacute cerebellar degeneration—opsoclonus*
  4. Optic neuritis—retinal degeneration
 B. Spinal cord
  1. Gray matter myelopathy
   a. Subacute motor neuropathy
   b. "Autonomic insufficiency"
  2. Subacute necrotic myelopathy
 C. Peripheral nerves and roots
  1. Subacute sensory neuronopathy (dorsal root ganglionitis)*
  2. Sensorimotor peripheral neuropathy
  3. Acute polyneuropathy, "Guillain-Barré" type
  4. Autonomic neuropathy
 D. Neuromuscular junction and muscle
  1. Polymyositis and dermatomyositis (dermatomyositis in older men*)
  2. "Myasthenic" syndrome
  3. Myasthenia gravis (thymoma)
  4. Neuromyotonia
II. Metabolic encephalopathy
 A. Destruction of vital organs
  1. Liver (hepatic coma)
  2. Lung (pulmonary encephalopathy)
  3. Kidney (uremia)
  4. Bone (hypercalcemia)
 B. Elaboration of hormonal substances by tumor
  1. "Parathormone" (hypercalcemia)
  2. "Corticotropin" (Cushing's syndrome)
  3. Antidiuretic hormone (water intoxication)

 C. Competition between tumor and brain for essential substrates
  1. Hypoglycemia (large retroperitoneal tumors)
  2. Tryptophan (carcinoid)
 D. Malnutrition
III. Infections (usually associated with lymphomas)
 A. Parasites
  1. Toxoplasma cerebral abscess
 B. Fungi
  1. Meningitis (cryptococcosis)
  2. Encephalitis (aspergillosis, mucormycosis)
 C. Bacteria
  1. Meningitis (*Listeria monocytogenes*)
 D. Viruses
  1. Herpes zoster (radiculitis, myelitis, encephalitis, granulomatous vasculitis)
  2. Progressive multifocal leukoencephalopathy
IV. Vascular disease
 A. Intracranial hemorrhage
  1. Subdural hematoma
  2. Subarachnoid hemorrhage
  3. Intracerebral hemorrhage
 B. Cerebral infarction
  1. Thrombotic (due to "hypercoagulability")
  2. Embolic nonbacterial thrombotic endocarditis
V. Side effects of therapy
 A. Chemotherapy
  1. Central nervous system
  2. Peripheral nervous system
 B. Radiation therapy
   See Table 123–3

* Neurologic disorders that may precede diagnosis of cancer and strongly suggest its presence.
From Posner JB: Nonmetastatic effects of cancer on the nervous system. In Wyngaarden JB, and Smith LH Jr (eds): Cecil Textbook of Medicine. 17th ed. Philadelphia, WB Saunders Co, 1985, pp 1081–1084.

neuronopathy, and the myasthenic syndrome. These are discussed in the paragraphs below.

Subacute cerebellar degeneration caused by cancer has a clinical picture sufficiently characteristic to suggest strongly that cancer is present even if the neurologic symptoms predate the appearance of the tumor. There is usually subacute onset of bilateral and symmetrical cerebellar dysfunction, the patient being equally ataxic in arms and legs. Severe dysarthria is usually present, and vertigo and diplopia are common, but nystagmus may be absent. Many patients have neurologic signs pointing to disease outside the cerebellum: extensor plantar responses are common; tendon reflexes may be either diminished or exaggerated; and dementia occurs in about half. The cerebrospinal fluid is usually normal, but there may be as many as 40 lymphocytes per cubic milliliter and an elevated protein content. The disease, which may be associated with any cancer, precedes the discovery of the neoplasm by periods of from weeks to three years in more than half the patients, and it tends to run a progressive course over weeks to months, rendering the patient severely disabled. Cerebellar atrophy may be seen on a CT scan, particularly if done late in the course of the illness. Characteristic pathologic

changes consist of diffuse or patchy loss of Purkinje cells in all areas of the cerebellum. There may be lymphocytic cuffs around blood vessels, particularly in the deep nuclei. This illness can be distinguished from cerebellar metastases by the symmetry of its signs and the absence of increased intracranial pressure, and from alcoholic-nutritional cerebellar degeneration because dysarthria and ataxia in the upper extremities are prominent in the carcinomatous cerebellar degenerations and are usually mild or absent in the alcoholic variety. The hereditary cerebellar degenerations rarely run so rapid a course. At times the disorder stabilizes or improves with successful treatment of the tumor. Antibodies to cerebellar Purkinje cells have been found in the serum of a few patients.

Another, less common cerebellar syndrome is that of *opsoclonus* (spontaneous, conjugate, chaotic eye movements most severe when voluntary eye movements are attempted). Opsoclonus is frequently associated with cerebellar ataxia and myoclonus of the trunk and extremities. It is most common in children as a remote effect of neuroblastoma. In children, the neurologic symptoms respond to adrenocorticosteroid therapy and to therapy of the tumor.

Subacute sensory neuronopathy is marked by loss of sensation with relative preservation of motor power. The illness sometimes precedes the appearance of the carcinoma and progresses over a few months, leaving the patient with a moderate or severe disability. The cerebrospinal fluid protein is usually elevated. Pathologically, there is destruction of posterior root ganglia with perivascular lymphocytic cuffing and wallerian degeneration of sensory nerves. Many of the patients have inflammatory and degenerative changes in brain and spinal cord as well. The entity is rare and there is no treatment. Some patients harbor an antibody that reacts with an antigen found in the nuclei of neurons throughout the central nervous system. Dorsal root ganglion cells also harbor the antigen.

The *myasthenic syndrome* occurs predominantly in men over 40 and is associated with intrathoracic tumors in 70 per cent of the patients (sometimes called the Lambert-Eaton syndrome). The patients complain of weakness and fatigability of proximal muscles, particularly of the pelvic girdle and thighs. The cranial nerves and respiratory muscles are less involved. In addition, patients complain of dryness of the mouth, impotence, pain in the thighs, and peripheral paresthesias. On examination, there is weakness of the proximal muscles, but strength increases over several seconds of a sustained contraction. The deep tendon reflexes are diminished or absent. The diagnosis is made by electromyographic studies in which repeated nerve stimulations at rates above ten per second cause a progressive increase in the size of the muscle action potential (the opposite of myasthenia gravis). The neuromuscular defect in this illness is believed to be deficient release of acetylcholine. Similar findings have been produced in experimental animals by injection of either serum IgG or extract of tumor in patients with the disorder, suggesting an autoimmune etiology. Plasmapheresis and immunosuppressant drugs may relieve symptoms. The illness responds poorly to anticholinesterase drugs but does respond to guanidine hydrochloride given in doses of 15 to 40 mg/kg/day.

INJURY FROM THERAPEUTIC RADIATION

When parts of the nervous system are included within an ionizing irradiation portal, adverse effects may result (Table 123–3). The likelihood of adverse effects is related to the total dose of radiation, the size of each fraction, the total duration over which the dose is received, and the volume of nervous system tissue irradiated. Other factors such as underlying nervous system disease (e.g., brain tumor, cerebral edema), previous surgery, concomitant use of chemotherapeutic agents, and individual susceptibility make it impossible to define precisely a safe dose for any given individual. However, general guidelines allow the radiation therapist to calculate generally safe nervous system doses. Adverse effects may involve any portion of the central or peripheral nervous system and may occur acutely or be delayed weeks to years following irradiation.

Clinical Manifestations

Acute encephalopathy may follow large radiation doses to patients with increased intracranial pressure, particularly in the absence of corticosteroid prophylaxis. Immediately following treatment, susceptible patients develop headache, nausea and vomiting, somnolence, fever, and occasionally worsening of neurologic signs, rarely culminating in cerebral herniation and death. Acute encephalopathy usually follows the first radiation fraction and becomes progressively less severe with each ensuing fraction. This disorder is believed to result from increased intracranial pressure and/or brain edema from radiation-induced alteration of the blood-brain barrier. It responds to corticosteroids. Acute worsening of neurologic symptoms does not occur after spinal cord irradiation.

Early delayed encephalopathy or myelopathy appears 6 to 16 weeks after therapy and persists for days to weeks. In children, the encephalopathy commonly follows prophylactic irradiation of the brain for leukemia and is called the "radiation somnolence syndrome." The disorder is characterized by somnolence, often associated with headache, nausea, vomiting, and sometimes fever. The electroencephalogram may be slow, but there are no focal signs. In adults, the syndrome usually follows whole-brain irradiation for brain tumors and is characterized by lethargy and worsening of focal neurologic signs. Both disorders usually respond to steroids but if untreated will resolve spontaneously. In adults, the syndrome may be distinguished from recurrent brain tumor by CT scan. In children, lumbar puncture rules out the potential diagnosis of meningeal leukemia. *Early*

TABLE 123–3. RADIATION INJURY TO THE NERVOUS SYSTEM

TIME AFTER RT	ORGAN AFFECTED	CLINICAL FINDINGS
Primary Injury		
Immediate (min to hrs)	Brain	Acute encephalopathy
Early delayed (6–16 wks)	Brain	Somnolence, focal signs
	Spinal cord	Lhermitte's sign
Late delayed (mos to yrs)	Brain	Dementia, focal signs
	Spinal cord	Transverse myelopathy
	Peripheral nerves	Paralysis, sensory loss
Secondary Injury (years)	Several	Brain, cranial, and/or peripheral nerve sheath tumors
	Arteries (atherosclerosis)	Cerebral infarction
	Endocrine organs	Metabolic encephalopathy

delayed myelopathy follows radiation therapy to the neck or upper thorax and is characterized by Lhermitte's sign (an electric shock–like sensation radiating into various parts of the body when the neck is flexed). The symptoms resolve spontaneously. Early delayed radiation syndromes are believed to result from demyelination, possibly due to radiation-induced damage to oligodendroglia.

Late delayed radiation injury appears months to years following radiation and may affect any part of the nervous system. In the brain, there are two clinical syndromes. The first follows whole-brain irradiation either to patients without brain tumors (prophylactic irradiation for oat cell carcinoma) or in some patients with primary and metastatic brain tumors. The disorder is characterized by dementia without focal signs. There is cerebral atrophy on CT scan and pathological changes are nonspecific, and there is no treatment. The second disorder affects patients who receive either focal brain irradiation during therapy of extracranial neoplasms or whole-brain irradiation for intracranial neoplasms. Neurological signs suggest a mass and include headache, focal or generalized seizures, and hemiparesis. Brain CT scans reveal a hypodense mass, sometimes with contrast enhancement (see Fig. 115–1). Neuropathological features include coagulative necrosis of white matter, telangiectasia, fibrinoid necrosis and thrombus formation, and glial proliferation and bizarre multinucleated astrocytes. The clinical and CT findings cannot be distinguished from brain tumor, and the diagnosis can be made only by biopsy. Corticosteroids sometimes ameliorate symptoms. The treatment, if the disorder is focal, is surgical removal. *Late delayed myelopathy* is characterized by progressive paralysis, sensory changes, and sometimes pain. A Brown-Sequard syndrome (weakness and loss of proprioception in the extremities of one side with loss of pain and temperature sensation on the other) is often present at onset. Patients occasionally respond transiently to steroids, and the disorder may stop progressing, but generally patients become paraplegic or quadriplegic. Pathological changes include necrosis of the spinal cord. *Late delayed neuropathy* may affect any cranial or peripheral nerve. Common disorders are blindness from optic neuropathy and paralysis of an upper extremity from brachial plexopathy after therapy for lung or breast cancer. The pathogenesis is probably fibrosis and ischemia of the plexus. There is no treatment.

Radiation-induced tumors, including meningiomas, sarcomas or, less commonly, gliomas, may appear years to decades after cranial irradiation and may follow even low-dose radiation therapy. Malignant or atypical nerve sheath tumors may follow irradiation of the brachial, cervical, and lumbar plexuses. The central nervous system may also be damaged when radiation alters extraneural structures. Radiation therapy accelerates *atherosclerosis*, and cerebral infarction associated with carotid artery occlusion in the neck may occur many years after neck irradiation. Endocrine (pituitary, thyroid, parathyroid) dysfunction from radiation may be associated with neurologic signs. Hypothyroidism or hyperparathyroidism from radiation may also cause an encephalopathy.

NON-NEOPLASTIC ALTERATIONS OF INTRACRANIAL PRESSURE

INTRODUCTION AND DEFINITIONS

Intracranial pressure is determined by rates of cerebrospinal fluid (CSF) formation and absorption and by cerebral venous pressure, the last a reflection of systemic venous pressure. Lumbar puncture pressure in the lateral decubitus position accurately reflects intracranial pressure in most instances. The normal CSF pressure is usually between 65 and 195 mm of CSF (5 to 15 mm Hg), although pressures as high as 250 mm of CSF have been reported in apparent normals. Nevertheless, pressures above 170 are suspect, and pressures above 200 should be considered abnormal until proved otherwise. CSF pressure is not affected by obesity. Elevated CSF pressure measured at lumbar puncture does not necessarily reflect neurologic disease; e.g., elevation of the head of the bed can raise the lumbar CSF pressure, although it lowers intracranial pressure. Elevation of systemic venous pressure, such as occurs acutely with coughing, straining, crying or chronically with congestive heart failure or venous obstruction (superior vena cava or jugular veins) raises intracranial pressure. Hypercapnia (e.g., pulmonary disease, excessive sedation) increases the cerebral blood volume and thus CSF pressure. Conversely, if the patient is positioned with the head down, lumbar puncture pressure will be lower, although intracranial pressure becomes higher. The loss of CSF around the needle hole between the time the needle enters the subarachnoid space and the manometer is placed also lowers intracranial pressure. When all of these artifactual causes of altered intracranial pressure are eliminated, the commonest cause of intracranial *hypertension* is intracranial tumor (p. 722) and the commonest cause of intracranial *hypotension* is a CSF leak following lumbar puncture or myelogram (p. 647). This section discusses several other disorders that can alter intracranial pressure.

INTRACRANIAL HYPERTENSION

Pseudotumor cerebri, as the name suggests, is a disorder characterized by increased intracranial pressure in the absence of a tumor or obvious obstruction of CSF pathways. The cause is usually not established, although a number of central nervous system or systemic illnesses appear to play an ·etiologic role. Pseudotumor can follow head trauma, middle ear disease, internal jugular vein ligation, oral contraceptive use, pregnancy, and polycythemia vera, all being conditions that suggest possible cerebral venous occlusion. In a few such patients, cerebral venograms do in fact show sagittal or lateral sinus occlusion. The disorder has also been reported in patients on prolonged corticosteroid therapy, after steroid withdrawal, with Addison's disease or hypoparathyroidism, and with ingestion of drugs such as vitamin A, nalidixic acid, and tetracycline. Most cases, however, are idiopathic.

The disorder usually affects young (ages 20 to 30), usually obese females, is characterized by headache, papilledema, and at times visual obscurations (sudden momentary, usually bilateral visual loss), and has a benign prognosis.

Most patients with pseudotumor present to the physician with headache and papilledema. In a few, headaches are absent and the disorder is discovered because of either visual obscurations or papilledema found on routine ophthalmological examination. Sometimes there is no papilledema or only unilateral papilledema even though intracranial pressure is grossly elevated. Visual obscurations do not portend visual loss. However, whether or not patients have visual obscurations, 10 to 15 per cent of patients lose some vision during the course of the disease, varying from small scotomata to total blindness. Other clinical symptoms that are less common but that may concern the physician include vomiting, diplopia, vertigo, tinnitus, neck pain and stiffness, orbital pain, drowsiness, and dysesthetic sensation. These false localizing signs probably result from minor shifts of normal structures engendered by the intracranial hypertension. The disorder usually runs a benign course, with the headache and papilledema resolving in several weeks to several months, although in many patients intracranial pressure as measured at lumbar puncture remains elevated for months to years.

The diagnosis is suspected clinically and established by the presence of elevated intracranial pressure in a patient with a normal CT scan. The CSF pressure is usually above 300 mm and its composition is otherwise normal, although in some patients there may be a relatively low protein (below 15 mg/dl). If venous obstruction is suspected, digital venous angiography should be performed. A few errors in diagnosis occur in patients with an anomalous elevation of the optic discs (pseudopapilledema) or, very rarely, in patients with diffuse infiltrating gliomas of the brain (gliomatosis cerebri). The first can be ruled out by appropriate ophthalmologic tests, including fluorescein angiography, and the second usually by MRI and time.

Treatment is symptomatic. Repeated lumbar punctures sometimes relieve the headaches, and some physicians believe that corticosteroids are helpful. Only if there is evidence of progressive visual loss is therapeutic intervention mandatory. In that instance, the best treatment appears to be shunting the CSF from the lumbar sac into the peritoneum.

Hydrocephalus refers to an enlargement of the cerebral ventricular system by an increase in the amount of ventricular fluid. Obstructive hydrocephalus can result from either stenosis or occlusion of CSF pathways within the ventricular system (noncommunicating) or from stenosis or occlusion of subarachnoid pathways outside the ventricular system (communicating). Nonobstructive hydrocephalus results from passive enlargement of the ventricular system because of atrophy of brain substance (hydrocephalus ex vacuo). Obstructive hydrocephalus is often but not always associated with intracranial hypertension and, when acute, may be rapidly fatal. The more chronic the hydrocephalus, the more likely the intracranial hypertension is to be either mild or undetectable (normal pressure hydrocephalus) and the more likely the symptoms are to be indolent.

Acute hydrocephalus, such as occurs with sudden obstruction of the ventricular system (e.g., colloid cyst of the third ventricle, subarachnoid or cerebellar hemorrhage), is characterized by sudden severe headache, vomiting, lethargy, and sometimes coma. If the system is not decompressed, herniation and death can occur in a short time. Subacute (subarachnoid hemorrhage, meningitis, leptomeningeal neoplasia) or chronic hydrocephalus (congenital aqueductal stenosis, spinal cord tumors, idiopathic normal pressure hydrocephalus) is usually characterized by progressive lethargy, apathy, and dementia, often associated with an unsteady gait and urgency incontinence of urine. There may be bilateral corticospinal tract signs, particularly in the lower extremities, with hyperactive knee and ankle jerks and extensor plantar responses. If the pressure is grossly elevated, patients may develop headache and papilledema, but these are uncommon.

The presence of enlarged ventricles is detected easily by CT scan. Unfortunately, it is not always easy to distinguish on the CT scan between obstructive hydrocephalus and hydrocephalus ex vacuo unless the cause (e.g., tumor) can be identified. A lumbar puncture revealing an elevated intracranial pressure assists in the diagnosis, but because some patients with obstructive hydrocephalus have a relatively normal intracranial pressure, that test likewise may not give a definitive diagnosis. In patients with classic symptoms of chronic hydrocephalus (i.e., dementia, gait unsteadiness, and incontinence), removal of CSF at lumbar puncture sometimes relieves symptoms, indicating both that CSF obstruction is producing the symptoms and that ventricular shunting will be therapeutic.

INTRACRANIAL HYPOTENSION

Intracranial hypotension usually follows lumbar puncture but occasionally results from spontaneous or traumatically induced tears of the dura, leading to leakage of subarachnoid fluid. The resulting low CSF pressure is characterized by headache beginning occipitally and radiating frontally when the patient assumes the erect posture. The headache is sometimes associated with nausea, vomiting, photophobia, and a stiff neck. Some patients develop diplopia from abducens nerve paralysis. Auditory symptoms such as tinnitus and vestibular symptoms such as dizziness also can occur. The symptoms probably result because the brain, unsupported by CSF, shifts downward when the erect posture is assumed. The diagnosis is easily made on clinical grounds if the patient has undergone a lumbar puncture or myelogram a few days previously, but can be established only by performing a lumbar puncture and noting the low CSF pressure if no such history is present. Symptoms usually resolve spontaneously but in a few instances may persist, in which case a search for the site of the leak should be made. Some investigators have recommended epidural injection of a few cc's of the patient's blood to patch a dural leak following lumbar puncture, and in a few instances of spontaneous or traumatic dural tears, surgical repair of the leak has been necessary.

REFERENCES

Gilbert HA, and Kagan AR (eds): Radiation Damage to the Nervous System. A Delayed Therapeutic Hazard. New York, Raven Press, 1980. *A comprehensive description of all of the nervous system side effects of therapeutic irradiation.*

Henson RA, and Urich H: Cancer and the Nervous System. Oxford, Blackwell Scientific, 1982. *Comprehensive and up-to-date descriptions of all of the paraneoplastic disorders affecting the nervous system.*

Rottenberg DA, and Posner JB: Intracranial pressure control. In Cottrell JE, and Turndorf H (eds): Anesthesia and Neurosurgery. St Louis, CV Mosby Co, 1980, pp 89–118. *This well-referenced chapter provides a quantitative description of the CSF system. Some familiarity with the subject is helpful.*

Shapiro K, Marmarou A, and Portnoy H (eds): Hydrocephalus. New York, Raven Press, 1984. *A multiauthored monograph on clinical, physiological, and therapeutic aspects of hydrocephalus.*

Shapiro WR: Treatment of neuroectodermal brain tumors. Ann Neurol 12:23, 1982

Walker MD (ed): Oncology of the Nervous System. Boston, Martinus Nijhoff, 1983. *An up-to-date multiauthored monograph on all aspects of CNS tumors.*

INFECTIOUS AND INFLAMMATORY DISORDERS OF THE NERVOUS SYSTEM

124

Despite its sequestration from the rest of the body by the blood-brain barrier, the central nervous system is subject to attack by many of the same infectious agents and antigen-antibody reactions that affect the remainder of the body. As with systemic infections, bacterial, fungal, and parasitic infections of the nervous system are particularly likely to occur when the body's resistive mechanisms have been breached. Viral infections of the nervous system are also common. Although more frequent in immunosuppressed hosts, many viruses (e.g., that causing herpes zoster) are neurotropic (i.e., have a predilection for invasion of the nervous system). Except for slow viruses, discussed in this section, virus diseases of the nervous system are described in Chapter 86. When managing inflammatory disease of the nervous system, one has the obligation not only to identify and treat the invading organism but to search for host factors that may predispose to further infections. Table 124–1 lists some of these factors.

BACTERIAL INFECTIONS OF THE BRAIN

Bacteria reach the nervous system from a prior site of infection in a systemic organ. The only exception occurs when a communication connects the central nervous system and the surface of the body, such as can follow central nervous system trauma, surgical procedures, or the development of spontaneous CSF fistulae. A careful search for the last is always warranted in a patient with repetitive central nervous system bacterial infections.

Bacterial infections of the central nervous system may be meningeal or parameningeal. The most common infection, acute bacterial meningitis, is discussed in detail in Chapter 86. Less common *parameningeal infections* include brain and spinal epidural abscesses and brain and spinal subdural abscesses (subdural empyema). This chapter discusses these, along with parenchymal brain and spinal abscesses and certain unusual neurologic complications of bacterial infections resulting from bacterial endocarditis, secondary venous sinus thrombosis, and malignant external otitis.

INTRACRANIAL ABSCESSES

Intracranial abscesses are pockets of pus localized to one of the intracranial compartments (i.e., the epidural space, the subdural space, or the brain itself). *Epidural abscesses* usually arise by

TABLE 124–1. IMMUNE DEFECTS AND SOME INFECTING ORGANISMS IN IMMUNOSUPPRESSED PATIENTS

	EXAMPLES	BACTERIA	FUNGI	PARASITES	VIRUSES
Neutrophil defects	Acute leukemia Chemotherapy	S. pyogenes S. aureus Enteric bacilli	Candida sp. Aspergillus sp. Mucor sp.		
Monocyte defects	Hodgkin's disease Chemotherapy	L. monocytogenes Salmonella sp. N. asteroides Mycobacterium sp.	C. neoformans Candida sp. H. capsulatum C. immitis	P. carinii T. gondii S. stercoralis	Cytomegalovirus Varicella-zoster H. simplex Vaccinia virus
Globulin defects	Multiple myeloma Chronic lymphocytic leukemia Chemotherapy	S. pneumoniae Enteric bacilli		P. carinii	Vaccinia virus
Interrupted integument	Finger or bone marrow punctures IV needles and catheters Bladder catheters	S. pyogenes S. aureus Enteric bacilli	Candida sp.		Vaccinia virus H. simplex
Infusion infections	Blood products IV fluids	Enteric bacilli Salmonella sp.	Candida sp.	Malaria sp. T. gondii	Hepatitis B Cytomegalovirus E.-B. virus
Surgical procedures	Tracheostomy Respiratory assistance Endoscopies	S. pyogenes S. aureus Enteric bacilli B. fragilis Salmonella sp.	Candida sp.		H. simplex

Modified from Armstrong D: Infectious complications of neoplastic disease: Their diagnosis and management—Part I. Clin Bull 6: 135–141, 1976.

direct extension from adjacent osteomyelitis, mastoiditis, or infection of the paranasal sinuses. In the early stages, signs and symptoms are usually those of infection of the extracranial site from which they arose. Thus, head pain and often local swelling and redness commonly overlie the site of the epidural abscess. Fever usually is present accompanied by leukocytosis with a preponderance of polymorphonuclear leukocytes. Focal neurologic signs are uncommon, and increased intracranial pressure is not usually present. In the early stage the cerebrospinal fluid usually contains at most a few lymphocytes with a slightly elevated protein. If the initial disorder is untreated, the infection may breach the dura to produce a subdural empyema, bacterial meningitis, or brain abscess. If the epidural inflammation lies close to a large venous sinus, thrombophlebitis with sinus occlusion (page 784) often complicates the infection. The extent of an epidural abscess is usually easily defined by CT scan, a contrast-enhancing mass being identified in the epidural space compressing the underlying brain. In their early stages, such abscesses can be treated successfully with appropriate antibiotics (the organism having been identified by culture of purulent material from the ear or sinuses). In some instances, particularly when the abscess is large or when it fails to shrink rapidly with antibiotic therapy, surgical drainage is required.

Subdural Abscess

Most subdural abscesses (subdural empyemas) arise from infection of paranasal sinuses or the middle ear (otitis media). Organisms from the primary infection follow cranial venous channels (often producing thrombophlebitis as they go) through the dura into the subdural space. Occasionally, traumatically induced subdural hematomas become secondarily infected to form subdural empyemas. The site of the empyema depends on the site of the primary infection. Those of the paranasal sinuses usually extend over the frontal lobe, while those from ear infections penetrate the skull posteriorly both above and below the tentorium. Inflammatory reaction excited by the organism may produce a membrane that completely walls off the collection of pus.

Most patients with subdural empyema suffer the signs and symptoms of sinusitis or otitis prior to the onset of the empyema. As the intracranial abscess develops, the pain of the primary process usually worsens, with more severe headache spreading widely from its original site. Fever, if not already present, develops, the white count rises, and patients often become drowsy and may vomit. Secondary thrombophlebitis of the brain often develops and causes focal neurologic signs of seizures or hemiparesis. Eventually the intracranial pressure rises, and a fulminant course may produce death within a few days if no treatment is undertaken. The diagnosis is suggested by a history of pre-existing infection combined with local physical abnormalities. CT scans define both the site of primary infection and the subdural collection of pus. If obtained, the cerebral spinal fluid is usually under increased pressure and may contain several hundred cells with an elevated protein but normal glucose concentration. Lumbar puncture, however, should not be performed in patients suspected of subdural empyema, since no organisms will be recovered and the rapidly increasing intracranial pressure threatens to produce cerebral herniation.

Subdural empyema almost always requires surgical drainage. Drainage combined with appropriate antibiotic therapy usually relieves the symptoms and cures the patient if the disease is detected in its earliest stages. Unfortunately, diagnosis is often delayed, resulting in a mortality of about 25 per cent. Most patients die as a result of venous sinus thrombosis with secondary cerebral infarction or meningitis.

Brain Abscess

Brain abscess is the commonest intracranial abscess. Like those of the epidural and subdural space, parenchymal abscesses of the brain can arise by direct extension along venous channels from infections in the paranasal sinuses or the ear. Currently, however, most arise by hematogenous spread from infections elsewhere in the body. Metastatic abscess probably originates from a transient bacteremia with organisms lodging in capillary vessels of the brain. Organisms then produce first a focal bacterial encephalitis, followed in days or weeks by encapsulation of pus to form a true abscess. Unlike epidural or subdural abscesses, in which one almost always can identify the primary site of the infection, in a substantial number of patients with brain abscesses the systemic infection may already have resolved without having produced symptoms. Some patients with brain abscess give a history of dental manipulation or mild urinary tract infection several weeks earlier; others have had lung infections. Congenital cyanotic heart disease and arteriovenous shunts in the lungs increase the risk of brain abscess because the lungs normally filter out circulating bacteria. Immunosuppressed patients often develop multiple rather than the single brain abscesses that most often affect patients with normal immunity.

The primary site of the infection determines the offending organism. Common agents include an aerobic or microaerophilic *Streptococcus* as well as enteric bacteria. In traumatic abscesses, staphylococci are common; *Clostridium* occasionally is present. Many of the infections are mixed. Rarer causes of abscesses include *Actinomyces and Nocardia*. Tuberculous abscesses are uncommon in the United States, but frequent in less developed countries.

The site of a brain abscess depends partly on its source. Those that originate in the middle ear generally invade the temporal lobe or cerebellum, those in the paranasal sinus penetrate the frontal lobe, and those from penetrating injuries involve the wound site. Hematogenous abscesses can affect any part of the brain, although most are in the distribution of the middle cerebral artery, the largest area.

Most abscesses produce symptoms similar to but more rapidly progressive than those of a brain tumor. It is uncommon for patients to suffer from fever, substantial tenderness of the skull, or an elevated white blood cell count. Instead, patients present with headache, signs of increased intracranial pressure, and focal signs that depend on the site of the lesion (see page 773). Focal or generalized seizures are a common accompaniment.

The major differential diagnosis usually lies with brain tumor and less often with stroke or nonlocalized infection. Abscess may be suspected almost immediately if a patient suffers one of the predisposing causes (e.g., immune suppression, cyanotic heart disease, arteriovenous shunting in the lungs) or if a systemic bacterial infection has occurred in the recent past. A history of a draining ear or evidence of otitis media, particularly when clinical symptoms and signs point to a lesion in the temporal lobe or cerebellum, strengthens the likelihood of brain abscess, as does a history of purulent sinusitis. If fever exists or the white blood cell count is elevated (neither usually is the case), the diagnosis favors abscess. Lumbar puncture should not be performed because of the risk of cerebral herniation. The CT scan is helpful but not always diagnostic. Abscess is characterized by a hypodense lesion surrounded by a contrast enhancing ring. The abnormality can resemble rings that sometimes rim primary and metastatic brain tumors as well as recent cerebral infarcts. A thin, smooth-walled ring suggests an abscess, whereas a thick, irregular ring is more common with brain tumor (Fig. 124–1). However, it usually requires surgical exploration to make the diagnosis.

The treatment begins with antibiotics. For abscesses 3 cm or smaller, antibiotics alone will usually suffice, the choice depending on the causal organism. If the organism is not known, a combination of penicillin and chloramphenicol in high doses for a period of about six weeks is usually effective. CT scanning helps greatly in judg-

FIGURE 124–1. CT scan showing a brain abscess. A woman presented to physicians after a focal seizure followed by headache and weakness of the arm. There had been a history of dental work performed several weeks before. CT scan revealed a contrast-enhanced ringlike mass surrounded by edema. It is not possible on this scan to differentiate tumor from abscess. At surgery a well-encapsulated abscess was encountered.

ing the effectiveness of antibiotic therapy and deciding when, if ever, surgical extirpation is necessary. Even after full recovery the contrast-enhancing ring may persist for many weeks and does not imply that the abscess is still active. Large abscesses, failure of the lesion to shrink or the patient to improve with antibiotic therapy, or the presence of a doubtful diagnosis mandate surgical removal or biopsy. With early detection and vigorous antimicrobial treatment most patients do not need surgery and recover with few sequelae other than a tendency to seizures, which can be controlled by anticonvulsants. This approach has reduced the mortality from brain abscesses in some series to about 5 per cent.

VENOUS SINUS AND CORTICAL THROMBOPHLEBITIS

Bacterial infections of the central nervous system may cause thrombophlebitis with secondary occlusion of the large dural sinuses. Similarly, occlusion of large dural sinuses may occur in the absence of infection in patients with disorders of clotting (see Table 120–5). The most common sites of infective sinus occlusion are the lateral sinus (a complication of acute or chronic otitis media), cavernous sinus (a complication of orbital or nasal sinus infection), and the superior sagittal sinus, usually occluded by direct extension of the infected clot from the first two. Cortical veins may be involved either by direct contact with an infection in the epidural or subdural space or by extension of infective clot from the sinuses.

The symptoms of lateral sinus occlusion depend on the rapidity of the occlusion and the im-

portance of that sinus in draining the brain's blood. Since the two lateral sinuses are often different sizes, slowly developing occlusion of the smaller one usually causes no symptoms at all. Occlusion of the dominant lateral sinus is often heralded by headache and papilledema (pseudotumor cerebri, also called, when otitis was a more common problem, otitic hydrocephalus). There are usually no focal signs unless the occlusion spreads to involve the jugular vein, in which case there may be pain, swelling, and a palpable cord in the neck. If the occlusion spreads to the inferior petrosal sinus, abducens and trigeminal nerve involvement (Gradenigo's syndrome) can be added and, if the jugular bulb is involved, dysarthria, dysphagia, and neck weakness (jugular foramen syndrome) ensue.

Cavernous sinus occlusion produces a more florid picture. Such occlusions often are caused by a staphylococcal infection of the face or sinus and begin with fever, headache, nausea, vomiting, and seizures. Proptosis affects the ipsilateral eye with chemosis and ophthalmoplegia, to which sensory loss in the distribution of the first division of the trigeminal nerve sometimes is added (all result from the third, fourth, fifth, and sixth nerves passing through the cavernous sinus). Papilledema is a late event.

Sagittal sinus occlusion is characterized by headache and, often, papilledema. If acute in onset and involving the posterior sinus, bilateral hemorrhagic infarction of the brain develops, sometimes producing bilateral hemiparesis more marked in the leg and proximal arm than in the hand and face.

The diagnosis of sinus occlusion or corticothrombophlebitis should be suspected in a patient with a head or neck infection who develops signs of increased intracranial pressure with or without focal neurologic signs. The diagnosis of sinus occlusion can easily be made by a digital intravenous angiogram (Fig. 124–2), although the test does not distinguish between infective and noninfective thromboses.

Infective sinus thrombosis is usually successfully treated with appropriate antibiotics; sometimes despite treatment the clot propagates to cause severe cerebral infarction and even death. Anticoagulation for sinus thrombosis is controversial. Many physicians fear that anticoagulants will lead to brain hemorrhage, and this is probably particularly true in infected cases.

MALIGNANT EXTERNAL OTITIS

This rare central nervous system infection deserves specific mention because it is potentially lethal but curable if diagnosed early. The disorder affects elderly diabetic patients and begins as an external auditory canal infection with *Pseudomonas aeruginosa*. The infection spreads from the ear to the soft tissue, invading the parotid gland, temporomandibular joint, masseter muscle, and temporal bone. Cranial nerves VI through XII often become involved. Although most cases produce pain in the ear, purulent drainage often re-

FIGURE 124–2. Digital venous angiogram (DIVA), lateral view patient facing left, in a patient with sagittal sinus occlusion. The procedure is generally more effective in demonstrating the cerebral venous system than is an arteriogram, because the cerebral hemispheres are filled with contrast material simultaneously. The patient had a bland occlusion of the posterior sagittal sinus (arrows). Inflammatory sinus occlusions have a similar appearance.

mains absent. Culture of the ear, however, reveals the *Pseudomonas* organism; the condition responds to intravenous carbenicillin and gentamicin.

Although not bacterial in origin, another rare intracranial infection in diabetics also deserves mention. This disorder, *rhinocerebral phycomycetes*, affects young diabetics with or without ketoacidosis. The disorder, caused by the fungus Phycomycetes (mucormycosis), begins as a focal infection of the nose or palate and spreads to involve the posterior orbit and cavernous sinus, leading to cavernous sinus occlusion. The often fulminant disease can lead to internal carotid artery as well as cavernous sinus occlusion. The rapid onset of proptosis and ocular palsies accompanied by high fever, headache, nausea, and prostration suggests the diagnosis. Careful inspection of the nose or palate often reveals a black necrotic patch, scrapings of which reveal the organism. Antifungal agents may help, but the disease is often fatal.

BACTERIAL ENDOCARDITIS

The disseminated emboli of subacute bacterial endocarditis affect the nervous system of a quarter to a third of patients (Table 124–2). The most common symptom is that of an embolic stroke characterized by the acute onset of focal motor weakness. Multiple small emboli may lead to a clinical picture resembling a toxic encephalopathy with confusion, hallucinations, and lethargy with or without fleeting focal signs. Infected emboli lodged in cerebral blood vessels may lead to aneurysm formation (mycotic aneurysm). These aneu-

rysms typically form in the distal portion of arteries in contradistinction to congenital aneurysms, which locate themselves more proximally. The aneurysms may rupture to cause severe cerebral or subarachnoid hemorrhage. Resolution of the aneurysms after antibiotic therapy has been reported, but in many patients surgical clipping is necessary to prevent recurrent hemorrhage. As in other disorders causing sepsis, brain abscesses can result from either acute or subacute bacterial endocarditis.

SPINAL INFECTIONS

The spinal leptomeninges contiguous with those of the intracranial cavity are bathed by the same cerebrospinal fluid and share in all of the meningeal infections and inflammatory processes that affect the brain. Subdural and epidural collections of pus, however, can be localized to the spinal canal and present with clinical pictures that differ from their counterparts in the intracranial cavity. Spinal cord parenchymal abscesses are exceedingly rare. They usually reach the spinal cord, as they do the brain, by hematogenous spread.

SPINAL ABSCESS

Most spinal epidural abscesses occur at either the cervical or lumbar level and extend from an infected focus in an adjacent vertebral body (osteomyelitis), *Staphylococcus aureus* being the most common organism. Other abscesses arise either by hematogenous spread to the epidural space or by direct extension from a paravertebral infected focus. Depending on the virulence of the

TABLE 124–2. NEUROLOGIC COMPLICATIONS OF BACTERIAL ENDOCARDITIS*

NEUROLOGIC COMPLICATION	PRESENTING COMPLICATION†	NO. OF TIMES NEUROLOGIC COMPLICATION OCCURRED†
Cerebral infarction in territory of middle cerebral arteries		34
Cerebral infarction in territory of vertebrobasilar arteries	22	4
Meningeal signs and symptoms	3	33
Seizures	5	24
Multiple microemboli		23
Microscopic brain abscesses		8
Visual disturbances	1	6‡
Cranial or peripheral neuropathy		5
Mycotic aneurysm		4
Subarachnoid hemorrhage (without identifiable mycotic aneurysm)	2	5
Cerebral infarcts in "watershed areas" due to hypotension		3
Intracerebral hemorrhage	2	4
Subdural hemorrhage	1	2
Macroscopic brain abscess		1
Psychiatric disturbance	3	4

* Modified from Pruitt AA, Rubin RH, Karchmer AW, and Duncan GW: Neurologic complications of bacterial endocarditis. Medicine 57:329–343, 1978.
† More than one complication was frequently observed in a single patient. Each complication is listed separately.
‡ Four patients developed retinal artery emboli, one a retinal artery hemorrhage, and one cortical blindness.

organism, clinical signs may develop either rapidly or slowly. In either case, neck or back pain is the most prominent symptom. The pain is usually severe and, in its early stages, well-localized. One finds marked tenderness of the spine over the site of the infection. As the illness develops, pain may spread in a dermatomal distribution as nerve roots are irritated by the inflammatory process. Unless effective treatment is started, the patient develops progressive weakness and sensory loss below the site of the lesion (myelopathy), which may lead to paraplegia in hours to days. Most patients with acute epidural abscesses are febrile and toxic, with an elevated white count. In the more chronic processes these findings may be absent, but the erythrocyte sedimentation rate is usually elevated. X-rays of the vertebral body may not become abnormal for several weeks following the onset of symptoms even when the patient is suffering from osteomyelitis. Traditionally, the diagnosis has been made by myelography. Spinal fluid obtained at the time of myelography is characterized by pleocytosis (up to several hundred white cells), elevated protein, and a normal glucose concentration; organisms are rarely cultured. In more chronic processes the pleocytosis may be absent. Recently, some workers have reported a high diagnostic accuracy using CT scans, which show an extradural lesion leading to either a complete or a partial block in most cases plus percutaneous tapping of the abscess for bacteriological diagnosis.

Spinal subdural empyemas, usually caused by *Staphylococcus aureus*, are more likely to be associated with meningitis and spinal cord infarction than are epidural abscesses but otherwise are similar in clinical presentation. The diagnostic and therapeutic approaches are also similar.

Antibiotic therapy should be started as soon as the diagnosis is suspected. In the past, surgical drainage has been considered imperative in acute abscesses. Recently, a nonsurgical approach similar to that employed in brain abscess has been suggested, but too few results yet exist to judge the effectiveness of this approach. Chronic abscesses sometimes respond to antibiotics alone, but if signs of myelopathy appear, the patient should be surgically decompressed. The outcome is usually satisfactory in patients who are not completely paralyzed at the time treatment is undertaken.

Acute or subacute spinal abscesses must be differentiated from acute (subacute) transverse myelitis (see p. 792) and from spinal epidural or subdural hematomas (usually a disorder of patients with abnormal coagulation). Chronic spinal abscesses must be distinguished from tumor. In the acute disorder, fever, toxicity, and a history of prior infection support the diagnosis of abscess, and a carefully done myelogram or CT scan reveals the lesion to be extradural. Acute transverse myelopathy is associated either with a normal myelogram or with swelling of the spinal cord itself. In the more chronic form, differentiation between tumor and abscess may be more difficult.

Both conditions can produce x-ray changes in the vertebral bodies, inflammation being more likely to affect two contiguous vertebral bodies across an intravertebral disc, whereas tumors are usually restricted to individual vertebral bodies. If the diagnosis is in doubt, biopsy of the vertebral body or decompression of the epidural space is necessary to make the differentiation.

OTHER BACTERIAL INFECTIONS

Two bacterial diseases of the nervous system, syphilis and tuberculosis, once common in the United States, are now rare, adding to the difficulty in making a definitive diagnosis when they are encountered. A discussion of the systemic manifestations of syphilis can be found on p. 587 and tuberculosis on p. 165.

SYPHILIS

The spirochete causing syphilis invades the central nervous system in most instances of systemic infection. The organism then may either be cleared by host defenses or persist to produce a more chronic infection expressed symptomatically only years later. The most common form of neurosyphilis is asymptomatic; patients harbor in the CSF a few white cells and have a positive serological test for syphilis. Symptomatic neurosyphilis can appear as acute or subacute meningitis (meningitic form) resembling that of other bacterial infections and usually occurring during the stage of secondary syphilis when there are cutaneous changes as well. The diagnosis is suspected by the history of syphilis as well as by the cutaneous changes, if present, and established by positive serological tests in the CSF. Patients respond promptly to antisyphilitic therapy.

Vascular syphilis begins two to ten years after the primary lesion. The disorder is characterized by both meningeal inflammation and a vasculitis of small arterial vessels, the latter leading to arterial occlusion. Clinically the disorder produces few signs of meningitis but results in monofocal or multifocal cerebral or spinal infarction. The disorder may be mistaken for an autoimmune vasculitis or even arteriosclerotic cerebral vascular disease. The early and prominent spinal cord signs should lead one to expect syphilis, while the findings in the CSF of pleocytosis, elevated gamma globulin, and a positive serological test for syphilis establish the diagnosis. Patients respond to antibiotic therapy, although recovery from focal abnormalities may be incomplete.

General paresis, once a common cause of admission to mental institutions, is now rare. The disorder results from syphilitic invasion of the parenchyma of the brain and begins clinically 10 to 20 years after the primary infection. Paresis is characterized by progressive dementia, sometimes with manic symptoms and megalomania and often with coarse tremors affecting facial muscles and tongue. The diagnostic clue is the presence of Argyll Robertson pupils (p. 692). The spinal fluid is always abnormal. The diagnosis is made by serological tests. Early treatment with antibiotics usually leads to improvement but not complete recovery.

Tabes dorsalis is a chronic infective process of the dorsal roots which appears 10 to 20 years after primary syphilitic infection. The disorder is characterized by lightning-like pains and a progressive sensory neuropathy affecting predominantly large fibers, more in the lower extremity than elsewhere. There is profound loss of vibration and position sense as well as areflexia. Autonomic fibers are also affected, causing postural hypotension, trophic ulcers of the feet, and traumatic arthropathy of joints. Argyll Robertson pupils are usually present. Spinal fluid serological tests are usually positive. The disorder responds only partially to treatment by antibiotics.

Rare complications of syphilis include *progressive optic atrophy, gumma* (a mass lesion in the brain), *congenital neurosyphilis,* and syphilitic infection of the *auditory* and *vestibular system.* Descriptions can be found in appropriate texts.

TUBERCULOSIS

Central nervous system tuberculosis can occur in several forms, sometimes without evidence of active infection elsewhere in the body. The most common form is *tuberculous meningitis.* This disorder is characterized by the subacute onset of headache, stiff neck, and fever. After a few days, affected patients become confused and disoriented. They often develop abnormalities of cranial nerve function, particularly hearing loss due to the marked inflammation at the base of the brain. Most patients if untreated lapse into coma and die within three to four weeks of onset. An accompanying arteritis may produce focal signs, including hemiplegia, during the course of the disorder. Tubercular meningitis must be distinguished from other causes of acute and subacute meningeal infection, a process that often is not easy even after examination of the spinal fluid. The pressure and cell count are elevated with up to a few hundred cells, a mixture of leukocytes and lymphocytes. The protein is elevated, usually above 100 mg/dl and often to very high levels, and the glucose is depressed. Smears for acid-fast bacilli are positive in only about 25 per cent of samples. Tuberculosis organisms will grow on culture, but only after several weeks. Recently, accurate CSF markers for the rapid diagnosis of the disease have been reported and are available through the Center for Disease Control in the United States. Pending complete availability and accuracy of such measures, patients with subacutely developing meningitis suspected of having tuberculosis should be treated with antituberculous agents prior to definitive diagnosis. Large samples of CSF should be sent for culture, and a careful search should be made for tuberculosis elsewhere in the body. Seventy-five per cent of such patients have a positive tuberculin skin test, and in most a careful search yields evidence of systemic tuberculosis.

Tuberculomas of the brain produce symptoms and signs either of the mass lesion or of meningitis, the tuberculomas being found incidentally. One or multiple lesions are identified on CT scan, but the scan itself does not distinguish tuberculomas from brain tumor or other brain abscesses. In the absence of evidence of meningeal or systemic tuberculosis, biopsy is necessary for diagnosis. Patients with tuberculomas, as those with tuberculous meningitis, respond to antituberculous therapy, but brain lesions may remain visible in the CT scan long after the patient has improved clinically; the clinical course and not the scan predicts the outcome.

Less common manifestations of tuberculosis include *chronic arachnoiditis* characterized by a low-grade inflammatory response in the spinal fluid and progressive pain with signs of either cauda equina or spinal cord dysfunction. The diagnosis of arachnoiditis is suggested by a myelogram showing evidence of fibrosis and compartmentalization instead of the usually smooth subarachnoid lining. The disorder responds poorly to treatment. *Tuberculous myelopathy* probably results from direct invasion of the organism from the subarachnoid space. Patients present with a subacutely developing myelopathy characterized by sensory loss either in the legs or in all four extremities, depending on the site of the spinal cord invasion. Many patients have additional signs of meningitis, including fever, headache, and stiff neck. The spinal fluid usually contains cells and tuberculous organisms. Myelogram may show evidence of arachnoiditis and frequently demonstrates an enlarged spinal cord or complete block to the passage of contrast material in the thoracic or cervical region.

SLOW AND LATENT VIRUS INFECTIONS OF THE NERVOUS SYSTEM

Acute viral meningitis and encephalitis are discussed on page 555. The term *slow virus infection* describes a group of transmissible disorders in which a long latent period separates the time between first inoculation and the subsequent development of disease in the host. *Latent infection* occurs with the herpes-varicella virus when, after an acute infection, the virus becomes quiescent (in sensory ganglia), only to become reactivated years later as herpes zoster.

Slow virus infections are of two kinds. One is caused by a transmissible agent not yet characterized that is highly resistant to usual sterilization procedures and thus far has escaped morphologic identification. The other results from conventional viral forms and is related to an abnormal host immune response. The illnesses caused by the first agents include kuru and Creutzfeldt-Jakob disease (CJD). The slow infections caused by otherwise typical viruses include subacute sclerosing panencephalitis, progressive rubella panencephalitis, and progressive multifocal encephalopathy. A chronic progressing or

TABLE 124–3. SOME CAUSES OF CNS VIRAL INFECTIONS*

VIRUS	MENINGITIS	ENCEPHALITIS
Enteroviruses	40	10
Mumps	12	14
Lymphochocytic choriomeningitis	6	9
Leptospira	3	2
Herpes simplex	1	10
Arboviruses	1	11
Other†	2	4

* Modified from Johnson RT: Viral meningitis and encephalitis. In Wyngaarden JB, and Smith LH Jr (eds): Cecil Textbook of Medicine. 17th ed. Philadelphia, WB Saunders Co, 1985, pp 2122–2126.

† Includes Epstein-Barr virus, measles, influenza, *Mycoplasma pneumoniae*, Rocky Mountain spotted fever, and fungal infections.

relapsing viral infection also has been proposed but never proved as a cause of several rare neurologic disorders, including chronic focal epilepsy, Mollaret's relapsing meningitis, Behçet's syndrome, and the Vogt-Koyanagi-Harada syndrome, all of which have some dimension of inflammation in their natural history. A slow virus cause also has been sought, so far unsuccessfully, in several other neurologic disorders, including multiple sclerosis, Parkinson's disease, and motor neuron disease. The 17th edition of the *Cecil Textbook of Medicine*, as well as the monograph by Johnson listed in the bibliography, discusses these conditions more extensively (Table 124–3).

Kuru, a disease of the primitive Fore tribe of New Guinea, provided the prototype for the existence of the nonimmunogenic infectious particle of subviral form. The illness causes a progressive ataxia, ophthalmoplegia, and dementia leading to death in 3 to 20 months. It appears to have been transmitted from person to person by tribal cannibalism. Passage of a similar disorder by inoculation of patient brain material into, at first, chimpanzees and subsequently several other mammalian species led to the discovery of the unique infectious agent. Since the Fore tribe has abolished ritual cannibalism, kuru has almost disappeared.

Creutzfeldt-Jakob disease develops mainly after age 40 in a worldwide distribution. The illness is characterized by progressive myoclonus, signs of upper motor neuron dysfunction, ataxia, and intellectual decline, all evolving rapidly over a period of weeks to a few months. Neither fever nor blood or spinal fluid abnormalities occur, but the EEG early on undergoes diffuse slowing and later shows repeated short bursts of sharp waves. Although CJD is relatively rare and sporadic in its distribution, a slight familial predisposition is observed. Like kuru, to which its cause may relate closely, the disorder can be transmitted to a variety of animal species. Medical personnel appear to carry little or no risk of contamination by affected patients, but person-to-person transmission has taken place via transplanted contaminated corneas or the successive use of intracerebral electrodes from affected persons and, apparently, via other neurosurgical instruments as well. There is no effective treatment.

FUNGAL AND PARASITIC CNS INFECTIONS

Fungal and parasitic infections of the central nervous system are less common than viral and bacterial infections and often affect immunosuppressed patients. Table 124–4 lists the more common of these infections and the setting in which they are likely to occur. Like bacterial infections, fungal and parasitic infections may cause either meningitis or parenchymal abscesses. The meningitides, when they occur, present with clinical symptoms that, while similar, are usually less severe and abrupt than those of acute bacterial meningitis. The common causes of meningitis are fungal and include especially cryptococcosis, coccidioidomycosis, and histoplasmosis. *Cryptococcal meningitis* is a sporadic infection that affects both immunosuppressed patients (50 per cent) and nonimmunosuppressed patients. The disorder is characterized by headache and sometimes fever and stiff neck. The clinical symptoms may evolve for periods as long as weeks or months; diagnosis can be made only by identifying the organism or its antigen in the cerebrospinal fluid. Histoplasma and coccidioidomycosis menigitis occur in endemic areas and often affect nonimmunosuppressed individuals. The diagnosis is suggested by a history of residence in the appropriate geographical area and confirmed by spinal fluid evaluation. Antifungal treatment, particularly in the nonimmunosuppressed patient, is usually effective.

Parasitic infections of the nervous system usually produce focal abscesses rather than diffuse meningitis. The commonest to affect the nonimmunosuppressed host is cysticercosis, a disorder caused by the *Taenia solium* tape worm contracted by eating inadequately cooked pork. The disorder is common in the underdeveloped world and parts of the United States having a large Hispanic population. The brain may be invaded in as many as 60 per cent of infected persons. Invasion of the brain leads to formation of either single or multiple cysts, which often lie in the parenchyma but sometimes reside in the ventricles or subar-

TABLE 124–4. SOME FUNGAL AND PARASITIC CAUSES OF CNS INFECTIONS

FUNGAL INFECTION	HELMINTHS PARASITIC INFECTION	PROTOZOAN INFECTION
Cryptococcosis	Trichinosis	Toxoplasmosis
Coccidioidomyocosis	Cysticercosis	Amebiasis
Aspergillosis	Echinococcosis	Malaria
Mucormycosis	Schistosomiasis	Chagas' disease
Actinomycosis	Angiostrongyliasis	Trypanosomiasis
Histoplasmosis	Ascariasis	(African)
Blastomycosis		
Candidiasis		

FIGURE 124–3. Toxoplasma abscesses in a patient with acquired immune deficiency syndrome (AIDS). *A*, CT scan shows one contrast-enhanced mass (arrow). *B*, Magnetic resonance image reveals multiple masses (arrows) not seen on CT scan, leading physicians to suspect abscesses rather than tumor.

achnoid space. Seizures and increased intracranial pressure are the most common clinical symptoms. CT scanning identifies small intracranial calcifications and hypodense cysts. Serum indirect hemagglutination tests are usually positive and confirm the diagnosis. Where cysts obstruct the ventricular system to cause symptoms, shunting procedures may be necessary. Recent evidence suggests that the anthelmintic praziquantel may be effective therapy.

Toxoplasmosis of the brain, when it occurs in the adult, is a manifestation of immunosuppression. Patients with abnormal cellular immunity may develop single or multiple abscesses (Fig. 124–3), which appear usually as ring-enhancing lesions on CT scan. The lesions cannot be distinguished from brain tumors or other infections, so that stereotactic directed needle biopsy often is required to make the diagnosis. Toxoplasma abscesses can be effectively treated with a combination of pyrimethamine and sulfadiazine.

CHRONIC MENINGITIS

Most cases of meningitis due to common viral and bacterial agents either resolve spontaneously or respond promptly to treatment. The diagnosis is usually rapidly established by appropriate CSF studies. Some patients, however, suffer from a subacute or chronic meningitis in which the diagnosis is not easily made. In addition to infectious agents, the clinical picture of subacute or chronic meningitis can be caused by neoplasms, sarcoidosis, or a variety of other illnesses of unknown cause. Table 124–5 lists the differential diagnosis of chronic meningitis. A definitive diagnosis can be established only by identifying definitive systemic manifestations of the underlying

disease or by repeatedly examining the spinal fluid for evidence of malignant cells, organisms, or abnormal antibodies or antigens. If a diagnosis cannot be made by lumbar puncture it often is useful to perform a cisternal puncture, since many inflammatory and granulomatous infections of the meninges are most prominent at the base of the brain. Careful search for illness outside the central nervous system may disclose the hilar adenopathy of sarcoidosis, or the genital ulcers of herpes simplex or the Behçet syndrome. In a few instances, one never ferrets out a diagnosis, and some patients suffer continuous or recurrent symptoms and signs of meningeal inflammation for months or years.

TABLE 124–5. SOME CAUSES OF SUBACUTE AND CHRONIC MENINGITIS

I. **Bacterial Infections**
 Partially treated acute bacterial meningitis
 Parameningeal infections
 Syphilis and tuberculous meningitis
II. **Viral Meningitis and Meningoencephalitis**
III. **Fungal and Parasitic Meningitis**
IV. **Neoplasm**
 Primary and metastatic leptomeningeal tumor
 Epidermoid cyst with rupture
V. **Vascular Lesions**
 Subdural hematoma
 Subarachnoid hemorrhage (late)
 Granulomatous arteritis
VI. **Unknown**
 Systemic lupus erythematosus
 Behçet's syndrome
 Mollaret's meningitis
 Sarcoidosis
 Vogt-Koyanagi-Harada syndrome
 Benign lymphocytic meningitis

DEMYELINATING AND OTHER CNS INFLAMMATORY DISORDERS OF PROBABLE IMMUNE CAUSE

Demyelinating Disorders

Several disorders that are believed to operate via abnormal immune mechanisms produce central nervous system dysfunction by damaging the myelin sheaths covering axons. The conditions appear to have their primary effect on the oligodendroglial cells, which are responsible for the production and maintenance of the myelin sheaths. The acute lesions of these demyelinating disorders usually contain inflammatory infiltrates, particularly lymphocytes, at the site of subsequent demyelination. There may be evidence of production of IgG within the central nervous system characterized by an elevated cerebrospinal fluid–to–serum IgG ratio. In their severe forms, the disorders also can damage other structures in demyelinated areas, including axons and astrocytic cells. Disorders with a relative predilection for damaging myelin are listed in Table 124–6. Those which have an immune basis are discussed here. Others, if they affect primarily adults, are found elsewhere in the text under appropriate headings.

Multiple Sclerosis (MS). The commonest of the presumed immune demyelinating disorders is multiple sclerosis. The disorder usually causes its first symptoms between the ages of about 20 and 40 years and is characterized by remissions and exacerbations of neurologic dysfunction from several different sites in the central nervous system over many years (lesions disseminated in space and time). Typically, an otherwise healthy person suffers an acute or subacute attack of unilateral loss of vision, true vertigo, ataxia, paresthesias, incontinence, diplopia, dysarthria, or paralysis (Table 124–7). The symptoms result from a "plaque" or myelin loss in the white matter of the brain (usually periventricular), brainstem, or

TABLE 124–6. DEMYELINATING DISORDERS*

A. Unknown Cause
  1. Multiple sclerosis
  2. Devic's disease
  3. Optic neuritis
  4. Acute transverse myelopathy
B. Parainfectious Disorders
  1. Acute disseminated encephalomyelitis
  2. Acute hemorrhagic leukoencephalopathy
C. Viral Infections
  1. Progressive multifocal leukoencephalopathy
  2. Subacute sclerosing panencephalitis
D. Nutritional Disorders
  1. Combined systems disease (vitamin B_{12} deficiency)
  2. Demyelination of the corpus callosum (Marchiafava-Bignami)
  3. Central pontine myelinolysis
E. Anoxic-Ischemic Sequelae
  1. Delayed postanoxic cerebral demyelination
  2. Progressive subcortical ischemic encephalopathy

* Modified from Silberberg DH: The demyelinating diseases. In Wyngaarden JB, and Smith LH Jr (eds): Cecil Textbook of Medicine. 17th ed. Philadelphia, WB Saunders Co, 1985, pp 2143–2149.

spinal cord, which is believed to prevent conduction of nerve impulses. The symptoms usually are painless, remain for several days to weeks, and then partially or completely resolve. After a period of relative freedom, new symptoms appear. Although individual frequencies vary widely, the average rate of exacerbations is about one every other year. In some patients the clinical course consists of progressive neurologic dysfunction; this usually takes the form of a slowly progressive myelopathy characterized by spasticity and ataxia, predominantly of the lower extremities. In other instances one or two attacks may characterize the disease of an entire lifetime, with significant disability never developing. On average, about 60 per cent of patients remain fully functional 10 years after the first attack, and 25 to 30 per cent remain functional 30 years after the

TABLE 124–7. SYMPTOMS AND SIGNS OF MULTIPLE SCLEROSIS*

SYMPTOM	PER CENT OF PATIENTS	SIGN	PER CENT OF PATIENTS
Muscle weakness	96	Spasticity or hyperreflexia, or both	98
Ocular disturbance	85	Babinski sign	92
Urinary disturbance	82	Absent abdominal reflexes	82
Gait ataxia	60	Dysmetria or intention tremor	79
Paresthesias	60	Nystagmus	71
Dysarthria or scanning speech	54	Impairment of vibratory sensation	61
Mental disturbance	47	Impairment of position sensation	52
Pain	19	Impairment of pain sensation	44
Vertigo	17	Facial weakness	42
Dysphagia	12	Impairment of touch sensation	29
Convulsions	6	Impairment of temperature sensation	17
Decreased hearing	6	Changes in state of consciousness	5
Tinnitus	5		

* Modified from Merritt's Textbook of Neurology. 7th ed. Philadelphia, Lea and Febiger, 1984.

onset. Statistically, the disorder does not greatly decrease life expectancy, although a few patients become severely disabled and die early from recurrent infections and the complications of being bedridden.

Certain characteristic symptoms suggest the diagnosis of multiple sclerosis. These include bilateral internuclear ophthalmoplegia (see p. 694), Lhermitte's sign (electric shock–like sensation radiating to the extremities initiated by neck flexion), and a marked exacerbation of neurologic symptoms associated with acute febrile illness. Although all neurologic dysfunction becomes worse with fever, raising the body temperature characteristically both exacerbates the present signs of multiple sclerosis and uncovers new signs not detected during normothermia.

The diagnosis depends upon identifying clinical or laboratory evidence of central nervous system lesions that are disseminated either in space or time, supplemented by laboratory evidence of immune dysfunction. Otherwise healthy persons who suffer relapsing and remitting neurologic dysfunction over a long period of time (e.g., diplopia in year one, sensory loss in an arm in year three, urgency incontinence in year five, etc.) almost certainly have multiple sclerosis. Furthermore, evidence of more than one widely spaced lesion in the nervous system (e.g., optic neuritis plus internuclear ophthalmoplegia) strongly suggests disseminated sclerosis in someone of the susceptible age group who lacks evidence of other disease. In patients with unifocal lesions, laboratory tests such as abnormal visual or auditory evoked responses may detect a subclinical lesion residing elsewhere in the nervous system.

The laboratory examination is helpful but not definitive. Most patients have an elevated gamma globulin in their spinal fluid, and separate, discrete (oligoclonal) bands are found in the gamma region on agarose or polyacrylamide gel electrophoresis in about 90 per cent of patients. Multiple oligoclonal bands (more than two) strongly support a diagnosis of multiple sclerosis in an appropriate clinical case, although inflammatory diseases of the nervous system can also produce oligoclonal bands. The CT scan may show hypodense areas or, during the acute stage, areas that enhance after contrast. These areas of demyelination characteristically occur in the periventricular areas of the brain, particularly around the lateral ventricles. Magnetic resonance imaging is considerably more sensitive than CT scan in bringing out discrete patches of increased signals in the periventricular area which strongly suggest the diagnosis (Fig. 124–4). A word of caution: periventricular areas of increased signals of no known significance are seen in many older patients.

The etiology of multiple sclerosis is unknown, although clues point to infectious (viral), immunological, and genetic factors. The disease is far more common in the northern and southern temperate latitudes than in the more equatorial regions. Furthermore, individuals who move before age five from a tropical to a temperate area in-

FIGURE 124–4. A magnetic resonance image from a patient with multiple sclerosis. Multiple lesions of the white matter (arrows) with a predilection for periventricular areas strongly supports the diagnosis of multiple sclerosis in a patient with an appropriate history and physical findings.

crease their likelihood of contracting multiple sclerosis. On the contrary, those leaving such regions after the age of 15 experience the low incidence of the region where they were born. The findings suggest an infective agent acquired early in life (a slow virus or exposure to a childhood infection?). An immune disorder is suggested not only by the inflammatory infiltrates sometimes seen in the perivascular areas of the demyelinated plaques but also by the fact that a decrease in suppressor lymphocytes in the serum usually precedes acute attacks. A relapsing encephalomyelitis resembling multiple sclerosis has been produced by injection of antigen into experimental animals. Genetic predisposition is suggested by the fact that haplotype DW2 is found in about 65 per cent of MS patients, compared with 15 per cent of control subjects. In addition, the disorder is uncommon in Orientals and African blacks and even in those with these ancestries who are born in the United States.

The diagnosis can be difficult, particularly in the absence of the typical remitting and exacerbating history, and when one cannot find evidence for widespread dissemination of lesions. Often in its early stages, the symptoms are primarily sensory, sometimes in bizarre and "nonanatomical" distribution, leading the physician to worry about a conversion reaction, particularly in younger patients. Occasionally signs in MS may be severe and apparently unifocal, so that they at first suggest a brain or spinal cord tumor or vascular disease. Particular difficulty arises with brain stem disorders. A small, single brain stem lesion can give rise to a multiplicity of cranial nerve, sensory, cerebellar, and motor signs, while similar findings can be caused by multifocal disease. To prove a disseminated disorder in a patient with prominent brain stem signs requires evidence of dysfunction of structures not represented in the brain stem (e.g., optic neuritis, visual field deficit, or aphasia). Visually evoked responses often help because the optic nerve is a common site of multiple sclerosis, causing abnormalities of conduction in the optic nerve, often without clinical symptoms. A particularly difficult differential diagnosis is between multiple sclerosis with remitting and exacerbating symptoms and small arteriovenous anomalies of the medulla or pons, which can produce by recurrent small hemorrhages remitting and exacerbating symptoms.

One can treat the symptoms of multiple sclerosis, but so far not the disease. Many physicians believe that acute bouts of neurologic dysfunction resolve more quickly when treated with short-term administration of corticosteroids. No evidence indicates that such treatment has a beneficial long-term effect. Some therapeutic trials suggest the potential efficacy of immunosuppressive agents in chronic progressive multiple sclerosis and of interferon given intrathecally in the treatment of remitting and exacerbating multiple sclerosis. Plasmapheresis has also been recommended by some. None of these treatments has been proven to be efficacious. Patients minimally affected by the disorder require no specific treatment. The illness understandably frightens patients, however, and sympathetic reassurance and follow-up provide considerable support. Patients severely disabled by late symptoms, which generally include spasticity and bladder and bowel dysfunction, often are best treated in multidisciplinary centers where physical therapy, psychological support, family counseling, and supportive medical therapy are all available.

Acute Disseminated Encephalomyelitis. This monophasic demyelinating inflammatory disorder can appear after viral infections or as a complication of vaccination. The disorder usually produces multifocal brain and spinal cord symptoms but may be restricted to one area, particularly optic nerve (acute optic neuropathy) or spinal cord (acute transverse myelopathy). When the disorder is related to an antecedant viral infection, it usually occurs 6 to 10 days after the appearance of the other systemic symptoms. When it follows vaccination, it usually begins 10 days to three weeks after the injections. At times a similar syndrome can appear in the absence of any identifiable exposure. The pathogenesis is believed to reside in an antigen-antibody response, the antigen being either the injected vaccination protein or the infecting virus. Clinically the disorder is usually characterized by the acute development of headache, fever, and multifocal neurologic signs. The most severely affected patients develop delirium, stupor, or coma. Seizures are relatively common. The spinal fluid is characterized by pleocytosis of 20 to 200 lymphocytes and usually an elevated gamma globulin. Protein concentration may be a little elevated, but glucose concentration is usually normal. Myelin basic protein can be identified in the spinal fluid in some of the patients. The electroencephalogram is usually diffusely abnormal, with widespread slowing, but does not have the characteristic focal slow and sharp wave activity of herpes simplex encephalitis.

Acute disseminated encephalomyelitis produces clinical and spinal fluid manifestations similar to those of acute viral encephalitis and cannot, in fact, be distinguished from that disorder by clinical findings. Since neither acute encephalomyelitis nor acute viral encephalitis, save for herpes simplex, can be treated definitively, such a differentiation is not valid. Despite its presumed immune mechanism, neither corticosteroids nor other immunosuppressive agents have proved efficacious in treatment.

Acute Transverse Myelopathy (Myelitis). Acute transverse myelopathy is a clinical syndrome characterized by the rapid onset of ascending or transverse spinal cord dysfunction, usually involving primarily the midthoracic or high thoracic cord. The disorder usually begins with fairly severe back pain and sometimes fever and malaise. In a matter of 12 to 24 hours, the patient complains of weakness and paresthesias in the lower extremities, sometimes associated with radicular pain at the level of the uppermost involved cord segments. Occasionally the disease is painless. In its severest form, complete paralysis and loss of sensation and autonomic function develop below the highest level of the lesion. In less severe forms there may be patchy loss of sensation with bilateral corticospinal tract signs predominating or a Brown-Sequard syndrome. In a few patients, the spinal cord signs ascend for hours to a week or two and reach a stable level, usually in the upper thoracic cord. In about half the patients there is a preceding history of banal infection, usually upper respiratory, or of a vaccination, the myelopathy presumably being a delayed immune response. Rarely, the illness is associated with an occult neoplasm.

The spinal fluid usually contains 50 to 100 white cells and a slightly elevated protein concentration. The diagnostic problem is to distinguish acute transverse myelopathy from parameningeal infection with secondary involvement of the cord. The history and findings in transverse myelopathy may mimic those of epidural or subdural infections. The diagnosis can always be established by myelography. In patients with acute transverse myelopathy, however, the spinal cord may be sufficiently swollen to produce a complete block to myelographic dye, so that care must be taken to distinguish the swollen cord from an epidural or subdural block. Magnetic resonance imaging eventually will replace myelography as the diagnostic test of choice. There is no effective treatment for the disorder. About one third of patients make a spontaneous recovery.

Acute hemorrhagic leukoencephalitis is a fatal, rare variant of acute encephalomyelitis. The illness usually occurs after an upper respiratory infection and is characterized by sudden headache, seizures, and rapid progression to coma. Patients often die within a few days. CSF often shows more polymorphonuclear leukocytes than lymphocytes. The brain at autopsy is swollen, with bilateral and asymmetrical hemorrhages scattered throughout the white matter. There is no known treatment.

Other Demyelinating Disease. Devic's disease (neuromyelitis optica) is a clinical syndrome characterized by transverse myelopathy and optic neuropathy. The two symptoms usually occur within days or weeks of each other. The disease is generally thought to be a variant of multiple sclerosis, but in many instances, particularly when the myelopathy is severe, there may be necrosis of the cord far more intense than the demyelinating plaques seen in most examples of multiple sclerosis.

Acute optic neuritis can either occur as a symptom of multiple sclerosis or arise in isolation independently. This disorder is described on p. 691.

Reye's Syndrome. Reye's syndrome is a parainfectious encephalopathy, primarily in children, which follows viral infection, usually influena type A or B or varicella. The syndrome is characterized by failure of liver and brain function and is thought to result from a mitochondrial disturbance of those organs, leading to metabolic derangements including serum hyperammonemia, lactic acidosis, and elevation of free fatty acids. Recent evidence suggests that in children with primary viral illness such as influenza and varicella, ingestion of aspirin may play a role in the pathogenesis. Reye's syndrome usually begins as the initial viral illness clears. The onset is with headache, intractable vomiting, and lethargy or stupor. Patients may rapidly become comatose. The diagnosis is confirmed by evidence of hepatic dysfunction without hyperbilirubinemia, elevated arterial ammonia level, and in children hypoglycemia (in the few cases reported in adults hypoglycemia has been uncommon). The CSF is normal save for increased pressure, and liver biopsy reveals a noninflammatory panlobular hepatocellular accumulation of lipid droplets and both histochemical and ultrastructural evidence of inflammation. At postmortem examination the brain shows marked swelling accompanied by ultrastructural changes in mitochondria similar to those found in liver. Mortality is high in comatose patients. Careful control of increased intracranial pressure using hyperosmolar agents and correction of hypoglycemia and electrolyte abnormalities may allow for recovery. Adults with the syndrome appear to have a lesser mortality than children.

REFERENCES

Enzmann DR: Origin of Infections and Inflammations of the Central Nervous System: Computed Tomography, Ultrasound and Nuclear Magnetic Resonance. New York, Raven Press, 1984. *A recent monograph with excellent illustrations devoted to the characteristics of intracranial infections recognized by various forms of imaging.*

Hallpike JF, Adams CWM, and Tourtellotte WW (eds): Multiple Sclerosis: Pathology, Diagnosis and Management. Baltimore, Williams and Wilkins, 1983. *A recent monograph encompassing many aspects of multiple sclerosis.*

Hooper DS, Pruitt AA, and Rubin RH: Central nervous system infection in the chronically immune suppressed. Medicine 61:166, 1982. *An analysis of opportunistic CNS infections along with a comprehensive literature review.*

Johnson RT: Viral Infections of the Nervous System. New York, Raven Press, 1982. *A comprehensive discussion of both common and rare viral CNS infections.*

Vinken PJ, and Bruyn GW: Handbook of Clinical Neurology. Vols. 33, 34, 35. Amsterdam, North-Holland Publishing Co, 1978. *Detailed chapters on bacterial (including syphilis and tuberculosis), viral, parasitic, and fungal infections of the central nervous system in man.*

INDEX

Note: Page numbers in italics represent illustrations; t indicates tables.

Electrocardiography (ECG) (*Continued*)
in ischemic heart disease, 26
in mitral regurgitation, 55–56
in myocardial contusion, 115
in myocardial infarction, 27t
in myxedema coma, 457
in pericarditis, *105*, 110, 573
in pleural effusions, 110
in syncope diagnosis, 101
in valvular heart disease, 52t–53t
long-term, for cardiac disorders, 31t
metabolic effects on, 27t
normal, 10
with exercise, 28
resting, for arrhythmias, 82
sine wave, in hyperkalemia, 198
Electroencephalography (EEG), 649–650
in absence seizure, 763
in epilepsy diagnosis, 765–766, *766*
normal, 765, *765*
Electrolyte(s), in pancreatic fluid, 312
disorders of, 194–201
repletion therapy with, for acute
diarrhea, 583–584
Electromechanical dissociation, features of,
103
Electromyography, 652
in myasthenia gravis, 712
in polymyositis and dermatomyositis,
622
normal and abnormal muscle on, *651*
Electronystagmography, 697
Electrophoresis, hemoglobin, patterns of,
366
protein, for detecting monoclonal
immunoglobulin, 388, *389*
in rheumatic diseases, 611
Electroshock, for depression, 667
Embolism, 119. See also *Thrombosis.*
obstructing aortic bifurcation, 117
of bacterial endocarditis, affecting brain,
785
of brain, from heart, 742
of coronary arteries, 64
"paradoxical," definition of, 119
pulmonary. See *Pulmonary embolism.*
renal, 243
risk of, in acute myocardial infarction,
73
"saddle," definition of, 119
systemic, direct current cardioversion
and, 87–88
with infective endocarditis, 568
surgery for, 571
Emory-Dreyfus dystrophy, 705–706
Emphysema, 141
clinical and laboratory findings in, 140t
compliance curves for, *128*
Empyema, 175
subdural, 782–783
spinal, 786
undrained, diagnosis of, 566
Empyema necessitatis, 175
Encephalitis, 555–557
herpes simplex virus, computed
tomography of, *556*
infectious organisms and, 555t
Encephalomyelitis, acute disseminated,
792
Encephalopathy, delayed post-traumatic,
758
hepatic. See *Hepatic encephalopathy.*
hypertensive, 746–747

Encephalopathy (*Continued*)
metabolic, acute, 655–656
laboratory tests in, 657t
pupillary responses in, *692*
radiation and, 778
Endarteritis, bacterial, 572
Endobronchial obstruction, 566
Endocarditis. See *Infective endocarditis.*
Endocrine disease, and hypoglycemia, **499**
and myopathies, 708
radiation and, 779
Endocrine neoplasia, multiple (MEN),
types of, 299, 508, 510
Endocrine system, effect of cancer on, 411
effect of end-stage renal disease on, 224
effect of liver disease on, 319t
female, function of, 472–480
Endoscopic injection sclerotherapy, for
variceal hemorrhage, 267, 332
Endoscopic retrograde
cholangiopancreatography, 289
for chronic pancreatitis, 316, *316*
for gallstones, 288
for jaundice, 284
percutaneous transhepatic
cholangiography vs., 289t
Endoscopy, fiberoptic, 288
for gastrointestinal bleeding, 266
for gastrointestinal diseases, 288–289
for inflammatory bowel disease, 302
for stomach carcinoma, 307
Endotheliosis, of toxemia, 251
Endotracheal tube, in adult respiratory
distress syndrome, 157
End-stage renal disease (ESRD). See also
Chronic renal failure; Uremia.
causes of, 219, 219t
clinical manifestations of, 221–225, 222t
neurological, 223–224
in diabetic glomerulopathy, 248–249
Entamoeba histolytica, and diarrhea, 280,
582
epidemiologic characteristics of, 581t
Enteritis, regional. See *Crohn's disease.*
Enteropathy, gluten-sensitive, 273–274
Enterotoxins, and diarrhea, 580–581
ingested with food, 581
Enterovirus, and infection, 543
Enthesopathy, definition of, 632–633
in ankylosing spondylitis, 633
in Reiter's syndrome, 636
Environment, and cancer, 409t
colon, 308
esophageal, 306
body heat lost to, 536
extremities damaged by, 119–120
Enzymes, adrenal, defects in, 470
cardiac, in acute myocardial infarction,
72, *72*
defective, in disorders of amino acid
metabolism, 435
in abnormal sexual differentiation. 473
inhibition of, in host defense against
viruses, 531
Eosinophilia, tropical, 149
with pulmonary infiltrates, 149
Ependymomas, 727, 771
Epidural abscesses, 781–782
Epidural hematoma, 727–728
Epigastric pain, in stomach carcinoma, 307
Epiglottitis, 560–561
Epilepsy, 760–770

Epilepsy (*Continued*)
definition of, 760
diagnosis of, 765
etiology of, 761
generalized, 763–770
convulsive, 764
nonconvulsive, 763
primary, 763–764
secondary, 763
incidence of, 761
management of, 767
partial continuous, 768
pathophysiology of, 761
postinfantile, clinical features of, 765t
post-traumatic, 758
primary (idiopathic), definition of, 760
reflex, 764
secondary (symptomatic), definition of,
760
temporal lobe, depersonalization
reactions vs., 670
Epileptic seizures, atonic-akinetic, 764
control of, 767
definition of, 760
focal, 761
generalized, 761
partial, 761
partial complex, 762–763, 762t
partial motor, 761–762
partial sensory, 762
patterns of, 761–763, 761t
primary motor (rolandic), 762
serial, 768
syncope vs., 766, 766t
tonic-clonic (grand mal), 764
Epinephrine, administered in life support,
103
function of, 471
in recovery from hypoglycemia, 491
Epithelial cells, bronchial, 565
squamous, in respiratory secretions, *564*
Epithelium, host defense function of, 528
Epstein-Barr virus, and mononucleosis,
548–549
Ergonovine, provocative testing with, in
variant angina, 71
Erysipelas, 577
Erythema chronicum migrans, 548
Erythema nodosum, with inflammatory
bowel disease, 302
Erythroblast, 345
Erythroblastosis fetalis, prevention of, 368
Erythrocyte(s), aplasia of, 349
appearance of, diagnostic value of, 348
in bone marrow, 344–345
in hemolytic anemia, 356
mass of, normal and polycythemic, *376*
transfusion of, 367
compatability testing for, 368
trauma to, and hemolysis, 361
Erythrocyte count, normal range of, 346–
347
Erythrocyte indices, 348
Erythrocyte sedimentation rate, 610, 610t
Erythromelalgia, 396
Erythromycin, for *Legionella* respiratory
infection, 165
Erythropoiesis, 345
Erythropoietin, function of, 345
Escape beat, definition of, 80
Escherichia coli, and colitis, 585
epidemiologic characteristics of, 581t
Esophageal rings, 292